Endocrinology

Series Editor
Andrea Lenzi
Chair of Endocrinology
Department of Experimental Medicine
Section of Medical Pathophysiology
Food Science and Endocrinology
Sapienza University of Rome
Rome, Italy

Series Co-Editor
Emmanuele A. Jannini
Chair of Endocrinology & Medical Sexology (ENDOSEX)
Department of Systems Medicine
University of Rome Tor Vergata
Rome, Italy

Within the health sciences, Endocrinology has an unique and pivotal role. This old, but continuously new science is the study of the various hormones and their actions and disorders in the body. The matter of Endocrinology are the glands, i.e. the organs that produce hormones, active on the metabolism, reproduction, food absorption and utilization, growth and development, behavior control and several other complex functions of the organisms. Since hormones interact, affect, regulate and control virtually all body functions, Endocrinology not only is a very complex science, multidisciplinary in nature, but is one with the highest scientific turnover. Knowledge in the Endocrinological sciences is continuously changing and growing. In fact, the field of Endocrinology and Metabolism is one where the highest number of scientific publications continuously flourishes. The number of scientific journals dealing with hormones and the regulation of body chemistry is dramatically high. Furthermore, Endocrinology is directly related to genetics, neurology, immunology, rheumatology, gastroenterology, nephrology, orthopedics, cardiology, oncology, gland surgery, sexology and sexual medicine, psychology, psychiatry, internal medicine, and basic sciences. All these fields are interested in updates in Endocrinology. The Aim of the MRW in Endocrinology is to update the Endocrinological matter using the knowledge of the best experts in each section of Endocrinology: basic endocrinology, neuroendocrinology, endocrinological oncology, pancreas with diabetes and other metabolic disorders, thyroid, parathyroid and bone metabolism, adrenals and endocrine hypertension, sexuality, reproduction and behavior.

More information about this series at: http://www.springer.com/series/14021

Antonino Belfiore • Derek LeRoith
Editors

Principles of Endocrinology and Hormone Action

With 125 Figures and 53 Tables

Springer

Editors
Antonino Belfiore
Magna Graecia University
Catanzaro, Italy

Derek LeRoith
Icahn School of Medicine at Mt. Sinai
New York, NY, USA

ISBN 978-3-319-44674-5 ISBN 978-3-319-44675-2 (eBook)
ISBN 978-3-319-45217-3 (print and electronic bundle)
https://doi.org/10.1007/978-3-319-44675-2

Library of Congress Control Number: 2017949669

Printed on acid-free paper

This Springer imprint is published by Springer Nature
The registered company is Springer International Publishing AG
The registered company address is: Gewerbestrasse 11, 6330 Cham, Switzerland

Series Preface

Is there an unmet need for a new MRW series in Endocrinology and Metabolism? It might not seem so! The vast number of existing textbooks, monographs and scientific journals suggest that the field of hormones (from genetic, molecular, biochemical and translational to physiological, behavioral, and clinical aspects) is one of the largest in biomedicine, producing a simply huge scientific output. However, we are sure that this new series will be of interest for scientists, academics, students, physicians and specialists alike.

The knowledge in Endocrinology and Metabolism limited to the two main (from an epidemiological perspective) diseases, namely hypo/hyperthyroidism and diabetes mellitus, now seems outdated and perhaps closer to the practical interests of the general practitioner than to those of the specialist. This has led to endocrinology and metabolism being increasingly considered as a subsection of internal medicine rather than an autonomous specialization. But endocrinology is much more than this.

We are proposing this series as the *manifesto* for **Endocrinology 2.0**, embracing the fields of medicine in which hormones play a major part but which, for various historical and cultural reasons, have thus far been "ignored" by endocrinologists. Hence, this MRW comprises "traditional" (but no less important or investigated) topics: from the molecular actions of hormones to the pathophysiology and management of pituitary, thyroid, adrenal, pancreatic and gonadal diseases, as well as less usual and common arguments. Endocrinology 2.0 is, in fact, the science of hormones, but it is also the medicine of sexuality and reproduction, the medicine of gender differences and the medicine of well-being. These aspects of Endocrinology have to date been considered of little interest, as they are young and relatively unexplored sciences. But this is no longer the case. The large scientific production in these fields coupled with the impressive social interest of patients in these topics is stimulating a new and fascinating challenge for Endocrinology.

The aim of the **MRW in Endocrinology** is thus to update the subject with the knowledge of the best experts in each field: basic endocrinology, neuroendocrinology, endocrinological oncology, pancreatic disorders, diabetes and other metabolic disorders, thyroid, parathyroid and bone metabolism, adrenal and endocrine hypertension, sexuality, reproduction and behavior. We are sure that this ambitious aim, covering for the first time the whole spectrum of Endocrinology 2.0, will be fulfilled in this vast Springer MRW in Endocrinology Series.

Andrea Lenzi
Emmanuele A. Jannini

Preface

The endocrine system involves a complex signaling network that regulates essential functions involved in growth, reproduction, and homeostasis. We are increasingly recognizing that this regulatory system comprises not only hormones secreted by the classical endocrine glands, but also hormones and regulatory factors produced by many organs and tissues, such as the heart, gut, bone, and adipose tissue, and that it involves extensive cross talk with the neural and immune system that are the other two crucial regulatory networks. At the same time, our knowledge of hormone synthesis, release, and transport as well as the molecular basis of hormone action has been greatly and rapidly expanded. Endocrine disorders include hormone deficiency or excess as well as peripheral resistance to selective hormones. Some of these disorders, such as thyroid diseases and type 2 diabetes mellitus, represent real social health problems for their high prevalence in the population and severe clinical complications. Several other disorders are less frequent but equally critical for health or otherwise important for their social implications, such as disorders involving impairment of growth or fertility. Emerging aspects include the notion that common endocrine disorders, such as insulin resistance and related conditions, may increase cancer risk and that the endocrine system contributes to regulate the process of aging.

Understanding the complexity of endocrine system physiology is crucial to prevent endocrine disorders and their complications, to improve the sensitivity of our diagnostic tools, and to provide the rationale for pharmacological, immunological, or genetic interventions.

Thanks to recent advances in this field, endocrine disorders can be now correctly assessed not only clinically but also by sensitive laboratory hormone measurements and by genetic and/or immunological testing as needed. Besides, as the endocrine system regulates the functions of all organs and apparatus, it is difficult to underestimate the relevance of endocrine physiology to all fields of Internal Medicine, including the prevention and treatment of common diseases such as cardiovascular diseases and cancer.

This volume has the ambitious aims to provide a comprehensive coverage of the current view of the physiology of the endocrine system and hormone synthesis and release, transport, and action at the molecular and cellular level. It is intended to provide essential as well as in depth information to the medical students, but also to specialists in Endocrinology, Gynecology, Pediatrics, and Internal Medicine.

Each chapter has been written by a recognized expert in the specific field, and we wish to warmly express our gratitude and appreciation to all the authors who enthusiastically agreed to contribute to this endeavor and have made a remarkable effort to provide a complete, updated, yet easy to read, and fresh overview of the current knowledge in endocrine physiology.

Contents

About the Editors

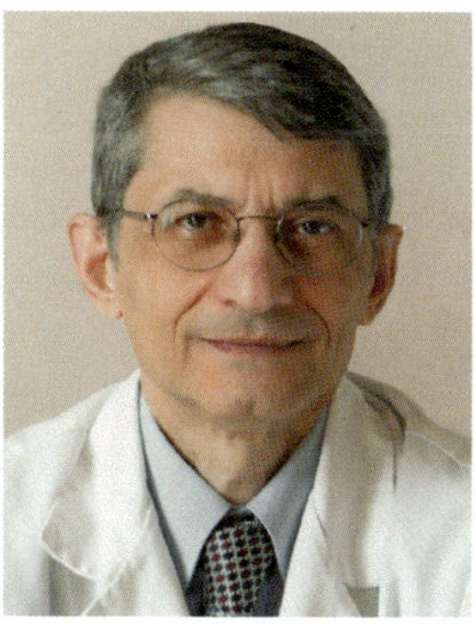

Antonino Belfiore is Professor of Endocrinology and Head of the Endocrine Unit at the University of Catanzaro, Italy. He obtained his M.D. degree at University of Catania, Italy, and graduated in Endocrinology and Metabolic Diseases (University of Catania) and Nuclear Medicine (University of Padoa). He completed his postgraduate training at the University of Naples (Ph.D.), at the University College of London, Clinical Immunology Department (1985–1987), and at the University of San Francisco, Diabetes Research Branch. He has been Assistant Professor in Endocrinology at the University of Catania till 1998, when he moved to the University of Catanzaro, first as Associate Professor, and from 2006 as Full Professor of Endocrinology.

Dr. Belfiore has a long-standing interest in the epidemiology, clinical aspects and biology of thyroid diseases, and in endocrine-related tumors. He is the Head of the research laboratory of Endocrinology at the University of Catanzaro, and current main interests of his research group concern the study of the IGF system dysregulation in human cancer, with particular focus on the role of the insulin receptor, its isoforms, and molecular modulators of these receptors in cancer.

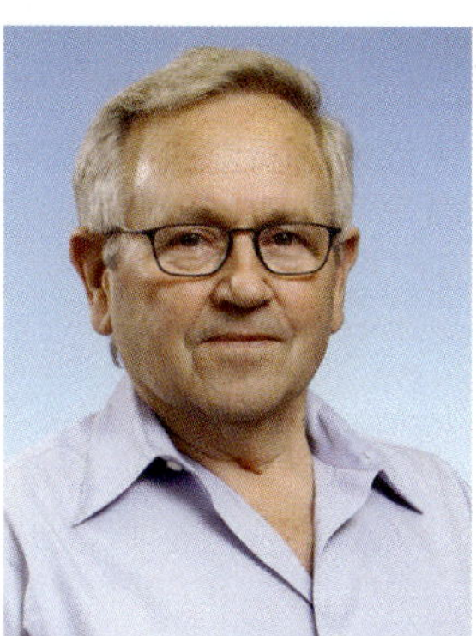

Derek LeRoith is currently Interim Chief and Director of Research in the Division of Endocrinology, Diabetes and Bone Disease, Icahn School of Medicine at Mount Sinai, New York.

Dr. LeRoith received his medical and research training at the University of Cape Town, South Africa, and completed his postgraduate training in London, United Kingdom. Subsequently, he was a member of the medical faculty at Ben-Gurion University Medical School in Israel.

Dr. LeRoith worked for the National Institutes of Health (NIH) from 1979 until 2005 in the field of endocrinology and diabetes, and he advanced to Diabetes Branch Chief at the NIH in Bethesda, Maryland. His research interests include the role of insulin and insulin-like growth factors in normal physiology and in disease states, including obesity, type 2 diabetes mellitus (T2DM), and cancer. His clinical interests primarily involve the pathophysiology and management of obesity and T2DM. Dr. LeRoith has published more than 600 research and review articles on these topics, as well editing numerous textbooks and is currently Editor in Chief of the AACE journal *Endocrine Practice*.

Contributors

Filippo Acconcia Department of Science, University Roma Tre, Rome, Italy

Erik K. Alexander The Thyroid Section, Department of Medicine, Brigham and Women's Hospital, Boston, MA, USA

Harvard Medical School, Boston, MA, USA

Hussain Alsaffar Department of Paediatric Endocrinology, Alder Hey Children's Hospital, Liverpool, UK

Trevor E. Angell The Thyroid Section, Department of Medicine, Brigham and Women's Hospital, Boston, MA, USA

Harvard Medical School, Boston, MA, USA

Antonio Aversa Department of Experimental and Clinical Medicine, Magna Graecia University of Catanzaro, Catanzaro, CZ, Italy

Joanne Blair Department of Paediatric Endocrinology, Alder Hey Children's Hospital, Liverpool, UK

Marco Boscaro Endocrinology Unit, Department of Medicine DIMED, University-Hospital of Padova, Padova, Italy

Andrew J. Brooks The University of Queensland Diamantina Institute, The University of Queensland, Translational Research Institute, Woolloongabba, QLD, Australia

The University of Queensland, Institute for Molecular Bioscience, Brisbane, QLD, Australia

John C. Burnett Jr. Department of Cardiovascular Diseases, Cardiorenal Research Laboratory, Rochester, MN, USA

Filippo Ceccato Endocrinology Unit, Department of Medicine DIMED, University-Hospital of Padova, Padova, Italy

Sheue-yann Cheng Laboratory of Molecular Biology, National Cancer Institute, Bethesda, MD, USA

Paul J. Davis Pharmaceutical Research Institute, Albany College of Pharmacy and Health Sciences, and Albany Medical College, Albany, NY, USA

Adolfo J. de Bold Department of Pathology and Laboratory Medicine, University of Ottawa, Faculty of Medicine, and the University of Ottawa, Heart Institute, Ottawa, ON, Canada

Farhad Dehkhoda The University of Queensland Diamantina Institute, The University of Queensland, Translational Research Institute, Woolloongabba, QLD, Australia

Carolina DiBlasi Division of Pediatric Endocrinology, Seattle Children's Hospital/ University of Washington, Seattle, WA, USA

Sara A. DiVall Division of Pediatric Endocrinology, Seattle Children's Hospital/ University of Washington, Seattle, WA, USA

Alan P. Farwell Section of Endocrinology, Diabetes, and Nutrition, Boston Medical Center, Boston, MA, USA

Department of Medicine, Boston University School of Medicine, Boston, MA, USA

Mathieu Ferron Institut de recherches cliniques de Montréal (IRCM), Montréal, QC, Canada

Giovanna Finzi Azienda Socio Sanitaria Territoriale Dei Sette Laghi (ASST), Varese, Italy

Franco Folli Department of Medicine, Division of Diabetes, University of Texas Health Science Center, San Antonio, TX, USA

Davide Francomano Department Experimental Medicine, Sapienza University of Rome, Rome, Italy

Alessandra Gambineri Division of Endocrinology, Department of Medical and Surgical Sciences, Centre for Applied Biomedical Research (C.R.B.A.), S. Orsola-Malpighi Hospital, Alma Mater Studiorum University of Bologna, Bologna, Italy

Jens Peter Goetze Department of Clinical Biochemistry, Rigshospitalet, and University of Aarhus, Copenhagen, Denmark

Department of Clinical Medicine, Aarhus University, Aarhus, Denmark

Javier González-Maeso Department of Physiology and Biophysics, Virginia Commonwealth University, Richmond, VA, USA

Shilpa Gupta Division of Hematology, Oncology, and Transplantation, Department of Medicine, Masonic Cancer Center, University of Minnesota, Minneapolis, MN, USA

David Hackney Department of Obstetrics and Gynecology, Case Western Reserve University, Cleveland, OH, USA

Department of Obstetrics and Gynecology, University Hospitals of Cleveland, Cleveland, OH, USA

Fady Hannah-Shmouni Section on Endocrinology and Genetics (SEGEN), National Institute of Child Health and Human Development (NICHD), National Institutes of Health (NIH), Bethesda, MD, USA

Stephen A. Huang Thyroid Program of the Division of Endocrinology, Boston Children's Hospital, Boston, MA, USA

Alessandro Ilacqua Free Lance, Rome, Italy

Sandra Incerpi Department of Sciences, University Roma Tre, Rome, Italy

Carolyn M. Klinge Department of Biochemistry and Molecular Genetics, Center for Genetics and Molecular Medicine, University of Louisville School of Medicine, Louisville, KY, USA

Noriyuki Koibuchi Department of Integrative Physiology, Gunma University Graduate School of Medicine, Maebashi, Gunma, Japan

Peter Kopp Division of Endocrinology, Metabolism and Molecular Medicine, Feinberg School of Medicine, Northwestern University, Chicago, IL, USA

Christopher S. Kovacs Faculty of Medicine – Endocrinology, Memorial University of Newfoundland, Health Sciences Centre, St. John's, Newfoundland, Canada

Birthe B. Kragelund Structural Biology and NMR Laboratory, Department of Biology, University of Copenhagen, Copenhagen, Denmark

Kelly Kuo Department of Obstetrics and Gynecology, Oregon Health and Science University, Portland, OR, USA

C. B. Lambalk Department of Obstetrics and Gynecology, VU Medical Center Amsterdam, Amsterdam, The Netherlands

Antonia Lanni Department of Environmental, Biological, Pharmaceutical Sciences and Technologies, Second University of Naples, Caserta, Italy

Changhan D. Lee Davis School of Gerontology, University of Southern California, Los Angeles, CA, USA

Angela M. Leung Division of Endocrinology, Department of Medicine, UCLA David Geffen School of Medicine, Los Angeles, CA, USA

Division of Endocrinology, Department of Medicine, VA Greater Los Angeles Healthcare System, Los Angeles, CA, USA

Valentina Lo Preiato Bologna, Italy

Valter D. Longo Davis School of Gerontology, University of Southern California, Los Angeles, CA, USA

IFOM, FIRC Institute of Molecular Oncology, Milano, Italy

Elizabeth Lowden Division of Endocrinology, Metabolism and Molecular Medicine, Feinberg School of Medicine, Northwestern University, Chicago, IL, USA

Noemi Malandrino National Institute of Diabetes and Digestive and Kidney Diseases Intramural Research Program, National Institutes of Health, Bethesda, MD, USA

Massimo Mannelli Department of Experimental and Clinical Biomedical Sciences "Mario Serio", University of Florence, Florence, Italy

Piero Marchetti Department of Clinical and Experimental Medicine, University of Pisa, Pisa, Italy

Maria Marino Department of Science, University Roma Tre, Rome, Italy

Lorella Marselli Department of Clinical and Experimental Medicine, University of Pisa, Pisa, Italy

Sam Mesiano Department of Reproductive Biology, Case Western Reserve University, Cleveland, OH, USA

Uberto Pagotto Division of Endocrinology, Department of Medical and Surgical Sciences, Centre for Applied Biomedical Research (C.R.B.A.), S. Orsola-Malpighi Hospital, Alma Mater Studiorum University of Bologna, Bologna, Italy

Gabriele Parenti Endocrinology Unit, Department of Medicine and Geriatrics, Azienda Ospedaliera-Universitaria di Careggi, Careggi Hospital, Florence, Italy

Jens Z. Pedersen Department of Biology, University of Rome Tor Vergata, Rome, Italy

Hanna Pincas Department of Neurology, Icahn School of Medicine at Mount Sinai, New York, NY, USA

Salvatore Piro Department of Clinical and Experimental Medicine, Division of Internal Medicine, Garibaldi-Nesima Hospital, University of Catania, Catania, Italy

Jens F. Rehfeld Department of Clinical Biochemistry, Rigshospitalet, University of Copenhagen, Copenhagen, Denmark

Linda Johnston Rohrbasser Paediatric Endocrinology and Diabetes Practice, Starnberg, Germany

Gian Paolo Rossi Clinica dell'Ipertensione Arteriosa – Department of Medicine, Internal Medicine 4 DIME, University of Padova, Padova, Italy

Frederique Ruf-Zamojski Department of Neurology, Icahn School of Medicine at Mount Sinai, New York, NY, USA

Carla Scaroni Endocrinology Unit, Department of Medicine DIMED, University-Hospital of Padova, Padova, Italy

Stuart C. Sealfon Department of Neurology, Icahn School of Medicine at Mount Sinai, New York, NY, USA

Robert J. Smith The Warren Alpert School of Medicine, Brown University, Providence, RI, USA

Constantine A. Stratakis Section on Endocrinology and Genetics (SEGEN), National Institute of Child Health and Human Development (NICHD), National Institutes of Health (NIH), Bethesda, MD, USA

Francesca Urbano Department of Clinical and Experimental Medicine, Division of Internal Medicine, Garibaldi-Nesima Hospital, University of Catania, Catania, Italy

Paul-Emmanuel Vanderriele Clinica dell'Ipertensione Arteriosa – Department of Medicine, Internal Medicine 4 DIME, University of Padova, Padova, Italy

Joseph G. Verbalis Division of Endocrinology and Metabolism, Georgetown University School of Medicine, Washington, DC, USA

M. O. Verhoeven Department of Obstetrics and Gynecology, VU Medical Center Amsterdam, Amsterdam, The Netherlands

Valentina Vicennati Bologna, Italy

Morris F. White Division of Endocrinology, Boston Children's Hospital, Harvard Medical School, Boston, MA, USA

Douglas Yee Division of Hematology, Oncology, and Transplantation, Department of Medicine, Masonic Cancer Center, University of Minnesota, Minneapolis, MN, USA

Xuguang Zhu Laboratory of Molecular Biology, Center for Cancer Research, National Cancer Institute, National Institutes of Health, Bethesda, MD, USA

Part I

Introduction to the Endocrine System

The Endocrine System

1

Angela M. Leung and Alan P. Farwell

Abstract

The endocrine system allows for the communication between the multiple cells and organs and is comprised of complex network of hormones, hormone receptors, carrier molecules, and signaling pathways. Characteristic of this system is that hormones generally act on cells that are physically separated from the secretory cell/gland, often traveling through the circulatory system to reach target tissues. Hormonal regulation is achieved by the ability of hormones to have specific biologic activity at their target tissues, important for energy production and metabolism, somatic growth and development, reproduction, and ability for the body to respond to internal and external stimuli. These complex interactions utilize controlled mechanisms of hormone synthesis and secretion and communication with other signaling molecules. Hormone deficiency or excess can each result from glandular or extraglandular processes and can be assessed clinically by laboratory testing that may include provocative testing if indicated.

Keywords

Endocrine • Hormone • Hormone receptor • Signaling

A.M. Leung (✉)
Division of Endocrinology, Department of Medicine, UCLA David Geffen School of Medicine, Los Angeles, CA, USA

Division of Endocrinology, Department of Medicine, VA Greater Los Angeles Healthcare System, Los Angeles, CA, USA
e-mail: AMLeung@mednet.ucla.edu

A.P. Farwell
Section of Endocrinology, Diabetes, and Nutrition, Boston Medical Center, Boston, MA, USA

Department of Medicine, Boston University School of Medicine, Boston, MA, USA
e-mail: Alan.Farwell@bmc.org; amleung@mednet.ucla.edu

A. Belfiore, D. LeRoith (eds.), *Principles of Endocrinology and Hormone Action*, Endocrinology, https://doi.org/10.1007/978-3-319-44675-2_1

Contents

Introduction

The *endocrine system* refers to the complex, interrelated mechanisms of communication between cells of an organism. The system is comprised of a diverse series of signaling mechanisms required for the regulation, processes, and functions required of multiple organs. Communication in the endocrine system is made possible by *hormones*, biologically active chemical substances that are secreted from ductless glands in the body and circulate through the bloodstream to act on target cells or organs. The actions of hormones in the endocrine system allow for the exquisite regulation of energy production and metabolism, somatic growth and development, reproduction, and responses to internal and external stimuli.

Hormone action can be classified into endocrine, paracrine, and autocrine actions (Fig. 1). The *endocrine action* of hormones refers to the transport of hormones in circulation to exert their metabolic actions at target tissues. Hormones can bind to carrier proteins in the circulatory system and thus exist in both their unbound (also termed free) and bound forms. However, in most cases, only the unbound/free hormone has biological activity. The differential affinity of binding proteins to hormones enables the precise availability of hormones in circulation and at target

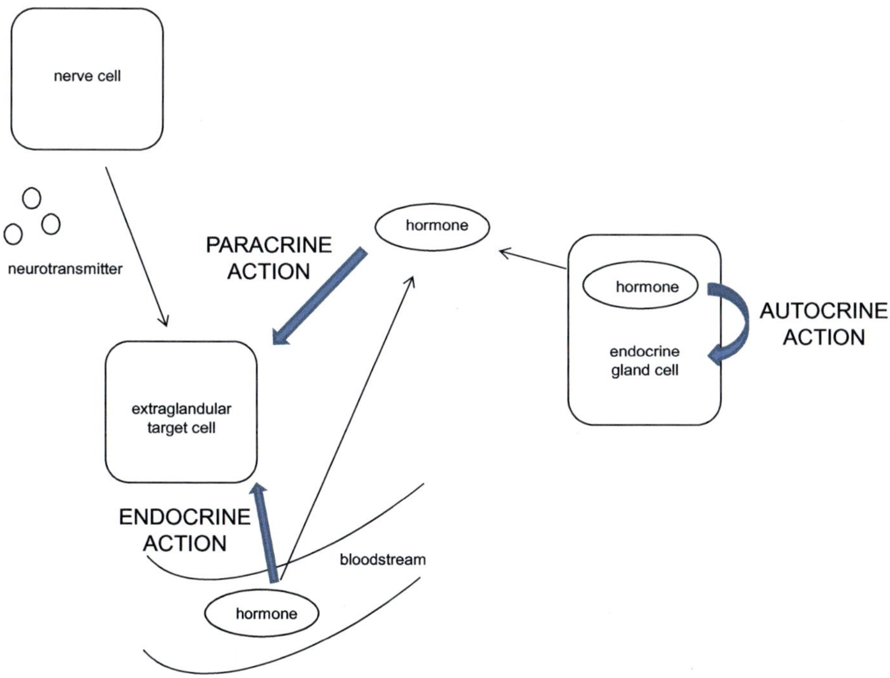

Fig. 1 Classes of hormone action

site(s). Once at their target sites, hormones interact with *hormone receptors*, proteins which recognize a unique binding site of the hormone. Hormone receptors facilitate the transmission of information carried by the hormone to generate a cellular response. Hormone receptors may be located on the target cell's surface or intracellularly, the latter which requires a mechanism of entry of the hormone into the cell to exert its action.

However, some hormones also or exclusively have *paracrine actions*, in which hormones are locally secreted to act upon surrounding cells. Examples of paracrine actions include the release of testosterone by the testes to control spermatogenesis, insulin-like growth factor in most tissues to control cell proliferation, somatostatin by the delta cells of the pancreatic islets to inhibit secretion of insulin from the beta cells and glucagon from the alpha cells, and growth factors in bone. Paracrine factors are usually produced and secreted in much smaller quantities than hormones which have endocrine action, given the specificity of the paracrine factor at local tissues and absence of the need to circulate throughout the body. Finally, a hormone can also act on its own cell of origin (*autocrine action*), such as the inhibitory action of insulin on its own secretion by the pancreatic beta cells.

The ability to achieve high hormone concentrations within a tissue is also facilitated by local diffusion of the hormone from its site of secretion. One example is the delivery of testosterone from the Leydig cells of the testes to the adjacent spermatogenetic tubules. Additionally, the local production of active hormone from a circulating hormone precursor can increase the intracellular concentration of a hormone. This is demonstrated by the conversion of testosterone to dihydrotestosterone (DHT) in the prostate and the production of 3,5,3′-triiodothyronine (T3) from the deiodination of thyroxine in the pituitary, within the brain, and in other tissues.

The above definitions are adequate to define the concepts of hormones and receptors in most cases. However, increased understanding of the actions of other molecules has led to some broadened definitions. Regulatory molecules that mainly act as *neurotransmitters*, such as catecholamines and acetylcholine, may also act as classic hormones. Conversely, small peptides, such as thyrotropin-releasing hormone (TRH) that is produced in the hypothalamus and acts on the anterior pituitary to release thyrotropin and prolactin, are also found in neurons throughout the body and can function as neurotransmitters.

The classic endocrine glands, whose primary function is hormone production, include the thyroid, pituitary, adrenal, and parathyroid glands and the pancreatic islets. However, not all hormones are produced by pure endocrine glands. The ovary and testes, which produce the sex hormones, also produce oocytes and sperm. The brain is a major source for many peptide hormones, including proopiomelanocortin (POMC), the precursor molecule for corticotropin (ACTH), endorphins, and melanocyte-stimulating hormone (MSH). Lipotropin is synthesized not only in the anterior pituitary but also in the placenta and the gastrointestinal tract. Other body systems that produce hormones, yet while serving other primary functions, include the heart (which secretes atrial natriuretic factor), the liver (which secretes insulin-like growth factor-I and angiotensinogen and enables the conversion of thyroxine (T4) into the metabolically active T3), the kidney (which secretes erythropoietin and the active form of vitamin D), and the gastrointestinal tract (which secretes gastrin, cholecystokinin, somatostatin, and other hormones).

Interrelationships with Other Systems

The functions and actions of the endocrine system overlap considerably with the nervous system and the immune system, which also have key roles in extracellular communication. Like the endocrine system, the nervous system has evolved to release regulatory substances from nerve cells that act across synaptic junctions to transmit a signal to adjacent cells. As noted above, these neurotransmitters may also function as true circulating hormones, while some hormones also function as neurogenic mediators in the central nervous system. Thus, if a regulatory molecule is released into the circulation to act, it is considered a hormone; if it is released from a nerve terminal to act locally, it is a neurotransmitter. The same regulatory molecule may therefore be both a hormone and a neurotransmitter.

The hypothalamus serves as a direct connection between the nervous and endocrine systems, as the source of both hormones that are stored in the posterior pituitary and releasing peptides that regulate hormone secretion from the anterior pituitary. The autonomic nervous system often exerts control over the function of endocrine tissues. The pituitary, pancreatic islets, renal juxtaglomerular cells, and the adrenal gland all respond to neural stimulation. Thus, the same cell can function as both an endocrine and a neural cell.

The immune system, initially thought to function autonomously, is now known to be subject to both neural and endocrine regulation. The cytokine regulators of the immune system are not usually considered hormones, but they clearly fit the definition as regulatory molecules that are secreted by one cell and influence another cell. The actions of cytokines are not limited to immunomodulation, as interleukins, interferons, and tumor necrosis factor produced by the immune system during systemic illness exert a major influence on hormone metabolism, especially that of thyroid hormone. Similarly, corticosteroids are major immunomodulators, as are the metabolic derangements produced by endocrine dysfunction, such as hyperglycemia in uncontrolled diabetes mellitus. Thus, while the central focus of endocrinology is on hormones, it is clear that not all hormones belong to the endocrine system and that there is considerable overlap between the endocrine, nervous, and immune systems.

Classes of Hormones

Hormones can be categorized into three classes according to their major components: peptide hormones, amino acid analogues, and steroid hormones (Table 1).

Peptide hormones are the most prevalent and diverse. They include hormones that are defined by a wide range of sizes, composition, number of chains, modification of groups, and mechanisms of production. Some examples are large single-chain peptides, such as the 192-amino acid growth hormone (GH), the cyclic peptide of TRH that is comprised of just three amino acids, and prolactin. The anterior pituitary hormones, thyrotropin (TSH), follicle-stimulating hormone (FSH), and luteinizing hormone (LH) are glycosylated and consist of two chains each, one of which is common to all three hormones (α chain), while the other is distinct and confers specificity to the hormone (β chain). Insulin is comprised of two chains that are derived from posttranslational cleavage of a single gene product (preproinsulin), while adrenocorticotropic hormone (ACTH), melanocyte-stimulating hormone (MSH), and β-endorphin are single-chain proteolytic products of a large precursor molecule, proopiomelanocortin (POMC).

The *amino acid analogue hormones* are water-soluble and derived from amino acids. Specifically, the *amines* are derived from tyrosine and secreted from the thyroid (these are termed *iodothyronines*) and adrenal medulla. The precursor of the iodothyronines is thyroglobulin, a 660,000-Da glycoprotein that is synthesized by the thyroid follicular cell containing >100 tyrosine residues. The iodothyronines are formed by iodination and coupling of two tyrosines and are the only iodinated compounds with significant biologic activity. In the adrenal catecholamine-secreting cells, tyrosine is converted sequentially to dopamine, norepinephrine, and epinephrine. Serotonin (5-hydroxytryptamine) is derived from tryptophan.

Steroid hormones are derivatives of cholesterol containing a similar core known as the cyclopentanoperhydrophenanthrene ring. Synthesis of the steroid hormones

Table 1 Classes of hormones

Peptide hormones	
Small peptides	Vasopressin (ADH)
	Oxytocin
	Melanocyte-stimulating hormone (MSH)
	Thyrotropin-releasing hormone (TRH)
	Gonadotropin-releasing hormone (GnRH)
Intermediate peptides	Insulin
	Glucagon
	Growth hormone (GH)
	Prolactin (PRL)
	Parathyroid hormone (PTH)
	Calcitonin
	Corticotropin (ACTH)
	Corticotropin-releasing hormone (CRH)
	β-Endorphin
	Gastrointestinal peptides
	Cytokines
	Growth factors
Glycoproteins	Proopiomelanocortin (POMC)
	Follicle-stimulating hormone (FSH)
	Luteinizing hormone (LH)
	Thyrotropin (TSH)
	Chorionic gonadotropin (CG)
Amino acid analogues	
Iodothyronines	Thyroxine (T4)
	3,5,3′-Triiodothyronine (T3)
	3′,5′,3-Triiodothyronine (rT3)
Amines	Dopamine
	Epinephrine
	Norepinephrine
	Melatonin
	Serotonin
Steroid hormones	
	Estrogens
	Progesterone (P)
	Testosterone (T)
	Dihydrotestosterone (DHT)
	Cortisol
	Aldosterone
	Vitamin D
	Retinoic acid
	Prostaglandins

occurs as a result of enzymatically induced changes to the cholesterol core. Synthesis of the adrenal and sex steroids occurs in the adrenal cortex and testes or ovaries, respectively.

Hormone-Receptor Binding

Hormone action requires binding of the hormone to a receptor at the target cell. This allows the hormone to be distinguished from all other substances and to activate a cellular response upon hormone binding. Further regulation is achieved by a variable number of hormone receptors per type of target cell. Hormones can be grouped into two categories according to the location of its receptor at the target cell: on the cell surface (*cell surface receptors*) or intracellularly at the level of the nucleus (*nuclear receptors*). Most peptide hormones bind to cell surface receptors, while the amino acid derivatives and steroid hormones are usually ligands for nuclear receptors. In some instances, mutational changes in the structure of a hormone receptor result in the constitutive inactivation or activation of the hormone binding, leading to clinical scenarios of hormone deficiency and excess, respectively.

Hormones Binding to Cell Surface Receptors

Cell surface receptors are glycoproteins that are highly mobile within the plasma membrane. Hydrophilic portions of the receptor are exposed at the cell surface, while the hydrophobic portions of the molecule are buried within the lipid bilayer. Cell surface receptors bind water-soluble hormones, such as peptide hormones, monoamines, and prostaglandins. Since these water-soluble hormones are not able to transverse the lipid bilayer to enter the cell, the cell surface receptor serves to transmit the hormonal "message" to the interior of the cell. The binding of the hormone to the cell surface receptor is reversible, allowing the receptor to be activated repeatedly, although the hormone-receptor complex may also be internalized, thus producing a single response from a single ligand-receptor interaction. Although there may be a variable number of cell surface receptors, the principal target tissues for a particular hormone generally contain the largest complement of receptor molecules and are exposed to the highest concentration of hormone.

The binding of a hormone to a cell surface receptor stimulates a cascade of complex events through the generation of second messengers. The activation of protein kinases results in phosphorylations and altered conformation of a diverse number of molecules, which then produces a series of metabolic effects. Posttranslational modifications of the receptor can affect downstream signaling pathways. Pathologic factors, such as genetics, autoimmune processes, and exogenous toxin exposures, may further contribute toward regulation of hormone sensitivity.

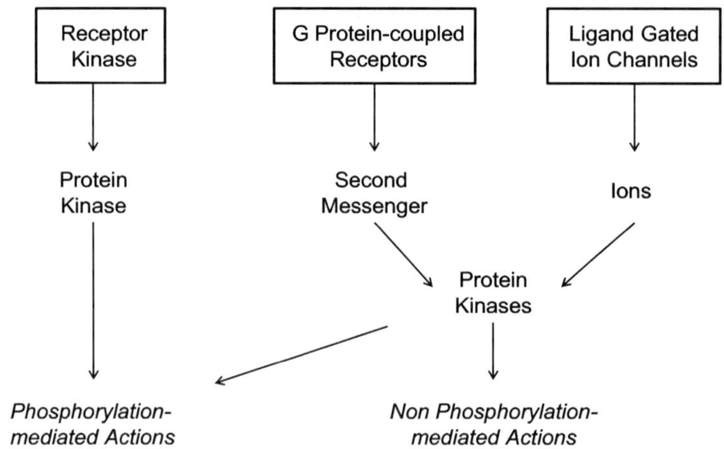

Fig. 2 Cell surface receptor response pathways

Cell surface receptors which trigger intracellular signaling pathways can be subcategorized by their different molecular mechanisms: ligand-gated ion channels, receptor tyrosine kinases, receptor serine/threonine kinases, receptor guanylate cyclase, G-protein-coupled receptors, and cytokine receptors (Fig. 2). The action of G-protein-coupled receptors and cytokine receptors depends on the recruitment of other molecules, while the remaining types of cell surface receptors can also function as ion channels or enzymes to achieve effector function. Thus, hormones may utilize a variety of intracellular mediators, and a given hormone may utilize one or more of these intracellular pathways. The metabolic events regulated by the activation of cell surface receptors may either be rapid alterations in ion or substrate flux across the plasma membrane or slower alterations in protein levels by modulation of gene transcription.

Hormones Binding to Nuclear Receptors

Lipid-soluble hormones are small ligands (molecular mass <1,000 Da) and thus able to penetrate the plasma membrane to interact with intracellular nuclear receptors, which are much larger proteins (molecular mass 50,000–100,000 Da) (Fig. 3). The classic nuclear receptors are those for the thyroid and steroid hormones, the latter which include aldosterone, cortisol, estradiol, progesterone, and testosterone. Vitamins A and D metabolites are other lipophilic signaling molecules that also utilize nuclear receptors.

While most lipid-soluble hormones enter cells by passive diffusion, the thyroid hormones utilize active transport proteins, such as monocarboxylate transporter 8 (MCT8), MCT10, and organic anion transporting polypeptide 1 (OATP1C1), to

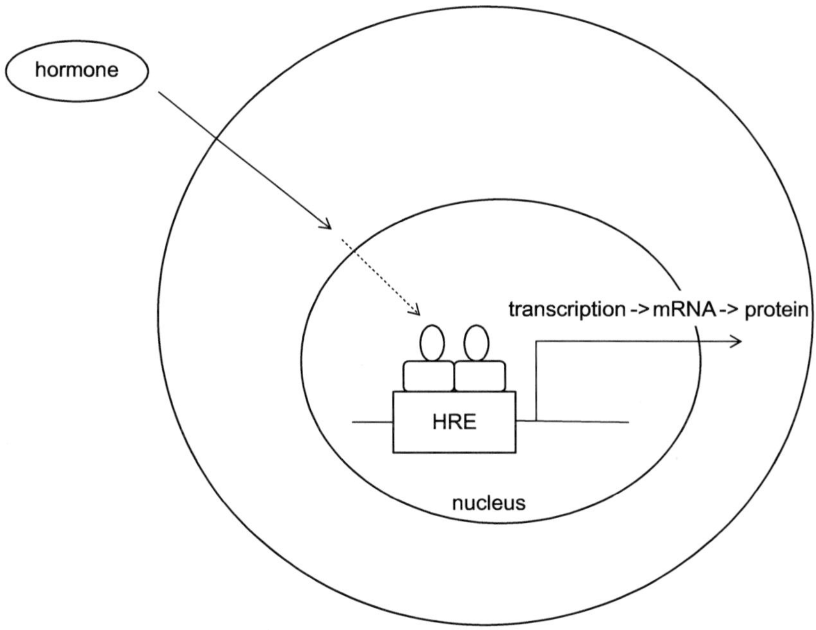

Fig. 3 Nuclear receptor signaling pathways

interact with the thyroid nuclear receptors. Vitamin A is stored in the liver and metabolized to retinoic acid, which acts as a ligand for the retinoic acid receptor (RARs) in the nucleus, or if converted to its isomer, another nuclear receptor termed the retinoid X receptor (RXR). Vitamin D3 is produced in the skin as a result of the action of ultraviolet radiation on 7-dehydrocholesterol. Vitamin D3 is transported to the liver, where it is converted to 25-hydroxy vitamin D, and then to the kidney tubule to be converted to its active form, 1,25-dihydroxy vitamin D. This active form of vitamin D binds to the vitamin D receptor (VDR) that is located in cells of almost all organs.

Nuclear hormone receptors can also be encoded by more than one gene, such as thyroid and estrogen; both of these receptors have an α and a β gene. Some receptors can also mediate the signals of more than one hormone, such as the androgen receptor that can interact with both DHT and testosterone.

Nuclear receptors bind to lipophilic ligands with high affinity. This binding is mediated by the C-terminal ligand-binding domain and domains D and E of the nuclear receptor. Meanwhile, specificity of ligand-receptor binding is accomplished by binding of the C domain of nuclear receptors to the hormone response element (HRE) gene sequences of the ligand. Most nuclear receptors bind to HREs as dimers. As the metabolic effects of these proteins are then produced by the translation products of the thyroid or steroid hormone-regulated mRNAs, the actions of these hormones are relatively slow, compared to cell surface receptors.

Roles of Hormones

Hormones have many roles that work together to achieve the exquisite regulation required of many body processes. This regulation by the endocrine system is often the result of different mechanisms at many targets, thereby allowing the body to respond to a diverse variety of concurrent physiologic changes and pathologic insults. The major body processes regulated by hormones include energy production, utilization and storage (intermediary metabolism), growth, development, reproduction, and maintenance of the internal environment (mineral and water metabolism and cardiovascular effects).

Energy Production

Hormones are the primary mediators of substrate flux and the conversion of food into energy production. The utilization of glucose and other fuels is regulated by a number of different hormones. Catecholamines, ghrelin, growth hormone, testosterone, and cortisol induce the breakdown of lipids and the hydrolysis of triglycerides into glycerol and free fatty acids (lipolysis). Glucocorticoids, catecholamines, growth hormone, cortisol, and glucagon promote hyperglycemia. Consistent with the occasional need for rapid mobilization of fuels, many of these catabolic hormones exert their actions by the activation of adenyl cyclase. In contrast, insulin and the insulin growth factors (IGFs) are anabolic hormones and store fuel for later use. Finally, the thyroid hormones directly affect energy production at the level of the mitochondria, which have their own specific thyroid hormone receptors.

Intermediary Metabolism, Growth, and Development

Hormones are crucial for normal somatic growth and development. The major hormones involved in development and growth are thyroid hormone, growth hormone, the sex steroids, insulin, and other growth factors. Thyroid hormone affects both growth and development and has a particularly critical role in early neurodevelopment. Growth hormone primarily regulates growth, and the sex steroids mainly regulate sexual development.

Androgens, estrogens, growth hormone, thyroid hormone, and prolactin can act as growth factors. The action of some of these is reliant on the availability of other hormones to act as growth factors. One example is growth hormone, which requires thyroid hormone for its normal synthesis and secretion, in part through the stimulation and action of IGF-1 by thyroid hormone. In contrast, glucocorticoids in excess and somatostatin inhibit the secretion of growth hormone and TSH.

Reproduction

Hormonal regulation is essential for normal reproductive processes. Hormones are required for both the production of ova and sperm from the gonads and the dimorphic anatomical, functional, and behavioral development of males and females that is essential for sexual reproduction. Regulation is achieved by the negative feedback within the hypothalamic-pituitary-gonadal axis. Gonadotropin-releasing hormone (GnRH) is secreted in pulsatile fashion from the hypothalamus to stimulate gonadotropin production in the pituitary. The gonadotropins are essential regulators of ovarian and testicular function and the subsequent secretion of the sex steroids from the gonads. The sex steroids control functions crucial for pregnancy and for sexual differentiation and development.

Mineral and Water Metabolism

Aldosterone, parathyroid hormone (PTH), and vitamin D have primary functions in ion regulation, while vasopressin (also termed antidiuretic hormone, ADH) regulates water metabolism. These hormones bind to specific receptors at various target tissues. Aldosterone binds to mineralocorticoid receptors (MRs) located in the kidney, distal colon, heart, central nervous system (hippocampus), brown adipose tissue, and sweat glands and is important for the regulation of extracellular volume and potassium homeostasis. The mineralocorticoid receptor (MR) can be stimulated by both aldosterone and cortisol. Parathyroid hormone binds to one of the two parathyroid hormone receptors: parathyroid hormone 1 receptor (PTH1R) is expressed in bone and kidney to increase serum calcium concentrations, while parathyroid hormone 2 receptor (PTH2R) is expressed in the central nervous system, pancreas, testes, and placenta. The nuclear vitamin D receptor (VDR), which binds 1,25-dihydroxy vitamin D, is more diverse and located in cells of almost all organs. In addition, several other hormones (insulin, glucagon, catecholamines, thyroid hormone, and glucocorticoids) have secondary effects on water and electrolyte metabolism.

Cardiovascular Functions

While not usually considered an endocrine organ, the heart, specifically the atria, produces atrial natriuretic peptide (ANP), which has extensive effects on the cardiovascular system. Important to the regulation of water, sodium, and potassium, ANP acts on the kidneys to decrease extracellular fluid volume, renal arterial pressure, and urinary potassium excretion.

Many other hormones also affect cardiovascular function, including catecholamines, thyroid hormone, mineralocorticoids, and the sex steroids. Catecholamines increase pulse, blood pressure, myocardial contractility, and cardiac conduction velocity. Thyroid hormones have an important role in maintaining heart rate, stroke volume, peripheral vascular resistance, and cardiac contraction. Mineralocorticoids maintain fluid and sodium homeostasis that is important within the cardiovascular system. Finally, the sex steroids have varied roles in cardiovascular health: testosterone stimulates the renin-angiotensin-aldosterone system, while estrogen inhibits this; progesterone has both vasodilatory and vasoconstrictive effects.

Tropic Actions

Some hormones have primary roles to regulate the production of other hormones (tropic effects), and many of these are produced in and secreted from the anterior pituitary. TSH regulates thyroid hormone production, LH regulates estrogen production in the female and testosterone production in the male, and ACTH regulates glucocorticoid production in the adrenal gland. These hormones share a similar mechanism by the activation of adenyl cyclase to increase the rate of hormone synthesis and secretion. They may also promote cell division to result in enlargement (hyperplasia) of the target gland.

Hormone Synthesis, Storage, and Secretion

Some hormones are secreted in their active forms, while others later undergo activation in order to be biologically active. The rates and mechanisms of hormone synthesis, storage, and secretion are generally different between the peptide and amine hormones, compared to the steroid hormones.

Peptide and Amine Hormones

Cells that synthesize peptide or amine hormones store the hormones in granules and, thus, have a readily releasable pool of hormone. Specific subcellular pathways consist of interactions between the endoplasmic reticulum (ER), Golgi apparatus, and secretory granules. Upon the appropriate stimulus, the storage granules migrate to the cell surface and fuse with the plasma membrane, and hormone is secreted into the extracellular space (exocytosis). In some cells, this process is dependent upon calcium influx into the cell. In the second pathway of intracellular hormone transport and secretion, vesicles instead mediate this process and enable the movement of hormone stored within them toward the cell surface.

In some pathways, the stimulus for hormone release also induces synthesis of new hormone, resulting in a biphasic secretion pattern. There is an early release of preformed hormone from secretory vesicles, followed by release of newly synthesized hormone.

Steroid Hormones

The release of steroid hormones provides the stimulus for increased synthesis of hormone. Secretion of steroid hormones follows simple bulk transfer pathways involving concentration gradients into the circulation. While the tropic hormones from the anterior pituitary are secreted in the microgram range, their corresponding peripheral hormone levels are usually produced in milligram amounts and have much longer half-lives. The classic steroid hormones are the thyroid hormones and corticosteroids (aldosterone, cortisol, estradiol, progesterone, and testosterone).

Thyroid hormone synthesis requires the uptake on iodine from circulation into the thyroid follicular cell. Iodine is transferred to the follicular lumen and becomes oxidized by thyroid peroxidase for the iodination of thyroglobulin to form the thyroid hormone precursors, MIT and DIT. Stimulation of the thyrocyte by TSH results in proteolysis of thyroglobulin and release of the thyroid hormones, T3 and T4, into circulation. However, despite a large amount of preformed hormone stored in the thyroid gland, secretion of thyroid hormone does not respond as quickly to the stimulus, in contrast to the peptide and amine hormones.

The corticosteroids are synthesized from cholesterol within the zona glomerulosa of adrenal cortical cells. Low-density lipoprotein (LDL) binds to LDL receptors on the cell surface of adrenal tissue, then undergoes endocytosis, and fuses with lysozymes to produce cholesterol. Cholesterol can also be synthesized within the adrenal cortex or be derived from other lipid subfractions. Cholesterol then undergoes various hydroxylations, methylations, and demethylation processes that ultimately result in the production of glucocorticoids, androgens, estrogen, and their derivatives. Most of the steroidogenic synthetic actions are mediated by cytochrome P450 enzymes.

Rates of Hormone Secretion

The secretion rates of hormones are dependent on usually multiple signals, including nutrient intake, stress, and adrenergic pathways. Pathways are interconnected with and adapt to the local environment. In general, only limited quantities of hormones are stored within the body, and even stores of peptide hormones are depleted within hours to days. Most peptide hormones are secreted in episodic bursts at irregular intervals on daily, hourly, or minute-by-minute frequencies.

The pattern of secretion of some hormones is dependent on local stimuli. Sleep-related release occurs with many hormones, including growth hormone (mostly secreted during slow-wave sleep) and prolactin from the anterior pituitary. Other hormones are subject to circadian variation (which is dependent on environmental cues, primarily light exposure), such as ACTH, and subsequent cortisol, secretion. Insulin is secreted upon nutrient intake and other signals. Prolactin secretion is relatively tonic, but peaks in episodic bursts when prompted by suckling. Parathyroid hormone secretion is stimulated by decreasing serum calcium concentrations. The frequency of pulses of secretion of some of the tropic hormones, such as the gonadotropins, determines whether these hormones will be stimulatory or inhibitory.

Ultimately, the rate of release of hormone is determined by its rate of synthesis. Two exceptions are thyroid hormone and vitamin D. Both hormones are stored in large amounts, providing a safeguard against long periods of iodine deficiency or absence of sunlight exposure, respectively. The thyroid gland contains an approximate 2-month supply of stored thyroid hormone for this purpose.

Transport of Hormones

For the most part, hormones must be transported some distance to their target organs. Thus, they must be synthesized in relatively higher concentrations, compared to their requirement at target cells. The primary transport medium is the plasma, although the lymphatic system and the cerebrospinal fluid are also important. Since delivery of the hormone to its target tissue is required before a hormone can exert its effects, the presence or absence of specific transport mechanisms plays a major role in mediating hormonal action.

The water-soluble hormones (peptide hormones, catecholamines) are transported in plasma in solution and require no specific transport mechanism. Because of this, the water-soluble hormones are generally short-lived, circulating in the plasma in concentrations in the femtomolar range. These properties allow for rapid shifts in circulating hormone concentrations, which is necessary with the pulsatile tropic hormones or the catecholamines. This is consistent with the rapid onset of action of the water-soluble hormones.

The lipid-soluble hormones (thyroid hormone, steroids) circulate in the plasma bound to specific carrier proteins. This ensures the appropriate distribution of the water-insoluble ligands and prevents the loss of the hormones through urine or bile excretion routes. Many of the proteins have a high affinity for a specific hormone, such as thyronine-binding globulin (TBG), sex hormone-binding globulin (SHBG), and cortisol-binding globulin (CBG). Nonspecific, low-affinity binding of these hormones to albumin also occurs.

Carrier proteins act as reservoirs of hormone, resulting in picomolar to micromolar circulating hormone concentrations. Since it is generally believed that only the free hormone can enter cells and, thus, can exert its biological actions, a dynamic equilibrium must exist between the bound and free hormone. The protein-bound hormones are in rapid equilibrium with the unbound, or free, fractions, thus ensuring the immediate availability of the free hormones to target cells. Thus, alterations in the amount of binding protein available or in the affinity of the hormone for the binding protein can markedly alter the total circulating pool of hormone without affecting the free concentration of hormone.

Carrier proteins act as buffers to both blunt sudden increases in hormone concentration and diminish degradation of the hormone once it is secreted. The half-life of hormones that utilize carrier proteins is thus longer than those that are not protein bound. Indeed, carrier proteins have a profound effect on the clearance rate of hormones; the greater the capacity for high-affinity binding of the hormone in the plasma, the slower the clearance rate. In some instance, the carrier proteins allow slow, tonic delivery of the hormone to its target tissue. This is consistent with the slower onset of action of the lipid-soluble hormones.

Hormone Metabolism

Clearance of hormones from the circulation plays a critical role in the modulation of hormone levels in response to varied physiologic and pathologic processes. The time required to reach a new steady-state concentration in response to changes in hormone release is dependent upon the half-life of the hormone in circulation. Thus, an increase in hormone release or administration will have a much more marked effect if the hormone is cleared rapidly from the circulation as opposed to one that is cleared more slowly.

Hormone metabolism is also linked to the processes that they regulate. For example, insulin and catecholamines participate in rapid cellular responses, and their short half-lives facilitate the wide swings in their levels that are essential for their regulatory actions. Conversely, hormones that participate in transcriptional regulation control more long-term cellular responses; their longer half-lives buffer rapid fluctuations in free hormone levels. Most peptide hormones have a plasma half-life measured in minutes, consistent with the rapid actions and pulsatile nature of secretion of these hormones.

Rapid clearance of hormone is achieved by the lack of protein binding in the plasma, degradation or internalization of the hormone at its site of action, and ready clearance of the hormone by the kidney. Binding to serum proteins markedly decreases hormone clearance, as is observed with the steroid hormones and the iodothyronines. Metabolism of the steroid hormones occurs primarily in the liver by reductions, conjugations, oxidations, and hydroxylations that serve to inactivate the hormone and increase their water solubility, facilitating their excretion in the urine and the bile. Metabolic transformation also may serve to activate an inactive hormone precursor, such as the deiodination of thyroxine to form T3 and the hydroxylation of vitamin D at the 1 and 25 positions.

Hormone metabolism is not as tightly regulated as hormone synthesis and release. However, alterations in the metabolic pathways may be clinically important. Drugs that increase activity of the liver P450 enzymes, such as phenytoin, rifampin, carbamazepine, and large doses of barbiturates also increase the turnover of steroid and thyroid hormones and may expose latent adrenal insufficiency or decreased thyroid reserve. More commonly, the administration of these drugs may require increases in the dose of steroids or thyroid hormone administered to achieve the same effect. Thus, large doses of barbiturates may decrease the effectiveness of oral contraceptives.

Alterations in the binding capacity of serum transport proteins also alter the dynamic equilibrium between bound and free hormone, leading to changes in hormone release or replacement requirements. For example, the estrogen-induced increase in TBG may be one possible explanation for the frequently observed increase in the administered dose of L-thyroxine required in the pregnant patient with hypothyroidism. Finally, starvation and illness markedly inhibit the activity of the 5′-deiodinase in the liver. This results in decreased serum T3 concentrations due to the impaired production of T3 from T4 and increased concentrations of the metabolically inactive 3,3′,5′- triiodothyronine (reverse T3) due to decreased clearance. This may be a physiologic response to conserve the body's energy stores.

Regulation of Hormone Secretion

A distinguishing characteristic of endocrine systems is the feedback regulation of hormone production. Two major influences that are essential to feedback control of hormone secretion are input from higher neural centers and changing plasma levels of hormone or other substances. These regulatory networks allow (1) hormone levels, and subsequent hormone action, to be controlled within relatively narrow parameters in the basal state, (2) the establishment of circadian rhythms for hormonal secretion, and (3) the stimulation or inhibition of hormone secretion in response to a variety of sensory inputs.

The classic paradigm for feedback regulation is the hypothalamic-pituitary-target gland axis, where the target gland is either the thyroid, adrenal, or the gonads (Fig. 4). Neural input from higher centers lead to the secretion of a releasing factor from the hypothalamus that acts upon the pituitary to release a tropic hormone. The tropic hormone then stimulates hormone production and release from the target gland. The increase in circulating hormone levels then inhibits further production of the hypothalamic releasing factor, the tropic hormone, or both. Other factors that exert feedback regulation on hormone production include ions (i.e., the effect of calcium on PTH secretion), metabolites (glucose on insulin and glucagon secretions), and osmolarity and fluid volume (vasopressin, renin, and aldosterone).

While most examples of feedback regulation are inhibitory, positive feedback systems also exist. Oxytocin release is stimulated by uterine contractions, which, in

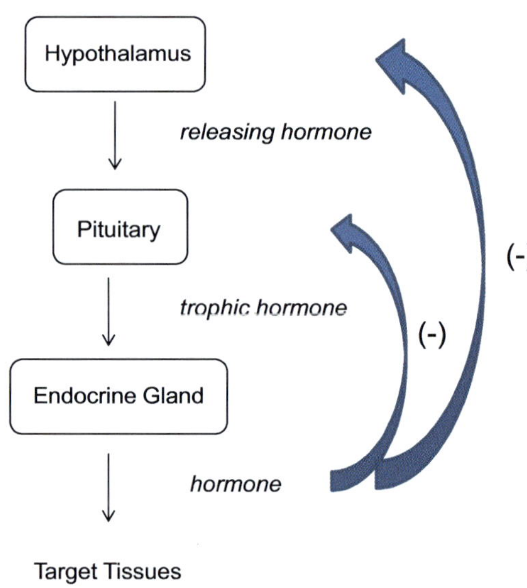

Fig. 4 Feedback regulation of the hypothalamic-pituitary-target gland axis

turn, stimulates further uterine contractions. The result of this positive feedback loop is eventual expulsion of the newborn from the uterus. During the menstrual cycle, the gonadotropins are subject to both positive and negative control. In general, estradiol exerts a negative influence on gonadotropin secretion. However, during the late follicular phase, estradiol concentrations reach a critical level and trigger the LH and FSH surges, leading to ovulation.

Disorders of the Endocrine System

The clinical consequences of dysfunction of the endocrine glands are primarily those associated with hormone deficiency or excess. The disorders that produce these clinical syndromes are diverse and occur by a variety of mechanisms. These include abnormalities with the endocrine glands themselves, including genetic defects, ectopic production of hormones, abnormal conversion of prohormones to their active form, diminished or enhanced response of target tissues to hormones, and iatrogenic factors. The few disorders of the endocrine glands that do not involve altered hormone secretion include simple goiter in the thyroid and nonfunctioning adenomas or carcinomas, which may occur at all endocrine glands.

The negative feedback regulation of many of the endocrine glands allows diagnosis of both overt dysfunction, which is often clinically apparent, and subclinical dysfunction, the management of which is often controversial. In addition, measurement of the levels of the components of the feedback loop will also provide information about the location of the abnormality. In the classical example of negative feedback involving the pituitary trophic hormones and the hormones secreted by the peripheral glands (thyroid, adrenal, testis), decreased peripheral hormone levels and increased pituitary hormone levels are consistent with primary gland deficiency, which is the typical cause of hormone deficiency. Conversely, if both the pituitary and peripheral hormones are low, a central (pituitary, hypothalamus) source is the likely cause of the deficiency. In the case of hormone excess, suppressed pituitary hormone levels indicate primary gland hyperactivity, while increased pituitary hormones suggest pituitary hypersecretion, a far less common condition. A similar example is seen with the PTH-calcium axis. Thus, the laboratory plays a significant role in the evaluation of endocrine dysfunction.

Hormone Deficiency Syndromes

Gland Dysfunction

The most common cause of hormone deficiency is autoimmune destruction of endocrine tissue. All endocrine glands are susceptible to autoimmune involvement, and some syndromes include dysfunction of more than a single gland.

Endocrine glands also may be injured or destroyed by infectious agents (tuberculosis of the adrenals), infection or hemorrhage (postpartum necrosis of the pituitary and adrenal hemorrhage), chemical or radiation exposure (testicular damage with chemotherapy, hypothyroidism after mantle irradiation for lymphoma, and, less commonly, hypopituitarism after brain irradiation), space-occupying lesions (hypopituitarism due to craniopharyngioma), primary or secondary neoplasia, or surgical removal.

Defects in embryogenesis can lead to absence or malformation of the endocrine glands, as seen with thyroid agenesis, sublingual thyroid, and chromosomal abnormalities leading to gonadal dysgenesis or agenesis (Turner's syndrome) or hyalinization of the seminiferous tubules and decreased testosterone production (Klinefelter's syndrome). Alternatively, gland development may be normal, but an enzyme necessary for hormone production may be absent, as in congenital adrenal hyperplasia and some forms of congenital goiter.

Finally, hormone production may be diminished or absent due to lack of a nutrient or an environmental factor, such as iodine-deficient goiter or vitamin D deficiency due to lack of exposure to sunlight or malabsorption.

Extraglandular Dysfunction

Extraglandular disorders can also result in hormone deficiency. These processes include the defective conversion of a prohormone to its active form (e.g., impaired conversions of 25-hydroxy vitamin D to 1,25-dihydroxy vitamin D in vitamin D-dependent rickets and chronic renal failure and absent or dysfunctional 5-α-reductase, which converts testosterone to dihydrotestosterone, resulting in androgen deficiency).

There may also be enhanced degradation of the hormone to result in hormone deficiency. Enhanced degradation of hormone usually affects the response to exogenously administered hormone, as in the phenytoin-induced increase in metabolism of steroid hormones in patients with adrenal insufficiency or L-thyroxine in patients with hypothyroidism, the increased metabolism of T3 and T4 in individuals with tumors expressing high levels of the iodothyronine deiodinase type 3 (D3) (consumptive hypothyroidism), and the unmasking of Addison's disease by the administration of thyroid hormone in individuals with Hashimoto's thyroiditis (Schmidt's syndrome).

Finally, a target tissue may be unable to respond to a hormone (hormone resistance). This may be due to either dysfunction or absence of hormone receptors or the production of substances that block access of the hormone to its receptor. Hormone resistance produces a clinical picture of hormone deficiency in the presence of normal or supernormal hormone secretion or administration.

Other examples of hormone resistance include those to a G-protein subunit α receptor (pseudohypoparathyroidism type 1A), GH receptor (Laron syndrome), insulin receptor (as in type 2 diabetes mellitus), TSH receptor (thyroid hormone resistance), and androgen receptor (androgen insensitivity syndrome). Albright and his colleagues first recognized hormone resistance in their characterization of pseudohypoparathyroidism in 1942. This disorder is now known to be a result of altered receptor signaling due to absent or subnormal amounts of a G-protein subunit which couples hormone-receptor binding to the activation of the catalytic subunit of adenyl cyclase. These individuals have hypocalcemia in the presence of high circulating levels of PTH. Presently, the most common disorder of hormone resistance occurs in obese patients with type 2 diabetes mellitus. The pathogenesis of this disorder is multifactorial and includes abnormal down-regulation of the insulin receptor as well as post-receptor defects. The absence of one or more of the thyroid hormone-receptor isoforms has been described in patients with generalized thyroid hormone resistance. Familial resistance to TSH, due to point mutations in the TSH receptor, the production of biologically less active TSH, or as yet undetermined abnormalities, may result in elevated serum TSH and normal or even low serum thyroid hormone concentrations. In androgen insensitivity syndrome, the absence of testosterone receptors results in female development, despite a 46XY karyotype and high circulating testosterone concentrations.

Finally, receptor antibodies may also rarely produce clinical hormone deficiency in the presence of elevated hormone concentrations and normal hormone receptors, as in rare forms of diabetes mellitus due to antibodies to the insulin receptor and hypothyroidism due to TSH receptor-blocking antibodies.

Hormone Excess Syndromes

Gland Dysfunction

Hyperfunctioning tumors of endocrine glands are usually well-differentiated adenomas which usually manifest clinically as excess hormone production. Despite their benign histopathology, endocrine adenomas can cause serious morbidity and mortality due to their excessive hormone secretion. A pheochromocytoma may cause death due to a catecholamine-induced hypertensive crisis. Acromegaly (due to excess growth hormone) and Cushing's disease (due to excess cortisol) may cause physical deformity, organ damage, and potentially lethal cardiovascular and metabolic perturbations. A pituitary macroadenoma, even though nonfunctional (not producing hormones), may cause visual loss due to damage of the optic chiasm caused by suprasellar extension and increased tumor growth.

More rarely, endocrine cells that continually produce excessive amounts of hormone can be also hyperplastic or neoplastic. While an autonomously functioning tumor (adenoma) is made up of a subset of cells in an endocrine gland, hyperplasia involves all of the cells in the gland. A potential mechanism for hyperplasia is the abnormal set point for the negative feedback control of hormone secretion, resulting in excess secretion of the tropic hormone and excess production of the target gland hormones. Examples of hyperplasia are hyperparathyroidism secondary to the chronically low serum calcium concentrations, as seen in end-stage renal disease (tertiary hyperparathyroidism), bilateral adrenal hyperplasia secondary to excess ACTH stimulation, and thyroid hyperplasia (goiter) in response to TSH stimulation among iodine-deficient individuals. The clinical syndromes caused by excess hormone production due to an autonomously functioning adenoma are often indistinguishable from that caused by gland hyperplasia.

Finally, virtually all endocrine cells have the potential to lose their responsiveness to normal regulatory mechanisms and undergo neoplastic change. Hormone-secreting carcinomas, while rare, can be lethal despite the presence of a hormone marker, as in adrenal and parathyroid carcinoma.

Extraglandular Dysfunction

Non-endocrine tumors, mainly carcinomas, can occasionally produce hormones in excess and present as an endocrine disorder. In most cases, the hormones produced ectopically are those that arise from a single gene, such as ACTH, PTH, erythropoietin, growth hormone, and serotonin. While a large number of non-endocrine cells can produce hormones, ectopic hormone production is primarily associated with APUD (amine precursor uptake and decarboxylation) cells. These cells are found in small cell lung carcinomas, carcinoid tumors, thymomas, and hormone-secreting tumors of the gastrointestinal system, among others.

Gland hyperplasia can occur in the absence of intrinsic glandular dysfunction if the hyperfunctioning gland is reacting appropriately to another stimulus. In Graves' disease, hypersecretion of thyroid hormone is caused by an antibody that binds to and activates the TSH receptor on the thyroid follicular cells. The chronic stimulation of the thyroid leads to follicular cell hyperplasia and hyperthyroidism.

While hormone resistance usually produces a clinical picture of hormone deficiency in the setting of hormone hypersecretion, thyrotoxicosis due to pituitary thyroid hormone resistance has also been described. The only abnormal or deficient T3 receptors are located in the pituitary in this disorder, making the pituitary resistant to the inhibitory feedback inhibition of T3. Most cases of thyroid hormone resistance are caused by mutations in the thyroid hormone-receptor β (THRB) gene, although in the past decade, novel mutations in also the thyroid hormone receptor α (THRA) gene have also been identified in a few individuals.

Not all causes of hormone excess syndromes are due to hyperfunctioning glands or tumors. Leakage of preformed thyroid hormone into the circulation following acute destruction of thyroid follicles may also produce thyrotoxicosis, whether due to a virus (e.g., subacute thyroiditis), an autoimmune-mediated process (e.g., postpartum thyroiditis), or manipulation of the neck, such as in rare cases following parathyroid or other neck surgery. In contrast to autonomous adenomas and hyperplasia, these disorders are usually transient.

Hormone excess states can also occur by the administration of supraphysiologic doses of hormones, both as overreplacement of a primary hormone-deficient disorder and as treatment of a non-endocrine disorder. Cushing's syndrome due to pituitary or adrenal dysfunction is relatively rare, while iatrogenic Cushing's syndrome is more common due to the widespread use of corticosteroids as therapeutic agents. Rarely, the administration of a nonhormonal substance can have hormonal effects, as in the case of licorice ingestion producing a syndrome indistinguishable from primary hyperaldosteronism and exposure to supraphysiologic doses of iodine resulting in iodine-induced thyrotoxicosis.

Evaluation of the Endocrine System

Clinical Evaluation

The evaluation of the endocrine patient, as with any medical patient, begins with the history and physical exam. Consistent with the systemic nature of endocrine disorders, all organ systems may be affected, some to a greater degree than others. Many signs and symptoms of hormone excess or deficiency, especially in long-standing or advanced cases, are readily apparent at the time of initial presentation. More often, the clinical presentation is subtle, and the use of laboratory testing is necessary to make a diagnosis.

However, with the advent of sensitive hormone assays, the concept of subclinical disease, defined as abnormal hormone levels in the absence of clinical symptoms or signs, relies exclusively upon the laboratory to establish a diagnosis. The presenting signs and symptoms of many endocrine disorders are sufficiently vague as to include endocrine dysfunction in the differential diagnosis of many common problems, such as weakness, fatigue, weight loss or gain, hypertension, and diarrhea or constipation. Furthermore, endocrine disorders may be secondary to other medical disorders that dominate the clinical presentation.

Laboratory Evaluation

The biochemical assessment is an integral part of the evaluation of an endocrine disorder. Assays are currently available to measure most, if not all, of the clinically important hormones. However, measurements must be obtained with regard to an understanding of their variability in relation to fasting status, environmental stress, age, gender, diurnal pattern, and pulsatility.

Immunoassays are the most common measurement techniques utilized by commercial laboratories. Using this technique, hormones are measured by assessing the ability of the hormone in the sample to compete with a known amount of labeled hormone for binding to a hormone-specific antibody. The initial assays utilized radioactive labeling of hormones for quantification (radioimmunoassay, RIA), but recently nonradioactive labels (such as enzymes in enzyme-linked immunosorbent assays [ELISA]) are being used that increase the sensitivity of the assay. Other techniques utilized for measurement of hormones include high-performance liquid chromatography (HPLC) and mass spectrometry (MS). The sensitivity and specificity of these various measurement techniques, particularly in relation to other coexisting clinical factors, influence their applicability.

Concentrations of free hormones can be measured or estimated by several methods. The most accurate method is by physically separating the free from the bound hormone, as is done by equilibrium dialysis, and measuring the free hormone directly. However, this is not routinely done due to the time-consuming, labor-intensive process required. Alternatively, measurement of the serum binding proteins will allow an estimate of free hormone. This may be done by direct measurement of the serum binding proteins or an indirect measurement achieved by assessing the saturation of the binding proteins. The latter approach is used frequently in the determination of free thyroid hormone concentrations.

In some instances, measurement of urinary hormones or metabolites may give an assessment of overall hormone production, particularly with hormones in which the plasma levels are subject to frequent variations, such as catecholamines and cortisol.

In hormone excess disorders where there is potentially more than one site of excess hormone secretion, plasma measurements of the specific hormone(s) do not define the site(s) of the excess production and are thus of limited utility. Measurement of hormone levels in samples obtained by cannulation of the venous outflow of a gland allows the termination of the site of hormone secretion. This is useful, for example, in evaluating adenoma vs. hyperplasia as the cause of hyperaldosteronism and in differentiating between Cushing's disease (pituitary ACTH secretion) and ectopic ACTH secretion. The use of imaging techniques such as magnetic resonance imaging (MRI), computerized tomography (CT), and specific isotope localization studies is often helpful in defining the tumor site.

Finally, common screening laboratory tests have identified some endocrine disorders before clinical symptoms arise. One example is the routine measurement of serum calcium in many patients, which has essentially eliminated the presentation of patients with advanced hyperparathyroidism. This practice has also resulted in identifying a large asymptomatic population of patients with primary hyperparathyroidism, some of whom may never manifest clinical symptoms associated with the disease.

Provocative Testing

Provocative testing in endocrinology is a means to assess the ability of an endocrine gland to dynamically respond to regulatory factors. It is especially useful when the static plasma or urinary levels are borderline abnormal. In the case of suspected hypofunction or decreased hormonal reserve, an agent is administered to stimulate hormone production and release. The ACTH stimulation test measures the cortisol response to an intravenous administration of a synthetic fragment of ACTH and is helpful in the evaluation of adrenal insufficiency, especially due to ACTH deficiency. Insulin-induced hypoglycemia, intravenous arginine infusion, and exercise are provocative tests to assess for growth hormone reserve. GnRH and TRH administration assess pituitary reserve for gonadotropin and thyrotropin secretion, respectively.

In suspected cases of excess hormone production, agents that instead suppress hormone secretion are used. The oral glucose tolerance test is useful in suppressing growth hormone secretion in the evaluation of acromegaly. Variations of the dexamethasone suppression test are used to determine the etiology of Cushing's syndrome, whether the defect is in the pituitary or hypothalamic or adrenal or rarely an ectopic ACTH-secreting tumor.

Summary

In this introduction, we have laid the foundation regarding the principles of endocrinology that will be detailed in the subsequent chapters of this book. These general principles are essential toward the examination of normal physiology or an evaluation of endocrine dysfunction. This solid understanding of endocrine pathophysiology provides a rational approach to the patient with endocrine disease and allows for a logical, cost-effective evaluation.

Part II

Hormone Synthesis, Secretion, and Transport

Synthesis, Secretion, and Transport of Peptide Hormones

2

Noemi Malandrino and Robert J. Smith

Abstract

Peptide hormones are composed of polypeptide chains with a size ranging from three to hundreds of amino acids. Peptide hormone synthesis involves several steps occurring in the nucleus and cytoplasm of secretory cells, including gene transcription into the precursor nuclear ribonucleic acid, posttranscriptional modifications of the precursor messenger ribonucleic acid transcript, translation of the mature messenger ribonucleic acid, and cotranslational and posttranslational modifications of the hormonal peptide. Synthesis of peptide hormones is regulated at one or more of the above-mentioned biosynthetic steps in order to meet the secretory requirements of endocrine glands. Once they are synthesized, peptide hormones are packaged into secretory granules until appropriate stimuli result in their secretion into the extracellular space. Secretion is not uniform, but rather follows pulsatile patterns and rhythmic changes which, in association with feedback mechanisms, ensure that hormone production is adequate and prevent the excessive release of hormones. Most peptide hormones are water soluble and therefore do not require carrier proteins to circulate in the blood stream. This property results in rapid hormone degradation by plasma proteases and a shorter half-life and duration of action compared to other types of hormones, such as steroid and thyroid hormones.

N. Malandrino
National Institute of Diabetes and Digestive and Kidney Diseases Intramural Research Program, National Institutes of Health, Bethesda, MD, USA
e-mail: noemimalandrino@gmail.com

R.J. Smith (✉)
The Warren Alpert School of Medicine, Brown University, Providence, RI, USA
e-mail: robert_j_smith@brown.edu

A. Belfiore, D. LeRoith (eds.), *Principles of Endocrinology and Hormone Action*, Endocrinology, https://doi.org/10.1007/978-3-319-44675-2_3

Keywords
Peptide hormone • Synthesis • Secretion • Transport • Gene transcription • Posttranscriptional processing • Translation • Posttranslational processing

Contents

General Characteristics of Peptide Hormones

Peptide hormones are molecules that have as their core structure one or more polypeptide chains ranging from three to hundreds of amino acids in size. The number of different peptide hormones exceeds that of the other major hormone classes, i.e., steroid and amine hormones. Peptide hormones can be synthesized and secreted by specialized cells of endocrine glands or by cells within tissues or organs whose main function is not the synthesis of hormones, e.g., gut, heart, kidneys, and adipose tissue (Table 1). After their synthesis, peptide hormones are stored in membrane-bound secretory vesicles, thus enabling their rapid secretion and onset of action when required. Once secreted, most peptide hormones are not bound to carrier proteins in the circulation. Thus, they are subject to rapid degradation by serum proteases, resulting in shorter half-life and duration of action compared to steroid hormones (Pocock et al. 2013).

Peptide hormones are water-soluble and, unlike steroid hormones, do not readily cross hydrophobic cell membranes. Most peptide hormones exert their actions by binding to specific receptors located on the surface of target cells. The binding of peptide hormones to the extracellular domain of plasma membrane receptors induces the initiation of intracellular signal transduction processes, leading to the opening of ion channels and/or activation of enzymes involved in the production of second messengers and phosphorylated proteins causing specific cellular responses (Pocock et al. 2013). A small number of peptide hormones, including epidermal growth factor, the parathyroid hormone-related protein, and possibly to some extent other hormones, are able to transmit signals by interacting with intracellular cytoplasmic or nuclear receptors through an intracrine mechanism (Re 1999).

Table 1 Examples of human peptide hormones and their sites of synthesis

Site of synthesis	Hormone
Hypothalamus	Arginine vasopressin
	Corticotropin-releasing hormone
	Growth hormone-releasing hormone
	Gonadotropin-releasing hormone
	Oxytocin
	Prolactin-releasing hormone
	Somatostatin
	Thyrotropin-releasing hormone
Anterior pituitary	Adrenocorticotropin hormone
	Follicle-stimulating hormone
	Luteinizing hormone
	Growth hormone
	Prolactin
	Thyroid-stimulating hormone
Parathyroid glands	Calcitonin
	Parathyroid hormone
Heart	Atrial natriuretic peptide
Gastrointestinal tract	Cholecystokinin
	Gastrin
	Ghrelin
	Glucagon-like peptides
	Glucose-dependent insulinotropic polypeptide
	Obestatin
	Oxyntomodulin
	Secretin
Liver and multiple other tissues	Insulin-like growth factor-1
Pancreas	Glucagon
	Insulin
	Amylin
	Pancreatic polypeptide
	Somatostatin
	Vasoactive intestinal peptide
Kidneys	Erythropoietin
	Renin
Adipose tissue	Adiponectin
	Leptin
	Resistin

This chapter will review the processes involved in the synthesis, secretion, and transport of peptide hormones, which, due to the specific characteristics of this category of hormones, differ from the mechanisms occurring for steroid and amine hormones.

Synthesis of Peptide Hormones

Peptide hormones typically are produced by secretory cells containing substantial amounts of rough endoplasmic reticulum (RER) and Golgi sacs, which represent the sites where peptide hormones are synthesized and packaged. These cells contain often highly abundant secretory vesicles, which are formed from the Golgi apparatus and store the synthesized hormones prior to their secretion in response to appropriate stimuli.

Most peptide hormones are composed of a single amino acid chain or the association of two or more peptide subunits encoded by a single gene. Conversely, some glycosylated (glycoprotein) peptide hormones, e.g., follicle-stimulating hormone (FSH), luteinizing hormone (LH), chorionic gonadotropin (hCG), and thyroid-stimulating hormone (TSH), consist of two noncovalently linked subunits encoded by separate genes on separate chromosomes (Gharib et al. 1990). While each individual peptide hormone has a distinct profile of molecular actions and physiological functions, many peptide hormones are recognized to belong to families that share genetic and peptide structural homologies in sites that are essential for aspects of their conformation and biological activity. Examples include the growth hormone family (growth hormone (GH), placental lactogen, and prolactin) (Cooke et al. 1980), the glycoprotein hormone family (FSH, LH, hCG, and TSH) (Gharib et al. 1990), and the insulin-insulin-like growth factor family (insulin, IGF-1, and IGF-2) (Blundell and Humbel 1980). The homologies in these peptide hormone families are thought to reflect their evolutionary emergence from a common ancestral gene.

The synthesis of peptide hormones often involves several steps occurring in the nucleus and cytoplasm of secretory cells. These steps include:

1. Gene transcription to form the precursor heterogeneous nuclear ribonucleic acid (hnRNA)
2. Posttranscriptional modifications of the hnRNA transcript
3. Translation of the mature messenger RNA (mRNA) into the encoded peptide chain
4. Cotranslational and posttranslational modifications of the peptide chains

Gene Transcription

The first stage in the synthesis of peptide hormones is the transcription of the genetic information contained in double-stranded deoxyribonucleic acid (DNA) to generate a single-stranded precursor RNA molecule, designated hnRNA. This process is mediated by the enzyme RNA polymerase II.

The regulation of gene transcription is an important determinant of the level of gene expression. As is the case for other structural genes, the genes encoding peptide hormones have both coding and regulatory regions. The coding regions consist of exons containing nucleotide sequences that are conserved in the mature mRNA, and intron sequences that are excised during posttranscriptional modifications of the hnRNA in the nucleus. The most important regulatory regions are located in a 5′-flanking region positioned immediately upstream of the first transcribed nucleotide, and include a promoter region, which is necessary for the accurate initiation and efficiency of transcription. Two functional domains are found in the promoter. The first consists of an initiator element, which includes the transcription start site and a TATA box, located 25–35 nucleotides upstream of the transcription start site. This domain is required for the correct initiation of transcription. The second domain, located immediately upstream of the transcription start site, contains regulatory sequences that play a pivotal role in determining the rate of transcription. These sequences, denoted cis-acting regulatory elements, interact with transcription factors, which are generally encoded by different genes and defined as trans-acting factors. Another group of regulatory elements, called enhancers, are usually located further upstream or downstream of the promoter region. The response elements are additional cis-acting elements found in the promoter regulatory regions, which serve as binding sites for multiple factors including hormones, resulting in the promotion or suppression of transcription of the genes they regulate.

The interaction of the TATA box with specific transcription factors (i.e., TFIID, TFIIA, TFIIB, TFIIF, TFIIE, TFIIH, TFIIJ) leads to the formation of a preinitiation complex, which regulates the correct initiation of transcription. After the preinitiation complex is formed, the trans-acting factors bind to the regulatory elements and contact the preinitiation complex with resulting increased or decreased transcription.

Once transcription of an RNA strand is initiated, the enzyme RNA polymerase II continues the elongation process of the transcript until a sequence is reached and transcribed that signals cleavage and polyadenylation of the RNA at the 3′ end of the encoded mRNA, leading to transcription termination (Lodish et al. 2008).

Posttranscriptional Modifications

The primary transcript hnRNA is a precursor of mature mRNA containing both exons and introns complementary to the DNA template. After the initiation of transcription, the hnRNA undergoes three major modifications in the nucleus that result in the formation of the mature mRNA. The first modification is cotranscriptional and consists of the addition of a 7-methylguanosine cap to the 5′ end of the nascent RNA strand. The 5′ cap protects the mRNA from degradation by ribonucleases and also mediates the nuclear transport of the mRNA and the binding and assembly of ribosomes at the 5′ end of the mRNA. A second modification involves the cleavage of the RNA strand at the 3′ end, downstream of the polyadenylation signal sequence AAUAAA, and the addition of a poly-A tail (200–250 adenylate residues) by the poly-A polymerase enzyme. This poly-A tail further protects the mRNA from degradation and regulates the transport of the mature mRNA to the cytoplasm. A third modification is the removal of the noncoding introns by splicing. This process is accomplished by spliceosomes, which are complexes composed of small ribonucleoproteins and associated nuclear proteins. Spliceosomes recognize and cut introns at specific 5′ and 3′ end sequences, which are denoted splice donor and acceptor sites,

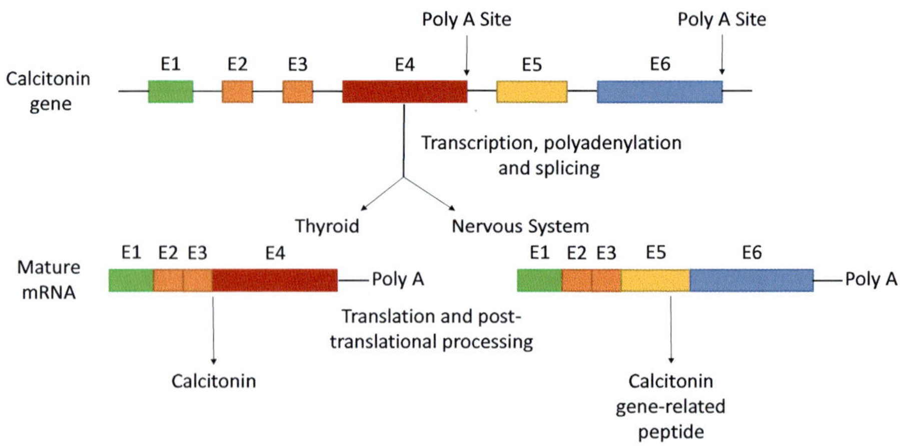

Fig. 1 Calcitonin and calcitonin gene-related peptide are encoded by a single gene which undergoes tissue-specific alternative splicing and polyadenylation of the RNA transcript to generate different hormone variants. *E* Exon

respectively. The two ends of the introns are brought together to form a loop structure which is rapidly degraded, and the two contiguous exons are joined together to assemble the coding region of the mature mRNA (Lodish et al. 2008).

Alternative splicing refers to optional splicing patterns for hnRNA transcripts and represents one of the several processes involved in the generation of biologic diversification of the genetic information. Alternative splicing is a process whereby the primary transcript can be spliced differently in the same or in different tissues, resulting in the synthesis of two or more variants of mRNA and the resulting protein from a single gene. An example of alternative splicing occurs in the processing of calcitonin/calcitonin gene-related peptide pre-mRNA. Both calcitonin and calcitonin gene-related peptide are encoded by the same gene. Splicing and polyadenylation of the pre-mRNA at the end of exon 4 results in the synthesis of calcitonin mRNA, which is mainly found in the thyroid gland. Excision of exon 4, binding of exon 3 and 5, and polyadenylation at the end of exon 6 result in the formation of calcitonin gene-related peptide mRNA, which is mainly found in the nervous system (Amara et al. 1982) (Fig. 1).

Translation of Mature mRNA

The transport of mature mRNA from the nucleus to the cytoplasm is mediated by a nuclear pore complex, which is a large structure located in the nuclear envelope composed of several copies of approximately 30 different proteins called nucleoporins.

In the cytoplasm, the mRNA is translated into the amino acid sequence of the respective peptide hormone. Each amino acid of the hormone peptide chain is specified in the mRNA by nucleotide triplets called codons. The first translated codon, or start codon, is usually AUG, which encodes methionine. At the 3′ end, the mRNA contains a stop codon (UAA, UAG, UGA) that serves to signal translation termination. The translation process includes three steps, initiation, elongation, and termination, and requires the interaction of the mRNA with two other types of RNA, namely ribosomal RNA (rRNA) and transfer RNA (tRNA). The rRNA is transcribed in the nucleolus where it combines with ribosomal proteins to form the ribosomes. These structures consist of two major subunits, designated 60S and 40S, and mediate the recognition between a codon of mRNA and the appropriate anticodon of tRNA. The tRNA is a cloverleaf-shaped molecule acting as an adapter delivering specific amino acids to the ribosomes. Each tRNA contains a trinucleotide anticodon sequence that is complementary to a specific mRNA codon sequence, thus resulting in a specific attachment site for the amino acid encoded by that mRNA codon. Binding of the appropriate amino acid to the cognate tRNA is mediated by a specific aminoacyl-tRNA synthetase. This reaction results in amino acid activation, characterized by the formation of a high-energy bond between the amino acid and the tRNA molecule. This bond will subsequently provide the energy necessary to form a peptide bond between adjacent amino acids as the peptide chain forms.

The first step in the initiation phase of mRNA translation is the formation of a preinitiation complex. This complex results from the association of the ribosome 40S subunit with an initiator tRNA carrying the amino acid methionine, in a process mediated by a group of proteins known as initiation factors. The preinitiation complex subsequently binds to the 5′ cap of mRNA, forming the initiation complex, and slides down the mRNA in the 3′ direction until the initiator tRNA carrying the amino acid methionine recognizes the start codon AUG. The ribosome 60S subunit then binds to the 40S subunit to initiate the translation. Once the complete ribosome is assembled, it contains two binding sites for tRNA, designated P and A sites. The initiator tRNA is initially bound at the P site. After the first peptide bond is formed, the P site binds the tRNA at the end of the growing peptide chain (peptidyl tRNA). The A site binds the tRNA carrying the subsequent amino acid to be added (aminoacyl tRNA).

In the elongation phase, the 60S subunit enzyme peptidyl transferase catalyzes peptide bond formation between the first amino acid methionine and the subsequent encoded amino acid. This reaction is followed by the transfer of the nascent polypeptide chain from the peptidyl tRNA to the amino acid bound to the aminoacyl tRNA. The transfer of the polypeptide chain results in the P site binding the now unacylated tRNA, while a new peptidyl tRNA occupies the A site. Due to a conformational change, the ribosome then translocates three nucleotides along the mRNA, displacing the unacylated tRNA into the cytosol. The new peptidyl tRNA is transferred from the A to the P site, and the next codon to be translated now occupies the A site to start a new elongation step. Similar to the initiation events, the elongation process is also mediated by a series of proteins designated elongation factors.

In the termination phase, after a stop codon is reached and recognized in the A site by specific proteins called release factors, the completed polypeptide chain is cleaved and released from the last tRNA in the P site. The binding between the two ribosomal subunits, terminal tRNA and mRNA is then released, and these molecules become available for reassembly and synthesis of another protein chain.

Translation of peptide hormones begins on ribosomes located within the cytoplasm. In order to be secreted outside of the producing cell, the nascent peptide hormone chains, while still being assembled, enter a secretory pathway that targets these proteins to the endoplasmic reticulum (ER) membrane. This process is mediated by an N-terminal signal sequence within the first segment of the nascent polypeptide chain. The signal sequence and the ribosome 60S subunit bind a signal-recognition particle (SRP), which is a cytosolic ribonucleoprotein complex. The interaction of the SRP with an SRP receptor complex located on the ER membrane results in the translocation of the ribosome and nascent polypeptide to the ER, where translation continues (Lodish et al. 2008).

Cotranslational and Posttranslational Modifications of Peptide Hormones

Most peptide hormones are initially synthesized as larger precursors, which then undergo several modifications. These modifications may occur during or after translation and lead to the formation of the mature hormones.

After the transfer of ribosomes from the cytoplasm to the ER membrane, as translation continues, the growing polypeptide chain enters the ER lumen and the signal sequence required for the transfer is rapidly cleaved by a signal peptidase. The peptide hormone precursors expressing the signal sequence are defined as pre-hormones or pre-prohormones. The release of the signal sequence results in the conversion of these precursors to hormones or prohormones, the latter requiring additional processing in the ER and Golgi complex to form mature active proteins. Examples of this process are shown for pregrowth hormone and preproinsulin in Fig. 2.

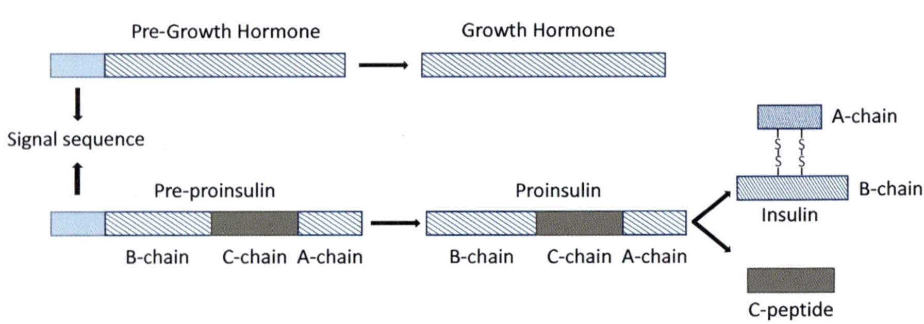

Fig. 2 After the translocation of the nascent polypeptide to the ER lumen, the N-terminal signal sequence is enzymatically cleaved from the peptide precursor, generating the final hormone product (e.g., growth hormone) or a prohormone (e.g., proinsulin), which requires further processing to be converted to the mature hormone

During translation in the ER lumen, nascent peptide hormones may be subjected to additional modifications, which contribute to the stability and folding of the final peptide hormone product. These modifications include: covalent addition of oligosaccharide side chains (glycosylation) to serine and threonine residues (O-linked oligosaccharides) or asparagine residues (N-linked oligosaccharides), disulfide bond formation, and appropriate folding and assembly of proteins.

Once translation is terminated and proper folding and assembly have occurred, the newly synthesized hormones are transferred to the Golgi apparatus, which consists of several membranous regions, including the cis-, medial-, and trans-Golgi regions and the trans-Golgi network. The transport of peptide hormones from the ER to the Golgi apparatus occurs via transport vesicles, which arise from the ER and fuse together to form the cis-Golgi cisternae. In the cis-Golgi, peptide hormones may undergo further proteolytic and N-linked carbohydrate modifications through processes that are completed in the medial- and trans-Golgi regions. Other posttranslation modifications occurring in the Golgi apparatus may include phosphorylation, acetylation, and acylation. Fully processed peptide hormones then enter the trans-Golgi network where they are incorporated into membranous vesicles, called secretory granules. Many peptide hormones in the secretory pathway are stored as inactive prohormones in the secretory granules, where they require a post-Golgi proteolytic cleavage mediated by a prohormone convertase to become active hormones. The peptide hormones are stored in the secretory granules until

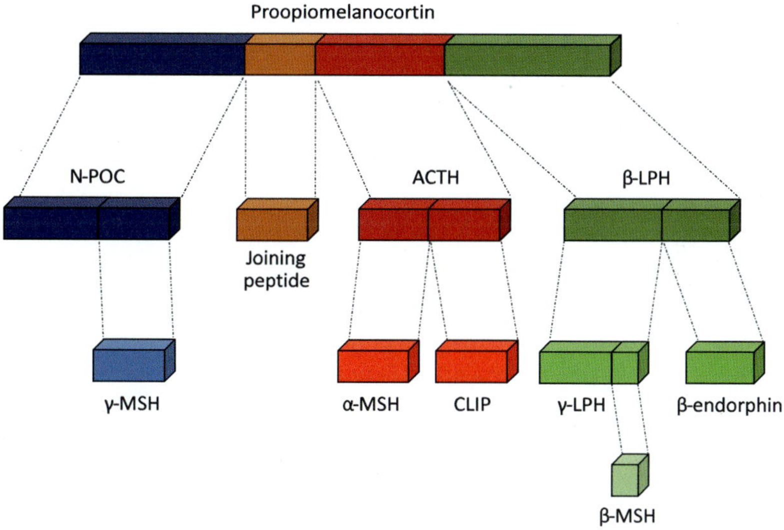

Fig. 3 Posttranslational processing of proopiomelanocortin peptide results in the production of several tissue- and species-specific hormones. *N-POC* N-proopiomelanocortin, *ACTH* adrenocorticotropin hormone, *β-LPH* β-lipotropin, *MSH* melanocyte stimulating hormone, *CLIP* corticotropin-like intermediate lobe peptide, *γ-LPH* γ-lipotropin

appropriate extracellular stimuli, including neural or hormonal signals, induce their release by fusion of the vesicles with the plasma membrane (Lodish et al. 2008).

The complexity of posttranslational processing is illustrated by the processing of the precursor peptide proopiomelanocortin (POMC), resulting in the generation of multiple tissue-specific and functionally distinct peptide hormones (Fig. 3). POMC cleavage in the human anterior pituitary gland generates adrenocorticotropin hormone (ACTH), N-proopiomelanocortin (N-POC), joining peptide (JP) and β-lipotropin (β-LPH). β-LPH may be then processed to β-endorphin (Gibson et al. 1993). In some nonhuman species, POMC is also expressed in the intermediate lobe of the pituitary gland, where ACTH, N-POC, and β-LPH are further cleaved into the smaller peptides α, β, and γ-melanocyte stimulating hormones (α-, β-, and γ-MSH), corticotropin-like intermediate lobe peptide (CLIP) and β-endorphin (Eipper and Mains 1980). α-MSH and β-endorphin are also generated in the hypothalamus (Pritchard et al. 2002), while α-MSH and ACTH are formed and secreted in the skin (Wintzen et al. 1996). This tissue-specific alternative posttranslational processing represents an additional mechanism by which polypeptide diversity is achieved.

Regulation of Peptide Hormone Synthesis

Synthesis of peptide hormones is finely regulated at one or more of the four biosynthetic steps involved in gene expression, thus assuring that production of specific peptide hormones matches the secretory requirements of endocrine glands under different physiological conditions (Darnell 1982). At the transcriptional level, for example, the interaction between DNA-binding proteins and regulatory elements influences the rate of production of the initial RNA transcript. Posttranscriptional alternative splicing in the nucleus and posttranslational modifications in the ER and Golgi apparatus regulate the synthesis of tissue-specific hormone variants. Additional examples of control points include the transport of RNA from the nucleus to the cytoplasm (Palazzo and Akef 2012), the regulation of mRNA stability and the resulting steady-state amount of the active mRNA in the cytoplasm, the formation of the initiation complex during translation, and the control of secretory granule release (Becker 2001).

Secretion of Peptide Hormones

As a result of changes in cytoplasmic calcium concentrations, peptide hormones are released from secretory granules by exocytosis, a process characterized by cytoskeletal protein-mediated migration of the granules toward the cell surface, followed by their fusion with the plasma membrane and delivery of the hormones into the extracellular space.

The secretion of peptide hormones from endocrine cells follows the so-called regulated secretory pathway, where hormones are not continuously secreted, but rather they are secreted acutely in response to a stimulus. In the absence of secretory stimuli, endocrine cells are able to store mature granules containing high concentrations of peptide hormones. When the appropriate signal occurs, endocrine cells then can rapidly release higher amounts of hormones than would be possible if this depended on de novo synthesis in response to the secretory signal (Griffin and Ojeda 2004; Lodish et al. 2008).

Peptide hormone secretion may be controlled by several stimulatory factors, including metabolites, hormones, and neuropeptides, which are released in response to modifications in the homeostatic balance. For example, hormones such as insulin and parathyroid hormone are secreted in response to increases in circulating levels of glucose and calcium, respectively. When these metabolites return to the normal range, insulin and parathyroid hormone secretion decreases. As an example of other secretory control mechanisms, the release of hypothalamic hormones results from the interaction between central nervous system stimuli that include stress, afferent stimuli, and neuropeptides. Once hypothalamic hormones are secreted, they cause the release of pituitary hormones, which in turn control the secretion of peripheral hormones in their respective target glands. Secretion of peptide hormones, such as insulin and glucagon, may be also directly regulated by the autonomic nervous system through postganglionic sympathetic nerves (Normal and Litwack 1997).

Circulating hormone concentrations are determined by the balance of hormone secretion and clearance rates, patterns of hormone secretion, and feedback mechanisms, thus ultimately achieving and maintaining hormone levels that are appropriate to stimulate a specific response from target tissues and re-establish or preserve homeostasis. Hormone secretion is not uniform, but rather it is characterized but a periodic pulsatile release, with rapid increase and subsequent decrease, which is hormone specific and induced by environmental or hormonal cues. Pulses may have variable frequency and amplitude. The frequency of bursts of release of most peptide hormones ranges from 4 to 30 min (e.g., for insulin, glucagon, and parathyroid hormone) to 45–180 min (e.g., for anterior pituitary hormones). The amplitude of pituitary hormone pulses may vary up to 1000-fold in the same individual on the same day, while insulin release shows lower pulse amplitude (Veldhuis et al. 2008).

In addition to pulsatile patterns, hormones may show rhythmic changes. Some of the rhythmic patterns are principally determined by environmental stimuli, such as the light-dark cycle or the sleep-wake cycle, while other patterns are regulated by an internal biological clock. Hormone secretion bursts occurring with a frequency of about 1 h are defined as *circhoral*. A frequency of secretion longer than 1 h, but shorter than 24 h is termed *ultradian*. The interaction between the retina and hypothalamic suprachiasmatic nuclei in response to light plays a major role in determining the *circadian* pattern of secretion, which shows a periodicity of about 24 h. ACTH is an example of peptide hormone with marked circadian rhythm, characterized by a sharp increase of its plasma levels during the early morning hours. A longer periodicity may be seen for other hormones, such as the gonadotropins, with preovulatory peaks occurring every 30 days during the menstrual cycle (Griffin and Ojeda 2004).

Hormone concentrations are also regulated by closed-loop feedback mechanisms, which are the responses of target cells to control levels of the hormones that originally stimulated them. *Negative feedback*, which inhibits the initial hormone signal, is the most common mechanism modulating hormone secretion. Conversely, *positive feedback* increases the initial stimulus. Three patterns of feedback may occur: long loop, short loop, and ultra-short loop. An example of negative feedback is the inhibition of the adeno-hypophyseal hormone ACTH and hypothalamic hormone corticotropin-releasing hormone (CRH) by cortisol. The secretion of cortisol is stimulated by ACTH and CRH in the adrenal gland. The control of ACTH and CRH by cortisol is a designated long feedback loop, because of the need for cortisol to travel from its site of secretion in the adrenals to the central nervous system located hypothalamus and pituitary gland. A short feedback loop is exemplified by the inhibition of CRH by ACTH (requiring the movement of ACTH between the spatially close pituitary and hypothalamus), whereas an ultra-short loop is exemplified by the feedback inhibition by CRH of its own secretion in the hypothalamus (Molina 2013). An example of positive feedback is the preovulatory surge of luteinizing hormone (LH) during the menstrual cycle. LH induces the secretion of estradiol by the ovary and, when estradiol reaches a threshold level, it induces a rapid increase in LH production, the so-called preovulatory surge of LH, which is a key driver of ovulation. This and other positive feedback mechanisms are self-limiting. After reaching a peak, LH levels progressively decline, even if estradiol levels are still elevated. This results from the limited capacity of secretory cells to produce LH, and the action of additional negative feedback loops (Griffin and Ojeda 2004). Feedback mechanisms are essential in preventing the excessive release of hormones, which could lead to pathologic conditions, and also in temporally balancing hormone secretion and levels to metabolic and environmental changes (Molina 2013).

Transport of Peptide Hormones

Most peptide hormones are soluble in aqueous solvents and do not require carrier proteins for transport in the blood stream. This makes them vulnerable to rapid protease degradation, resulting in a short plasma half-life and duration of action. By contrast, the nonpeptide steroid and thyroid hormones circulate in association with specific binding proteins and have relatively long plasma half-lives (Pocock et al. 2013). A small number of peptide hormones do circulate in association with binding proteins, including growth hormone (GH), insulin-like growth factors (IGF-1 and IGF-2), and CRH.

The GH-binding protein (GHBP) is a soluble form of the membrane-bound GH receptor (GHR), composed of a part of the extracellular domain of the GHR. It is generated by a metalloproteinase proteolytic cleavage and binds approximately 50 percent of circulating GH (Nussey and Whitehead 2001). The function of GHBP is not completely understood, however it may serve to increase GH half-life in the circulation or reduce GH availability to membrane-bound GHR (Fisker 2006).

IGFs are also bound to high-affinity carrier proteins in the circulation and in the extracellular space. IGF-binding proteins (IGFBPs) are a family of six proteins sharing homologies in gene and protein structure. All IGFBPs, with the exception of IGFBP-6, bind IGF-1 and IGF-2 with similar affinity. IGFBP-6 binds IGF-2 with a 40-fold higher affinity than IGF-1. By binding IGFs, IGFBPs regulate their transport in the blood and access to the extravascular space, their half-lives and metabolic clearance, their tissue and cell-type distributions, and their interactions with IGF receptors, and thereby modulate tissue-specific biological actions of the IGFs (Jones and Clemmons 1995). IGFBP-3 is the most abundant form of IGFBP in plasma. Binding of IGF-1 to IGFBP-3 provides a stable reservoir of the hormone in the circulation, which can be released in a more active form at cell surface sites of IGF-1 action. The high affinity binding of IGFs to IGFBPs and the low percentage of IGF circulating in free unbound form results in relatively stable concentrations and a longer half-life of IGF-1 in comparison, for example, with GH, which is much less extensively protein bound (Nussey and Whitehead 2001).

CRH-binding protein (CRHBP) is thought to have important functions in the regulation of CRH action. CRHBP may decrease CRH action by decreasing the availability of CRH for binding with its cellular receptors. The complex also influences CRH signaling activity that may include a role in terminating CRH signaling by accelerating its clearance, enhancing activity by protecting CRH from degradation under other conditions, and increasing signaling by contributing to the transport of CRH to target tissues (Seasholtz et al. 2002).

Summary

Peptide hormones are composed of polypeptide chains that are generated through a complex of synthesis and processing in the nucleus and cytoplasm of secretory cells. After synthesis is completed, peptide hormones are packaged into secretory granules and then secreted into the extracellular space in response to specific stimuli. Secretion follows pulsatile patterns and rhythmic changes, which, in association with feedback mechanisms, ensure appropriate hormone production. Unlike steroid and thyroid hormones, most peptide hormones do not require carrier proteins to circulate in the blood, therefore resulting in short half-life and duration of action.

Endocrine disease states typically result when these processes are disrupted. For example, endocrine disorders result when inherited traits or acquired events result in dysregulation of peptide hormone synthesis and secretion (increased or decreased synthesis and secretion by cells normally producing a hormone, or ectopic production by other cell types), insufficiency or overabundance of secretory cells, genetic modifications in hormone structure that cause increased or decreased stability or activity at target cells, changes in hormone binding proteins resulting in increased or decreased hormone stability or action, abnormalities in other pathways controlling the duration of hormone action, or abnormalities in cellular receptors for hormones or in cellular pathways activated or inhibited as a part of normal hormone action. An understanding of these underlying disease mechanisms can be valuable in establishing effective approaches to the prevention, treatment, or cure of endocrine diseases.

References

Amara SG, Jonas V, Rosenfeld MG, Ong ES, Evans RM. Alternative RNA processing in calcitonin gene expression generates mRNAs encoding different polypeptide products. Nature. 1982;298(5871):240–4.

Becker KL. Principles and practice of endocrinology and metabolism. 3rd ed. Philadelphia: Lippincott Williams & Wilkins; 2001.

Blundell TL, Humbel RE. Hormone families: pancreatic hormones and homologous growth factors. Nature. 1980;287(5785):781–7.

Cooke NE, Coit D, Weiner RI, Baxter JD, Martial JA. Structure of cloned DNA complementary to rat prolactin messenger RNA. J Biol Chem. 1980;255(13):6502–10.

Darnell Jr JE. Variety in the level of gene control in eukaryotic cells. Nature. 1982;297(5865):365–71.

Eipper BA, Mains RE. Structure and biosynthesis of pro-adrenocorticotropin/endorphin and related peptides. Endocr Rev. 1980;1:1–27.

Fisker S. Physiology and pathophysiology of growth hormone-binding protein: methodological and clinical aspects. Growth Hormon IGF Res. 2006;16(1):1–28.

Gharib SD, Wierman ME, Shupnik MA, Chin WW. Molecular biology of the pituitary gonadotropins. Endocr Rev. 1990;11(1):177–99.

Gibson S, Crosby SR, White A. Discrimination between beta- endorphin and beta-lipotrophin in human plasma using two-site immunoradiometric assays. Clin Endocrinol. 1993;39:445–53.

Griffin JE, Ojeda SR. Textbook of endocrine physiology. 5th ed. New York: Oxford University Press; 2004.

Jones JI, Clemmons DR. Insulin like growth factor and their binding proteins: biologic actions. Endocr Rev. 1995;16:3–34.

Lodish H, Berk A, Kaiser CA, Krieger M, Scott MP, Bretscher A, et al. Molecular cell biology. 6th ed. New York: W.H. Freeman & Company; 2008.

Molina PE. Endocrine physiology. 4th ed. New York: Mc Graw Hill; 2013.

Normal AW, Litwack G. Hormones. 2nd ed. New York: Academic Press; 1997.

Nussey S, Whitehead S. Endocrinology: an integrated approach. Oxford: BIOS Scientific Publishers; 2001.

Palazzo AF, Akef A. Nuclear export as a key arbiter of "mRNA identity" in eukaryotes. Biochim Biophys Acta. 2012;1819(6):566–77.

Pocock G, Richards CD, Richards D. Human physiology. 4th ed. Oxford: Oxford University Press; 2013.

Pritchard LE, Turnbull AV, White A. Pro-opiomelanocortin processing in the hypothalamus: impact on melanocortin signalling and obesity. J Endocrinol. 2002;172:411–21.

Re R. The nature of intracrine peptide hormone action. Hypertension. 1999;34:534–8.

Seasholtz AF, Valverde RA, Denver RJ. Corticotropin-releasing hormone-binding protein: biochemistry and function from fishes to mammals. J Endocrinol. 2002;175(1):89–97.

Veldhuis JD, Keenan DM, Pincus SM. Motivations and methods for analyzing pulsatile hormone secretion. Endocr Rev. 2008;29(7):823–64.

Wintzen M, Yaar M, Burbach JP, Gilchrest BA. Proopiomelanocortin gene product regulation in keratinocytes. J Invest Dermatol. 1996;106:673–8.

Steroid Hormones: Synthesis, Secretion, and Transport

3

Filippo Acconcia and Maria Marino

Abstract

In mammalian systems, there are six families of steroid hormones that can be classified on both a chemical and a biological basis. They are the estrogens, progesterone, androgens, mineralocorticoids, glucocorticoids, and vitamin D. These steroid hormones play a critical role in numerous physiological and pathophysiological processes and consequently garnered substantial research interest over the last century. The vast majority of circulating steroids in mammals come from the endocrine activity of the gonads and adrenal glands, which metabolize the lipid cholesterol to generate the steroid repertoire. Numerous investigations spanning decades have painstakingly elucidated the molecular enzymes and reactions of steroidogenesis distributed throughout the mitochondrial and microsomal compartments of steroidogenic cells. This chapter deals with the biosynthetic pathways, release, and transport of the major classes of steroid hormones in mammals. In particular, steroidogenesis is discussed as a single process that is repeated in each gland with cell type-specific variations on a single theme. Moreover, the homeostatic mechanisms that regulate the secretion or release of the steroid hormones and precursor hormone by feedback loops or by biological rhythms have been also discussed. Finally, the role of steroid-specific plasma transport proteins and the local inactivation of the excess of active steroids inside the cells are reported in order to obtain a clear picture on how the concentrations of active steroid hormones are regulated.

Keywords

Cholesterol • Steroidogenic enzymes • Steroid hormones • Steroid-binding proteins • Steroidogenic glands • Non-steroidogenic tissues

---

F. Acconcia • M. Marino (✉)
Department of Science, University Roma Tre, Rome, Italy
e-mail: maria.marino@uniroma3.it

A. Belfiore, D. LeRoith (eds.), *Principles of Endocrinology and Hormone Action*, Endocrinology, https://doi.org/10.1007/978-3-319-44675-2_4

Contents

Introduction

Steroids play a critical role in numerous physiological and pathophysiological processes and consequently garnered substantial research interest over the last century. The first steroid hormone, estrone, was isolated in 1929 at a time before the characteristic ring structure of the steroid nucleus had been elucidated (Miller 1988). Today well over 230 naturally occurring steroids have been isolated and chemically characterized. In addition, an uncountable number of steroids and steroid analogs have been chemically synthesized and evaluated for their pharmacological properties. The basis of these recent developments is to be found in the papers authored by Professor Adolf O.R. Windaus (1876–1959) a German chemist who defined the structural determination of cholesterol. Professor Windaus was awarded with Nobel Prize in Chemistry in 1928 "for the services rendered through his research into the constitution of the sterols and their connection with the vitamins" (Miller 1988).

Steroids have a complicated structure of fused rings, which can be subjected to a wide array of modifications by the introduction of hydroxyl or carbonyl substituents and unsaturation (double or triple bonds). In addition, heteroatoms such as nitrogen or sulfur can replace the ring carbons, and halogens and sulfhydryl or amino groups may replace steroid hydroxyl moieties. Furthermore, the ring size can be expanded or contracted by the addition or removal of carbon atoms. An important structural feature of any steroid is recognition of the presence of asymmetric carbon atoms and designation in the formal nomenclature of the structural isomer that is present. Steroids are

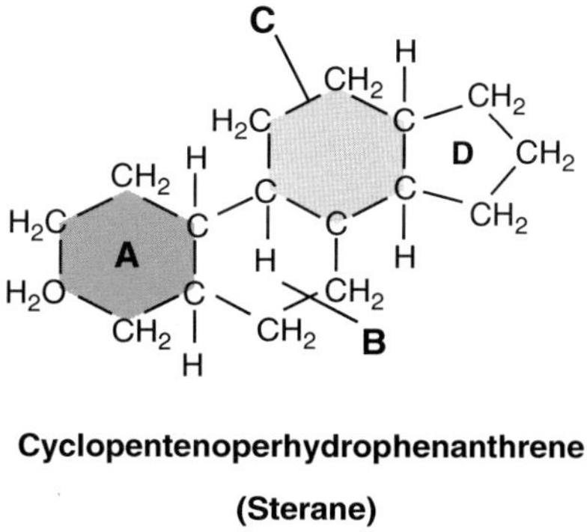

Fig. 1 Ring structure of the completely hydrogenated, cyclopentanoperhydrophenanthrene, also known as sterane. The structure illustrates the 17 carbons and the convention for the *A–D* labels for the four rings

Table 1 Class of steroid hormones

Steroid class	N° of C atoms	Principal active steroid in humans	Systematic name IUPAC
Estrogens	18	17β-Estradiol	(8R,9S,13S,14S,17S)-13-methyl-6,7,8,9,11,12,14,15,16,17-Decahydrocyclopenta[a] phenanthrene-3,17-diol
Androgens	19	Testosterone	(8R,9S,10R,13S,14S,17S)-17-Hydroxy-10,13-dimethyl-1,2,6,7,8,9,11,12,14,15,16,17-dodecahydrocyclopenta[a] phenanthren-3-one
		Dihydrotestosterone	(5S,8R,9S,10S,13S,14S,17S)-17-Hydroxy-10,13-dimethyl-1,2,4,5, 6,7,8,9,11,12,14,15,16,17-tetradecahydrocyclopenta [a] phenanthren-3-one
Progestins	21	Progesterone	Pregn-4-ene-3,20-dione
Glucocorticoids	21	Cortisol	11β-11,17,21-Trihydroxypregn-4-ene-3,20-dione
Mineralocorticoids	21	Aldosterone	11β-11,21-Dihydroxy-3,20-dioxopregn-4-en-18-al
Vitamin D	27	1,25-Dihydroxy vitamin D3 (cholecalciferol)	9,10-Seco-5,7,10 (19)-Cholestatriene-3β-ol
Bile acid	24	Cholic acid	3α,7α,12α-Trihydroxy-5β-cholan 24-oic acid

derived from a phenanthrene ring structure to which a pentane ring has been attached; this yields in the completely hydrogenated form, cyclopentanoperhydrophenanthrene, or the sterane ring structure (Fig. 1). The three six-carbon cyclohexane rings are designated A, B, and C rings, and the five-carbon cyclopentane ring is denoted as the D ring. The six-carbon atoms of a cyclohexane ring are not fixed rigidly in space, but are capable of interchanging through turning and twisting between several structural arrangements in space (chair and boat conformations). The approach of steroid conformational analysis has been of great value to the organic chemistry as a tool to predict or understand the course of synthetic organic chemical reactions. It is also known that conformational considerations play an increasingly useful role in the understanding of steroid hormone–receptor interactions (Fieser and Fieser 1959).

The diversity of steroid structures ranges from insect steroid hormones (ecdysone) to the world of plant growth regulators (brassinolides). In mammalian systems, there are six families of steroid hormones that can be classified on both a chemical (structure) and a biological (hormonal) basis (see Table 1). They are the estrogens, progestins, androgens, mineralocorticoids, glucocorticoids, and vitamin D. In addition, the bile acids are structurally related to cholesterol and thus could constitute a seventh member of the steroid family.

This chapter deals with the biosynthetic pathways, release, and transport of the major classes of steroid hormones in mammals.

Steroid Biosynthesis

Steroidogenesis entails processes by which cholesterol is converted to biologically active steroid hormones. Historically, steroid hormone synthesis only occurred in the steroidogenic glands (i.e., adrenal glands, gonads, and placenta). A significant number of studies have now challenged this view by demonstrating that several organs, including the brain, adipose tissue, and intestine, are capable of producing steroid hormones. These are called non-steroidogenic or intracrine tissues. Intracrine tissues do not have the ability to transform cholesterol into active steroid hormones, but depending on enzymes that are expressed in the tissues, active steroids are produced from various steroid precursors (Luu-The 2013). Whereas most endocrine texts discuss adrenal, ovarian, testicular, placental, and other steroidogenic processes in a gland-specific fashion, according to Walter L. Miller's view, steroidogenesis is better understood as a single process that is repeated in each gland with cell type-specific variations on a single theme (Miller and Auchus 2011). Thus, in this paragraph, an overview of cholesterol uptake and steroidogenic enzymes will precede the description of the synthesis of specific hormones in both steroidogenic and non-steroidogenic tissues.

Cholesterol

All of mammalian steroids are biologically derived from cholesterol. The cholesterol is the most prevalent steroid in all animals and has multiple physiological roles that include its structural presence in all membranes. Cholesterol also is the starting point in the biosynthesis of all steroid hormones, vitamin D and its steroid hormone daughter metabolite, 1α,25-dihydroxy vitamin D ($1\alpha,25(OH)_2D$), and the bile acids. The level of the total body cholesterol is determined by a complex interplay of dietary available cholesterol, de novo synthesis of cholesterol, and excretion of cholesterol and bile salts. The liver and intestine together account for more than 60% of the body's daily biosynthesis of this sterol from acetate via a complex pathway primarily found in the endoplasmic reticulum, but most steroidogenic cholesterol is derived from circulating lipoproteins (Chang et al. 2006). High-density lipoproteins (HDLs) may be taken up via scavenger receptor B1 (SR-B1), and low-density lipoproteins (LDLs) are taken up by receptor-mediated endocytosis via LDL receptors. LDL can suppress the rate-limiting enzyme in cholesterol synthesis, 3-hydroxy-3-methylglutaryl coenzyme A reductase. Although rodents preferentially use the HDL/SR-B1 pathway, the principal human source to obtain steroidogenic cholesterol is receptor-mediated endocytosis of LDL. After circulating LDL is internalized by receptor-mediated endocytosis, the resulting endocytic vesicles fuse with lysosomes, where the LDL proteins are degraded by proteolysis, liberating the cholesteryl esters, which are then hydrolyzed to "free" cholesterol by lysosomal acid lipase (Horton et al. 2002; Brown et al. 1979; Kraemer 2007). However, cholesterol is never truly free, as its solubility is only about 20 μmol/L, so that the term "free cholesterol" refers to cholesterol that is bound to proteins or membranes, but lacks a covalently linked group. Free cholesterol may be used by the cell or stored in lipid droplets following reesterification by acyl coenzyme A-cholesterol-acyltransferase. Similarly, HDL cholesteryl esters that enter the cell via SR-B1 are elaborated by hormone-sensitive neutral lipase, following which the free cholesterol may also be used or reesterified for storage. Intracellular cholesterol transport may be vesicular (mediated by membrane fusion) or non-vesicular (bound to proteins) (Chang et al. 2006). Both vesicular and non-vesicular cholesterol transport occur in steroidogenic cells, but non-vesicular transport involving high-affinity cholesterol-binding steroidogenic acute regulatory protein (StAR)-related lipid transfer (START) domain proteins appears to be the principal means of cholesterol transport from lipid droplets to the outer mitochondrial membrane (OMM). Movement of cholesterol from the OMM to the inner mitochondrial membrane (IMM) requires a multi-protein complex on the OMM (Chang et al. 2006).

Steroidogenic Enzymes

Numerous investigations have elucidated the molecular enzymes and reactions of steroidogenesis distributed throughout the mitochondrial and microsomal compartments of steroidogenic cells (Miller and Auchus 2011). Six P450 enzymes participate in steroidogenesis, and at least three more participate in the processing of vitamin D; five of these are found in mitochondria. The first step of steroidogenesis occurs in the mitochondria, where the cytochrome P450 side-chain cleavage enzyme (P450scc, *CYP11A1* gene) cleaves the aliphatic tail of cholesterol. The final product of this first reaction common to all steroidogenic pathways is the pregnenolone (Miller and Auchus 2011). The expression of the *CYP11A1* gene and, thus, the pregnenolone synthesis render a cell "steroidogenic." P450scc and its cofactors are localized on the matrix face of the inner mitochondrial membrane. Although P450scc is known to be the rate-limiting enzyme for adrenal and gonadal steroid hormones, it is not the catalytic process of the cholesterol side-chain cleavage enzyme that is rate limiting. Rather, the presence and properties of the StAR transporter at the OMM facilitate the movement of cholesterol across the OMM to the IMM site of the P450scc. Indeed, StAR facilitates the actions of cholesterol side-chain cleavage that result in the production of mineralocorticoids and glucocorticoids, in the adrenals, and of estrogens or androgens in the gonads (Stocco et al. 2005). The most convincing evidence for the essential nature of StAR is that mutations of the *StAR* gene can result in a defect associated with the disease known as lipoid congenital adrenal hyperplasia characterized by a deficiency of both adrenal and gonadal steroid hormones (Stocco et al. 2005; Riegelhaupt et al. 2010).

Once pregnenolone is produced from cholesterol, it may undergo 17-α-hydroxylation to 17OH-pregnenolone that ultimately leads in the adrenal cortex to the synthesis of aldosterone and cortisol, in the ovarian *theca* and *granulosa* cells to progesterone, and in the testes into testosterone. 3β-hydroxysteroid dehydrogenase (3βHSD) converts pregnenolone to progesterone. The hydroxysteroid dehydrogenase, 290–380 amino acids (35–45 kDa), may be found both in the mitochondria and in the endoplasmic reticulum; it utilizes the nicotinamide adenine dinucleotide ($NADH/NAD^+$ or $NADPH/NADP^+$) as electron acceptors or electron donors. Although rodents contain multiple 3βHSD isoforms, the human genome has only two active genes and several pseudogenes. The type 1 enzyme catalyzes 3βHSD activity in the placenta, breast, liver, brain, and some other tissues. This isoform is required for placental progesterone production during pregnancy. In contrast, the type 2 enzyme (3βHSD2) is the principal isoform in the adrenals and gonads. Alternatively, pregnenolone may exit the mitochondrion and become the substrate for P450c17 in the endoplasmic reticulum. Pregnenolone appears to exit the mitochondrion unaided; no transport protein has been found, and physiologic evidence does not suggest the presence of such a transporter (Miller and Auchus 2011).

The subsequent steps in steroid biosynthesis (see next paragraphs) are synthesized by a family of homologous oxidative enzymes (~57 human enzymes) collectively known as the cytochrome P450 hydroxylases. Each individual P450 enzyme is composed of about 500 amino acids and has a single heme (protoporphyrin ring with a single chelated Fe^{2+} group). The cytochrome moiety is structurally analogous to the hemoprotein cytochromes of the electron transport chain present in mitochondria that are dedicated to the production of ATP. All contain some kind of covalently bound protoporphyrin ring coordinatcly bound to onc atom of iron, which can be reversibly oxidized and reduced. As a class, most of these P450 enzymes are subject to inhibition by the presence of carbon monoxide. Cytochrome P450 steroid enzymes are known to be present in the liver, adrenal cortex, ovary, testis, kidney, placenta, lungs, intestinal mucosa, and selected regions of the brain. Each P450 hydroxylase has a substrate-binding domain that is comparable in its ability to define substrate specificity to that of the ligand-binding domains of steroid receptors and plasma transport proteins for steroid hormones. Thus, the three-dimensional structure of the substrate-binding domain of a P450 hydroxylase determines which of the some 22–27 carbons of the substrate will acquire a new hydroxyl group (Miller and Auchus 2011).

Catalysis by P450scc and other mitochondrial P450 enzymes requires two electron-transfer intermediates, ferredoxin reductase and ferredoxin. Ferredoxin, which has ~116 amino acids (14 kDa), is a sulfur/iron electron shuttle protein in the mitochondrial electron transport process associated with steroid hydroxylation. The ferredoxin protein acts as a shuttle, accepting electrons from ferredoxin oxidoreductase, which then diffuses in the mitochondrial matrix to a P450 hydroxylase where it donates a pair of electrons. Ferredoxin oxidoreductase is an inner mitochondrial membrane-bound flavoprotein with a molecular weight of 51,100. It is responsible for the transfer of electrons from NADPH to ferredoxin and is widely expressed in many human tissues (Miller and Auchus 2011).

Glucocorticoid and Mineralocorticoid Hormone Synthesis

The naturally occurring cortisol is the most prevalent member of the family of glucocorticoids and binds tightly to the glucocorticoid receptor, but in vitro it has a high affinity for mineralocorticoid receptor (MR) (Cooper and Stewart 2009). Whenever the blood concentration of cortisol falls below the normal circulating concentration of 6–20 μg/100 mL, additional cortisol will be produced. The daily secretory rate of cortisol is 10–20 mg/day. In addition, when an individual experiences significant levels of stress, there will be an increased production of cortisol reaching 200 μg/100 mL. Cortisol's most important action is to increase and maintain blood glucose levels via the biochemical process of gluconeogenesis in the combined actions of muscle cells, fat cells, and liver cells. Mineralocorticoids are a class of steroid hormones that regulate salt and water balances. Aldosterone is the primary mineralocorticoid. Mineralocorticoids promote sodium and potassium transport, usually followed by changes in water balance. Cells of the adrenal zona fasciculata and zona reticularis synthesize and secrete the glucocorticoid cortisol (Fig. 2). The adrenal zona glomerulosa cells preferentially synthesize and secrete aldosterone (Fig. 3) (Ehrhart-Bornstein et al. 1998).

In these adrenal zones, progesterone is converted to 11-deoxycorticosterone by 21-hydroxylase (P450c21), which catalyzes the 21-hydroxylation of both glucocorticoids and mineralocorticoids. The final steps in the synthesis of both glucocorticoids and mineralocorticoids again take place in the mitochondria, where two proteins that share 93% sequence identity, 11β-hydroxylase (P450c11β, *CYP11B1*) and aldosterone synthase (P450c11AS, *CYP11B2*), reside (Figs. 2 and 3). P450c11β catalyzes the 11β-hydroxylation of 11-deoxycortisol to cortisol, and P450c11AS catalyzes the 11β-hydroxylation, 18-hydroxylation, and 18-methyl oxidation to convert deoxycorticosterone to aldosterone.

The interconversion of active cortisol and hormonally inactive glucocorticoids such as cortisone and dehydrocorticosterone is mediated by the two isozymes of 11β-hydroxysteroid dehydrogenase (11βHSD) (Fig. 2). Both enzymes are hydrophobic, membrane-bound proteins that bind cortisol/cortisone and corticosterone/

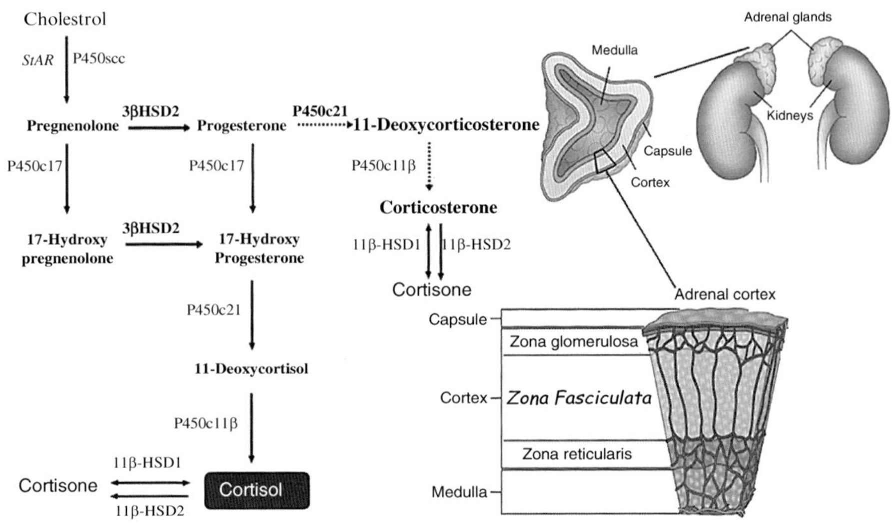

Fig. 2 Major steroidogenic pathways in the adrenal zona fasciculata. This zona express P450c17, so pregnenolone is hydroxylated to 17β-hydroxypregnenolone (or progesterone to 17-hydroxyprogesterone). 3βHSD2 and P450c17 generate 17-hydroxyprogesterone, the preferred substrate for P450c21, yielding 11-deoxycortisol. P450c11β, which is unique to the zona fasciculata, completes the synthesis of cortisol. Corticosterone is normally a minor product (*dashed arrows*) derived from a parallel pathway without the action of P450c17. The kidney, as well as other non-steroidogenic tissues, expresses 11βHSD1, which interconverts hormonally active glucocorticoids such as cortisol and corticosterone in their inactive counterpart cortisone and dehydrocorticosterone

11-dehydrocorticosterone, but otherwise their properties and physiological roles differ substantially. The type 1 enzyme (11βHSD1) is a dimer of 34 kDa subunits expressed mainly in glucocorticoid-responsive tissues such as the liver, testis, lung, fat, and kidney proximal tubule. The type 1 enzyme catalyzes both the oxidation of cortisol to cortisone using $NADP^+$ as cofactor and the reduction of cortisone to cortisol using NADPH cofactor. Thus, the net flux of steroid driven by 11βHSD1 depends on the relative concentrations of available NADPH and $NADP^+$, which usually favors reduction in cells. The 41 kDa type 2 enzyme (11βHSD2) has only 21% sequence identity with 11βHSD1 and catalyzes only the oxidation of cortisol to cortisone using NAD+; whether or not 11βHSD2 catalyzes reductive reactions remains undemonstrated. 11βHSD2 is expressed in mineralocorticoid-responsive tissues and thus serves to prevent cortisol from overwhelming renal or placenta mineralocorticoid receptors. The placenta also has abundant $NADP^+$ favoring the oxidative action of 11βHSD1, so that in placenta both enzymes protect the fetus from high maternal concentrations of cortisol (Cooper and Stewart 2009; Miller and Auchus 2011). In vitro, cortisol has a high affinity for mineralocorticoid receptor (MR), but its inactivation to cortisone (which is unable to bind the MR) enables aldosterone to bind to the MR. The expression of 11βHSD1 is constitutive in a range of tissues including the liver, white adipose tissue, bone, and the central nervous system. However, it also has inducible expression in many other tissues

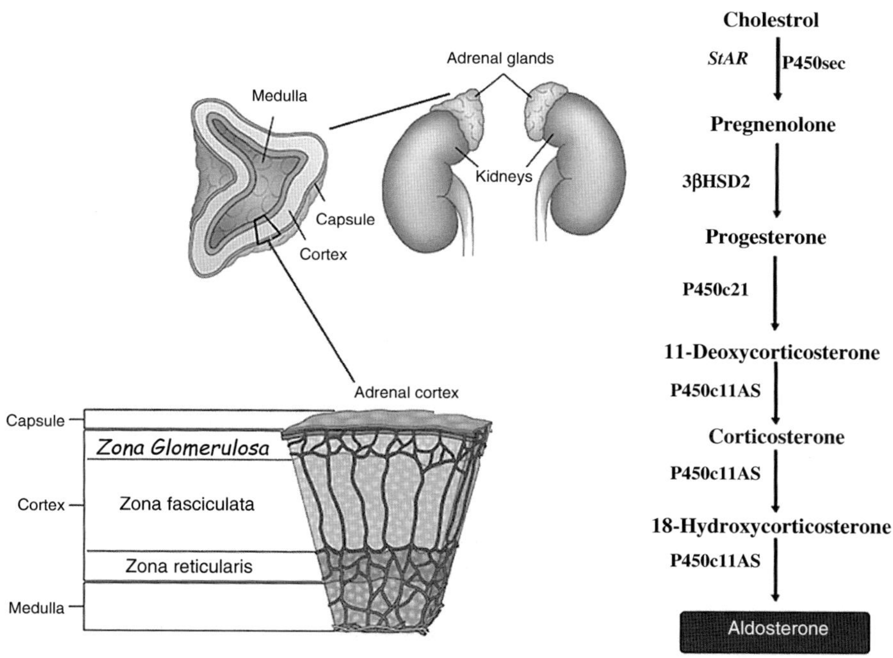

Fig. 3 Major steroidogenic pathways in the adrenal zona glomerulosa. The conversion of cholesterol to pregnenolone by P450scc is common to all three zones. 3βHSD2 converts pregnenolone to progesterone. P450c17 is absent, but P450c21 produces deoxycorticosterone, which is a substrate for P45011AS. P45011AS catalyzes 11-hydroxylations, which completes aldosterone synthesis

including fibroblasts, skeletal and smooth muscle, and immune cells (Cooper and Stewart 2009).

Comparison of the subcellular localization of the various hydroxylase enzymes with the sequence of steroid movement through a metabolic pathway indicates the important role of cellular compartmentalization. Thus, in the conversion of cholesterol into cortisol in the adrenal cortex, the steroid must move sequentially from the mitochondria (side-chain cleavage) to the endoplasmic reticulum (17α- and 21-hydroxylation) and then back to the mitochondria (11β-hydroxylation). Histologic and electron microscopic examination of steroidogenic cells suggests that domains of the endoplasmic reticulum containing the steroidogenic P450 enzymes come close to the OMM during hormonally induced steroidogenesis, forming a steroidogenic complex, so that the movement of steroidal intermediates from the mitochondrion to the endoplasmic reticulum involves very small distances (Miller and Auchus 2011; Miller 2013).

Androgen Hormone Synthesis

Testosterone is the principal male androgen (300–1100 ng/dl plasma). An important biologically active metabolite of testosterone, produced in certain target tissues, is

5α-dihydrotestosterone. The biological actions of androgens can be divided into those directed toward the development and maintenance of the male reproductive system and those that have anabolic effects on several other organs including skeletal muscle and brain.

In the adrenal gland, both 17α-dihydroxypregnenolone and 17α-dihydroxyprogesterone can be converted to the 19-carbon androgen precursors dehydroepiandrosterone (**DHEA**) and androstenedione by the 17,20-lyase activity of P450c17 (Fig. 4). The rate of the lyase reaction can be increased more than tenfold by cytochrome b5 (b5) which promotes the electron transfer for the lyase reaction. Cytochrome b5 is a small (12–17 kDa) hemoprotein found as a membrane-bound protein in the liver and as a soluble protein lacking the *C*-terminal membrane anchor in erythrocytes. The adrenal zona reticularis expresses large amounts of P450c17 and cytochrome b5, maximizing 17,20-lyase activity, so that DHEA is produced, much of which is sulfated to DHEAS by cytosolic sulfotransferase (SULT2A1) enzyme. The adrenal zona reticularis produces abundant DHEA. As DHEA accumulates, small amounts are converted to androstenedione, and very small amounts of this androstenedione are

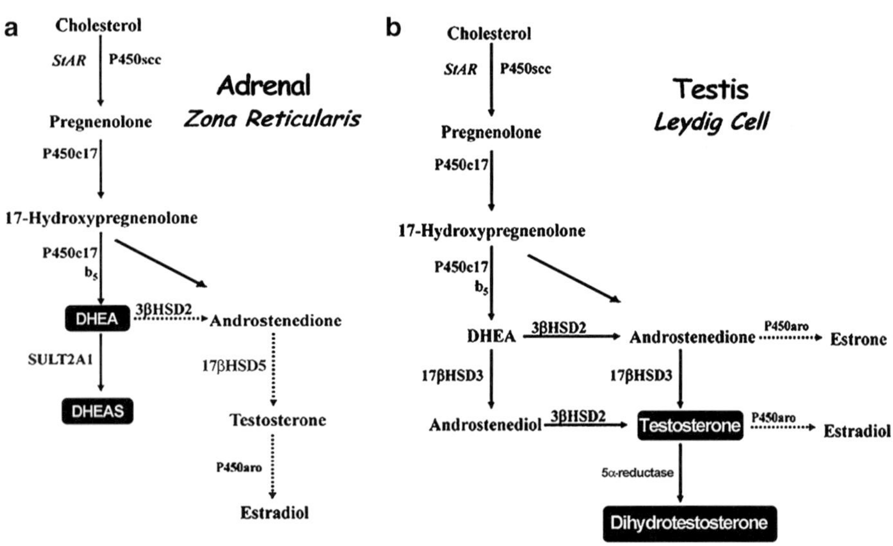

Fig. 4 Major steroidogenic pathways of DHEA and testosterone synthesis. (**a**) The adrenal zona reticularis has large amounts of P450c17 and cytochrome b5 (b5) but little 3βHSD2, so that pregnenolone is sequentially oxidized to 17-hydroxypregnenolone and then DHEA. The adrenal zona fasciculata contains little b5, minimizing the 17,20-lyase activity of P450c17, and little DHEA is produced from 17β-hydroxypregnenolone. SULT2A1 sulfates DHEA, and resulting DHEAS is released to circulation for non-steroidogenic tissues. Testosterone and estradiol synthesis are minor pathways (*dashed arrows*). (**b**) In testicular Leydig cells, cholesterol is converted to DHEA by the same enzymes using the same cofactors as in the adrenal zona reticularis. Leydig cells contain abundant 17βHSD3, so that Leydig cells efficiently produce testosterone, via androstenedione and/or androstenediol. Estradiol synthesis is a minor pathway (*dashed arrows*) in Leydig cells

converted to testosterone (Auchus and Rainey 2004). Up to 30 mg of DHEA is secreted daily by the adrenal cortex, and the blood levels of this prohormone and its sulfate derivative (DHEAS) are high. DHEA is considered a weak androgen that can be converted to testosterone and androstenediol or to estrogens in other steroidogenic (ovary, testis) and non-steroidogenic tissues (adipose tissue, brain) (Auchus and Rainey 2004; Miller and Auchus 2011). A group of dehydrogenases catalyzes the conversions DHEA to androstenedione and testosterone, estrone and estradiol, and others. These enzymes are collectively known as the 17-β-hydroxysteroid dehydrogenases (17βHSDs), sometimes also termed 17-oxidoreductases or 17-ketosteroid reductases. There are at least 14 human 17βHSD isoforms, which vary widely in size, structure, substrate specificity, cofactor utilization, and physiological functions. The most important in normal steroidogenesis are 17βHSD1, 17βHSD3, and 17βHSD5. The reactions in which these enzymes are involved are reported in Figs. 4 and 5.

In the testis, the cleavage of cholesterol side chain is confined to the mitochondria of the Leydig cells in which the role of the StAR protein is the same as in other steroidogenic cells. DHEA produced in the testis is not sulfated but is readily converted to androstenedione and then testosterone. Testicular testosterone synthesis, as reflected in plasma hormone levels, changes throughout the life of a normal human male. Testosterone production has two peaks during the second trimester in utero and another during the 6 months after birth. The relative quiescence of the androgen synthetic pathway persists throughout childhood until the beginning of the pubertal period. Plasma testosterone rises to adult levels by the end of puberty and begins to decline in middle age (andropause) (Auchus and Rainey 2004; Miller and Auchus 2011). In many target tissues, unmodified testosterone interacts with the androgen receptor (AR) to bring about the appropriate biological responses. In others, not limited to the prostate and hair follicles, testosterone is reduced at the 5α position to form 5α-dihydrotesterone (DHT), which has a greater affinity for the AR than testosterone; this is sometimes referred to as the amplification pathway. In some tissues, exemplified by the bone and brain, the active derivative of testosterone is estradiol, produced locally by aromatase, which then interacts with the estrogen receptors (ERs). This has been referred to as the diversification pathway (Miller and Auchus 2011).

The enzyme responsible for the conversion of testosterone to DHT is a Δ4-3-ketosteroid-5α-oxidoreductase (5α-reductase) that requires NADPH as a cofactor (Fig. 4). In rodents and humans, there are two forms of 5α-reductase. The two reductases are encoded by separate genes and share about 50% amino acid homology. The two 5α-reductase subtypes are important beyond the context of male genital differentiation and androgen action because both enzymes reduce a variety of steroids in degradative pathways. Progesterone, 17-dihydroxyprogesterone, and related C21 steroids are excellent substrates for both 5α-reductases, particularly the type 1; cortisol, cortisone, corticosterone, and related compounds are also good substrates. Such 5α-reduced steroids may be metabolized further and conjugated for excretion in the urine (Russell and Wilson 1994).

Aromatization of testosterone to estradiol by P450 aromatase (see below) occurs in several tissues of the adult male, including the adipose, testis (Sertoli cells and

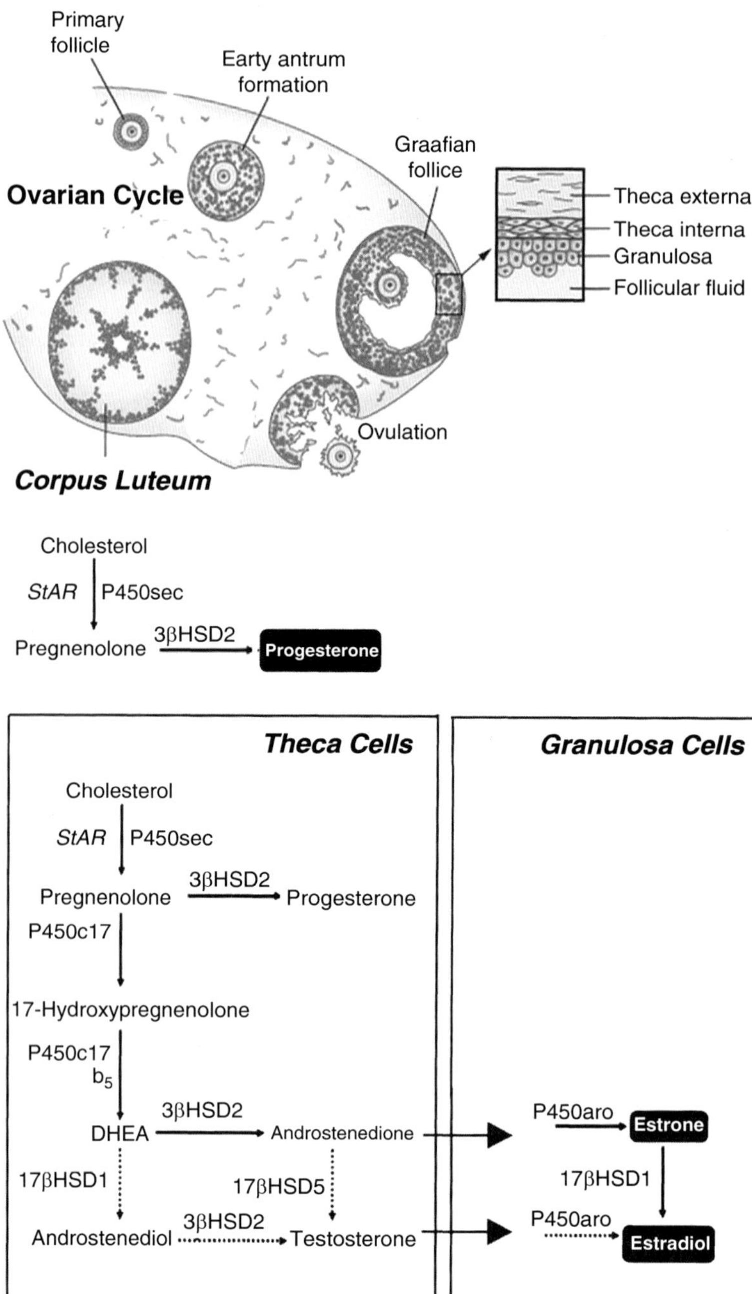

Fig. 5 Major steroidogenic pathways of ovarian steroid hormones. The ovarian theca cells express StAR, P450scc, and P450c17 and hence produce C19 androgens. Theca cells do not express aromatase (P450aro); hence, androstenedione and testosterone must return to the granulosa cells, which contain

Leydig cells), brain, bone, breast, liver, and blood vessels. In these tissues androstenedione can also be aromatized, yielding the weak estrogen estrone, which can then be metabolized to estradiol through reduction of the 17-keto group by 17β-hydroxysteroid dehydrogenase (Fig. 4) (Normington and Russell 1992).

Studies of fetal androgen biosynthesis and mechanisms of virilization in the tammar wallaby have revealed the presence of a novel, alternative, so-called backdoor pathway that leads from 17-hydroxyprogesterone to DHT without going through androstenedione or testosterone as intermediate steroids. This pathway is initiated when either progesterone or 17-hydroxyprogesterone is reduced by 5α-reductase. This pathway is an alternative, backdoor pathway to DHT, by which DHT is produced without utilizing DHEA, androstenedione, and testosterone as intermediates. Consequently, the presence of 5α-reductases in steroidogenic and non-steroidogenic cells does not preclude the production of C19 steroids, but rather paradoxically enhances the production of DHT. Originally described in marsupials, the backdoor pathway is relevant to human steroidogenesis (Miller and Auchus 2011). Human enzymes catalyze all of the reactions required to complete this alternative route to DHT, and good evidence documents production of 5α-reduced androgens by the fetal adrenal, at least in some pathological states.

Estrogen and Progesterone Hormone Synthesis

The two most important steroid hormones of the adult female are 17β-estradiol (estradiol) and progesterone. In addition, two metabolites of estradiol, estrone (E1) and estriol (E3), circulate at high levels at certain phases of menstrual cycle and during pregnancy. El and E3 have been thought to be the inactive metabolites of estradiol, but E3 has significant effects on the immune system, and a closer examination of the physiological functions of these two steroids is warranted. As for androgens, the biological actions of E2 can be divided into those directed toward the development and maintenance of the female reproductive system and those that have effects on several other organs including the cardiovascular system, metabolism, and brain.

The naturally occurring estrogens are typically 18-carbon steroids that have an aromatic A ring with a phenolic hydroxyl; the naturally occurring progestin, progesterone, has 21 carbons, with another one additional oxygenation (oxo) on both C-3 and C-20. Ovarian estrogen synthesis, as reflected in plasma hormone levels, pulsates every month, during different phases of the menstrual cycle, and changes throughout the life of a normal human female. The peak of estrogen synthetic pathway during the 6 months after birth is followed by the relative quiescence throughout childhood until the beginning of the pubertal period. Plasma estrogen pulsates at adult levels by the end of

Fig. 5 (continued) abundant aromatase and 17βHSD1, completing the synthesis of estradiol (the two cell model of ovarian steroidogenesis). In the luteal phase, 3βHSD2 in the corpus luteum metabolizes nascent pregnenolone to progesterone, the final product. Minor pathways are shown with *dashed arrows*

Table 2 Production rates of ovarian steroid hormones during the ovary cycle

Hormones	Early follicular μg/day	Ovulation μg/day	Luteal μg/day
17β-Estradiol	70	400–800	300
Estrone	80	300–600	200
Progesterone	1000	4000	24,000

puberty and begins to decline in middle age (menopause). The amounts of estradiol, estrone, and progesterone produced by the ovary and circulating during different phases of the menstrual cycle are shown in Table 2.

The enzymatic steps of estradiol synthesis are partitioned between the granulosa and theca cells of the ovary, which surround the oocyte and form a follicle (Fig. 5). The cells of the theca interna express cholesterol side-chain cleavage activity (P450scc) and StAR (Tian et al. 2015). Pregnenolone is converted to androstenedione by the removal of carbons 20 and 21. Androstenedione diffuses across the basement membrane of the follicle into the follicular fluid from which it is taken up by granulosa cells. The endoplasmic reticulum of granulosa cells expresses P450 aromatase that converts androstenedione to estrone (Tian et al. 2015). All circulating estrone and estradiol are produced by the aromatization of androgens, including those derived from adrenal and placental steroidogenesis. In addition, P450 aromatase is expressed in non-steroidogenic tissues, especially fat and bone. A single gene on chromosome 15q21.1 encodes P450 aromatase. This gene contains five different transcriptional start sites with individual promoters that permit the tissue-specific regulation of its expression in diverse tissues. Estradiol is further synthesized by the action of 17βHSD1 (see previous paragraph) that converts estrone to estradiol (Fig. 5). This enzyme is also expressed in the liver and placenta where it reduces 16α-hydroxyestrone to estriol (E3), the characteristic estrogen of pregnancy. As a whole, in order for sufficient amounts of estrogen to be synthesized for maturation and ovulation of the follicle, both granulosa cells and theca cells must be functional.

Following ovulation, the major steroid produced by the luteinized cells of the corpus luteum is progesterone, although estrogen continues to be synthesized and secreted as well (Fig. 5).

Vitamin D Synthesis

Vitamin D and its metabolites are not technically steroids in the strict chemical sense, as the B ring of cholesterol is opened (secosteroid). Nevertheless, these sterols are derived from cholesterol, assume shapes that are very similar to steroids, and bind to a nuclear receptor (Norman 1998; Miller and Auchus 2011).

In the human skin, ultraviolet radiation at 270–290 nm directly cleaves the 9–10 carbon–carbon bonds of the cholesterol B ring, converting 7-dehydro-cholesterol to cholecalciferol (vitamin D3) (Norman 1998). Plants and yeast produce ergocalciferol (vitamin D2), which has essentially the same properties as cholecalciferol. Both calciferols are biologically inactive prohormones that are then activated, and subsequently inactivated, by mitochondrial P450 enzymes. The initial step in the activation of vitamin D is its hepatic 25-hydroxylation to 25(OH)D, which may be catalyzed by 25-hydroxylase (*CYP2R1*). The active, hormonal form of vitamin D, $1,25(OH)_2D$ (calcitriol), is produced in the kidney proximal tubule by the hydroxylation of 25(OH)D by the mitochondrial 1α-hydroxylase, P450c1α, encoded by the *CYP27B1* gene. 1α-hydroxylation is the rate-limiting step in the activation of vitamin D. These chemical transformations can occur in the absence of further ultraviolet exposure. The resulting vitamin D3 is then transported in the general circulatory system by the 50 kDa vitamin D-binding protein (DBP). $1,25(OH)_2D$ in the circulation derives primarily from the kidney, but 1α-hydroxylase activity is also found in keratinocytes, macrophages, osteoblasts, and placenta (Norman 1998; Miller and Auchus 2011).

Control of Steroid Hormone Synthesis and Release

The production and/or secretion of most hormones are regulated by highly specific homeostatic mechanisms. The secretion or release of the hormone is normally related to the requirement for the biological response(s) generated by the specific hormone. Because of their hydrophobic nature, steroid hormones and precursors can leave the steroidogenic cell easily and are not stored. Thus, steroidogenesis (excluding vitamin D metabolites) is regulated primarily at the first step in their synthesis (the cleavage of the side chain of cholesterol) and at the level of steroidogenic enzyme gene expression and activity (Miller and Auchus 2011).

Once the biological response has been generated, the secretion of the hormone is restrained to prevent an overresponse. Thus, a characteristic feature of most endocrine systems is the existence of a feedback loop that limits or regulates the secretion of the hormone. Two general categories of endocrine feedback systems have been described (Fig. 6): those in which the function achieved by the hormone directly feeds back upon the endocrine gland that secretes the hormone (positive or negative loops) and those involving the inputs from internal and external environments to the central nervous system (CNS) and hypothalamus (generally negative long loops). This latter category of endocrine feedback is organized into endocrine axes, which contain three levels of hormonal output. The highest level of hormonal output is neurohormonal and relies on the release of neurohormones, called releasing hormones, from hypothalamic nuclei into the portal vessels between the hypothalamus and the pituitary gland. The cells of the adenohypophysis make up the intermediate level of an endocrine axis releasing the tropic or stimulating hormones, which, in turn, stimulate the peripheral endocrine glands/cells (including steroidogenic cells) to produce the final, biologically active hormone (Fig. 6). Throughout the hypothalamus/pituitary/gland axes, the CNS exerts the control of hormone synthesis and release, and it realizes the integration of body functions (Molina 2010). Another contributor to the biological availability of steroid hormones that deserve mention here is the control exerted by biological rhythms on steroid hormone production (Lin et al. 2015).

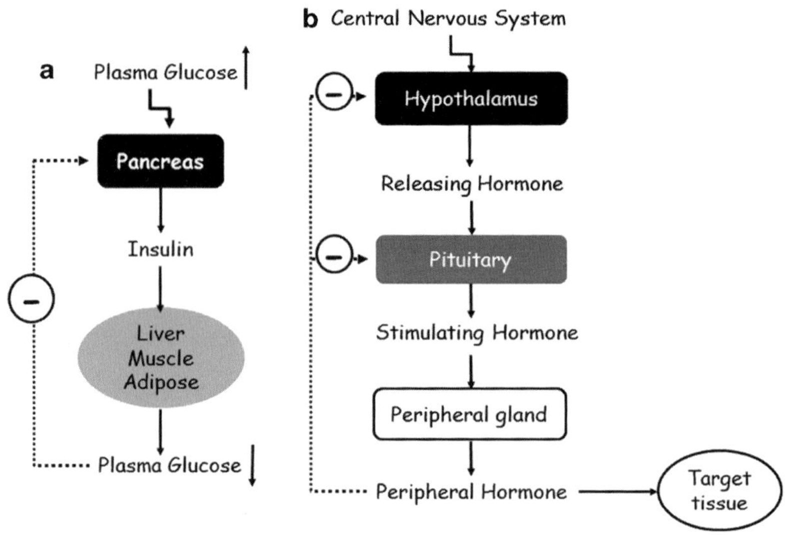

Fig. 6 Feedback regulation of hormone synthesis. Two general categories of endocrine feedback systems have been described: those in which the function achieved by the hormone directly feeds back upon the endocrine gland that secretes the hormone (**a**) and those involving the central nervous system (CNS) and hypothalamus (**b**)

Hypothalamus/Pituitary/Adrenal (HPA) Axis and Cortisol Synthesis and Release

The endocrine axis that controls the cortisol synthesis from the steroidogenic cells of adrenal zona fasciculata begins from the release of corticotropin-releasing hormone (CRH) from the hypothalamic neurons. CRH, a peptide of 41 amino acids, binds to its cognate receptors (a G protein-coupled receptor associated to a Gs/cAMP/PKA signaling pathway) on corticotrope cells to the pituitary. CRH acutely stimulates the release of adrenocorticotropin hormone (ACTH) into the circulatory system. ACTH, a 39-amino acid peptide, binds to the melanocortin-2 receptor (MC2R) located on the cells in the zona fasciculata of adrenal cortex (Gaffey et al. 2016). Within minutes upon ACTH binds to MC2R, cellular cholesterol is rapidly mobilized and transported to mitochondria. ACTH rapidly increases the expression and the activity of StAR through PKA-dependent phosphorylation resulting in the increase of pregnenolone levels. Over a period of several hours, ACTH increases the transcription of the gene encoding the steroidogenic enzymes (e.g., P450scc and the 11β-hydroxylase) and their coenzymes crucial to the production of cortisol as well as the expression of LDL receptor, thus increasing cholesterol uptake and its utilization to produce high level of cortisol (Miller and Auchus 2011).

The cortisol released into bloodstream inhibits both the release of CRH from hypothalamic neurons and ACTH secretion from pituitary corticotrope cells. There is a long negative feedback loop of cortisol, which is initiated by cortisol release from the adrenal zona fasciculata that then travels through the entire circulatory system to engage with the glucocorticoid receptor (GR) in target cells. Some cortisol will cross the blood–brain barrier and send a negative signal to both the brain cortex and the hippocampus, so that the hypothalamus diminishes the CRH signal sent from the hypothalamus to the pituitary. This then lowers the rate of secretion of ACTH by the pituitary. The overall feedback inhibition of ACTH is implemented very rapidly. The feedback on the hippocampus may shut off further electrical activity responsible for the release of CRH and the subsequent release of ACTH. These actions are mediated by GR located in these cells that operate transcriptionally (Wood 2013).

The release of CRH, and hence of ACTH, is pulsatile with about 7–15 episodes per day. The stimulation of cortisol release occurs within 15 min of the surge of ACTH. An important feature in the release of cortisol is that in addition to being pulsatile, it follows a circadian rhythm, with a peak in early morning and a nadir in late afternoon (see paragraph in section "Regulatory Feedback of Vitamin D Synthesis and Release"). However, many types of stress, neurogenic (e.g., emotional like fear), pathological (e.g., infection), and metabolic (e.g., hypoglycemia), overtake both the regulation exerted by circadian rhythm and the negative feedback from cortisol levels driving to the extensive secretion of ACTH, which will further elevate the circulating concentrations of cortisol. This means that hypothalamus could reset the "set point" of the HPA axis in response to stress (Lin et al. 2015; Gaffey et al. 2016).

Stress is anything that throws the body out of homeostatic balance – for example, an injury, an illness, or exposure to extreme heat or cold. Stress thus occurs when the body is exposed to a "stressor," which threatens homeostasis, and the "stress response" is the attempt of the body to counteract the stressor and reestablish homeostasis (allostasis). There are two key aspects of stress response. On the one hand, the body responds to short-term stressor by releasing epinephrine (and norepinephrine) from the adrenal medulla, as well as cortisol secretion from the adrenal cortex that increases heart rate, blood pressure, and glucose availability. These mediators promote adaptation to an acute stressor, as well as to simple acts like getting out of bed in the morning or climbing a flight of stairs. On the other hand, chronic elevation of stressors, e.g., intensive cold, prolonged loud noise, serious injury, burns, surgery, and significant changes in the environment that chronically increased heart rate and blood pressure, can cause pathophysiological changes, for example, in the cardiovascular system. These stressful circumstances necessitate the response adaptation, which is not well granted by a single mediator. Rather, the combination of multiple mediators (e.g., vasopressin, CRH, cortisol) addresses the specific aspects of a stressor that culminate in the breakdown of glycogen necessary to enable escape or survive the "fight or flight" or provide "nervous energy." Both types of stress responses usually occur simultaneously; one change in operation does not preclude the utilization of the other pathway. There are, however, certain conditions that can cause the pathways to operate separately. The sympathetic system generating epinephrine and norepinephrine is activated when the organism attempts to escape from or deal with the environmental challenge or the fight or flight. On the other hand, the HPA axis, ending in cortisol release from the adrenal gland, is also operative when the individual becomes immobile, passive, and depressed. A chronic emotional reaction of passivity and defeat to a stressful situation can produce dire consequences, as the adrenal hypertrophy and levels of cortisol continue to increase. This can generate a Cushingoid-like bodily reaction in which visceral fat accumulates and blood pressure becomes elevated, and arteriosclerosis and type 2 diabetes eventually develop. Sequential episodes of elevated glucocorticoids cause sufficient repression of glucose uptake in peripheral cells to involve insulin release from the β-cells of the pancreas (Gaffey et al. 2016).

The Control of Mineralocorticoid and Androgen Release from Adrenals

In contrast to glucocorticoids, which are under exclusive neuroendocrine regulation by HPA, aldosterone synthesis and release in the adrenal zona glomerulosa are predominantly regulated by angiotensin II and extracellular K^+ and, to a lesser extent, by ACTH. Aldosterone is part of the renin-angiotensin-aldosterone system, which is responsible for preserving circulatory homeostasis in response to a loss of salt and water. Renin is an enzyme secreted by the granular cells associated with the Bowman's capsule of the kidney's nephron in response to a drop in blood pressure and/or a decrease in blood Na^+ concentration. Renin's substrate is the blood protein angiotensinogen (57 kDa) secreted by the liver and then localized within the capillaries of the lungs. The hormone angiotensin II is an octapeptide produced by the angiotensin converting enzyme (ACE) acting on the precursor, angiotensin I, the product of renin activity. Angiotensin II is a hormone that acts on the zona glomerulosa of the adrenal cortex where it stimulates the production and secretion of aldosterone (Molina 2010). Aldosterone binds to its receptor (MR) in the kidney's collecting duct where it increases the reabsorption of both Na^+ and water and, also, increases secretion of H^+ and K^+ into the urine, thus leading to an increased blood volume, which increases blood pressure until it has returned to normal. Although both angiotensin II and K^+ stimulate aldosterone release by increasing intracellular Ca^{2+} concentrations, they achieve this result through different mechanisms (Molina 2010). Angiotensin II binds to G protein-coupled receptor resulting in activation of phospholipase C, which results in the production of two second messengers: diacylglycerol and inositol 1,4,5-trisphosphate which, respectively, activate protein kinase C activity and stimulate the release of Ca^{2+} from the endoplasmic reticulum stores. K^+, on the other hand, mediates an influx of extracellular Ca^{2+} via voltage-gated L- and T-type Ca^{2+} channels. The surge of intracellular Ca^{2+} concentration increases calcium/calmodulin activity in the zona glomerulosa that promotes transcription of genes for steroidogenic enzymes, especially the gene encoding P450scc, thus increasing the amounts of the steroidogenic enzymes involved in aldosterone synthesis (Clyne et al. 1997; Bassett et al. 2004).

The control and regulation of the release of adrenal androgens (DHEA) depends on ACTH. However, it is known that adrenal secretion of DHEA increases in children at the age of 6–8 years (adrenarche) and peak between the ages of 20 and 30 years. Thereafter, serum levels of DHEA decrease markedly during the aging process. This is not paralleled by a similar decrease in ACTH or cortisol production (Wood 2013).

Hypothalamus/Pituitary/Testis Axis and Testosterone Synthesis and Release

The hypothalamic decapeptide gonadotrophin-releasing hormone (GnRH) released by secretory granules of the GnRH hypothalamic neurons is required for the male and female reproductive function. In the absence of GnRH, secretion of the two pituitary gonadotrophic hormones is either completely (luteinizing hormone, LH) or greatly (follicle-stimulating hormone, FSH) diminished.

The secretion of GnRH is characterized by its pulsatile nature. The amplitude and frequency of GnRH pulses are restrained from the age of 4 to 6 months until the onset of puberty, at which time the increase in both amplitude and frequency of GnRH (and therefore gonadotrophin) secretion is the hallmark of the onset of reproductive maturation. Furthermore, the two gonadotrophins show pulse frequency discrimination, with LH responding to faster frequencies of the GnRH pulse and FSH to slower frequencies. The pulse generator for GnRH secretion is now thought to lie in neurons of the preoptic area that contain a triad of neuropeptides, kisspeptin, neurokinin B, and dynorphin, which project into the cell bodies and terminals of GnRH neurons of the hypothalamus. Although kisspeptin is thought to be an important component of the GnRH pulse generator, the exact mechanism by which this occurs and the role of other neuropeptides such as neurokinin B are still under intense study (Plant 2008; Molina 2010; Chevrier et al. 2011).

Although the first steps of hypothalamus/pituitary/gonad axis are similar between sexes, the effects exerted by pituitary tropic hormones are different in male and in female. The testicular target of LH, the Leydig cells, serves two principal functions: (a) they are the site of production of testosterone, producing, in adult males, approximately 7 mg daily for systemic transport to distal target tissues, and (b) they have paracrine interactions with the immediately adjacent seminiferous tubules to support spermatogenesis. LH-mediated stimulation of testosterone synthesis and secretion is initiated by the binding of LH to specific receptors on the plasma membranes of the Leydig cell. An increased level of cAMP within the Leydig cell activates PKA (cyclic AMP-dependent protein kinase) which, through phosphorylation of specific transcription factors, induces the synthesis of StAR. Under prolonged stimulation, LH increases the expression and activities of other enzymes in the pathway from pregnenolone to testosterone (Miller and Auchus 2011). In the adult male, FSH in conjunction with testosterone acts on the Sertoli cells of the seminiferous tubule to initiate sperm production. In humans, FSH is required for normal spermatogenesis throughout adult life. FSH binds to its specific G protein-coupled receptor on the Sertoli cell to increase, through a cAMP-dependent mechanism, the synthesis of specific proteins, including the androgen-binding protein (ABP) and inhibin. ABP is thought to function to concentrate androgens in the seminiferous tubules and deliver the steroid hormone to developing spermatocytes and spermatids (Molina 2010). ABP is now known to be a homolog of sex hormone-binding globulin, SHBG, the serum-binding protein for androgens and estrogens (see next chapter).

Testosterone can exert negative feedback on the axis through three possible levels: the kisspeptin neurons of the arcuate nucleus, which regulate the output of GnRH neurons, the GnRH neurons themselves, and the pituitary gonadotrope cells. The relative contribution of each of these components to overall LH and FSH secretion varies with species, but each probably contributes to the negative feedback effect of testosterone in humans. Although kisspeptin neurons contain both androgen (AR) and estrogen (ERs) receptors, testosterone represses kisspeptin expression and GnRH secretion via AR activity. In the pituitary, testosterone decreases the expression and release of LH and FSH only after the aromatization of testosterone to estrogen. Thus, in contrast to the situation in kisspeptin neurons, pituitary estrogen and ERs play an important role in the negative feedback that controls testosterone synthesis (Plant 2008; Molina 2010; Chevrier et al. 2011).

The adult human male produces approximately 45 μg of estradiol per day, mostly from aromatization of testosterone in the adipose tissue, bone, brain, breast, blood vessels, liver, and both the Sertoli and Leydig cells of the testes. The aromatization of testosterone is a critical step in its action in several tissues. In bone, estrogen mediates the closure of the epiphyseal plate during puberty and decreases bone mineral resorption; in the spermatozoa, where it mediates the cell motility; in prostate, where ERs are necessary for water resorbing and gland maturation; and in the brain where estrogen participates in the negative feedback inhibition of testosterone on GnRH secretion. Estradiol produced from testosterone affects other areas of brain affecting mood and cognitive function. In a small number of cases of inactivating mutations of aromatase in men, observations have included tall stature, low bone mineral density, and changes in carbohydrate and lipid metabolism (Miller and Auchus 2011).

Hypothalamus/Pituitary/Ovary Axis and Synthesis and Release of Estrogen and Progesterone

Reproductive function in females is pulsatile being characterized by cycles of follicle development, ovulation, and preparation of the uterine endometrium for implantation of the blastocyst resulting from a fertilized egg (Plant 2008). The hormones that constitute the hypothalamic-pituitary-ovarian axis orchestrate and synchronize these events. There are two differences that distinguish this system from its male counterpart: (1) there are two distinct phases of the cycle, follicular and luteal; (2) at one brief specific point in the cycle, the pituitary and hypothalamic centers respond.

During the majority of thc follicular phase (first half) of the cycle, the theca cells are the target of LH, while the granulosa cells are the FSH target. The type of receptor each cell expresses determines this responsiveness. The cells of the theca interna express receptors for LH, the response to which is an increase in steroid acute regulatory protein (StAR) and the cleavage of the side chain of cholesterol. Androstenedione diffuses across the basement membrane of the follicle into the follicular fluid from which it is taken up by granulosa cells. These cells express the FSH receptor which, when activated by FSH, brings about, through adenyl cyclase activation, the synthesis of aromatase that converts androstenedione to estrone.

Action of 17β-hydroxysteroid dehydrogenase (17-ketosteroid reductase; HSD17B1) converts estrone to estradiol. Thus, unlike the male, both gonadotrophins must be secreted in appropriate amounts to assure estrogen synthesis. Following ovulation, when theca and granulosa cells of the follicle have differentiated into the corpus luteum, LH from the pituitary is required for the production of progesterone, which is necessary for the growth of the uterine endometrium (Plant 2008; Miller and Auchus 2011).

The sex steroid hormones, estrogens and progesterone, control gonadotrophin secretion. Both estradiol and progesterone exert negative feedback inhibition on GnRH secretion by the hypothalamus as well as by direct inhibition of gonadotrophin secretion at the pituitary (Plant 2008). The latter involves alterations in the expression of the genes required for LH and FSH synthesis as well as modulation of the sensitivity of pituitary gonadotrophs to GnRH. The negative feedback effect of estrogen predominates during the follicular phase of the reproductive cycle and that of progesterone, synthesized in large amounts by the corpus luteum, predominates during the luteal phase. However, the surge of estrogen hormones, typical of ovulation, exerts a positive feedback on GnRH and LH secretion further increasing estrogen synthesis in the ovary. A group of kisspeptin-1 neurons in the hypothalamic anteroventral periventricular nucleus mediates this estrogen-positive stimulus. These cells respond to the rapid rise in estrogens produced by the maturing follicle with increased Kiss-1 secretion and stimulation of GnRH secretion that drives the midcycle LH surge. The positive feedback of estrogen on LH (and FSH) secretion is also exerted at the pituitary gland and involves enhancement of the sensitivity to GnRH. The relative role of the pituitary, as opposed to changes in GnRH secretion, in mediating the ovulatory LH surge varies with species. In primates, including humans, the pituitary appears to be the predominant site of this regulatory event. The molecular mechanism of the switch from negative to positive feedback by estrogen is not understood, but it is probably related to the different effects exerted by different estrogen concentrations on the levels of their cognate receptors (Molina 2010).

Androgens play important roles in the reproductive functions of females. Indeed, testosterone and androstenedione are the substrates for aromatase and obligatory intermediates in the production of estradiol and estrone, respectively. Adrenal androgens play a critical role in female puberty bringing about the changes in pubic and axillary hair (adrenarche). Excessive exposure to androgens during uterine life can bring about masculinization of a female fetus, depending on the timing and extent of the exposure. Excess androgens at any point in adult life can have masculinizing effects on the female, manifested as excess hair growth, voice changes, and changes in body composition (Miller and Auchus 2011).

Regulatory Feedback of Vitamin D Synthesis and Release

The regulation of vitamin D synthesis and release is a good example of endocrine feedback systems in which the function achieved by the hormone directly feeds back upon the endocrine gland that secretes the hormone (positive or negative loops).

Indeed, the production of 1,25$(OH)_2$D by 1α-hydroxylase in the kidney is a tightly regulated process and is a central factor in the feedback regulation of calcium homeostasis. The production of the active form of vitamin D [1,25$(OH)_2$D or calcitriol] is under negative feedback regulation by plasma Ca^{2+} levels. A rise in plasma Ca^{2+} levels inhibits the hydroxylation at C-1 and favors hydroxylation at C-24, leading to the synthesis of an inactive metabolite of vitamin D (24,25$(OH)_2$D). In addition, the parathyroid hormone, released from parathyroid glands, stimulates the activity of kidney 1α-hydroxylase, favoring an increase in synthesis of the active form of vitamin D. Vitamin D, as well as high Ca^{2+} levels, suppresses the activity of 1α-hydroxylase, decreasing its own synthesis and favoring the synthesis of 24,25 $(OH)_2$D. Vitamin D increases intestinal Ca^{2+} absorption and suppresses the synthesis and release of parathyroid hormone from the parathyroid glands completing the endocrine feedback system (Khundmiri et al. 2016).

Hormonal Rhythms

The profound environmental changes brought about by the rotation of the Earth around its axis allowed the evolution of endogenous timekeepers that enable an organism to reliably predict the time of day and adjust behavior and physiology accordingly. Not surprisingly, large aspects of our endocrine system, including hormone synthesis and release, are tightly connected to the circadian clock. In 1970s it was discovered that information about the external light–dark cycle provide photic data to both classical retinal photoreceptors – cone and rod cells – as well as to melanopsin-containing retinal ganglion cells. Through the retino-hypothalamic tract (RHT), this information is passed to an anatomical entity underlining the mammalian circadian, the suprachiasmatic nucleus (SCN). The SCN is a bilaterally paired structure with high cell body density located adjacent to the third ventricle and directly atop the optic chiasm. The current model suggests that the central mechanism of the mammalian molecular clock is composed of a set of clock genes intertwined with a delayed interlocking transcriptional–translational feedback loop, coupled to several auxiliary mechanisms reinforcing robustness and stability. The functional molecular clockwork does not exist only in SCN neurons, but (almost) every single cell in the brain and periphery is capable of oscillating in a circadian manner. Molecular clock rhythms have been shown even in cultured cells, such as immortalized fibroblast cells, which display robust oscillations of clock gene expression. One major function of the SCN is to synchronize internal biological processes to external time cues. To do this, SCN innervates other regions of the brain, in particular the hypothalamic nuclei which are important integrating centers for energy homeostasis and control of steroid hormone synthesis. Indeed, cortisol represents the best-studied steroid hormone that is subject to direct and dominant regulation by the circadian clock (Lin et al. 2015; Barclay et al. 2012).

Blood levels of cortisol display a robust circadian rhythm. The circadian rise of cortisol is phase-locked to the time of awakening, peaking at few hours before the onset of the active phase, i.e., the early morning for diurnal animals such as humans and the evening for nocturnal animals such as rodents. This cortisol rise promotes arousal and boosts performance during the early active phase. Importantly, cortisol rhythms persist under constant environmental conditions, suggesting that the endogenous circadian clock drives them. Surgical ablation of the SCN completely abolishes the circadian rhythm of cortisol in blood, indicating that the SCN is the origin of cortisol rhythmicity. Well before the discovery of clock genes or peripheral clocks, it was shown that adrenal glands when isolated and cultured in vitro display a robust circadian rhythm of metabolism and steroid secretion. In line with this, researchers have provided evidence that a local adrenocortical clock imposes a circadian gating mechanism altering ACTH sensitivity during the course of the day. Thus, while the SCN is indispensable for the circadian rhythm of cortisol secretion, the adrenal clock provides an additional level of control to modulate the proficiency of cortisol production across the circadian cycle, and further clocks along the HPA axis may be involved. Adrenalectomy shortens re-entrainment in the SCN, lung, and kidney following phase shifts, suggesting that GCs may serve to stabilize the phase of peripheral clocks against external noise. In the case of jetlag-induced circadian desynchronization, it was shown that manipulation of the cortisol rhythm could speed up or slow down activity adaptation to the new light–dark cycles, depending on the intervention time (Lin et al. 2015; Barclay et al. 2012).

Circadian rhythms, which do influence GnRH and gonadotrophin secretion in other mammalian species, do not have a strong influence in humans, but sleep itself appears to have direct effects on the nature of LH secretion, which vary with the reproductive status of the individual (Lin et al. 2015; Barclay et al. 2012).

Steroid Secretion and Transport

Steroid hormones, like other hormones, are chemical messengers that send a signal within a physiological system from point A (secretion) to point B (biological action). Steroid hormones are synthesized, but not stored, within specific endocrine cells that could be associated with an anatomically defined endocrine gland.

Upon the receipt of an appropriate physiological signal, which may take the form of either a change in the concentration of some component in the blood (e.g., another hormone, Ca^{2+}, stressors) or a neural signal, the hormones are released into the circulation. They are transported in the bloodstream to one or more target cells, which are defined as targets by the presence of the specific high-affinity receptors, members of nuclear receptor superfamily located either on the membrane or within the cell (endocrine system) (Fig. 7) (Molina 2010; Norman and Henry 2015).

A type of hormonal communication system does not involve the circulatory system at all. In paracrine systems, hormones secreted from the steroidogenic cells interact with their cognate receptors in neighboring cells, which are reached by diffusion (Fig. 7). As with endocrine system, the nearby target cells may be all the same type or may differ from each other. Several, if not all, of the steroid hormones

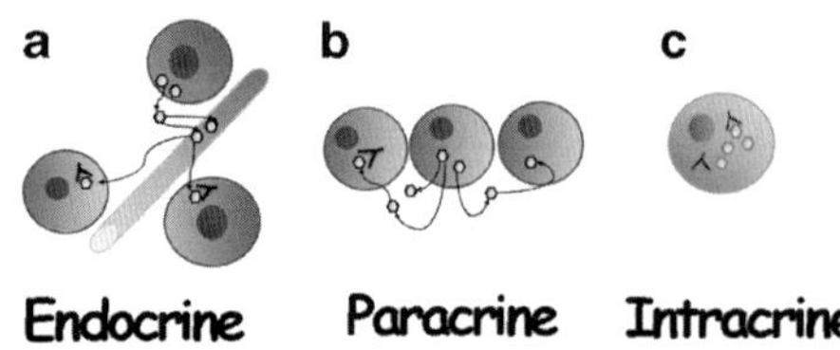

Fig. 7 Type of hormonal communication system. These systems may involve (**a**) or not (**b**, **c**) the circulatory system

act by paracrine in addition to endocrine mechanisms. For example, in the testis, testosterone not only is released into the blood from the interstitial cells in which it is produced but also diffuses to nearby seminiferous tubules to support the production of sperm (see previous paragraphs).

Finally, some cells both produce the same hormone and respond to it. This type of system is referred to as autocrine for all class of hormones excluding steroid hormones. The appearance during evolution of the repertoire of cell-specific steroidogenic enzymes (see previous chapter) permits to produce steroid hormones intracellularly according to the local needs without biologically significant release of active sex steroids in the circulation. This type of system, specific for steroid hormones, is referred to as intracrine (Fig. 7). Examples of intracrine system involve androgen/estrogen synthesis in non-steroidogenic tissues during andropause and menopause. All tissues, except the endometrium, possess the intracrine enzymes able to transform DHEA into androgens and/or estrogens. Humans, along with other primates, are unique among animal species in having adrenals that secrete large amounts of the inactive precursor steroid DHEA, which is converted at various levels into active androgens and/or estrogens in specific peripheral tissues according to the mechanisms of intracrinology. It is very important to mention that an essential aspect of intracrinology is that the active sex steroids are not only made locally but that they are also inactivated locally at exactly the same site where synthesis takes place. In fact, the sex steroids made from DHEA in peripheral tissues are essentially released outside the cells as inactive compounds. DHEA of adrenal, ovarian, or exogenous (e.g., drugs) origin is distributed by the general circulation to all tissues indiscriminately. The transformation of DHEA into estrogens/androgens, however, is tissue specific, ranging from none in the endometrium to various cell-specific levels in the other tissues of the human body. Most importantly, approximately 95% of the active estrogens and androgens are inactivated locally before being released in the blood as inactive metabolites, thus avoiding inappropriate exposure of the other tissues (Luu-The 2013; Labrie 2015). As a whole, the intracrine process that is typical for steroid hormones binding to nuclear receptors is thus equivalent to autocrine and paracrine processes activated by hormones binding to transmembrane receptors. Although the terms autocrine and paracrine are used for both nuclear and transmembrane receptors, it is important to make the distinction, especially because nuclear steroid receptors could be also found extrinsically linked to the plasma membrane and act in an extranuclear manner (Molina 2010; Norman and Henry 2015).

Steroid-Binding Proteins

Most steroid hormones have limited solubility in plasma due to their intrinsic hydrophobic nature; accordingly, steroid hormones are largely (99%) bound to specific plasma transport proteins, which are synthesized in the liver. All steroid hormones, except one, have their cognate plasma-binding protein. The exception is aldosterone; 50% of aldosterone is believed to circulate as the free steroid in the plasma compartment. Each transport protein has a specific ligand-binding domain for its cognate hormone, which displays little amino acid sequence homology with the ligand binding of the cognate receptors. The Kd of a steroid hormone for its plasma transport is always "looser," e.g., $1–100 \times 10^{-8}$ M, than that of the Kd of the nuclear receptor. Thus, the tighter binding of the steroid hormone to its target receptor when it has arrived at a target tissue allows the hormone to be concentrated inside the target cell. The current view is that it is the "free" form of steroid hormones and not the complex of the hormone with its plasma transport proteins that interacts with receptors in or on the target cells to begin the sequence of steps that result in the generation of a biological response (Molina 2010; Norman and Henry 2015).

In the plasma compartment, the steroid hormones move through the circulatory system bound to their partner transport protein. However, an important issue concerns the details of the mode of delivery of steroid hormones to their target cells. Because the "free" form of the steroid hormone is believed to be the form of steroid that moves across the outer plasma membrane of a target cell, it has been postulated that the steroid ligand dissociates from its plasma transport protein and then diffuses first through the capillary wall and then through the outer wall membrane of target cells. However, it is apparent that the endothelial wall of capillaries contains fenestrations. Thus, it is also possible for the plasma steroid transport protein (with bound steroid hormone) to exit the capillary bed via a fenestration and move to be immediately adjacent to the outer cell membrane of the appropriate target cell for the steroid hormone in question. Here the steroid hormone will dissociate from the transport protein, diffuse through the plasma membrane, and then bind to an unoccupied partner steroid receptor.

A corticosteroid-binding globulin (CBG) is present in blood. This protein is also referred to as transcortin. It is synthesized in the liver and exported to the circulation. This protein binds cortisol with relatively high affinity (binding constant $\cong$ 108 M−1; the dissociation constant for the reaction, CBG + cortisol $\leftrightarrow$ CBG – cortisol, is about 10^{-8} M cortisol). Because of the affinity of the protein for cortisol, most of the hormone circulates in the bound form as reflected in the equilibrium, which favors the complex: CBG + cortisol $\leftrightarrow$ CBG-cortisol.

There is only a small amount of the free steroid hormone in a target cell. Nevertheless, at the target cell, the free steroid enters the cell plasma membrane, probably by a free diffusion process. The driving force behind the movement of free hormone in the target cell appears, in part, to be proportionate to the number of unoccupied cortisol hormone-specific nuclear receptor molecules that have moved from the nucleus of the target cell out to the cytoplasm that still have empty ligand-binding sites (unoccupied receptors). The affinity of the nuclear receptor for cortisol is similar (20 nM) to that of the circulating CBG-cortisol complex. Steroid hormones cycle into and out of a target cell, and the number of unoccupied nuclear receptors determines the proportion of molecules retained in the cell.

Of the total testosterone in the circulation, 0.5–3% is free (not bound to protein), 54–68% is bound to albumin with relatively low affinity, and the remainder is bound to sex hormone-binding globulin, SHBG, with high affinity. SHBG, synthesized in the liver, is a dimeric glycosylated protein with a molecular mass of 84 kDa. SHBG has a preference for steroids with a 17β-hydroxyl [Kd ≅ (1–5) × 10–10 M], so it binds testosterone, DHT, and estradiol, but not, for example, progesterone or cortisol. Thus, it serves as the specific transport protein for both testosterone and estradiol. Plasma levels of SHBG are twofold greater in nonpregnant women than in men. The synthesis, and therefore the plasma concentration, of SHBG is increased in pregnancy and hyperthyroidism and is decreased by androgens, glucocorticoids, insulin, and growth hormone.

The plasma contains the vitamin D-binding protein (DBP) that is utilized to transport vitamin D secosterols. DBP resembles the corticosteroid-binding globulin, which carries glucocorticoids, and the steroid hormone-binding globulin. DBP is a slightly acidic (pH = 5.2) monomeric glycoprotein of 53,000 Da, which is synthesized and secreted by the liver as a major plasma constituent.

DBP is a multifunctional protein in that it binds both vitamin D and its metabolites. One molecule of DBP has only one ligand-binding domain-binding site for secosterols of the vitamin D family. Thus, while a single DBP can carry only one ligand, the relatively high concentration of DBP molecules present in the blood compartment permits the DBP population as a whole to bind the hydrophobic parent, vitamin D3, as well as the hydrophobic daughter metabolites, $25(OH)D_3$, $1\alpha,25(OH)_2D_3$, and $24,25(OH)D_3$. Since the total plasma concentration of vitamin D sterols is only ~0.2 μM, while DBP circulates at 9–13 μM, under normal circumstances only a very small proportion of the sterol-binding sites on DBP are occupied.

For some endocrine systems, the concentration of the plasma transport protein can be subject to physiological regulation; that is, the concentration of plasma transport proteins can be either increased or decreased. Thus, changes for plasma transport proteins can alter the amount of free hormone in the blood, as well as affect the total amount of hormone in the blood. This role of the binding proteins in the availability of steroid hormones can be of considerable physiological relevance in clinical situations (Molina 2010; Norman and Henry 2015).

Steroid Hormone Metabolism

The effective concentration of a hormone is determined by the rates of its production, delivery to the target tissue, and degradation. The excess of steroids that are not bound to the receptors will be inactivated into the target cell, and hormone metabolites will be secreted in the circulation. In addition, the local inactivation of the excess of active steroids inside the cells is an important manner to regulate active steroid concentration (Molina 2010; Norman and Henry 2015).

The hydrophobic steroid hormones and the vitamin D are filtered by the kidney and generally reabsorbed. About 1% of the cortisol produced daily ends up in the urine. Steroid hormones are ordinarily handled by metabolizing them to inactive and to water-soluble forms that are more effectively eliminated. The free steroid fraction is accessible to the metabolic inactivation. The inactivation is accomplished by converting hydroxyl groups to keto groups, reducing double bounds, and conjugating the steroids with glucuronide and sulfate groups. These processes occur in the liver through phase I and phase II biotransformation reactions. Over 50 different steroid metabolites have been described.

Cortisol is reversibly inactivated by conversion to cortisone and to tetrahydrocortisol and tetrahydrocortisone in the liver and kidney. These metabolites are referred to as 17-hydroxycorticosteroids, and their determination in 24 h urine collections is used to assess the status of adrenal steroid production. As discussed before, localized tissue metabolism contributes to modulation of the cortisol biological effects by the isoforms of the enzymes 11βHSD1 and 11βHSD2.

Aldosterone is metabolized in the liver to tetrahydroglucuronide derivative and excreted in the urine. A fraction of aldosterone is metabolized to aldosterone 18-glucuronide, which can be hydrolyzed back to free aldosterone under low pH conditions.

In the liver, testosterone undergoes 5β-reduction, followed by 3α-reduction and reduction of the 17-keto group. DHT undergoes 3α- and 17β-reduction. Both reduced catabolites are then conjugated with glucuronic acid or, to a lesser extent, sulfate, released back into the circulation and removed from the body in the urine or bile.

Estrogens are metabolized by sulfation or glucuronidation, and the conjugates are excreted into the urine. Estrogen can also be metabolized through hydroxylation and subsequent methylation to form catechol and methoxy estrogens.

$1,25(OH)_2D$ may be inactivated by the principal hepatic drug-metabolizing enzyme, microsomal CYP3A4, or by its 24-hydroxylation by vitamin D 24-hydroxylase (P450c24), encoded by the CYP24A1 gene. This mitochondrial enzyme can catalyze the 24-hydroxylation of $25(OH)D_3$ to $24,25(OH)_2D_3$ and of $1,25(OH)_2D_3$ to $1,24,25(OH)_3D_3$, primarily in the kidney and intestine, thus inactivating vitamin D (Norman and Henry 2015).

Conclusions

Steroid hormones regulate a wide variety of developmental and physiological processes from fetal life to adulthood. Important functions of these hormones include regulation of the mammalian stress response, electrolyte and fluid homeostasis, and the development and maintenance of both primary and secondary sexual characteristics. Despite efforts to correlate steroid structures with their activities, this area was not understood until the various steroid hormone receptors were identified and cloned. Thus, the contemporary definition of each class of steroid is based on the nuclear receptor(s) to which it binds, rather than on the chemical structure of the steroid. In addition, disorders of steroid hormone synthesis were formerly thought to be confined to rare genetic lesions; consequently, more study has been devoted to steroid hormone action than to steroid hormone synthesis. Work in the past 30 years has identified the steroidogenic enzymes and their genes, reinvigorating studies of steroid biosynthesis by discoveries of roles for altered regulation of steroidogenesis in common disorders such as hypertension and the polycystic ovary syndrome and by discoveries of steroid-modifying enzymes in target tissues that mediate some forms of apparent tissue specificity of hormone action.

Summary

Steroidogenesis entails processes by which cholesterol is converted to biologically active steroid hormones. Six classes of steroid hormones, all of which are indispensable for mammalian life, are made from cholesterol via complex biosynthetic pathways that are initiated by specialized, tissue-specific enzymes found in mitochondria and endoplasmic reticulum. These hormones include glucocorticoids (cortisol, corticosterone) and mineralocorticoids (aldosterone) produced in the adrenal cortex; estrogens (estradiol), progestins (progesterone), and androgens (testosterone, dihydrotestosterone) produced in the gonads; and calciferols (1,25-dihydroxy vitamin D [$1,25OH_2D_3$]) produced in the kidney. Historically, steroid hormone synthesis only occurred in the steroidogenic glands (i.e., adrenal glands, gonads, and placenta). A significant number of studies have now challenged this view by demonstrating that several organs, including the brain, adipose tissue, and intestine, are capable of producing steroid hormones. These are called non-steroidogenic or intracrine tissues.

The production and/or secretion of most hormones are regulated by the homeostatic mechanisms, which operate in that particular endocrine system. The secretion or release of the hormone is normally related to the requirement for the biological response(s) generated by the specific hormone. Because of their hydrophobic nature, steroid hormones and precursors can leave the steroidogenic cell easily and are not stored. Thus, steroidogenesis is regulated primarily at the first step in their synthesis (the cleavage of the side chain of cholesterol) and at the level of steroidogenic enzyme gene expression and activity. Once the biological response has been generated, the secretion of the hormone is restrained to prevent an overresponse. Thus, a characteristic feature of most endocrine systems is the existence of a feedback loop (either direct or multistep) that limits or regulates the secretion of the hormone. Another contributor to the biological availability of steroid hormones is the control exerted by biological rhythms on steroid hormone production.

Steroid hormones are synthesized, but not stored, within specific endocrine cells from which they are easily secreted in the plasma. However, most steroid hormones have limited solubility in plasma due to their intrinsic hydrophobic nature; accordingly, steroid hormones are largely bound to specific plasma transport proteins, which are synthesized in the liver. All steroid hormones, except aldosterone, have their cognate plasma-binding protein.

The excess of steroids that are not released or bound to the receptors will be inactivated into the cell, and hormone metabolites will be secreted in the circulation. This local inactivation of the excess of active steroids inside the cells is an important manner to regulate active steroid concentration.

As a whole, the key determinants of the steroid hormone response are the presence of a response system (receptors and signaling transduction pathways in target cells) and hormone blood concentration. The effective concentration of a steroid hormone is determined by the rates at which the steroid is biosynthesized and enters the body pools, the "tightness" of binding of the steroid to its plasma carrier protein, and the rate at which the steroid is biologically inactivated by catabolism and removed from body pools.

Cross-References

► Growth Hormones and Aging
► Ovarian Physiology
► Steroid Hormone Receptors and Signal Transduction Processes
► The Adrenal Glands
► The Endocrine Control of Human Pregnancy
► The Endocrinology of Puberty
► The Hypothalamus–Pituitary Axis
► The Parathyroids
► The Physiology of the Testis
► The Posterior Pituitary

References

Auchus RJ, Rainey WE. Adrenarche–physiology, biochemistry and human disease. Clin Endocrinol (Oxf). 2004;60:288.

Barclay JL, Tsang AH, Oster H. Interaction of central and peripheral clocks in physiological regulation. Prog Brain Res. 2012;199:163.

Bassett MH, White PC, Rainey WE. The regulation of aldosterone synthase expression. Mol Cell Endocrinol. 2004;217:67.

Brown MS, Kovanen PT, Goldstein JL. Receptor-mediated uptake of lipoprotein-cholesterol and its utilization for steroid synthesis in the adrenal cortex. Rec Prog Horm Res. 1979;35:215.

Chang TY, Chang CC, Ohgami N, Yamauchi Y. Cholesterol sensing, trafficking and esterification. Annu Rev Cell Dev Biol. 2006;22:129.

Chevrier L, Guimiot F, de Roux N. GnRH receptor mutations in isolated gonadotropic deficiency. Mol Cell Endocrinol. 2011;346:21.

Clyne CD, Zhang Y, Slutsker L, Mathis JM, White PC, Rainey WE. Angiotensin II and potassium regulate human CYP11B2 transcription through common cis-elements. Mol Endocrinol. 1997;11:638.

Cooper MS, Stewart PM. 11Beta-hydroxysteroid dehydrogenase type 1 and its role in the hypothalamus-pituitary-adrenal axis, metabolic syndrome, and inflammation. J Clin Endocrinol Metab. 2009;94:4645.

Ehrhart-Bornstein M, Hinson JP, Bornstein SR, Scherbaum WA, Vinson GP. Intraadrenal interactions in the regulation of adrenocortical steroidogenesis. Endocr Rev. 1998;19:101.
Fieser LF, Fieser M. Steroids. New York: Reinhold Publishing Corp; 1959. p. 1–945.
Gaffey AE, Bergeman CS, Clark LA, Wirth MM. Aging and the HPA axis: Stress and resilience in older adults. Neurosci Biobehav Rev. 2016;68:928.
Horton JD, Goldstein JL, Brown MS. SREBPs: activators of the complete program of cholesterol and fatty acid synthesis in the liver. J Clin Invest. 2002;109:1125.
Khundmiri SJ, Murray RD, Lederer E. PTH and Vitamin D. Compr Physiol. 2016;6:561.
Kraemer FB. Adrenal cholesterol utilization. Mol Cell Endocrinol. 2007;42:265–6.
Labrie F. All sex steroids are made intracellularly in peripheral tissues by the mechanisms of intracrinology after menopause. J Steroid Biochem Mol Biol. 2015;145:133.
Lin XW, Blum ID, Storch KF. Clocks within the Master Gland: Hypophyseal Rhythms and Their Physiological Significance. J Biol Rhythms. 2015;30:263.
Luu-The V. Assessment of steroidogenesis and steroidogenic enzyme functions. J Steroid Biochem Mol Biol. 2013;137:176.
Miller WL. Molecular biology of steroid hormone synthesis. Endocr Rev. 1988;9:295.
Miller WL. Steroid hormone synthesis in mitochondria. Mol Cell Endocrinol. 2013;379:62.
Miller WL, Auchus RJ. The molecular biology, biochemistry, and physiology of human steroidogenesis and its disorders. Endocr Rev. 2011;32:81.
Molina PE. Endocrine physiology. 3rd ed. New York: McGraw-Hill Company; 2010. p. 1–303.
Norman AW. Sunlight, season, skin pigmentation, vitamin D, and 25-1100 hydroxyvitamin D: integral components of the vitamin D endocrine system. Am J Clin Nutr. 1998;67:1108.
Norman AW, Henry HL. Hormones. 3rd ed. London: Elsevier; 2015. p. 1–413.
Normington K, Russell DW. Tissue distribution and kinetic characteristics of rat steroid 5-reductase enzymes. Evidence for distinct physiological functions. J Biol Chem. 1992;267:19548.
Plant TM. Hypothalamic control of the pituitary–gonadal axis in higher primates: key advances over the last two decades. J Neuroendocrinol. 2008;20:719.
Riegelhaupt JJ, Waase MP, Garbarino J, Cruz DE, Breslow JL. Targeted disruption of steroidogenic acute regulatory protein D4 leads to modest weight reduction and minor alterations in lipid metabolism. J Lipid Res. 2010;51:1134.
Russell DW, Wilson JD. Steroid 5-reductase: two genes/two enzymes. Ann Rev Biochem. 1994;63:25.
Stocco DM, Wang X, Jo Y, Manna PR. Multiple signaling pathways regulating steroidogenesis and steroidogenic acute regulatory protein expression: more complicated than we thought. Mol Endocrinol. 2005;19:2647.
Tian Y, Shen W, Lai Z, Shi L, Yang S, Ding T, Wang S, Luo A. Isolation and identification of ovarian theca-interstitial cells and granulose cells of immature female mice. Cell Biol Int. 2015;39:584.
Wood CE. Development and programming of the hypothalamus-pituitary-adrenal axis. Clin Obstet Gynecol. 2013;56:610.

Further Reading

d'Anglemont de Tassigny X, Colledge WH. The role of kisspeptin signaling in reproduction. Physiology (Bethesda). 2010;25:207–17.
Miller WL. Disorders in the initial steps of steroid hormone synthesis. J Steroid Biochem Mol Biol. 2017;165:18–37. pii: S0960-0760(16)30055-3.
Rahmani B, Ghasemi R, Dargahi L, Ahmadiani A, Haeri A. Neurosteroids; potential underpinning roles in maintaining homeostasis. Gen Comp Endocrinol. 2016;225:242–50.
Tsang AH, Barclay JL, Oster H. Interactions between endocrine and circadian systems. J Mol Endocrinol. 2013;52:R1–16.

Molecular Mechanisms of Thyroid Hormone Synthesis and Secretion

4

Noriyuki Koibuchi

Abstract

Thyroxine (T_4) and triiodothyronine (T_3), collectively called as thyroid hormones, are synthesized in the thyroid gland. Another molecule called reverse T_3 (rT_3), whose function is unknown, is also secreted from the thyroid gland. T_4 is the major molecule synthesized and secreted from the thyroid gland, whereas other molecules are mainly generated in extrathyroidal tissues by deiodination of T_4. The thyroid hormone synthetic pathway comprises the following steps: (1) thyroglobulin synthesis and secretion into the follicular lumen; (2) iodine uptake into the follicular epithelial cells; (3) iodine transport and efflux into the follicular lumen; (4) oxidation of iodine, iodination of thyroglobulin tyrosine residues, and coupling of iodotyrosines; (5) endocytosis of the thyroglobulin-thyroid hormone complex into follicular epithelial cells; (6) hydrolysis of the complex; and (7) secretion of thyroid hormone. Thyroid-stimulating hormone (thyrotropin) stimulates thyroid hormone synthesis. In this chapter, the outline of the thyroid hormone synthetic pathway is discussed. The mechanisms regulating thyroid hormone synthesis is briefly described. Furthermore, the clinical aspects of altered thyroid hormone synthesis and secretion induced by immunological or genetic abnormalities are also discussed.

Keywords

Thyroxine • Triiodothyronine • Thyroid gland • Follicle • Iodine • Na^+/I^- symporter • Thyroglobulin • Thyroid peroxidase • Dual oxidase

Conflict of Interest: The author does not have any conflict of interest.

N. Koibuchi (✉)
Department of Integrative Physiology, Gunma University Graduate School of Medicine, Maebashi, Gunma, Japan
e-mail: nkoibuch@gunma-u.ac.jp

A. Belfiore, D. LeRoith (eds.), *Principles of Endocrinology and Hormone Action*, Endocrinology, https://doi.org/10.1007/978-3-319-44675-2_5

Contents

Chemical Structure of Thyroid Hormones

Thyroid hormones play a major role in development and functional maintenance of many organs (Koibuchi and Chin 2000). They are a group of hormones synthesized and secreted from the thyroid gland, which is located in front of the trachea, below the thyroid cartilage. In general, two compounds, thyroxine (3,5,3′,5′-tetra-iodo-L-thyronine, T_4) and triiodothyronine (3,5,3′-tri-iodo-L-thyronine, T_3), are considered thyroid hormones. In addition, another compound called reverse T_3 (3,3′,5′-tri-iodo-L-thyronine, rT_3) is secreted from the thyroid gland. Their chemical structures are shown in Fig. 1. The essential molecular structure comprises two iodinated benzene rings connected by ether linkage. T_4 is the major hormone secreted from the thyroid gland, whereas the other hormones are mainly generated by the deiodination of T_4 in extrathyroidal tissues. The ratio of the secretion of T4:T3:rT3 from the thyroid gland is approximately 100:5:2.5. T_3, a bioactive thyroid hormone, is mainly produced by the deiodination of T_4 in thyroid hormone target tissues.

Synthesis and Secretion of Thyroglobulin into the Follicular Lumen

In the thyroid gland, thyroid hormone is synthesized within the unique structure called the thyroid follicle, which comprises a layer of follicular epithelial cells (also known as thyroid follicular cells or thyrocytes) surrounding a follicular lumen. Notably, the unique feature of the thyroid hormone synthetic pathway is that thyroid hormone is produced in the follicular lumen and not inside the follicular epithelial cells. No other hormone is produced outside the cell. The outline of the thyroid hormone synthetic pathway is shown in Fig. 2.

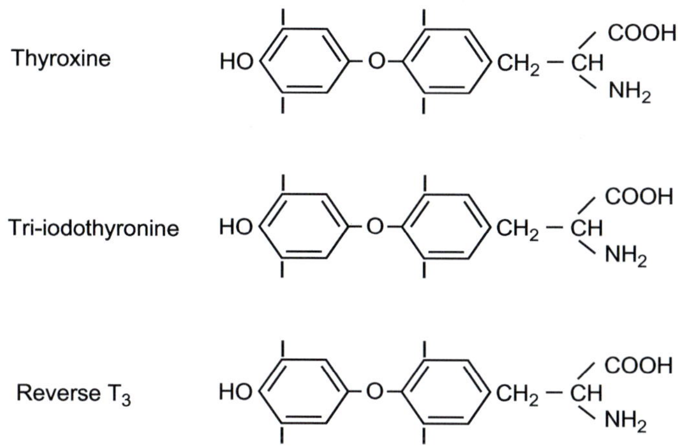

Fig. 1 Chemical structure of thyroid hormones

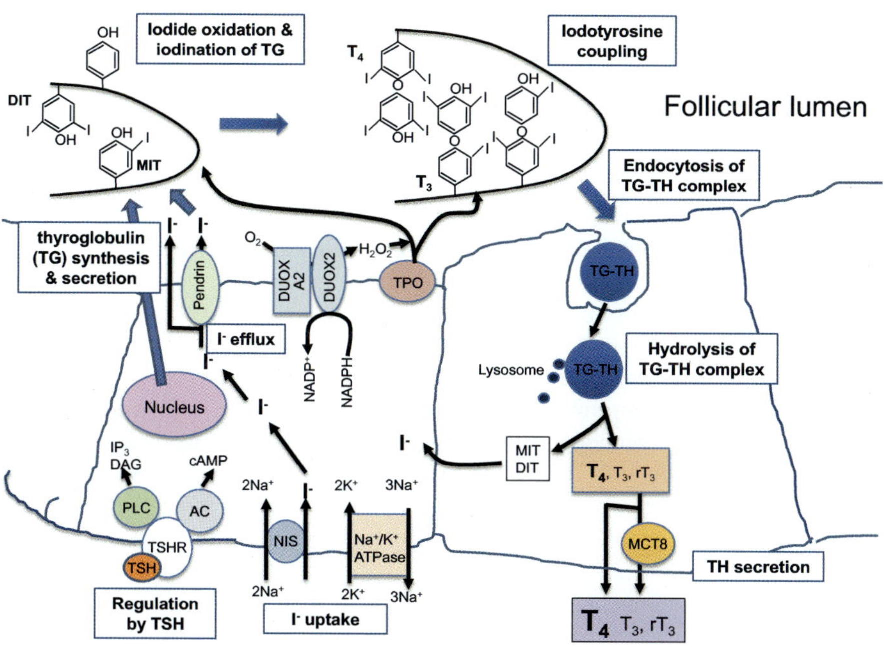

Fig. 2 Thyroid hormone (TH) synthetic pathway. AC, adenyl cyclase; DIT, diiodotyrosine; DUOX, dual oxidase; MCT8, monocarboxylate transporter; MIT, monoiodotyrosine; NIS, Na+/I-symporter; PLC, phospholipase C; TPO, thyroid peroxidase; TSH, thyrotropin; TSHR, thyrotropin receptor

The follicular lumen is filled with a glycoprotein called thyroglobulin (TG) that is specific to the thyroid gland. Human TG is a large glycoprotein containing 2,748 amino acids. It is synthesized within follicular epithelial cells and secreted by exocytosis into the lumen, where it forms a homodimer. TG contains 123 tyrosine residues. Among these residues, those located close to the N- and C-termini are utilized to synthesize thyroid hormones. Although these residues play a major role in thyroid hormone synthesis, other residues may also be important to form an appropriate secondary structure for effective hormone synthesis. Only a missense mutation (G2320R) in the TG gene induces severe hypothyroidism (Shimokawa et al. 2014).

Iodine Uptake into Follicular Epithelial Cells

The iodine concentration in follicular epithelial cells is 40-fold higher than that in plasma. Thus, iodine in plasma must be transported against a high concentration gradient. Iodine is transported as iodide (I^-) by secondary active transport. The transporter called Na^+/I^- symporter (NIS) is located on the basal membrane of thyroid epithelial cells (Portulano et al. 2014). Human NIS comprises 643 amino acids and has 13 transmembrane domains. NIS cotransports a single I^- molecule with two Na^+ molecules using a Na^+ electrochemical gradient generated by Na^+/K^+ ATPase. Thyroid-stimulating hormone (TSH, thyrotropin) stimulates iodine uptake mainly by stimulating NIS transcription. In contrast, high dose of intracellular I^- transiently inhibits thyroid hormone synthesis through the inhibition of iodine organification (Wolff-Chaikoff effect).

Iodine Transport and Efflux into the Follicular Lumen

After uptake by NIS, I^- is transported toward the apical membrane. I^- secretion into the follicular lumen is not mediated by NIS but by other transporters. Previous studies have shown that a transporter called pendrin, an anion exchange protein, plays a major role in transporting I^- into the lumen (Kopp et al. 2008). Pendrin is a highly hydrophobic membrane protein comprising 780 amino acids and contains 12 transmembrane domains. In addition to I^-, it transports other anions, such as Cl^- and HCO_3^-. However, although pendrin plays a major role in I^- efflux into the lumen, several other proteins may also be involved in I^- transport (Bizhanova and Kopp 2011).

Iodine Oxidization and Organification and Coupling of TG Iodotyrosine Residues

After efflux into the follicular lumen, I^- is oxidized to I, which is then linked to TG tyrosine residues by covalent bonds. Next, two mono- or di-iodinated tyrosine (iodotyrosine) residues are coupled to form ether bonds to generate iodothyronines.

The coupling of two diiodotyrosines forms T_4, whereas, with lesser degree, that of monoiodotyrosine and diiodotyrosine forms either T_3 or rT_3. Both synthesis steps are catalyzed by thyroid peroxidase (TPO) (Ruf and Carayon 2006), which belongs to the heme peroxidase family. Human TPO comprises 933 amino acids and is anchored at the apical membrane of follicular epithelial cells via a C-terminal transmembrane domain. Being a heme peroxidase, TPO requires hydrogen peroxide (H_2O_2) as the final electron acceptor. H_2O_2 is produced at the apical membrane by a membrane-bound NADPH-dependent flavoprotein called dual oxidase (DUOX) (Grasberger 2010). Two paralogs, DUOX1 and 2 (1,551 and 1,548 amino acids in humans, respectively), are located in the apical membrane. To localize in the apical membrane, they form heterodimers with another group of transmembrane proteins called DUOX maturation factors (DUOXA). Two human thyroid-specific DUOXA paralogs, DUOXA1 and 2 (483 and 320 amino acids, respectively), have been identified. Because TPO is not activated by phosphorylation, H_2O_2 production by DUOX is critical for both tyrosine residue iodination and coupling. Thus, failure to produce H_2O_2 causes severe hypothyroidism (Amano et al. 2016). DUOX is activated by increased intracellular calcium. TSH, upon binding to the TSH receptor, activates DUOX by intracellular calcium mobilization through the $G_{q/11}$-phospholipase C pathway.

Uptake of TG-Thyroid Hormone Complex by Endocytosis

After iodotyrosine coupling, thyroid hormone does not dissociate from the TG molecule in the follicular lumen. TG-thyroid hormone complexes are endocytosed by follicular epithelial cells by endocytosis. This process is also activated by TSH.

Thyroid Hormone Production by TG Molecule Hydrolysis

Internalized vesicles containing TG-thyroid hormone complex fuse with lysosomes, resulting in complex breakdown and thyroid hormone release. This also produces iodotyrosines (monoiodotyrosine and diiodotyrosine). TG is further degraded to produce amino acids. Iodotyrosines are deiodinated by iodotyrosine dehalogenase to produce free iodine and are recycled in the follicular epithelial cells.

Secretion of Thyroid Hormone

After TG degradation, thyroid hormone (mainly T_4) is secreted into the bloodstream at the basal membrane. Although the precise mechanisms of thyroid hormone secretion have not yet been completely clarified, thyroid hormone transporters, particularly monocarboxylate transporter (MCT) 8, may play a major role in secretion (Di Cosmo et al. 2010). MCT8 comprises 539 amino acids in humans and contains 12 transmembrane domains. It promotes the uptake and secretion of thyroid hormone. However, MCT8 disruption cannot completely inhibit thyroid hormone secretion, indicating that additional mechanisms may be involved.

Effect of TSH on Thyroid Hormone Synthesis

TSH, a glycoprotein hormone, is secreted from the anterior pituitary. It comprises an α-subunit, which is common to other glycoprotein hormones such as luteinizing hormone and follicle-stimulating hormone, and a β-subunit, which is unique to TSH. It binds to the TSH receptor (TSHR), a G-protein-coupled receptor. It is translated into a protein comprising 764 amino acids, followed by cleavage of a 352–366-amino acid peptide, resulting in the formation of extracellular A and B subunits containing seven transmembrane domains (Rapoport and McLachlan 2016).

The effects of TSH on the thyroid hormone synthetic pathway are shown in Table 1. TSHR activates both the G_s-adenyl cyclase-cAMP and $G_{q/11}$-phospholipase C-β signaling pathways (Kleinau et al. 2013). The cAMP pathway regulates many steps in the synthesis and secretion of thyroid hormone, such as the expression of NIS, TG, and TPO, iodide uptake, and hormone secretion, whereas $G_{q/11}$-phospholipase C-β pathway activates iodine organification (activation of H_2O_2 production, see above) by stimulating intracellular calcium mobilization and iodide efflux from the apical membrane. TSH also stimulates follicular epithelial cell proliferation.

Defects of Thyroid Hormone Synthesis and Secretion in Adults (Clinical Aspects)

Clinical disorders of thyroid hormone synthesis and secretion are commonly observed in adults. In the United States, hyperthyroidism has a prevalence of 1.3% of the population, whereas hypothyroidism has a prevalence of 4.6% (Hollowell et al. 2002). The prevalence is higher in East Asia such as Japan (hyperthyroidism, 2.9%; hypothyroidism, 6.5%) (Kasagi et al. 2009). In both hyper- and hypothyroid cases, the prevalence is higher in females. The most common cause of these disorders is an autoimmune thyroid disease. Autoimmune disease affects the thyroid gland more than any other organ (McLeod and Cooper 2012). Hyperthyroidism is mainly caused by Graves' disease, which is caused by a unique autoantibody to TSHR acting as a TSHR agonist. On the other hand, more than 90% of adult-onset hypothyroidism in countries with iodine sufficiency is caused by Hashimoto disease, which is caused by T-cell-mediated follicular epithelial cell injury, causing decreased secretion of the thyroid hormone. Autoantibodies against TG, TPO, and TSHR (blocking antibody) are found in patients. The mechanism causing autoimmune thyroid disease has not yet been fully clarified. In particular, the mechanism generating TSH receptor stimulating autoantibody needs to be clarified. Trials to clarify such mechanisms are currently underway by many researchers.

Table 1 Effects of TSH on the thyroid hormone synthetic pathway

Function	G-protein	Action
Iodine mobilization	G_s	Iodine uptake (induction of NIS expression and its translocation to basal membrane)
	$G_{q/11}$, G_s	Iodine efflux to follicular lumen
Hormone synthesis	G_s	TG and TPO expression
	$G_{q/11}$	H_2O_2 production
	$G_{q/11}$	TG iodination
Hormone secretion	G_s	Iodinated TG uptake into follicular epithelial cells
	G_s	Thyroid hormone secretion
Other	G_s, $G_{q/11}$	Follicular epithelial cell proliferation

Another important cause of decreased synthesis and secretion of thyroid hormone is iodine deficiency. Because iodine is an essential component of the thyroid hormone, its deficiency results in impairment of the thyroid hormone synthesis (Zimmermann 2013). Although programs to control iodine deficiency, such as providing iodized salt, have been effective, it is still a major concern to the human health, particularly among children and pregnant women in many countries (de Benoist et al. 2008).

The signs and symptoms caused by hyper- and hypothyroidism are described in another chapter (Cheng, S. ▶ Chap.9, "Thyroid Hormone Nuclear Receptors and Molecular Actions" Part III).

Congenital Defects in Thyroid Hormone Synthesis and Secretion

Because the thyroid hormone is essential for normal growth, development, and functional maintenance of many organs, deficiency of the thyroid hormone induced by thyroid gland dysgenesis or thyroid dyshormonogenesis results in various abnormalities in many organs known as cretinism in humans. The role of thyroid hormone during development has been discussed in more detail in another chapter (Cheng, S. Part III) and a previous article (Koibuchi and Chin 2000). Most congenital thyroid dysgenesis and thyroid dyshormogenesis are caused by mutation of genes that regulate thyroid development or thyroid hormone synthesis (Park and Chatterjee 2005). Another important factor that may cause congenital thyroid dyshormogenesis is iodine deficiency (see above).

Various genes are involved in inducing congenital hypothyroidism. In particular, thyroid agenesis or dysgenesis is caused by mutations in thyroid transcription factors (TTFs) such as NKX2-1, FOXE1, and PAX 8 (Fernández et al. 2015). A homeobox protein, NKX2-1, which was previously called TTF-1, is expressed in multiple tissues in addition to the thyroid gland, e.g., lung, pituitary, and hypothalamus. In the thyroid gland, NKX2-1 may play an important role in maintaining thyroid follicular structure and follicular epithelial cell survival. Mutation of this gene in humans results in thyroid agenesis or hypoplasia and respiratory distress. Forkhead box protein, FOXE1, which was previously called TTF-2, is expressed in the thyroid gland as well as in other tissues that are derived from the pharyngeal arches and wall, e.g., tongue, palate, and esophagus. It may regulate migration of thyroid precursor cells. Mutation of FOXE1 in humans results in ectopy, agenesis or hypoplasia of the thyroid gland, and cleft palate. Paired box protein, PAX8, is expressed in the developing thyroid gland, kidney, and brain. This protein may be essential for thyroid precursor cell survival possibly by inhibiting apoptosis. Mutation of PAX8 in humans results in ectopy, agenesis, or hypoplasia of the thyroid gland, problems in the urogenital tract, and, rarely, unilateral kidney. In addition to mutation of these transcription factors, mutation of TSH receptor sometimes results in hypoplasia of the thyroid gland, because TSH regulates the proliferation of thyroid follicular cells (Kleinau et al. 2013).

Thyroid dyshormonogenesis is caused by the mutations in genes that play critical roles in thyroid hormone synthetic pathway. Such genes include TG (Targovnik et al. 2010), TPO (Ruf and Carayon 2006), and DUOX (Grasberger 2010). The role of these factors on thyroid hormone synthesis has been discussed above.

Summary

The thyroid hormone synthetic pathway is quite unique, in that, although it is a relatively small molecule comprising two iodinated phenol rings, it is synthesized by the breakdown of a large protein, TG. Furthermore, most synthetic process occurs in the extracellular space (follicular lumen).

The research on thyroid hormone synthesis began early compared with that on other hormones. In addition, many genes that induce congenital hypothyroidism have been reported. Nevertheless, many questions remain to be answered. In particular, the mechanisms generating TSHR-stimulating autoantibody and the role of TTFs on the thyroid gland development remain unclarified. Additional novel approaches may be required to solve such questions.

Cross-References

▶ The Thyroid
▶ Thyroid Hormone Nuclear Receptors and Molecular Actions

References

Amano I, Takatsuru Y, Toya S, Haijima A, Iwasaki T, Grasberger H, Refetoff S, Koibuchi N. Aberrant cerebellar development in mice lacking dual oxidase maturation factors. Thyroid. 2016;26:741–52.

Bizhanova A, Kopp P. Controversies concerning the role of pendrin as an apical iodide transporter in thyroid follicular cells. Cell Physiol Biochem. 2011;28:485–90.

de Benoist B, McLean E, Andersson M, Rogers L. Iodine deficiency in 2007: global progress since 2003. Food Nutr Bull. 2008;29:195–202.

Di Cosmo C, Liao X-H, Dumitrescu AM, Philp NJ, Weiss RE, Refetoff S. Mice deficient in MCT8 reveal a mechanism regulating thyroid hormone secretion. J Clin Invest. 2010;120:3377–88.

Fernández LP, López-Márquez A, Santisteban P. Thyroid transcription factors in development, differentiation and disease. Nat Rev Endocrinol. 2015;11:29–42.

Grasberger H. Defects of thyroidal hydrogen peroxidase generation in congenital hypothyroidism. Mol Cell Endocrinol. 2010;322:99–106.

Hollowell JG, Staehling NW, Flanders WD, Hannon WH, Gunter EW, Spencer CA, Braverman LE. Serum TSH, T(4), and thyroid antibodies in the United States population (1988 to 1994): National Health and Nutrition Examination Survey (NHANES III). J Clin Endocrinol Metab. 2002;87:489–99.

Kasagi K, Takahashi N, Inoue G, Honda T, Kawachi Y, Izumi Y. Thyroid function in Japanese adults as assessed by a general health checkup system in relation with thyroid-related antibodies and other clinical parameters. Thyroid 2009;19:937–44.

Kleinau G, Neumann S, Grüters A, Krude H, Biebermann H. Novel insights on thyroid-stimulating hormone receptor signal transduction. Endocr Rev. 2013;34:691–724.

Koibuchi N, Chin WW. Thyroid hormone action and brain development. Trends Endocrinol Metab. 2000;11:123–8.

Kopp P, Pesce L, Solis JC. Pendred syndrome and iodide transport in the thyroid. Trend Endocrinol Metab. 2008;19:260–8.

McLeod DSA, Cooper DS. The incidence and prevalence of thyroid autoimmunity. Endocrine. 2012;42:252–65.

Park SM, Chatterjee VK. Genetics of congenital hypothyroidism. J Med Genet. 2005;42:379–89.

Portulano C, Paroder-Belenitsky M, Carrasco N. The Na^{+}/I^{-} symporter (NIS): mechanism and medical impact. Endocr Rev. 2014;35:106–49.

Rapoport B, McLachlan SM. TSH receptor cleavage into subunits and shedding of the a-subunit. Endocr Rev. 2016;37:114–34.

Ruf J, Carayon P. Structural and functional aspects of thyroid peroxidase. Arch Biochem Biophys. 2006;445:269–77.

Shimokawa N, Yousefi B, Morioka S, Yamaguchi S, Ohsawa A, Hayashi H, et al. Altered cerebellum development and dopamine distribution in a rat genetic model with congenital hypothyroidism. J Neuroendocrinol. 2014;26:164–75.

Targovnik HM, Esperante SA, Rivolta CM. Genetics and phenomics of hypothyroidism and goiter due to thyroglobulin mutations. Mol Cell Endocrinol. 2010;322:44–55.

Zimmermann MB. Iodine deficiency and endemic cretinism. In: Braverman LE, Cooper D, editors. The thyroid. A fundamental and clinical text. Philadelphia: Lippincott; 2013. p. 217–41.

Further Reading

Koibuchi N, Yen PM, editors. Thyroid hormone disruption and neurodevelopment contemporary clinical neuroscience series. New York: Springer-Verlag; 2016. ISBN 978-1-4939-3737-0.

Part III

Hormone Receptors and Signal Transduction Processes

G Protein-Coupled Receptors

5

Hanna Pincas, Javier González-Maeso, Frederique Ruf-Zamojski, and Stuart C. Sealfon

Abstract

G protein-coupled receptors (GPCRs) include one of the largest gene families in the mammalian genome. The diversity of receptor binding sites and coupling mechanisms provides the signaling specificity necessary to maintain homeostasis. Various G protein-coupled receptors are critical for the functioning of every endocrine system in health and disease, and these proteins are the predominant targets of therapeutic drugs. GPCRs are grouped by primary sequence into different families that all have a canonical seven alpha helical transmembrane domain structure. In recent years, solving the crystal structure for an increasing number of these receptors has helped to resolve the molecular mechanisms of ligand interaction and activation. Despite their name, they couple to cellular signaling via both heterotrimeric G proteins and G protein-independent mechanisms. Receptor and signaling regulatory mechanisms contribute to controlling the level of the cellular responses elicited. A variety of endocrine and systemic diseases are caused by specific receptor mutations.

Keywords

Crystallography • Pharmacology • Signal transduction • Genetics • Regulation

Contents

H. Pincas • F. Ruf-Zamojski • S.C. Sealfon (✉)
Department of Neurology, Icahn School of Medicine at Mount Sinai, New York, NY, USA
e-mail: hanna.pincas@mssm.edu; frederique.ruf-zamojski@mssm.edu; Stuart.Sealfon@mssm.edu

J. González-Maeso
Department of Physiology and Biophysics, Virginia Commonwealth University, Richmond, VA, USA
e-mail: Javier.maeso@vcuhealth.org

A. Belfiore, D. LeRoith (eds.), *Principles of Endocrinology and Hormone Action*, Endocrinology, https://doi.org/10.1007/978-3-319-44675-2_6

Introduction

Homeostasis is maintained via a plethora of extracellular factors that coordinate activity among organs and cell types. These mediators include hormones, peptides, neurotransmitters, proteins, ions, and lipids that act via specific receptors to elicit cellular responses. The functional classification of receptors includes at least three general types of cell surface receptors: G protein-coupled receptors

(GPCRs), ion channel receptors, and enzyme-associated receptors. The GPCRs form the largest and most diverse mammalian receptor group. This extreme diversity of binding sites serves the role of GPCRs throughout the endocrine system to maintain signaling specificity with hormones transmitted through the bloodstream and portal circulations. GPCRs are also promising therapeutic targets. In fact, 40–50% of drugs currently available on the market target GPCRs (Stewart and Fisher 2015).

GPCRs share a topology of seven α-helical transmembrane domains (Fig. 1). This structural template shows wide evolutionary conservation. Members of the largest rhodopsin-like GPCR family can be found in yeast, slime mold, plants, and protozoa. The rhodopsin-like GPCR family comprises one of the largest gene families known. GPCRs account for more than 1% of total cellular protein.

The term GPCR refers to the association with and signaling through heterotrimeric (α-, β-, and γ-subunit) G proteins. Although ligand-bound GPCRs were originally thought to activate downstream effectors only via G protein dissociation into G_α and $G_{\beta\gamma}$ subunits, many other heterotrimeric G protein-independent transduction mechanisms have been characterized. Hence, GPCRs interact with various GPCR regulatory proteins, multidomain scaffolding proteins, and chaperone molecules. Additional factors that affect signal transduction and specificity are GPCR homo- and heterodimerization. The diversity of GPCRs, of their signaling cascades, and of their regulatory factors underlies the specificity of the cellular response required for endocrine processes.

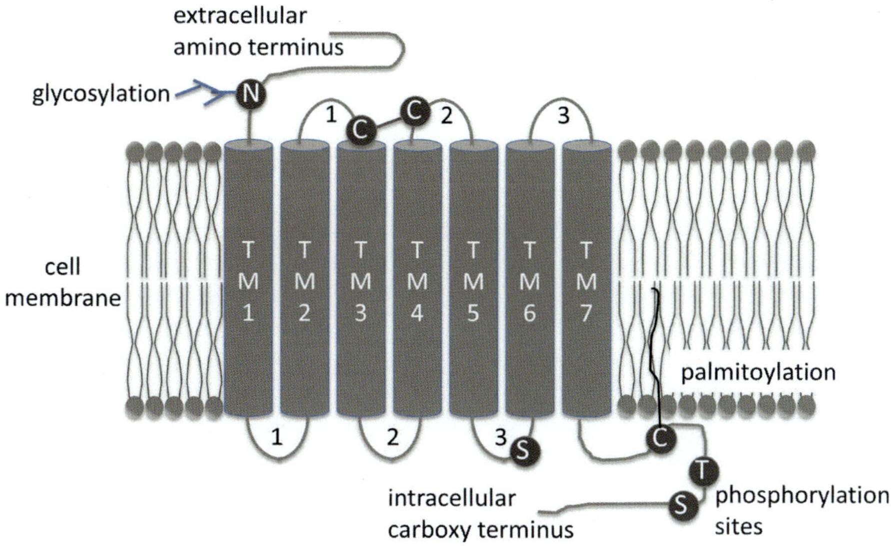

Fig. 1 Schematic of GPCR structure. Sites for extracellular glycosylation and disulfide bond formation as well as intracellular palmitoylation and phosphorylation are indicated

Classification of G Protein-Coupled Receptors

The visual pigment opsin and the β-adrenergic receptor were the first GPCRs resolved at the primary amino acid sequence level by molecular cloning in the mid-1980s. Approximately 800 GPCRs have been identified in the human genome (Davenport et al. 2013). Based on both physiological and structural features, GPCRs have been grouped into either five families (rhodopsin, adhesion, secretin, glutamate, frizzled) (Lee et al. 2015) or four classes (A, B, C, F) (Kolakowski 1994). Class A represents by far the largest group (for review, see Venkatakrishnan et al. 2014). Class A receptors have various functions, such as vision, olfaction, and regulation of immune response, and include most of the receptors for hormones. Class B comprises 47 receptors that are notably involved in glucose homeostasis and includes receptors for the hormones secretin, glucagon, and corticotropin-releasing factor. Class C consists of 15 receptors that are notably involved in synaptic transmission and includes the glutamate receptors. Class F receptors (11 members) participate in the Wnt and hedgehog signal transduction pathways. While the different GPCR classes lack significant sequence homology across families, the heptahelical transmembrane domain structure is preserved among all GPCR classes.

The structure of class A/rhodopsin family receptors has been the most studied, with the prototype rhodopsin structure being the first determined by X-ray crystallography, followed by the β_2-adrenergic receptor (β_2AR), and other class A receptors including the ternary structure of the agonist-bound (β_2AR)–Gs complex (Figs. 2 and 3). The crystal structure of the 7-transmembrane (7TM) domain has been obtained for two class B/secretin family GPCRs, the glucagon receptor (GCGR) and the corticotropin-releasing factor receptor type 1, and for two class C/glutamate family GPCRs, metabotropic glutamate receptors 1 and 5 (for review, see Lee et al. 2015).

Structural Features of G Protein-Coupled Receptors

All GPCRs share the same general structural organization, with seven hydrophobic transmembrane (7TM) α-helices interconnected by three extracellular loops (ECL) and three intracellular loops (ICL), an extracellular N-terminus, and a C-terminus located intracellularly (Fig. 1). While the size of each TM segment is conserved, varying from 20 to 27 residues, the N-terminus, loops, and C-terminus show considerable variability in length, typically ranging from tens to several hundreds of residues.

In order to compare similar amino acid sequences among different receptors, the most accepted consensus is the Ballesteros and Weinstein method. In this approach, the most conserved single residue in each transmembrane helical domain is assigned the arbitrary number 50, and each residue is numbered according to its position relative to this conserved residue. For example, 4.57 indicates an amino acid located in transmembrane segment 4, seven residues further along the sequence than the most conserved amino acid in helix 4, Trp(4.50). The most conserved amino acids of

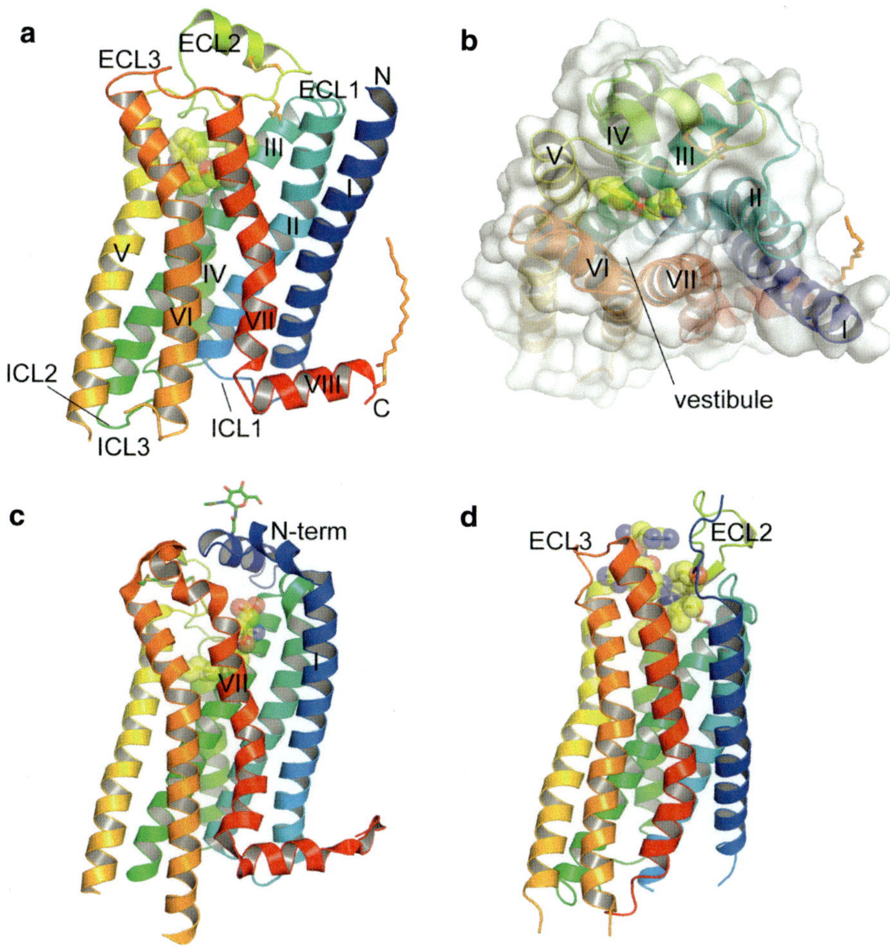

Fig. 2 Diversity of class A GPCR structures and binding sites. (**a**, **b**) Structure of the β_2-adrenergic receptor bound to the agonist carazolol from transmembrane and extracellular views. (**c**) Sphingosine-1-phosphate receptor structure bound to the antagonist ML056. (**d**) Neurotensin-bound neurotensin receptor structure. Disulfide bonds, palmitoylation, and N-terminus glycans are included (Reprinted from Lee et al. (2015))

each transmembrane segment in rhodopsin and rhodopsin-like GPCRs are $Asn^{1.50}$, $Asp^{2.50}$, $Arg^{3.50}$, $Trp^{4.50}$, $Pro^{5.50}$, $Pro^{6.50}$, and $Pro^{7.50}$. Implicit in this numbering scheme is the hypothesis that many relatively conserved amino acids at corresponding positions serve analogous structural and functional roles.

Bovine rhodopsin was the first GPCR whose crystal structure was determined, confirming the existence of seven transmembrane helices. The seven transmembrane domains form a structural core, which is involved in ligand binding and in signal transduction through structural rearrangements. The N-terminus and extracellular

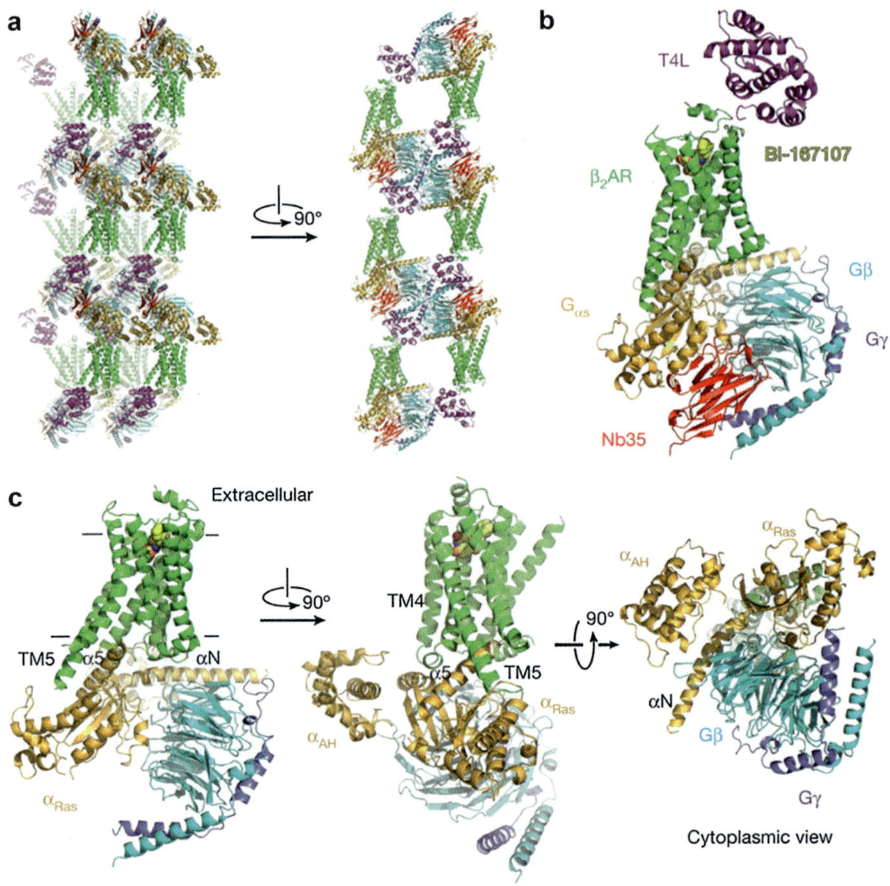

Fig. 3 **Structure of the β_2AR–Gs complex**. (**a**) Alternating layers of receptor and G protein within the crystal are shown. (**b**) The overall structure showing the β_2AR in *green* bound to an agonist (*yellow* spheres) and interacting with Gαs (*orange*). Gβ is *cyan* and Gγ is *purple*. A G_S binding nanobody (*red*) and T4 lysozyme (*magenta*) fused to the amino terminus of the receptor were included to facilitate crystallization. (**c**) The biological complex omitting nanobody and T4 lysozyme (Reprinted from Rasmussen et al. (2011))

loops play fundamental roles in processes related to ligand recognition and ligand access. The intracellular loops interact physically with heterotrimeric G proteins, G protein-coupled receptor kinases (GRKs), and other downstream signaling components (for review, see Zhang et al. 2015).

Crystallographic studies over the past decade and a half have confirmed the hypothesis that, although transmembrane regions display high sequence variability among GPCRs, they share conserved residues at key topological positions (for review, see Venkatakrishnan et al. 2014). One of the most conserved motifs among class A GPCRs is the D[E]$R^{3.50}$Y motif, which frequently forms an "ionic lock" via a salt bridge with D/E$^{6.30}$. This ionic lock was identified in the rhodopsin structure (Palczewski et al. 2000). It was proposed as a domain involved in the inactive conformation of GPCRs, hindering G protein coupling at the cytoplasmic region. W$^{6.48}$xP is also described as one of the components that switch conformations between the active and inactive state of the receptor. A third conserved motif involved in GPCR activation is the NP$^{7.50}$xxY motif. Besides the transmembrane domains, extracellular loops also have some conserved motifs. Hence, most GPCRs harbor a highly conserved Cys$^{3.25}$ disulfide bond between the extracellular tip of the third transmembrane domain and a cysteine residue in the second extracellular loop. This disulfide bond stabilizes the conformation of extracellular domains and constrains the structural arrangement forming the entrance to the ligand-binding pocket. Similarly, the conformation of the intracellular loops is relatively conserved, which may be related to the limited range of GPCR binding partners.

The secondary structures in the extracellular loop region vary considerably between different receptors. For instance, the second extracellular loop has an α-helical structure in adrenergic GPCRs and a hairpin structure in all peptide GPCRs. In contrast, the first and third extracellular loops are relatively shorter and do not show distinct secondary structures.

Posttranslational Modifications

Glycosylation

Most GPCRs have at least one glycosylation site in their N-terminal domain (Wheatley and Hawtin 1999). A few GPCRs, such as the α_{2B}-adrenoceptor, lack identifiable glycosylation sites. In GPCRs that are glycosylated, complex or hybrid high-mannose oligosaccharides are linked to the Asn side chain (N-linked glycosylation).

The effects of glycosylation differ in specific GPCRs. Glycosylation is important for the stability of the GnRH and vasopressin V_{1a} receptors, but does not affect ligand binding. Glycan chains are essential for folding and trafficking of the TRH receptor, the FSH receptor, and the vasoactive intestinal peptide (VIP) 1 receptor. For the TRH, somatostatin, β_2-adrenergic, and gastrin-releasing peptide receptors, glycosylation contributes to high-affinity ligand binding and may also influence receptor–G protein coupling. For many GPCRs however, no function for glycosylation has been identified.

Palmitoylation

Covalent lipid modifications that interact with the cytoplasmic face of the cell membrane serve to anchor numerous signaling proteins (Qanbar and Bouvier 2003).

Protein fatty acylation may occur either through thioester linkages (S-acylation) or amide linkages (N-acylation). N-Acylation occurs on the amino-terminal glycines and S-acylation occurs on cysteine residues. Palmitate is the most commonly used S-linked fatty acid. Protein palmitoylation is reversible and can be regulated.

Many GPCRs are palmitoylated at cysteine residues in the intracellular C-terminal tail. Palmitoylation of GPCRs anchors the C-terminal tail to the plasma membrane, creating in effect a fourth intracellular loop. The elimination of palmitoylation sites attenuates G protein coupling of endothelin ET_B, β_2-adrenoceptors, and somatostatin SST_5 receptors (Qanbar and Bouvier 2003). The palmitoylation state governs receptor internalization by regulating accessibility to the arrestin-mediated internalization pathway (Charest and Bouvier 2003; Ponimaskin et al. 2005).

GPCR phosphorylation, which is crucial for regulation of receptor activity, is described in a later section.

Diversity of Receptor–Ligand Interaction

The cumulative resolution of structures of class A, B, C, and F receptors (for review, see Cooke et al. 2015) has not only allowed to better grasp the mechanistic details of ligand recognition, including diverse ligand-binding modes, but also improved strategies for structure-based drug design. Variations in the location and size of the ligand-binding sites are found among class A receptors (Venkatakrishnan et al. 2013) (Fig. 2). Furthermore, the antagonist CP-376395 of the class B corticotropin-releasing factor receptor 1 (CRF1) binds to a much deeper pocket than any class A receptor ligand (Hollenstein et al. 2014). The ligand-binding pocket of the negative allosteric modulator (NAM) in class C metabotropic glutamate GluR5 is narrow and located in the transmembrane region, halfway between those of class A and class B receptors (Dore et al. 2014). In contrast, the ligand-binding pocket of the class F receptor smoothened (SMO) is closer to the extracellular space than those of class A receptors, interacting with the second and third extracellular loops (Wang et al. 2013).

The physicochemical properties of the binding sites help to make ligand-binding predictions and thus have implications in drug discovery. The two main attributes of binding sites are the presence of hydrogen bonds or ionic interactions and the presence of lipophilic hotspots. Computational methods can evaluate the relative energies of water molecules and determine which ones favor or reduce ligand binding. To illustrate this, the GPCR CXCR4 has a small-molecule binding site with a single lipophilic hotspot high in the ligand-binding pocket and an unfavorable ionic interaction due to more solvent exposure. By contrast, the dopamine D3 ligand eticlopride binds at lipophilic hotspots deep in the pocket, thus dislodging several water molecules (for review, see Cooke et al. 2015).

Mechanism of Receptor Activation

In the classical model of GPCR activation, receptors are in equilibrium between an inactive (R) and an active (R*) state. Thus, a small fraction of receptors in the active state account for GPCR basal or constitutive activity (i.e., activity in the absence of agonist). In accordance with the two-state model, agonists shift the equilibrium toward the active state, whereas inverse agonists displace it toward the inactive state. Partial agonists shift the equilibrium toward the active state less strongly. Pure antagonists inhibit agonists in a competitive manner, without altering the equilibrium. However, a multi-state model has emerged, where the receptor can assume multiple distinct active and inactive states and a ligand is proposed to stabilize specific conformational states of a given GPCR (for review, see Sato et al. 2016). This multi-state model explains the existence of the phenomenon of biased agonism, described below.

The high-resolution crystal structures of the GPCR–G protein (Fig. 3) and several GPCR-agonist complexes have provided insights into the molecular mechanisms of ligand binding and the conformational changes induced by the ligand (for review, see Zhang et al. 2015). Receptor activation involves conserved motifs, called molecular microswitches, that are involved in the transitions between inactive and active states. For instance, the ionic lock involved in the inactive conformation of rhodopsin is broken during receptor activation. Transmembrane helices 3 and 6 form an ionic lock via interaction of R135 and E134 of the conserved E(D)$R^{3.50}$Y motif (TM3) and E247 and T251 of TM6. Similarly, ligand interaction induces a conformational change within the side chain of $W^{6.48}$ in the $CW^{6.48}$xP motif, resulting in the sixth transmembrane segment moving outward with subsequent GPCR activation (Park et al. 2008; Scheerer et al. 2008).

Another important feature of GPCR activation is the rearrangement of the transmembrane helices around proline bends. Class A GPCRs have highly conserved prolines in TM5, TM6, and TM7. The activation of class A GPCRs involves helical rearrangement, such as a proline-induced deformation of TM5, rotation and translation of TM6, and inward repositioning of TM7 (for review, see Venkatakrishnan et al. 2014). Classes B and F GPCRs have prolines at similar positions in TM4 and TM5, and class C receptors have two conserved prolines in TM6 and TM7 (see Venkatakrishnan et al. 2014). It is hypothesized that these prolines also contribute to conformational changes occurring during receptor activation.

Biased Agonism

Many GPCRs activate multiple downstream signaling pathways. Different agonists acting at the same GPCR may induce very different relative activation of these multiple signaling pathways coupled to that receptor. The signaling selectivity represented by this biased agonism (originally called “stimulus trafficking”) can contribute to the effects of therapeutic agonists and is important in drug discovery (for review, see Violin et al. 2014).

Agonist bias is believed to result from GPCRs having distinct active conformations that differ in their activation of different signaling pathways and from the capacity of certain agonists to stabilize a particular pattern of active GPCR conformations. An example of agonist bias is the signaling effects of psychedelic or non-psychedelic serotonin 5-HT$_{2A}$ receptor agonists (Gonzalez-Maeso et al. 2007; Schmid and Bohn 2010). Additional findings that support the fundamental role of biased agonism in whole animal models include the modulation of circadian glucocorticoid oscillation via CXCR7 receptors recruiting β-arrestin-dependent signaling by intermediate peptides (Ikeda et al. 2013), as well as the recent discovery of an opioid analgesic (PZM21) that activates Gi proteins with high selectivity for the μ-opioid receptor and minimal β-arrestin-2 recruitment (Manglik et al. 2016). Considering that morphine and other opioids induce respiratory depression via μ-opioid through the β-arrestin interaction, whereas their analgesic effects are G protein-dependent, these findings may provide the basis for the development of new opioid ligands with improved analgesic and less unwanted respiratory effects.

Receptor–G Protein Coupling and Selectivity

The binding of a ligand to a GPCR induces a conformational change that promotes the formation of active Gα-GTP and the release of Gβγ dimer (Fig. 4). The G proteins in turn stimulate downstream effectors including enzymes (adenylate cyclases, phospholipases), ion channels, and protein kinases (for review, see Stewart and Fisher 2015) (Fig. 5).

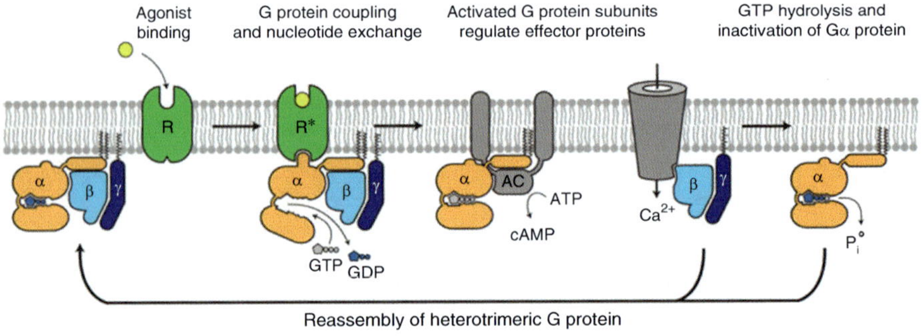

Fig. 4 **G protein cycle**. Agonist binding to the receptor leads to conformational rearrangements of the cytoplasmic ends of transmembrane segments that enable the G$_s$ heterotrimer (α, β, and γ) to bind the receptor. GDP is released from the α-subunit upon formation of GPCR–G protein complex. GTP binds to α-subunit resulting in dissociation of the α- and βγ-subunits from the receptor. The subunits regulate their respective effector proteins. The G protein heterotrimer reassembles from α- and βγ-subunits following hydrolysis of GTP to GDP by the intrinsic GTPase activity of the α-subunit (Reprinted from Rasmussen et al. (2011))

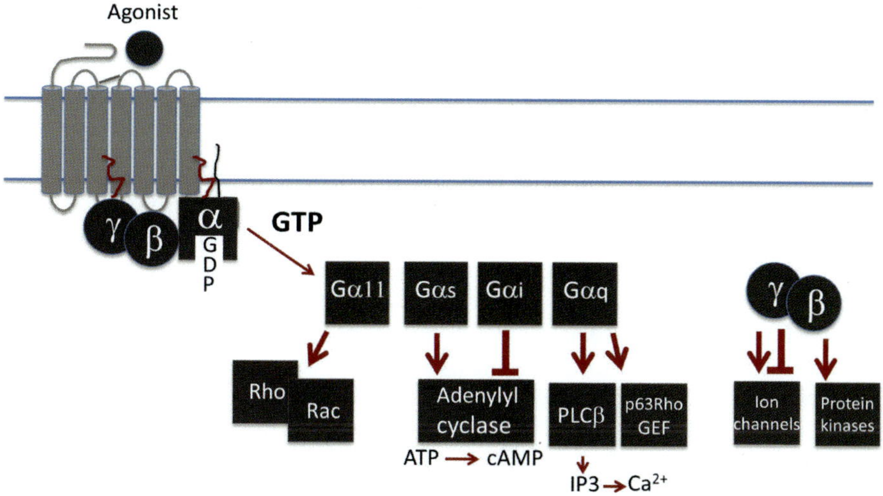

Fig. 5 Diversity of G protein signaling mechanisms. Heterotrimeric G proteins stimulate second messengers such as Ca^{2+}, cAMP, protein kinase activity, and ion channel activity. In conjunction with additional non-G protein mechanisms, these signals generate an integrated cellular response

Heterotrimeric G Proteins

Gilman and Rodbell received the Nobel Prize in Physiology in 1994 for the discovery of G proteins and their role in signal transduction. In the 1990s, scientists characterized the crystal structures of G proteins such as Gαs, Gαt, Gαi, Gβγ dimer, and Gαβγ heterotrimer (for review, see Duc et al. 2015).

G proteins bind and cause the hydrolysis of guanine nucleotides. Heterotrimeric G proteins are composed of three subunits (α, β, and γ) (Milligan and Kostenis 2006; Oldham and Hamm 2008). In its inactive state, the Gα subunit binds guanosine diphosphate (GDP), and in its active state, it binds guanosine triphosphate (GTP). The β- and γ-subunits are tightly bound to each other to form a dimer. The exchange of GDP for GTP is facilitated by the conformational change induced by the agonist binding to the GPCR. The GTP-bound Gα subunit and the βγ-dimer each activate downstream effectors (Fig. 4).

Twenty-one Gα, 6 Gβ, and 12 Gγ subunits are found in humans. Most Gα subunits are expressed ubiquitously. The four major classes (Gs, Gi/o, Gq/11, and G12/13) of G proteins are based on Gα subunit sequence similarities (Baltoumas et al. 2013). The various heterotrimeric complexes generated by combining these different Gα, Gβ, and Gγ subunits influence the specificity of both GPCRs and their downstream signal transduction (Oldham and Hamm 2008).

Crystallography revealed that the Gα subunit consists of two domains, a domain similar to Ras-like small GTPases with binding sites for $G_{\beta\gamma}$ and an α-helical domain, which is thought to segregate the guanine nucleotide in the GTP-binding domain; the guanine nucleotide-binding pocket is positioned between the Ras-like and the helical domains (for review, see Duc et al. 2015; Stewart and Fisher 2015). The Gβ subunit includes an N-terminal α-helix and a seven-bladed β-propeller motif. The Gγ subunit is composed of two α-helices connected by a linker loop. Gβ dimerizes with Gγ via a coiled-coil interaction between the N-terminal helix of Gβ and the N-terminal helix of Gγ (Sondek et al. 1996).

How a G protein gets activated and transmits the signal from a GPCR to its effectors can be recapitulated as follows: ligand binding to the GPCR induces a conformational change in the receptor, as described earlier, that promotes G protein binding and the release of GDP from the Gα G protein subunit. Next, GTP binds to Gα, which induces the dissociation of Gα from the Gβγ dimer. Both GTP-bound Gα and the released Gβγ dimer can then activate downstream effector molecules. Deactivation of the G protein occurs via the GTPase activity of Gα, which hydrolyzes GTP into GDP and leads to heterotrimer reassociation (Fig. 4). The rate of hydrolysis varies among the different classes of G proteins (for review, see Duc et al. 2015; Stewart and Fisher 2015).

Molecular Basis of Receptor–G Protein Coupling

Although GPCRs are numerous and diverse, and G proteins exhibit some degree of variety, GPCRs interact only with a few G proteins, as defined by their Gα subunit (Milligan and Kostenis 2006; Oldham and Hamm 2008). Accordingly, GPCRs are typically distinguished by their $G_{i/o}$, G_s, or $G_{q/11}$ coupling (Table 1).

In 2011, the Kobilka group elucidated how a GPCR activates a G protein when they determined the X-ray crystal structure of the β_2-adrenoceptor-G protein complex (Fig. 3). They observed a major displacement of the α-helical domain of Gα relative to the Ras-like domain upon receptor binding, causing the opening of the nucleotide-binding pocket (Rasmussen et al. 2011). The main interactions between the receptor and Gαs involve the rotation and movement of the C-terminal α5-helix of the Gαs Ras-like domain toward the β_2-adrenergic receptor, which propagates the conformational changes from the agonist-bound receptor to the nucleotide-binding pocket. With regard to the GPCR regions involved in the GPCR–G protein interface, the X-ray crystal structure of receptor–Gs complex revealed that the binding regions of the receptor comprise transmembrane domains 3, 5, and 6 and intracellular loops 2 and 3. The C-terminus of Gαs, which contacts TM3, TM5, TM6, and parts of ICL2 (Rasmussen et al. 2011), may provide the selectivity of the GPCR–G protein coupling. Other G protein regions may interact with GPCRs (Mnpotra et al. 2014; Rasmussen et al. 2011).

Regulation of Receptor–G Protein Coupling by RNA Editing

RNA editing is a molecular process that creates diversity both at the RNA and at the protein level. Deamination of adenosine into inosine (A to I) is a typical RNA editing

Table 1 Classification of selected GPCRs relevant to endocrinology, according to the current IUPHAR database

GPCR class	Family name	Ligand	Principal transduction
A (rhodopsin-like)	5-Hydroxytryptamine receptors	5-Hydroxytryptamine	$G_{i/o}$ (subtypes 1A, 1B, 1D, 1E, 1F), $G_{q/11}$ (subtypes 2A, 2B, 2C), G_s (subtypes 4, 6, 7), G_i/G_o (subtype 5A)
	Acetylcholine receptors (muscarinic)	Acetylcholine	$G_{q/11}$ (subtypes M1, M3, M5), $G_{i/o}$ (subtypes M2, M4)
	Angiotensin receptors	Angiotensin	$G_{q/11}$ (subtype 1), G_i/G_o, Tyr and Ser/Thr phosphatases (subtype 2)
	Apelin receptor	Apelin-36, apelin-13, apelin-17; apelin receptor early endogenous ligand	$G_{i/o}$
	Bradykinin receptors	Bradykinin, kallidin, T-kinin	$G_{q/11}$ (B1 and B2 receptors)
	Galanin receptors	Galanin, galanin-like peptide	$G_{i/o}$ (subtypes 1, 3), $G_{i/o}$, $G_{q/11}$ (subtype 2)
	Ghrelin receptor	Ghrelin	$G_{q/11}$
	Glycoprotein hormone receptors	FSH, hCG, LH, TSH	G_s (FSH receptor), G_s, $G_{q/11}$ (LH receptor), all four families of G proteins (TSH receptor)
	Gonadotropin-releasing hormone receptors	GnRH I, GnRH II	$G_{q/11}$ (subtypes 1, 2)
	G protein-coupled estrogen receptor	17β-estradiol	G_s, $G_{i/o}$
	Kisspeptin receptor	Kisspeptin-10, kisspeptin-13, kisspeptin-14, kisspeptin-54	$G_{q/11}$
	Neurotensin receptors	Large neuromedin N, large neurotensin, neuromedin N, neurotensin	$G_{q/11}$
	Orexin receptors	Orexin-A, orexin-B	$G_{q/11}$
	Prolactin-releasing peptide receptor	PrRP-20, PrRP-31	$G_{q/11}$
	Somatostatin receptors	CST-17, SRIF-14, SRIF-28	G_i
	Thyrotropin-releasing hormone receptors	TRH	G_q
	Vasopressin and oxytocin receptors	Oxytocin, vasopressin	$G_{q/11}$ (subtypes V_{1A}, V_{1B}), G_s (subtype V_2), $G_{q/11}$, $G_{i/o}$ (subtype OT)

(*continued*)

Table 1 (continued)

GPCR class	Family name	Ligand	Principal transduction
B (secretin receptor family)	Calcitonin receptors	Amylin, calcitonin, α-CGRP, β-CGRP, etc.	G_s
	Corticotropin-releasing factor receptors	Corticotropin-releasing hormone, urocortin 1, 2, 3	G_s
	Glucagon receptor family	GHRH, gastric inhibitory polypeptide, glucagon, secretin, etc.	G_s
	Parathyroid hormone receptors	PTH	G_s, $G_{q/11}$
	VIP and PACAP receptors	PACAP-38, PACAP-27, PHM, PHV, VIP	G_s
C (metabotropic glutamate)	Calcium-sensing receptors	Ca^{2+}, Mg^{2+}	$G_{q/11}$, $G_{i/o}$, $G_{12/13}$ (CaS receptor), unknown ($GPRC_6$ receptor)
	Class C orphans	Unknown	Unknown
	$GABA_B$ receptors	GABA	$G_{i/o}$
	Metabotropic glutamate receptors	L-Glutamic acid	$G_{q/11}$ (subtypes 1, 5), $G_{i/o}$ (subtypes 2, 3, 4, 6, 7, 8)
F (frizzled/ smoothened)	Class frizzled GPCRs	WNTs	Unknown

event that affects precursor and mature mRNAs and results in an alteration of amino acid sequences (as inosine is recognized as guanosine during translation). Transcripts of the human serotonin 2C receptor, for example, are subject to A-to-I RNA editing, thereby generating multiple receptor isoforms that vary in constitutive activity and G protein coupling efficacy (for review, see O'Neil and Emeson 2012). RNA editing also can increase receptor diversity. 5-HT_{2C} transcripts have five A-to-I editing sites, with predicted amino acid sequence alterations affecting the second intracellular loop; up to 24 receptor isoforms can be produced.

Effect of Posttranslational Modifications on Receptor–G Protein Coupling Selectivity

The best defined GPCR regulatory mechanisms are mediated by G protein-coupled receptor kinases (GRKs), arrestins, and regulator of G protein signaling (RGS) proteins.

The standard allosteric two-state (off–on) model of GPCR activation has evolved into a complex paradigm of functional selectivity based on multisite phosphorylation. G protein-coupled receptor kinases (GRKs) are recruited to the receptor and phosphorylate cytosolic segments, thereby recruiting β-arrestins, which besides sterically hindering the G protein interaction also can serve as signal transducers (Lefkowitz and Shenoy 2005). Based on mass spectrometry analyses, β_2AR has 13 serine/threonine phosphorylation sites in the third intracellular loop and the C-terminal tail, which are phosphorylated by multiple kinases. GRK2 and GRK6, which have different phosphorylation sites on the receptor, induce distinct conformations of β-arrestin upon its recruitment to the receptor and subsequently distinct patterns of downstream signaling. Overall, evidence suggests that the different phosphorylation patterns of GRKs establish a "barcode" that ultimately determines different β-arrestin functional capabilities (for review, see Prabakaran et al. 2012).

Regulators of G Protein Signaling Proteins (RGS Proteins)

RGS proteins are negative regulators of G protein signaling. They accelerate the GTPase activity of Gα, thereby promoting the reassociation of the heterotrimeric complex with the GPCR and the termination of signaling to downstream effectors (Fig. 6). Thus, RGS proteins determine the extent of the cellular response to GPCR stimulation (for review see Stewart and Fisher 2015).

There are 20 mammalian RGS proteins that function as GTPases, accelerating proteins or GAPs for $G\alpha_{i/o}$, $G\alpha_{q/11}$, or both. Another 20 RGS proteins contain non-functional RGS homology domains that frequently serve as an interface with GPCRs or Gα subunits. Resolution of the crystal structure of the RGS protein–Gα complex has revealed the mechanism by which RGS catalyzes GTP hydrolysis by Gα by stabilizing the transition state of Gα for nucleotide hydrolysis (Berman et al. 1996; Tesmer et al. 1997). As they can compete for effector binding, RGS proteins also have the ability to modulate adenylate cyclase, MAPK, IP_3/Ca^{2+} signaling, K^+ conductance, and visual signaling (Neubig and Siderovski 2002; Yan et al. 1997).

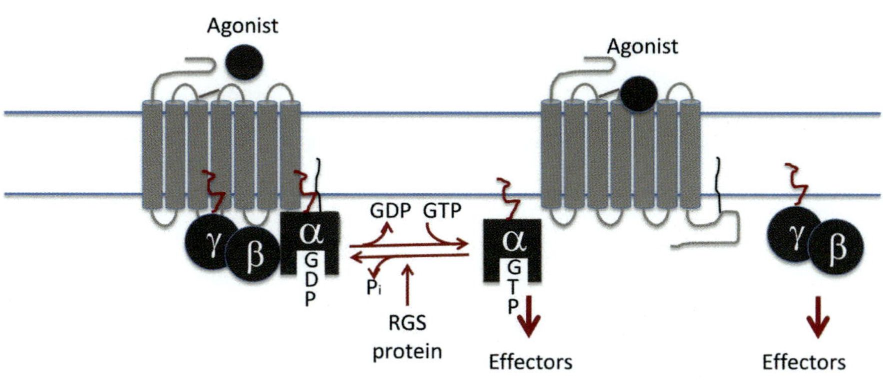

Fig. 6 G protein regulation by RGS proteins. RGS proteins accelerate the intrinsic GTPase activity of Gα and promote reassociation of the heterotrimeric complex with the receptor at the cell membrane, thereby terminating signaling

Activators of G Protein Signaling (AGS)

AGS proteins, in contrast with RGS proteins, use diverse mechanisms to activate G proteins. They are organized in four groups: group I, guanine nucleotide exchange factors (GEFs); group II, guanine nucleotide dissociation inhibitors (GDIs); group III, *G*βγ binding proteins; and group IV, Gα16 binding proteins (for review, see Park 2015).

Group I AGS proteins, which facilitate the exchange of GDP for GTP on Gα, do so in the absence of GPCRs (for review, see Blumer and Lanier 2014). They also demonstrate selectivity in their interaction with G proteins. Group II AGS proteins carry one to four GPR motifs that stabilize GDP-bound Gα. Group III are *G*βγ-interacting proteins that show nonselectivity for Gα. The fourth group comprises AGS11–13 that are selective for Gα16, but their mechanism of action remains to be elucidated. Groups I–III are thought to act together in a core signaling triad (GEF/GαGPR/*G*βγ-interacting proteins) that is akin to the one formed by GPCR/Gαβγ/effector.

G Protein-Dependent Signaling Effectors

GPCRs generate a variety of cellular responses, ranging from intracellular production of cAMP to induction of gene transcription. GPCRs can stimulate different families of G proteins ($G\alpha_s$, $G\alpha_i$, $G\alpha_q$, and $G\alpha_{12/13}$ in mammals). Receptors that interact predominantly with $G\alpha_s$ stimulate adenylate cyclase as the downstream effector, while those coupled to $G\alpha_{q/11}$ activate phospholipase C, which increases intracellular Ca^{2+} levels (Fig. 5). Some GPCRs transduce extracellular signals in the absence or nearly absence of G protein activation (Brzostowski and Kimmel 2001; DeWire et al. 2007).

Adenylyl Cyclase Signaling

The discovery of adenylate cyclases (Manning and Gilman 1983) preceded that of G proteins. There are nine membrane adenylate cyclase isoforms (AC1–AC9) in mammals. They consist of two transmembrane hydrophobic domains and two cytosolic domains, C1 and C2, which represent the enzyme catalytic core and are significantly homologous (for review, see Seifert et al. 2012). Although all ACs are activated by stimulatory G proteins, AC5 and AC6 are also negatively regulated by inhibitory G proteins (for review, see Bodmann et al. 2015). Hence, Gilman's group and others established the direct interaction of adenylate cyclases with Gαs and Gαi by protein biochemistry (Dessauer et al. 1998; Sunahara et al. 1997). In particular, six subtypes of inhibitory G proteins ($G\alpha i_{1,2,3}$, $G\alpha o_{A,B}$, and Gαz) were shown to bind AC5 and AC6 (Dessauer et al. 1998).

Phospholipase C Signaling

Phospholipase C-β (PLC-β) is the major effector of $G\alpha_q$, and it also displays a GTPase-activating protein (GAP) function that is selective for $G\alpha_q$ (for review, see Litosch 2016). Rapid hydrolysis of phosphatidylinositol-4,5-bisphosphate (PIP_2) by PLC-β results in the accumulation of inositol-1,4,5-trisphosphate (IP_3) and diacylglycerol (DAG). IP3 induces the release of cytosolic Ca^{2+} from intracellular stores, while DAG activates protein kinase C (PKC). There are four PLC-β isoforms (β1–β4), which are activated by $G\alpha_q$ with variable efficiencies (Smrcka and Sternweis 1993). The amplitude of the signal transmitted from the agonist-bound receptor to the effector is determined by the relative rates of the receptor-promoted activation of $G\alpha_q$ and the GTPase-activating protein (GAP) activity of PLC-β (Biddlecome et al. 1996; Mukhopadhyay and Ross 1999).

Thirteen PLC family members have been cloned. They belong to six classes, β , γ , δ , ε , η, and ζ (for review, see Vines 2012). Although the residues are poorly conserved between members, there is 40–50% homology for the N-terminal pleckstrin homology domain (PH), the EF hand, the X and Y domains, and the C2 domain. Except for PLC-ζ, all PLC family members have a PH domain, which is implicated in signal transduction. The EF hand, X, Y, and C2 domains form the catalytic core.

Other $G\alpha_q$ effectors include p63RhoGEF, G protein-regulated kinase 2 (GRK2), as well as type 1A phosphatidylinositol-3-kinase (PI3K) and tetratricopeptide repeat 1 (TPR1). The guanine nucleotide exchange factor (GEF) activity of p63RhoGEF catalyzes the exchange of bound GDP for GTP on Rho GTPases, which in turn control key cellular processes such as regulation of actin cytoskeleton (for review, see Sanchez-Fernandez et al. 2014). Interestingly, p63RhoGEF and PLC-β_2 compete with each other following $G\alpha_q$ activation. GRK2 acts as a suppressor of $G\alpha_q$ signaling via binding and most likely sequestration of activated $G\alpha_q$ (Carman et al. 1999). PI3K, which is involved in the regulation of the Akt pathway, is inhibited by activated $G\alpha_q$ via a direct interaction (Ballou et al. 2003). TPR1 is a scaffold protein that functions as an adaptor between $G\alpha_{16}$ and Ras (Marty et al. 2003). Two other atypical effectors, PKCζ and MEK5, associate with $G\alpha_q$ upon GPCR activation to activate the ERK5 MAPK in a PLC-β-independent manner (Garcia-Hoz et al. 2010).

Ion Channel Signaling

Ion channel activation is mediated by G proteins following GPCR ligand binding, thereby inducing specific downstream signaling cascades. The activation of ion channels by G proteins can either be direct or indirect via a second messenger. Examples of direct interactions with G proteins include high-voltage N-type calcium channels/Gαo (inhibition) and L-type calcium channels/Gαs (stimulation; for review, see Luttrell 2006). Moreover, the Gβγ heterodimer can also activate ion channels, as in the case of the inward-rectifying muscarinic-gated potassium channel.

Voltage-gated calcium channels (VGCC) are modulated by a variety of GPCRs following agonist activation. Hence, presynaptic N, P/Q, and R-type calcium channels are negatively regulated by GPCRs, while the sodium leak channels non-selective (NALCN) are activated by the acetylcholine M3 muscarinic receptor (M3R) (for review, see Altier 2012).

G Protein-Coupled Receptor Signaling Networks

In the early model of GPCR signaling, receptor activation leads to dissociation of heterotrimeric G proteins into α- and βγ-subunits that activate effector molecules, including second messenger systems. Activation of these pathways modulates cellular responses in the target cells. However, the number of effectors is much smaller than the number of GPCRs. Cells express multiple different GPCRs, leading to integration and cross regulation among the different signaling pathways. The presence of G protein-independent signaling pathways further increases the complexity of GPCR regulation of signaling and cell responses.

Multiple G Protein Coupling

Although GPCRs usually preferentially stimulate one G protein type, many receptors can activate several different G protein classes (Hermans 2003). The α_2-adrenoceptor can suppress or activate adenylate cyclase activity via $G_{i/o}$ or G_s, with the signaling altered according to agonist concentration. Promiscuous coupling (the capacity for a receptor to couple to more than one G protein type) has also been demonstrated using receptor–G protein fusion proteins, in which a G_α subunit is fused to the receptor (Milligan et al. 2004).

Membrane Microdomains and GPCR Signaling

Different GPCRs that signal through the same G protein in a single cell type have been found to sometimes activate different cellular responses (Ostrom 2002). The concept of random mixing of receptors and signaling components cannot easily account for these observations because it does not include compartmentalization of molecules in cells (Gonzalez-Maeso et al. 2002; Remmers et al. 2000). The compartmentalization of receptors and effectors in membrane microdomains is an important determinant of receptor signaling (Ostrom 2002; Ostrom et al. 2000).

Caveolae are plasma membrane microdomains enriched in caveolins, cholesterol, and sphingolipids (Insel et al. 2005). Several GPCRs, G proteins, and other signaling proteins are located in caveolae (Ostrom 2002). This compartmentalization may cause receptor coupling to multiple effect systems, increase signaling, or influence which pathway is activated.

Cross Talk Between GPCRs

One mechanism of integration of signaling of different GPCRs occurs through modulation of signaling pathways of one GPCR by activation of a different GPCR on the same cell (Hur and Kim 2002; Jordan et al. 2000; Neves et al. 2002). For example, activation of phospholipase C by purinergic P2Y_2 receptors via G_q proteins inhibits cAMP synthesis stimulated by β-adrenoceptors via G_s proteins (Suh et al. 2001).

In addition to modulating other GPCR-signaling pathways, signaling pathways activated by GPCRs also influence the signaling of other structural classes of receptors. Epidermal growth factor receptors, for example, can be transactivated by stimulation of a number of GPCRs (Hur and Kim 2002). GPCRs may also cause cross talk regulation of downstream signaling pathways. For example, vasopressin and bombesin (acting at G_q-coupled receptors) act synergistically with several growth factors to stimulate growth. Morphine desensitization, internalization, and downregulation of the $G_{i/o}$-coupled μ-opioid receptor are facilitated by activation of the $G_{q/11}$-coupled 5-HT_{2A} receptor (Lopez-Gimenez et al. 2008). Another important area of cross talk is via heterodimerization of different GPCRs, discussed in a subsequent section.

G Protein-Coupled Receptor Interacting Proteins

Besides GRKs, arrestins, RGS and AGS, additional GPCR-interacting proteins (GIPs) including other GPCRs (via homo- or heterodimerization), scaffolding, and accessory proteins have been identified. Dimerization plays an important role in ligand recognition, signaling, and receptor trafficking. GIPs assist nascent receptors in correct folding, target them to the appropriate subcellular compartments, and accomplish their signaling tasks. GIPs include receptor activity-modifying proteins (RAMPs), PDZ domain-containing proteins, various ions, lipids, and peptides that act as allosteric modulators (for review, see Brady and Limbird 2002; Maurice et al. 2011; van der Westhuizen et al. 2015). Thus, GIPs are involved in the regulation of GPCR function, may play a role in pathophysiology, and represent potential targets for drug development.

Receptor Activity-Modifying Proteins (RAMPs)

RAMPs are a family of accessory proteins that alter the ligand pharmacology or signaling of several GPCRs (Gingell et al. 2016). Structurally, they contain an extracellular N-terminal domain, a single transmembrane-spanning domain, and a short intracellular C-terminal domain. RAMPs were initially characterized as coupling partners for the class B calcitonin receptor-like receptor (CRLR). Hence, the induction of cAMP production by the calcitonin gene-related peptide (CGRP) receptor is dependent on RAMP1 expression. Additionally, RAMPs act as molecular chaperones in receptor trafficking, as it is the case with CRLR and the class C extracellular calcium-sensing receptor (CaSR). Based on in vivo studies, RAMPs play major roles in the cardiovascular, renal, and respiratory systems, as well as in inflammation. In terms of drug development, RAMPs and the RAMP–GPCR interface both represent promising targets.

Interestingly, the receptor component protein (RCP) is a small intracellular peripheral membrane protein that is critical for CGRP signaling, as loss of RCP expression results in a decrease in CGRP-induced cAMP production. A functional CGRP receptor thus consists of the receptor itself, the chaperone RAMP, and RCP that couples the receptor to downstream effectors (for review, see Brady and Limbird 2002).

Melanocortin Receptor Accessory Proteins (MRAPs)

Like RAMPs, MRAPs are also single transmembrane-spanning proteins, which modulate the expression, trafficking, and signaling of members of the melanocortin receptor (MCR) family. Without MRAP, the melanocortin 2 receptor MC2R stays in the ER (for review, see Maurice et al. 2011).

Homer Family Proteins

The Homer proteins, which contain a PDZ-like domain in their N-terminal region, bind the C-terminal tail of the metabotropic glutamate receptors $mGlu_1$ and $mGlu_5$ at huge postsynaptic membrane-associated protein complexes termed postsynaptic densities (PSD) and thus contribute to postsynaptic signaling and plasticity (for review, see Maurice et al. 2011). In neurons, the ratio between Homer1a and Homer1b regulates the cell surface expression of $mGlu_5$ and thus the calcium signaling response of the receptor.

Cytoskeleton-Associated Proteins

Numerous proteins modulate GPCR intracellular trafficking by playing the role of adaptors between the receptors and cytoskeleton-associated proteins. Examples include the dynein light chain Tctex-1 (t-complex testis expressed 1), which is critical for the apical surface targeting of rhodopsin (for review, see Maurice et al. 2011). Filamin A is an actin-binding protein that controls GPCR trafficking. The interaction of D2 and D3 dopamine receptors with protein 4.1N is crucial for their localization at the neuronal plasma membrane. Conversely, binding of protein 4.1G to the metabotropic glutamate receptor subtype 1 diminishes its anchoring to the cell surface membrane.

PDZ Domain-Containing Proteins

GPCRs interact with a number of PDZ domain-containing proteins that act as adaptors of multimeric complexes and modulate signaling (Maurice et al. 2011).

Hence, the sodium–hydrogen exchanger regulatory factors, NHERF-1 (also known as EBP50) and NHERF-2, bind to several GPCRs; β_2AR binding of NHERF-1 is involved in the receptor-mediated regulation of Na+/H+ exchange. NHERF-2 regulates P2Y1 purinergic receptor-induced calcium signaling. MUPP1 is a multi-PDZ domain protein that interacts with the melatonin MT_1 receptor and stimulates its coupling to the G_i/adenylate cyclase pathway.

Other GPCR-Interacting Proteins and Allosteric Modulators

Various other GIPs as well as ion, lipid, and peptide allosteric modulators have been reported. Details can be found in recent reviews (Brady and Limbird 2002; Maurice et al. 2011; van der Westhuizen et al. 2015).

G Protein-Independent Signaling by G Protein-Coupled Receptors

The traditional GPCR-mediated signaling transduction involves activation of downstream effectors via the catalysis of heterotrimeric G protein dissociation into G_α and $G_{\beta\gamma}$ subunits. However, the heptahelical receptors have the ability to stimulate G protein-independent signaling pathways, such as mitogen-activated protein kinase (MAPK) cascades.

Although β-arrestins are classically known for desensitizing GPCRs, they also have the ability to mediate the activation of MAPK signaling via the recruitment of signaling molecules distinct from G protein-mediated signaling, thus setting off a second wave of signaling (for review, see Smith and Rajagopal 2016). Hence, β-arrestins function as adaptors that bind both the nonreceptor tyrosine kinase c-Src and ligand-bound β_2AR, causing c-Src recruitment to the membrane and the GPCR sequestration, which results in Ras-dependent activation of the MAPKs ERK1 and ERK2 (Luttrell et al. 1999). In the case of angiotensin II type 1a receptors (AT1aR), the receptor, β-arrestin-2, and components of the ERK cascade form a multiprotein complex. β-arrestins act as scaffolds that enhance c-Raf-1 and MEK-dependent activation of ERK2 (Luttrell et al. 2001). β-arrestins were also shown to scaffold JNK1/2 and thus promote their activation (Kook et al. 2013). β-arrestins mediate p38 MAPK activation, yet the underlying molecular mechanism remains to be elucidated (Sun et al. 2002).

G Protein-Coupled Receptor Dimerization

In addition to the plethora of GIPs that include scaffolding and accessory proteins modulating GPCRs, GPCRs can form homo-, heterodimers, or larger oligomers. GPCR homo-/heterodimerization and hetero-oligomerization have been implicated in the regulation of GPCR function, trafficking, and ligand pharmacology (for review, see Milligan 2009). This phenomenon has important biological implications, i.e., the modulation of GPCR signaling and the mediation of cross talk between GPCR pathways. Clinically, GPCR heterodimers may be exploited as potential drug targets. While most studies have relied on expressing recombinant receptors in heterologous cells, very few have demonstrated the existence of GPCR heteromers in native tissues or in vivo. Probing close physical relationships between two GPCRs is technically challenging. Recent progress, notably in the development of proximity-based assays, may help to better evaluate the presence and function of GPCR heteromers in native tissues (for review, see Gomes et al. 2016). On the whole, there has been accumulating evidence supporting heteromerization between GPCRs, yet the underlying molecular mechanisms and functional effects of heteromerization remain to be elucidated.

Homodimerization

Although GPCRs were originally thought to function as monomers, co-expression and co-immunoprecipitation studies, reported nearly two decades ago, provided evidence for the existence of multiple copies of each of the β_2AR, the dopamine D2 receptor, and the δ-opioid peptide (DOP) receptor within a complex (for review, see Milligan 2009). Although DOP receptor dimerization was inhibited by specific agonists (Cvejic and Devi 1997), agonist-induced dissociation of the homomultimer was not corroborated by resonance energy transfer techniques (McVey et al. 2001), highlighting the need for independent confirmation. The dopamine D_2 receptor was shown to homodimerize as well as to heterodimerize with the 5-hydroxytryptamine 5-HT_{1B} receptor; furthermore, ligand selectivity was demonstrated for the receptor monomer vs. the dimer (Ng et al. 1996). More recent research on the β_2AR contradicted earlier work suggesting that the dimer, but not the monomer, was involved in G protein activation and receptor function (Whorton et al. 2007). Similarly, when rhodopsin is incorporated into a reconstituted phospholipid bilayer particle, it is monomeric and activates transducin (Whorton et al. 2008). Accordingly, it seems unlikely that GPCR dimerization is necessary for G protein activation and signal transduction.

Some GPCR dimers were previously described in crystal structure studies. For instance, the β_2AR dimer is formed via lipids composed of two cholesterol and two palmitic acid molecules in the carboxy-terminal region (Rasmussen et al. 2007). The CXCR4 homodimer involves interactions via helices V and VI (Wu et al. 2010). Overall, a number of studies have reported GPCR dimerization or oligomerization in heterologous systems, yet there is still a lack of physiological or pathological evidence.

Heterodimerization

The occurrence and significance of GPCR heterodimerization have remained elusive. Previous heterologous expression studies and/or yeast two-hybrid studies revealed that the $GABA_B$ receptors $GABA_BR1$ and $GABA_BR2$ form heterodimers via their intracellular C-terminal tails and that these heterodimers are fully functional (White et al. 1998). Similarly, the amino acid taste receptor, T1R1+3, was characterized as a heterodimer of taste-specific T1R1 and T1R3 GPCRs (Nelson et al. 2002). GPCR heterodimerization is thought to happen early during protein synthesis and to be involved in the receptor delivery to the cell surface. Hence, the C-terminal endoplasmic reticulum (ER) retention motif of $GABA_{B1}$ is key in the cell surface delivery of a functional $GABA_B$ receptor heterodimer (Margeta-Mitrovic et al. 2000). Co-expression of the β_2AR with an altered β_2AR harboring the C-terminal tail of $GABA_{B1}$ results in intracellular ER retention of both the mutant and the wild-type receptor (Salahpour et al. 2004). In cells co-expressing the cannabinoid CB1 receptor and the orexin OX1 receptor, the CB1 receptor antagonist causes a redistribution of both receptors to the cell surface; likewise, the selective OX1 receptor antagonist causes a redistribution of both receptors to the cell surface when they are co-expressed, indicating that the two receptors most likely form stable heterodimers that are regulated by both CB1 and OX1 receptor ligands (Ellis et al. 2006). Thus, selective ligands may trigger co-trafficking of heterodimerized GPCRs.

With regard to pharmacology of a GPCR heterodimer, the effect of a selective ligand on the conformation of a GPCR can be relayed to G protein activation via the other GPCR, implying the induction of a conformational change of the other GPCR in the absence of direct ligand binding. This is illustrated with the neurotransmitter GABA, which binds to the N-terminal region of $GABA_{B1}$ within the $GABA_B$ receptor heterodimer $GABA_{B1}$–$GABA_{B2}$. Additionally, a ligand with no affinity for a given GPCR can regulate the function of that GPCR if it forms a heterodimer with a receptor for which the ligand has affinity. As an example, in cells co-expressing the human DOP opioid and chemokine CXCR2 receptors, a CXCR2 antagonist enhanced the function of DOP receptor agonists, although it had no affinity for the DOP receptor alone (Parenty et al. 2008). Thus, the CXCR2 antagonist functions as an allosteric modulator of a GPCR heterodimer.

GPCR heterodimers may be implicated in disease etiology and/or represent potential targets for disease treatment. Hallucinogenic drug models of psychosis have some similitudes with characteristics of schizophrenia, and the contribution of the 5-hydroxytryptamine 5-HT_{2A} receptor $G_{i/o}$-mediated signaling pathway is essential for distinguishing hallucinogenic from non-hallucinogenic agonists of this receptor (Gonzalez-Maeso et al. 2007). Gonzalez-Maeso and his collaborators carried out co-immunoprecipitation experiments in human brain tissues and RET-based assays in transfected cells to demonstrate that the 5-HT_{2A} receptor (2AR) interacts with the $mGlu_2$ but not the $mGlu_3$ receptor (Gonzalez-Maeso et al. 2008). The 2AR–mGluR2 complex may be involved in the altered cortical processes of schizophrenia.

Identifying small-molecule ligands that target specific GPCR heterodimers may enable researchers to study heterodimer expression and function in native tissues or cells and in vivo, as well as to ultimately treat diseases. The opioid agonist 6′-guanidinonaltrindole, which activates the DOP–KOP receptor heterodimer (but not homomers), is the best heterodimer-selective ligand described so far (Waldhoer et al. 2005). In most cases of reported heterodimers, however, either data validation in native cells has been missing, or data observed in native tissues have not replicated those obtained in heterologous systems. Investigators have proposed the following criteria for claiming evidence of heterodimerization in endogenous systems: (i) heterodimer components should colocalize and physically interact; (ii) heterodimers should have biochemical properties that differ from those of their individual components; (iii) heterodimer disruption should result in a loss of heterodimer-specific properties (for review, see Gomes et al. 2016).

Mechanisms of G Protein-Coupled Receptor Desensitization

Receptor desensitization occurs when there is a rapid decline in the receptor response to repeated or sustained agonist stimulation. By contrast, receptor downregulation, which is a decrease in the number of receptors on the cell surface, is a slower process that extends over hours (for review, see Smith and Rajagopal 2016).

GPCR desensitization entails (i) receptor phosphorylation and subsequent uncoupling of the receptor from its cognate G protein and (ii) receptor internalization to intracellular compartments. Receptor desensitization can be separated into homologous mechanisms, in which the activated receptor is desensitized, and heterologous densensitization, in which downstream signaling such as adenylate cyclase activation leads to desensitization of any GPCRs with cAMP-activated protein kinase A phosphorylation sites. Homologous desensitization typically involves the sequential actions of G protein-coupled receptor kinases (GRKs) and β-arrestins (Ferguson 2001; Krupnick and Benovic 1998) (for review, see Walther and Ferguson 2013).

Uncoupling of Receptors from G Proteins

β-Arrestins are thought to suppress G protein signaling by preventing the G protein–GPCR interaction at the second (ICL2) and third (ICL3) intracellular loops of the receptor (DeGraff et al. 2002; Marion et al. 2006). This competition between arrestin and G protein for receptor binding results in desensitization of the downstream effector pathways (for review, see Smith and Rajagopal 2016). β-Arrestin binding requires (i) activation of the GPCR by its ligand and (ii) GRK-mediated receptor phosphorylation, as previously reported for β_2AR (Krasel et al. 2005).

GPCR phosphorylation can either target the ligand-bound receptor (homologous desensitization) or various GPCRs throughout the cell (heterologous desensitization). While phosphorylation of the GPCR intracellular residues is predominantly mediated by GRKs in homologous desensitization, heterologous desensitization is often mediated by PKA or PKC. In both cases, the residues that are phosphorylated are serine and threonine.

β-Arrestins were originally proposed to be involved in β_2AR desensitization and were found to share homology with the retinal visual arrestin (for review, see Smith and Rajagopal 2016). Visual arrestin (arrestin-1) blocks rhodopsin signaling in the retina. The arrestin family consists of four members: two visual arrestins, arrestin-1 (visual arrestin) and arrestin-4 (cone arrestin), and two nonvisual arrestins, β-arrestin-1 and β-arrestin-2 (also referred to as arrestin-2 and arrestin-3). The structurally related α-arrestins have been implicated in receptor endocytosis (Patwari and Lee 2012). Based on high-resolution crystallography and mutagenesis experiments, visual arrestin comprises an N-terminal and a C-terminal domain, each of which is organized as a seven-strand β-sandwich. The N-terminal domain is responsible for recognition of the activated receptor, while the C-terminal domain contains a secondary receptor-binding region (Luttrell and Lefkowitz 2002).

There are seven human GRKs (GRK1–7). GRK1 and GRK7 are expressed in the eye; GRK2, GRK3, GRK5, and GRK6 are ubiquitous; and GRK4 is predominantly in the reproductive tract (Premont and Gainetdinov 2007). GRKs have similar structures, with an N-terminal RGS-like domain involved in receptor recognition, a central catalytic domain, and a C-terminal domain that facilitates the translocation of the kinase to the plasma membrane. Besides targeting the C-terminal tail of the GPCR for phosphorylation (e.g., for rhodopsin and β_2AR), GRK can target other intracellular GPCR sites such as ICL3 (e.g., for α2-adrenergic receptor and M2 muscarinic receptor (Liggett et al. 1992; Pals-Rylaarsdam and Hosey 1997)).

Unlike GRK phosphorylation, which depends on receptor activation by its ligand, PKA- or PKC-mediated phosphorylation of the receptor is dependent upon the increase in second messenger intracellular concentration (e.g., cAMP or DAG). Hence, besides their classical function in signal transduction via phosphorylation of downstream effectors, PKA and PKC are involved in a negative feedback mechanism, namely, heterologous receptor desensitization, through GPCR phosphorylation.

Endocytosis and Internalization of G Protein-Coupled Receptors

Receptor internalization can lead to either receptor resensitization or degradation (for review, see Walther and Ferguson 2013). Besides their role in receptor desensitization through the uncoupling of GPCRs from G proteins, arrestins target GPCRs for internalization via clathrin-coated pits (for review, see Lee et al. 2016). Additionally, they indirectly regulate GPCR trafficking by coordinating their ubiquitination and deubiquitination.

Arrestins represent an adaptor between the GPCR and key components of the internalization machinery. They bind to trafficking proteins (clathrin, clathrin adaptor protein 2 AP2), thus functioning as scaffolds in the receptor-mediated endocytosis pathway (Gurevich and Gurevich 2015). Mechanistically, binding of nonvisual arrestins to GPCR stimulates the release of the arrestin C-terminal tail, which contains binding sites for clathrin and AP2. Binding of clathrin and AP2 to those C-terminal sites induces receptor internalization via coated pits. This is exemplified by β_2AR, whose internalization is promoted by arrestin-2 and arrestin-3 (Goodman et al. 1996).

Arrestin-Independent Internalization

GPCRs use more than one internalization pathway. In the muscarinic M2 receptor, mutation of the two clusters of serine/threonine residues that are required for arrestin binding and receptor desensitization does not block receptor endocytosis, suggesting that the receptor internalizes in an arrestin-independent manner (Pals-Rylaarsdam et al. 1997). Similarly, while wild-type protease-activated receptor 2 (PAR2) internalizes in a β-arrestin-dependent manner, mutation of all the serine/threonine in the receptor C-tail results in β-arrestin-independent internalization (Ricks and Trejo 2009). The type II GnRH receptor can internalize both in an arrestin-dependent and arrestin-independent fashion (Ronacher et al. 2004). Alternatively, GPCRs can internalize in a β-arrestin-independent manner via caveolae (for review, see Walther and Ferguson 2013). Hence, β1AR mutants lacking GRK phosphorylation sites are internalized via caveolae following PKA phosphorylation, independently of β-arrestin, suggesting that PKA- and GRK-mediated phosphorylation influence β1AR internalization in an additive fashion (Rapacciuolo et al. 2003). Although diverse internalization mechanisms have been reported, β-arrestin and clathrin dependent, β-arrestin and clathrin independent, β-arrestin independent and clathrin dependent, and β-arrestin dependent and clathrin independent (Marchese et al. 2003), the majority of GPCRs are internalized via the β-arrestin-dependent, clathrin-mediated internalization pathway.

Stability of the GPCR/β-Arrestin Complex and GPCR Intracellular Fate

Distinct β-arrestins differentially regulate GPCR internalization. For instance, β-arrestin-2 promotes β_2AR internalization 100 times more efficiently than β-arrestin-1 (Kohout et al. 2001). Thus, GPCRs have been grouped into two categories based on the strength of the GPCR/arrestin interaction, which is thought to determine whether they are preferentially recycled or degraded. One class of receptors (e.g., β_2AR, μ-opioid receptors, dopamine D1A receptors) has a higher affinity for β-arrestin-2, and their association with arrestins is transient, resulting in their transfer to endosomes and their recycling to the plasma membrane and their resensitization. Conversely, other receptors (e.g., V2 vasopressin, neurotensin 1, angiotensin II type 1a receptors) bind β-arrestin-1 and β-arrestin-2 with comparable affinity, and their association with arrestins remains steady through endocytosis, predominantly resulting in lysosomal degradation (for review, see Walther and Ferguson 2013).

Alternate Role of Arrestins in GPCR Signaling

Although β-arrestins are known for regulating GPCR signaling, they can also mediate signaling via the recruitment of signaling molecules distinct from G protein-mediated signaling, thus setting off a second wave of signaling (Luttrell et al. 1999, 2001). In the case of angiotensin II type 1a receptors (AT1aR), β-arrestins act as scaffolds to enhance ERK2 activation. Interestingly, there is a correlation between the affinity of the GPCR/arrestin complex and the degree of β-arrestin–ERK binding, as the class of GPCRs forming stable receptor–β-arrestin complexes activates ERK more persistently than those forming transient receptor–β-arrestin complexes (Tohgo et al. 2003).

G Protein-Coupled Receptor Ubiquitination

To recapitulate the principal functions of arrestins, they are implicated in GPCR desensitization, GPCR internalization, and GPCR post-endocytic trafficking. Both arrestin ubiquitination and GPCR ubiquitination regulate GPCR trafficking (for review, see Gurevich and Gurevich 2015). Upon agonist stimulation, both GPCR and arrestin are ubiquitinated. While arrestin ubiquitination may affect the stability of the GPCR/arrestin complex (Shenoy and Lefkowitz 2003) and appears to be required for receptor internalization (Shenoy et al. 2001), GPCR ubiquitination is dependent upon arrestin and may mediate lysosomal sorting (Marchese and Benovic 2001; Shenoy et al. 2001). However, one study reports that agonist-stimulated ubiquitination of arrestin-2 by E3 ubiquitin ligase Mdm2 has no effect on β_2AR internalization (Ahmed et al. 2011). Notably, the pattern of β-arrestin ubiquitination correlates with the stability of the GPCR/β-arrestin complex, as receptors forming a stable complex are linked with persistent ubiquitination (Shenoy and Lefkowitz 2003).

Downregulation of G Protein-Coupled Receptors

Lysosomal targeting leads to a decline in the number of receptors on the cell surface. Gurevich's group has proposed two distinct models for the recycling versus degradation of GPCRs. According to the first model, the longer time the GPCR spends in the endosome, the higher the likelihood that it will be targeted to lysosomal degradation. This hypothesis is in agreement with the fate of internalized receptors being determined by the stability of GPCR/arrestin interaction (see above). The second model speculates that only phosphorylated forms of the receptor are targeted to lysosomes for degradation (Pan et al. 2003) (for review, see Gurevich and Gurevich 2015). It is based on studies indicating that GPCR dephosphorylation may be necessary for its recycling to the cell surface (Hsieh et al. 1999). Indeed, Gurevich's group previously showed that arrestin-2 mutants, which bind to activated GPCRs independently of receptor phosphorylation, prevent β_2AR downregulation (Pan et al. 2003).

G Protein-Coupled Receptor Signaling and Disease

The GPCR superfamily represents the most prevalent group of transmembrane receptors, thus mediating the majority of physiological responses to hormones, neurotransmitters, ions, light, and odors. Consequently, impairment of GPCR function can cause a wide range of diseases, including blindness, cancers, cardiovascular diseases, neuropsychiatric, and metabolic disorders. A large variety of endocrine diseases are due to GPCR mutations (Table 2).

Naturally occurring GPCR mutations may cause alterations in ligand binding, G protein coupling, receptor desensitization, and receptor recycling in a variety of

Table 2 GPCR mutations causing endocrine disease. Partial list of the large number of endocrine diseases caused by specific GPCR mutations

Receptor mechanism	Disease	Receptor
Adrenocorticotropin receptor (ACTHR/MC2R)	Isolated glucocorticoid deficiency	Loss of function
Arginine vasopressin receptor 2 (AVPR2)	Nephrogenic diabetes insipidus	Loss of function
Calcium-sensing receptor (CASR)	Familial hypocalciuric hypercalcemia	Loss of function
	Neonatal severe hyperparathyroidism	Loss of function
Ghrelin receptor	Short stature	Loss of basal activity
Gonadotropin-releasing hormone	Idiopathic hypogonadotropic	Reduced/loss of function
Hormone receptor (GnRHR)	Hypogonadism	
Growth hormone-releasing hormone	Short stature	Loss of function
Follicle-stimulating hormone receptor (FSHR)	Ovarian dysgenesis	Loss of function
KISS1 receptor	Central hypogonadotropic hypogonadism	Loss of function
Luteinizing hormone/chorionic gonadotropin receptor (LHCGR)	Familial male precocious puberty	Constitutive activity
	Leydig cell hyperplasia	Constitutive activity
Melanocortin 4 receptor (MC4R)	Autosomal dominant obesity	Loss of function
Parathyroid hormone receptor	Jansen's chondrodysplasia	Constitutive activity
	Blomstrand's chondrodysplasia	Lack of adenylyl cyclase signaling
Thyroid-stimulating hormone	Non-autoimmune	Constitutive activity
Receptor (TSHR)	Thyroiditis	
	Toxic adenoma	Constitutive activity
	Congenital hypothyroidism	Loss of function
	Familial gestational hyperthyroidism	Activation by HCG

human genetic diseases (for review, see Thompson et al. 2008b). Loss-of-function mutations result in reduced ligand binding, while gain-of-function mutations lead to constitutive activation or enhanced binding. As an example, polycystic kidney disease is an inherited disorder that can result in progressive loss of renal function. Genetic variants in the *PKD1* gene, which encodes the GPCR polycystin-1 (PC-1), are the predominant factor associated with the disease in nearly two-thirds of patients (Hama and Park 2016).

A large number of genetic endocrine disorders affecting every endocrine system result from specific GPCR mutations. Hence, mutations in the LH receptor (LHCGR) result in a constitutively active receptor and are linked to familial male precocious puberty. An FSH receptor (FSHR) mutation that causes decreased affinity for its ligand is associated with ovarian dysgenesis. GnRHR reduced or loss-of-function mutations are associated with idiopathic hypogonadotropic hypogonadism (IHH). TSH receptor (TSHR) mutations lead to constitutive activity causing non-autoimmune thyroiditis as well as adenomas. Loss-of-function mutations in the calcium-sensing receptor (CASR) are responsible for familial hypocalciuric hypercalcemia and neonatal severe hyperparathyroidism. Loss-of-function mutations in the melanocortin 4 receptor (MC4R), which is involved in energy homeostasis, are associated with severe autosomal dominant obesity. A mutation in the high-affinity binding site of the thyrotropin-stimulating hormone receptor has been identified as a cause of familial gestational hyperthyroidism. The altered receptor can be activated by chorionic gonadotropin as well as its native agonist, thyrotropin-stimulating hormone. Elevated levels of chorionic gonadotropin during pregnancy lead to unregulated activation of the thyrotropin-stimulating hormone receptor, resulting in clinical hyperthyroidism occurring only during pregnancy.

Genes encoding accessory proteins for GPCRs (e.g., G protein, RGS, AGS, GRK) are also disrupted in various hereditary diseases (Thompson et al. 2008a). Termination of GPCR signaling relies on the hydrolysis of GTP by the intrinsic GTPase activity of Gα. If impaired, this process can bring about a number of diseases. Hence, cholera toxin, which is produced by *Vibrio cholerae* upon infection, prevents GTP hydrolysis by covalently modifying an arginine residue located in the nucleotide-binding pocket of Gαs. This causes prolonged activation of GPCR signaling and thus elevated cAMP levels in mucous intestinal cells, leading to secretory diarrhea. In some pituitary tumors, mutation of the same arginine residue in the gene encoding Gαs also results in prolonged GPCR signaling and enhanced secretion of growth hormone (Vallar et al. 1987). Inactivating Gαs variants are associated with a form of pseudohypoparathyroidism called Albright's hereditary osteodystrophy (Spiegel 1990), whereas activating mutations are observed in patients with McCune–Albright syndrome and in various tumors (Turan and Bastepe 2015). RGS2 SNPs are linked to hypertension in African Americans, and GRK4 mutations that increase GRK4 activity are associated with hypertension and sodium sensitivity. Aberrant upregulation of GRK2 and/or GRK5, which interferes with GPCR signaling, can lead to cardiovascular diseases, neurodegenerative disorders, and cancer (Penela 2016). Moreover, epigenetic modulation of GPCR signaling has been associated with CNS disorders as well as pain disorders (Dogra et al. 2016).

Summary

G protein-coupled receptors (GPCRs) include one of the largest gene families in the mammalian genome. About 800 human GPCRs have been identified. The specificity provided by the diversity of GPCR receptor binding sites leads to their playing crucial roles in every endocrine system, and GPCRs represent the predominant target of therapeutic drugs. The term GPCR refers to the classical coupling of these receptors via heterotrimeric G proteins. In addition, they can also couple via many other non-heterotrimeric G protein interactions.

GPCRs are grouped by primary sequence similarity into different families that all have a canonical seven alpha helical transmembrane domain structure. Covalent modifications of these receptors include extracellular glycosylation and intracellular palmitoylation and phosphorylation. By far, the largest family, class A, comprises the rhodopsin-like GPCRs that have over 700 members including the majority of receptors for hormones and neurotransmitters. A distinct gene family, class B, also includes receptors for hormones including secretin, glucagon, and corticotropin-releasing factor.

In recent years, the crystal structure has been solved for an increasing number of GPCRs. The increasing number of solved crystal structures for GPCRs includes rhodopsin, the β_2-adrenergic receptor, the glucagon receptor, the corticotropin-releasing factor receptor, and two metabotropic receptors. The agonist-bound crystal structure of the β_2-adrenergic receptor has clarified the mechanism of activation of the receptor, which involves helical movement around proline bends in the transmembrane helices. The crystal structures from the different classes reveal distinct location of the ligand-binding pockets both across and within classes.

Despite their name, they couple to cellular signaling via both heterotrimeric G proteins and G protein-independent mechanisms. Specific heterotrimeric G proteins can signal by regulating different mediators, including adenylyl cyclase, phospholipase C, and ion channel activity. A specific GPCR may couple to more than one heterotrimeric G protein, and agonists can influence the relative coupling to different pathways activated by the same receptor, a phenomenon called biased agonism. The activity of GPCRs can be modulated by regulators of G protein signaling proteins (RGS) and activators of G protein signaling (AGS). Receptor activity may also be modified by interaction with receptor activity-modifying proteins (RAMP) as well as a variety of other signal-transducing or signal-modulating proteins. GPCR activity can be regulated by phosphorylation by protein kinases. Receptor dimerization and cross dimerization of different GPCR subtypes contribute to creating functional diverse receptor complexes.

Hundreds of endocrine and systemic diseases are caused by specific receptor mutations. Examples include cases of male precocious puberty due to LH receptor mutations, idiopathic hypogonadotropic hypogonadism due to GnRH receptor mutations, and autoimmune thyroid disease due to TSH receptor mutations.

Cross-References

▶ Cytokine Receptors
▶ Genetic Disorders of Adrenocortical Function
▶ Molecular Mechanisms of Thyroid Hormone Synthesis and Secretion
▶ Principles of Endocrine Diseases
▶ Synthesis, Secretion, and Transport of Peptide Hormones

References

Ahmed MR, Zhan X, Song X, Kook S, Gurevich VV, Gurevich EV. Ubiquitin ligase parkin promotes Mdm2-arrestin interaction but inhibits arrestin ubiquitination. Biochemistry. 2011;50(18):3749–63.

Altier C. GPCR and voltage-gated calcium channels (VGCC) signaling complexes. Subcell Biochem. 2012;63:241–62.

Ballou LM, Lin HY, Fan G, Jiang YP, Lin RZ. Activated G alpha q inhibits p110 alpha phosphatidylinositol 3-kinase and Akt. J Biol Chem. 2003;278(26):23472–9.

Berman DM, Kozasa T, Gilman AG. The GTPase-activating protein RGS4 stabilizes the transition state for nucleotide hydrolysis. J Biol Chem. 1996;271(44):27209–12.

Biddlecome GH, Berstein G, Ross EM. Regulation of phospholipase C-beta1 by Gq and m1 muscarinic cholinergic receptor. Steady-state balance of receptor-mediated activation and GTPase-activating protein-promoted deactivation. J Biol Chem. 1996;271(14):7999–8007.

Blumer JB, Lanier SM. Activators of G protein signaling exhibit broad functionality and define a distinct core signaling triad. Mol Pharmacol. 2014;85(3):388–96.

Bodmann EL, Wolters V, Bunemann M. Dynamics of G protein effector interactions and their impact on timing and sensitivity of G protein-mediated signal transduction. Eur J Cell Biol. 2015;94(7–9):415–9.

Baltoumas FA, Theodoropoulou MC, Hamodrakas SJ. Interactions of the alpha-subunits of heterotrimeric G-proteins with GPCRs, effectors and RGS proteins: a critical review and analysis of interacting surfaces, conformational shifts, structural diversity and electrostatic potentials. J Struct Biol. 2013;182(3):209–18.

Brady AE, Limbird LE. G protein-coupled receptor interacting proteins: emerging roles in localization and signal transduction. Cell Signal. 2002;14(4):297–309.

Brzostowski JA, Kimmel AR. Signaling at zero G: G-protein-independent functions for 7-TM receptors. Trends Biochem Sci. 2001;26(5):291–7.

Carman CV, Parent JL, Day PW, Pronin AN, Sternweis PM, Wedegaertner PB, et al. Selective regulation of Galpha(q/11) by an RGS domain in the G protein-coupled receptor kinase, GRK2. J Biol Chem. 1999;274(48):34483–92.

Charest PG, Bouvier M. Palmitoylation of the V2 vasopressin receptor carboxyl tail enhances beta-arrestin recruitment leading to efficient receptor endocytosis and ERK1/2 activation. J Biol Chem. 2003;278(42):41541–51.

Cooke RM, Brown AJ, Marshall FH, Mason JS. Structures of G protein-coupled receptors reveal new opportunities for drug discovery. Drug Discov Today. 2015;20(11):1355–64.

Cvejic S, Devi LA. Dimerization of the delta opioid receptor: implication for a role in receptor internalization. J Biol Chem. 1997;272(43):26959–64.

Davenport AP, Alexander SP, Sharman JL, Pawson AJ, Benson HE, Monaghan AE, et al. International Union of Basic and Clinical Pharmacology. LXXXVIII. G protein-coupled receptor list: recommendations for new pairings with cognate ligands. Pharmacol Rev. 2013;65(3):967–86.

DeGraff JL, Gurevich VV, Benovic JL. The third intracellular loop of alpha 2-adrenergic receptors determines subtype specificity of arrestin interaction. J Biol Chem. 2002;277(45):43247–52.

Dessauer CW, Tesmer JJ, Sprang SR, Gilman AG. Identification of a gialpha binding site on type V adenylyl cyclase. J Biol Chem. 1998;273(40):25831–9.

DeWire SM, Ahn S, Lefkowitz RJ, Shenoy SK. Beta-arrestins and cell signaling. Annu Rev Physiol. 2007;69:483–510.

Dogra S, Sona C, Kumar A, Yadav PN. Epigenetic regulation of G protein coupled receptor signaling and its implications in psychiatric disorders. Int J Biochem Cell Biol. 2016;77 (Pt B):226–39.

Dore AS, Okrasa K, Patel JC, Serrano-Vega M, Bennett K, Cooke RM, et al. Structure of class C GPCR metabotropic glutamate receptor 5 transmembrane domain. Nature. 2014;511 (7511):557–62.

Duc NM, Kim HR, Chung KY. Structural mechanism of G protein activation by G protein-coupled receptor. Eur J Pharmacol. 2015;763(Pt B):214–22.

Ellis J, Pediani JD, Canals M, Milasta S, Milligan G. Orexin-1 receptor-cannabinoid CB1 receptor heterodimerization results in both ligand-dependent and -independent coordinated alterations of receptor localization and function. J Biol Chem. 2006;281(50):38812–24.

Ferguson SS. Evolving concepts in G protein-coupled receptor endocytosis: the role in receptor desensitization and signaling. Pharmacol Rev. 2001;53(1):1–24.

Garcia-Hoz C, Sanchez-Fernandez G, Diaz-Meco MT, Moscat J, Mayor F, Ribas C. G alpha(q) acts as an adaptor protein in protein kinase C zeta (PKCzeta)-mediated ERK5 activation by G protein-coupled receptors (GPCR). J Biol Chem. 2010;285(18):13480–9.

Gingell J, Simms J, Barwell J, Poyner DR, Watkins HA, Pioszak AA, et al. An allosteric role for receptor activity-modifying proteins in defining GPCR pharmacology. Cell Discov. 2016;2:16012.

Gomes I, Ayoub MA, Fujita W, Jaeger WC, Pfleger KD, Devi LA. G protein-coupled receptor heteromers. Annu Rev Pharmacol Toxicol. 2016;56:403–25.

Gonzalez-Maeso J, Rodriguez-Puertas R, Meana JJ. Quantitative stoichiometry of G-proteins activated by mu-opioid receptors in postmortem human brain. Eur J Pharmacol. 2002;452(1):21–33.

Gonzalez-Maeso J, Weisstaub NV, Zhou M, Chan P, Ivic L, Ang R, et al. Hallucinogens recruit specific cortical 5-HT(2A) receptor-mediated signaling pathways to affect behavior. Neuron. 2007;53(3):439–52.

Gonzalez-Maeso J, Ang RL, Yuen T, Chan P, Weisstaub NV, Lopez-Gimenez JF, et al. Identification of a serotonin/glutamate receptor complex implicated in psychosis. Nature. 2008;452 (7183):93–7.

Goodman Jr OB, Krupnick JG, Santini F, Gurevich VV, Penn RB, Gagnon AW, et al. Beta-arrestin acts as a clathrin adaptor in endocytosis of the beta2-adrenergic receptor. Nature. 1996;383 (6599):447–50.

Gurevich VV, Gurevich EV. Arrestins: critical players in trafficking of many GPCRs. Prog Mol Biol Transl Sci. 2015;132:1–14.

Hama T, Park F. Heterotrimeric G protein signaling in polycystic kidney disease. Physiol Genomics. 2016;48(7):429–45.

Hermans E. Biochemical and pharmacological control of the multiplicity of coupling at G-protein-coupled receptors. Pharmacol Ther. 2003;99(1):25–44.

Hollenstein K, de Graaf C, Bortolato A, Wang MW, Marshall FH, Stevens RC. Insights into the structure of class B GPCRs. Trends Pharmacol Sci. 2014;35(1):12–22.

Hsieh C, Brown S, Derleth C, Mackie K. Internalization and recycling of the CB1 cannabinoid receptor. J Neurochem. 1999;73(2):493–501.

Hur EM, Kim KT. G protein-coupled receptor signalling and cross-talk: achieving rapidity and specificity. Cell Signal. 2002;14(5):397–405.

Ikeda Y, Kumagai H, Skach A, Sato M, Yanagisawa M. Modulation of circadian glucocorticoid oscillation via adrenal opioid-CXCR7 signaling alters emotional behavior. Cell. 2013;155 (6):1323–36.

Insel PA, Head BP, Ostrom RS, Patel HH, Swaney JS, Tang CM, et al. Caveolae and lipid rafts: G protein-coupled receptor signaling microdomains in cardiac myocytes. Ann N Y Acad Sci. 2005;1047:166–72.

Jordan JD, Landau EM, Iyengar R. Signaling networks: the origins of cellular multitasking. Cell. 2000;103(2):193–200.

Kohout TA, Lin FS, Perry SJ, Conner DA, Lefkowitz RJ. Beta-arrestin 1 and 2 differentially regulate heptahelical receptor signaling and trafficking. Proc Natl Acad Sci U S A. 2001;98(4):1601–6.

Kolakowski LF Jr. GCRDb: a G-protein-coupled receptor database. Receptors Channels. 1994;2 (1):1–7

Kook S, Zhan X, Kaoud TS, Dalby KN, Gurevich VV, Gurevich EV. Arrestin-3 binds c-Jun N-terminal kinase 1 (JNK1) and JNK2 and facilitates the activation of these ubiquitous JNK isoforms in cells via scaffolding. J Biol Chem. 2013;288(52):37332–42.

Krasel C, Bunemann M, Lorenz K, Lohse MJ. Beta-arrestin binding to the beta2-adrenergic receptor requires both receptor phosphorylation and receptor activation. J Biol Chem. 2005;280(10):9528–35.

Krupnick JG, Benovic JL. The role of receptor kinases and arrestins in G protein-coupled receptor regulation. Annu Rev Pharmacol Toxicol. 1998;38:289–319.

Lee SM, Booe JM, Pioszak AA. Structural insights into ligand recognition and selectivity for classes A, B, and C GPCRs. Eur J Pharmacol. 2015;763(Pt B):196–205.

Lee MH, Appleton KM, Strungs EG, Kwon JY, Morinelli TA, Peterson YK, et al. The conformational signature of beta-arrestin2 predicts its trafficking and signalling functions. Nature. 2016;531(7596):665–8.

Lefkowitz RJ, Shenoy SK. Transduction of receptor signals by beta-arrestins. Science. 2005;308 (5721):512–7.

Liggett SB, Ostrowski J, Chesnut LC, Kurose H, Raymond JR, Caron MG, et al. Sites in the third intracellular loop of the alpha 2A-adrenergic receptor confer short term agonist-promoted desensitization. Evidence for a receptor kinase-mediated mechanism. J Biol Chem. 1992;267(7):4740–6.

Litosch I. Decoding Galphaq signaling. Life Sci. 2016;152:99–106.

Lopez-Gimenez JF, Vilaro MT, Milligan G. Morphine desensitization, internalization, and down-regulation of the mu opioid receptor is facilitated by serotonin 5-hydroxytryptamine2A receptor coactivation. Mol Pharmacol. 2008;74(5):1278–91.

Luttrell LM. Transmembrane signaling by G protein-coupled receptors. Methods Mol Biol. 2006;332:3–49.

Luttrell LM, Lefkowitz RJ. The role of beta-arrestins in the termination and transduction of G-protein-coupled receptor signals. J Cell Sci. 2002;115(Pt 3):455–65.

Luttrell LM, Ferguson SS, Daaka Y, Miller WE, Maudsley S, Della Rocca GJ, et al. Beta-arrestin-dependent formation of beta2 adrenergic receptor-Src protein kinase complexes. Science. 1999;283(5402):655–61.

Luttrell LM, Roudabush FL, Choy EW, Miller WE, Field ME, Pierce KL, et al. Activation and targeting of extracellular signal-regulated kinases by beta-arrestin scaffolds. Proc Natl Acad Sci U S A. 2001;98(5):2449–54.

Manglik A, Lin H, Aryal DK, McCorvy JD, Dengler D, Corder G, et al. Structure-based discovery of opioid analgesics with reduced side effects. Nature. 2016;537(7619):185–90.

Manning DR, Gilman AG. The regulatory components of adenylate cyclase and transducin. A family of structurally homologous guanine nucleotide-binding proteins. J Biol Chem. 1983;258 (11):7059–63.

Marchese A, Benovic JL. Agonist-promoted ubiquitination of the G protein-coupled receptor CXCR4 mediates lysosomal sorting. J Biol Chem. 2001;276(49):45509–12.

Marchese A, Chen C, Kim YM, Benovic JL. The ins and outs of G protein-coupled receptor trafficking. Trends Biochem Sci. 2003;28(7):369–76.

Margeta-Mitrovic M, Jan YN, Jan LY. A trafficking checkpoint controls GABA(B) receptor heterodimerization. Neuron. 2000;27(1):97–106.

Marion S, Oakley RH, Kim KM, Caron MG, Barak LS. A beta-arrestin binding determinant common to the second intracellular loops of rhodopsin family G protein-coupled receptors. J Biol Chem. 2006;281(5):2932–8.

Marty C, Browning DD, Ye RD. Identification of tetratricopeptide repeat 1 as an adaptor protein that interacts with heterotrimeric G proteins and the small GTPase Ras. Mol Cell Biol. 2003;23 (11):3847–58.

Maurice P, Guillaume JL, Benleulmi-Chaachoua A, Daulat AM, Kamal M, Jockers R. GPCR-interacting proteins, major players of GPCR function. Adv Pharmacol. 2011;62:349–80.

McVey M, Ramsay D, Kellett E, Rees S, Wilson S, Pope AJ, et al. Monitoring receptor oligomerization using time-resolved fluorescence resonance energy transfer and bioluminescence resonance energy transfer. The human delta -opioid receptor displays constitutive oligomerization at the cell surface, which is not regulated by receptor occupancy. J Biol Chem. 2001;276 (17):14092–9.

Milligan G. G protein-coupled receptor hetero-dimerization: contribution to pharmacology and function. Br J Pharmacol. 2009;158(1):5–14.
Milligan G, Kostenis E. Heterotrimeric G-proteins: a short history. Br J Pharmacol. 2006;147 Suppl 1:S46–55.
Milligan G, Feng GJ, Ward RJ, Sartania N, Ramsay D, McLean AJ, et al. G protein-coupled receptor fusion proteins in drug discovery. Curr Pharm Des. 2004;10(17):1989–2001.
Mnpotra JS, Qiao Z, Cai J, Lynch DL, Grossfield A, Leioatts N, et al. Structural basis of G protein-coupled receptor-Gi protein interaction: formation of the cannabinoid CB2 receptor-Gi protein complex. J Biol Chem. 2014;289(29):20259–72.
Mukhopadhyay S, Ross EM. Rapid GTP binding and hydrolysis by G(q) promoted by receptor and GTPase-activating proteins. Proc Natl Acad Sci U S A. 1999;96(17):9539–44.
Nelson G, Chandrashekar J, Hoon MA, Feng L, Zhao G, Ryba NJ, et al. An amino-acid taste receptor. Nature. 2002;416(6877):199–202.
Neubig RR, Siderovski DP. Regulators of G-protein signalling as new central nervous system drug targets. Nat Rev Drug Discov. 2002;1(3):187–97.
Neves SR, Ram PT, Iyengar R. G protein pathways. Science. 2002;296(5573):1636–9.
Ng GY, O'Dowd BF, Lee SP, Chung HT, Brann MR, Seeman P, et al. Dopamine D2 receptor dimers and receptor-blocking peptides. Biochem Biophys Res Commun. 1996;227(1):200–4.
O'Neil RT, Emeson RB. Quantitative analysis of 5HT(2C) receptor RNA editing patterns in psychiatric disorders. Neurobiol Dis. 2012;45(1):8–13.
Oldham WM, Hamm HE. Heterotrimeric G protein activation by G-protein-coupled receptors. Nat Rev Mol Cell Biol. 2008;9(1):60–71.
Ostrom RS. New determinants of receptor-effector coupling: trafficking and compartmentation in membrane microdomains. Mol Pharmacol. 2002;61(3):473–6.
Ostrom RS, Post SR, Insel PA. Stoichiometry and compartmentation in G protein-coupled receptor signaling: implications for therapeutic interventions involving G(s). J Pharmacol Exp Ther. 2000;294(2):407–12.
Palczewski K, Kumasaka T, Hori T, Behnke CA, Motoshima H, Fox BA, et al. Crystal structure of rhodopsin: a G protein-coupled receptor. Science. 2000;289(5480):739–45.
Pals-Rylaarsdam R, Hosey MM. Two homologous phosphorylation domains differentially contribute to desensitization and internalization of the m2 muscarinic acetylcholine receptor. J Biol Chem. 1997;272(22):14152–8.
Pals-Rylaarsdam R, Gurevich VV, Lee KB, Ptasienski JA, Benovic JL, Hosey MM. Internalization of the m2 muscarinic acetylcholine receptor. Arrestin-independent and -dependent pathways. J Biol Chem. 1997;272(38):23682–9.
Pan L, Gurevich EV, Gurevich VV. The nature of the arrestin x receptor complex determines the ultimate fate of the internalized receptor. J Biol Chem. 2003;278(13):11623–32.
Parenty G, Appelbe S, Milligan G. CXCR2 chemokine receptor antagonism enhances DOP opioid receptor function via allosteric regulation of the CXCR2-DOP receptor heterodimer. Biochem J. 2008;412(2):245–56.
Park F. Activators of G protein signaling in the kidney. J Pharmacol Exp Ther. 2015;353(2):235–45.
Park JH, Scheerer P, Hofmann KP, Choe H-W, Ernst OP. Crystal structure of the ligand-free G-protein-coupled receptor opsin. Nature. 2008;454(7201):183–7.
Patwari P, Lee RT. An expanded family of arrestins regulate metabolism. Trends Endocrinol Metab. 2012;23(5):216–22.
Penela P. Chapter three – ubiquitination and protein turnover of G-protein-coupled receptor kinases in GPCR signaling and cellular regulation. Prog Mol Biol Transl Sci. 2016;141:85–140.
Ponimaskin E, Dumuis A, Gaven F, Barthet G, Heine M, Glebov K, et al. Palmitoylation of the 5-hydroxytryptamine4a receptor regulates receptor phosphorylation, desensitization, and beta-arrestin-mediated endocytosis. Mol Pharmacol. 2005;67(5):1434–43.
Prabakaran S, Lippens G, Steen H, Gunawardena J. Post-translational modification: nature's escape from genetic imprisonment and the basis for dynamic information encoding. Wiley Interdiscip Rev Syst Biol Med. 2012;4(6):565–83.

Premont RT, Gainetdinov RR. Physiological roles of G protein-coupled receptor kinases and arrestins. Annu Rev Physiol. 2007;69:511–34.

Qanbar R, Bouvier M. Role of palmitoylation/depalmitoylation reactions in G-protein-coupled receptor function. Pharmacol Ther. 2003;97(1):1–33.

Rapacciuolo A, Suvarna S, Barki-Harrington L, Luttrell LM, Cong M, Lefkowitz RJ, et al. Protein kinase A and G protein-coupled receptor kinase phosphorylation mediates beta-1 adrenergic receptor endocytosis through different pathways. J Biol Chem. 2003;278(37):35403–11.

Rasmussen SG, Choi HJ, Rosenbaum DM, Kobilka TS, Thian FS, Edwards PC, et al. Crystal structure of the human beta2 adrenergic G-protein-coupled receptor. Nature. 2007;450 (7168):383–7.

Rasmussen SG, DeVree BT, Zou Y, Kruse AC, Chung KY, Kobilka TS, et al. Crystal structure of the beta2 adrenergic receptor-Gs protein complex. Nature. 2011;477(7366):549–55.

Remmers AE, Clark MJ, Alt A, Medzihradsky F, Woods JH, Traynor JR. Activation of G protein by opioid receptors: role of receptor number and G-protein concentration. Eur J Pharmacol. 2000;396(2–3):67–75.

Ricks TK, Trejo J. Phosphorylation of protease-activated receptor-2 differentially regulates desensitization and internalization. J Biol Chem. 2009;284(49):34444–57.

Ronacher K, Matsiliza N, Nkwanyana N, Pawson AJ, Adam T, Flanagan CA, et al. Serine residues 338 and 339 in the carboxyl-terminal tail of the type II gonadotropin-releasing hormone receptor are critical for beta-arrestin-independent internalization. Endocrinology. 2004;145(10):4480–8.

Salahpour A, Angers S, Mercier JF, Lagace M, Marullo S, Bouvier M. Homodimerization of the beta2-adrenergic receptor as a prerequisite for cell surface targeting. J Biol Chem. 2004;279 (32):33390–7.

Sanchez-Fernandez G, Cabezudo S, Garcia-Hoz C, Beninca C, Aragay AM, Mayor Jr F, et al. Galphaq signalling: the new and the old. Cell Signal. 2014;26(5):833–48.

Sato J, Makita N, Iiri T. Inverse agonism: the classic concept of GPCRs revisited [review]. Endocr J. 2016;63(6):507–14.

Scheerer P, Park JH, Hildebrand PW, Kim YJ, Krauß N, Choe H-W, et al. Crystal structure of opsin in its G-protein-interacting conformation. Nature. 2008;455(7212):497–502.

Schmid CL, Bohn LM. Serotonin, but not N-methyltryptamines, activates the serotonin 2A receptor via a ß-arrestin2/Src/Akt signaling complex in vivo. J Neurosci Off J Soc Neurosci. 2010;30 (40):13513–24.

Seifert R, Lushington GH, Mou TC, Gille A, Sprang SR. Inhibitors of membranous adenylyl cyclases. Trends Pharmacol Sci. 2012;33(2):64–78.

Shenoy SK, Lefkowitz RJ. Trafficking patterns of beta-arrestin and G protein-coupled receptors determined by the kinetics of beta-arrestin deubiquitination. J Biol Chem. 2003;278 (16):14498–506.

Shenoy SK, McDonald PH, Kohout TA, Lefkowitz RJ. Regulation of receptor fate by ubiquitination of activated beta 2-adrenergic receptor and beta-arrestin. Science. 2001;294 (5545):1307–13.

Smith JS, Rajagopal S. The beta-arrestins: multifunctional regulators of G protein-coupled receptors. J Biol Chem. 2016;291(17):8969–77.

Smrcka AV, Sternweis PC. Regulation of purified subtypes of phosphatidylinositol-specific phospholipase C beta by G protein alpha and beta gamma subunits. J Biol Chem. 1993;268(13):9667–74.

Sondek J, Bohm A, Lambright DG, Hamm HE, Sigler PB. Crystal structure of a G-protein beta gamma dimer at 2.1A resolution. Nature. 1996;379(6563):369–74.

Spiegel AM. Albright's hereditary osteodystrophy and defective G proteins. N Engl J Med. 1990;322(20):1461–2.

Stewart A, Fisher RA. Introduction: G protein-coupled receptors and RGS proteins. Prog Mol Biol Transl Sci. 2015;133:1–11.

Suh BC, Kim JS, Namgung U, Han S, Kim KT. Selective inhibition of beta(2)-adrenergic receptor-mediated cAMP generation by activation of the P2Y(2) receptor in mouse pineal gland tumor cells. J Neurochem. 2001;77(6):1475–85.

Sun Y, Cheng Z, Ma L, Pei G. Beta-arrestin2 is critically involved in CXCR4-mediated chemotaxis, and this is mediated by its enhancement of p38 MAPK activation. J Biol Chem. 2002;277(51):49212–9.

Sunahara RK, Dessauer CW, Whisnant RE, Kleuss C, Gilman AG. Interaction of Gsalpha with the cytosolic domains of mammalian adenylyl cyclase. J Biol Chem. 1997;272(35):22265–71.

Tesmer JJ, Berman DM, Gilman AG, Sprang SR. Structure of RGS4 bound to AlF4 – activated G (i alpha1): stabilization of the transition state for GTP hydrolysis. Cell. 1997;89(2):251–61.

Thompson MD, Cole DE, Jose PA. Pharmacogenomics of G protein-coupled receptor signaling: insights from health and disease. Methods Mol Biol. 2008a;448:77–107.

Thompson MD, Percy ME, McIntyre Burnham W, Cole DE. G protein-coupled receptors disrupted in human genetic disease. Methods Mol Biol. 2008b;448:109–37.

Tohgo A, Choy EW, Gesty-Palmer D, Pierce KL, Laporte S, Oakley RH, et al. The stability of the G protein-coupled receptor-beta-arrestin interaction determines the mechanism and functional consequence of ERK activation. J Biol Chem. 2003;278(8):6258–67.

Turan S, Bastepe M. GNAS spectrum of disorders. Curr Osteoporos Rep. 2015;13(3):146–58.

Vallar L, Spada A, Giannattasio G. Altered Gs and adenylate cyclase activity in human GH-secreting pituitary adenomas. Nature. 1987;330(6148):566–8.

van der Westhuizen ET, Valant C, Sexton PM, Christopoulos A. Endogenous allosteric modulators of G protein-coupled receptors. J Pharmacol Exp Ther. 2015;353(2):246–60.

Venkatakrishnan AJ, Deupi X, Lebon G, Tate CG, Schertler GF, Babu MM. Molecular signatures of G-protein-coupled receptors. Nature. 2013;494(7436):185–94.

Venkatakrishnan AJ, Flock T, Prado DE, Oates ME, Gough J, Madan BM. Structured and disordered facets of the GPCR fold. Curr Opin Struct Biol. 2014;27:129–37.

Vines CM. Phospholipase C. Adv Exp Med Biol. 2012;740:235–54.

Violin JD, Crombie AL, Soergel DG, Lark MW. Biased ligands at G-protein-coupled receptors: promise and progress. Trends Pharmacol Sci. 2014;35(7):308–16.

Waldhoer M, Fong J, Jones RM, Lunzer MM, Sharma SK, Kostenis E, et al. A heterodimer-selective agonist shows in vivo relevance of G protein-coupled receptor dimers. Proc Natl Acad Sci U S A. 2005;102(25):9050–5.

Walther C, Ferguson SS. Arrestins: role in the desensitization, sequestration, and vesicular trafficking of G protein-coupled receptors. Prog Mol Biol Transl Sci. 2013;118:93–113.

Wang C, Wu H, Katritch V, Han GW, Huang XP, Liu W, et al. Structure of the human smoothened receptor bound to an antitumour agent. Nature. 2013;497(7449):338–43.

Wheatley M, Hawtin SR. Glycosylation of G-protein-coupled receptors for hormones central to normal reproductive functioning: its occurrence and role. Hum Reprod Update. 1999;5(4):356–64.

White JH, Wise A, Main MJ, Green A, Fraser NJ, Disney GH, et al. Heterodimerization is required for the formation of a functional GABA(B) receptor. Nature. 1998;396(6712):679–82.

Whorton MR, Bokoch MP, Rasmussen SG, Huang B, Zare RN, Kobilka B, et al. A monomeric G protein-coupled receptor isolated in a high-density lipoprotein particle efficiently activates its G protein. Proc Natl Acad Sci U S A. 2007;104(18):7682–7.

Whorton MR, Jastrzebska B, Park PS, Fotiadis D, Engel A, Palczewski K, et al. Efficient coupling of transducin to monomeric rhodopsin in a phospholipid bilayer. J Biol Chem. 2008;283(7):4387–94.

Wu B, Chien EY, Mol CD, Fenalti G, Liu W, Katritch V, et al. Structures of the CXCR4 chemokine GPCR with small-molecule and cyclic peptide antagonists. Science. 2010;330(6007):1066–71.

Yan Y, Chi PP, Bourne HR. RGS4 inhibits Gq-mediated activation of mitogen-activated protein kinase and phosphoinositide synthesis. J Biol Chem. 1997;272(18):11924–7.

Zhang D, Zhao Q, Wu B. Structural studies of G protein-coupled receptors. Mol Cells. 2015;38(10):836–42.

Receptor Tyrosine Kinases and the Insulin Signaling System

6

Morris F. White

Abstract

Protein tyrosine kinases (PTKs) are encoded by a large multigene family. PTKs regulate many aspects of metabolism, growth, and cancer progression – including cell proliferation, differentiation, and survival, adhesion and motility, and systemic nutrient homeostasis (Schlessinger 2014; Robinson et al. 2000; Lemmon and Schlessinger 2010). Of the approximately 90 unique PTKs in the human genome, 58 are cell-surface RTKs (receptor tyrosine kinases), which pass once through the plasma membrane (Fig. 1). The extracellular ligand-binding domains translate the rise and fall of circulating polypeptide growth factors, cytokines, and hormones into unique patterns of intracellular signals (Lemmon and Schlessinger 2010); cell-cell interactions regulate some RTK family members. In the first part of this chapter, I will summarize the RTK landscape and describe how deep understanding of the EGFR (epidermal growth factor receptor) set the stage to understand RTK signaling. In the second part, I focus upon the insulin receptor signaling cascade and its heterologous regulation, because it has a broad role in metabolic regulation and is my principle interest for the past 30 years.

Keywords

Protein tyrosine kinase receptor signaling • Insulin signaling • IRS1 • IRS2 • EGF signaling

M.F. White (✉)
Division of Endocrinology, Boston Children's Hospital, Harvard Medical School, Boston, MA, USA
e-mail: morris.white@childrens.harvard.edu

A. Belfiore, D. LeRoith (eds.), *Principles of Endocrinology and Hormone Action*, Endocrinology, https://doi.org/10.1007/978-3-319-44675-2_7

Contents

Introduction

Ligand binding usually promotes the formation of RTK dimers – or in a few cases modifies a preexisting dimer – which activates the intracellular catalytic domain to transfer γ-phosphate from ATP onto specific tyrosyl residues of the RTK complex. This autophosphorylation reaction – which usually occurs in "trans" – is the first response to ligand-induced dimerization. Heterologous adapter proteins and enzymes recruited to the autophosphorylated sites can also be tyrosine phosphorylated. Depending upon their distribution in space and duration in time, these diverse proximal signals generate or regulate downstream effectors that control cytoplasmic and nuclear events – including the production of phospholipid mediators, GTP/GDP cycles, the activity or location of transcription factors, or cascades of Ser/Thr phosphorylation.

RTKs dysregulated by mutations, toxins, or challenging lifestyles can promote acute or chronic disease – including cancer, obesity, cardiometabolic disease, and diabetes. The life-threatening sequelae of dysregulated or amplified RTKs – such as ERBB2 (HER2, human epidermal growth factor receptor 2) – drive the development of new drugs to block RTK activity with enough specificity to prevent the progression of disease with minimal off-target consequences (Lemmon and Schlessinger 2010).In the subset of human cancers associated with an amplified ERBB2 gene – breast, ovary, stomach, lung, and salivary gland – the ERBB2-blocking antibody Herceptin (trastuzumab) can be beneficial (Mates et al. 2015).

The RTK Landscape

Introduction

Years before the discovery of PTKs, early work established the existence of specific cell-surface receptors for insulin, EGF, NGF (nerve growth factor), and other factors. The families of RTKs grew rapidly upon identification of the EGFR tyrosine kinase (Schlessinger 2014). In 1980, Ushiro and Cohen discovered that EGF treatment ofA431 cell membrane preparations activates immediately a cAMP/cGMP-independent protein kinase activity (Carpenter et al. 1979). The specificity of the EGF-sensitive kinase toward tyrosine residues was revealed by new electrophoretic methods to separate phosphotyrosine from phosphothreonine developed during the investigation of v-Src phosphorylation (the transforming PTK encoded by the *Rous sarcoma virus* (Hunter and Sefton 1980; Ushiro and Cohen 1980). During the next few years, phosphotyrosine was detected in the presumptive receptors for insulin and PDGF (platelet-derived growth factor), which indicated strongly that cell metabolism and growth might be regulated by RTKs (Kasuga et al. 1982a, b; Ek and Heldin 1982; Ek et al. 1982). Regardless, the prototype RTK was not established definitively until biochemical analysis of the EGFR revealed partial amino acid sequences with strong similarities to the v-erbB oncogene, and cDNA cloning provided the complete deduced amino acid sequence of the tyrosine kinase domain (Ullrich et al. 1984; Ullrich and Schlessinger 1990).Work during the next 10 years – including the full sequence of human genomes – revealed 20 families of human RTKs (Robinson et al. 2000). The family members are type I transmembrane proteins anchored in the plasma membrane by a single hydrophobic sequence, which separates the highly variable extracellular ligand-binding domain from the highly conserved intracellular tyrosine kinase (Fig. 1).

Each RTK family displays common and unique biological properties owing to its tissue specificity and timing of expression; intracellular trafficking, degradation, and recycling; the cohort of downstream signaling proteins recruited to the autophosphorylated receptor; and feedback mechanisms that modulate the signal intensity and duration. In many cases, multiple receptor isoforms can form heterologous

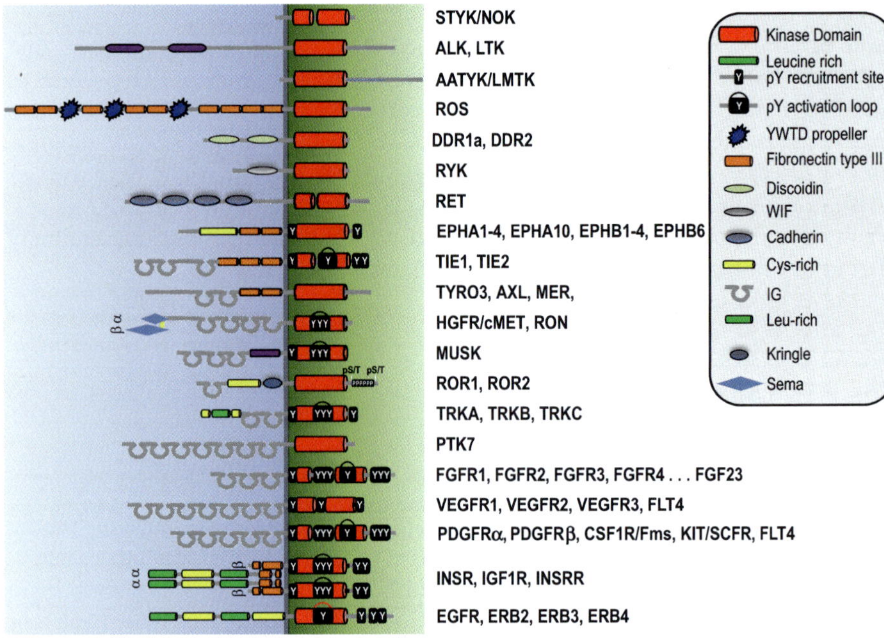

Fig. 1 The 20 families of human RTKs (receptor tyrosine kinases). The extracellular region is illustrated to the *left* on the *blue-shaded* background; the intracellular tyrosine kinase is illustrated to the *right* on the *green-shaded* background. Functional domains are defined in the *gray box*

receptor dimers with many ligands to generate distinct downstream signals. The ERBB family is the prototype RTKs. Its structural and functional features provide a solid framework to understand the mechanisms of regulated and dysregulated signal transduction (Lemmon et al. 2016). Although the function of most RTKs is still poorly understood at both the molecular and systemic level, the search for specific activators and inhibitors – some of which are already clinically available or in clinical trials – has been underway for years.

ERBB Family

EGFR is the prototype ERBB family member (Fig. 1) (Schlessinger 2014).EGFR binds several ligands in addition to EGF – including TGFα (transforming growth factor-α), HBEGF (heparin-binding EGF-like growth factor), AREG (amphiregulin), BTC (betacellulin), EREG (epiregulin), and (EPGN (epigen) (Schneider and Wolf 2009). By comparison, ERBB2 lacks a known ligand but dimerizes with the other ERBB members to generate a signal. ERBB3 binds neuregulin but lacks an active kinase domain; neuregulins are a family of four structurally related proteins and spliced isoforms with diverse functions in the development of the nervous system, cardiac development, Schwann cell and oligodendrocyte differentiation, and formation of neuromuscular synapses

(Burden and Yarden 1997). ERBB4 is activated by neuregulin-2 and neuregulin-3, HBEGF, and BTC. The tyrosyl-phosphorylated EGFR has multiple interaction partners, including SHC (SRC homology 2 domain containing), CBL (casitas B-lineage lymphoma), PTPN11 (protein-tyrosine phosphatase 1D (PTP-1D), STAT5 (signal transducer and activator of transcription 5), CRK (v-crk avian sarcoma virus), and several sites for GRB2 (growth factor receptor-bound protein 2) (Schulze et al. 2005). SHC is the major interaction partner for ERBB2; ERBB3 interacts mainly with the PI3K (class 1A phosphatidylinositol 3-kinase); and ERBB4 has many partners (Schulze et al. 2005).Insufficient ERBB signaling associates with neurodegenerative diseases, schizophrenia, and amyotrophic lateral sclerosis, whereas excess ERBB signaling promotes solid tumors (Lemmon and Schlessinger 2010).

Insulin Receptor Family

The receptors for insulin (InsR) and insulin-like growth factors (IGF1 and IGF2) occur as preexisting but inactive dimers linked by disulfide bonds (Fig. 1). The InsR plays a key role in nutrient homeostasis and the IGFR controls tissue and body growth. These tetrameric receptors are synthesized as single polypeptides which upon cleavage at a furin site generate disulfide-linked α- and β-subunits ($\alpha\beta^{IR}$ or $\alpha\beta^{IGF1R}$). These dimers assemble with additional disulfide bonds to form the InsR ($\alpha\beta^{IR}\bullet\alpha\beta^{IR}$), IGF1R ($\alpha\beta^{IGF1R}\bullet\alpha\beta^{IGF1R}$), or hybrid receptors ($\alpha\beta^{IR}\bullet\ \alpha\beta^{IGF1R}$) (Benyoucef et al. 2007). Since the InsR occurs in two isoforms, a total of five receptors subtypes can be produced from the InsR and IGF1R genes (Blanquart et al. 2008). Dysfunctional INSRs cause rare forms of severe insulin resistance, metabolic disease, and growth abnormalities (Kahn et al. 1976). The IRS (insulin receptor substrate) proteins are the principle targets phosphorylated by the insulin receptor family, which provides a platform for multiple downstream signals that can be regulated through feedback and heterologous mechanisms (see details below).

Platelet-Derived Growth Factor Family

The PDGFR family has five members that are important for regulating cell proliferation, cellular differentiation, cell growth, development, and cancer (Fig. 1). The extracellular regions of these receptors contain five immunoglobulin-like domains, whereas the intracellular region contains a distinctive tyrosine kinase domain with a relatively long "kinase insert region." The PDGFR isoforms – PDGFRα and PDGFRβ – can dimerize with four PDGF isoforms (PDGFA, PDGFB, PDGFC, and PDGFD). PDGFs contain a conserved region, which remains noncovalently associated after processing to form a dimer that binds and activates two PDGFRs (Shim et al. 2010). The four PDGF ligands (PDGFA, PDGFB, PDGFC, PDGFD) are under independent genetic control, which gives the signaling system a high degree of flexibility – including the generation of PDGF homo- or heterodimers (PDGFAA, PDGFAB, PDGFBB,

PDGFCC, PDGFDD) and the formation of three dimeric receptors αα, ββ, and αβ. Sites of tyrosine autophosphorylation in the PDGFβ receptor recruit signaling molecules to the juxtamembrane domain (SHC, STAT5, SRC), the kinase insert region (GRB2, PI3K, SHC, NCK, SHP2, RasGAP, STAT5), and the C-terminal tail (PLCγ, SHP2) (Kazlauskas and Cooper 1989). Phosphorylation of a single tyrosine residue in the second kinase domain promotes the catalytic activity of this RTK (Heldin and Lennartsson 2013). Enhanced PDGF•PDGFR signaling is a hallmark of a variety of diseases, including cancers, atherosclerosis, pulmonary fibrosis, and restenosis (Ostman 2004).

Fibroblast Growth Factor Receptor Family

FGFRs (fibroblast growth factor receptors) consist of four members that bind to the largest family of growth factors, including 22 distinct FGFs (Fig. 1). FGFs are a family of growth factors, with members involved in angiogenesis, wound healing, embryonic development, and various endocrine signaling pathways. Most FGFs are key players in tissue-specific proliferation and differentiation – especially during development – because they signal at the site of secretion owing to specific binding to cell-surface-associated heparan sulfate proteoglycans that restrict their diffusion into the circulation. Like the insulin receptor, FGFRs recruit adapter molecules for tyrosyl phosphorylation that add diversity to the signaling complexes (Lemmon and Schlessinger 2010). A few FGFs– including FGF19, FGF21, and FGF23 – escape the site of secretion because they lack a heparin-binding domain and can enter the circulation to signal at distant sites (Fisher and Maratos-Flier 2016; Reitman 2007).Without heparin binding, Fgf21 signals via FGFR1 and FGFR2 in complex with the co-receptor βKlotho (KLB) (Fisher and Maratos-Flier 2016). Circulating Fgf21 is produced almost entirely by PPARα-mediated transcription in the liver (Badman et al. 2007; Markan et al. 2014), where Fgf21 cell autonomously promotes fatty acid oxidation (Fisher et al. 2014).Cold exposure and β-adrenergic agonists stimulate Fgf21 secretion within the adipose tissue to promote energy expenditure and metabolic health by uncoupling BAT mitochondria (Hondares et al. 2011; Chartoumpekis et al. 2011) and "browning" inguinal white adipose tissue (Fisher et al. 2012).

Vascular Endothelial Growth Factor Receptor Family

VEGFR-1, VEGFR-2, and VEGFR-3 are important for monocytes/macrophages and blood vascular endothelial and lymphatic endothelial cells in both physiology and cancer (Claesson-Welsh 2016).Hypoxia induces VEGFR1 expression through a hypoxia-inducible enhancer element in the VEGFR1 promoter (Nomura et al. 1995). Five mammalian dimeric VEGF polypeptides (VEGFA, VEGFB, VEGFC, and VERGFD) and PIGF (placenta growth factors) are spliced (VEGFA, VEGFB, and VEGFC) or processed (VEGFC and VEGFD) to generate a wide range of isoforms that dimerize to activate the VEGFRs. Moreover, signaling is further diversified by neuropilins, heparan sulfate, and integrins, which act as VEGF co-receptors (Koch et al. 2011). Upon ligand-induced dimerization, the VEGFR1 activates the PKCγ→PKC cascade that produces mild MAPK (mitogen-activated protein kinase) activity. It also activates the PI3K→AKT cascade (Koch et al. 2011; Shibuya 2006). Since the RTK activity of VEGFR1 is comparatively weak, it displays mild activity toward migration/proliferation.

Hepatocyte Growth Factor Receptor

HGFR (hepatocyte growth factor receptor, cMet) is similar structurally to the insulin receptor. The HGF pro-peptide is cleaved to generate a disulfide-stabilized α-β dimer that dimerizes to activate the HGFR (Fajardo-Puerta et al. 2016). Kinase activation promotes autophosphorylation, which recruits GRB2, SHC, PI3-kinase, PLCγ, STAT3, and GAB1 (Grb2-associated binding protein 1). The downstream signaling pathways generate diverse cellular responses, including proliferation, survival, motility, invasion, and angiogenesis (Fig. 1). HGFR is essential for embryonic development, organogenesis, and wound healing, whereas its abnormal activation is associated with cancer of the kidney, liver, stomach, breast, and brain (Zhang and Babic 2016). Since HGF is the only known ligand, the HGF→HGFR axis is an attractive drug target for activation or inhibition. A hybrid receptor created through the interaction of the HGFR with the InsR might promote tyrosine phosphorylation and activation of the InsR→Irs signaling revealing a role in metabolic control (Fafalios et al. 2011).

TRK Family

TRKA, TRKB, and TRKC (tropomyosin receptor kinases) regulate synaptic strength and plasticity in the mammalian nervous system. TRK receptors affect neuronal survival and differentiation and promote the functional properties of neurons. Homodimeric neurotrophins are the common ligands of the TRKRs: NGF (nerve growth factor) and NT3 (neurotrophin-3) bind TRKA; brain-derived neurotrophic factor (BDNF), NT3, and NT4 (neurotrophin-4) bind TRKB; and NT3 binds TRKC. A member of the tumor necrosis factor receptor superfamily $p75^{NTR}$ (p75 neurotrophin receptor) affects the binding affinity and specificity of TRK receptor activation by neurotrophins (Bothwell 2016). This selectivity can produce complex results as illustrated with sympathetic neurons, which express TRKA and $p75^{NTR}$, but not TRKB (Bothwell 2016). Neurotrophin binding promotes dimerization and activation of the TRKRs, which undergo trans-autophosphorylation on three tyrosine residues in the "activation loop," and at other sites to recruit SHC, SH2B (SH2B adapter protein 2), GRB2, PI3K, STAT, and PLCγ (Huang and Reichardt 2003). Regardless, a system level understanding is largely incomplete (Bothwell 2016).

Erythropoietin-Producing Hepatocellular Receptor Family

EPHRs (erythropoietin-producing human hepatocellular receptors) form the largest known subfamily of RTKs with a complicated signaling mechanism. EPHRs are classified into nine EPHA or five EPHB subfamilies depending upon whether they bind to glycophosphatidylinositol-linked (ephrin-As) or transmembrane (ephrin-Bs) ligands (Kania and Klein 2016). EPHRs are composed of a Cys-rich domain, two fibronectin (FN) domains, and an NH_2-terminal extracellular ligand-binding domain (LBD) that binds to the extracellular domain of membrane-tethered ephrins. The signaling mechanisms are complex because EPHRs and ephrins can act simultaneously as receptors and ligands, leading to bidirectional – parallel or antiparallel – signaling. Crystal structures of ephrin↔EPHR interactions reveal complex and alternative patterns of oligomerization. Forward ephrin→EPHR signaling requires autophosphorylation in the EPHR intracellular juxtamembrane domain (Kania and Klein 2016; Kullander et al. 2001), which recruits various adapters and enzymes – including Nck1 (non-catalytic region of tyrosine kinase adaptor protein 1) and Nck2, PI3K, Src family kinases, and Vav2/Vav3 (guanine nucleotide exchange factors for the Rho family of GTP-binding proteins). For reverse signaling, intracellular domains of ephrin-B are tyrosine phosphorylated by Src PTKs, which can recruit the Grb4•Pak1•Dock180 complex (Kania and Klein 2016; Palmer et al. 2002). Together this signaling mechanism regulates cell proliferation, repulsion, migration, and adhesion, which are important in developmental processes such as pattern formation and morphogenesis of segmented structures and neural connections (Kania and Klein 2016). Bidirectional ephrin↔EPHR signaling also controls energy metabolism as it mediates communication between pancreatic islet β-cells to regulate insulin secretion: EphrinA→EPHRA forward signaling inhibits insulin secretion, whereas reverse signaling stimulates it (Konstantinova et al. 2007). First identified in an erythropoietin-producing hepatoma cell line, ephrin↔EPHR also promotes cancer and other diseases.

TAM-Receptor Family

TYRO3, AXL, and MERTK (tyrosine-protein kinase Mer) are homologous RTKs that are essential for immune homeostasis (Rothlin et al. 2015). TAM RTKs have sequence similarity to the insulin receptor, cMET, and RON tyrosine kinase subdomains (Rothlin et al. 2015). TAM RTKs are activated by PROS1 (protein S) or GAS6 (growth arrest-specific gene 6) and differentially modulated by the presence of apoptotic cells, phosphatidylserine-containing lipid vesicles, and enveloped virus (Tsou et al. 2014). AXL can be activated by conventional ligand-dependent dimerization with GAS6, ligand-independent dimerization, interaction between two monomers on neighboring cells, or heteromeric dimerization (Janssen et al. 1991). The TAM family regulates cell proliferation, survival, adhesion migration, blood clot stabilization, and regulation of inflammatory cytokine release (Janssen et al. 1991). Autophosphorylation of MERTK provides docking sites for GRB2 or PLCG2 and induces phosphorylation of MAPK1, MAPK2, FAK/PTK2, or RAC1. MERTK signaling plays a role in various processes such as macrophage clearance of apoptotic cells, platelet aggregation, cytoskeleton reorganization, and engulfment. Deficiencies in TAM signaling associate with chronic inflammatory and broad-spectrum autoimmunity involving a severe lymphoproliferative disorder (Lu and Lemke 2001).

Tyrosine Kinase with Immunoglobulin-Like and EGF-Like Domains

TIE1 and TIE2 (tyrosine kinase with immunoglobulin-like and EGF-like domains) are cell-surface receptors that are activated by ANG1, ANG2, ANG3, and ANG4(angiopoietins). TIERs consist of three Ig-like domains, three EGF domains, and three FNIII (fibronectin type III) repeats in the extracellular region. The catalytic domain of TIERs displays 45% sequence identity with the FGFR1 and is activated by receptor tetramerization facilitated by the multimeric angiopoietin ligands (Barton et al. 2014). Similar to ErbB receptors, the activation loop in TIE2R adopts an overall "active conformation" independent of phosphorylation; however, the carboxy-terminal tail acts as a substrate mimetic to inhibit autophosphorylation. Tyrosine phosphorylation in the C-terminus recruits Grb2, PI3K, PTPN11, and DOK2 (Barton et al. 2014). ANG→TIER signaling is essential during embryonic vessel assembly and maturation and functions as a key regulator of adult vascular homeostasis. ANG2 antagonizes the activation of TIER by ANG1, whereas alone ANG2 can activate TIERs. Like PDGFR, TIERs contain a kinase insert region with autophosphorylation sites that bind and activate the PI3K→AKT cascade. Mice lacking either ANG1 or TIE2 die before birth (Suri et al. 1996). By contrast, dysregulated ANG→TIER axis can promote malignant neoplasia by inducing angiogenesis (Hilbert and Klaschik 2015).

RYK and ROR Families

Ryk (related to receptor tyrosine kinase) and Ror (receptor tyrosine kinase-like orphan receptor) families were classified initially as orphan RTKs but are now known to contain extracellular WNT (wingless)-binding domains (Green et al. 2014). ROR and RYK display extracellular membrane-proximal Kringle domains that can mediate protein-protein interactions and Frizzled-like CDRs (cysteine-rich domains) that bind WNT. RYK displays a second WNT-binding module called the WIF (WNT-inhibitory factor) domain. WNT ordinarily activates Frizzled, a family of G protein-coupled receptors, which regulate cell proliferation and differentiation. RYK and ROR are mostly associated with polarized cell migration. ROR1 and RYK might be pseudo kinases, whereas

ROR2 contains a functional intracellular tyrosine kinase domain related to the Trk-family (Oishi et al. 2003). Interestingly, both $Ror2^{-/-}$ and $Wnt5a^{-/-}$mice exhibit dwarfism, facial abnormalities, short limbs and tails, dysplasia of lungs and genitals, and ventricular septal defects. Together with interaction studies, these physiological results suggest that RORs act as receptors for Wnt5a to activate non-canonical WNT signaling (Green et al. 2014).The phosphorylation of ROR1 might be mediated by complexes with the EGFR or HGFR (Borcherding et al. 2014). In lung carcinoma and gastric carcinoma cell lines, ROR1 is phosphorylated by MET, and silencing ROR1 impairs cell growth. Since ROR1 is absent in most adult tissue, it might be druggable target for some cancer therapies.

Discoidin Domain Receptor Family

DDR1 (discoidin domain receptor tyrosine kinase 1) and DDR2 (Vogel et al. 1997) are expressed in normal and transformed epithelial cells and activated by various types of collagen, which stimulate tyrosine autophosphorylation to promote poorly defined cell-collagen interactions (Fu et al. 2013). Alternative splicing of the DDR genes results in multiple transcript that are expressed mainly in the kidney, lung, gastrointestinal tract, and brain; and overexpressed in human tumors from the breast, ovary, esophagus, and brain. DDRs are major cellular sensors of environmental cues and appear critical for normal development as revealed by the phenotype of DDR-deficient mice (Fu et al. 2013). Phosphorylation of tyrosine residues in the intracellular domains – including an NPXY motif in the juxtamembrane region – generates docking sites for SH2 and PTB (phosphotyrosine binding) domain-containing proteins, respectively, which promote the activation of the PI3K → AKT and SHC → Ras → MAPK cascades (Fu et al. 2013).

RET Family

RET (rearranged during transfection) proto-oncogene encodes an RTK for the glial cell line-derived neurotrophic factor family (GDNF, neurturin, artemin, and persephin) that supports the survival of dopaminergic and motor neurons (Knowles et al. 2006; Oppenheim et al. 1995).Loss-of-function mutations in RET are implicated in Hirschsprung disease, a congenital condition owing to missing nerve cells in the colon that impairs colon motility. Activating RET mutations occur in human cancers, including familial medullar thyroid carcinoma and multiple endocrine neoplasia 2A and 2B (Knowles et al. 2006). Structural studies suggest that the canonical activation loop resides in a phosphorylation independent "open" conformation, suggesting that a novel mechanism might controls RET signaling (Knowles et al. 2006). Regardless, phosphorylation at several tyrosine residues (two of them in the activation loop) are important for signaling (Coulpier et al. 2002).

Tyrosine-Protein Kinase-Like 7 Family

PTK7 (tyrosine-protein kinase-like 7) is a RTK that was discovered originally in colon cancer (Mossie et al. 1995). PTK7 functions in various processes including embryonic morphogenesis and epidermal wound repair (Peradziryi et al. 2012). It functions as a co-receptor in Wnt, semaphorin/plexin, and VEGF signaling pathways. Although PTK7 does not contain a canonical WNT-binding domain, it appears to interact with some WNTs to inhibit WNT→β-catenin signaling (Peradziryi et al. 2011). PTK7 recruits Dsh (Dishevelled), which regulates canonical (β-catenin) and non-canonical Wnt signaling pathways. Although the kinase homology domain is largely conserved, it lacks amino acid motifs critical for catalytic activity (Peradziryi et al. 2012). Thus, PTK7→Dsh might be mediated by RACK1 (receptor for activated C kinase 1) that interacts with protein kinase C and the kinase domain of PTK7.

Muscle-Specific Kinase Family

MuSK (muscle-specific kinase) is a RTK required for the formation and maintenance of the neuromuscular junction. The ligand for MuSK is LRP4 (low-density lipoprotein receptor-related protein-4), a transmembrane protein in muscle whose binding affinity for MuSK is potentiated by a neuronally derived heparan sulfate proteoglycan called AGRIN. AGRIN is a component of the basal lamina that causes the aggregation of acetylcholine receptors on cultured muscle fibers (Rupp et al. 1991). MuSK undergoes trans-autophosphorylation on three tyrosine residues in the activation loop (Y750, Y654, Y755), which increases kinase activity and biological function (Bergamin et al. 2010). Interestingly, phosphorylation of the $NPXY_{553}$ motif in the juxtamembrane binds to the PTB domain of the adapter protein DOK7. DOK7 serves as a substrate of MuSK and as a cytoplasmic ligand to stabilize the MuSK dimer facilitating trans-autophosphorylation in the activation loop (Bergamin et al. 2010). Thus, LRP4, AGRIN, and DOK7 cooperate to fully activate MuSK to induce clustering of acetylcholine receptors (AChR) essential for the postsynaptic structures. Failure of AChR clustering is associated with disorders in neuromuscular transmission, including congenital myasthenic syndrome and myasthenia gravis (Okada et al. 2006).

Apoptosis-Associated Tyrosine Kinase 1/Lemur Kinase Family

AATYK1 (apoptosis-associated tyrosine kinase 1)/LMTK (Lemur kinase) family of RTKs is expressed predominantly in the nervous system where they can regulate neurite extension and apoptosis (Gaozza et al. 1997). Although the kinase domain of AATYK is most like the PTK families, AATYKs display serine phosphorylation that might be mediated by Cdk5 (cell division protein kinase 5) (Tomomura et al. 2007).

Recent work suggests that LMTK1 negatively controls dendritic formation by regulating Rab11A (Ras-related protein Rab-11A)-positive endosomal trafficking in a Cdk5-dependent manner (Takano et al. 2014).

Serine/Threonine/Tyrosine Kinase)/Novel Oncogene with Kinase Domain Family

STYK (serine/threonine/tyrosine kinase)/NOK (novel oncogene with kinase domain) is 30% homologous with members of the FGFR/PDGFR family on the intracellular tyrosine kinase domain (Liu et al. 2004). Although the 422-amino acid protein contains an N-terminal transmembrane domain and a C-terminal RTK, it lacks an extracellular domain for ligand binding, suggesting that it might be a co-receptor. STYK1 can activate MAPK and PI3K pathways and promotes cell proliferation, differentiation, and survival. STYK1 is dysregulated in several human malignancies including breast, lung, ovary, blood, prostate, and colorectal cancer (Hu et al. 2015).

Anaplastic Lymphoma Kinase Family

ALK (anaplastic lymphoma kinase) and LTK (leukocyte receptor tyrosine kinase) are expressed throughout the adult mammalian hippocampus CA1 and CA3 regions (Weiss et al. 2012). ALK contains an extracellular binding site for the basic heparin-binding growth factors pleiotrophin (neurite growth-promoting factor 1, NEGF1) and midkine (neurite growth-promoting factor 2, NEGF2). Both factors distribute similarly to ALK in the nervous system during fetal development. NEGGF2 is a developmentally important retinoic acid-responsive gene product strongly induced during mid-gestation – hence the name midkine. The intracellular regions of both ALK and LTK are related to the insulin receptor family (Grande et al. 2011). The intracellular juxtamembrane region contains a binding site for the PTB (phosphotyrosine binding) domain of IRS1 (insulin receptor substrate-1); and the catalytic domain contains three autophosphorylation sites in the activation loop followed by the C-terminal domain with interaction sites for PLCγ and SHC (Tartari et al. 2008). Interestingly, inhibition of ALK in mammals enhances cognitive performance (Weiss et al. 2012). By comparison, alterations in the ALK gene, including mutations, overexpression, amplification, translocations, or other structural rearrangements are implicated in human cancer (Grande et al. 2011; Schonherr et al. 2012). ALK activates many interconnected and overlapping pathways, including PI3K, AKT, ERK, and STAT3 (Grande et al. 2011).

ROS Family

ROS1 (ROS proto-oncogene) belongs to the drosophila sevenless subfamily of tyrosine kinase genes, and is related closely to ALK and LTK. The extracellular domain contains sequences that are analogous to sequences found in cell adhesion molecules and extracellular matrix proteins. ROS might be involved in cellular attachment, as a soluble ligand is unknown. Activated ROS promotes signaling through PLCγ, PI3K→AKT, STAT3, VAV3, and ERK. ROS1 rearrangements are detected in a variety of human cancers, including glioblastoma, non-small cell lung cancer, ovarian cancer, gastric adenocarcinoma, and colorectal cancer (Davies and Doebele 2013).

EGFR Dimerization and Activation

RTK dimers or higher order oligomers are probably required, but not always sufficient for signal transduction (Lemmon and Schlessinger 2010). The exact steady-state distribution between monomer and oligomer depends upon the intrinsic structure of each RTK and the effect of ligand binding. At one extreme, the receptors for insulin and IGF1 (insulin-like growth factor 1) exist as inactive covalently linked tetramers before ligand binding. However, for others the unliganded receptors exist in a steady-state distribution between monomer and dimer. The steady-state distribution probably depends upon the concentration of the RTK and any homologous partners in the plasma membrane, the basal ligand concentration, and the concentration of any auxiliary components or inhibitory factors (Lemmon et al. 2016). Extracellular ligand binding stabilizes the RTK dimer, which facilitates additional steps toward full activation usually involving juxtaposition of the adjacent catalytic domains to promote trans-autophosphorylation of tyrosine residues in the kinase activation loop (A-loop) and phosphorylation of tyrosine residues outside the catalytic domain to recruit heterologous signaling proteins (Schlessinger 2000; Burgess et al. 2003).

Remarkable progress during the past decades reveals a general framework to understand the regulation of RTKs upon extracellular ligand binding. The detailed mechanisms can differ between the families of RTKs; however, extensive cell biology, analysis of receptor mutants and orthologs, and crystal structures of EGFRs revealed a clear picture of the effect of EGF binding on receptor dimerization (Burgess et al. 2003). The extracellular EGFR resolves into four subdomains – designated I–IV (Fig. 2). The monomeric inactive EGFR has a bent configuration held together by intramolecular interactions between the dimerization arm (II) and the tethering arm (IV) (Ferguson et al. 2003). This "tethered conformation" separates the two EGF-binding sites and occludes the extracellular dimerization surfaces; however, a rare "extended conformation" exposes the dimerization arm (II) and juxtaposes the two EGF-binding sites (Fig. 2a and b) (Burgess et al. 2003). EGF binds with low affinity to the "tethered conformation" because it can only touch one binding surface (Fig. 2c), whereas EGF binds with high affinity to the "extended conformation" that exposes the binding sites in subdomains I and III (Fig. 2d). As the concentration of receptors in the extended conformation rises, more receptor dimerization surfaces are also available to promote receptor dimerization (Fig. 2e). Contrary to many other RTKs, the bound EGF molecules never interact in the dimer as

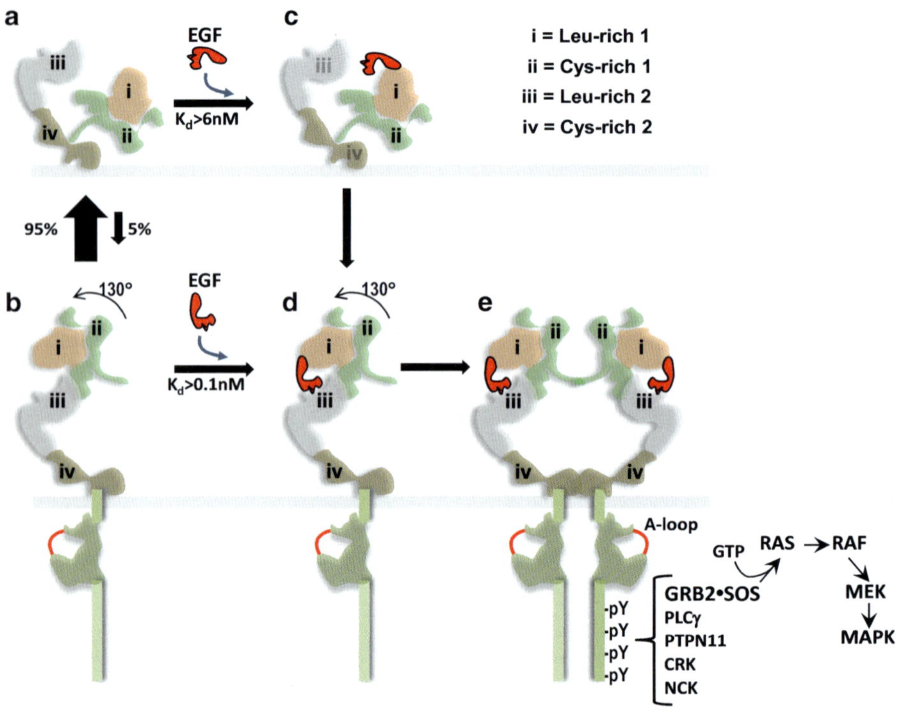

Fig. 2 Activation of the EGF receptor and downstream signaling. The extracellular EGFR contains four subdomains designated i, ii, iii, and iv. (**a**) The monomeric inactive EGFR is stabilized by interactions between domain ii and domain iv, which separates the two EGF-binding sites in domains I and iii, and occludes the extracellular dimerization surfaces of domains ii and iv: (c) EGF binds with low affinity to a single site in this conformation. (**b**) The inactive monomer exists in an unstable conformation that juxtaposes the EGF-binding sites in subdomains i and iii, which promote high-affinity binding and (**d**) dimerization. (**e**) Autophosphorylation of the juxtaposed intracellular domains recruits signaling protein, which generates various signals, including the MAPK cascade

the high-affinity binding sites in the dimerized receptor are never adjacent. Although well separated, the EGF-binding sites in the assembled dimer are not equivalent and develop some asymmetry – possibly related to changes that occur around the plasma membrane during autophosphorylation – which leads to negative cooperative EGF binding (Pike 2012).

A single hydrophobic transmembrane spanning segment separates the intracellular catalytic domain of all RTKs from the extracellular ligand-binding domain (Fig. 1) (Schlessinger 2014). Dimerization per se and subsequent conformational changes promote tyrosine autophosphorylation, suggesting that this is the first step in signal transduction. All RTKs contain 1–3 tyrosine residues in the activation loop (A-loop) of the intracellular catalytic domain where the first autophosphorylation occurs after ligand binding. Autophosphorylation of these residues stabilizes the

A-loop in an "open" configuration, which facilities ATP binding and phosphorylation of other tyrosine residues in the receptor or in heterologous substrates. Most of the tyrosine residues that become autophosphorylated on RTKs are in non-catalytic regions of the cytoplasmic domain, including the juxtamembrane region (e.g., PDGFR and KIT), the kinase insert region (e.g., FGFR and KIT), or the carboxyl terminal tail.

The EGFR is the prototype of the ErbB family of RTKs. By contrast to most RTKs, the A-loop of the EGFR resides constitutively in the open configuration usually reserved for phosphorylated A-loops, suggesting that kinase activation is not a regulatory event of EGF binding. EGFR trans-autophosphorylation mainly targets tyrosine residues in the adjacent carboxy-terminal tail of the receptor, which generates SH2 (Src homology-2) domain-binding sites that recruit signaling enzymes (PLCγ, Shp2, SOS) or adapters (GRB2, CRK, NCK).Thus, after dimer-mediated trans-autophosphorylation, the EGFR and its family members are platforms for assembly of multicomponent intracellular signaling pathways (Fig. 2e). Each RTKs has adapted its own version of this mechanism to link extracellular ligand binding to intracellular signal transduction.

The Insulin Receptor Family

Insulin has physiologic effects everywhere in the body, but it is secreted only from pancreatic β-cells. Insulin is synthesized as a single polypeptide (proinsulin) that is processed by PCSK1 (prohormone convertase-1/convertase-3) into the bioactive disulfide-linked A and B chains and the excised "C-peptide." Human IGF1 and IGF2 display high sequence similarity with both the A and B chains of insulin but retain the connecting peptide along with a C-terminal extension called the "D domain" (Brzozowski et al. 2002). Extensive analysis of natural insulin mutations supplemented with hypothesis-driven site-directed mutagenesis reveals two asymmetric receptor-binding surfaces called "S1" (the classical site) and "S2" (the novel site) (Fig. 3) (De Meyts 2008). Together both sites generate high-affinity insulin binding that activates the insulin receptor tyrosine kinase.

The insulin receptor (IR) is encoded by a 150-kb gene on human chromosome 19p13.3–p13.2 that contains 22 exons. Exon-11 is alternatively spiced depending upon the tissue and developmental stage to produce two InsR isoforms: IRA lacks the residues encoded by exon-11; IRB includes the 12 amino acid residues encoded by exon-11 (De Meyts 2008; Yang Feng et al. 1985; Seino and Bell 1989). IRB binds only insulin with high affinity, whereas IRA binds both insulin and IGF2 with moderate affinity (Belfiore et al. 2009). The homologous IGF1R is assembled without alternative splicing from a 19-exon gene located on human chromosome 15. The IGF1R binds IGF1 and IGF2 with high affinity but binds insulin weakly. A high-affinity ligand is unknown for the third member of the family called the IRR (insulin receptor-related receptor) (Shier and Watt 1989). The IRR appears to sense alkali conditions in the kidney to modulate systemic bicarbonate concentrations (Deyev et al. 2011).

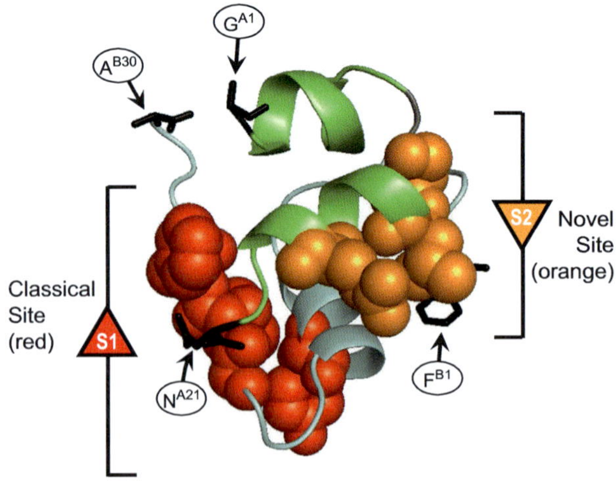

Fig. 3 The conformation of insulin and its receptor-binding site. Insulin structure showing the position of some critical amino acids that compose the two binding surfaces (*S1* and *S2*) that interact with the L1•CR•CT and $Fn_3$1•$Fn_3$2 regions of the insulin receptor, respectively. The A chain is shown in *green* and the B chain is shown in *blue*, and some amino acids composing each binding site are shown as space filling residues in *red* (*S1*) or *orange* (*S2*). The amino and carboxyl terminal residues of each chain are labeled in *black*

The insulin and IGF1 receptor precursors have similar structures, which are processed to form holoreceptors composed of two α-subunits and two β-subunits. The process is best characterized for the IR, which is synthesized as a single protein with a classical amino-terminal signal sequence followed by well-defined extracellular modules – including two leucine-rich motifs (L1 and L2) flanking a cysteine-rich (CR) region followed by three fibronectin III motifs ($Fn_3$1, $Fn_3$2, and $Fn_3$3) ending with a hydrophobic transmembrane spanning domain and the intracellular tyrosine kinase (Fig. 4). $Fn_3$2 is interrupted by a 120-amino-acid insert containing a furin cleavage site that generates upon cleavage the α- and β-subunits of the holoreceptor. Depending upon relative expression levels, the pro-receptors for insulin and IGF1 assemble either as disulfide-linked homodimers – IR ($\alpha\beta^{IR}$•$\alpha\beta^{IR}$) or the IGF1R ($\alpha\beta^{IGF1R}$•$\alpha\beta^{IGF1R}$) – or as hybrid receptors ($\alpha\beta^{IR}$• $\alpha\beta^{IGF1R}$) with approximate molecular masses of 350,000 by SDS-PAGE (Benyoucef et al. 2007). Since the insulin receptor occurs in two isoforms, five receptor types can be produced from the co-expressed receptor genes (Blanquart et al. 2008). Upon reduction of the disulfide bonds, SDS-PAGE resolves the InsR and IGF1R into the α- and β-subunits that migrate near 135-kDa and 95-kDa, respectively (Kasuga et al. 1982c; Hedo et al. 1983). Hybrid receptors can be detected by specific immunoblotting strategies (Benyoucef et al. 2007).

Like the EGFR, each insulin receptor α-subunit contains two insulin-binding sites, but unlike the EGFR a functional high-affinity site is created between adjacent α-subunits. Insulin binding begins through interactions between "S2" on insulin with the $Fn_3$1•$Fn_3$2 interface in the α-subunit (De Meyts et al. 2004). Sixteen amino acid

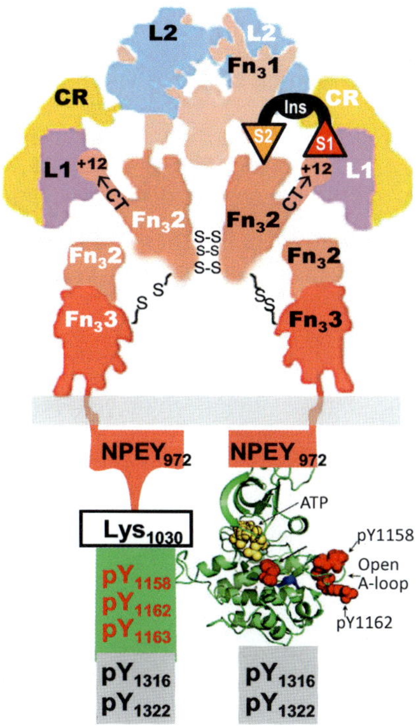

Fig. 4 A diagram of the activated insulin receptor. Diagram of the mature insulin receptor composed of two extracellular a-subunits and two intracellular b-subunits. Contiguous modules of the two α subunits are indicated by *black* or *white* labels and dashed tracings. The holoreceptor is stabilized extracellularly by disulfide bonds between cysteine residues (S-S) in the α- and β-subunits, as well as by noncovalent interactions. Two regions within the α-subunit contribute to insulin binding – including L1•CR (and the extra 12 amino acids encoded by exon-11 in the B form of the insulin receptor) that binds S1 of insulin and the junction between $Fn_3 1$ (the first fibronectin III domain) and $Fn_3 2$ that S2 of insulin. The β-subunit contains the tyrosine kinase catalytic domain with an ATP-binding site (Lys_{1030}) and several tyrosine phosphorylation sites, including those in the juxtamembrane region (pY_{972}), activation loop ($pY_{1158,\ 1162,\ 1163}$), and carboxyl terminal regions

residues at the COOH-terminus (CT) of $Fn_3 2$ interact with the L1•CR-region to create a composite insulin-binding site – L1 → CR → CT – that interacts with "S1" on insulin (Figs. 3 and 4). Although the α-subunits are arranged symmetrically in the dimer, there is a sharp bend between the L2 and $Fn_3 1$ → $Fn_3 2$ regions that juxtaposes the L1 → CR → CT domain antiparallel to $Fn_3 1$ → $Fn_3 2$ (Fig. 4) (Lawrence et al. 2007; Ward et al. 2007; McKern et al. 2006; Hubbard 2013; Vashisth and Abrams 2013). Insulin binds to the L1 → CR → CT domain of one α-subunit and to the $Fn_3 1$ → $Fn_3 2$ region of the adjacent α-subunit to create the cross-link that activates the kinase (Hubbard 2013). Only one insulin molecule can bind with high affinity (Lawrence et al. 2007; McKern et al. 2006; Kiselyov et al. 2009). Inclusion of exon-11 in IRB lengthens the CT-region by 12 amino acids, which modifies the

L1•CR•CT domain to exclude IGF2 binding and reduce strongly IGF1 affinity, while promoting high insulin-binding affinity. These details have been described in detail (Vashisth and Abrams 2013; Menting et al. 2013).

Structure and Regulation of the INSR Tyrosine Kinase

The discovery that rare cases of severe insulin resistance in humans associated with INSR mutations that inactivate the tyrosine kinase – without altering insulin binding – reveals tyrosyl phosphorylation as the principle signal that drives insulin signaling (Taylor 1999). The intracellular portion of the insulin receptor β-subunit is composed of three distinct regions that contain tyrosyl phosphorylation sites (numbered as in IRB): Y_{965} and Y_{972} in the juxtamembrane region between the transmembrane helix and the cytoplasmic tyrosine kinase domain; Y_{1158}, Y_{1162}, and Y_{1163} in the activation loop (A-loop) of the catalytic core; and Y_{1328} and Y_{1334} in the COOH-terminus (Ullrich et al. 1985; White et al. 1988; Rajagopalan et al. 1991) (Fig. 4). As summarized in the previous sections, most receptor tyrosine kinases are activated by ligand-induced dimerization, which brings two intracellular catalytic domains together to mediate tyrosine phosphorylation of the A-loop and the other sites that recruit cellular substrates (Schlessinger 2000). Since the homologous InsR and IGF1R reside in the plasma membrane as preformed but inactive covalent dimers, high-affinity insulin or IGF binding adds a transient cross-link to induce and stabilize structural transitions within the receptor that activate the intracellular catalytic site (Hubbard 2013).

Before insulin stimulation, the unphosphorylated Tyr_{1162} – the second of the three A-loop tyrosine residues – is positioned near the catalytic site, while the amino-terminal end of the A-loop (D_{1150}FG-motif) folds into the ATP-binding site elevating the apparent K_m for ATP (Hubbard 2013; Cann and Kohanski 1997; Hubbard et al. 1994). Since the closed A-loop exists in equilibrium with an open conformation, ATP occasionally gains access to mediate basal autophosphorylation (Till et al. 2001). Infrequent oscillation from the "closed" to an "open" conformation in the basal state might be coupled to complementary changes in the α-subunits, which can be stabilized by insulin binding to accelerate ATP entry and accelerate trans-autophosphorylation of Tyr_{1162}. Once initiated, the autophosphorylation cascade progresses to Tyr_{1158} but more slowly to Tyr_{1163}, which stabilizes the open conformation to allow unrestricted access by Mg-ATP and protein substrates (Hubbard 2013). This model of kinase regulation is supported by activation of the kinase upon substitution of Asp_{1161} with alanine in the middle of the A-loop, which shifts the steady-state conformation of the unphosphorylated A-loop toward the open configuration (Till et al. 2001). Substitution of Tyr_{1162} with phenylalanine also increases basal autophosphorylation, consistent with its role to stabilize the closed conformation or compete with ATP and protein substrates for binding at the kinase active site (Ellis et al. 1986; Wilden et al. 1992). Whether other kinases can activate the insulin receptor by phosphorylation of A-loop tyrosine residues independently of insulin is an open question that deserves attention.

The Insulin Receptor Substrates

Following discovery of the RTKs, many investigators searched for cellular proteins that might mediate downstream signals (Kasuga et al. 1982a; Kasuga et al. 1982b). The "substrate" hypothesis was an attractive mechanism from the beginning, but it was difficult to establish because beyond the RTKs themselves, only proteins with unlikely signaling potential were found initially (Cooper et al. 1983). The first evidence for a substrate of any RTK came from anti-phosphotyrosine antibody immunoprecipitates that revealed a 185-kDa phosphoprotein (pp185) in insulin-stimulated hepatoma cells (White et al. 1985). This protein displayed many features expected for a biologically important insulin receptor substrate – including immediate phosphorylation upon insulin stimulation and no phosphorylation by catalytically inactive or biologically inactive insulin receptors (White et al. 1988). Together these data provided the first clue that receptor autophosphorylation followed closely by substrate phosphorylation could be the initial step in signal transduction.

Purification and molecular cloning of pp185 revealed the first of a large family of signaling scaffolds and the first insulin receptor substrate called IRS1 (Sun et al. 1991). Four IRS-protein genes exist in rodents, but only three (IRS1, IRS2 and IRS4) are expressed in humans (Bjornholm et al. 2002). IRS1 and IRS2 are broadly expressed in mammalian tissues, whereas IRS4 is largely restricted to the hypothalamus (Numan and Russell 1999; Sadagurski et al. 2014). The IRS proteins are arguably the most important adapter molecules linking the InsR and IGF1R to downstream signaling cascades and heterologous regulatory components used by many signaling systems. Moreover, work with transgenic mice reveals that all insulin responses – especially those that are associated with somatic growth; carbohydrate, protein, and lipid metabolism; hepatic, adipose, skeletal muscle, and cardiovascular physiology; pancreatic β-cell function; and central nutrient homeostasis – are mediated through IRS1, IRS2, or both (White 2003).

IRS proteins are composed of tandem structurally similar PH and PTB domains followed by a long unstructured tail of tyrosine phosphorylation sites that coordinate the insulin/IGF signal. During insulin and IGF1 stimulation, some tyrosine residues in the tail are phosphorylated and recruit the SH2 domains of various signaling proteins, especially the 85 kDa regulatory subunit of the PI3K (White and Myers 2001). The interaction between IRS1 and PI3K was the first insulin signaling cascade to be reconstituted successfully in vivo and in vitro (Backer et al. 1992).

Specific insulin-stimulated tyrosine phosphorylation of the IRS protein is accomplished through at least two mechanisms – including specific recruitment of IRS to the juxtamembrane region of the InsR followed by recognition of preferred phosphorylation motifs by the "open" catalytic domain. Several motifs have been identified as optimal insulin receptor-mediated phosphorylation sites in IRS1 – including several YMXM-motifs and the YVNI-, YIDL-, and YASI-motifs (Songyang and Cantley 1995; Songyang et al. 1995; Shoelson et al. 1992; Hubbard 1997). These motifs are targeted by the InsR catalytic domain as antiparallel β-strands relative to

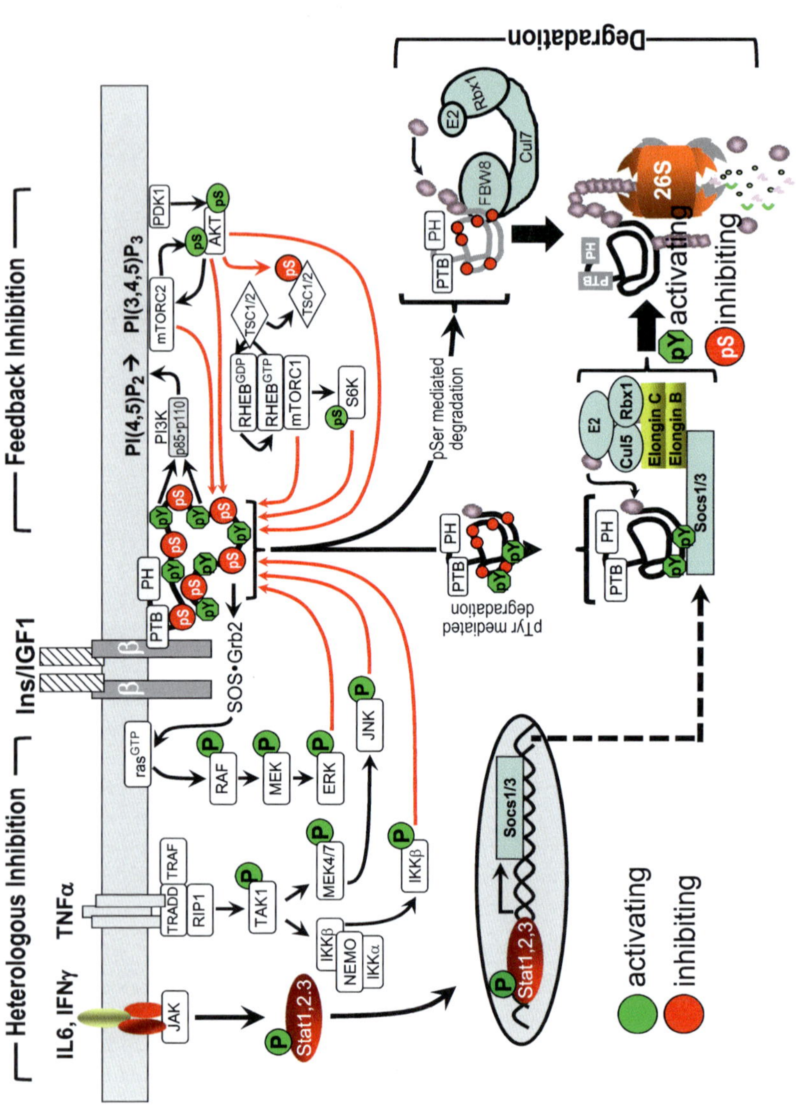

Fig. 5 (continued)

the COOH-terminal end of the open A-loop. This orientation positions the hydrophobic side chain in the Y^{+1} and Y^{+3} positions into two hydrophobic pockets on the activated kinase (Hubbard 1997).

The selective and regulated recruitment of IRS to the juxtamembrane region of the activated InsR and IGF1R is important for signaling specificity. The juxtamembrane region is about 35 residues long and connects the transmembrane helix of the IRβ subunit to the kinase domain (Figs. 4 and 5). Autophosphorylation of Tyr_{972} in the juxtamembrane region creates a docking site (...$NPEpY_{972}$...) for the PTB (phosphotyrosine binding) domain in the IRS proteins and in another signaling protein called SHC (White et al. 1988; Pelicci et al. 1992; Eck et al. 1996). The $NPEpY_{972}$-motif fills an L-shaped cleft on the PTB domain, while the N-terminal residues of the bound peptide form an additional strand in the β-sandwich (Eck et al. 1996). The $NPEpY_{972}$-motif is a low-affinity binding site for the PTB domain of IRS1 ($K_d \sim 87$ μM), owing to a destabilizing effect of E_{971} that facilitates autophosphorylation of Y_{972} by the insulin receptor (Hubbard 2013; Farooq et al. 1999). By comparison, the PTB domain of SHC binds to $NPEpY_{972}$ with a much higher affinity ($K_d \sim 4$ μM).

Regardless, the PH domain immediately upstream of the PTB domain helps recruit the IRSs to the InsR (Fig. 3) (Yenush et al. 1996). The PH domain is structurally similar but functionally distinct from the PTB domain (Dhe-Paganon et al. 1999). Although the PH domain promotes the interaction between IRS and the IR, its mechanism of action remains poorly understood as it does not bind phosphotyrosine. PH domains are generally thought to bind phospholipids, but the PH domains in IRS1 and IRS2 are poor examples of this binding specificity (Lemmon et al. 1996, 2002). These PH domains bind to negative patches in various proteins, which might be important for InsR recruitment (Burks et al. 1997). Regardless, the PH domain in IRS plays an important and specific role as it can be interchanged among the IRS-proteins without noticeable loss of bioactivity, whereas heterologous PH domains reduce IRS1 function when substituted for the IRS1 PH domain (Burks et al. 1998).

IRS2 utilizes an additional mechanism to interact with the insulin receptor, which is absent in IRS1. Amino acid residues 591 and 786 – especially Tyr_{624} and Tyr_{628} – in IRS2 mediate a strong interaction with the activated InsR catalytic site (Sawka-Verhelle et al. 1996, 1997). This binding region in IRS2 was originally called the

Fig. 5 Schematic diagram of heterologous and feedback inhibition of insulin signaling mediated by pS/T^{IRS1} or degradation. Various kinases in the insulin signaling cascade are implicated in this feedback mechanism, including PKB, mTOR, S6 K, ERK, AKT, and atypical PKC isoforms. Other IRS kinases are activated by heterologous signals, including lipids, TNFα, or other cytokines. Serine phosphorylation of IRS1 can recruit CRL7 ubiquitinylation complex to mediate degradation of IRSs through the 26S proteasome. Proinflammatory cytokines that cause insulin resistance also induce the expression of SOCS family members, which contain an NH_2-terminal SH2 domain and a COOH-terminal SOCS box (216,217). SOCS1 or SOCS3 can target phosphotyrosine residues in IRS1 or IRS2 for ubiquitinylation and degradation, because the SOCS box associates with elongin BC-containing ubiquitin ligase E3

kinase regulatory-loop binding (KRLB) domain because tris-phosphorylation of the A-loop was required to observe the interaction (Sawka-Verhelle et al. 1996). Structure analysis reveals an essential functional part of the KRLB domain – residues 620–634 in murine IRS2 – that fits into the "open" catalytic site of the insulin receptor (Wu et al. 2008). With the A-loop out of the catalytic site – by autophosphorylation or other means – Tyr_{621} of IRS2 inserts into the receptor ATP-binding pocket while Tyr_{628} aligns for phosphorylation. This interaction might attenuate signaling by blocking ATP access to the catalytic site, or it might promote signaling by opening the catalytic site before tris-autophosphorylation. Interestingly, the KRLB-motif does not bind to the IGF1R possibly explaining signaling differences between InsR and IGF1R, as well as the receptor hybrids (Wu et al. 2008).

Transcriptional Regulation of Insulin Signaling Components

Over a decade of genetic experiments in mice establishes that changes in the relative function of a broad array of insulin signaling components, nutrient sensors, and their downstream metabolic effectors can have profound effects upon insulin sensitivity and nutrient homeostasis. While this work is remarkably informative, the complexity and tissue specificity of heterologous regulation complicate the identification and design of strategies for the treatment of insulin resistance and its pathological sequela. Although the list of insulin signaling components and their interactions continues to grow, the IRSs retain a special place as the common integrating node that coordinates insulin responses in all tissues and cells. Indeed, a 50% reduction in the concentration of the IR, IRS1, and IRS2 achieved by genetic methods causes growth deficits and diabetes in mice (Kido et al. 2000). We are now aware of many heterologous pathways that regulate the concentration and function of these proximal insulin signaling components, but how dysregulation of these mechanisms contributes to the progression in humans of insulin resistance, metabolic disease, and type 2 diabetes is not understood well enough to guide the development of efficacious and safe treatments.

At the genomic level, various components in the insulin signaling cascade are regulated byYY1 (Yin Yang 1) – including IGF1 and IGF2, IRS1 and IRS2, and AKT1, AKT2, and AKT3 in skeletal muscle (Blattler et al. 2012). Although the concerted repression of multiple signaling components can have strong effects, reduced expression of individual signaling molecules can also lead to insulin resistance. Although decreased expression of IRS1 in patients and rodents is associated with diabetes, few studies have investigated whether dysregulated transcription of IRS1 might be involved. By contrast, IRS2 transcription is regulated by multiple factors, including CREB (cAMP response element-binding protein) and its coactivator CRTC2 (CREB-regulated transcription coactivator 2,), FOXO1/FOXO3, NFAT (nuclear factor of activated T-cells), TFE3 (transcription factor E3), HIF2α (hypoxia-inducible factor-2α encoded by Epas1), and SREBP1 (sterol regulatory element-binding protein 1) (Thorpe et al. 2015;

Antonetti et al. 1996). Under fasting conditions, the cAMP-responsive CREB coactivator CRTC2 promotes glucose homeostasis by stimulating gluconeogenesis in the liver upon assembly of CREB•CRTC2 dimers on relevant CRE promoter sites, including a half-CRE on IRS2 (Antonetti et al. 1996). The induction of hepatic IRS2 during fasting appears to modulate glucose homeostasis as it mediates a feedback response that limits glucose output from the liver even when the insulin concentration is low.

A transcriptional mechanism regulates IRS2 in pancreatic β-cells. Since β-cells are always exposed to insulin and IGF, the insulin/IGF signaling cascade appears to be regulated through the coordinate action of FOXO1/FOXO3, NFAT, and CREB•CRTC2 (Tsunekawa et al. 2011; Demozay et al. 2011; Jhala et al. 2003; Li et al. 2008). Since β-cell mass and function must be protected during the challenge of chronic nutrient excess, heterologous mechanisms – including glucose-stimulated Ca^{2+} influx and cAMP production – defend IRS2 expression. In addition to its immediate role in insulin secretion, Ca^{2+} activates calcineurin which dephosphorylates NFAT to facilitate its entry into the nucleus where it induces expression of IRS2 and other genes (Demozay et al. 2011). Glucose, glucagon-like peptide-1, and other GPCR agonists also increase the cAMP concentration in β-cells, which has many important effects, including the activation of CREB•CRTC2 that promotes IRS2 transcription (Assmann et al. 2009; Park et al. 2006). Through this mechanism, the responsibility for insulin/IGF1 itself to trigger downstream insulin/IGF signaling in β-cells has been replaced by indirect control through glucose, incretins, or neuronal signals – the physiologically relevant regulators of pancreatic β-cell function. Whether drugs can be found to modulate this mechanism to promote β-cell function needs to be further investigated (Kuznetsova et al. 2016).

Regulation of Insulin Signaling by Proteolysis

Proteasome-mediated degradation regulates many biological processes including signal transduction, gene transcription, and cell cycle progression (Kirschner 1999). Proteins targeted for destruction by the 26S proteasome are polyubiquitinylated by various complexes containing ubiquitin-activating enzymes (E1), ubiquitin-conjugating enzymes (E2), and ubiquitin-protein ligases (E3). IRS1 and IRS2 can be polyubiquitinylated during chronic inflammatory states, nutrient excess, and hyperinsulinemia through various tissue-specific mechanisms (Rui et al. 2001).

One of these regulatory pathways is associated with proinflammatory cytokine-mediated upregulation of SOCS1/SOCS3 (suppressors of cytokine signaling) (Fig. 5).In another mechanism, the cullin-RING E3 ubiquitin ligase 7 (CRL7) can mediate IRS1 degradation downstream of feedback serine phosphorylation signals generated by PI3K→AKT→mTORC1 cascade (Xu and Sarikas 2008) (Fig. 5). Chronic consumption of high-calorie diets upregulates CBLB (Cbl proto-oncogene B), a RING-type E3 ubiquitin ligase that belongs to the casitas B-lineage lymphoma family of proteins (Samuel and Shulman 2012). CBL proteins share a conserved NH_2-terminal region containing a tyrosine kinase-binding domain and a RING-finger domain to facilitate E3 ubiquitin ligase activity. Calorie excess induces ChREBP (carbohydrate-responsive element-binding protein) and SREBP1c, which upregulates MSTN (myostatin) in murine muscle and liver-inducing CBLB to drive insulin resistance through the polyubiquitinylation and degradation of IRS1 (Bonala et al. 2014). Finally, MG53 (Mitsugumin 53), a TRIM (tripartite motif-containing) family E3 ubiquitin ligase, can promote IRS1 and InsR degradation in muscle during calorie excess.

Heterologous Regulation of IRS1 by Ser/Thr Phosphorylation

IRS1 and IRS2 are regulated by a complex mechanism involving phosphorylation of more than 50 serine/threonine residues (pS/T^{IRS1} or pS/T^{IRS2}) located in the tail regions (see Fig. 5) (Copps and White 2012). Understanding how phospho-S/Ts regulate signaling is a difficult problem because so many sites and phosphorylation/dephosphorylation mechanisms can be involved. Heterologous signaling cascades initiated by proinflammatory cytokines or metabolic excess – including TNFα (tumor necrosis factor-α), endothelin-1, angiotensin II, excess nutrients (free fatty acids, ceramides, amino acids, and glucose), or endoplasmic reticulum stress – are implicated in pS/T^{IRS1} (Zick 2003; Gual et al. 2005) (Fig. 5). Many biochemical and genetic experiments in cell-based systems suggest that various pS/T^{IRS1} sites are associated with a 50% reduction of insulin-stimulated tyrosine phosphorylation (Zick 2005). Based upon genetic experiments, this level of inhibition is sufficient to cause glucose intolerance that could progress to diabetes, especially if pancreatic β-cells also fail to provide adequate compensatory hyperinsulinemia (Kido et al. 2000).

A few studies have investigated directly the function of pS/T^{IRS1} in transgenic mice or genetic knock-in to augment or replace endogenous (wild-type) IRS1 with a mutant version. Transgenic expression in mice of a triple Ser→Ala mutant of IRS1 ($S{\rightarrow}A302^{Irs1}$; $S{\rightarrow}A307^{Irs1}$; $S{\rightarrow}A612^{Irs1}$) expressed in skeletal muscle suggest that phosphorylation at these serine residues can promote insulin resistance (Morino et al. 2008). Regardless, genetic knock-in experiments to replace wild-type IRS1 in mice with a single mutant ($S{\rightarrow}A307^{IRS1}$) do not support this result (Copps et al. 2010). Contrary to the sensitizing effect of the $A307^{IRS1}$ mutation in cell-based assays, homozygous $A307^{IRS1}$ mice show increased fasting insulin, mild glucose intolerance, and decreased PI3K binding (p85 and p110) compared against control mice. Moreover, homozygous $A302^{IRS1}$ mice display normal insulin signaling, even though $S302^{Irs1}$ is a major insulin-stimulated site in skeletal muscle (Copps et al. 2016). It is possible that multiple phospho-S/Ts work together to inhibit insulin signaling.

pS/T^{IRS1} is usually considered to be associated with the progression of insulin resistance; however, recent work suggests that it might also be an important physiological feedback mechanism to control the intensity of insulin signaling. Using monoclonal antibodies against more than 25 pS/T^{IRS1}, we noted that all the observed phosphorylation events increase during insulin stimulation (Hancer et al. 2014). Moreover, these pS/T^{IRS1} are downstream of the PI 3-kinase and AKT, whereas some of the phosphorylation sites are also sensitive to mTorc1, S6 k, or some stress-activated kinases (Hancer et al. 2014). While inhibition of various kinases reduce pS/T^{IRS1}, they increase insulin-stimulated pY^{Irs1}. Thus, pS/T^{IRS1}appears to be an integrated mechanism to modulate insulin-stimulated pY^{IRS1} by feedback or heterologous inflammatory cascades.

Dephosphorylation of pS/T^{IRS1} Couples GPCRs to the PI3K→AKT Cascade

Recent work suggests that pS/T^{IRS1} might be an important mechanism coupling GPCRs (G-protein-coupled receptors) to the PI3K → AKT cascade.PI3Ks are lipid kinases central to numerous signaling pathways, which are organized into three classes – class I, class II, and class III (Thorpe et al. 2015). RTKs usually regulate the class IA PI3Ks, which are composed of one catalytic subunit (p110α or p110β) inhibited and stabilized by a regulatory subunit (p85α, p85β, p55α, p50α, or p55γ) (Antonetti et al. 1996; Taniguchi et al. 2006; Ueki et al. 2002). The regulatory subunits contain 2 SH2 (src homology 2) domains that bind phosphorylated YMPM-motifs in IRS1/IRS2 to disinhibit the catalytic domain that produces PI P_3 (phosphatidylinositol 3,4,5-trisphosphate) (Thorpe et al. 2015; Vanhaesebroeck et al. 2012; Cantley 2002). The p110γ isoform does not bind to a p85 subunit but binds to the unrelated p101 regulatory subunit linking p110γ to $G_{\beta\gamma}$ subunits released from heterotrimeric G-proteins downstream of GPCRs (G-protein-coupled receptors) (Vanhaesebroeck et al. 2012).

Regardless, we found that pS/T^{IRS1}also has a role in the regulation of PI3K→AKT signaling by GPCRs (G-protein-coupled receptors) (Law et al. 2016). This mechanism was discovered during experiments investigating the activation of AKT by FSH (follicle-stimulated hormone). FSH binds to its GPCR, which activates PKA (protein kinase A) upon adenylyl cyclase-mediated cAMP production (Hunzicker-Dunn and Maizels 2006), but how this mechanism couples to PI3K → AKT has been difficult to understand (Srinivas et al. 1997; Balasubramanian et al. 1997). Interestingly, ovarian granulosa cells secrete low levels of IGF1 that activate constitutively the IGF1R through a paracrine mechanism. However, IGF1 fails to stimulate IRS1 tyrosine phosphorylation or recruit PI3K before FSH stimulation (Law and Hunzicker-Dunn 2016).

In ovarian granulosa cells and some other cell types, GPCRs → PKA can phosphorylate MYPT1 (myosin phosphatase-targeting subunit 1) – a regulatory subunit of PP1 (protein phosphatase 1). Importantly, the phosphorylated and activated MYPT1•PP1 complex associates with the IGF1R•IRS1 complex where it can dephosphorylate at least four (and possibly more) pS/T^{IRS1} – including $S318^{IRS1}$, $Ser346^{IRS1}$, $Ser612^{IRS1}$, and $S789^{IRS1}$. Regulated dephosphorylation of pS/T^{IRS1}promotes IRS1 tyrosine phosphorylation, which activates the PI3K→AKT cascade (Fig. 6). In this model, activation of PI3K requires both PKA-mediated relief

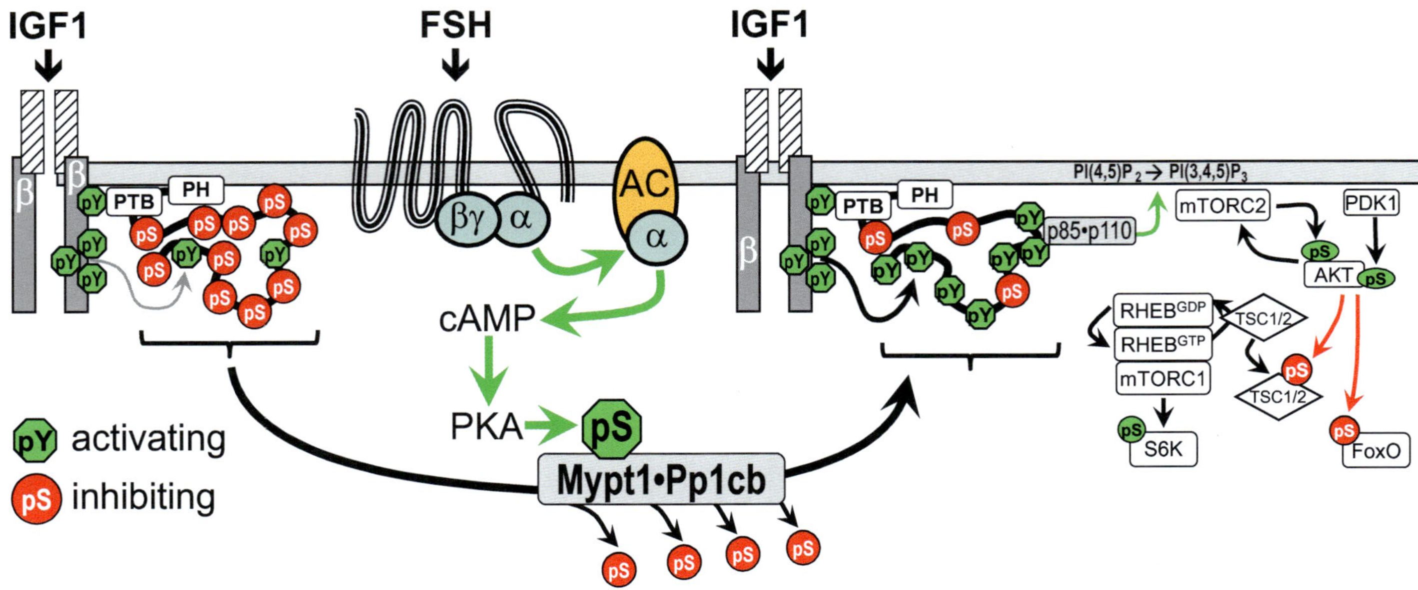

Fig. 6 FSH (follicle-stimulating hormone) GPCR-activated PI3K → AKT via PP1-mediated dephosphorylation of pS/T^{IRS1}. Endogenous IGF1 secreted from cells activates the IGF1R but fails to stimulate IRS1 tyrosine phosphorylation to recruit and activate the PI3K, owing to excess pS/T^{IRS1}. PKA-activated by upstream GPCRs – in this case the FSH receptor coupled to Gas – phosphorylate and activate MYPT1, a regulatory subunit for PP1. Activated PP1 dephosphorylates pS/T^{IRS1}, which facilitates IGF1R-dependent IRS1 tyrosine phosphorylation to activate the PI3K → AKT cascade and downstream targets

of IRS1 inhibition and IGF1R-mediated tyrosine phosphorylation of IRS1. Together these effects couple GPCR → cAMP signaling to the AKT—| FOXO1 (fork head box O1) to drive synergistic expression of genes that underlies follicle maturation (Law et al. 2016). PP1 activation to relieve IRS1 inhibition might be a general mechanism by which GPCRs act with the insulin and IGF receptors or possibly other receptors to activate PI3K → AKT cascade.

Summary and Perspectives

The investigation of the RTKs reveals a highly integrated multisystemic network that plays critical roles in cellular growth, differentiation, development and metabolism. When receptor tyrosine kinases fail, life threatening diseases develop, especially cancer but also progressive metabolic disease. Importantly, when a mutation constitutively activates a RTK (i.e. EGFR) cell growth can accelerate in unpredictable locations. On the other hand, loss of function can disrupt metabolic homeostasis (i.e. IR). Since the network of signaling pathways controlled by RTKs are similar across the families, drugs to modulate dysregulated signaling to control disease progression can have unintended consequences. For example, efforts to suppress the PI3K cascade to stop cancer growth might also cause severe glucose intolerance and life-threatening diabetes. Innovative ways to modulate dysregulated RTK—perhaps with targeted antibodies or other engineered binding proteins—can provide ways to leverage RTKs for the cure of disease.

Cross-References

- ▶ Cytokine Receptors
- ▶ Principles of Endocrine Diseases
- ▶ Synthesis, Secretion, and Transport of Peptide Hormones
- ▶ Targeting of Steroid Hormone Receptor Function in Breast and Prostate Cancer
- ▶ The Endocrine Pancreas
- ▶ The Endocrine Regulation of Energy and Body Weight

Literature Cited

Antonetti DA, Algenstaedt P, Kahn CR. Insulin receptor substrate 1 binds two novel splice variants of the regulatory subunit of phosphatidylinositol 3-kinase in muscle and brain. Mol Cell Biol. 1996;16:2195–203.

Assmann A, Ueki K, Winnay JN, Kadowaki T, Kulkarni RN. Glucose effects on beta-cell growth and survival require activation of insulin receptors and insulin receptor substrate 2. Mol Cell Biol. 2009;29(11):3219–28.

Backer JM, Myers Jr MG, Shoelson SE, Chin DJ, Sun XJ, Miralpeix M, et al. Phosphatidylinositol 3′-kinase is activated by association with IRS-1 during insulin stimulation. EMBO J. 1992;11 (9):3469–79.

Badman MK, Pissios P, Kennedy AR, Koukos G, Flier JS, Maratos-Flier E. Hepatic fibroblast growth factor 21 is regulated by PPAR alpha and is a key mediator of hepatic lipid metabolism in ketotic states. Cell Metab. 2007;5(6):426–37.

Balasubramanian K, LaVoie HA, Garmey JC, Stocco DM, Veldhuis JD. Regulation of porcine granulosa cell steroidogenic acute regulatory protein (StAR) by insulin-like growth factor I: synergism with follicle-stimulating hormone or protein kinase A agonist. Endocrinology. 1997;138(1):433–9.

Barton WA, Dalton AC, Seegar TC, Himanen JP, Nikolov DB. Tie2 and Eph receptor tyrosine kinase activation and signaling. Cold Spring Harb Perspect Biol. 2014;6(3):a009142.

Belfiore A, Frasca F, Pandini G, Sciacca L, Vigneri R. Insulin receptor isoforms and insulin receptor/insulin-like growth factor receptor hybrids in physiology and disease. Endocr Rev. 2009;30(6):586–623.

Benyoucef S, Surinya KH, Hadaschik D, Siddle K. Characterization of insulin/IGF hybrid receptors: contributions of the insulin receptor L2 and Fn1 domains and the alternatively spliced exon 11 sequence to ligand binding and receptor activation. Biochem J. 2007;403(3):603–13.

Bergamin E, Hallock PT, Burden SJ, Hubbard SR. The cytoplasmic adaptor protein Dok7 activates the receptor tyrosine kinase MuSK via dimerization. Mol Cell. 2010;39(1):100–9.

Bjornholm M, He AR, Attersand A, Lake S, Liu SC, Lienhard GE, et al. Absence of functional insulin receptor substrate-3 (IRS-3) gene in humans. Diabetologia. 2002;45(12):1697–702.

Blanquart C, Achi J, Issad T. Characterization of IRA/IRB hybrid receptors using bioluminescence resonance energy transfer. Biochem Pharmacol. 2008;6286–96.

Blattler SM, Cunningham JT, Verdeguer F, Chim H, Haas W, Liu H, et al. Yin Yang 1 deficiency in skeletal muscle protects against rapamycin-induced diabetic-like symptoms through activation of insulin/IGF signaling. Cell Metab. 2012;15(4):505–17.

Bonala S, Lokireddy S, McFarlane C, Patnam S, Sharma M, Kambadur R. Myostatin induces insulin resistance via Cblb-mediated degradation of IRS1 in response to high calorie diet intake. J Biol Chem. 2014;289:7654–70.

Borcherding N, Kusner D, Liu GH, Zhang W. ROR1, an embryonic protein with an emerging role in cancer biology. Protein Cell. 2014;5(7):496–502.

Bothwell M. Recent advances in understanding neurotrophin signaling. F1000Res. 2016;5. pii: F1000 Faculty Rev-1885. doi: 10.12688/f1000research.8434.1.

Brzozowski AM, Dodson EJ, Dodson GG, Murshudov GN, Verma C, Turkenburg JP, et al. Structural origins of the functional divergence of human insulin-like growth factor-I and insulin. Biochemistry. 2002;41(30):9389–97.

Burden S, Yarden Y. Neuregulins and their receptors: a versatile signaling module in organogenesis and oncogenesis. Neuron. 1997;18(6):847–55.

Burgess AW, Cho HS, Eigenbrot C, Ferguson KM, Garrett TP, Leahy DJ, et al. An open-and-shut case? Recent insights into the activation of EGF/ErbB receptors. Mol Cell. 2003;12(3):541–52.

Burks DJ, Pons S, Towery H, SmithHall J, Myers MG, Yenush L, et al. Heterologous pleckstrin homology domains do not couple IRS-1 to the insulin receptor. J Biol Chem. 1997;272 (44):27716–21.

Burks DJ, Wang J, Towery H, Ishibashi O, Lowe D, Riedel H, et al. IRS pleckstrin homology domains bind to acidic motifs in proteins. J Biol Chem. 1998;273(47):31061–7.

Cann AD, Kohanski RA. Cis-autophosphorylation of juxtamembrane tyrosines in the insulin receptor kinase domain. Biochemistry. 1997;36(25):7681–9.

Cantley LC. The phosphoinositide 3-kinase pathway. Science. 2002;296(5573):1655–7.

Carpenter G, King Jr LE, Cohen S. Rapid enhancement of protein phosphorylation in A431 cell membrane preparations by epidermal growth factor. J Biol Chem. 1979;254:4884–91.

Chartoumpekis DV, Habeos IG, Ziros PG, Psyrogiannis AI, Kyriazopoulou VE, Papavassiliou AG. Brown adipose tissue responds to cold and adrenergic stimulation by induction of FGF21. Mol Med. 2011;17(7–8):736–40.

Claesson-Welsh L. VEGF receptor signal transduction - A brief update. Vascul Pharmacol. 2016;86:14–7.

Cooper JA, Reiss NA, Schwartz RJ, Hunter T. Three glycolytic enzymes are phosphorylated at tyrosine in cells transformed by Rous sarcoma virus. Nature. 1983;302(5905):219–23.

Copps KD, White MF. Regulation of insulin sensitivity by serine/threonine phosphorylation of insulin receptor substrate proteins IRS1 and IRS2. Diabetologia. 2012;55(10):2565–82.

Copps KD, Hancer NJ, Opare-Ado L, Qiu W, Walsh C, White MF. Irs1 serine 307 promotes insulin sensitivity in mice. Cell Metab. 2010;11(1):84–92.

Copps KD, Hancer NJ, Qiu W, White MF. Serine 302 phosphorylation of mouse insulin receptor substrate 1 (Irs1) is dispensable for normal insulin signaling and feedback regulation by hepatic S6 kinase. J Biol Chem. 2016;291:8602–17.

Coulpier M, Anders J, Ibanez CF. Coordinated activation of autophosphorylation sites in the RET receptor tyrosine kinase: importance of tyrosine 1062 for GDNF mediated neuronal differentiation and survival. J Biol Chem. 2002;277(3):1991–9.

Davies KD, Doebele RC. Molecular pathways: ROS1 fusion proteins in cancer. Clin Cancer Res. 2013;19(15):4040–5.

De Meyts P. The insulin receptor: a prototype for dimeric, allosteric membrane receptors? Trends Biochem Sci. 2008;33(8):376–84.

De Meyts P, Palsgaard J, Sajid W, Theede AM, Aladdin H. Structural biology of insulin and IGF-1 receptors. Novartis Found Symp. 2004;262:160–71.

Demozay D, Tsunekawa S, Briaud I, Shah R, Rhodes CJ. Specific glucose-induced control of insulin receptor substrate-2 expression is mediated via Ca^{2+}-dependent calcineurin/NFAT signaling in primary pancreatic islet beta-cells. Diabetes. 2011;60(11):2892–902.

Deyev IE, Sohet F, Vassilenko KP, Serova OV, Popova NV, Zozulya SA, et al. Insulin receptor-related receptor as an extracellular alkali sensor. Cell Metab. 2011;13(6):679–89.

Dhe-Paganon S, Ottinger EA, Nolte RT, Eck MJ, Shoelson SE. Crystal structure of the pleckstrin homology-phosphotyrosine binding (PH-PTB) targeting region of insulin receptor substrate 1. Proc Natl Acad Sci USA. 1999;96(15):8378–83.

Eck MJ, Dhe-Paganon S, Trub T, Nolte RT, Shoelson SE. Structure of the IRS-1 PTB domain bound to the juxtamembrane region of the insulin receptor. Cell. 1996;85(5):695–705.

Ek B, Heldin CH. Characterization of a tyrosine-specific kinase activity in human fibroblast membranes stimulated by platelet-derived growth factor. J Biol Chem. 1982;257(17):10486–92.

Ek B, Westermark B, Wasteson A, Heldin CH. Stimulation of tyrosine-specific phosphorylation by platelet-derived growth factor. Nature. 1982;295(5848):419–20.

Ellis L, Clauser E, Morgan DO, Edery M, Roth RA, Rutter WJ. Replacement of insulin receptor tyrosine residues 1162 and 1163 compromises insulin-stimulated kinase activity and uptake of 2-deoxyglucose. Cell. 1986;45(5):721–32.

Fafalios A, Ma J, Tan X, Stoops J, Luo J, Defrances MC, et al. A hepatocyte growth factor receptor (Met)-insulin receptor hybrid governs hepatic glucose metabolism. Nat Med. 2011;17 (12):1577–84.

Fajardo-Puerta AB, Mato Prado M, Frampton AE, Jiao LR. Gene of the month: HGF. J Clin Pathol. 2016;69(7):575–9.

Farooq A, Plotnikova O, Zeng L, Zhou MM. Phosphotyrosine binding domains of Shc and insulin receptor substrate 1 recognize the NPXpY motif in a thermodynamically distinct manner. J Biol Chem. 1999;274(10):6114–21.

Ferguson KM, Berger MB, Mendrola JM, Cho HS, Leahy DJ, Lemmon MA. EGF activates its receptor by removing interactions that autoinhibit ectodomain dimerization. Mol Cell. 2003;11(2):507–17.

Fisher FM, Maratos-Flier E. Understanding the physiology of FGF21. Annu Rev Physiol. 2016;78:223–41.

Fisher FM, Kleiner S, Douris N, Fox EC, Mepani RJ, Verdeguer F, et al. FGF21 regulates PGC-1alpha and browning of white adipose tissues in adaptive thermogenesis. Genes Dev. 2012;26(3):271–81.

Fisher FM, Chui PC, Nasser IA, Popov Y, Cunniff JC, Lundasen T, et al. Fibroblast growth factor 21 limits lipotoxicity by promoting hepatic fatty acid activation in mice on methionine and choline-deficient diets. Gastroenterology. 2014;147(5):1073–83. e6.

Fu HL, Valiathan RR, Arkwright R, Sohail A, Mihai C, Kumarasiri M, et al. Discoidin domain receptors: unique receptor tyrosine kinases in collagen-mediated signaling. J Biol Chem. 2013;288(11):7430–7.
Gaozza E, Baker SJ, Vora RK, Reddy EP. AATYK: a novel tyrosine kinase induced during growth arrest and apoptosis of myeloid cells. Oncogene. 1997;15(25):3127–35.
Grande E, Bolos MV, Arriola E. Targeting oncogenic ALK: a promising strategy for cancer treatment. Mol Cancer Ther. 2011;10(4):569–79.
Green J, Nusse R, van Amerongen R. The role of Ryk and Ror receptor tyrosine kinases in Wnt signal transduction. Cold Spring Harb Perspect Biol. 2014;6(2):a009175.
Gual P, Le Marchand-Brustel Y, Tanti JF. Positive and negative regulation of insulin signaling through IRS-1 phosphorylation. Biochimie. 2005;87(1):99–109.
Hancer NJ, Qiu W, Cherella C, Li Y, Copps KD, White MF. Insulin and metabolic stress stimulate multisite serine/threonine phosphorylation of insulin receptor substrate 1 and inhibit tyrosine phosphorylation. J Biol Chem. 2014;289(18):12467–84.
Hedo JA, Kahn CR, Hayoshi M, Yamada KM, Kasuga M. Biosynthesis and glycosylation of the insulin receptor. Evidence for a single polypeptide precursor of the two major subunits. J Biol Chem. 1983;258:10020–6.
Heldin CH, Lennartsson J. Structural and functional properties of platelet-derived growth factor and stem cell factor receptors. Cold Spring Harb Perspect Biol. 2013;5(8):a009100.
Hilbert T, Klaschik S. The angiopoietin/TIE receptor system: focusing its role for ischemia-reperfusion injury. Cytokine Growth Factor Rev. 2015;26(3):281–91.
Hondares E, Iglesias R, Giralt A, Gonzalez FJ, Giralt M, Mampel T, et al. Thermogenic activation induces FGF21 expression and release in brown adipose tissue. J Biol Chem. 2011;286 (15):12983–90.
Hu L, Chen HY, Cai J, Zhang Y, Qi CY, Gong H, et al. Serine threonine tyrosine kinase 1 is a potential prognostic marker in colorectal cancer. BMC Cancer. 2015;15:246.
Huang EJ, Reichardt LF. Trk receptors: roles in neuronal signal transduction. Annu Rev Biochem. 2003;72:609–42.
Hubbard SR. Crystal structure of the activated insulin receptor tyrosine kinase in complex with peptide substrate and ATP analog. EMBO J. 1997;16(18):5572–81.
Hubbard SR. The insulin receptor: both a prototypical and atypical receptor tyrosine kinase. Cold Spring Harb Perspect Biol. 2013;5(3):1–12.
Hubbard SR, Wei L, Ellis L, Hendrickson WA. Crystal structure of the tyrosine kinase domain of the human insulin receptor. Nature. 1994;372:746–54.
Hunter T, Sefton BM. Transforming gene product of Rous sarcoma virus phosphorylates tyrosine. Proc Natl Acad Sci U S A. 1980;77(3):1311–5.
Hunzicker-Dunn M, Maizels ET. FSH signaling pathways in immature granulosa cells that regulate target gene expression: branching out from protein kinase A. Cell Signal. 2006;18 (9):1351–9.
Janssen JW, Schulz AS, Steenvoorden AC, Schmidberger M, Strehl S, Ambros PF, et al. A novel putative tyrosine kinase receptor with oncogenic potential. Oncogene. 1991;6(11):2113–20.
Jhala US, Canettieri G, Screaton RA, Kulkarni RN, Krajewski S, Reed J, et al. cAMP promotes pancreatic beta-cell survival via CREB-mediated induction of IRS2. Genes Dev. 2003;17 (13):1575–80.
Kahn CR, Flier JS, Bar RS, Archer JA, Gorden P, Martin MM, et al. The syndromes of insulin resistance and acanthosis nigricans: insulin receptor disorders in man. N Engl J Med. 1976;294:739–45.
Kania A, Klein R. Mechanisms of ephrin-Eph signalling in development, physiology and disease. Nat Rev Mol Cell Biol. 2016;17(4):240–56.
Kasuga M, Karlsson FA, Kahn CR. Insulin stimulates the phosphorylation of the 95,000-dalton subunit of its own receptor. Science. 1982a;215(4529):185–7.
Kasuga M, Zick Y, Blithe DL, Crettaz M, Kahn CR. Insulin stimulates tyrosine phosphorylation of the insulin receptor in a cell-free system. Nature. 1982b;298:667–9.

Kasuga M, Hedo JA, Yamada KM, Kahn CR. The structure of the insulin receptor and its subunits: evidence for multiple non-reduced forms and a 210K possible proreceptor. J Biol Chem. 1982c;257:10392–9.

Kazlauskas A, Cooper JA. Autophosphorylation of the PDGF receptor in the kinase insert region regulates interactions with cell proteins. Cell. 1989;58(6):1121–33.

Kido Y, Burks DJ, Withers D, Bruning JC, Kahn CR, White MF, et al. Tissue-specific insulin resistance in mice with mutations in the insulin receptor, IRS-1, and IRS-2. J Clin Invest. 2000;105(2):199–205.

Kirschner M. Intracellular proteolysis. Trends Cell Biol. 1999;9(12):M42–5.

Kiselyov VV, Versteyhe S, Gauguin L, De Meyts P. Harmonic oscillator model of the insulin and IGF1 receptors' allosteric binding and activation. Mol Syst Biol. 2009;5:243.

Knowles PP, Murray-Rust J, Kjaer S, Scott RP, Hanrahan S, Santoro M, et al. Structure and chemical inhibition of the RET tyrosine kinase domain. J Biol Chem. 2006;281(44):33577–87.

Koch S, Tugues S, Li X, Gualandi L, Claesson-Welsh L. Signal transduction by vascular endothelial growth factor receptors. Biochem J. 2011;437(2):169–83.

Konstantinova I, Nikolova G, Ohara-Imaizumi M, Meda P, Kucera T, Zarbalis K, et al. EphA-Ephrin-A-mediated beta cell communication regulates insulin secretion from pancreatic islets. Cell. 2007;129(2):359–70.

Kullander K, Mather NK, Diella F, Dottori M, Boyd AW, Klein R. Kinase-dependent and kinase-independent functions of EphA4 receptors in major axon tract formation in vivo. Neuron. 2001;29(1):73–84.

Kuznetsova A, Yu Y, Hollister-Lock J, Opare-Addo L, Rozzo A, Sadagurski M, et al. Trimeprazine increases IRS2 in human islets and promotes pancreatic beta cell growth and function in mice. JCI Insight. 2016;1(3):1–20.

Law NC, Hunzicker-Dunn ME. Insulin receptor substrate 1, the hub linking follicle-stimulating hormone to phosphatidylinositol 3-kinase activation. J Biol Chem. 2016;291(9):4547–60.

Law NC, White MF, Hunzicker-Dunn ME. G protein-coupled receptors (GPCRs) that signal via protein kinase A (PKA) cross-talk at insulin receptor substrate 1 (IRS1) to activate the PI3K/AKT pathway. J Biol Chem. 2016;291(53):27160–9.

Lawrence MC, McKern NM, Ward CW. Insulin receptor structure and its implications for the IGF-1 receptor. Curr Opin Struct Biol. 2007;17(6):699–705.

Lemmon MA, Schlessinger J. Cell signaling by receptor tyrosine kinases. Cell. 2010;141(7):1117–34.

Lemmon MA, Ferguson KM, Schlessinger J. PH domains: diverse sequences with a common fold recruit signaling molecules to the cell surface. Cell. 1996;85(5):621–4.

Lemmon MA, Ferguson KM, Abrams CS. Pleckstrin homology domains and the cytoskeleton. FEBS Lett. 2002;513(1):71–6.

Lemmon MA, Freed DM, Schlessinger J, Kiyatkin A. The dark side of cell signaling: positive roles for negative regulators. Cell. 2016;164(6):1172–84.

Li D, Yin X, Zmuda EJ, Wolford CC, Dong XC, White MF, et al. The repression of IRS2 gene by ATF3, a stress-inducible gene, contributes to pancreatic beta-cell apoptosis. Diabetes. 2008;57(3):635–44.

Liu L, Yu XZ, Li TS, Song LX, Chen PL, Suo TL, et al. A novel protein tyrosine kinase NOK that shares homology with platelet- derived growth factor/fibroblast growth factor receptors induces tumorigenesis and metastasis in nude mice. Cancer Res. 2004;64(10):3491–9.

Lu Q, Lemke G. Homeostatic regulation of the immune system by receptor tyrosine kinases of the Tyro 3 family. Science. 2001;293(5528):306–11.

Markan KR, Naber MC, Ameka MK, Anderegg MD, Mangelsdorf DJ, Kliewer SA, et al. Circulating FGF21 is liver derived and enhances glucose uptake during refeeding and overfeeding. Diabetes. 2014;63(12):4057–63.

Mates M, Fletcher GG, Freedman OC, Eisen A, Gandhi S, Trudeau ME, et al. Systemic targeted therapy for her2-positive early female breast cancer: a systematic review of the evidence for the 2014 cancer care Ontario systemic therapy guideline. Curr Oncol. 2015;22(Suppl 1):S114–22.

McKern NM, Lawrence MC, Streltsov VA, Lou MZ, Adams TE, Lovrecz GO, et al. Structure of the insulin receptor ectodomain reveals a folded-over conformation. Nature. 2006;443 (7108):218–21.
Menting JG, Whittaker J, Margetts MB, Whittaker LJ, Kong GK, Smith BJ, et al. How insulin engages its primary binding site on the insulin receptor. Nature. 2013;493(7431):241–5.
Morino K, Neschen S, Bilz S, Sono S, Tsirigotis D, Reznick RM, et al. Muscle-specific IRS-1 Ser->Ala transgenic mice are protected from fat-induced insulin resistance in skeletal muscle. Diabetes. 2008;57(10):2644–51.
Mossie K, Jallal B, Alves F, Sures I, Plowman GD, Ullrich A. Colon carcinoma kinase-4 defines a new subclass of the receptor tyrosine kinase family. Oncogene. 1995;11(10):2179–84.
Nomura M, Yamagishi S, Harada S, Hayashi Y, Yamashima T, Yamashita J, et al. Possible participation of autocrine and paracrine vascular endothelial growth factors in hypoxia-induced proliferation of endothelial cells and pericytes. J Biol Chem. 1995;270(47):28316–24.
Numan S, Russell DS. Discrete expression of insulin receptor substrate-4 mRNA in adult rat brain. Brain Res Mol Brain Res. 1999;72(1):97–102.
Oishi I, Suzuki H, Onishi N, Takada R, Kani S, Ohkawara B, et al. The receptor tyrosine kinase Ror2 is involved in non-canonical Wnt5a/JNK signalling pathway. Genes Cells. 2003;8 (7):645–54.
Okada K, Inoue A, Okada M, Murata Y, Kakuta S, Jigami T, et al. The muscle protein Dok-7 is essential for neuromuscular synaptogenesis. Science. 2006;312(5781):1802–5.
Oppenheim RW, Houenou LJ, Johnson JE, Lin LF, Li L, Lo AC, et al. Developing motor neurons rescued from programmed and axotomy-induced cell death by GDNF. Nature. 1995;373 (6512):344–6.
Ostman A. PDGF receptors-mediators of autocrine tumor growth and regulators of tumor vasculature and stroma. Cytokine Growth Factor Rev. 2004;15(4):275–86.
Palmer A, Zimmer M, Erdmann KS, Eulenburg V, Porthin A, Heumann R, et al. EphrinB phosphorylation and reverse signaling: regulation by Src kinases and PTP-BL phosphatase. Mol Cell. 2002;9(4):725–37.
Park S, Dong X, Fisher TL, Dunn S, Omer AK, Weir G, et al. Exendin-4 uses Irs2 signaling to mediate pancreatic beta cell growth and function. J Biol Chem. 2006;281(2):1159–68.
Pelicci GL, Lanfrancone L, Grignani F, McGlade J, Cavallo F, Forni G, et al. A novel transforming protein (SHC) with an SH2 domain is implicated in mitogenic signal transduction. Cell. 1992;70 (1):93–104.
Peradziryi H, Kaplan NA, Podleschny M, Liu X, Wehner P, Borchers A, et al. PTK7/Otk interacts with Wnts and inhibits canonical Wnt signalling. EMBO J. 2011;30(18):3729–40.
Peradziryi H, Tolwinski NS, Borchers A. The many roles of PTK7: a versatile regulator of cell-cell communication. Arch Biochem Biophys. 2012;524(1):71–6.
Pike LJ. Negative co-operativity in the EGF receptor. Biochem Soc Trans. 2012;40(1):15–9.
Rajagopalan M, Neidigh JL, McClain DA. Amino acid sequences Gly-Pro-Leu-Tyr and Asn-Pro-Glu-Tyr in the submembranous domain of the insulin receptor are required for normal endocytosis. J Biol Chem. 1991;266:23068–73.
Reitman ML. FGF21: a missing link in the biology of fasting. Cell Metab. 2007;5(6):405–7.
Robinson DR, Wu YM, Lin SF. The protein tyrosine kinase family of the human genome. Oncogene. 2000;19(49):5548–57.
Rothlin CV, Carrera-Silva EA, Bosurgi L, Ghosh S. TAM receptor signaling in immune homeostasis. Annu Rev Immunol. 2015;33:355–91.
Rui L, Fisher TL, Thomas J, White MF. Regulation of insulin/insulin-like growth factor-1 signaling by proteasome-mediated degradation of insulin receptor substrate-2. J Biol Chem. 2001;276 (43):40362–7.
Rupp F, Payan DG, Magill-Solc C, Cowan DM, Scheller RH. Structure and expression of a rat agrin. Neuron. 1991;6(5):811–23.
Sadagurski M, Dong XC, Myers Jr MG, White MF. Irs2 and Irs4 synergize in non-LepRb neurons to control energy balance and glucose homeostasis. Mol Metab. 2014;3(1):55–63.

Samuel VT, Shulman GI. Mechanisms for insulin resistance: common threads and missing links. Cell. 2012;148(5):852–71.

Sawka-Verhelle D, Tartare-Deckert S, White MF, Van Obberghen E. Insulin receptor substrate-2 binds to the insulin receptor through its phosphotyrosine-binding domain and through a newly identified domain comprising amino acids 591–786. J Biol Chem. 1996;271 (11):5980–3.

Sawka-Verhelle D, Baron V, Mothe I, Filloux C, White MF, Van Obberghen E. Tyr624 and Tyr628 in insulin receptor substrate-2 mediate its association with the insulin receptor. J Biolo Chem. 1997;272(26):16414–20.

Schlessinger J. Cell signaling by receptor tyrosine kinases. Cell. 2000;103(2):211–25.

Schlessinger J. Receptor tyrosine kinases: legacy of the first two decades. Cold Spring Harb Perspect Biol. 2014;6(3):a008912.

Schneider MR, Wolf E. The epidermal growth factor receptor ligands at a glance. J Cell Physiol. 2009;218(3):460–6.

Schonherr C, Hallberg B, Palmer R. Anaplastic lymphoma kinase in human cancer. Crit Rev Oncog. 2012;17(2):123–43.

Schulze WX, Deng L, Mann M. Phosphotyrosine interactome of the ErbB-receptor kinase family. Mol Syst Biol. 2005;1:2005.0008.

Seino S, Bell GI. Alternative splicing of human insulin receptor messenger RNA. Biochem Biophys Res Commun. 1989;159:312–6.

Shibuya M. Vascular endothelial growth factor receptor-1 (VEGFR-1/Flt-1): a dual regulator for angiogenesis. Angiogenesis. 2006;9(4):225–30. discussion 31.

Shier P, Watt VM. Primary structure of a putative receptor for a ligand of the insulin family. J Biol Chem. 1989;264:14605–8.

Shim AH, Liu H, Focia PJ, Chen X, Lin PC, He X. Structures of a platelet-derived growth factor/ propeptide complex and a platelet-derived growth factor/receptor complex. Proc Natl Acad Sci U S A. 2010;107(25):11307–12.

Shoelson SE, Chatterjee S, Chaudhuri M, White MF. YMXM motifs of IRS-1 define substrate specificity of the insulin receptor kinase. Proc Natl Acad Sci U S A. 1992;89(6):2027–31.

Songyang Z, Cantley LC. Recognition and specificity in protein tyrosine kinase-mediated signaling. TIBS. 1995;20:470–5.

Songyang Z, Carraway III KL, Eck MJ, Harrison SC, Feldman RA, Mohammadi M, et al. Catalytic specificity of protein-tyrosine kinases is critical for selective signalling. Nature. 1995;373:536–9.

Srinivas G, Vennison SJ, Sudha SN, Balasubramanian P, Sekar V. Unique regulation of crystal protein production in Bacillus thuringiensis subsp. yunnanensis is mediated by the cry protein-encoding 103-megadalton plasmid. Appl Environ Microbiol. 1997;63(7):2792–7.

Sun XJ, Rothenberg P, Kahn CR, Backer JM, Araki E, Wilden PA, et al. Structure of the insulin-receptor substrate Irs-1 defines a unique signal transduction protein. Nature. 1991;352(6330):73–7.

Suri C, Jones PF, Patan S, Bartunkova S, Maisonpierre PC, Davis S, et al. Requisite role of angiopoietin-1, a ligand for the TIE2 receptor, during embryonic angiogenesis. Cell. 1996;87 (7):1171–80.

Takano T, Urushibara T, Yoshioka N, Saito T, Fukuda M, Tomomura M, et al. LMTK1 regulates dendritic formation by regulating movement of Rab11A-positive endosomes. Mol Biol Cell. 2014;25(11):1755–68.

Taniguchi CM, Kondo T, Sajan M, Luo J, Bronson R, Asano T, et al. Divergent regulation of hepatic glucose and lipid metabolism by phosphoinositide 3-kinase via Akt and PKClambda/zeta. Cell Metab. 2006;3(5):343–53.

Tartari CJ, Gunby RH, Coluccia AM, Sottocornola R, Cimbro B, Scapozza L, et al. Characterization of some molecular mechanisms governing autoactivation of the catalytic domain of the anaplastic lymphoma kinase. J Biol Chem. 2008;283(7):3743–50.

Taylor SI. Deconstructing type 2 diabetes. Cell. 1999;97:9–12.

Thorpe LM, Yuzugullu H, Zhao JJ. PI3K in cancer: divergent roles of isoforms, modes of activation and therapeutic targeting. Nat Rev Cancer. 2015;15(1):7–24.

Till JH, Ablooglu AJ, Frankel M, Bishop SM, Kohanski RA, Hubbard SR. Crystallographic and solution studies of an activation loop mutant of the insulin receptor tyrosine kinase: insights into kinase mechanism. J Biol Chem. 2001;276(13):10049–55.

Tomomura M, Morita N, Yoshikawa F, Konishi A, Akiyama H, Furuichi T, et al. Structural and functional analysis of the apoptosis-associated tyrosine kinase (AATYK) family. Neuroscience. 2007;148(2):510–21.

Tsou WI, Nguyen KQ, Calarese DA, Garforth SJ, Antes AL, Smirnov SV, et al. Receptor tyrosine kinases, TYRO3, AXL, and MER, demonstrate distinct patterns and complex regulation of ligand-induced activation. J Biol Chem. 2014;289(37):25750–63.

Tsunekawa S, Demozay D, Briaud I, McCuaig J, Accili D, Stein R, et al. FoxO feedback control of basal IRS-2 expression in pancreatic beta-cells is distinct from that in hepatocytes. Diabetes. 2011;60(11):2883–91.

Ueki K, Yballe CM, Brachmann SM, Vicent D, Watt JM, Kahn CR, et al. Increased insulin sensitivity in mice lacking p85beta subunit of phosphoinositide 3-kinase. Proc Natl Acad Sci USA. 2002;99(1):419–24.

Ullrich A, Schlessinger J. Signal transduction by receptors with tyrosine kinase activity. Cell. 1990;61(2):203–12.

Ullrich A, Coussens L, Hayflick JS, Dull TJ, Gray A, Tam AW, et al. Human epidermal growth factor receptor cDNA sequence and aberrant expression of the amplified gene in A431 epidermoid carcinoma cells. Nature. 1984;309(5967):418–25.

Ullrich A, Bell JR, Chen EY, Herrera R, Petruzzelli LM, Dull TJ, et al. Human insulin receptor and its relationship to the tyrosine kinase family of oncogenes. Nature. 1985;313:756–61.

Ushiro H, Cohen S. Identification of phosphotyrosine as a product of epidermal growth factor-activated protein kinase in A-431 cell membranes. J Biol Chem. 1980;255:8363–5.

Vanhaesebroeck B, Stephens L, Hawkins P. PI3K signalling: the path to discovery and understanding. Nat Rev Mol Cell Biol. 2012;13(3):195–203.

Vashisth H, Abrams CF. All-atom structural models of insulin binding to the insulin receptor in the presence of a tandem hormone-binding element. Proteins. 2013;81(6):1017–30.

Vogel W, Gish GD, Alves F, Pawson T. The discoidin domain receptor tyrosine kinases are activated by collagen. Mol Cell. 1997;1(1):13–23.

Ward CW, Lawrence MC, Streltsov VA, Adams TE, McKern NM. The insulin and EGF receptor structures: new insights into ligand-induced receptor activation. Trends Biochem Sci. 2007;32 (3):129–37.

Weiss JB, Xue C, Benice T, Xue L, Morris SW, Raber J. Anaplastic lymphoma kinase and leukocyte tyrosine kinase: functions and genetic interactions in learning, memory and adult neurogenesis. Pharmacol Biochem Behav. 2012;100(3):566–74.

White MF. Insulin signaling in health and disease. Science. 2003;302(5651):1710–1.

White MF, Myers Jr MG. The molecular basis of insulin action. In: DeGroot LJ, Jameson JL, editors. Endocrinology. 4th ed. Philadelphia: W.B. Saunders Co.; 2001. p. 712–27.

White MF, Maron R, Kahn CR. Insulin rapidly stimulates tyrosine phosphorylation of a Mr 185,000 protein in intact cells. Nature. 1985;318:183–6.

White MF, Livingston JN, Backer JM, Lauris V, Dull TJ, Ullrich A, et al. Mutation of the insulin receptor at tyrosine 960 inhibits signal transmission but does not affect its tyrosine kinase activity. Cell. 1988;54:641–9.

Wilden PA, Siddle K, Haring E, Backer JM, White MF, Kahn CR. The role of insulin-receptor kinase domain autophosphorylation in receptor-mediated activities – analysis with insulin and antireceptor antibodies. J Biol Chem. 1992;267(19):13719–27.

Wu J, Tseng YD, Xu CF, Neubert TA, White MF, Hubbard SR. Structural and biochemical characterization of the KRLB region in insulin receptor substrate-2. Nat Struct Mol Biol. 2008;15(3):251–8.

Xu X, Sarikas A. as-Santagata DC, Dolios G, Lafontant PJ, Tsai SC, et al. The CUL7 E3 ubiquitin ligase targets insulin receptor substrate 1 for ubiquitin-dependent degradation. Mol Cell. 2008;30(4):403–14.

Yang Feng TL, Francke U, Ullrich A. Gene for human insulin receptor: localization to site on chromosome 19 involved in pre-B-cell leukemia. Science. 1985;228:728–31.

Yenush L, Makati KJ, SmithHall J, Ishibashi O, Myers MG, White MF. The pleckstrin homology domain is the principle link between insulin receptor and IRS-1. J Biol Chem. 1996;271 (39):24300–6.

Zhang J, Babic A. Regulation of the MET oncogene: molecular mechanisms. Carcinogenesis. 2016;37(4):345–55.

Zick Y. Role of Ser/Thr kinases in the uncoupling of insulin signaling. Int J Obes Relat Metab Disord. 2003;27(Suppl 3):S56–60.

Zick Y. Ser/Thr phosphorylation of IRS proteins: a molecular basis for insulin resistance. Sci STKE. 2005;2005(268):1–3.

Cytokine Receptors

7

Andrew J. Brooks, Farhad Dehkhoda, and Birthe B. Kragelund

Abstract

Cytokine receptors initiate intracellular signaling that regulate a diverse range of biological and medically important functions including metabolism control, neural stem cell activation, inflammatory responses, bone development, as well as blood cell and immune cell development and growth. The unifying feature of these receptors is their ability to activate the JAK-STAT pathway; however, they are grouped into two structurally related classes, known as class I and class II. Class I cytokine receptors have over 30 members including receptors for erythropoietin (EPO), prolactin (PRL), growth hormone (GH), thrombopoietin (TPO), leptin, (LEP), granulocyte-macrophage colony-stimulating factor (GM-CSF), leukemia inhibitory factor (LIF), interleukin-3 (IL-3), IL-5, IL-6, and IL-7. The class II cytokine receptor family includes the interferon receptors, IL-10 receptor, and number of more recently discovered cytokine receptors for IL-19, IL-20, IL-22, IL-24, IL-26, and IL-29. This chapter will review the structure, activation mechanism, and signaling of cytokine receptors.

A.J. Brooks (✉)
The University of Queensland Diamantina Institute, The University of Queensland, Translational Research Institute, Woolloongabba, QLD, Australia

The University of Queensland, Institute for Molecular Bioscience, Brisbane, QLD, Australia
e-mail: a.brooks@uq.edu.au

F. Dehkhoda
The University of Queensland Diamantina Institute, The University of Queensland, Translational Research Institute, Woolloongabba, QLD, Australia
e-mail: farhad.dehkhoda@uq.edu.au

B.B. Kragelund
Structural Biology and NMR Laboratory, Department of Biology, University of Copenhagen, Copenhagen, Denmark
e-mail: bbk@bio.ku.dk

A. Belfiore, D. LeRoith (eds.), *Principles of Endocrinology and Hormone Action*, Endocrinology, https://doi.org/10.1007/978-3-319-44675-2_8

Keywords
Cytokine Receptors • JAK-STATs • Growth Hormone Receptor • Prolactin Receptor • Class I Cytokine Receptors • Class II Cytokine Receptors

Contents

Introduction

Cytokine receptors play pivotal roles in many cellular processes. They initiate signaling cascades that regulate a vast range of vital physiological functions, including metabolism control, neural stem cell activation, inflammatory responses, bone development, as well as blood cell and immune cell development and growth. They are also involved in reproduction, lactation, postnatal growth, and body composition. One of the most defining and indeed unifying features of this diverse group of receptors is their ability to activate Janus kinase (JAK) tyrosine kinases to initiate signaling. The cytokine receptors are grouped into two classes based on sequence homology and structural features. The class I cytokine receptor family (Fig. 1) comprises more than 30 members including receptors for erythropoietin (EPO), prolactin (PRL), growth hormone (GH), thrombopoietin (TPO), leptin (LEP), granulocyte-macrophage colony-stimulating factor (GM-CSF), leukemia inhibitory factor (LIF), interleukin-3 (IL-3), IL-5, IL-7, and IL-6 (Waters and Brooks 2015). The class II receptors initially included the interferon receptors and IL-10 receptor; however, due to the discovery of further cytokines and their receptors, this class has expanded to include others such as IL-19, IL-20, IL-22, IL-24, IL-26, and IL-29 (Renauld 2003). Only some class I cytokine receptors have ligands that are considered hormones and are directly involved in the endocrine system. These are GH, PRL, and LEP.

Cytokines

Cytokines are a group of pleiotropic small soluble polypeptides that exhibit a wide range of actions. They can affect cells from which they are secreted in an autocrine fashion, on other cells in near vicinity in a paracrine fashion, or on distant target cells

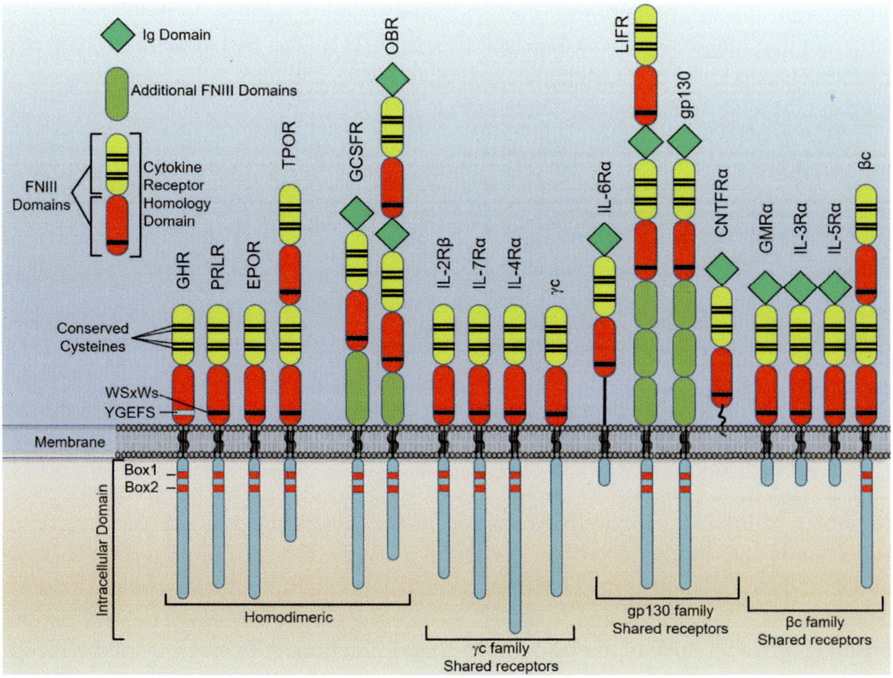

Fig. 1 Domain organization of class I cytokine receptors. Illustration showing domains of examples of homodimeric receptors and of the γc, gp130, and βc family of receptors

in an endocrine fashion. Cytokines bind to their cognate transmembrane receptors and initiate downstream signaling leading to multiple functions including induction of immune responses, cell proliferation, altered metabolism, and differentiation.

Class I cytokines (activate class I cytokine receptors) are characterized by their four-α-helix bundle protein structures. The four α-helices of hematopoietic cytokines fold in an "up-up-down-down" orientation with the two first helices (A and B) being parallel to each other and antiparallel to the other two (C and D), and they are connected by two long, overhand loops (Kossiakoff and De Vos 1998). Based on the length of these helices, they are classified into two groups: a "short-chain" group and a "long-chain" group (Wells and de Vos 1996). Members of the "long-chain" group possess 160–200 residues and long helices (~25 residues) with an angle of about 18° between the AD and BC helix pairs (Sprang and Bazan 1993). Based on structural evidence, growth hormone (GH), interleukin-6 (IL-6), granulocyte colony-stimulating factor (G-CSF), leukemia inhibitory factor (LIF), erythropoietin (EPO), and prolactin (PRL) (Kossiakoff and De Vos 1998) belong to the long-chain cytokine group. Analogously, cytokines that belong to the short-chain group are shorter (105–145 residues) with shorter helices (~15 residues) and a wider AD/BC packing angle of 35°. Members of this family include granulocyte-macrophage colony-stimulating factor (GM-CSF), macrophage colony-stimulating factor (M-CSF), IL-2, IL-3, IL-4, IL-5, IL-7, IL-9, and IL-13 (Wells and de Vos 1996).

In addition, the short-chain group of cytokines contains β-sheets in their structure, a structure that long-chain cytokines lack (Sprang 1993). The first structure solved of a cytokine was porcine GH (Abdel-Meguid et al. 1987), and later the crystal structure of human GM-CSF was reported (Walter et al. 1992).

Class II cytokines were originally confined to interferons (IFNs) and IL-10; however, with the discovery of new cytokines, this has forced a reorganization of the classifications. Based on current classification, class II cytokines are grouped into four different types including type I, II, and III IFNs and the IL-10 family of cytokines. Although these cytokines share common structural features, they induce various and diverse responses on their target cells (Pestka et al. 2004b).

Cytokine Receptors

Class I Cytokine Receptors

Members of the class I cytokine receptor family (also known as the hematopoietin superfamily) are fundamentally important in a diverse range of biological processes, and their dysregulation is implicated in roles in cancers, inflammatory bowel disease, osteoporosis, multiple sclerosis, as well as disorders related to blood cell formation, postnatal growth, obesity, lactation, and neural function. All class I cytokine receptors employ receptor-associated Janus kinases (JAK1, JAK2, JAK3, and TYK2) bound to a conserved "Box1" motif of the intracellular domain of the receptor to initiate intracellular signaling (Waters and Brooks 2015). Generally this is predominantly transmitted through activation of signal transducers and activators of transcription (STATs), of which several different types exist (STAT1, STAT2, STAT3, STAT4, STAT5a, STAT5b, and STAT6). In addition to the associated JAKs, several members of the class I receptor family have now been shown to associate with and activate Src family kinases (SFKs), and for some receptors, this has been further defined to be independent of receptor interaction with, and activations of, JAK (Ingley 2012; Kobayashi et al. 1993; Perugini et al. 2010; Rowlinson et al. 2008).

The cytokine receptors are single-pass transmembrane receptors with an N-terminal extracellular domain (ECD) and a C-terminal intracellular domain (ICD) (Fig. 1). Great insight into the mechanism of these receptors has been obtained through solving the extracellular domain structures that bind their ligand. ECD structures of many members of this receptor family have now been solved including that of GHR (Brown et al. 2005; de Vos et al. 1992), EPOR (Livnah et al. 1998, 1999), PRLR (Broutin et al. 2010; Dagil et al. 2012), GM-CSFR (Hansen et al. 2008a), IL-3Rα (Broughton et al. 2014), IL-6R (Boulanger et al. 2003; Skiniotis et al. 2005), IL-7Rα (McElroy et al. 2009), and LIFR (Huyton et al. 2007; Skiniotis et al. 2008). There are currently no high-resolution structures of a full-length class I cytokine receptor; however, there is a low-resolution EM structure of the full-length IL-6 receptor with bound JAK1 (Lupardus et al. 2011), and recently a full structural model was presented of full-length PRLR (Bugge et al. 2016b). A few NMR structures of the transmembrane domains (TMDs) have been solved which show

how these are α-helical (Bugge et al. 2016b; Kim et al. 2007; Li et al. 2014, 2015), and a recent in-depth review has described the details of these structures, including their dimers (Bugge et al. 2016a). The only structural analysis of the intracellular domain for class I cytokine receptors has shown that the ICDs of the GHR and PRLR are intrinsically disordered throughout their entire length and appears to contain disordered lipid interaction domains (Bugge et al. 2016b; Haxholm et al. 2015).

The extracellular domain of class I cytokine receptors is characterized by an approximately 200-amino acid residue-long modular region known as a cytokine receptor homology (CRH) domain (de Vos et al. 1992) that comprises a cytokine-binding region (Fig. 1). The CRH module possesses two fibronectin type III (FNIII) domains connected via a short, rather inflexible linker region. The N-terminal domain of the CRH (upper FNIII) carries four conserved cysteine residues that form two disulfide bonds. The membrane-proximal C-terminal domain (lower FNIII) contains a conserved WSxWS motif, with the exception of GHR which possesses the homologous sequence YGeFS (Waters and Brooks 2011). The WSxWS motif is not necessary for cytokine binding; however, it is important for the receptor expression and stability (Hilton et al. 1995) and has been speculated to form a binding site for ligands of the extracellular matrix (Olsen and Kragelund 2014). The WSxWS motif appears not to be directly involved in binding the ligand (Dagil et al. 2012; Olsen and Kragelund 2014), but undergoes conformational changes of importance for activation (see below for PRLR) (Dagil et al. 2012). The WSxWS motif and conserved cysteine residues are defining features of the class I cytokine receptor family (Bazan 1990; Liongue and Ward 2007). Some class I cytokine receptors such as GHR, PRLR, and EPOR have a single CRH which is sufficient to mediate cytokine binding and receptor activation, while other members of this family carry additional membrane-proximal (FNIII) domains or immunoglobulin III (IgIII) domains and may possess even more than one CRH (Fig. 1) (Liongue and Ward 2007; Waters and Brooks 2015). Class I cytokine receptors that possess two CRHs include LIFR, leptin receptor (LEPR or OBR), TPO receptor (TPOR or MPL), and the common beta chain (βc) (Liongue and Ward 2007; Sato and Miyajima 1994).

Each FNIII domain of the CRH possesses seven β-strands that are sequentially named A, B, C, C′, E, F, and G, where these strands form a sandwich of two antiparallel β-sheets, one with three strands (A, B, and E) and the other with four strands C, C′, F, and G (Bagley et al. 1997; de Vos et al. 1992; Wang et al. 2009). The four conserved cysteine residues are buried deep in the core of the N-terminal FNIII domain of a CRH and form two disulfide bonds that connect strands A to B and C′ to E. The GHR possesses an additional cysteine residue in the C-terminal E strand of the CRH that forms a disulfide bond with strand F, the cysteine of which is also present in other class I receptors as a reduced cysteine (Bagley et al. 1997; de Vos et al. 1992; Wang et al. 2009). The linker between the two domains is short, rather inflexible, and via a short turn formation, it generates an angle between the domains. This arrangement secures that two tryptophans, one from each FNIII domain, are presented toward the incoming ligand where they form prominent parts of the binding site.

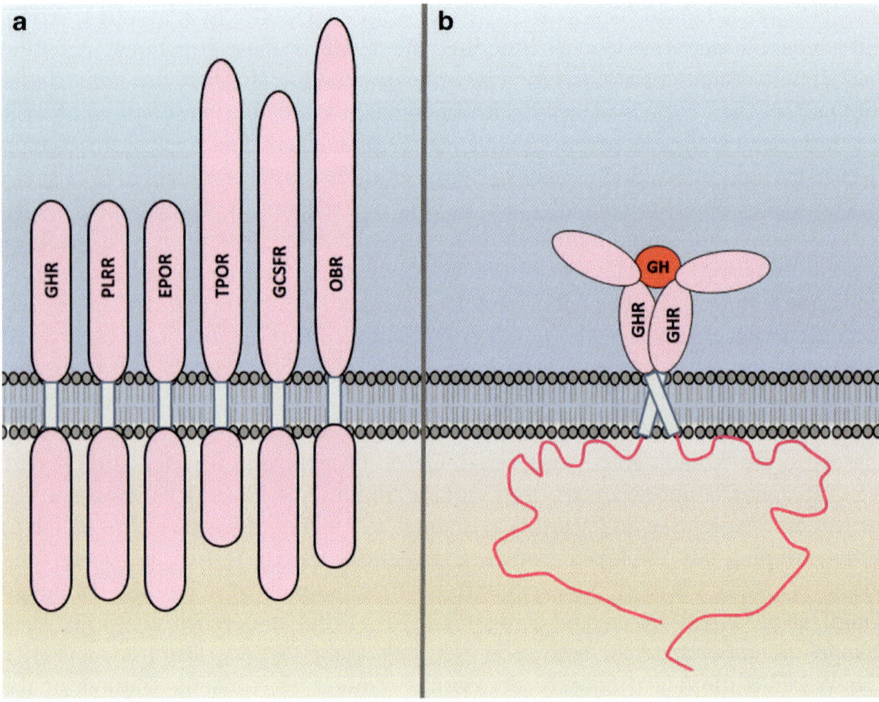

Fig. 2 The homodimeric class I cytokine receptors. Illustration showing ECD, TMD, and ICD for each member (**a**) and an example of a ligand-bound active receptor shown for GHR bound to GH (**b**)

Some members of the class I cytokine receptor family, including GHR, PRLR, EPOR, and LEPR, are homodimers when bound to their activating ligand (Fig. 2). Other receptor members form a complex of two receptor subunits and in some cases three receptor subunits, where one subunit is shared between different cytokine receptor complexes. There are three shared class I cytokine receptor subunits: GP130 (also known as CD130, IL-6ST, or IL-6β), common beta chain (βc), and common gamma chain (γc) (Broughton et al. 2015; McElroy et al. 2012; Miyajima et al. 1992; Ozaki and Leonard 2002; Skiniotis et al. 2008). These shared receptors do not typically show substantial affinity toward cytokines; however, in the presence of cytokine-specific α-receptors, they form high-affinity cytokine receptor complexes that initiate intracellular signaling (Hercus et al. 2013; Nicola and Hilton 1998; Wang et al. 2009).

The ICDs of cytokine receptors have properties that characterize them as intrinsically disordered (ID) (Dunker et al. 2001; Sigalov 2011; Tantos et al. 2012; Wright and Dyson 1999), at least in the absence of bound signaling proteins (Bugge et al. 2016b; Haxholm et al. 2015; Skiniotis et al. 2008). Intrinsically disordered proteins (IDPs) or regions (IDR) can fold upon binding (Dyson and Wright 2005), but very often they exploit short linear sequence motifs (SLiM) for interactions (Davey et al. 2012;

Fuxreiter et al. 2007; Neduva et al. 2005) that may or may not fold into a helix or a strand when bound (Fuxreiter 2012; Fuxreiter et al. 2004; Mohan et al. 2006; Vacic et al. 2007). Thus, the mere length of the ICDs of the cytokine receptors has the potential to carry numerous small interaction motifs, which is the prerequisite for their generally large interactome. The intracellular proline-rich Box1 motif, which is a perfect example of a SLiM, is located a short distance from the cell membrane and is an essential feature of this class of cytokine receptors. A less conserved Box2 sequence consisting of acidic, hydrophobic, and aromatic residues is located close to but C-terminal of the Box1 motif (Bagley et al. 1997; Waters and Brooks 2015). The Box1 motif is essential for signal transduction to JAKs and acts as a high-affinity binding site for a cognate JAK, while the Box2 also appears to play an important role in the interaction with, and signal transduction to, JAKs (Bagley et al. 1997; Usacheva et al. 2002). Activation of the receptor results in JAK phosphorylation followed by further phosphorylation of multiple tyrosine residues in the ICD of the receptor (Brooks and Waters 2010; Shuai and Liu 2003). This provides a scaffold for binding of STAT members, especially STAT5a and STAT5b, which are subsequently phosphorylated by the receptor-bound JAK. The phosphorylated STATs are then transported to the nucleus where they drive the transcriptional regulation aspect of the cytokine/hormone action (Baker et al. 2007; Brooks et al. 2008; Shuai and Liu 2003). The JAK members are not restricted to phosphorylation of certain tyrosine residues in a cytoplasmic domain of a cytokine receptor as they can directly phosphorylate other signal-transducing protein substrates. Accordingly, STAT1 and STAT3 can be activated directly by JAK2 without binding to the cytokine receptor. The SFKs, Ras/extracellular signal-regulated kinase (ERK), phosphoinositol (PI)-3 kinase/Akt, and nuclear factor kappa-light-chain-enhancer of activated B cell (NF-κB) pathways are shown to be activated for GHR, PRLR, and other cytokine receptors (Chin et al. 1998; Fresno Vara et al. 2000; Rawlings et al. 2004; Slavova-Azmanova et al. 2014; Waters and Brooks 2011).

Homodimeric Class I Cytokine Receptors

The homodimeric class I cytokine receptors include the simplest members of this family with a single CRH (GHR, PRLR, and EPOR) and more complex receptors such as LEPR and TPOR with two CRHs (Fig. 2). The simple homodimeric receptors have been extensively studied at the structural and functional level and have become archetypes for understanding the mechanism of activation and signal transduction. The GHR and PRLR will be discussed in detail due to their importance in endocrinology and the large amount of structural and functional data available.

Growth Hormone Receptor (GHR)

Activation of GHR by GH mediates a diverse range of physiological actions, particularity metabolic and growth-related actions. These actions can be directly mediated by GH or indirectly by insulin-like growth factor 1 (IGF-1) (Brooks and Waters 2010; Lichanska and Waters 2008). There is considerable evidence for an important role for GH signaling in cancer, including a role for nuclear-localized GHR (Brooks et al. 2008; Chhabra et al. 2011; Conway-Campbell et al. 2007, 2008).

The GHR signals through the well-characterized JAK-STAT signaling pathway and also through ERK1/ERK2 signaling via SFKs (Brooks and Waters 2010). The extracellular domain of GHR is cleaved by proteolysis from the full-length membrane-bound form, generating a soluble protein that retains GH-binding ability. This protein is known as the growth hormone-binding protein (GHBP) and can be found in humans and other species (Barnard et al. 1989; Baumann 2002). There is strong evidence that GHBP plays important functional roles in modulating GH action (Herington and Brooks 2014).

The GHR is a 638-amino acid residue-long homodimeric class I cytokine receptor with one CRH, a single-pass transmembrane domain, and a 350-residue-long cytoplasmic intracellular domain. The GHR was the first class I cytokine receptor to be cloned and the first to have its extracellular domain structure solved. This crystal structure was in complex with the ligand GH and showed two receptors bound to a single hormone (de Vos et al. 1992). Elegant biophysical studies showed that GH first bound one receptor with high affinity at a site known as site 1 and then subsequently bound the second receptor with lower affinity in what is known as site 2 (Cunningham et al. 1991; Fuh et al. 1992). The residues that contribute with major binding energy in the hormone/receptor complex are Trp^{104} and Trp^{169}, one from each site with Trp^{104} playing a key role in the weaker site 2 interaction (Clackson et al. 1998; Walsh et al. 2004). The lower cytokine receptor domain of each receptor interacts and thus is also termed the dimerization domain or site 3 with significant contribution to the overall stability of the ternary complex (Chen et al. 1997; Waters and Brooks 2011).

Prolactin Receptor (PRLR)

The biological functions of PRLR signaling include, in addition to its regulation of lactation, growth and differentiation of the mammary gland, modulation of cell proliferation, and survival (Freeman et al. 2000; Horseman and Gregerson 2014; Oakes et al. 2008). Although it remains controversial, a link between PRL signaling and cancer, especially breast and prostate cancers, has been proposed (Bogorad et al. 2008; Ginsburg and Vonderhaar 1995; Tworoger et al. 2013; Wennbo et al. 1997). Activation of the PRLR by PRL, which is produced by the pituitary gland or locally in certain tissues such as the breast and prostate, activates primarily the JAK2/STAT5, the PI3K/Akt, and the mitogen-activated protein kinase (MAPK) pathways, for the latter mainly ERK1/ERK2 and p38 MAPK (Clevenger 2003; Clevenger et al. 2009). In addition, SFKs including Fyn and Src, focal adhesion kinase (FAK), and a Vav2-Nek3-Rac signaling axis are activated (Acosta et al. 2003; Clevenger and Medaglia 1994; Miller et al. 2007). PRLR regulates the transcription of numerous genes, including receptor activator of NF-κB ligand (RANKL), important for mammary gland development (Srivastava et al. 2003), and suppressor of cytokine signaling-3 (SOCS3), a negative feedback regulator of cytokine signaling (Barclay et al. 2009); see below.

The many physiological functions of the PRLR may also be associated with its rare ability to bind other hormones than its cognate ligand PRL, and under different physiological conditions, it can signal in responses to GH and placental lactogen

(PL) (Bole-Feysot et al. 1998; Fu et al. 1992). Although the GH, PRL, and PL are structurally homologous (Teilum et al. 2005), different residues have been shown to be responsible for providing the energy and specificity of the interaction in complex with PRLR (Broutin et al. 2010; Elkins et al. 2000; Somers et al. 1994). Interestingly, the different complexes are variably sensitive to environmental factors such as pH (Keeler et al. 2004).

Similar to the GHR, the PRLR forms trimeric complexes with the hormones; whereas the binding site 1 and 2 affinities of the GH/GHR complex are both in the nM range (Cunningham et al. 1991; Uchida et al. 1999), binding of PRL to PRLR occurs through a much lower combined site 2 and site 3 interactions with just ~30 μM affinity (Jomain et al. 2007). This indeed has consequences for the lifetime of the complex and is manifested in a signaling network, similar to but also different from GHR.

As an archetype and simple class I receptor, the PRLR has only a single CRH on its extracellular side, and in addition to the defining cysteine bridges, the WSxWS motif possesses different additional molecular switches within the lower FNIII domain of relevance to its signaling properties. Based on structural and other biophysical studies, it was found that the WSxWS motif adopted a significantly different conformation in the unbound state of the receptor compared to that of the complex. In the unbound state, the two side chains of the two tryptophans Trp^{191} and Trp^{194} arrange in a T-stack that stabilizes an *off-state* of the receptor in which the dimerization surface of the receptor (site 3) is not mature (Dagil et al. 2012). Binding of the hormone leads to a conformational change that reorients the tryptophans into a tryptophan-arginine ladder (Olsen and Kragelund 2014) with measureable local effects in the receptor dimerization site (site 3). Thus, in PRLR, and potentially in other receptors, the lower FNIII domain acts to stabilize the receptor *off-state*, a role that is supported by a constitutive signaling of a prostate cancer-identified variant that lacks this domain (ΔS2) (Tan et al. 2013), as well as a constitutive active variants, $Ile^{146} \rightarrow Leu^{146}$, identified in a breast cancer cohort (Bogorad et al. 2008). Furthermore, a second motif, forming a quartet of residues, and only important in the second receptor in the complex, was seen to control the duration of intracellular MAPK signaling (Zhang et al. 2015). Thus, together these data highlight the very interesting notion that the extracellular domains of class I receptors are not just mere ligand-binding domains that act to capture these in the surrounding solute, but they may exert more sophisticated tasks in modulating the onset as well as the timing of intracellular signaling.

The PRL/PRLR receptor system has been structurally characterized both using x-ray crystallography and solution-state NMR spectroscopy, and the portfolio of structures includes structures of PRL (Teilum et al. 2005), the 1:1 and 1:2 complexes of PRL:PRLR-ECD (Broutin et al. 2010) and of PL:PRLR-ECD (van Agthoven et al. 2010), and the 1:1 complex of a PRL-based antagonist and the PRLR-ECD (Svensson et al. 2008). Besides structures of the complexes, the NMR structure of the unbound PRLR-ECD-D2 domain (C-terminal FNIII domain) has been solved (Dagil et al. 2012), and thorough NMR and biophysical characterization have characterized the hPRLR-ICD as being intrinsically disordered throughout its length

(Haxholm et al. 2015). Recently, combining NMR and computation, a full structural model of the human PRLR was described, which was the first full structure of any cytokine receptor (Bugge et al. 2016b). This structure highlighted that the extracellular domain merely is the tip of a huge molecular iceberg with a long and extended capture radius of the disordered ICD. Interestingly, the structure of the transmembrane helix, which was solved in a membrane mimic detergent, was seen to be equally as long as one FNIII domain, and since this domain carries much of the responsibility for the dimerization process as well as acts as transducers of the signal across the lipid bilayer, this holds the key to the mechanistic understanding.

gp130 Family of Shared Cytokine Receptors

The gp130 is the founding member of the tall cytokine receptors (>1 CRH) and serves as a signal-transducing subunit for IL-6, IL-11, IL-27, LIFR, oncostatin-M (OSM), ciliary neurotropic factor (CNTF), cardiotrophin-1 (CT-1), cardiotrophin-like cytokine (CLC), and others (Fig. 3). The roles played by the gp130 family of cytokines are diverse and include immune responses, neural growth, maintenance of stem cell pluripotency, and cardiovascular functions through signaling via IL-6, CNTF, LIF, and CT-1, respectively. The gp130 cytokines form a dimerization complex through three different combinations of receptor subunits and engage in oligomeric signaling complexes (Wang et al. 2009). The first combination is the formation of a gp130 homodimer following cytokine (IL-6 or IL-11) binding to the specific α-receptors IL-6Rα and IL-11Rα (Matadeen et al. 2007; Schuster et al. 2003; Xu et al. 2010). The second gp130-receptor combination is the formation of a heterodimer with the shared LIFR induced by multiple cytokines such as OSM, CLC, LIF, CNTF, or CT-1 (Pflanz et al. 2004; Skiniotis et al. 2008). Of these cytokines, LIF and OSM can directly interact with gp130 or LIFR with no need to bind any specific α-receptor. However, other cytokines (CLC, CNTF, and CT-1) need to be recognized by a nonsignaling CNTFα receptor (CNTFRα) to form a quaternary signaling complex with gp130 and LIFR (Elson et al. 2000). The third gp130 complex is with the OSM receptor. OSM is the only cytokine that can induce LIFR/gp130- and OSMR/gp130-receptor combinations (Heinrich et al. 1998; Wang et al. 2009).

IL-6 is a pleiotropic cytokine that exhibits both inflammatory and anti-inflammatory functions dependent on its cellular context. It also plays a substantial role in hematopoiesis, regeneration, and tumor formation (Jenkins et al. 2007; Scheller et al. 2011). IL-6Rα contains three domains (D1-D3), where D2 and D3 comprise one CRH (Fig. 3). The IL-6/gp130-receptor complex is initiated by binding of IL-6 to its specific nonsignaling receptor (IL-6Rα) via site 1 interaction. Following binary (IL-6/IL-6Rα) complex formation, this competent complex binds to the CRH of gp130 (situated at D2-D3) via site 2 interactions to form an intermediate nonsignaling ternary complex (Boulanger et al. 2003; Skiniotis et al. 2005). This complex then dimerizes with another ternary complex via interactions in site 3 and with gp130 D1 to form a signaling-competent hexamer (Fig. 3). The hexamer complex contains a membrane-distal "headpiece" and a membrane-proximal "leg" region. A single-particle EM imaging of the ECD of gp130 in a hexameric complex

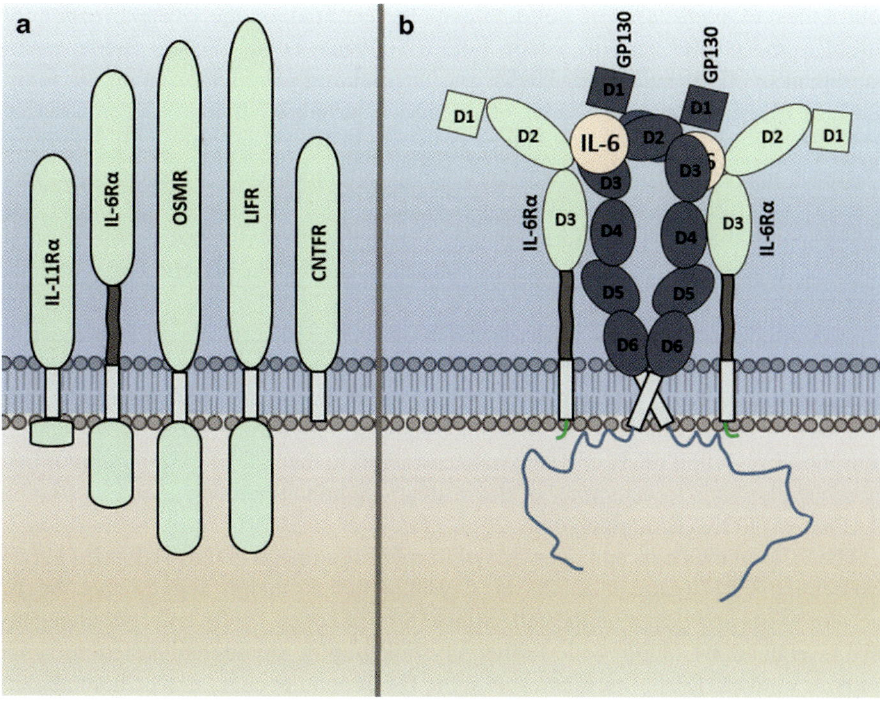

Fig. 3 The gp130 family of shared cytokine receptors. Illustration showing the ECD, TMD, and ICD for each receptor α-subunit (**a**); an example of a ligand-bound active receptor is shown for the hexameric domain structure of gp130/IL-6/IL-6Rα (**b**)

with IL-6/IL-6Rα revealed that the C-terminal FNIII domain "legs" (D6 domains) are brought into proximity on the cell surface upon cytokine binding to allow transphosphorylation of receptor-associated JAKs (Skiniotis et al. 2005). This was also supported by a later higher-resolution crystallography study of the entire ectodomain of gp130 (Xu et al. 2010).

The β_C Family of Shared Cytokine Receptors

Members of the family of the beta common (βc) cytokines including IL-3, IL-5, and GM-CSF are produced by activated T cells and play import roles in production, survival, and activation of many hematopoietic cells (Broughton et al. 2012). Some other cell types such as macrophages and epithelial cells can produce GM-CSF (Wang et al. 2014). IL-3 is the most pleiotropic cytokine among these family members as it stimulates production and function of hematopoietic stem cells, mast cells, and basophils (Broughton et al. 2015; Dahl et al. 2004). Contrary to IL-3, IL-5 is the most specific cytokine of this family and stimulates only the production and activation of eosinophils (Broughton et al. 2015; Lopez et al. 1988). Recent studies have demonstrated that IL-3 and GM-CSF can have actions outside the hematopoietic system. Preclinical studies suggested that GM-CSF contributes to metastasis of solid tumors by stimulating the overexpression of vascular endothelial growth factor (VEGF) (Wang et al. 2014), matrix metalloproteinase (Gutschalk et al. 2013), and chemokines (Broughton et al. 2015; Su et al. 2014). On the other hand, other studies proposed that overexpression of GM-CSF by human colorectal tumor cells might be an indication of improved prognosis and/or extended patient survival in colorectal cancer patients (Nebiker et al. 2014; Urdinguio et al. 2013).

The βc is the main signaling subunit shared by the cytokines of this family; however, it does not by itself bind to cytokines, but in the presence of a specific receptor α-chain, high-affinity complexes are formed where the bound cytokine makes close contacts with residues of the βc (Hercus et al. 2013). In a similar manner to initiation of signaling by the gp130 family, cytokines need first to bind to their specific α-receptor followed by binding to the βc receptor, which then completes a signaling-competent complex that activates associated JAK2s. Activation of the JAK2s results in transphosphorylation of six crucial tyrosine residues in the ICD of the β_C receptor that subsequently leads to activation of downstream signaling pathways such as STATs, MAPK, and PI3K (Broughton et al. 2012; Hercus et al. 2009).

The ECD of the βc receptor consists of four FNIII domains (D1-D4) divided in two consecutive CRH (Carr et al. 2001). Crystallographic studies suggest that the βc receptor exists as a dimer on the cell surface (Stomski et al. 1998), and later mutagenesis investigations along with further crystallography studies suggested that the cytokine binds to D1 of one chain and to the D4 of another chain in a βc homodimer, which thereby join in an antiparallel fashion (Murphy et al. 2003; Wang et al. 2009).

Of the three cytokines that signal through the βc receptor, only binding of the GM-CSF is discussed in details. The GM-CSF is a typical four α-helix bundle class I cytokine that binds to its specific α-subunit GMRα. The GMRα is comprised of three FNIII domains constituting an N-terminal domain (NTD), D2, and D3, the latter two constituting the CRH. Similar to other complexes, the GM-CSF binds to the GMRα in the elbow region between D2 and D3 forming a binary complex (Hansen et al. 2008b). The crystal structure of the binary complex has recently been solved, and comparison of this structure with the crystal structure of the ternary complex shows rotations of the membrane-proximal GHRα and βc receptor subunits (Broughton et al. 2016). It was suggested that such movements might reorient the transmembrane domains upon cytokine binding supporting that a receptor activation mechanism similar to what has been proposed for the GHR may exist. The GM-CSF ternary complex crystal structure also showed that two binary complexes bind to a βc dimer to form a hexameric complex (Hercus et al. 2013). In the ternary complex, the GMRα receptor binds to the D4 domain of the βc receptor via its D3 domain to form a third interaction site (site 3) (Hansen et al. 2008b). The structure of the βc receptor enables it to be assembled into a unique higher-order signaling complex that has not been seen in other cytokine receptors. The crystal lattice of the ternary complex forms an unexpected dodecamer complex (Fig. 4) comprised of two hexamers oriented in a head-to-head fashion (Hansen et al. 2008a, b). Three additional interaction sites were apparent from the dodecamer complex (Broughton et al. 2015). First is a large interaction surface "site 4" with major contributions from

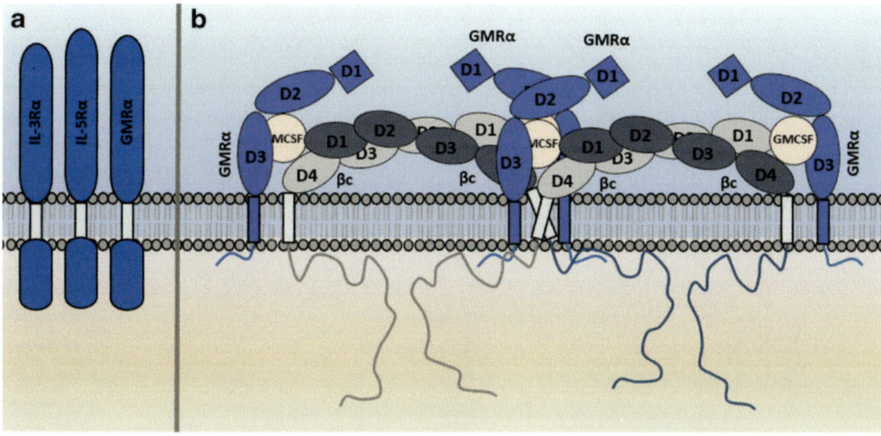

Fig. 4 The βc family of shared cytokine receptors with the higher-order signaling complex shown for GM-CSFR. Illustration showing the ECD, TMD, and ICD for each receptor α-subunit (**a**); an example of a ligand-bound active receptor is shown for the dodecameric GM-CSFR (**b**)

two central D4 domains of the βc receptor of each hexamer and minor contributions from interactions between the GMRα of one hexamer and the D4 domain of βc receptor of another hexamer. Second, interactions between two GM-CSF molecules in the center of the dodecamer complex were designated as site 5. Third, a possible site 6 interaction formed between the NTD domains of two GMRα subunits in the overlapping region of two hexamers was suggested (Broughton et al. 2012; Hercus et al. 2013). Formation of the dodecamer has been proposed to be critical for forming a competent receptor signaling complex (Hercus et al. 2009). Whether such higher-order complexes are possible for other cytokine receptors is currently not known.

The γc Family of Shared Cytokine Receptors

The γc receptor is a shared receptor subunit for a subset of class I cytokines (Fig. 5) including IL-2, IL-4, IL-7, IL-9, IL-15, and IL-21 (Walsh 2012). Cytokines of this family play a significant role in maintaining normal functions of the cells of the immune system. Survival and proliferation of natural cell precursors, B, and T cells have been shown to be upregulated in the bone marrow and thymus via cytokines of this family (Masse et al. 2007). Different forms of severe combined immunodeficiency (SCID) diseases, which are the most severe forms of primary immune deficiencies so far, have been linked to mutations in γc receptor such as X-linked SCID (XSCID) resulting in the absence of NK and T cells in patients (Noguchi et al. 1993; Rochman et al. 2009).

A signaling-competent γc receptor complex is composed of one of the specific cytokines mentioned above, a cytokine-specific α- or β-specific chain and a γc chain. Among the γc family of cytokines, IL-2 and IL-15 form receptor complexes comprised of three different receptor subunits in which they share IL-2Rβ and γc chains. IL-2 binds to IL-2Rβ, IL-2Rα, and γc to induce signaling, while IL-15 binds to IL-2Rβ, IL-15Rα,

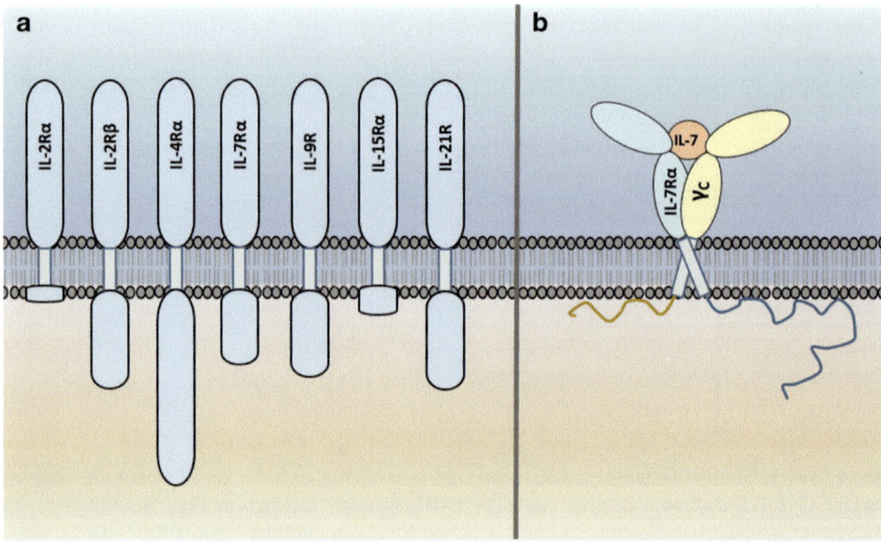

Fig. 5 The γc family of shared cytokine receptors. Illustration showing the ECD, TMD, and ICD for each receptor α-subunit (**a**); an example of a ligand-bound active receptor is shown for the heterodimeric domain structure of IL-7Rα/IL-7/γc (**b**)

and γc. IL-4, IL-7, IL-9, and IL-21 bind to their specific α-receptors and to the γc receptor for signaling (Kovanen and Leonard 2004; Wang et al. 2009). The γc receptor is not required for all receptor signaling complexes for this subset of cytokines as IL-13Rα heterodimerizes with IL-4Rα, which can be activated by IL-13 or IL-4 (Oh et al. 2010; Wang et al. 2009). Thus, it is currently not clear what determines the promiscuity of the different receptors and to what extent the ligand is deterministic.

The γc possesses a relatively short cytoplasmic domain (86 amino acid residues) compared to other signaling subunits of class I cytokine receptors, and it also lacks the classical Box1 or Box2 motif (Lai et al. 1996; Wang et al. 2009). However, despite the short cytoplasmic domain and lack of archetypal JAK-binding motif, the γc receptor retains the ability to bind JAK3 via its membrane-proximal region and is also known to be the only receptor that mediates JAK3-dependent signaling (Nelson et al. 1996; Suzuki et al. 2000; Wu and Sun 2012). Cytokine binding to γc receptor complexes results in activation of the γc-associated JAK3 and a different JAK family member bound to the opposing receptor subunit (Ghoreschi et al. 2009; Oh et al. 2010; Wang et al. 2009).

Class II Cytokine Receptors

The class II cytokine receptors are distinguished from class I cytokine receptors by several features including different arrangement of their conserved four cysteine residues and lack of the WSxWS motif in their ECD. Initially six receptors were described as class II cytokine receptors; however, discoveries of new cytokines led to the addition of further six new receptors which have resulted in a total of 12 class II cytokine receptors described to date (Langer et al. 2004; Liongue et al. 2016; Renauld 2003).

Cytokines for class I receptors were originally defined as interferons and IL-10, but with the discovery of more cytokines, this has expanded the class of IL-10-like (or IFN-like) cytokines. Interferons were initially discovered as antiviral agents during virus interference (Samuel 2001). The interferons are divided into three groups: types I, II, and III. Type I IFNs include IFN-α and IFN-β which are the best characterized and the most broadly expressed cytokines. However, other members such as IFN-δ (interferon-delta), IFN-ϵ (interferon-epsilon), IFN-κ (interferon-kappa), IFN-ν (interferon-nu), IFN-τ (interferon-tau), and IFN-ω (interferon-omega) are not ubiquitously expressed but are instead tissue specific (Finter 1996; Trinchieri 2010). Type I IFNs signal through heterodimeric receptor complexes composed of IFNAR1 and IFNAR2. The type II IFNs only possess the sole member IFN-γ which signals through the IFNGRI/IFNGR2 receptor complex (Liongue et al. 2016; Pestka et al. 2004a). Type III IFNs include IL-28A or IL-28α (IFN-λ2), IL-28B or IL-28β (IFN-λ3), and IL-29 (IFN-λ1) (Fox et al. 2009) and are also distantly related to IL-10-like family of cytokines. These cytokines unveil antiviral activity similar to type I IFNs with epithelial cells as their primary targets (Kotenko et al. 2003). This family of cytokines assembles signaling complexes through binding to IFN-λR1 (IL-28R) and IL-10R2 (Donnelly et al. 2004).

IL-10 is a prominent member of the class II cytokine family and exhibits a different mode of action compared to the other members. IL-10 is an anti-inflammatory cytokine that protects cells from effects of excessive inflammatory response (Zhang and An 2007). Other members of this family are IL-19, IL-20, IL-22, IL-24, and IL-26, which have protective roles on epithelial cells against pathogens such as bacteria and yeast (Liongue et al. 2016; Renauld 2003; Sa et al. 2007). Also, IL-20 has been reported to possess wound healing effects and maintaining homeostasis and tissue integrity at the time of infection (Ouyang et al. 2011). Signaling-competent receptor complexes of this family include a cytokine, R1 or a receptor α-chain, and R2 or a receptor β-chain. The R2 chains usually possess shorter intracellular domains, while R2 chains have longer cytoplasmic chains and can bind to other signal transduction protein such as STATs (Kotenko et al. 1997). IL-10 exclusively binds to the IL-10R1 and signals through a heterodimeric IL-10R1/IL-10R2 complex. The IL-10R2 is a shared signaling subunit for other IL-10-related cytokines such as IL-22 and IL-26 where IL-22R1/IL-10R2 and IL-20R1/IL-10R2 complexes are formed, respectively (Sheikh et al. 2004; Wang et al. 2002; Xie et al. 2000). IL-19, IL-20, and IL-24 form signaling complexes via binding to IL-20R1 and IL-20R2. In addition, IL-20 and IL-24 form functioning receptor complexes with IL-22R1 and IL-20R2 (Sabat 2010).

Mechanism of Cytokine Receptor Activation

Activation of JAK

Unlike the family of receptor tyrosine kinases (RTKs) such as fibroblast growth factor receptor (FGFR) or epidermal growth factor receptor (EGFR) (Lemmon and Schlessinger 2010; Singleton et al. 2013), cytokine receptors lack intrinsic tyrosine kinase activity and are critically dependent on association with members of the nonreceptor protein tyrosine kinases (PTKs) family of JAKs and SFKs for their signal transduction (Waters and Brooks 2015; Watowich et al. 1996). Binding of the cytokine to its cognate receptor(s) activates the receptor(s) and results in the activation of the associated specific JAK. There are four different mammalian JAKs: JAK1, JAK2, JAK3, and tyrosine kinase 2 (TYK2) (Darnell 1997). All members of the JAK family are ubiquitously expressed in mammals except for JAK3, which is primarily expressed in hematopoietic cells (Ghoreschi et al. 2009; Rane and Reddy 1994). A receptor complex may activate a single member of the JAK family or a combination of different JAK members (Ghoreschi et al. 2009). The JAKs are large (~1150 amino acid residues) multi-domain proteins that were initially classified into seven sequential JAK homology (JH) domains (JH1-7) (Wilks et al. 1991). Further structural studies suggested that JAKs contain an N-terminal band 4.1, ezrin, radixin, moesin (FERM) domain and a Src homology 2 (SH2) domain, followed by C-terminal pseudokinase (JH2 domain) and tyrosine kinase (JH1 domain) domains (Fig. 6) (Girault et al. 1999). The FERM and SH2 domains are critical for binding the receptor where the conserved Box1 motif is an essential component of this interaction (Ferrao et al. 2016; Haan et al. 2006; Wallweber et al. 2014). The notion that the pseudokinase inhibits basal activity of the kinase arose when experiments showed that deletion of the pseudokinase domain in full-length JAK resulted in constitutive activity of the kinase independent of ligand stimulation (Chen et al. 2000; Saharinen and Silvennoinen 2002). This was supported from studies showing that addition of the pseudokinase domain in trans suppressed kinase activity (Hammaren et al. 2015; Saharinen et al. 2003; Sanz Sanz et al. 2014). A recent study demonstrated a weak kinase activity for the pseudokinase domain which appears to be responsible for autophosphorylation of two inhibitory sites: Ser^{523} in the SH2-JH2 linker region and Tyr^{570} in the pseudokinase N lobe (Ungureanu et al. 2011). However, this feature was not conserved in other JAK family members (Toms et al. 2013). Following cytokine stimulation, two key tyrosine residues (Tyr^{1007} and Tyr^{1008}) in the activation loop of the JAK2 kinase domain become phosphorylated *in trans*, which results in full catalytic activity due to and seemingly enhanced by phosphorylation of additional sites in the domain (Silvennoinen and Hubbard 2015).

The activation of the receptor-bound JAKs in return phosphorylates multiple tyrosine residues in the intracellular region of the receptor which act as docking sites for SH2 domain-containing proteins such as STATs (Levy and Darnell 2002). Based on the activated cytokine receptor and its phosphorylated sites in the cytoplasmic domain, any one or more of six STAT family members (STAT1–STAT6)

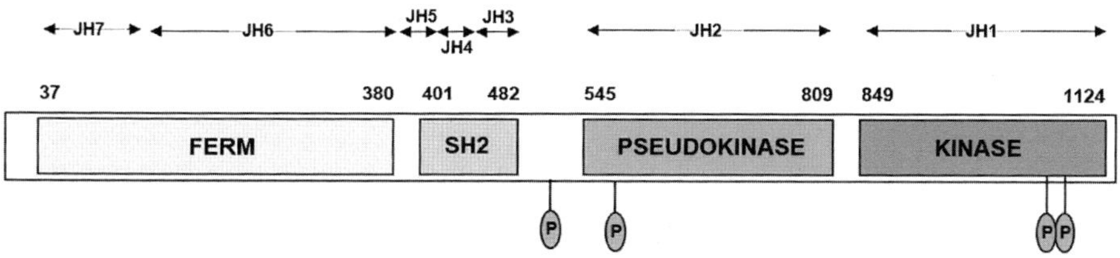

Fig. 6 JAK2 domain structure. Residue ranges of each domain are shown above, and phosphorylation sites important in activation are depicted below (*P*)

may be recruited via their SH2 domain (Babon et al. 2014). The STATs are subsequently phosphorylated by the active JAKs. The phosphorylation of the STATs is commonly thought to result in dimerization of the STATs; however, evidence shows that the STATs can exist as dimers in their unphosphorylated form (Braunstein et al. 2003; Shuai and Liu 2003). Phosphorylation of STATs leads to their DNA binding, nuclear accumulation, and action as transcription factors thereby regulating gene expression (Babon et al. 2014; Iyer and Reich 2008).

Our understanding of the activation mechanism of cytokine receptors has predominantly been due to studies of the simple homodimeric class I receptors and in particular the GHR which has become an archetype for this receptor class as it was the first member to be cloned (Leung et al. 1987) and the first to have its extracellular domain crystal structure solved in complex with its ligand (de Vos et al. 1992). The original mechanism for cytokine receptor activation was proposed from studies over 20 years ago (Wells and Kossiakoff 2014). This receptor activation paradigm proposed that ligand-free receptors existed on cell membranes as monomers and that cytokine binding induced receptor dimerization by first binding to the high-affinity site 1 on one receptor and subsequently binding to the lower-affinity site 2 on the second receptor. It was this ligand-mediated receptor dimerization that was proposed to be responsible for activation of the associated kinases by bringing them into close proximity. More recently a new paradigm of cytokine receptor activation has been proposed by using a range of different technologies to study the mechanism of GHR activation. Studies supporting the new paradigm show that the cytokine receptors exist predominantly as ligand-independent preformed dimers on the cell surface prior to cytokine binding and that cytokine binding induces a structural reorientation of the receptor dimers resulting in repositioning of the associated kinases leading to their activation (Brooks and Waters 2015; Wells and Kossiakoff 2014). The key features of this model is that upon activation, the extracellular juxtamembrane parts of the receptors move into close proximity, the transmembrane dimer interactions then reorient from a parallel interaction to a left-handed crossover dimer, and the intracellular juxtamembrane and Box1 sequences separate (Brooks et al. 2014; Brown et al. 2005). Prior to cytokine binding, the JAKs are proposed to be held in an inactive state where the kinase domain from one JAK is inhibited by the pseudokinase domain of a second JAK bound to the other receptor in the receptor dimer (Fig. 7). The receptor movements upon cytokine binding separate the JAKs and remove the

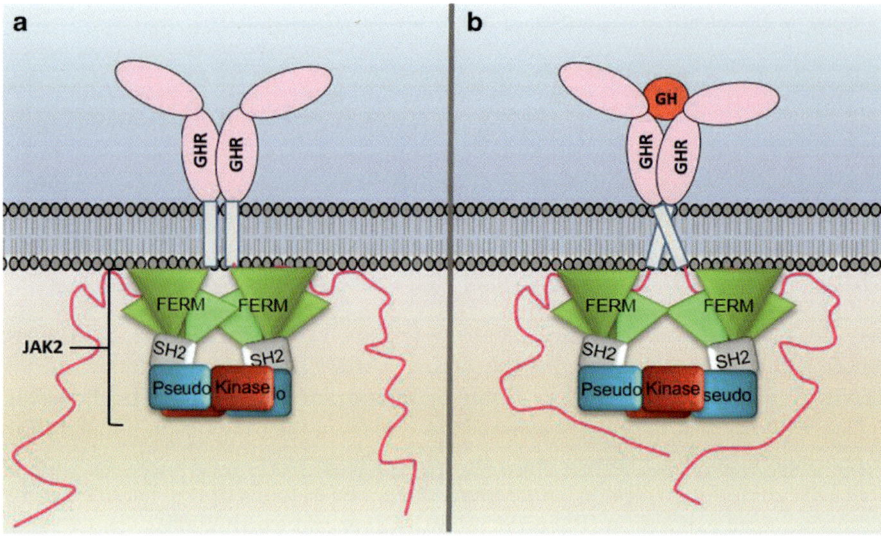

Fig. 7 Cytokine receptor activation mechanism. Model of receptor activation illustrated for GHR. Inactive dimeric receptors prior to ligand binding (**a**) and ligand-bound active receptors with repositioning of the TMD, ICD, and associated JAK2 resulting in kinase activation (**b**)

trans-inhibition bringing the kinase domains in close proximity resulting in *trans*-activation (Brooks et al. 2014; Waters and Brooks 2015). Although well supported by data for the GHR, further studies are indeed required to confirm if this mechanism is common to all cytokine receptors or if variations to the mechanism exist. Indeed structures of the transmembrane domains in dimeric states would be helpful in this respect.

Activation of SFKs

In addition to the associated JAKs, several cytokine receptors have been shown to associate with and activate SFKs. For some cytokine receptors, the activation of SFKs has been further described to be independent of receptor interaction with JAKs and/or activation of JAKs (Ingley 2012; Kobayashi et al. 1993; Perugini et al. 2010; Rowlinson et al. 2008). Much less is known about the activation mechanism of SFKs by cytokine receptors or if all cytokine receptors utilize SFKs; however, their activation predominantly leads to activation of the ERK1/ERK2 signaling pathway (Brooks and Waters 2010; Waters and Brooks 2015).

Receptor Cross Talk with the Membrane

For both GHR and PRLR, it has been discovered that their ICD has affinity for hallmark lipids of the inner leaflet of the plasma membrane, forming one (GHR) or three (PRLR) separate lipid interaction domains (LIDs). Similar to the T-cell immunoreceptors, interactions with the lipids in the common membrane-proximal LID were seen governed by SLiMs, which had resemblance to the so-called immunoreceptor tyrosine-based activation motifs (ITAMs). Some of these ITAM-like motifs in GHR and PRLR harbor tyrosines, which are potential targets for phosphorylation by SFKs, potentially regulating the membrane interaction. However, phosphorylation of such a tyrosine Tyr^{283} in PRLR was independent of lipid interaction and did not abolish the interaction. In addition to the ITAM-like motifs, positively charged residues played similar roles in lipid interaction, and mutation of either motif did not abolish membrane interaction (Bugge et al. 2016b; Haxholm et al. 2015). Thus, this suggests that the positive charges act to attract the LID to the membrane where the ITAM-like motifs anchor the ICD in the membrane via the hydrophobic side chains of the motif.

The role played by the lipid/cytokine receptor cross talk is currently incompletely understood. There may be several reasons to why cytokine receptors arrange part of their ICD along the bilayer normally. First, many kinases that partake in signaling are either themselves anchored in the bilayer through modification by acylation (Patwardhan and Resh 2010; Rawat et al. 2013; Rawat and Nagaraj 2010) or have a lipid interaction site in a domain, such as a phosphoinositide-binding site within the FERM domain of several tyrosine kinases (Bompard et al. 2003; Feng and Mertz 2015; Hamada et al. 2000) or within the SH2 domain of Src-type kinases (Park et al. 2016; Sheng et al. 2016). Thus, membrane interactions may aid the co-localization of the signaling proteins and thereby enhance signaling efficiency. How this is orchestrated mechanistically is not understood, and further studies are indeed needed to fully deconvolute the function of the LIDs.

Negative Regulation of Cytokine Receptor Signaling

There are three classes of major negative regulators of cytokine-mediated JAK-STAT signaling. These are the suppressor of cytokine signaling (SOCS), protein tyrosine phosphatases (PTPs), and protein inhibitors of activated STATs (PIAS). The SOCS provides a negative feedback loop as their expression is directly induced by STATs. SOCS can block signaling by binding to phosphorylated tyrosines on the receptor and blocking recruitment of further signaling molecules, they can directly inhibit JAK signaling by binding directly to the JAK kinase domain, and they can also induce ubiquitylation-mediated proteasomal degradation (Alexander and Hilton 2004; Babon et al. 2014; Linossi et al. 2013). The PIAS act by binding to activated STAT dimers, thereby blocking them from binding DNA (Rawlings et al. 2004; Shuai and Liu 2003). In addition, the protein LNK (SH2B3), a member of the SH2B/Lnk/APS family of adapter proteins, binds to JAK2 and has been shown to be an important inhibitor of JAK2 activation (Babon et al. 2014; Gery et al. 2009).

Cross-References

▶ Receptor Tyrosine Kinases and the Insulin Signaling System
▶ Targeting of Steroid Hormone Receptor Function in Breast and Prostate Cancer

References

Abdel-Meguid SS, Shieh HS, Smith WW, Dayringer HE, Violand BN, Bentle LA. Three-dimensional structure of a genetically engineered variant of porcine growth hormone. Proc Natl Acad Sci USA. 1987;84(18):6434–7.

Acosta JJ, Munoz RM, Gonzalez L, Subtil-Rodriguez A, Dominguez-Caceres MA, Garcia-Martinez JM, et al. Src mediates prolactin-dependent proliferation of T47D and MCF7 cells via the activation of focal adhesion kinase/Erk1/2 and phosphatidylinositol 3-kinase pathways. Mol Endocrinol. 2003;17(11):2268–82.

Alexander WS, Hilton DJ. The role of suppressors of cytokine signaling (SOCS) proteins in regulation of the immune response. Annu Rev Immunol. 2004;22:503–29.

Babon JJ, Lucet IS, Murphy JM, Nicola NA, Varghese LN. The molecular regulation of Janus kinase (JAK) activation. Biochem J. 2014;462(1):1–13.

Bagley CJ, Woodcock JM, Stomski FC, Lopez AF. The structural and functional basis of cytokine receptor activation: lessons from the common beta subunit of the granulocyte-macrophage colony-stimulating factor, interleukin-3 (IL-3), and IL-5 receptors. Blood. 1997;89(5):1471–82.

Baker SJ, Rane SG, Reddy EP. Hematopoietic cytokine receptor signaling. Oncogene. 2007; 26(47):6724–37.

Barclay JL, Anderson ST, Waters MJ, Curlewis JD. SOCS3 as a tumor suppressor in breast cancer cells, and its regulation by PRL. Int J Cancer. 2009;124(8):1756–66.

Barnard R, Quirk P, Waters MJ. Characterization of the growth hormone-binding protein of human serum using a panel of monoclonal antibodies. J Endocrinol. 1989;123(2):327–32.

Baumann G. Growth hormone binding protein. The soluble growth hormone receptor. Minerva Endocrinol. 2002;27(4):265–76.

Bazan JF. Structural design and molecular evolution of a cytokine receptor superfamily. Proc Natl Acad Sci USA. 1990;87(18):6934–8.

Bogorad RL, Courtillot C, Mestayer C, Bernichtein S, Harutyunyan L, Jomain JB, et al. Identification of a gain-of-function mutation of the prolactin receptor in women with benign breast tumors. Proc Natl Acad Sci USA. 2008;105(38):14533–8.

Bole-Feysot C, Goffin V, Edery M, Binart N, Kelly PA. Prolactin (PRL) and its receptor: actions, signal transduction pathways and phenotypes observed in PRL receptor knockout mice. Endocr Rev. 1998;19(3):225–68.

Bompard G, Martin M, Roy C, Vignon F, Freiss G. Membrane targeting of protein tyrosine phosphatase PTPL1 through its FERM domain via binding to phosphatidylinositol 4,5-biphosphate. J Cell Sci. 2003;116(Pt 12):2519–30.

Boulanger MJ, Chow DC, Brevnova EE, Garcia KC. Hexameric structure and assembly of the interleukin-6/IL-6 alpha-receptor/gp130 complex. Science. 2003;300(5628):2101–4.

Braunstein J, Brutsaert S, Olson R, Schindler C. STATs dimerize in the absence of phosphorylation. J Biol Chem. 2003;278(36):34133–40.

Brooks AJ, Waters MJ. The growth hormone receptor: mechanism of activation and clinical implications. Nat Rev Endocrinol. 2010;6(9):515–25.

Brooks AJ, Waters MJ. Rewriting the mechanism of JAK2 activation. Cell Cycle. 2015; 14(3):285–6.

Brooks AJ, Wooh JW, Tunny KA, Waters MJ. Growth hormone receptor; mechanism of action. Int J Biochem Cell Biol. 2008;40(10):1984–9.

Brooks AJ, Dai W, O'Mara ML, Abankwa D, Chhabra Y, Pelekanos RA, et al. Mechanism of activation of protein kinase JAK2 by the growth hormone receptor. Science. 2014;344(6185): 1249783.

Broughton SE, Dhagat U, Hercus TR, Nero TL, Grimbaldeston MA, Bonder CS, et al. The GM-CSF/IL-3/IL-5 cytokine receptor family: from ligand recognition to initiation of signaling. Immunol Rev. 2012;250(1):277–302.

Broughton SE, Hercus TR, Hardy MP, McClure BJ, Nero TL, Dottore M, et al. Dual mechanism of interleukin-3 receptor blockade by an anti-cancer antibody. Cell Rep. 2014;8(2):410–9.

Broughton SE, Nero TL, Dhagat U, Kan WL, Hercus TR, Tvorogov D, et al. The beta c receptor family – structural insights and their functional implications. Cytokine. 2015;74 (2):247–58.

Broughton SE, Hercus TR, Nero TL, Dottore M, McClure BJ, Dhagat U, et al. Conformational changes in the GM-CSF receptor suggest a molecular mechanism for affinity conversion and receptor signaling. Structure. 2016;24(8):1271–81.

Broutin I, Jomain JB, Tallet E, van Agthoven J, Raynal B, Hoos S, et al. Crystal structure of an affinity-matured prolactin complexed to its dimerized receptor reveals the topology of hormone binding site 2. J Biol Chem. 2010;285(11):8422–33.

Brown RJ, Adams JJ, Pelekanos RA, Wan Y, McKinstry WJ, Palethorpe K, et al. Model for growth hormone receptor activation based on subunit rotation within a receptor dimer. Nat Struct Mol Biol. 2005;12(9):814–21.

Bugge K, Lindorff-Larsen K, Kragelund BB. Understanding single-pass transmembrane receptor signaling from a structural viewpoint – what are we missing? FEBS J. 2016a. doi:10.1111/ febs.13793.

Bugge K, Papaleo E, Haxholm GW, Hopper JT, Robinson CV, Olsen JG, et al. A combined computational and structural model of the full-length human prolactin receptor. Nat Commun. 2016b;7:11578.

Carr PD, Gustin SE, Church AP, Murphy JM, Ford SC, Mann DA, et al. Structure of the complete extracellular domain of the common beta subunit of the human GM-CSF, IL-3, and IL-5 receptors reveals a novel dimer configuration. Cell. 2001;104(2):291–300.

Chen C, Brinkworth R, Waters MJ. The role of receptor dimerization domain residues in growth hormone signaling. J Biol Chem. 1997;272(8):5133–40.

Chen M, Cheng A, Candotti F, Zhou YJ, Hymel A, Fasth A, et al. Complex effects of naturally occurring mutations in the JAK3 pseudokinase domain: evidence for interactions between the kinase and pseudokinase domains. Mol Cell Biol. 2000;20(3):947–56.

Chhabra Y, Waters MJ, Brooks AJ. Role of the growth hormone–IGF-1 axis in cancer. Expert Rev Endocrinol Metab. 2011;6:71–84.

Chin H, Arai A, Wakao H, Kamiyama R, Miyasaka N, Miura O. Lyn physically associates with the erythropoietin receptor and may play a role in activation of the Stat5 pathway. Blood. 1998; 91(10):3734–45.

Clackson T, Ultsch MH, Wells JA, de Vos AM. Structural and functional analysis of the 1:1 growth hormone:receptor complex reveals the molecular basis for receptor affinity. J Mol Biol. 1998;277(5):1111–28.

Clevenger CV. Nuclear localization and function of polypeptide ligands and their receptors: a new paradigm for hormone specificity within the mammary gland? Breast Cancer Res. 2003; 5(4):181–7.

Clevenger CV, Medaglia MV. The protein tyrosine kinase P59fyn is associated with prolactin (PRL) receptor and is activated by PRL stimulation of T-lymphocytes. Mol Endocrinol. 1994; 8(6):674–81.

Clevenger CV, Gadd SL, Zheng J. New mechanisms for PRLr action in breast cancer. Trends Endocrinol Metab. 2009;20(5):223–9.

Conway-Campbell BL, Wooh JW, Brooks AJ, Gordon D, Brown RJ, Lichanska AM, et al. Nuclear targeting of the growth hormone receptor results in dysregulation of cell proliferation and tumorigenesis. Proc Natl Acad Sci U S A. 2007;104(33):13331–6.

Conway-Campbell BL, Brooks AJ, Robinson PJ, Perani M, Waters MJ. The extracellular domain of the growth hormone receptor interacts with coactivator activator to promote cell proliferation. Mol Endocrinol. 2008;22(9):2190–202.

Cunningham BC, Ultsch M, De Vos AM, Mulkerrin MG, Clauser KR, Wells JA. Dimerization of the extracellular domain of the human growth hormone receptor by a single hormone molecule. Science. 1991;254(5033):821–5.

Dagil R, Knudsen MJ, Olsen JG, O'Shea C, Franzmann M, Goffin V, et al. The WSXWS motif in cytokine receptors is a molecular switch involved in receptor activation: insight from structures of the prolactin receptor. Structure. 2012;20(2):270–82.

Dahl C, Hoffmann HJ, Saito H, Schiotz PO. Human mast cells express receptors for IL-3, IL-5 and GM-CSF; a partial map of receptors on human mast cells cultured in vitro. Allergy. 2004; 59(10):1087–96.

Darnell Jr JE. STATs and gene regulation. Science. 1997;277(5332):1630–5.

Davey NE, Van Roey K, Weatheritt RJ, Toedt G, Uyar B, Altenberg B, et al. Attributes of short linear motifs. Mol BioSyst. 2012;8(1):268–81.

de Vos AM, Ultsch M, Kossiakoff AA. Human growth hormone and extracellular domain of its receptor: crystal structure of the complex. Science. 1992;255(5042):306–12.

Donnelly RP, Sheikh F, Kotenko SV, Dickensheets H. The expanded family of class II cytokines that share the IL-10 receptor-2 (IL-10R2) chain. J Leukoc Biol. 2004;76(2):314–21.

Dunker AK, Lawson JD, Brown CJ, Williams RM, Romero P, JS O, et al. Intrinsically disordered protein. J Mol Graph Model. 2001;19(1):26–59.

Dyson HJ, Wright PE. Intrinsically unstructured proteins and their functions. Nat Rev Mol Cell Biol. 2005;6(3):197–208.

Elkins PA, Christinger HW, Sandowski Y, Sakal E, Gertler A, de Vos AM, et al. Ternary complex between placental lactogen and the extracellular domain of the prolactin receptor. Nat Struct Biol. 2000;7(9):808–15.

Elson GC, Lelievre E, Guillet C, Chevalier S, Plun-Favreau H, Froger J, et al. CLF associates with CLC to form a functional heteromeric ligand for the CNTF receptor complex. Nat Neurosci. 2000;3(9):867–72.

Feng J, Mertz B. Novel phosphatidylinositol 4,5-bisphosphate binding sites on focal adhesion kinase. PLoS One. 2015;10(7):e0132833.

Ferrao R, Wallweber HJ, Ho H, Tam C, Franke Y, Quinn J, et al. The structural basis for class II cytokine receptor recognition by JAK1. Structure. 2016;24(6):897–905.

Finter NB. The naming of cats-and alpha-interferons. Lancet. 1996;348(9024):348–9.

Fox BA, Sheppard PO, O'Hara PJ. The role of genomic data in the discovery, annotation and evolutionary interpretation of the interferon-lambda family. PLoS One. 2009;4(3):e4933.

Freeman ME, Kanyicska B, Lerant A, Nagy G. Prolactin: structure, function, and regulation of secretion. Physiol Rev. 2000;80(4):1523–631.

Fresno Vara JA, Carretero MV, Geronimo H, Ballmer-Hofer K, Martin-Perez J. Stimulation of c-Src by prolactin is independent of Jak2. Biochem J. 2000;345(Pt 1):17–24.

Fu YK, Arkins S, Fuh G, Cunningham BC, Wells JA, Fong S, et al. Growth hormone augments superoxide anion secretion of human neutrophils by binding to the prolactin receptor. J Clin Invest. 1992;89(2):451–7.

Fuh G, Cunningham BC, Fukunaga R, Nagata S, Goeddel DV, Wells JA. Rational design of potent antagonists to the human growth hormone receptor. Science. 1992;256(5064):1677–80.

Fuxreiter M. Fuzziness: linking regulation to protein dynamics. Mol BioSyst. 2012;8(1):168–77.

Fuxreiter M, Simon I, Friedrich P, Tompa P. Preformed structural elements feature in partner recognition by intrinsically unstructured proteins. J Mol Biol. 2004;338(5):1015–26.

Fuxreiter M, Tompa P, Simon I. Local structural disorder imparts plasticity on linear motifs. Bioinformatics. 2007;23(8):950–6.

Gery S, Cao Q, Gueller S, Xing H, Tefferi A, Koeffler HP. Lnk inhibits myeloproliferative disorder-associated JAK2 mutant, JAK2V617F. J Leukoc Biol. 2009;85(6):957–65.

Ghoreschi K, Laurence A, O'Shea JJ. Janus kinases in immune cell signaling. Immunol Rev. 2009;228(1):273–87.

Ginsburg E, Vonderhaar BK. Prolactin synthesis and secretion by human breast cancer cells. Cancer Res. 1995;55(12):2591–5.

Girault JA, Labesse G, Mornon JP, Callebaut I. The N-termini of FAK and JAKs contain divergent band 4.1 domains. Trends Biochem Sci. 1999;24(2):54–7.

Gutschalk CM, Yanamandra AK, Linde N, Meides A, Depner S, Mueller MM. GM-CSF enhances tumor invasion by elevated MMP-2, −9, and −26 expression. Cancer Med. 2013;2(2):117–29.

Haan C, Kreis S, Margue C, Behrmann I. Jaks and cytokine receptors – an intimate relationship. Biochem Pharmacol. 2006;72(11):1538–46.

Hamada K, Shimizu T, Matsui T, Tsukita S, Hakoshima T. Structural basis of the membrane-targeting and unmasking mechanisms of the radixin FERM domain. EMBO J. 2000; 19(17):4449–62.

Hammaren HM, Ungureanu D, Grisouard J, Skoda RC, Hubbard SR, Silvennoinen O. ATP binding to the pseudokinase domain of JAK2 is critical for pathogenic activation. Proc Natl Acad Sci USA. 2015;112(15):4642–7.

Hansen G, Hercus TR, McClure BJ, Stomski FC, Dottore M, Powell J, et al. The structure of the GM-CSF receptor complex reveals a distinct mode of cytokine receptor activation. Cell. 2008a;134(3):496–507.

Hansen G, Hercus TR, Xu Y, Lopez AF, Parker MW, McKinstry WJ. Crystallization and preliminary X-ray diffraction analysis of the ternary human GM-CSF receptor complex. Acta Crystallogr Sect F: Struct Biol Cryst Commun. 2008b;64(Pt 8):711–4.

Haxholm GW, Nikolajsen LF, Olsen JG, Fredsted J, Larsen FH, Goffin V, et al. Intrinsically disordered cytoplasmic domains of two cytokine receptors mediate conserved interactions with membranes. Biochem J. 2015;468(3):495–506.

Heinrich PC, Behrmann I, Muller-Newen G, Schaper F, Graeve L. Interleukin-6-type cytokine signalling through the gp130/Jak/STAT pathway. Biochem J. 1998;334(Pt 2):297–314.

Hercus TR, Thomas D, Guthridge MA, Ekert PG, King-Scott J, Parker MW, et al. The granulocyte-macrophage colony-stimulating factor receptor: linking its structure to cell signaling and its role in disease. Blood. 2009;114(7):1289–98.

Hercus TR, Dhagat U, Kan WL, Broughton SE, Nero TL, Perugini M, et al. Signalling by the betac family of cytokines. Cytokine Growth Factor Rev. 2013;24(3):189–201.

Herington AC, Brooks AJ. Growth hormone-binding proteins. Ref Module Biomed Res. 2014; http://dx.doi.org/10.1016/B978-0-12-801238-3.04053-8.

Hilton DJ, Watowich SS, Murray PJ, Lodish HF. Increased cell surface expression and enhanced folding in the endoplasmic reticulum of a mutant erythropoietin receptor. Proc Natl Acad Sci USA. 1995;92(1):190–4.

Horseman ND, Gregerson KA. Prolactin actions. J Mol Endocrinol. 2014;52(1):R95–106.

Huyton T, Zhang JG, Luo CS, Lou MZ, Hilton DJ, Nicola NA, et al. An unusual cytokine:Ig-domain interaction revealed in the crystal structure of leukemia inhibitory factor (LIF) in complex with the LIF receptor. Proc Natl Acad Sci USA. 2007;104(31):12737–42.

Ingley E. Functions of the Lyn tyrosine kinase in health and disease. Cell Commun Signal. 2012;10(1):21.

Iyer J, Reich NC. Constitutive nuclear import of latent and activated STAT5a by its coiled coil domain. FASEB J. 2008;22(2):391–400.

Jenkins BJ, Roberts AW, Greenhill CJ, Najdovska M, Lundgren-May T, Robb L, et al. Pathologic consequences of STAT3 hyperactivation by IL-6 and IL-11 during hematopoiesis and lymphopoiesis. Blood. 2007;109(6):2380–8.

Jomain JB, Tallet E, Broutin I, Hoos S, van Agthoven J, Ducruix A, et al. Structural and thermodynamic bases for the design of pure prolactin receptor antagonists: X-ray structure of Del1-9-G129R-hPRL. J Biol Chem. 2007;282(45):33118–31.

Keeler C, Hodsdon ME, Dannies PS. Is there structural specificity in the reversible protein aggregates that are stored in secretory granules? J Mol Neurosci. 2004;22(1–2):43–9.

Kim MJ, Park SH, Opella SJ, Marsilje TH, Michellys PY, Seidel HM, et al. NMR structural studies of interactions of a small, nonpeptidyl tpo mimic with the thrombopoietin receptor extracellular juxtamembrane and transmembrane domains. J Biol Chem. 2007;282(19):14253–61.

Kobayashi N, Kono T, Hatakeyama M, Minami Y, Miyazaki T, Perlmutter RM, et al. Functional coupling of the src-family protein tyrosine kinases p59fyn and p53/56lyn with the interleukin 2 receptor: implications for redundancy and pleiotropism in cytokine signal transduction. Proc Natl Acad Sci USA. 1993;90(9):4201–5.

Kossiakoff AA, De Vos AM. Structural basis for cytokine hormone-receptor recognition and receptor activation. Adv Protein Chem. 1998;52:67–108.

Kotenko SV, Krause CD, Izotova LS, Pollack BP, Wu W, Pestka S. Identification and functional characterization of a second chain of the interleukin-10 receptor complex. EMBO J. 1997; 16(19):5894–903.

Kotenko SV, Gallagher G, Baurin VV, Lewis-Antes A, Shen M, Shah NK, et al. IFN-lambdas mediate antiviral protection through a distinct class II cytokine receptor complex. Nat Immunol. 2003;4(1):69–77.

Kovanen PE, Leonard WJ. Cytokines and immunodeficiency diseases: critical roles of the gamma (c)-dependent cytokines interleukins 2, 4, 7, 9, 15, and 21, and their signaling pathways. Immunol Rev. 2004;202:67–83.

Lai SY, Xu W, Gaffen SL, Liu KD, Longmore GD, Greene WC, et al. The molecular role of the common gamma c subunit in signal transduction reveals functional asymmetry within multimeric cytokine receptor complexes. Proc Natl Acad Sci U S A. 1996;93(1):231–5.

Langer JA, Cutrone EC, Kotenko S. The Class II cytokine receptor (CRF2) family: overview and patterns of receptor-ligand interactions. Cytokine Growth Factor Rev. 2004;15(1):33–48.

Lemmon MA, Schlessinger J. Cell signaling by receptor tyrosine kinases. Cell. 2010; 141(7):1117–34.

Leung DW, Spencer SA, Cachianes G, Hammonds RG, Collins C, Henzel WJ, et al. Growth hormone receptor and serum binding protein: purification, cloning and expression. Nature. 1987;330(6148):537–43.

Levy DE, Darnell Jr JE. Stats: transcriptional control and biological impact. Nat Rev Mol Cell Biol. 2002;3(9):651–62.

Li Q, Wong YL, Huang Q, Kang C. Structural insight into the transmembrane domain and the juxtamembrane region of the erythropoietin receptor in micelles. Biophys J. 2014; 107(10):2325–36.

Li Q, Wong YL, Yueqi Lee M, Li Y, Kang C. Solution structure of the transmembrane domain of the mouse erythropoietin receptor in detergent micelles. Sci Rep. 2015;5:13586.

Lichanska AM, Waters MJ. New insights into growth hormone receptor function and clinical implications. Horm Res. 2008;69(3):138–45.

Linossi EM, Babon JJ, Hilton DJ, Nicholson SE. Suppression of cytokine signaling: the SOCS perspective. Cytokine Growth Factor Rev. 2013;24(3):241–8.

Liongue C, Ward AC. Evolution of class I cytokine receptors. BMC Evol Biol. 2007;7:120.

Liongue C, Sertori R, Ward AC. Evolution of cytokine receptor signaling. J Immunol. 2016; 197(1):11–8.

Livnah O, Johnson DL, Stura EA, Farrell FX, Barbone FP, You Y, et al. An antagonist peptide-EPO receptor complex suggests that receptor dimerization is not sufficient for activation. Nat Struct Biol. 1998;5(11):993–1004.

Livnah O, Stura EA, Middleton SA, Johnson DL, Jolliffe LK, Wilson IA. Crystallographic evidence for preformed dimers of erythropoietin receptor before ligand activation. Science. 1999; 283(5404):987–90.

Lopez AF, Sanderson CJ, Gamble JR, Campbell HD, Young IG, Vadas MA. Recombinant human interleukin 5 is a selective activator of human eosinophil function. J Exp Med. 1988; 167(1):219–24.

Lupardus PJ, Skiniotis G, Rice AJ, Thomas C, Fischer S, Walz T, et al. Structural snapshots of full-length Jak1, a transmembrane gp130/IL-6/IL-6Ralpha cytokine receptor complex, and the receptor-Jak1 holocomplex. Structure. 2011;19(1):45–55.

Masse GX, Corcuff E, Decaluwe H, Bommhardt U, Lantz O, Buer J, et al. gamma(c) cytokines provide multiple homeostatic signals to naive CD4(+) T cells. Eur J Immunol. 2007; 37(9):2606–16.

Matadeen R, Hon WC, Heath JK, Jones EY, Fuller S. The dynamics of signal triggering in a gp130-receptor complex. Structure. 2007;15(4):441–8.

McElroy CA, Dohm JA, Walsh ST. Structural and biophysical studies of the human IL-7/IL-7Ralpha complex. Structure. 2009;17(1):54–65.

McElroy CA, Holland PJ, Zhao P, Lim JM, Wells L, Eisenstein E, et al. Structural reorganization of the interleukin-7 signaling complex. Proc Natl Acad Sci U S A. 2012;109(7):2503–8.

Miller SL, Antico G, Raghunath PN, Tomaszewski JE, Clevenger CV. Nek3 kinase regulates prolactin-mediated cytoskeletal reorganization and motility of breast cancer cells. Oncogene. 2007;26(32):4668–78.

Miyajima A, Hara T, Kitamura T. Common subunits of cytokine receptors and the functional redundancy of cytokines. Trends Biochem Sci. 1992;17(10):378–82.

Mohan A, Oldfield CJ, Radivojac P, Vacic V, Cortese MS, Dunker AK, et al. Analysis of molecular recognition features (MoRFs). J Mol Biol. 2006;362(5):1043–59.

Murphy JM, Ford SC, Wiedemann UM, Carr PD, Ollis DL, Young IG. A novel functional epitope formed by domains 1 and 4 of the human common beta-subunit is involved in receptor activation by granulocyte macrophage colony-stimulating factor and interleukin 5. J Biol Chem. 2003;278(12):10572–7.

Nebiker CA, Han J, Eppenberger-Castori S, Iezzi G, Hirt C, Amicarella F, et al. GM-CSF production by tumor cells is associated with improved survival in colorectal cancer. Clin Cancer Res. 2014;20(12):3094–106.

Neduva V, Linding R, Su-Angrand I, Stark A, de Masi F, Gibson TJ, et al. Systematic discovery of new recognition peptides mediating protein interaction networks. PLoS Biol. 2005;3(12):e405.

Nelson BH, Lord JD, Greenberg PD. A membrane-proximal region of the interleukin-2 receptor gamma c chain sufficient for Jak kinase activation and induction of proliferation in T cells. Mol Cell Biol. 1996;16(1):309–17.

Nicola NA, Hilton DJ. General classes and functions of four-helix bundle cytokines. Adv Protein Chem. 1998;52:1–65.

Noguchi M, Yi H, Rosenblatt HM, Filipovich AH, Adelstein S, Modi WS, et al. Interleukin-2 receptor gamma chain mutation results in X-linked severe combined immunodeficiency in humans. Cell. 1993;73(1):147–57.

Oakes SR, Rogers RL, Naylor MJ, Ormandy CJ. Prolactin regulation of mammary gland development. J Mammary Gland Biol Neoplasia. 2008;13(1):13–28.

Oh CK, Geba GP, Molfino N. Investigational therapeutics targeting the IL-4/IL-13/STAT-6 pathway for the treatment of asthma. Eur Respir Rev. 2010;19(115):46–54.

Olsen JG, Kragelund BB. Who climbs the tryptophan ladder? On the structure and function of the WSXWS motif in cytokine receptors and thrombospondin repeats. Cytokine Growth Factor Rev. 2014;25(3):337–41.

Ouyang W, Rutz S, Crellin NK, Valdez PA, Hymowitz SG. Regulation and functions of the IL-10 family of cytokines in inflammation and disease. Annu Rev Immunol. 2011;29:71–109.

Ozaki K, Leonard WJ. Cytokine and cytokine receptor pleiotropy and redundancy. J Biol Chem. 2002;277(33):29355–8.

Park MJ, Sheng R, Silkov A, Jung DJ, Wang ZG, Xin Y, et al. SH2 domains serve as lipid-binding modules for pTyr-signaling proteins. Mol Cell. 2016;62(1):7–20.

Patwardhan P, Resh MD. Myristoylation and membrane binding regulate c-Src stability and kinase activity. Mol Cell Biol. 2010;30(17):4094–107.

Perugini M, Brown AL, Salerno DG, Booker GW, Stojkoski C, Hercus TR, et al. Alternative modes of GM-CSF receptor activation revealed using activated mutants of the common beta-subunit. Blood. 2010;115(16):3346–53.
Pestka S, Krause CD, Sarkar D, Walter MR, Shi Y, Fisher PB. Interleukin-10 and related cytokines and receptors. Annu Rev Immunol. 2004a;22:929–79.
Pestka S, Krause CD, Walter MR. Interferons, interferon-like cytokines, and their receptors. Immunol Rev. 2004b;202:8–32.
Pflanz S, Hibbert L, Mattson J, Rosales R, Vaisberg E, Bazan JF, et al. WSX-1 and glycoprotein 130 constitute a signal-transducing receptor for IL-27. J Immunol. 2004;172(4):2225–31.
Rane SG, Reddy EP. JAK3: a novel JAK kinase associated with terminal differentiation of hematopoietic cells. Oncogene. 1994;9(8):2415–23.
Rawat A, Nagaraj R. Determinants of membrane association in the SH4 domain of Fyn: roles of N-terminus myristoylation and side-chain thioacylation. Biochim Biophys Acta. 2010; 1798(10):1854–63.
Rawat A, Harishchandran A, Nagaraj R. Fatty acyl chain-dependent but charge-independent association of the SH4 domain of Lck with lipid membranes. J Biosci. 2013;38(1):63–71.
Rawlings JS, Rosler KM, Harrison DA. The JAK/STAT signaling pathway. J Cell Sci. 2004; 117(Pt 8):1281–3.
Renauld JC. Class II, cytokine receptors and their ligands: key antiviral and inflammatory modulators. Nat Rev Immunol. 2003;3(8):667–76.
Rochman Y, Spolski R, Leonard WJ. New insights into the regulation of T cells by gamma(c) family cytokines. Nat Rev Immunol. 2009;9(7):480–90.
Rowlinson SW, Yoshizato H, Barclay JL, Brooks AJ, Behncken SN, Kerr LM, et al. An agonist-induced conformational change in the growth hormone receptor determines the choice of signalling pathway. Nat Cell Biol. 2008;10(6):740–7.
Sa SM, Valdez PA, Wu J, Jung K, Zhong F, Hall L, et al. The effects of IL-20 subfamily cytokines on reconstituted human epidermis suggest potential roles in cutaneous innate defense and pathogenic adaptive immunity in psoriasis. J Immunol. 2007;178(4):2229–40.
Sabat R. IL-10 family of cytokines. Cytokine Growth Factor Rev. 2010;21(5):315–24.
Saharinen P, Silvennoinen O. The pseudokinase domain is required for suppression of basal activity of Jak2 and Jak3 tyrosine kinases and for cytokine-inducible activation of signal transduction. J Biol Chem. 2002;277(49):47954–63.
Saharinen P, Vihinen M, Silvennoinen O. Autoinhibition of Jak2 tyrosine kinase is dependent on specific regions in its pseudokinase domain. Mol Biol Cell. 2003;14(4):1448–59.
Samuel CE. Antiviral actions of interferons. Clin Microbiol Rev. 2001;14(4):778–809. table of contents.
Sanz Sanz A, Niranjan Y, Hammaren H, Ungureanu D, Ruijtenbeek R, Touw IP, et al. The JH2 domain and SH2-JH2 linker regulate JAK2 activity: a detailed kinetic analysis of wild type and V617F mutant kinase domains. Biochim Biophys Acta. 2014;1844(10):1835–41.
Sato N, Miyajima A. Multimeric cytokine receptors: common versus specific functions. Curr Opin Cell Biol. 1994;6(2):174–9.
Scheller J, Chalaris A, Schmidt-Arras D, Rose-John S. The pro- and anti-inflammatory properties of the cytokine interleukin-6. Biochim Biophys Acta. 2011;1813(5):878–88.
Schuster B, Meinert W, Rose-John S, Kallen KJ. The human interleukin-6 (IL-6) receptor exists as a preformed dimer in the plasma membrane. FEBS Lett. 2003;538(1–3):113–6.
Sheikh F, Baurin VV, Lewis-Antes A, Shah NK, Smirnov SV, Anantha S, et al. Cutting edge: IL-26 signals through a novel receptor complex composed of IL-20 receptor 1 and IL-10 receptor 2. J Immunol. 2004;172(4):2006–10.
Sheng R, Jung DJ, Silkov A, Kim H, Singaram I, Wang ZG, et al. Lipids regulate Lck activity through their interactions with the Lck SH2 domain. J Biol Chem. 2016;291(34):17639–50.
Shuai K, Liu B. Regulation of JAK-STAT signalling in the immune system. Nat Rev Immunol. 2003;3(11):900–11.

Sigalov AB. Cells diversify transmembrane signaling through the controlled chaos of protein disorder. Self Nonself. 2011;2(2):75–9.

Silvennoinen O, Hubbard SR. Molecular insights into regulation of JAK2 in myeloproliferative neoplasms. Blood. 2015;125(22):3388–92.

Singleton KR, Kim J, Hinz TK, Marek LA, Casas-Selves M, Hatheway C, et al. A receptor tyrosine kinase network composed of fibroblast growth factor receptors, epidermal growth factor receptor, v-erb-b2 erythroblastic leukemia viral oncogene homolog 2, and hepatocyte growth factor receptor drives growth and survival of head and neck squamous carcinoma cell lines. Mol Pharmacol. 2013;83(4):882–93.

Skiniotis G, Boulanger MJ, Garcia KC, Walz T. Signaling conformations of the tall cytokine receptor gp130 when in complex with IL-6 and IL-6 receptor. Nat Struct Mol Biol. 2005; 12(6):545–51.

Skiniotis G, Lupardus PJ, Martick M, Walz T, Garcia KC. Structural organization of a full-length gp130/LIF-R cytokine receptor transmembrane complex. Mol Cell. 2008;31(5):737–48.

Slavova-Azmanova NS, Kucera N, Louw A, Satiaputra J, Handoko A, Singer P, et al. Lyn kinase plays important roles in erythroid expansion, maturation and erythropoietin receptor signalling by regulating inhibitory signalling pathways that control survival. Biochem J. 2014; 459(3):455–66.

Somers W, Ultsch M, De Vos AM, Kossiakoff AA. The X-ray structure of a growth hormone-prolactin receptor complex. Nature. 1994;372(6505):478–81.

Sprang SR, Bazan JF. Cytokine structural taxonomy and mechanisms of receptor engagement. Curr Opin Struct Biol. 1993;3(6):815–27.

Srivastava S, Matsuda M, Hou Z, Bailey JP, Kitazawa R, Herbst MP, et al. Receptor activator of NF-kappaB ligand induction via Jak2 and Stat5a in mammary epithelial cells. J Biol Chem. 2003;278(46):46171–8.

Stomski FC, Woodcock JM, Zacharakis B, Bagley CJ, Sun Q, Lopez AF. Identification of a Cys motif in the common beta chain of the interleukin 3, granulocyte-macrophage colony-stimulating factor, and interleukin 5 receptors essential for disulfide-linked receptor heterodimerization and activation of all three receptors. J Biol Chem. 1998;273(2):1192–9.

Su S, Liu Q, Chen J, Chen J, Chen F, He C, et al. A positive feedback loop between mesenchymal-like cancer cells and macrophages is essential to breast cancer metastasis. Cancer Cell. 2014; 25(5):605–20.

Suzuki K, Nakajima H, Saito Y, Saito T, Leonard WJ, Iwamoto I. Janus kinase 3 (Jak3) is essential for common cytokine receptor gamma chain (gamma(c))-dependent signaling: comparative analysis of gamma(c), Jak3, and gamma(c) and Jak3 double-deficient mice. Int Immunol. 2000;12(2):123–32.

Svensson LA, Bondensgaard K, Norskov-Lauritsen L, Christensen L, Becker P, Andersen MD, et al. Crystal structure of a prolactin receptor antagonist bound to the extracellular domain of the prolactin receptor. J Biol Chem. 2008;283(27):19085–94.

Tan D, Tan S, Zhang J, Tang P, Huang J, Zhou W, et al. Histone trimethylation of the p53 gene by expression of a constitutively active prolactin receptor in prostate cancer cells. Chin J Physiol. 2013;56(5):282–90.

Tantos A, Han KH, Tompa P. Intrinsic disorder in cell signaling and gene transcription. Mol Cell Endocrinol. 2012;348(2):457–65.

Teilum K, Hoch JC, Goffin V, Kinet S, Martial JA, Kragelund BB. Solution structure of human prolactin. J Mol Biol. 2005;351(4):810–23.

Toms AV, Deshpande A, McNally R, Jeong Y, Rogers JM, Kim CU, et al. Structure of a pseudokinase-domain switch that controls oncogenic activation of Jak kinases. Nat Struct Mol Biol. 2013;20(10):1221–3.

Trinchieri G. Type I, interferon: friend or foe? J Exp Med. 2010;207(10):2053–63.

Tworoger SS, Eliassen AH, Zhang X, Qian J, Sluss PM, Rosner BA, et al. A 20-year prospective study of plasma prolactin as a risk marker of breast cancer development. Cancer Res. 2013; 73(15):4810–9.

Uchida H, Banba S, Wada M, Matsumoto K, Ikeda M, Naito N, et al. Analysis of binding properties between 20 kDa human growth hormone (hGH) and hGH receptor (hGHR): the binding affinity for hGHR extracellular domain and mode of receptor dimerization. J Mol Endocrinol. 1999; 23(3):347–53.
Ungureanu D, Wu J, Pekkala T, Niranjan Y, Young C, Jensen ON, et al. The pseudokinase domain of JAK2 is a dual-specificity protein kinase that negatively regulates cytokine signaling. Nat Struct Mol Biol. 2011;18(9):971–6.
Urdinguio RG, Fernandez AF, Moncada-Pazos A, Huidobro C, Rodriguez RM, Ferrero C, et al. Immune-dependent and independent antitumor activity of GM-CSF aberrantly expressed by mouse and human colorectal tumors. Cancer Res. 2013;73(1):395–405.
Usacheva A, Sandoval R, Domanski P, Kotenko SV, Nelms K, Goldsmith MA, et al. Contribution of the Box 1 and Box 2 motifs of cytokine receptors to Jak1 association and activation. J Biol Chem. 2002;277(50):48220–6.
Vacic V, Oldfield CJ, Mohan A, Radivojac P, Cortese MS, Uversky VN, et al. Characterization of molecular recognition features, MoRFs, and their binding partners. J Proteome Res. 2007; 6(6):2351–66.
van Agthoven J, Zhang C, Tallet E, Raynal B, Hoos S, Baron B, et al. Structural characterization of the stem-stem dimerization interface between prolactin receptor chains complexed with the natural hormone. J Mol Biol. 2010;404(1):112–26.
Wallweber HJ, Tam C, Franke Y, Starovasnik MA, Lupardus PJ. Structural basis of recognition of interferon-alpha receptor by tyrosine kinase 2. Nat Struct Mol Biol. 2014;21(5):443–8.
Walsh ST. Structural insights into the common gamma-chain family of cytokines and receptors from the interleukin-7 pathway. Immunol Rev. 2012;250(1):303–16.
Walsh ST, Sylvester JE, Kossiakoff AA. The high- and low-affinity receptor binding sites of growth hormone are allosterically coupled. Proc Natl Acad Sci U S A. 2004;101(49):17078–83.
Walter MR, Cook WJ, Ealick SE, Nagabhushan TL, Trotta PP, Bugg CE. Three-dimensional structure of recombinant human granulocyte-macrophage colony-stimulating factor. J Mol Biol. 1992;224(4):1075–85.
Wang M, Tan Z, Zhang R, Kotenko SV, Liang P. Interleukin 24 (MDA-7/MOB-5) signals through two heterodimeric receptors, IL-22R1/IL-20R2 and IL-20R1/IL-20R2. J Biol Chem. 2002; 277(9):7341–7.
Wang X, Lupardus P, Laporte SL, Garcia KC. Structural biology of shared cytokine receptors. Annu Rev Immunol. 2009;27:29–60.
Wang Y, Han G, Wang K, Liu G, Wang R, Xiao H, et al. Tumor-derived GM-CSF promotes inflammatory colon carcinogenesis via stimulating epithelial release of VEGF. Cancer Res. 2014;74(3):716–26.
Waters MJ, Brooks AJ. Growth hormone receptor: structure function relationships. Horm Res Paediatr. 2011;76(Suppl 1):12–6.
Waters MJ, Brooks AJ. JAK2 activation by growth hormone and other cytokines. Biochem J. 2015;466(1):1–11.
Watowich SS, Wu H, Socolovsky M, Klingmuller U, Constantinescu SN, Lodish HF. Cytokine receptor signal transduction and the control of hematopoietic cell development. Annu Rev Cell Dev Biol. 1996;12:91–128.
Wells JA, de Vos AM. Hematopoietic receptor complexes. Annu Rev Biochem. 1996;65:609–34.
Wells JA, Kossiakoff AA. Cell biology. New tricks for an old dimer. Science. 2014; 344(6185):703–4.
Wennbo H, Gebre-Medhin M, Gritli-Linde A, Ohlsson C, Isaksson OG, Tornell J. Activation of the prolactin receptor but not the growth hormone receptor is important for induction of mammary tumors in transgenic mice. J Clin Invest. 1997;100(11):2744–51.
Wilks AF, Harpur AG, Kurban RR, Ralph SJ, Zurcher G, Ziemiecki A. Two novel protein-tyrosine kinases, each with a second phosphotransferase-related catalytic domain, define a new class of protein kinase. Mol Cell Biol. 1991;11(4):2057–65.

Wright PE, Dyson HJ. Intrinsically unstructured proteins: re-assessing the protein structure-function paradigm. J Mol Biol. 1999;293(2):321–31.

Wu W, Sun XH. Janus kinase 3: the controller and the controlled. Acta Biochim Biophys Sin Shanghai. 2012;44(3):187–96.

Xie MH, Aggarwal S, Ho WH, Foster J, Zhang Z, Stinson J, et al. Interleukin (IL)-22, a novel human cytokine that signals through the interferon receptor-related proteins CRF2-4 and IL-22R. J Biol Chem. 2000;275(40):31335–9.

Xu Y, Kershaw NJ, Luo CS, Soo P, Pocock MJ, Czabotar PE, et al. Crystal structure of the entire ectodomain of gp130: insights into the molecular assembly of the tall cytokine receptor complexes. J Biol Chem. 2010;285(28):21214–8.

Zhang JM, An J. Cytokines, inflammation, and pain. Int Anesthesiol Clin. 2007;45(2):27–37.

Zhang C, Cherifi I, Nygaard M, Haxholm GW, Bogorad RL, Bernadet M, et al. Residue 146 regulates prolactin receptor folding, basal activity and ligand-responsiveness: potential implications in breast tumorigenesis. Mol Cell Endocrinol. 2015;401:173–88.

Steroid Hormone Receptors and Signal Transduction Processes

8

Carolyn M. Klinge

Abstract

Steroid hormones, *i.e.*, androgens, estrogens, glucocorticoids, mineralocorticoids, and progestins, bind with high affinity to their respective steroid hormone receptors (SR). SRs are members of a family of nuclear receptors (NR). Ligand-activated SRs dissociate from hsp90 chaperone complexes in the cytoplasm and enter the nucleus where they bind to specific DNA sequences: hormone response elements (HREs). SRs interact with coregulator proteins (coactivators and corepressors) as well as chromatin remodeling complexes to regulate target gene expression. In addition, some SRs are also associated with the plasma membrane (PM) and PM proteins. Hormone binding to PM-associated SRs activates G-protein coupled receptors (GPCR) and intracellular signaling pathways ultimately regulating gene transcription and other downstream sequelae. This chapter will review of SR/NR including protein structure, ligand activation, gene regulation, examples of rapid "non-genomic" signaling, and the roles of these receptors in human health and disease.

Keywords

Steroid hormones • Nuclear receptors • Androgen receptor • Estrogen receptor • Glucocorticoid receptor • Progesterone receptor • Mineralocorticoid receptor

Contents

C.M. Klinge (✉)
Department of Biochemistry and Molecular Genetics, Center for Genetics and Molecular Medicine, University of Louisville School of Medicine, Louisville, KY, USA
e-mail: carolyn.klinge@louisville.edu

A. Belfiore, D. LeRoith (eds.), *Principles of Endocrinology and Hormone Action*, Endocrinology, https://doi.org/10.1007/978-3-319-44675-2_9

Introduction

Steroid hormones, i.e., androgens, estrogens, glucocorticoids, mineralocorticoids, and progestins, regulate diverse processes in tissues throughout the body and in the brain. Steroid hormones bind with high affinity to proteins called steroid hormone receptors (SRs). These steroid receptors are primarily located intracellularly and act as ligand-activated transcription factors within the nucleus to regulate target gene expression. Depending on the tissue, a small proportion of these receptors, perhaps 5–10%, are associated with the plasma membrane (PM) and PM proteins such that ligand binding activates G protein-coupled receptors (GPCRs) and intracellular signaling pathways ultimately culminating in activation or repression of gene transcription and physiological effects. Sequence comparison has revealed that steroid hormone receptors belong to a diverse family of ligand-activated gene regulators called nuclear receptors (NRs) that share a highly conserved structure and common mechanisms affecting gene transcription (Laudet 1997). The evolutionary relationship among the SRs/NRs has been deduced by the high conservation in their DNA-binding domains (DBDs) and in their less-conserved ligand-binding domains (LBDs) and indicates that this large group of proteins arose from a common ancestral molecule (Laudet 1997; Thornton 2001; Thornton et al. 2003).

The steroid/nuclear hormone receptor superfamily (Table 1) includes 48 receptors for the gonadal and adrenal steroids; nonsteroidal ligands, e.g., thyroid hormones (T3, T4); vitamin D (1,25-dihydroxyvitamin D3 (1,25$(OH)_2$D3)); retinoic acid (RA); and fatty acids (FA), as well as "orphan" receptors. Some "orphan" receptors have been

Table 1 Members of the human steroid hormone and nuclear receptor gene superfamily. This table lists the receptor, common abbreviation of the receptor, and gene name and provides review articles for further reading. Additional information is located at the NURSA website: https://www.nursa.org

Ligands for receptors	Abbreviation/ Gene name	References
Receptors with known ligand(s)		
Estrogen α	(ERα, ESR1)	Reviewed in Hewitt et al. (2005), Patel and Skafar 2015, and Wang and Yin (2015)
Estrogen β	(ERβ, ESR2)	Reviewed in Dey et al. (2013) and Huang et al. (2015)
Androgen	(AR, AR)	Reviewed in Mikkonen et al. (2010)
Progesterone	(PR, PGR)	Reviewed in Jacobsen and Horwitz (2012))
Glucocorticoid	(GR, NR3C1)	Reviewed in Granner et al. (2015) and Meijsing (2015)
Mineralocorticoid	(MR, NR3C2)	Reviewed in Le Menuet and Lombès (2014) and Viengchareun et al. (2007)
Nuclear receptors with ligands		
Vitamin D	(VDR, VDR)	Reviewed in Christakos et al. (2016)
Thyroid hormone	TRβ (THRB)	Reviewed in Cheng et al. (2010) and Zhang and Lazar (2000)
	TRα (THRA)	
Retinoic acid	RARα (RARA)	Reviewed in Giguere (1994) and Mangelsdorf and Evans (1995a)
	RARα (RARA)	
	RARγ (RARG)	
Retinoid X receptor	RXRα (RXRA)	Reviewed in Evans and Mangelsdorf 2014) and Lefebvre et al. (2010)
	RXRβ (RXRB)	First described Mangelsdorf et al. (1990)
	RXRγ (RXRG)	First described Leid et al. (1992)
Peroxisome proliferator-activated receptors (PPARs)	PPARα (PPARA)	Reviewed in Fan and Evans (2015), Lee and Kim (2015), and Sauer (2015)
	PPARβ/ PPARδ (PPARD)	Reviewed in Pawlak et al. (2015)
	PPARγ (PPARG)	Reviewed in Giordano Attianese and Desvergne (2015)
		Reviewed in Shao et al. (2015)
Farnesoid X receptors	FXRα (NR1H4)	Bile acid receptors reviewed in Chiang (2002), Jiang et al. (2014), and Parks et al. (1999)
	FXRβ NR1H5)	First described Otte et al. (2003)

(*continued*)

Table 1 (continued)

Ligands for receptors	Abbreviation/ Gene name	References
Orphan receptors and their identified ligands		
Constitutive androstane receptor is a xenobiotic receptor	CAR (NR1I3)	Reviewed in Mullican et al. (2013)
		Reviewed in Banerjee et al. (2013, 2015), Chai et al. (2013), Cherian et al. (2015), Kobayashi et al. (2015), and Swanson et al. (2013)
Chicken ovalbumin upstream promoter transcription factors (COUP-TFs)	COUP-TFI (NR2F1)	Reviewed in Cooney et al. (2001) and Lin et al. (2011)
	COUP-TFII (NR2F2)	Reviewed in Litchfield et al. (2012)
	REV-ERBβ EAR2 (NR2F6)	Reviewed in Riggins et al. (2010), Safe et al. (2014), and Zhang and Dufau (2001)
Dosage-sensitive sex reversal-adrenal hypoplasia congenita critical region on the X chromosome, gene 1, DAX-1 NR0B1 lacks the zinc finger DBD, reviewed in Jadhav et al. (2011), McCabe (2007), Muscatelli et al. (1994), and Suntharalingham et al. (2015)		
Estrogen receptor-related receptors (ERRs)	ERRα (NR3B1)	Reviewed in Audet-Walsh et al. (2015), Deblois and Giguere (2011), Deblois et al. 2013), Huss et al. (2015)
	ERRβ (NR3B2)	Reviewed in Michalek et al. (2011)
	ERRγ (NR3B3)	
REV-ERBα, EAR1 (NR1D1)	Binds heme reviewed in Yin et al. (2010)	
Germ cell nuclear factor 1	Reviewed in Wang and Cooney (2013)	
Hepatocyte nuclear factor	GCNF	First characterized Greschik et al. (1999) and Hirose et al. (1995)
	HNF1α (HNF1A)	Reviewed in Yamagata (2014)
	HNF4α (HNF4A)	Reviewed in Drewes et al. (1996) and Walesky and Apte (2015)
	HNF4γ (HNF4G)	Reviewed in Cattin et al. (2009)
Liver receptor homolog-1 (LRH-1) (NR5A2)	Reviewed in Stein and Schoonjans (2015)	
Neuron-derived orphan receptor 1 (NOR1) (NR4A3)	Reviewed in Kurakula et al. (2014)	
NUR77, NGFI-B, GFRP1, NP10, TR3 (NR4A1)	Reviewed in Hawk et al. (2012), Lee et al. (2014), Mathisen et al. (2011), Mohan et al. (2012), Nakajima et al. (2012), Safe et al. (2016), Safe et al. (2014), Xue et al. (2012), and Zhao and Bruemmer (2010b)	
Pregnane X receptor (PXR)/ steroid X receptor (SXR) (NR1I2)	Reviewed in Banerjee et al. (2015) and Ma et al. (2015)	

(*continued*)

Table 1 (continued)

Ligands for receptors	Abbreviation/ Gene name	References
Photoreceptor-specific nuclear receptor (PNR) (NR2E2) retinal NR	Reviewed in Schorderet and Escher (2009) and Tan et al. (2013)	
RAR-related orphan receptors	Reviewed in Cook et al. (2015), Kojetin and Burris (2014), and Solt and Burris (2012)	
RORα (RORA)		
RORβ (RORB)		
ROR^{γ} (RORC)		
Steroidogenic factor 1 (SF-1, NR5A1)	Reviewed in Mizutani et al. (2015) and Suntharalingham et al. (2015)	
	First described in Wong et al. (1996)	
Small heterodimeric partner (SHP, NR0B2)	Reviewed in Goodwin et al. (2000) and Zhang et al. (2011)	
	First described in Seol et al. (1996) and (1997)	
TLX (NR2E1)	Reviewed in Islam and Zhang (2015) and Wang and Xiong (2016)	

"adopted" when their ligands were identified. Other "orphan" receptors whose endogenous ligands, if necessary, are as yet unknown; perhaps because they are regulated by other mechanisms, e.g., phosphorylation, expression, and location (Benoit et al. 2004; Mullican et al. 2013; Willson and Moore 2002). The SRs are considered class I members of the NR superfamily while the other NRs are class II receptors (Mangelsdorf et al. 1995b). This chapter will provide a review of these SRs/NRs including protein structure, ligand activation (as warranted), gene regulation, examples of rapid "nongenomic" signaling, and the roles of these receptors in human health and disease.

Steroid Hormones in Circulation and Entry into Target Cells

Steroid hormones are small hydrophobic and lipid-soluble cholesterol derivatives. In blood they circulate either free or bound (95%) to plasma carrier proteins (Thompson 1995). Sex hormone-binding globulin (SHBG), also known as testosterone-estradiol-binding globulin (TeBG), and androgen-binding protein (ABP) are encoded by the same gene (Danzo and Joseph 1994), but they differ in tissue expression and glycosylation (Hammond and Bocchinfuso 1995). SHBG is a glycated homodimeric plasma transport protein synthesized primarily in the liver and binds testosterone and dihydrotestosterone (DHT), with higher affinity than estradiol (E_2) and regulates free sex hormone bioavailability (Le et al. 2012). ABP is produced by the Sertoli cells of the testis (Joseph 1994). Corticosteroid-binding globulin (CBG or transcortin) binds glucocorticoids and progesterone, with differing affinities. When circulating levels of steroid hormones exceed the binding capacity of their respective binding proteins, they bind nonspecifically, and with low affinity, to albumin, from which they can readily dissociate and enter target cells (Westphal 1986).

SHBG binds to a specific cell membrane receptor called sex hormone-binding globulin receptor (SHBG-R) and activates adenylyl cyclase, thus increasing intracellular cAMP (Joseph 1994). Binding of SHBG to SHBG-R results in receptor-mediated endocytosis (Hammes et al. 2005). The interaction of SHBG with SHBG-R was shown to be inhibited when steroids are bound to SHBG, suggesting that SHBG is an allosteric protein (Porto et al. 1995). However, if unliganded SHBG is allowed to bind to its receptor on intact cells, and an appropriate steroid hormone then is introduced, adenylate cyclase is activated, and intracellular cAMP increases (Rosner et al. 1991). Several members of the organic anion-transporting polypeptide (OATP) family of proteins mediate the sodium and ATP-independent uptake of dehydroepiandrosterone (3β-hydroxy-5-androsten-17-one, DHEA), pregnenolone, and estrone into tissues including the breast and prostate and are overexpressed in tumors in these tissues (Cho et al. 2014). Once the steroid hormone is in the cytoplasm, it is not yet clear whether a transport protein is required for movement of the hydrophobic steroid molecule through the aqueous cytoplasm to the receptor, regardless of whether the receptor is cytoplasmic or nuclear in location. The current model is that the steroid hormone diffuses freely in the cytoplasm.

Structure/Function of the Domains of Steroid Hormone/Nuclear Receptors

The androgen, estrogen, glucocorticoid, progesterone, and mineralocorticoid receptors (AR, ER, GR, PR, and MR) share a common protein structure with the other NR, as shown here the thyroid receptors α and β (TRα and TRβ). As shown in Fig. 1, SRs/NRs contain several key structural elements which enable the high-affinity binding of their respective ligands, recognize and bind to discrete DNA response elements in some proximity to target genes with high affinity and specificity, and regulate gene transcription (Evans 2005; Evans and Mangelsdorf 2014). The receptor proteins have five or six domains lettered A–F from N- to C-terminus, encoded by eight to nine exons. The receptors contain three major functional domains:

1. A variable N-terminus (domains A and B) modulates transcription in a gene- and cell-specific manner through its N-terminal activation function 1 (AF-1) which acts in a ligand-dependent manner when expressed without the ligand-binding domain (LBD) (reviewed in Germain et al. 2006). For some receptors, including estrogen receptor α (ERα), AF-1 is regulated by phosphorylation (reviewed in Lannigan 2003; Rajbhandari et al. 2012).
2. A central DNA-binding domain (DBD, consisting of the C domain) is composed of two functionally distinct cys-cys zinc fingers and two α-helices through which the receptor physically interacts directly with the DNA helix (reviewed in Germain et al. 2006). The DBD is the most conserved domain.
3. The ligand-binding domain (LBD, domains E and in some receptors F) contains activation function 2 (AF-2). The F domain of ERα plays a role in distinguishing estrogen agonists versus antagonists, perhaps through interaction with cell-specific

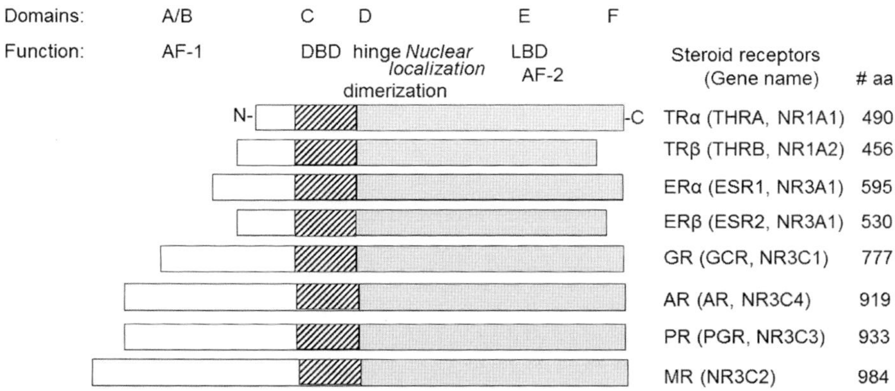

Fig. 1 Protein domain structure of the steroid hormone nuclear receptors and thyroid hormone receptors. Domains A- FF and function of each domain is shown schematically as linearized proteins from amino (N)- to carboxy (C)- terminals with common structural and functional domains. Variability between members of the steroid hormone receptors (NR3C family) is due primarily to differences in aa sequence of the amino (N)-terminal domain. Abbreviations: AF-1 = activation function-1; AF-2 = activation function-2; DBD= DNA binding domain contains two C4zinc fingers; LBD= ligand binding domain

factors (Patel and Skafar 2015). Domain-swapping experiments in which the DBD of ERα was switched with that of the GR produced a chimeric receptor that bound to specific DNA sequences bound by GR, but stimulated the transcription of glucocorticoid-responsive target genes when cells were treated with E_2 (Green and Chambon 1987), thus demonstrating the specificity of the DBD in target gene regulation.

The N-terminus is the least conserved part of SR/NR in length and amino acid composition. Deletion of the C-terminal LBD of the GR yields constitutive (hormone-independent) transcriptional activation, implying that the N-terminal regions harbor autonomous transcriptional activation functions that is regulated by phosphorylation (Carruthers et al. 2015). These and other experiments with other steroid receptors indicated that AF-1 is involved in activation of gene transcription, but is independent of ligand binding. GR is unique in that it "transrepresses" gene transcription by physically interacting with DNA-bound transcriptional activators, e. g., NF-κB, activator protein 1 (AP-1), and STAT3, to repress their downstream target genes (Ratman et al. 2013). The anti-inflammatory effects of glucocorticoids are ascribed to tethered transrepression (Cruz-Topete and Cidlowski 2015; Surjit et al. 2011). Recent studies from Pierre Chambon's lab show that SUMOylation of the GR NTD and formation of an NCoR1/SMRT/HDAC3 repressing complex are required for glucocorticoid-induced negative GRE-mediated direct transrepression, but does *not* affect positive GRE-mediated transactivation (Hua et al. 2016).

Some steroid receptors exist as isoforms, encoded by the same gene, but differing in their N-terminus. PR and AR exist in two distinct forms, A and B, synthesized from the same mRNA by alternate splicing. In addition PR-C (60 kDa) is co-expressed with PR-A and PR-B from the same gene (Lange 2008). The PR-A and PR-B isoforms differ by 128 amino acids in the N-terminal region, yielding PR-A = 90 kDa and PR-B = 120 kDa, which have differing capacities to regulate transcription (Daniel et al. 2015; De Amicis et al. 2009; Lydon and Edwards 2009). For example, PR-A expression is a negative prognostic indicator in breast cancer likely due to its ability to increase the expression of a subset of genes associated with invasion and breast tumor progression (McFall et al. 2015). In contrast, AR-A and AR-B isoforms show minimal differences in activation of a reporter gene in response to androgen agonists or antagonists in transiently transfected cells (Gao and McPhaul 1998).

The DBD is highly conserved and shows 60–95% homology among steroid receptors (Acconcia et al. 2005). The DBD varies in size from 66 to 70 aa and is hydrophilic due to its high content of basic aa (Evans 1988). The major function of this region is to bind to specific hormone response elements (HREs) of the target gene. DNA binding is achieved through the tetrahedral coordination of zinc (Zn) by four cysteine residues (C4) in each of two extensions that form two structurally distinct "Zn fingers" (Klug and Schwabe 1995). Zn fingers are common among gene regulatory proteins, with most C2H2 zinc finger transcription factors (Tadepally et al. 2008). Specificity of HRE binding is determined by the more highly conserved hydrophilic first Zn finger (C1) (Benoit et al. 2004), while the second Zn finger (C2) is involved in dimerization and stabilizing DNA binding by ionic interactions with the phosphate backbone of the DNA (O'Malley 1990). The D box is involved in HRE half-site spacing recognition. The highly conserved DBD shared by AR, GR, MR, and PR enables them to bind to the same HRE, called the glucocorticoid response element (GRE). The more C-terminal part of the C2 Zn finger and aa within the hinge region are involved in receptor dimerization in coordination with aa in the hinge region and the LBD.

The hinge region or D domain is a 40–50-amino acid sequence separating the DNA-binding and ligand-binding domains that contains sequences for receptor dimerization and ligand-dependent and ligand-independent nuclear localization sequences (NLSs) (Picard et al. 1990; Safer et al. 1998). The hinge region interacts with nuclear corepressor proteins (Safer et al. 1998) and with L7/SPA, a 27 kDa protein that increases the partial agonist activity of certain antagonist-liganded steroid hormone receptors, i.e., tamoxifen-liganded ERα, RU486-occupied PR, or RU486-occupied GR (Jackson et al. 1997). The hinge region of ERα is regulated by posttranslational modifications including methylation (Zhang et al. 2013), acetylation (Fu et al. 2004), and SUMOylation (Sentis et al. 2005). Site-directed mutational analysis of the D region of ERα demonstrated the contribution of the bipartite NLS to ERα's activation of AP-1-mediated gene transcription, indicating a role for this region in transactivation of other transcription factors (Burns et al. 2011).

The carboxy (C)-terminal or LBD is poorly conserved among members of the SR/NR superfamily, ranging from 218 to 264 aa in length and is hydrophobic, as would be expected for binding lipophilic metabolites of cholesterol, i.e., steroid hormones. Greater structural similarity between steroid hormones generally indicates greater aa sequence homology in the LBD. Sequences within the LBD form the binding site for hsp90 that blocks the DBD in the cytosolic, non-liganded GR

(Charn et al. 2010). Information from the x-ray crystal structures of the LBDs of the retinoic acid receptor (RAR), thyroid hormone receptor (TR), and ERα in the presence or absence of their cognate ligands has shown that the LBD has a compact structure consisting of 12 α-helices with a "pocket" into which the ligand fits (Bourguet et al. 1995, 2000; Renaud et al. 1995; Wagner et al. 1995). Binding of the ligand within the pocket alters the conformation of the LBD with helix 12 forming a "lid" over the pocket, trapping the ligand in a hydrophobic environment, and forming a surface on the LDB with which coactivator proteins interact. Helix 12 is indispensable for AF-2 function (Danielian et al. 1992; Durand et al. 1994). For ERα, 17β-estradiol (E_2) and the antiestrogen, or select ER modulator (SERM), raloxifene, form different aa contacts within the pocket (Brzozowski et al. 1997). This results in different positioning of helix 12 in the LBD that is thought to permit interaction with coactivators, e.g., SRC-1, in the presence of E_2, but not raloxifene, or by inference antiestrogens, such as tamoxifen (Brzozowski et al. 1997).

The C-terminal AF-2 transactivation domain is highly conserved within the nuclear receptor superfamily (Danielian et al. 1992) and is recognized by various transcriptional coregulators, also referred to as coactivators or corepressors (reviewed in Dasgupta et al. 2014; Klinge et al. 2004; O'Malley et al. 2012). AF-2 is localized to the most C-terminal end of the E domain. In ERα it constitutes aa # 530–553 (Seielstad et al. 1995). A third transactivation domain called AF-2a or tau2 has been localized to the N-terminal region of the LBD of ERα (Danielian, et al. 1992) and GR (Hollenberg and Evans 1988). Deletion experiments revealed a role for AF-2a and the DBD in targeting rat GR to the nuclear matrix (Tang et al. 1998), an interconnected ribonuclear-protein network within the nucleus that is thought to play important roles in transcription of active genes by stabilizing the assembly of the transcriptional machinery (Coelho et al. 2016). GR tau2 interacted with Hic-5 (hydrogen peroxide-inducible clone-5, TGFβ1I1) and coactivator GRIP1 to target GR to the nuclear matrix (Yang et al. 2000). Further studies revealed that Hic-5 acted as a gene-specific coactivator of unliganded GRα and as a corepressor of ligand-occupied GRα (Chodankar et al. 2014). More recent studies showed that Hic-5 also interacted with ERα, although more weakly than GRα, and selectively modulated ERα gene occupancy and expression in U2OS osteosarcoma cells (Chodankar et al. 2015).

While discussing the various domains of the SRs/NRs, it is important to note that the N- and C- terminals of ERα (Metivier et al. 2001), MR (Rogerson and Fuller 2003), AR (Zboray et al. 2015), PR (Goswami et al. 2014), and GR (Khan et al. 2012) interact in a ligand-dependent manner to modulate interaction with coregulators and thus either enhance or inhibit target gene transcription. Hormone-dependent phosphorylation of steroid hormone receptors may play an important role in binding of the receptor to its specific response element on the gene and subsequent activation of transcription. PR, GR, ERα, and vitamin D receptor(VDR) are all phosphorylated after binding to their respective ligands (reviewed in Lannigan 2003). In addition to phosphorylation, ERα and ERβ are acetylated, SUMOylated, glycosylated, and ubiquitinylated (reviewed in Le Romancer et al. 2011). These posttranslational modifications of SR/NR affect their interaction with other proteins including coregulators, thus impacting gene transcription.

Intracellular Location of Steroid/Nuclear Receptors

The overall distribution of SRs/NRs between plasma membrane, cytoplasm, mitochondria, and nucleus remains controversial. This controversy is the result of studies using different techniques, e.g., immunoprecipitation from different cell fractions and immunocytochemical staining, to examine receptor localization in different cells and tissues. Reports published before 1984 suggested that prior to hormone treatment, steroid receptors were located predominantly in the cytosolic fraction of target tissues in large protein complexes of 300–400 kDa based on sucrose density gradient and radioisotope steroid hormone labeling, e.g., ER in Gorski et al. (1973). Following hormone treatment, receptors were detected primarily in the nuclear fraction (Jensen and DeSombre 1973). Thus, early models assumed that unoccupied steroid receptors were in the cytoplasm with the receptor held in an inactive conformation by chaperone proteins, including hsp90 and hsp70 (Pratt and Toft 1997), until ligand binding "activated" the receptor, causing conformational changes. The complex of proteins associated with unliganded SRs is now called the "foldosome" complex (reviewed in Querol Cano et al. 2013). The general model of activation of a steroid receptor is shown in Fig. 2a. The conformational changes resulting from ligand binding result in receptor homodimerization and exposure of the nuclear localization domain, thus facilitating receptor dimer translocation to the nucleus. More recent studies demonstrate localization and even movement of ERα and ERβ between nuclear, mitochondrial, and cytoplasmic compartments (Cammarata et al. 2004; Simpkins et al. 2008).

Current models suggest that some proportion of unliganded SR and all the class II NR reside in the nucleus, bound to DNA (Fig. 2b). The exceptions are the GR and MR, which reside in the cytoplasm in association with hsp90, hsp70, and a variety of receptor-associated proteins in the absence of ligand (Gehring 1998). The hsp90 complex of proteins has chaperonin activity that facilitates hormone binding and subsequent proper folding of the GR (Dittmar et al. 1997). Upon activation by hormone-binding, GR conformational changes release hsp90 and the other proteins, and the ligand-occupied GR dimer translocates the nucleus (Hutchison et al. 1996). In contrast to GR, immunohistochemical localization experiments showed that ERα (King and Greene 1984), ERβ (Kuiper et al. 1996), PR (Perrot-Applanat et al. 1986), and AR (Husmann et al. 1990) are primarily nuclear in the absence of hormone treatment. All classes of NR are located in the nucleus, bound to DNA, in the absence of ligand (Mangelsdorf et al. 1995b). It is important to note that type II NR, e.g., TR, VDR, RAR, and RXR, do not interact with hsp90. These receptors are bound to DNA in the absence of ligand and are associated with corepressor proteins, e.g., NCoR and SMRT (Huang et al. 2000; Rosenfeld and Glass 2001, Rosenfeld et al.2006). Corepressor proteins NCoR and SMRT are associated with a complex of proteins that have histone deacetylase (HDAC) activity that repress gene expression by maintaining chromatin in a more condensed conformation (Rosenfeld and Glass 2001, Rosenfeld et al. 2006).

SR enters the nucleus by two processes: (1) passive diffusion through an "ever opened" central channel of the nuclear pore or (2) active transport that is mediated by interaction of the NLSs on the receptor proteins with the NLS receptor-hsp90

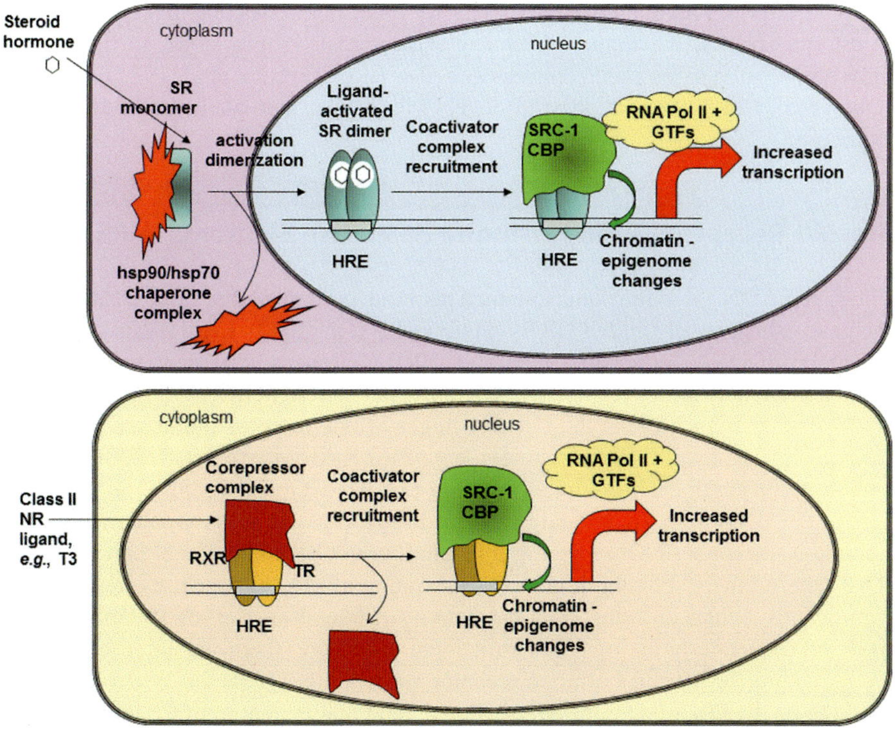

Fig. 2 General model of steroid hormone receptor (SR) and nuclear receptor (NR) activation of gene transcription. Target cells express SR and NRs. (**a**) Asteroid hormone, e.g., DHT, E_2, or cortisol, enters the nucleus and binds to the inactivate receptor monomer which is in the cytoplasm in a hsp90/hsp70 chaperone complex. Activation is described in the text. The ligand- activated SR homodimer enters the nucleus, binds to its cognate hormone response element, recruits coactivator proteins, *e.g.,* SRC-1 and CBP, which have HAT activity, and exist in complexes, e.g., ATP-dependent chromatin remodeling complexes. Chromatin modifications lead to enhanced RNA pol II recruitment and increased gene transcription. (**b**) For class II NRs, the receptor heterodimer is held in an inactive conformation by a corepressor complex including NCoR or SMART which interact with HDAC complexes. Ligand binding causes conformational changes the release the corepressor and recruit coactivators

complex (Guiochon-Mantel et al. 1996). The NLS-SR-NLS receptor-hsp90 complex binds to the nuclear pore complex via nucleoporins in an ATP-dependent process (DeFranco 1997; Elbi et al. 2004). The receptor is then trapped by binding to intranuclear components (Guiochon-Mantel et al. 1996). SR complexes associate with nuclear membranes and with chromatin components including histones, non-histone basic proteins, DNA and ribonucleoproteins (Ruh et al. 2004), and with nuclear matrix (Matsuda et al. 2002; Stenoien et al. 2001).

Steroid hormones generally autoregulate their receptor levels (Horwitz and McGuire 1978). The half-life of steroid hormone receptors ranges from 2 to 4 h for ERα (Kastner et al. 1990; Valley et al. 2008) and 4 h for AR (Syms et al. 1985), 7–10 h for PR (Nardulli et al. 1988), and 19 h for GR (McIntyre and Samuels 1985).

Steroid hormones regulate receptor levels for other hormones, e.g., E_2 increases PR in estrogen-responsive tissues (Clemens et al. 1998). Progesterone, in return, not only downregulates its own receptors but also ERα (Okulicz et al. 1981) and ERβ (Okret et al. 1991). Regulation of SR levels will, in turn, regulate cognate target gene expression.

Steroid Receptors Bind Hormone Response Elements (HREs)

The specific DNA-binding sites to which SR bind, conferring hormone sensitivity to the gene, are generally called HREs (Stedronsky et al. 2002). Core HREs consist of 13–15 bp of DNA. When first identified HRE consensus sequences were derived from alignment of genes responsive to a particular steroid hormone. HREs have two "half-sites" that each binds the C1 zinc finger of one receptor monomer. SR binds DNA as homodimers (or heterodimers, e.g., ERα/ERβ (Monroe et al. 2005; Powell and Xu 2008) with each monomer binding to adjacent major grooves on the same side of the DNA helix (Klug and Schwabe 1995). Class II NRs may interact with a retinoid X receptor (RXR) forming a heterodimer. RXR binds the 5′ half-site with RXR heterodimers showing higher DNA-binding affinity and stability, resulting in significantly enhanced transcriptional activity (Mangelsdorf et al. 1995b). On the basis of sequence homology and functional similarity, there are three classes of HREs within the steroid hormone receptor superfamily (Table 2). When SRs/NRs bind DNA, the DNA is deformed, causing a bend that is important for the assembly of coactivator/chromatin remodeling complex and facilitates interactions between components of the transcription complex and promotes DNA looping. ERα binding to an ERE results in a bend of the DNA toward the major groove (Nardulli et al. 1993; Sabbah et al. 1992). GR (Petz et al. 1997) and PR (Prendergast et al. 1996) also induce DNA bending. Similarly, class II NRs including TR and RXR induce DNA bending (e.g., Shulemovich et al. 1995).

The response elements for the AR, PR, MR, and GR are closely related and are collectively referred to as the glucocorticoid response element (GRE) consisting of a palindromic (symmetrical) sequence 5′-GGTACAnnnTGTTCT-3′, where n = any nucleotide (Beato et al. 1989). AR, PR, GR, and MR show subtle differences in DNA base contact points to GREs (Beato et al. 1989). Examples of genes containing one or more GREs whose transcription is upregulated by glucocorticoids include the much studied mouse mammary tumor virus (MMTV) promoter (Archer et al. 1995; Kinyamu et al. 2000), tyrosine aminotransferase (Jantzen et al. 1987), and enzymes involved in gluconeogenesis (Cole et al. 1993; De Martino et al. 2004; Feige and Auwerx 2007; Rodgers et al. 2005). Examples of genes that are specifically inhibited by glucocorticoids through "negative GREs" include pro-opiomelanocortin (Drouin et al. 1993), interleukin-1beta (Zhang et al. 1997), gonadotropin-releasing hormone (GnRH) (Chandran et al. 1996), and prolactin (PRL)(Subramaniam et al. 1997).

The minimal consensus estrogen response element (ERE) sequence is also palindromic, 5′-GGTCAnnnTGACC-3′ (Klein-Hitpass et al. 1988), and differs in only 2 bp from the GRE (Klock et al. 1987). Extension of the length of the ERE

Table 2 Hormone response element (HRE)-binding sites for steroid/nuclear receptors. Response elements for the class II nuclear receptors are direct repeats (DR), inverted repeats (IR), or everted repeats (EvR) of the indicated half-site with the letter following the DR or IR indicating the number of nucleotides separating the half-sites, e.g., DR5 is 5′-AGGTCAnnnnnAGGTCA-3′

Steroid/nuclear receptor	Consensus HRE	Reference
AR, GR, MR, and PR	ARE, GRE, MRE, PRE: 5′-AGAACAnnnTGTTCT-3′	Beato et al. (1989) and Geserick et al. (2005)
ERα and ERβ	ERE: 5′-AGGTCAnnnTGACCT-3′	Klinge (2001)
Class II NRs (PPAR, RAR, RXR, TR, and VDR)	DR: 5′-AGGTCA-3′	Stunnenberg (1993)
RAR homodimer	IR0	Helsen and Claessens (2014)
RXR/RAR	DR5, DR2, DR1	Bastien and Rochette-Egly (2004)
RXR/TR	DR4	Aumais et al. (1996)
TR homodimer	DR4, IR6	Helsen and Claessens (2014)
RXR/VDR or VDR homodimer	DR3	DeLuca and Zierold (1998)
RXR/PPAR	DR1	Willson et al. (2000)

palindrome, e.g., 5′-CAGGTCAnnnTGACCTG-3′, and the sequences immediately flanking the ERE helped determine ERα binding affinity (Anolik et al. 1993, 1995, 1996; Driscoll et al. 1996, 1998; Klinge 2001; Klinge et al. 1992a, b). One of the major advances in the field of transcriptional regulation by SR/NR has been the use of chromatin immunoprecipitation (ChIP) and ChIP-seq to identify receptor-binding sites in different types of cells with various treatments. We now appreciate that while SRs bind their consensus response elements (Table 2) with high affinity, these sites are located throughout the genome, not only in 5′ enhancer regions. Early experiments used human chromosome tiling arrays to identify ERα-binding sites throughout the human genome (Carroll and Brown 2006a, Carroll et al. 2006b; Eeckhoute et al. 2006, 2007; Kwon et al. 2007; Liu et al. 2008; Lupien et al. 2008; Tan-Wong et al. 2008). These studies were performed in MCF-7 human breast cancer cells with endogenous ERα and demonstrated that with E_2 treatment, ERα was recruited not only to the anticipated EREs in the 5′ promoter of known target genes but to ERES located in the 3′UTR and at great distances from established genes in the human genome (Carroll and Brown 2006a, Carroll et al. 2006b; Kwon et al. 2007; Lin et al. 2007; Liu et al. 2008; Stender et al. 2010; Welboren et al. 2009a, b). This provided new support for the idea of chromatin looping between distant sites allowing the assembly of a dynamic "transcriptional machine" that increases the efficiency of chromatin remodeling and facilitates gene transcription. Further studies have also demonstrated chromatin looping between promoter, intron, and 3′UTR regions of genes is regulated positively and negatively by E_2 (Eeckhoute et al. 2007; Tan-Wong et al. 2008). Overall, the interpretation of the vast amounts of data generated by global nuclear run-on sequencing (GRO-seq) and NGS is that E_2 increases transcription from both DNA strands and the ~30,000 transcripts regulated in MCF-7 cells include not only mRNA, rRNA, tRNA, and miRNA but also antisense, divergent, enhancer, and intergenic RNAs that may play roles in transcriptional regulation (Hah and Kraus 2014; Lam et al. 2014; Li et al. 2013).

In addition to EREs, ERα also occupies half-site EREs and AP-1 sites (Kininis et al. 2007) as well as sites for PAX2, FOXA1, AP2, TCF, PAX6, BACH1, MEF3, and LUN1 (Charn et al. 2010). In silico analysis revealed E_2-induced genes are enriched in binding sites for E2F1, NRF-1, and NF-Y transcription factors in ZR-75.1 breast cancer cells (Scafoglio et al. 2006). ERα-binding sites are cell specific: less than 20% of were common between E_2-treated ECC-1 endometrial and T47D breast cancer cells (Gertz et al. 2012). Together, these data and other studies reveal cell-specific, time-dependent ERα-, ERβ-, and apparent ERα/ERβ heterodimer DNA interactions throughout the genome resulting in different transcriptomes in the presence or absence of E_2 and other ligands.

The response elements for the various class II NRs, e.g., TR, RAR, RXR, and VDR, are composed of direct repeats of the half-site 5′-AGGTCA-3′ either with no space in between the half-sites (DR0) or separated by a gap of 1–5 nucleotides (DR1–DR5) (Umesono et al. 1991). The number of nucleotides separating the half-sites determines the specificity of class II NR binding (Mangelsdorf et al. 1995b). Many class II NR require RXR for hormonal activation of transcription (Mangelsdorf and Evans 1995a). The synergistic interaction between NRs and other transcription factors bound to regulatory cis-acting elements permits fine-tuning of the rates of transcription of target genes in response to the local cellular and hormonal milieu.

Regulation of Gene Transcription by Steroid Hormone Receptors

Initiation of transcription is a complex event occurring through the cooperative interaction of multiple factors at the target gene promoter. When bound to the specific HRE on the DNA, the hormone-receptor complex interacts with basal transcription factors and with other proteins to stabilize basal transcription factor binding and promote the assembly of the transcription initiation complex. Once the transcription initiation complex is in place, the enzyme RNA polymerase II is recruited to the transcription start site where it begins transcribing the DNA sequence into mRNA.

By binding to DNA, steroid hormone receptors regulate the transcription of RNA. Historically, we have considered the regulation of gene transcription in a positive manner by the steroid receptors, i.e., an SR binding to its HRE increased the levels of mRNA of the target gene. Transcriptional regulation was envisioned as involving SR-HRE interaction as a "cis"-acting element interaction since the HRE was located on the same DNA as the gene itself, generally located near the 5′ end (beginning) of the gene, upstream to the gene promoter with other transcription factor-binding elements, forming an upstream enhancer (Greenblatt 1997). The promoter, essential for gene activation, sets the basal rate of transcription and controls the accuracy of transcription initiation (Sauer and Tjian 1997). That view of how SRs regulate transcription has changed greatly in light of information from ChIP-seq studies described, as an example for ERα above, and the Encyclopedia of DNA Elements (ENCODE) project.

Data from Encyclopedia of DNA Elements (ENCODE, http://www.nature.com/encode/) revealed that ~75% of the human genome is transcribed and of that ~1% is mRNA, suggesting that other RNA transcripts, including long noncoding RNAs (lncRNAs) and small RNAs, including four major classes, small nuclear (sn)RNAs, small nucleolar (sno)RNAs, micro- (mi)RNAs, and transfer (t)RNAs, have regulatory functions (Djebali et al. 2012). Of the ~25,000 protein-coding genes in the human genome, only about half are expressed in any cell type due to cell-specific epigenomic signatures regulating a subset of enhancers controlling gene expression at a long range (Romanoski et al. 2015). Next-generation sequencing (NGS) by RNA sequencing (RNA-seq) identifies the cellular transcriptome, i.e., all the RNAs in that source (mRNA, rRNA, tRNA), the noncoding RNAs (ncRNAs), miRNAs, enhancer RNAs (eRNAs), endogenous small-interfering RNAs (siRNAs), PIWI-interacting RNAs (piRNAs), and lncRNAs, ranging from 1,000 to >90,000 bases (Marrone et al. 2014). The pervasiveness of transcription and the function of these transcripts are of keen interest (reviewed in Capobianco 2014).

ChIP-chip and ChIP-seq studies examining RNA pol II, coactivator, other transcription factor, and histone marks in E_2 treated MCF-7 cells have revealed that FoxA1 (Carroll et al. 2005), PBX, TLE1 (Holmes et al. 2012), AP2γ, and GATA3 (Theodorou et al. 2013) act as "pioneer factors" that remodel condensed chromatin to facilitate ERα binding (reviewed in Magnani and Lupien 2014). Pioneer factor interaction with nucleosomes coordinates the binding of other transcription factors, coregulators, and chromatin-modifying and remodeling complexes – all leading to increased transcription (reviewed in Iwafuchi-Doi and Zaret 2014).

Interaction of Steroid/Nuclear Receptors with Coactivators (Coregulators That Increase Transcriptional Activity)

DNA is complexed with histones, wound around nucleosomes, and condensed into a higher order helical fiber of 30 nm diameter that is decondensed for transcription (reviewed in Hübner et al. 2013). Studies have identified cell-specific ordering of chromatin into chromosome territories with each chromosome occupying a region of the nucleus with changes in chromatin topology, e.g., looping involved in gene transcription (Hübner et al. 2013). Epigenetic modifications to the N-terminal tails of core histones, i.e., lysine acetylation, lysine and arginine methylation, and serine and threonine phosphorylation, impact dynamics of chromatin structure and accessibility of transcription factor binding (Wang et al. 2004). Activation of gene transcription involves a network of interactions among transcription factors, histone-modifying enzymes, epigenetic readers, and components of RNA polymerase II. The human genome has >1 million enhancers (Heintzman et al. 2009). Enhancers were first identified as DNase I hypersensitive sites and are now defined as high H3K4me1 and H3K27Ac and low H3K4me3 by ChIP assays (reviewed in Palstra and Grosveld 2012).

Acetylation and methylation decrease histone's affinity for DNA to induce changes in nucleosomal structure that allows access to the DNA by nucleosomal sliding, histone exchange, or histone displacement (reviewed in Galvani and Thiriet 2015).

SRs interact with multiple proteins both when bound to DNA or in solution in vitro. Early experiments showed that overexpression of one type of steroid hormone receptor could inhibit or "squelch" the activation of transcription mediated by a different SR, hinting that steroid receptors compete for limited amounts of a factor(s) required for transcription (Meyer et al. 1989). Over the past 20 years, numerous coactivators have been identified (reviewed in Stashi et al. 2014; York and O'Malley 2010). Initially some of these proteins were called receptor-interacting proteins (RIPs) and receptor-associated proteins (RAPs); however, not all RIPs are coactivators. By definition, coactivators are considered to interact directly with the steroid/nuclear receptor and enhance transcription. Thus, the first coactivators for steroid receptors to be discovered, the SWI/SNF proteins (Yoshinaga et al. 1992), while not strictly coactivators, serve as bridging factors that interact between coactivators and basal transcription factors. Several coactivators have "general" transcriptional activator function, since they enhance transcription by different types of transcription factors, including steroid receptors.

Coactivator proteins contain one or more copies of an NR-binding motif, also called the NR box, consisting of the aa = LXXLL, which physically interacts with the steroid/nuclear receptors. Steroid receptors show different affinities for the various coactivators (Ding et al. 1998) and use different amino acids to contact the coactivators (Eng et al. 1998). Some coactivators, e.g., SRC-1 (NCOA1), SRC-1 (AIB1, NCOA3), and CREB/p300/CBP, have histone acetyltransferase (HAT) activity (Dallas et al. 1998; Shang et al. 2000; Spencer et al. 1997) providing a mechanism by which "coactivation" occurs. HATs acetylate lysine residues on the N-terminal tails of histones H3 and H4 in chromatin, resulting in a weaker association of histones with DNA, thus altering nucleosomal conformation and stability in a manner that facilitates transcriptional activation by RNA polymerase II (Sternglanz 1996). SRC-1, CBP/p300, CREB, and other coactivators form a ternary complex with liganded SR to increase gene transcription (Shibata et al. 1997). Thus, several HAT activities may be tethered to hormone-activated receptors on the promoter, yielding synergistic transactivation. Electron cryo-electron microscopy (cryo-EM) revealed the quaternary structure of an ERα, SRC-3 (AIB1), and p300, bound to the 700 bp plasmid, containing four tandem EREs, at a resolution of ~25 Å which indicated each ERα monomer bound one SRC-3 coactivator (two SRC-3s, two ERαs, and one p300 were visualized in the complex) with p300 bridging the two SRC-3 proteins (Yi et al. 2015). SRs/NRs show different affinities of interaction with coactivators (Zhou et al. 1998). There is a complex "histone code" regulating gene transcription that includes not only histone acetylation but methylation, ubiquitinylation, and other modifications that lead to a combinatorial epigenomic signature which enhances transcription (reviewed in Fischle et al. 2015; Gardner et al. 2011). Target cells express different levels of coactivators and corepressors which, along with the amount of receptor protein and ligand, allows fine-tuning of target gene transcription in response to steroid hormones (Smith and O'Malley 2004).

General Model of SR Nuclear Transcription Factor Activity

Steroid hormones are small hydrophobic and lipid-soluble molecules derived from cholesterol. They circulate in blood either free or bound (95%) to plasma carrier proteins (Thompson 1995). Sex hormone-binding globulin (SHBG), also known as testosterone-estradiol-binding globulin (TeBG), and androgen-binding protein (ABP) are encoded by the same gene (Danzo and Joseph 1994), but differ in tissue expression and glycosylation (Hammond and Bocchinfuso 1995). ABP is produced by the Sertoli cells of the testis, and SHBG is produced by the liver and is present in the circulatory system (Joseph 1994). SHBG binds most gonadal steroids, and corticosteroid-binding globulin (CBG or transcortin) binds glucocorticoids and progesterone, with differing affinities. When circulating levels of steroid hormones exceed the binding capacity of their respective binding proteins, they bind non-specifically, and with low affinity, to albumin, from which they can readily dissociate and enter target cells (Westphal 1986).

SHBG binds to a specific cell membrane receptor called sex hormone-binding globulin receptor (SHBG-R) and activates adenylyl cyclase, thus increasing intra-cellular cAMP (Joseph 1994). Binding of SHBG to SHBG-R also transfers SHBG into the cell as a consequence of receptor-mediated endocytosis (Hammes et al. 2005). The interaction of SHBG with SHBG-R was shown to be inhibited when steroids are bound to SHBG, suggesting that SHBG is an allosteric protein (Porto et al. 1995). However, if unliganded SHBG is allowed to bind to its receptor on intact cells, and an appropriate steroid hormone then is introduced, adenylate cyclase is activated and intracellular cAMP increases (Rosner et al. 1991). Several members of the organic anion-transporting polypeptide (OATP) family of proteins mediate the sodium and ATP-independent uptake of DHEA, pregnenolone, and estrone into tissues including the breast and prostate and are overexpressed in tumors in these tissues (Cho et al. 2014). Once the steroid hormone is in the cytoplasm, it is not yet clear whether a transport protein is required for movement of the hydrophobic steroid molecule through the aqueous cytoplasm to the receptor, regardless of whether the receptor is cytoplasmic or nuclear in location. The current model is that the steroid hormone diffuses freely in the cytoplasm.

Regulation of Gene Transcription by Interaction of Steroid/ Nuclear Receptors with Other Transcription Factors Bound to DNA (Tethering)

Steroid receptors interact directly with different transcription factors and alter target gene transcription without the steroid receptor interacting directly with DNA. The best studied example of this “transcriptional cross talk” is the interaction of the AP-1 transcription factor with GR (reviewed in Gottlicher et al. 1998). Depending on the cell type (Maroder et al. 1993) and the composition of the AP-1 complex, GR synergizes with AP-1 (Jun-Jun homodimer) or suppresses the Fos-Jun heterodimer (Diamond et al. 1990). In vitro assays demonstrated that ERα interacts with the

Fos-Jun AP-1 heterodimer and that the selective ER modulators (SERMs) raloxifene and tamoxifen are more potent agonists than E_2 at AP-1 sites (Cheung et al. 2005). For example tamoxifen-activated ERα activated the human collagenase gene through an AP-1 site (Webb et al. 1995). Tamoxifen agonism at AP-1 sites is cell-type specific, i.e., occurring in cell lines of the uterine, but not of breast origin. The DBD of ERα is required for tamoxifen activation at AP-1 sites. Conversely, the AP-1 components cJun and cFos inhibited E_2-dependent ERα-stimulated reporter gene activity in transiently transfected MCF-7 or CV-1 cells transfected with ERα (Tzukerman et al. 1991). DNA-binding experiments revealed that ERα-ERE binding was inhibited by the cJun protein and that ERα inhibited cJun-DNA binding (Tzukerman et al. 1991).

E_2 differentially regulates gene transcription through ERα and ERβ from an AP-1 site: with ERα, E_2-activated transcription, whereas with ERβ, E_2 inhibited transcription (Paech et al. 1997). Moreover, in contrast to ERα, the antiestrogens tamoxifen, raloxifene, and ICI 164,384 were potent transcriptional activators with ERβ at an AP-1 site. Thus, the two ERs differ in how they respond to ligand and response element, suggesting that ERα and ERβ may play different roles in gene regulation (Paech et al. 1997).

Sp1 is another transcription factor with which ERα interacts to activate gene transcription (reviewed in Safe and Kim 2008). A number of estrogen-responsive genes are activated by ERα-Sp1 interaction including cathepsin D (Krishnan et al. 1994), RARα (Rishi et al. 1996), VEGF (Stoner et al. 2004), and c-*fos* (Duan et al. 1998). ERα and Sp1 physically interact in a manner that requires both the N-terminal and C-terminal regions of ERα (Porter et al. 1997). The interaction of the Sp1 and ERα and the resulting increase in Sp1-DNA binding are observed in the presence or absence of E_2, whereas transactivation of promoter-reporter constructs is E_2 dependent. These results indicate that transcriptional activation requires more than ERα-Sp1 interaction and increased DNA binding. A likely interpretation is that coactivators are required.

NF-κB, a transcription factor dimer involved in regulation of inflammatory genes, also interacts directly with ERα, ERβ, and GR, and inhibition of NF-κB was demonstrated to stimulate ERβ and GR transcriptional activity in cells (Chu et al. 2004). More recent studies using circular chromosome conformation capture coupled with next-generation sequencing and high-resolution chromatin interaction analysis by paired-end tag sequencing have identified long-range chromatin interactions of GR, NF-κB, and p300 in HeLa cells (Kuznetsova et al. 2015).

Actions of SR in the Plasma Membrane

While most of the effects of steroid hormones are mediated through their interaction with their cognate receptors and subsequent effects on target gene transcription, certain rapid effects of steroid hormones and nuclear receptor ligands are incompatible with a transcriptional mechanism. A small proportion of classical steroid receptors, i.e., AR (Migliaccio et al. 2011), ERα (Watson et al. 2002Watson and

Lange 2005b), PR (Kowalik et al. 2013), GR (Song and Buttgereit 2006), and MR (Dooley et al. 2012), have been reported in the plasma membrane of various target cell types. In general, treatment of target cells containing SR in plasma membrane-associated complexes rapidly, within seconds, activates intracellular signaling pathways, e.g., MAPK, PI3K, JNK, that lead ultimately to alterations in gene expression and cell phenotypes. Computational modeling studies have identified two transmembrane helices (TMH) within the LBD of PRB, AR, ERα, and ERβ (Morrill et al. 2015).

Extranuclear Activities of GR and MR

GR can bind to cytoskeletal structures (Scherrer and Pratt 1992), and glucocorticoids stimulate the rapid onset of polymerization of actin in a nongenomic manner that involves decreased intracellular cAMP (Koukouritaki et al. 1997). GR has also been found in mitochondria in hepatic cells where it may activate mitochondrial gene expression (Demonacos et al. 1996), and in leukemic cells sensitivity to glucocorticoids-induced apoptosis appears to be regulated by translocation of GR into mitochondria (Sionov et al. 2006). Aldosterone rapidly actives protein kinase C (PKC), protein kinase D (PKD), and mitogen-activated protein kinase (MAPK) signaling cascades through transactivation of epidermal growth factor receptor (EGFR) and the tyrosine kinase c-Src (reviewed in Dooley et al. 2012).

Membrane-Initiated Progestin Signaling

Membrane progesterone receptors were initially characterized in amphibian oocytes, in fish, and in spermatids, reviewed in Baulieu and Robel (1995)Baulieu and Schumacher 1997), Braun and Thomas (2004), Hawkins and Thomas (2004), Maller (2003), Thomas et al. (2004), and Zhu et al. (2003a, b). There are three subtypes of membrane PR: α, β, and γ, with each a GPCR that is linked to inhibition of adenylate cyclase (Josefsberg Ben-Yehoshua et al. 2007; Thomas 2008; Zhu et al. 2003a; b). A novel PR that mediates rapid changes in Ca^{+2} conductance was reported in human sperm plasma membrane, reviewed in Revelli et al. (1998). A single transmembrane protein progesterone receptor membrane component 1 (PGMRC1) that has a MW 26–28 kDa was first purified from pig livers and has subsequently been identified in a variety of other tissues, including granulosa and luteal cells (Thomas 2008). PGMRC1 can bind to other molecules including heme, cholesterol metabolites, and proteins (Thomas 2008). In granulosa cells, progesterone activation of PGMRC1 results in antimitotic and anti-apoptotic action, and altered PGRMC1 expression correlates with premature ovarian failure, polycystic ovarian syndrome, and infertility (reviewed in Peluso and Pru 2014). Progesterone activation of PM-associated PGMRC1 activates ERK5 and increases BDNF release providing neuroprotection in the brain (reviewed in Singh et al. 2013). Higher MW oligomeric forms of PGMRC1 locate in the nucleus where PGMRC1 generally functions as a repressor of transcription in a human granulosa/luteal cell line (hGL5 cells) (Peluso et al. 2012). In addition, metabolites of progesterone and deoxycorticosterone act as positive allosteric modulators of the gamma-aminobutyric acid (GABA)A receptor complex in the cortex of rat brain, increasing the affinity of GABA binding to the GABAA receptor (Hawkinson et al. 1994). The neuroprotective effects of progesterone and its actions through GABAA receptor and PGRMC1 were recently reviewed (Guennoun et al. 2015). There is clearly a need for further research to elucidate the roles of membrane PRs in mediating progestin activity in various tissues

Membrane-Associated ER Signaling

E_2 has "nongenomic, extranuclear, or membrane-initiated" effects, i.e., independent of ER-mediated transcription, that occur within minutes after E_2 administration (reviewed in Levin 2015; Pietras and Marquez-Garban 2007; Watson et al. 2010). Tissues in which rapid effects of E_2 have been reported include the brain (reviewed in Toran-Allerand 2004), cardiovascular tissues (reviewed in Kim et al. 2014), and oocytes (Tesarik and Mendoza 1997). A generalized model for the activities of PM-associated ERs, which include dimeric full-length ERα, palmitoylated ERα46, N-terminal-truncated ERα36, and GPER, is shown in Fig. 3. ERα interacts with cavelolin-1 which functions as a scaffold for a number of signaling proteins, including Src kinase, Gα, EGFR, PKC, PELP1, and other signaling molecules (reviewed in Boonyaratanakornkit 2011; Girard et al. 2014).

One well-characterized system for the study of endogenous membrane ERα is the rat GH3/B6 pituitary tumor cell line in which ~10% of ERα localizes in the plasma membrane (Bulayeva et al. 2004a, b, c; Pappas et al. 1995; Watson et al. 1995, 2002, 2005a). Treatment of GH3/B6 pituitary cells to E_2 elicited a rapid (within 5 min) release of prolactin (PRL). GH3/B6 pituitary cells also show small amounts of membrane-associated ERβ and GPER (Watson et al. 2012). This model system has been used to characterize the rapid effects of environmentally relevant concentrations of endocrine-disrupting chemicals (EDCs) including bisphenol A and bisphenol S which include activation of JNK and MAPK and inhibition of E_2-induced PRL release (Vinas and Watson 2013).

A comparison of nuclear and membrane localization of recombinant ERα and ERβ in transfected CHO cells (considered to be ER null) showed that both ERα and ERβ were expressed predominantly in the nucleus with ~5% of each ER subtype located in the cell membrane (Razandi et al. 1999). E_2 treatment of these transfected CHO cells activated Gαq and Gαs proteins in the membrane and rapidly stimulated corresponding inositol phosphate production and adenylate cyclase activity (Razandi et al. 1999). Interestingly, membrane ERα and ERβ showed a distinct difference in their activities: cJun N-terminal kinase (JNK) activity was stimulated by E_2 in ERβ-expressing CHO, but was inhibited in CHO-ERα cells (Razandi et al. 1999). Plasma membrane ERα is a dimer that interacts with caveolin-1 (Cav-1) which interacts with G proteins, Src, Grb7, Raf, Ras, MEK, and the EGFR in MCF-7

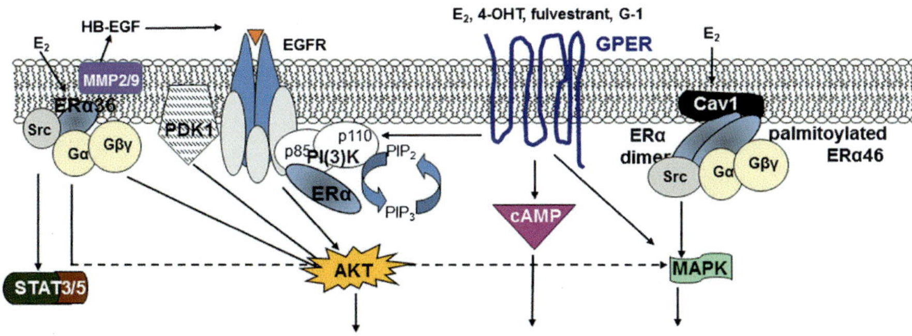

Fig. 3 Rapid activation of membrane-associated ERa, ERa46, ERa36, and GPER activates intracellular signaling pathways

cells and triggers the release of HB-EGF into the culture medium that, in turn, activates the EGFR and downstream signaling leading to activation of ERK1/2 (MAPK) and PI3K/AKT signaling cascades (Pedram et al. 2006; Razandi et al. 2003). Palmitoylation of ERα is important for its membrane localization (Acconcia et al. 2005; Pedram et al. 2007).

In MCF-7 cells, E_2 rapidly increased PIP2-phospholipase C activity (Graber et al. 1993), mobilized intracellular Ca^{2+}, and activated the MAPK (Improta-Brears et al. 1999) and PI3K/AKT pathways (Stoica et al. 2003). Since ERα lacks a transmembrane domain, how it gets to the plasma membrane (PM) has been controversial, but it appears to involve palmitoylation (Moriarty et al. 2006). In MCF-7 cells, the adaptor protein Shc shuttles ERα from the nucleus to the PM where ERα interacts with the IGF-1 receptor (IGF-1R) (Song et al. 2004). Similarly, another scaffold protein, called modulator of nongenomic activity of ER (MNAR), was reported to mediate ERα-cSrc interaction and MAPK signaling (Barletta et al. 2004; Cheskis 2004; Greger et al. 2006). A role for a membrane caveola-localized ERα variant (ERα46) in rapid NO release via PI3K/Akt-activated endothelial nitric oxide synthase (eNOS) in EC has been reported (Flototto et al. 2004; Hisamoto and Bender 2005; Kim and Bender 2005; Li et al. 2003).

Direct interactions between plasma membrane-associated ERα and Gαi have been implicated in eNOS activation and NO production in COS-7 cells transfected with ERα and specific Gαi proteins (Chambliss et al. 2010). E_2 stimulated the direct interaction of ERα with Gαi via ERα-striatin interaction in MCF-7 and other cells (Wu et al. 2013). Likewise, E_2 rapidly activates the G protein-coupled signal cascades in MCF-7 and other breast cancer cell lines.

GPER/GPR30

GPER (originally called GPR30) is an integral plasma membrane coupled to Gαs in its inactive state and, when activated, causes heterotrimeric G proteins that stimulate adenylate cyclase, Src, and EGFR signaling (Gaudet et al. 2015; Prossnitz and

Barton 2014). GPER is also associated with endoplasmic reticulum, likely from endocytic recycling. GPER is activated not only by E_2 but also by tamoxifen, raloxifene, fulvestrant, xenoestrogens, endocrine disruptors, synthetic, specific ligand G-1 (Gaudet et al. 2015), and DHEA (Teng et al. 2015). E_2 binds GPER with high affinity (Kd = 2.7 nM) and activates adenylate cyclase, AKT, and MAPK signaling (Filardo and Thomas 2012). Overexpression of FLAG-GPER in HeLa cells revealed that physiological concentrations (10 nM–1 μM) of E_2 stimulated FLAG-GPER translocation from the plasma membrane to the cytoplasm and that intracellular Ca^{++} was elevated within several seconds after the addition of E_2 in these cells (Funakoshi et al. 2006). Two synthetic GPER antagonists G-15 and G-36 are used in experiments to examine downstream signaling (Gaudet et al. 2015). GPER is thought to be the membrane receptor for aldosterone (Feldman 2014; Feldman and Gros 2013). GPER has been implicated in a variety of physiological processes in tissues including the brain, vascular endothelium, cardiovascular, lung, skeletal muscle, and bone and in processes including metabolism, immune regulation, neurotransmission, water reabsorption, and cancer progression in many tumor types (reviewed in Barton and Prossnitz 2015; Gaudet et al. 2015; Prossnitz and Barton 2014).

Summary Comments on the Functional Roles of Steroid Receptors

Androgen Receptor

AR is expressed in the male reproductive tract and in the female reproductive tract as well as many other tissues (reviewed in Chang et al. 2013). A number of AR knockout (ARKO) mice have been created for system or cell-specific knockout (reviewed in Chang et al. 2013). These studies revealed critical roles for AR not only for male reproductive tract function but also for folliculogenesis, fertility, and mammary gland development. AR and its regulation of gene transcription and rapid effects on cell signaling are best characterized in prostate cancer (reviewed in Green et al. 2012). The NTD of AR has polyglutamine (Poly-Q), polyproline (Poly-P), and polyglycine (Poly-G) repeats. The Poly-Q displays high variability, ranging in length from 18 to 22 repeats (normal) to over 40 repeats. There are a number of alternatively spliced AR variants, i.e., AR-V3, AR-V4, AR-V7, and AR-V12 that are constitutively active and thought to play a role in castration-resistant prostate cancer (CRPC) (Schweizer and Yu 2015). Overexpression and AR gene amplification as well as nucleotide mutations are found in AR in CRPC (reviewed in Waltering et al. 2012). Rapid signaling by androgens involves AR-Src interaction which may play a role in CRPC (Zarif et al. 2015). AR also contributes to breast cancer with current studies examining its contribution to triple-negative (Zhang et al. 2015) and endocrine-resistant breast cancer (Rechoum et al. 2014). Early clinical trials indicate a benefit for antiandrogen (enzalutamide) in breast cancer patients (Traina 2015), but further studies are needed.

There are five different AR knockout mouse lines with different exon deletions, and differences in these models and as a result of mouse strain background have been observed (reviewed in Rana et al. 2014). Early studies reported that male AR knockout (ARKO) mice are phenotypically female with an 80% reduction in testes size, and serum testosterone concentrations are lower than in wild-type (wt) mice (Yeh et al. 2002). ARKO mice displayed small hearts in relation to body weight with impaired contraction (reviewed in Rana et al. 2014). The male ARKO mice have reduced spermatogenesis and cancellous bone volumes. Female ARKO mice have reduced fertility (Yeh et al. 2002). The mice also have specific skeletal muscle defects (Altuwaijri et al. 2004). Creation of transgenic mice with conditional knockout of AR only in prostate epithelia (pes-ARKO) revealed that these mice lacked external phenotypic differences seen in the ARKO mice, but that they showed increased prostate epithelial cell proliferation (Wu et al. 2007). Other insights from the pes-ARKO mice have been reviewed (Rana et al. 2014).

Estrogen Receptors (ERs)

Until late 1996, only one ER was thought to mediate the physiological effects of estrogens. However, a second gene encoding a closely related, but distinct, ER, called ERβ, was first identified in rat prostate (Kuiper et al. 1996) and later in humans (Mosselman et al. 1996). The original ER was renamed ERα. ERα (*ESR1*, NR3A1) and ERβ (*ESR2*, NR3A2) can form heterodimers as well as homodimers in vitro and in vivo (Ogawa et al. 1998). Both ERs bind estrogens, estradiol (E2), estrone (E1), and estriol with high affinity in the nM range (Kuiper et al. 1997). In addition to full-length, wild-type ERα, a 66 kDa protein, a number of splice variants of ERα have been identified (reviewed in Herynk and Fuqua 2004). Among them, ERα46 (reviewed in Pietras and Marquez-Garban 2007; Toran-Allerand 2004) and ERα36 (reviewed in Wang and Yin 2015) are associated with membrane-initiated estrogen signaling. Likewise, ERβ splice variants have genomic and "nongenomic" activities and subcellular distribution (Davies et al. 2004; Thomas and Gustafsson 2011; Weiser et al. 2008). These splice variants can dimerize with wt ERα and ERβ, but the functional significance of such heterodimerization is not yet known.

The tissue distribution of ERα and ERβ overlaps, but often one subtype is dominant in a particular tissue. ERα is more highly expressed in the liver, mammary gland, pituitary, hypothalamus, uterus, and vagina than ERβ; ERβ is dominant in the colonic epithelium, prostate, ovary, and lung (reviewed in Hamilton et al. 2014; Zhao et al. 2010a). Studies in knockout mouse models provide evidence that ERα and ERβ play unique physiological roles (reviewed in Couse et al. 2000; Couse and Korach 1998, 1999; Hewitt et al. 2005). To the surprise of the investigators and others, global knockout of ERα expression was not lethal and had no effects on the ratio of male/female mice born (Couse et al. 1995). ERαKO mice survived to adulthood and developed grossly normal external genitalia, but both sexes were infertile (Lubahn et al. 1993). Reproductive findings in both ERαKO and ERαKO mice have been reviewed (Hamilton et al. 2014). Mammary glands of adult ERαKO female mice lack branching and terminal end bud formation (Korach et al. 2003). Disruption of ERα signaling in ERKO mice leads to an obese phenotype (Musatov et al. 2007; Ohlsson et al. 2000).

Because ERα is the best prognostic indicator for breast cancer patients and is the most successful molecular target in the history of cancer drug discovery (Zhou and Slingerland 2014), much is known about the molecular mechanisms of ERα in breast cancer. ERα is expressed at elevated levels in ~75% of clinical breast cancer samples (McGuire et al. 1986). In cell-based studies, ERβ is a dominant negative inhibitor of ERα-mediated transcriptional activity (reviewed in Böttner et al. 2014). Antiestrogens, e.g., tamoxifen, and aromatase inhibitors (AIs), e.g., letrozole, are used as adjuvant therapy to prevent disease recurrence in breast cancer patients whose tumors are ERα/PR+ (Freedman et al. 2015). Indeed, because of its disease relevance, more papers have been published on ERα than any other NR or transcription factor (Vaquerizas et al. 2009).

Glucocorticoid Receptors

GR is activated by cortisol from the adrenal in response to activation of the hypothalamic-pituitary-adrenal (HPA) axis and release of ACTH to stimulate the adrenal. The systemic effects of glucocorticoids are vast (reviewed in Talabér et al. 2013). GR exists in two isoforms GRα and GRβ, identical from the N-terminus to aa 727, with splice variants of each (reviewed in Lu and Cidlowski 2004). GR knockout or GR loss-of-function transgenic mice show that GR signaling controls glucose metabolism in the liver, skeletal muscle, and pancreas and regulates it (reviewed in Rose and Herzig 2013). GR regulates the transcription of circadian clock genes that are important for glucose and lipid homeostasis (reviewed in Dickmeis et al. 2013). Total GR knockout in mice causes postnatal death due to respiratory failure, whereas mice lacking GR in hepatocytes show profound hypoglycemia after prolonged fasting due to their lack of GR stimulation of genes involved in gluconeogenesis, i.e., phosphoenolpyruvate carboxykinase (PEPCK), pyruvate carboxylase, and glucose-6-phosphatase (reviewed in Rose and Herzig 2013). Glucocorticoids are clinically used to inhibit inflammation. GR represses the transcription of inflammatory genes by tethering to NFκB, AP-1, and STAT3 and inhibiting transcription by unknown mechanisms involving competition for coactivators and recruitment of HDACs (reviewed in Chinenov et al. 2013). To my knowledge, only four papers address the GR cistrome (Kadiyala et al. 2016a, b; Okun et al. 2015; Paakinaho et al. 2014). These studies indicate that GR actions depend on cellular and chromatin context. Future RNA-seq and cistrome studies are necessary to elucidate the mechanisms of the cell-specific functions.

Mineralocorticoid Receptors

Aldosterone activation of MR regulates renal sodium reabsorption and potassium excretion, thus playing a major role in blood pressure regulation and extracellular volume regulation. MR also binds cortisol, but the conformation of MR elicited upon cortisol binding is different from that when aldosterone binds, and this results in differences in intramolecular and coregulator interactions (reviewed in Fuller 2015). In addition to its expression in aldosterone-sensitive distal nephrons of the kidney, MR is expressed in vascular smooth muscle cells, venous endothelial cells, atrial cardiomyocytes, and subcutaneous adipocytes and in epidermis and hair follicle from the skin (reviewed in Jaisser and Farman 2016). MR is also expressed in specific areas of the brain at higher levels than GR, e.g., hippocampus (reviewed in Talabér et al. 2013). MR is expressed in a range of inflammatory cells, particularly the monocyte-macrophage lineage (reviewed in Fuller 2015). There has been an exponential increase in reports implicating MR in a variety of diseases and beneficial effects of MR agonists in a variety of tissues including eye and immune system (reviewed in Jaisser and Farman 2016).

Targeted disruption of MR resulted in neonatal death in homozygous MR knockout mice with death 8–13 days after birth due to dehydration by renal sodium and water loss (Berger et al. 1998). The MR-/- mice showed severe dehydration, hyperkalemia, hyponatremia, and high plasma levels of renin, angiotensin II, and aldosterone (Hubert et al. 1999). Cardiomyocyte-selective MR knockout or overexpression studies in mice showed that cardiomyocyte MR-null mice were protected from cardiac dilatation and failure in an infarct model (reviewed in Young and Rickard 2015). Whether inhibition of MR by therapeutic intervention will benefit patients with cardiovascular disease is of keen interest.

Only one paper has examined the cistromes of MR in aldosterone-treated human renal cells (Le Billan et al. 2015). ChIP for AR identified the consensus MRE (5′-AGxACAnnnTGTxCT-3′) and binding sites for early growth response protein 1 (EGR1), forkhead box (FOX), paired box protein 5 (PAX5), and activated protein 1 (AP-1), suggesting cooperation of MR with these transcription factors. Additional studies are needed to understand MR regulation of gene transcription.

Progesterone Receptors

Studies have shown that PR-A is required for reproductive function and uterine development while PR-B is required for normal mammary gland development (Lange 2008). Most PR-positive cells in humans express PR-A and PR-B, including the uterus, mammary gland, brain, bone, ovary, testes, pancreas, and tissues of the lower urinary tract (reviewed in Scarpin et al. 2009). Nongenomic/extranuclear effects of progesterone in human tissues/cells include acrosome reaction/capacitation, immunoregulatory function in T lymphocytes, platelet aggregation, and intestinal smooth muscle contraction (reviewed in Taraborrelli 2015). Clinical data from the Women's Health Initiative (WHI) trial indicated that medroxyprogesterone acetate (MPA) increased breast cancer risk, and a variety of in vitro studies support a stimulatory role of progestins in breast cancer (reviewed in Lange 2008). Antiprogestins are of clinical interest in breast cancer treatment (reviewed in Knutson and Lange 2014).

There were no effects on the viability or sexual differentiation of homozygous PR gene-disrupted mice (Lydon et al. 1995). The female homozygous for PR disruption are completely infertile while males exhibit no apparent effects on fertility. Serum LH levels in PRKO mice ~twofold higher (metestrus) than in wild-type mice (Chappell et al. 1997). However, basal FSH and LHRH levels were unaffected. Basal levels of E_2 and progesterone in serum were likewise similar in the two groups. Basal PRL levels were slightly higher in PRKO versus wild-type mice. These results confirm the essential role of PR in regulating the hypothalamic and/or pituitary axis that governs gonadotropin secretion (Chappell et al. 1997).

The transcriptome and cistromes of PR which have been examined in human endometrial stromal cells showed that FOSL2 is an important coregulator of PR-mediated stromal cell decidualization, which is required to establish and maintain pregnancy (Mazur et al. 2015). Much less is known about the PR cistromes than ERα cistrome.

Summary

Over the past 30 years, we have gained insight into the molecular mechanisms of the action of steroid hormones and their receptors. Yet, what we have learned from a wide range of techniques from targeted disruption in animal models, molecular cloning and overexpression studies in cells and animals, ChIP, ChIP-seq, NGS, GRO-seq, and chromatin capture experiments is that we still do not fully understand how this complex system works in vivo to maintain homeostasis and the precise mechanisms of endocrine disease. We know that steroid hormones and other ligands mediate their biological activities by binding to a superfamily of related receptors that share a common modular structure. Studies have revealed that unliganded and hormone-occupied SRs interact with specific binding sites throughout the genome and regulate transcription bidirectionally. We know that SRs interact with numerous coregulatory proteins that assist in chromatin remodeling and other epigenomic alterations that alter transcription initiation and elongation. We know that SRs also interact with other nuclear transcription factors bound to their response element to regulate gene transcription. We know that SRs exist in complexes of proteins with chromatin remodeling activity that bring distant regions together in a "chromatin kissing" model to regulate gene transcription. The nucleosome remodeling activity of SR coactivators and corepressors and their associated proteins has revealed the importance of the dynamic nature of chromatin structure in hormone-induced gene transcription. The importance of multiple levels of "cross talk" between cell membrane-bound SRs and other PM receptors, e.g., EGFR, acting via second messenger phosphorylation cascades, and nuclear SRs and between different classes of transcriptional enhancer proteins indicates the overall complexity involved in specific gene regulation. Finally, recent developments in the analysis of SR mutants and their function have enhanced our potential for clinical diagnosis and treatment of endocrine disorders.

Cross-References

▶ Genetic Disorders of Adrenocortical Function
▶ Molecular Mechanisms of Thyroid Hormone Synthesis and Secretion
▶ Ovarian Physiology
▶ Targeting of Steroid Hormone Receptor Function in Breast and Prostate Cancer
▶ The Adrenal Glands
▶ The Endocrine Regulation of Blood Pressure
▶ The Endocrinology of Puberty
▶ The Physiology of the Testis
▶ Thyroid Hormone Nuclear Receptors and Molecular Actions

References

Acconcia F, Ascenzi P, Bocedi A, Spisni E, Tomasi V, Trentalance A, Visca P, Marino M. Palmitoylation-dependent estrogen receptor {alpha} membrane localization: regulation by 17{beta}-Estradiol. Mol Biol Cell. 2005;16:231–7.

Altuwaijri S, Lee DK, Chuang KH, Ting HJ, Yang Z, Xu Q, Tsai MY, Yeh S, Hanchett LA, Chang HC, Chang C. Androgen receptor regulates expression of skeletal muscle-specific proteins and muscle cell types. Endocrine. 2004;25:27–32.

Anolik JH, Klinge CM, Bambara RA, Hilf R. Differential impact of flanking sequences on estradiol- *versus* 4-hydroxytamoxifen-liganded estrogen receptor binding to estrogen responsive element DNA. J Steroid Biochem Mol Biol. 1993;46:713–30.

Anolik JH, Klinge CM, Hilf R, Bambara RA. Cooperative binding of estrogen receptor to DNA depends on spacing of binding sites, flanking sequence, and ligand. Biochemistry (Mosc). 1995;34:2511–20.

Anolik JH, Klinge CM, Brolly CL, Bambara RA, Hilf R. Stability of the ligand of estrogen response element-bound estrogen receptor depends on flanking sequences and cellular factors. J Steroid Biochem Mol Biol. 1996;59:413–29.

Archer TK, Fryer CJ, Lee H-L, Zaniewski E, Liang T, Mymryk JS. Steroid hormone receptor status defines the MMTV promoter chromatin structure *in vivo*. J Steroid Biochem Mol Biol. 1995;53:421–9.

Audet-Walsh E, Giguere V. The multiple universes of estrogen-related receptor alpha and gamma in metabolic control and related diseases. Acta Pharmacol Sin. 2015;36:51–61.

Aumais JP, Lee HS, DeGannes C, Horsford J, White J. Function of directly repeated half sites as response elements for steroid hormones. J Biol Chem. 1996;271:12568–77.

Banerjee M, Robbins D, Chen T. Modulation of xenobiotic receptors by steroids. Molecules (Basel, Switzerland). 2013;18:7389–406.

Banerjee M, Robbins D, Chen T. Targeting xenobiotic receptors PXR and CAR in human diseases. Drug Discov Today. 2015;20:618–28.

Barletta F, Wong CW, McNally C, Komm BS, Katzenellenbogen B, Cheskis BJ. Characterization of the interactions of estrogen receptor and MNAR in the activation of cSrc. Mol Endocrinol. 2004;18:1096–108.

Barton M, Prossnitz ER. Emerging roles of GPER in diabetes and atherosclerosis. Trends Endocrinol Metab. 2015;26:185–92.

Bastien J, Rochette-Egly C. Nuclear retinoid receptors and the transcription of retinoid-target genes. Gene. 2004;328:1–16.

Baulieu EE, Robel P. Non-genomic mechanisms of action of steroid hormones. Ciba Found Symp. 1995;191:24–37.

Baulieu EE, Schumacher M. Neurosteroids, with special reference to the effect of progesterone on myelination in peripheral nerves. Mult Scler. 1997;3:105–12.

Beato M, Chalepakis G, Schauer M, Slater EP. DNA regulatory elements for steroid hormones. J Steroid Biochem. 1989;32:737–47.

Benoit G, Malewicz M, Perlmann T. Digging deep into the pockets of orphan nuclear receptors: insights from structural studies. Trends Cell Biol. 2004;14:369–76.

Berger S, Bleich M, Schmid W, Cole TJ, Peters J, Watanabe H, Kriz W, Warth R, Greger R, Schutz G. Mineralocorticoid receptor knockout mice: pathophysiology of Na+ metabolism. Proc Natl Acad Sci U S A. 1998;95:9424–9.

Boonyaratanakornkit V. Scaffolding proteins mediating membrane-initiated extra-nuclear actions of estrogen receptor. Steroids. 2011;76:877–84.

Böttner M, Thelen P, Jarry H. Estrogen receptor beta: tissue distribution and the still largely enigmatic physiological function. J Steroid Biochem Mol Biol. 2014;139:245–51.

Bourguet W, Ruff M, Chambon P, Gronemeyer H, Moras D. Crystal structure of the ligand-binding domain of the human nuclear receptor RXRα. Nature. 1995;375:377–82.

Bourguet W, Germain P, Gronemeyer H. Nuclear receptor ligand-binding domains: three-dimensional structures, molecular interactions and pharmacological implications. Trends Pharmacol Sci. 2000;21:381–8.

Braun AM, Thomas P. Biochemical characterization of a membrane androgen receptor in the ovary of the atlantic croaker (Micropogonias undulatus). Biol Reprod. 2004;71:146–55.

Brzozowski AM, Pike AC, Dauter Z, Hubbard RE, Bonn T, Engstrom O, Ohma L, Greene GL, Gustafsson JA, Carlquist M. Molecular basis of agonism and antagonism in the oestrogen receptor. Nature. 1997;389:753–8.

Bulayeva NN, Watson CS. Xenoestrogen-induced ERK-1 and ERK-2 activation via multiple membrane-initiated signaling pathways. Environ Health Perspect. 2004;112:1481–7.

Bulayeva NN, Gametchu B, Watson CS. Quantitative measurement of estrogen-induced ERK 1 and 2 activation via multiple membrane-initiated signaling pathways. Steroids. 2004a;69:181–92.

Bulayeva NN, Wozniak A, Lash LL, Watson CS. Mechanisms of membrane estrogen receptor-{alpha}-mediated rapid stimulation of Ca2+ levels and prolactin release in a pituitary cell line. Am J Physiol Endocrinol Metab. 2004b. doi:10.1152/ajpendo.00349.2004.

Burns KA, Li Y, Arao Y, Petrovich RM, Korach KS. Selective mutations in estrogen receptor α D-domain alters nuclear translocation and non-estrogen response element gene regulatory mechanisms. J Biol Chem. 2011;286:12640–9.

Cammarata PR, Chu S, Moor A, Wang Z, Yang S-H, Simpkins JW. Subcellular distribution of native estrogen receptor [alpha] and [beta] subtypes in cultured human lens epithelial cells. Exp Eye Res. 2004;78:861–71.

Capobianco E. RNA-Seq data: a complexity journey. Comput Struct Biotechnol J. 2014;11:123–30.

Carroll JS, Brown M. Estrogen receptor target gene: an evolving concept. Mol Endocrinol. 2006;20:1707–14.

Carroll JS, Liu XS, Brodsky AS, Li W, Meyer CA, Szary AJ, Eeckhoute J, Shao W, Hestermann EV, Geistlinger TR, Fox EA, Silver PA, Brown M. Chromosome-wide mapping of estrogen receptor binding reveals long-range regulation requiring the forkhead protein FoxA1. Cell. 2005;122:33–43.

Carroll JS, Meyer CA, Song J, Li W, Geistlinger TR, Eeckhoute J, Brodsky AS, Keeton EK, Fertuck KC, Hall GF, Wang Q, Bekiranov S, Sementchenko V, Fox EA, Silver PA, Gingeras TR, Liu XS, Brown M. Genome-wide analysis of estrogen receptor binding sites. Nat Genet. 2006;38:1289–97.

Carruthers CW, Suh JH, Gustafsson J-A, Webb P. Phosphorylation of glucocorticoid receptor tau1c transactivation domain enhances binding to CREB binding protein (CBP) TAZ2. Biochem Biophys Res Commun. 2015;457:119–23.

Cattin AL, Le Beyec J, Barreau F, Saint-Just S, Houllier A, Gonzalez FJ, Robine S, Pincon-Raymond M, Cardot P, Lacasa M, Ribeiro A. Hepatocyte nuclear factor 4alpha, a key factor for homeostasis, cell architecture, and barrier function of the adult intestinal epithelium. Mol Cell Biol. 2009;29:6294–308.

Chai X, Zeng S, Xie W. Nuclear receptors PXR and CAR: implications for drug metabolism regulation, pharmacogenomics and beyond. Expert Opin Drug Metab Toxicol. 2013;9:253–66.

Chambliss KL, Wu Q, Oltmann S, Konaniah ES, Umetani M, Korach KS, Thomas GD, Mineo C, Yuhanna IS, Kim SH, Madak-Erdogan Z, Maggi A, Dineen SP, Roland CL, Hui DY, Brekken RA, Katzenellenbogen JA, Katzenellenbogen BS, Shaul PW. Non-nuclear estrogen receptor alpha signaling promotes cardiovascular protection but not uterine or breast cancer growth in mice. J Clin Invest. 2010;120:2319–30.

Chandran UR, Attardi B, Friedman R, Zheng ZW, Roberts JL, DeFranco DB. Glucocorticoid repression of the mouse gonadotropin-releasing hormone gene is mediated by promoter elements that are recognized by heteromeric complexes containing glucocorticoid receptor. J Biol Chem. 1996;271:20412–20.

Chang C, Lee SO, Wang R-S, Yeh S, Chang T-M. Androgen receptor (AR) physiological roles in male and female reproductive systems: lessons learned from AR-knockout mice lacking AR in selective cells. Biol Reprod. 2013;89(21):1–16.

Chappell PE, Lydon JP, Conneely OM, O'Malley BW, Levine JE. Endocrine defects in mice carrying a null mutation for the progesterone receptor gene. Endocrinology. 1997;138:4147–52.

Charn TH, Liu ET-B, Chang EC, Lee YK, Katzenellenbogen JA, Katzenellenbogen BS. Genome-wide dynamics of chromatin binding of estrogen receptors {alpha} and {beta}: mutual restriction and competitive site selection. Mol Endocrinol. 2010;24:47–59.

Cheng S-Y, Leonard JL, Davis PJ. Molecular aspects of thyroid hormone actions. Endocr Rev. 2010;31:139–70.

Cherian MT, Chai SC, Chen T. Small-molecule modulators of the constitutive androstane receptor. Expert Opin Drug Metab Toxicol. 2015;11:1099–114.

Cheskis BJ. Regulation of cell signalling cascades by steroid hormones. J Cell Biochem. 2004;93:20–7.

Cheung E, Acevedo ML, Cole PA, Kraus WL. Altered pharmacology and distinct coactivator usage for estrogen receptor-dependent transcription through activating protein-1. Proc Natl Acad Sci U S A. 2005;102:559–64.

Chiang JY. Bile acid regulation of gene expression: roles of nuclear hormone receptors. Endocr Rev. 2002;23:443–63.

Chinenov Y, Gupte R, Rogatsky I. Nuclear receptors in inflammation control: repression by GR and beyond. Mol Cell Endocrinol. 2013;380:55–64.

Cho E, Montgomery RB, Mostaghel EA. Minireview: SLCO and ABC transporters: a role for steroid transport in prostate cancer progression. Endocrinology. 2014;155:4124–32.

Chodankar R, Wu DY, Schiller BJ, Yamamoto KR, Stallcup MR. Hic-5 is a transcription coregulator that acts before and/or after glucocorticoid receptor genome occupancy in a gene-selective manner. Proc Natl Acad Sci U S A. 2014;111:4007–12.

Chodankar R, Wu DY, Gerke DS, Stallcup MR. Selective coregulator function and restriction of steroid receptor chromatin occupancy by Hic-5. Mol Endocrinol. 2015;29:716–29.

Christakos S, Dhawan P, Verstuyf A, Verlinden L, Carmeliet G. Vitamin D: metabolism, molecular mechanism of action, and pleiotropic effects. Physiol Rev. 2016;96:365–408.

Chu S, Nishi Y, Yanase T, Nawata H, Fuller PJ. Transrepression of estrogen receptor {beta} signaling by nuclear factor-{kappa}B in ovarian granulosa cells. Mol Endocrinol. 2004;18:1919–28.

Clemens JW, Robker RL, Kraus WL, Katzenellenbogen BS, Richards JS. Hormone induction of progesterone receptor (PR) messenger ribonucleic acid and activation of PR promoter regions in ovarian granulosa cells: evidence for a role of cyclic adenosine 3′,5′-monophosphate but not estradiol. Mol Endocrinol. 1998;12:1201–14.

Coelho MB, Attig J, Ule J, Smith CWJ. Matrin3: connecting gene expression with the nuclear matrix. Wiley Interdiscip Rev: RNA. 2016. doi:10.1002/wrna.1336,n/a-n/a.

Cole TJ, Blendy JA, Schmid W, Strahle U, Schutz G. Expression of the mouse glucocorticoid receptor and its role during development. J Steroid Biochem Mol Biol. 1993;47:49–53.

Cook DN, Kang HS, Jetten AM. Retinoic acid-related orphan receptors (RORs): regulatory functions in immunity, development, circadian rhythm, and metabolism. Nucl Recept Res. 2015;2:2314.

Cooney AJ, Lee CT, Lin SC, Tsai SY, Tsai MJ. Physiological function of the orphans GCNF and COUP-TF. Trends Endocrinol Metab. 2001;12:247–51.

Couse JF, Korach KS. Exploring the role of sex steroids through studies of receptor deficient mice. J Mol Med. 1998;75:497–511.

Couse JF, Korach KS. Estrogen receptor null mice: what have we learned and where will they lead us? Endocr Rev. 1999;20:358–417.

Couse JF, Curtis SW, Washburn TF, Lindzey J, Golding TS, Lubahn DB, Smithies O, Korach KS. Analysis of transcription and estrogen insensitivity in the female mouse after targeted disruption of the estrogen receptor gene. Mol Endocrinol. 1995;9:1441–54.

Couse JF, Curtis Hewitt S, Korach KS. Receptor null mice reveal contrasting roles for estrogen receptor alpha and beta in reproductive tissues. J Steroid Biochem Mol Biol. 2000;74:287–96.

Cruz-Topete D, Cidlowski JA. One hormone, two actions: anti- and pro-inflammatory effects of glucocorticoids. Neuroimmunomodulation. 2015;22:20–32.

Dallas PB, Cheney IW, Liao D-W, Bowrin V, Byam W, Pacchione S, Kobayashi R, Yaciuk P, Moran E. p300/CREB binding protein-related protein p270 is a component of mammalian SWI/SNF complexes. Mol Cell Biol. 1998;18:3596–603.

Daniel AR, Gaviglio AL, Knutson TP, Ostrander JH, D'Assoro AB, Ravindranathan P, Peng Y, Raj GV, Yee D, Lange CA. Progesterone receptor-B enhances estrogen responsiveness of breast cancer cells via scaffolding PELP1- and estrogen receptor-containing transcription complexes. Oncogene. 2015;34:506–15.

Danielian PS, White R, Lees JA, Parker MG. Identification of a conserved region required for hormone dependent transcriptional activation by steroid hormone receptors. EMBO J. 1992;11:1025–33.

Danzo BJ, Joseph DR. Structure-function relationships of rat androgen – binding protein/human sex-hormone binding globulin: the effect of mutagenesis on steroid- binding parameters. Endocrinology. 1994;135:157–67.

Dasgupta S, Lonard DM, O'Malley BW. Nuclear receptor coactivators: master regulators of human health and disease. Annu Rev Med. 2014;65:279–92.

Davies MPA, O'Neill PA, Innes H, Sibson DR, Prime W, Holcombe C, Foster CS. Correlation of mRNA for oestrogen receptor beta splice variants ER{beta}1, ER{beta}2/ER{beta}cx and ER {beta}5 with outcome in endocrine-treated breast cancer. J Mol Endocrinol. 2004;33:773–82.

De Amicis F, Zupo S, Panno ML, Malivindi R, Giordano F, Barone I, Mauro L, Fuqua SAW, Ando S. Progesterone receptor B recruits a repressor complex to a half-pre site of the estrogen receptor {alpha} gene promoter. Mol Endocrinol. 2009;23:454–65.

De Martino MU, Bhattachryya N, Alesci S, Ichijo T, Chrousos GP, Kino T. The glucocorticoid receptor and the orphan nuclear receptor chicken ovalbumin upstream promoter-transcription factor II interact with and mutually affect each other's transcriptional activities: implications for intermediary metabolism. Mol Endocrinol. 2004;18:820–33.

Deblois G, Giguere V. Functional and physiological genomics of estrogen-related receptors (ERRs) in health and disease. Biochim Biophys Acta. 2011;1812:1032–40.

Deblois G, St-Pierre J, Giguere V. The PGC-1/ERR signaling axis in cancer. Oncogene. 2013;32:3483–90.

DeFranco DB. Subnuclear trafficking of steroid receptors. Biochem Soc Trans. 1997;25:592–7.

DeLuca HF, Zierold C. Mechanisms and functions of vitamin D. Nutr Rev. 1998;56:S4–10. discussion S 54–75.

Demonacos CV, Karayanni N, Hatzoglou E, Tsiriyiotis C, Spandidos DA, Sekeris CE. Mitochondrial genes as sites of primary action of steroid hormones. Steroids. 1996;61:226–32.

Dey P, Barros RPA, Warner M, Ström A, Gustafsson J-Å. Insight into the mechanisms of action of estrogen receptor β in the breast, prostate, colon, and CNS. J Mol Endocrinol. 2013;51:T61–74.

Diamond MI, Miner JN, Yoshinaga SK, Yamamoto KR. Transcription factor interactions: selectors of positive or negative regulation from a single DNA element. Science. 1990;249:1266–72.

Dickmeis T, Weger BD, Weger M. The circadian clock and glucocorticoids – interactions across many time scales. Mol Cell Endocrinol. 2013;380:2–15.

Ding XF, Anderson CM, Ma H, Hong H, Uht RM, Kushner PJ, Stallcup MR. Nuclear receptor-binding sites of coactivators glucocorticoid receptor interacting protein 1 (GRIP1) and steroid receptor coactivator 1 (SRC-1): multiple motifs with different binding specificities. Mol Endocrinol. 1998;12:302–13.

Dittmar KD, Demady DR, Stancato LF, Krishna P, Pratt WB. Folding of the glucocorticoid receptor by the heat shock protein (hsp) 90-based chaperone machinery: the role of p23 is to stabilize receptor.hsp90 heterocomplexes formed by hsp90.p60.hsp70. J Biol Chem. 1997;272:21213–20.

Djebali S, Davis CA, Merkel A, Dobin A, Lassmann T, Mortazavi A, Tanzer A, Lagarde J, Lin W, Schlesinger F, Xue C, Marinov GK, Khatun J, Williams BA, Zaleski C, Rozowsky J, Roder M, Kokocinski F, Abdelhamid RF, Alioto T, Antoshechkin I, Baer MT, Bar NS, Batut P, Bell K, Bell I, Chakrabortty S, Chen X, Chrast J, Curado J, Derrien T, Drenkow J, Dumais E, Dumais J, Duttagupta R, Falconnet E, Fastuca M, Fejes-Toth K, Ferreira P, Foissac S, Fullwood MJ, Gao H, Gonzalez D, Gordon A, Gunawardena H, Howald C, Jha S, Johnson R, Kapranov P, King B, Kingswood C, Luo OJ, Park E, Persaud K, Preall JB, Ribeca P, Risk B, Robyr D, Sammeth M, Schaffer L, See L-H, Shahab A, Skancke J, Suzuki AM, Takahashi H, Tilgner H, Trout D, Walters N, Wang H, Wrobel J, Yu Y, Ruan X, Hayashizaki Y, Harrow J, Gerstein M, Hubbard T, Reymond A, Antonarakis SE, Hannon G, Giddings MC, Ruan Y, Wold B, Carninci P, Guigo R, Gingeras TR. Landscape of transcription in human cells. Nature. 2012;489:101–8.

Dooley R, Harvey BJ, Thomas W. Non-genomic actions of aldosterone: from receptors and signals to membrane targets. Mol Cell Endocrinol. 2012;350:223–34.

Drewes T, Senkel S, Holewa B, Ryffel GU. Human hepatocyte nuclear factor 4 isoforms are encoded by distinct and differentially expressed genes. Mol Cell Biol. 1996;16:925–31.

Driscoll MD, Klinge CM, Hilf R, Bambara RA. Footprint analysis of estrogen receptor binding to adjacent estrogen response elements. J Steroid Biochem Mol Biol. 1996;58:45–61.

Driscoll MD, Sathya G, Muyan M, Klinge CM, Hilf R, Bambara RA. Sequence requirements for estrogen receptor binding to estrogen response elements. J Biol Chem. 1998;273:29321–30.

Drouin J, Sun YL, Chamberland M, Gauthier Y, De Lean A, Nemer M, Schmidt TJ. Novel glucocorticoid receptor complex with DNA element of the hormone- repressed POMC gene. EMBO J. 1993;12:145–56.

Duan R, Porter W, Safe S. Estrogen-induced c-fos protooncogene expression in MCF-7 human breast cancer cells: role of estrogen receptor Sp1 complex formation. Endocrinology. 1998;139:1981–90.

Durand B, Saunders M, Gaudon C, Roy B, Losson R, Chambon P. Activation function 2 (AF-2) of retinoic acid receptor and 9-cis retinoic acid receptor: presence of a conserved autonomous constitutive activating domain and influence of the nature of the response element on AF-2 activity. EMBO J. 1994;13:5370–82.

Eeckhoute J, Carroll JS, Geistlinger TR, Torres-Arzayus MI, Brown M. A cell-type-specific transcriptional network required for estrogen regulation of cyclin D1 and cell cycle progression in breast cancer. Genes Dev. 2006;20:2513–26.

Eeckhoute J, Keeton EK, Lupien M, Krum SA, Carroll JS, Brown M. Positive cross-regulatory loop ties GATA-3 to estrogen receptor {alpha} expression in breast cancer. Cancer Res. 2007;67:6477–83.

Elbi C, Walker DA, Romero G, Sullivan WP, Toft DO, Hager GL, DeFranco DB. Molecular chaperones function as steroid receptor nuclear mobility factors. Proc Natl Acad Sci U S A. 2004;101:2876–81.

Eng FCS, Barsalou A, Akutsu N, Mercier I, Zechel C, Made S, White JH. Different classes of coactivators recognize distinct but overlapping binding sites on the estrogen receptor ligand binding domain. J Biol Chem. 1998;273:28371–7.
Evans RM. The steroid and thyroid hormone receptor superfamily. Science. 1988;240:889–95.
Evans RM. The nuclear receptor superfamily: a rosetta stone for physiology. Mol Endocrinol. 2005;19:1429–38.
Evans RM, Mangelsdorf DJ. Nuclear receptors, RXR, and the Big Bang. Cell. 2014;157:255–66.
Fan W, Evans R. PPARs and ERRs: molecular mediators of mitochondrial metabolism. Curr Opin Cell Biol. 2015;33:49–54.
Feige JN, Auwerx J. Transcriptional coregulators in the control of energy homeostasis. Trends Cell Biol. 2007;17:292–301.
Feldman RD. Aldosterone and blood pressure regulation: recent milestones on the long and winding road from electrocortin to KCNJ5, GPER, and beyond. Hypertension. 2014;63:19–21.
Feldman RD, Gros R. Vascular effects of aldosterone: sorting out the receptors and the ligands. Clin Exp Pharmacol Physiol. 2013. doi:10.1111/1440-1681.12157,n/a-n/a.
Filardo EJ, Thomas P. Minireview: G protein-coupled estrogen receptor-1, GPER-1: its mechanism of action and role in female reproductive cancer, renal and vascular physiology. Endocrinology. 2012;153:2953–62.
Fischle W, Mootz HD, Schwarzer D. Synthetic histone code. Curr Opin Chem Biol. 2015;28:131–40.
Flototto T, Niederacher D, Hohmann D, Heimerzheim T, Dall P, Djahansouzi S, Bender HG, Hanstein B. Molecular mechanism of estrogen receptor (ER)[alpha]-specific, estradiol-dependent expression of the progesterone receptor (PR) B-isoform. J Steroid Biochem Mol Biol. 2004;88:131–42.
Freedman OC, Fletcher GG, Gandhi S, Mates M, Dent SF, Trudeau ME, Eisen A. Adjuvant endocrine therapy for early breast cancer: a systematic review of the evidence for the 2014 Cancer Care Ontario systemic therapy guideline. Curr Oncol (Toronto, Ont). 2015;22: S95–s113.
Fu M, Wang C, Zhang X, Pestell RG. Acetylation of nuclear receptors in cellular growth and apoptosis. Biochem Pharmacol. 2004;68:1199–208.
Fuller PJ. Novel interactions of the mineralocorticoid receptor. Mol Cell Endocrinol. 2015;408:33–7.
Funakoshi T, Yanai A, Shinoda K, Kawano MM, Mizukami Y. G protein-coupled receptor 30 is an estrogen receptor in the plasma membrane. Biochem Biophys Res Commun. 2006;346:904–10.
Galvani A, Thiriet C. Nucleosome dancing at the tempo of histone tail acetylation. Genes. 2015;6:607–21.
Gao T, McPhaul MJ. Functional activities of the A and B forms of the human androgen receptor in response to androgen receptor agonists and antagonists. Mol Endocrinol. 1998;12:654–63.
Gardner KE, Allis CD, Strahl BD. OPERating ON chromatin, a colorful language where context matters. J Mol Biol. 2011;409:36–46.
Gaudet HM, Cheng SB, Christensen EM, Filardo EJ. The G-protein-coupled estrogen receptor, GPER: the inside and inside-out story. Mol Cell Endocrinol. 2015;418:207–19.
Gehring U. Steroid hormone receptors and heat shock proteins. Vitam Horm. 1998;54:167–205.
Germain P, Staels B, Dacquet C, Spedding M, Laudet V. Overview of nomenclature of nuclear receptors. Pharmacol Rev. 2006;58:685–704.
Gertz J, Reddy TE, Varley KE, Garabedian MJ, Myers RM. Genistein and bisphenol A exposure cause estrogen receptor 1 to bind thousands of sites in a cell type-specific manner. Genome Res. 2012;22:2153–62.
Geserick C, Meyer H-A, Haendler B. The role of DNA response elements as allosteric modulators of steroid receptor function. Mol Cell Endocrinol. 2005;236:1–7.
Giguere V. Retinoic acid receptors and cellular retinoid binding proteins: complex interplay in retinoid signaling. Endocr Rev. 1994;15:61–79.

Giordano Attianese GM, Desvergne B. Integrative and systemic approaches for evaluating PPARbeta/delta (PPARD) function. Nucl Recept Signal. 2015;13, e001.

Girard BJ, Daniel AR, Lange CA, Ostrander JH. PELP1: a review of PELP1 interactions, signaling, and biology. Mol Cell Endocrinol. 2014;382:642–51.

Goodwin B, Jones SA, Price RR, Watson MA, McKee DD, Moore LB, Galardi C, Wilson JG, Lewis MC, Roth ME, Maloney PR, Willson TM, Kliewer SA. A regulatory cascade of the nuclear receptors FXR, SHP-1, and LRH-1 represses bile acid biosynthesis. Mol Cell. 2000;6:517–26.

Gorski J, Williams D, Giannopoulos G, Stancel G. The continuing evolution of an estrogen-receptor model. Adv Exp Med Biol. 1973;36:1–14.

Goswami D, Callaway C, Pascal BD, Kumar R, Edwards DP, Griffin PR. Influence of domain interactions on conformational mobility of the progesterone receptor detected by hydrogen/deuterium exchange mass spectrometry. Structure. 2014;22:961–73.

Gottlicher M, Heck S, Herrlich P. Transcriptional cross-talk, the second mode of steroid hormone receptor action. J Mol Med. 1998;76:480–9.

Graber R, Sumida C, Vallette G, Nunez EA. Rapid and long-term effects of 17 beta-estradiol on PIP2-phospholipase C-specific activity of MCF-7 cells. Cell Signal. 1993;5:181–6.

Granner DK, Wang JC, Yamamoto KR. Regulatory actions of glucocorticoid hormones: from organisms to mechanisms. Adv Exp Med Biol. 2015;872:3–31.

Green S, Chambon P. Oestradiol induction of a glucocorticoid-responsive gene by a chimaeric receptor. Nature. 1987;325:75–8.

Green SM, Mostaghel EA, Nelson PS. Androgen action and metabolism in prostate cancer. Mol Cell Endocrinol. 2012;360:3–13.

Greenblatt J. RNA polymerase II holoenzyme and transcriptional regulation. Curr Opin Cell Biol. 1997;9:310–9.

Greger JG, Guo Y, Henderson R, Ross JF, Cheskis BJ. Characterization of MNAR expression. Steroids. 2006;71:317–22.

Greschik H, Jean-Marie Wurtz PH, Köhler F, Moras D, Schüle R. Characterization of the DNA-binding and dimerization properties of the nuclear orphan receptor germ cell nuclear factor. Mol Cell Biol. 1999;19:690–703.

Guennoun R, Labombarda F, Gonzalez Deniselle MC, Liere P, De Nicola AF, Schumacher M. Progesterone and allopregnanolone in the central nervous system: response to injury and implication for neuroprotection. J Steroid Biochem Mol Biol. 2015;146:48–61.

Guiochon-Mantel A, Delabre K, Lescop P, Milgrom E. Intracellular traffic of steroid hormone receptors. J Steroid Biochem Mol Biol. 1996;56:1–6.

Hah N, Kraus WL. Hormone-regulated transcriptomes: lessons learned from estrogen signaling pathways in breast cancer cells. Mol Cell Endocrinol. 2014;382:652–64.

Hamilton KJ, Arao Y, Korach KS. Estrogen hormone physiology: reproductive findings from estrogen receptor mutant mice. Reprod Biol. 2014;14:3–8.

Hammes A, Andreassen TK, Spoelgen R, Raila J, Hubner N, Schulz H, Metzger J, Schweigert FJ, Luppa PB, Nykjaer A, Willnow TE. Role of endocytosis in cellular uptake of sex steroids. Cell. 2005;122:751–62.

Hammond GL, Bocchinfuso WP. Sex hormone-binding globulin/androgen-binding protein: steroid-binding and dimerization domains. J Steroid Biochem Mol Biol. 1995;53:543–52.

Hawk JD, Bookout AL, Poplawski SG, Bridi M, Rao AJ, Sulewski ME, Kroener BT, Manglesdorf DJ, Abel T. NR4A nuclear receptors support memory enhancement by histone deacetylase inhibitors. J Clin Invest. 2012;122:3593–602.

Hawkins MB, Thomas P. The unusual binding properties of the third distinct teleost estrogen receptor subtype ERbetaa are accompanied by highly conserved amino acid changes in the ligand binding domain. Endocrinology. 2004;145:2968–77.

Hawkinson JE, Kimbrough CL, Belelli D, Lambert JJ, Purdy RH, Lan NC. Correlation of neuroactive steroid modulation of [35S]t- butylbicyclophosphorothionate and [3H]

flunitrazepam binding and gamma aminobutyric acidA receptor function. Mol Pharmacol. 1994;46:977–85.
Heintzman ND, Hon GC, Hawkins RD, Kheradpour P, Stark A, Harp LF, Ye Z, Lee LK, Stuart RK, Ching CW, Ching KA, Antosiewicz-Bourget JE, Liu H, Zhang X, Green RD, Lobanenkov VV, Stewart R, Thomson JA, Crawford GE, Kellis M, Ren B. Histone modifications at human enhancers reflect global cell-type-specific gene expression. Nature. 2009;459:108–12.
Helsen C, Claessens F. Looking at nuclear receptors from a new angle. Mol Cell Endocrinol. 2014;382:97–106.
Herynk MH, Fuqua SAW. Estrogen receptor mutations in human disease. Endocr Rev. 2004;25:869–98.
Hewitt SC, Harrell JC, Korach KS. Lessons in estrogen biology from knockout and transgenic animals. Annu Rev Physiol. 2005;67:285–308.
Hirose T, O'Brien DA, Jetten AM. RTR: a new member of the nuclear receptor superfamily that is highly expressed in murine testis. Gene. 1995;152:247–51.
Hisamoto K, Bender JR. Vascular cell signaling by membrane estrogen receptors. Steroids. 2005;70:382–7.
Hollenberg SM, Evans RM. Multiple and cooperative trans-activation domains of the human glucocorticoid receptor. Cell. 1988;55:899–906.
Holmes KA, Hurtado A, Brown GD, Launchbury R, Ross-Innes CS, Hadfield J, Odom DT, Carroll JS. Transducin-like enhancer protein 1 mediates estrogen receptor binding and transcriptional activity in breast cancer cells. Proc Natl Acad Sci. 2012;109:2748–53.
Horwitz KB, McGuire WL. Nuclear mechanisms of estrogen action. Effects of estradiol and anti-estrogens on estrogen receptors and nuclear receptor processing. J Biol Chem. 1978;253:8185–91.
Hua G, Paulen L, Chambon P. GR SUMOylation and formation of an SUMO-SMRT/NCoR1-HDAC3 repressing complex is mandatory for GC-induced IR nGRE-mediated transrepression. Proc Natl Acad Sci. 2016;113:E626–34.
Huang EY, Zhang J, Miska EA, Guenther MG, Kouzarides T, Lazar MA. Nuclear receptor corepressors partner with class II histone deacetylases in a Sin3-independent repression pathway. Genes Dev. 2000;14:45–54.
Huang B, Warner M, Gustafsson J-Å. Estrogen receptors in breast carcinogenesis and endocrine therapy. Mol Cell Endocrinol. 2015;418:240–4. Part 3.
Hubert C, Gasc J-M, Berger S, Günther Schütz G, Corvol P. Effects of mineralocorticoid receptor gene disruption on the components of the renin-angiotensin system in 8-day-old mice. Mol Endocrinol. 1999;13:297–306.
Hübner MR, Eckersley-Maslin MA, Spector DL. Chromatin organization and transcriptional regulation. Curr Opin Genet Dev. 2013;23:89–95.
Husmann DA, Wilson CM, McPhaul MJ, Tilley WD, Wilson JD. Antipeptide antibodies to two distinct regions of the androgen receptor localize the receptor protein to the nuclei of target cells in the rat and human prostate. Endocrinology. 1990;126:2359–68.
Huss JM, Garbacz WG, Xie W. Constitutive activities of estrogen-related receptors: transcriptional regulation of metabolism by the ERR pathways in health and disease. Biochim Biophys Acta. 2015;1852:1912–27.
Hutchison KA, Dittmar KD, Stancato LF, Pratt WB. Ability of various members of the hsp70 family of chaperones to promote assembly of the glucocorticoid receptor into a functional hetero-complex with hsp90. J Steroid Biochem Mol Biol. 1996;58:251–8.
Improta-Brears T, Whorton AR, Codazzi F, York JD, Meyer T, McDonnell DP. Estrogen-induced activation of mitogen-activated protein kinase requires mobilization of intracellular calcium. Proc Natl Acad Sci U S A. 1999;96:4686–91.
Islam MM, Zhang C-L. TLX: a master regulator for neural stem cell maintenance and neurogenesis. Biochim Biophys Acta (BBA) – Gene Regul Mech. 2015;1849:210–6.
Iwafuchi-Doi M, Zaret KS. Pioneer transcription factors in cell reprogramming. Genes Dev. 2014;28:2679–92.

Jackson TA, Richer JK, Bain DL, Takimoto GS, Tung I, Horwitz KB. The partial agonist activity of antagonist-occupied steroid receptors is controlled by a novel hinge domain-binding coactivator L7/SPA and the corepressors N-CoR or SMRT. Mol Endocrinol. 1997;11:693–705.

Jacobsen BM, Horwitz KB. Progesterone receptors, their isoforms and progesterone regulated transcription. Mol Cell Endocrinol. 2012;357:18–29.

Jadhav U, Harris RM, Jameson JL. Hypogonadotropic hypogonadism in subjects with DAX1 mutations. Mol Cell Endocrinol. 2011;346:65–73.

Jaisser F, Farman N. Emerging roles of the mineralocorticoid receptor in pathology: toward new paradigms in clinical pharmacology. Pharmacol Rev. 2016;68:49–75.

Jantzen HM, Strahle U, Gloss B, Stewart F, Schmid W, Boshart M, Miksicek R, Schutz G. Cooperativity of glucocorticoid response elements located far upstream of the tyrosine aminotransferase gene. Cell. 1987;49:29–38.

Jensen EV, DeSombre ER. Estrogen-receptor interaction. Science. 1973;182:126–34.

Jiang C, Xie C, Li F, Zhang L, Nichols RG, Krausz KW, Cai J, Qi Y, Fang ZZ, Takahashi S, Tanaka N, Desai D, Amin SG, Albert I, Patterson AD, Gonzalez FJ. Intestinal farnesoid X receptor signaling promotes nonalcoholic fatty liver disease. J Clin Invest. 2014. doi:10.1172/jci76738.

Josefsberg Ben-Yehoshua L, Lewellyn AL, Thomas P, Maller JL. The role of xenopus membrane progesterone receptor {beta} in mediating the effect of progesterone on oocyte maturation. Mol Endocrinol. 2007;21:664–73.

Joseph DR. Structure, function, and regulation of androgen-binding protein/sex hormone-binding globulin. Vitam Horm. 1994;49:197–280.

Kadiyala V, Sasse SK, Altonsy MO, Berman R, Chu HW, Phang TL, Gerber AN. Cistrome-based cooperation between airway epithelial glucocorticoid receptor and nf-kappab orchestrates anti-inflammatory effects. J Biol Chem. 2016a. doi:10.1074/jbc.M116.721217.

Kadiyala V, Sasse SK, Altonsy MO, Phang TL, Gerber AN. Cistrome analysis of glucocorticoid receptor activity in bronchial epithelial cells defines novel mechanisms of steroid efficacy. Ann Am Thorac Soc. 2016b;13 Suppl 1:S103.

Kastner P, Krust A, Turcotte B, Stropp U, Tora L, Gronemeyer H, Chambon P. Two distinct estrogen-regulated promoters generate transcripts encoding the two functionally different human progesterone receptor forms A and B. EMBO J. 1990;9:1603–14.

Khan SH, Awasthi S, Guo C, Goswami D, Ling J, Griffin PR, Simons Jr SS, Kumar R. Binding of the N-terminal region of coactivator TIF2 to the intrinsically disordered AF1 domain of the glucocorticoid receptor is accompanied by conformational reorganizations. J Biol Chem. 2012;287:44546–60.

Kim KH, Bender JR. Rapid, estrogen receptor-mediated signaling: why is the endothelium so special? Sci STKE. 2005;2005:pe28.

Kim KH, Young BD, Bender JR. Endothelial estrogen receptor isoforms and cardiovascular disease. Mol Cell Endocrinol. 2014;389:65–70.

King WJ, Greene GL. Monoclonal antibodies localize oestrogen receptor in the nuclei of target cells. Nature. 1984;307:745–7.

Kininis M, Chen BS, Diehl AG, Isaacs GD, Zhang T, Siepel AC, Clark AG, Kraus WL. Genomic analyses of transcription factor binding, histone acetylation, and gene expression reveal mechanistically distinct classes of estrogen-regulated promoters. Mol Cell Biol. 2007;27:5090–104.

Kinyamu HK, Fryer CJ, Horwitz KB, Archer TK. The mouse mammary tumor virus promoter adopts distinct chromatin structures in human breast cancer cells with and without glucocorticoid receptor. J Biol Chem. 2000;275:20061–8.

Klein-Hitpass L, Ryffel GU, Heitlinger E, Cato AC. A 13 bp palindrome is a functional estrogen responsive element and interacts specifically with estrogen receptor. Nucleic Acids Res. 1988;16:647–63.

Klinge CM. Estrogen receptor interaction with estrogen response elements. Nucleic Acids Res. 2001;29:2905–19.

Klinge CM, Bambara RA, Hilf R. Antiestrogen-liganded estrogen receptor interaction with estrogen responsive element DNA *in vitro*. J Steroid Biochem Mol Biol. 1992a;43:249–62.

Klinge CM, Peale Jr FV, Hilf R, Bambara RA, Zain S. Cooperative estrogen receptor interaction with consensus or variant estrogen responsive elements in vitro. Cancer Res. 1992b;52:1073–81.

Klinge CM, Jernigan SC, Mattingly KA, Risinger KE, Zhang J. Estrogen response element-dependent regulation of transcriptional activation of estrogen receptors alpha and beta by coactivators and corepressors. J Mol Endocrinol. 2004;33:387–410.

Klock G, Strahle U, Schutz G. Oestrogen and glucocorticoid responsive elements are closely related but distinct. Nature. 1987;329:734–6.

Klug A, Schwabe JWR. Zinc fingers. FASEB J. 1995;9:597–604.

Knutson TP, Lange CA. Tracking progesterone receptor-mediated actions in breast cancer. Pharmacol Ther. 2014;142:114–25.

Kobayashi K, Hashimoto M, Honkakoski P, Negishi M. Regulation of gene expression by CAR: an update. Arch Toxicol. 2015;89:1045–55.

Kojetin DJ, Burris TP. REV-ERB and ROR nuclear receptors as drug targets. Nat Rev Drug Discov. 2014;13:197–216.

Korach KS, Emmen JMA, Walker VR, Hewitt SC, Yates M, Hall JM, Swope DL, Harrell JC, Couse JF. Update on animal models developed for analyses of estrogen receptor biological activity. J Steroid Biochem Mol Biol. 2003;86:387–91.

Koukouritaki SB, Margioris AN, Gravanis A, Hartig R, Stournaras C. Dexamethasone induces rapid actin assembly in human endometrial cells without affecting its synthesis. J Cell Biochem. 1997;65:492–500.

Kowalik MK, Rekawiecki R, Kotwica J. The putative roles of nuclear and membrane-bound progesterone receptors in the female reproductive tract. Reprod Biol. 2013;13:279–89.

Krishnan V, Wang X, Safe S. Estrogen receptor-SP1 complexes mediate estrogen-induced cathepsin D gene expression in MCF-7 human breast cancer cells. J Biol Chem. 1994;269:15912–7.

Kuiper GG, Enmark E, Pelto-Huikko M, Nilsson S, Gustafsson J-A. Cloning of a novel estrogen receptor expressed in rat prostate and ovary. Proc Natl Acad Sci U S A. 1996;93:5925–30.

Kuiper GG, Carlsson B, Grandien J, Enmark E, Haggblad J, Nilsson S, Gustafsson J-A. Comparison of the ligand binding specificity and transcript tissue distribution of estrogen receptors α and β. Endocrinology. 1997;138:863–70.

Kurakula K, Koenis DS, van Tiel CM, de Vries CJM. NR4A nuclear receptors are orphans but not lonesome. Biochim Biophys Acta (BBA) – Mol Cell Res. 2014;1843:2543–55.

Kuznetsova T, Wang SY, Rao NA, Mandoli A, Martens JH, Rother N, Aartse A, Groh L, Janssen-Megens EM, Li G, Ruan Y, Logie C, Stunnenberg HG. Glucocorticoid receptor and nuclear factor kappa-b affect three-dimensional chromatin organization. Genome Biol. 2015;16:264.

Kwon Y-S, Garcia-Bassets I, Hutt KR, Cheng CS, Jin M, Liu D, Benner C, Wang D, Ye Z, Bibikova M, Fan J-B, Duan L, Glass CK, Rosenfeld MG, Fu X-D. Sensitive ChIP-DSL technology reveals an extensive estrogen receptor {alpha}-binding program on human gene promoters. Proc Natl Acad Sci U S A. 2007;104:4852–7.

Lam MTY, Li W, Rosenfeld MG, Glass CK. Enhancer RNAs and regulated transcriptional programs. Trends Biochem Sci. 2014;39:170–82.

Lange CA. Integration of progesterone receptor action with rapid signaling events in breast cancer models. J Steroid Biochem Mol Biol. 2008;108:203–12.

Lannigan DA. Estrogen receptor phosphorylation. Steroids. 2003;68:1–9.

Laudet V. Evolution of the nuclear receptor superfamily: early diversification from an ancestral orphan receptor. J Mol Endocrinol. 1997;19:207–26.

Le Billan F, Khan JA, Lamribet K, Viengchareun S, Bouligand J, Fagart J, Lombès M. Cistrome of the aldosterone-activated mineralocorticoid receptor in human renal cells. FASEB J. 2015;29:3977–89.

Le Menuet D, Lombès M. The neuronal mineralocorticoid receptor: from cell survival to neurogenesis. Steroids. 2014;91:11–9.

Le Romancer M, Poulard C, Cohen P, Sentis S, Renoir JM, Corbo L. Cracking the estrogen receptor's posttranslational code in breast tumors. Endocr Rev. 2011;32:597–622.

Le TN, Nestler JE, Strauss Iii JF, Wickham Iii EP. Sex hormone-binding globulin and type 2 diabetes mellitus. Trends Endocrinol Metab. 2012;23:32–40.

Lee WS, Kim J. Peroxisome proliferator-activated receptors and the heart: lessons from the past and future directions. PPAR Res. 2015;2015:271983.

Lee S-O, Jin U-H, Kang JH, Kim SB, Guthrie AS, Sreevalsan S, Lee J-S, Safe S. The orphan nuclear receptor NR4A1 (Nur77) regulates oxidative and endoplasmic reticulum stress in pancreatic cancer cells. Mol Cancer Res. 2014;12:527–38.

Lefebvre P, Benomar Y, Staels B. Retinoid X receptors: common heterodimerization partners with distinct functions. Trends Endocrinol Metab. 2010;21:676–83.

Leid M, Kastner P, Lyons R, Nakshatri H, Saunders M, Zacharewski T, Chen JY, Staub A, Garnier JM, Mader S, et al. Purification, cloning, and RXR identity of the HeLa cell factor with which RAR or TR heterodimerizes to bind target sequences efficiently. Cell. 1992;68:377–95.

Levin ER. Extranuclear steroid receptors are essential for steroid hormone actions. Annu Rev Med. 2015;66:271–80.

Li L, Haynes MP, Bender JR. Plasma membrane localization and function of the estrogen receptor alpha variant (ER46) in human endothelial cells. Proc Natl Acad Sci U S A. 2003;100:4807–12.

Li W, Notani D, Ma Q, Tanasa B, Nunez E, Chen AY, Merkurjev D, Zhang J, Ohgi K, Song X, Oh S, Kim HS, Glass CK, Rosenfeld MG. Functional roles of enhancer RNAs for oestrogen-dependent transcriptional activation. Nature. 2013;498:516–20.

Lin CY, Vega VB, Thomsen JS, Zhang T, Kong SL, Xie M, Chiu KP, Lipovich L, Barnett DH, Stossi F, Yeo A, George J, Kuznetsov VA, Lee YK, Charn TH, Palanisamy N, Miller LD, Cheung E, Katzenellenbogen BS, Ruan Y, Bourque G, Wei CL, Liu ET. Whole-genome cartography of estrogen receptor alpha binding sites. PLoS Genet. 2007;3, e87.

Lin F-J, Qin J, Tang K, Tsai SY, Tsai M-J. Coup d'Etat: an orphan takes control. Endocr Rev. 2011. doi:10.1210/er.2010-0021,er.2010-0021.

Litchfield LM, Riggs KA, Hockenberry AM, Oliver LD, Barnhart KG, Cai J, Pierce Jr WM, Ivanova MM, Bates PJ, Appana SN, Datta S, Kulesza P, McBryan J, Young LS, Klinge CM. Identification and characterization of nucleolin as a COUP-TFII coactivator of retinoic acid receptor β transcription in breast cancer cells. PLoS One. 2012;7, e38278.

Liu Y, Gao H, Marstrand TT, Strom A, Valen E, Sandelin A, Gustafsson J-A, Dahlman-Wright K. The genome landscape of ER{alpha}- and ER{beta}-binding DNA regions. Proc Natl Acad Sci. 2008. doi:10.1073/pnas.0712085105,0712085105.

Lu NZ, Cidlowski JA. The origin and functions of multiple human glucocorticoid receptor isoforms. Ann N Y Acad Sci. 2004;1024:102–23.

Lubahn DB, Moyer JS, Golding TS, Couse JF, Korach KS, Smithies O. Alteration of reproductive function but not prenatal sexual development after insertional disruption of the mouse estrogen receptor gene. Proc Natl Acad Sci U S A. 1993;90:11162–6.

Lupien M, Eeckhoute J, Meyer CA, Wang Q, Zhang Y, Li W, Carroll JS, Liu XS, Brown M. FoxA1 translates epigenetic signatures into enhancer-driven lineage-specific transcription. Cell. 2008;132:958–70.

Lydon JP, Edwards DP. Finally! A model for progesterone receptor action in normal human breast. Endocrinology. 2009;150:2988–90.

Lydon JP, DeMayo FJ, Funk CR, Mani SK, Hughes AR, Montgomery CAJ, Shyamala G, Conneely OM, O'Malley BW. Mice lacking progesterone receptor exhibit pleiotropic reproductive abnormalities. Genes Dev. 1995;9:2266–78.

Ma X, Chen J, Tian Y. Pregnane X receptor as the "sensor and effector" in regulating epigenome. J Cell Physiol. 2015;230:752–7.

Magnani L, Lupien M. Chromatin and epigenetic determinants of estrogen receptor alpha (ESR1) signaling. Mol Cell Endocrinol. 2014;382:633–41.

Maller JL. Signal transduction. Fishing at the cell surface. Science. 2003;300:594–5.

Mangelsdorf DJ, Evans RM. The RXR heterodimers and orphan receptors. Cell. 1995;83:841–50.

Mangelsdorf DJ, Ong ES, Dyck JA, Evans RM. Nuclear receptor that identifies a novel retinoic acid response pathway. Nature. 1990;345:224–9.

Mangelsdorf DJ, Thummel C, Beato M, Herrlich P, Schutz G, Umesono K, Blumberg B, Kastner P, Mark M, Chambon P, Evans RM. The nuclear receptor superfamily: the second decade. Cell. 1995;83:835–9.

Maroder M, Farina AR, Vacca A, Felli MP, Meco D, Screpanti I, Frati L, Gulino A. Cell-specific bifunctional role of Jun oncogene family members on glucocorticoid receptor-dependent transcription. Mol Endocrinol. 1993;7:570–84.

Marrone AK, Beland FA, Pogribny IP. Noncoding RNA response to xenobiotic exposure: an indicator of toxicity and carcinogenicity. Expert Opin Drug Metab Toxicol. 2014: 1–14 doi: 10.1517/17425255.2014.954312

Mathisen GH, Fallgren ÅB, Strøm BO, Boldingh Debernard KA, Mohebi BU, Paulsen RE. Delayed translocation of NGFI–B/RXR in glutamate stimulated neurons allows late protection by 9-cis retinoic acid. Biochem Biophys Res Commun. 2011;414:90–5.

Matsuda K, Ochiai I, Nishi M, Kawata M. Colocalization and ligand-dependent discrete distribution of the estrogen receptor (ER)alpha and ERbeta. Mol Endocrinol. 2002;16:2215–30.

Mazur EC, Vasquez YM, Li X, Kommagani R, Jiang L, Chen R, Lanz RB, Kovanci E, Gibbons WE, DeMayo FJ. Progesterone receptor transcriptome and cistrome in decidualized human endometrial stromal cells. Endocrinology. 2015;156:2239–53.

McCabe ERB. DAX1: increasing complexity in the roles of this novel nuclear receptor. Mol Cell Endocrinol. 2007;265–266:179–82.

McFall T, Patki M, Rosati R, Ratnam M. Role of the short isoform of the progesterone receptor in breast cancer cell invasiveness at estrogen and progesterone levels in the pre- and post-menopausal ranges. Oncotarget. 2015;6:33146–64.

McGuire WL, Clark GM, Dressler LG, Owens MA. Role of steroid hormone receptors as prognostic factors in primary breast cancer. NCI Monogr. 1986;1986:19–23.

McIntyre WR, Samuels HH. Triamcinolone acetonide regulates glucocorticoid-receptor levels by decreasing the half-life of the activated nuclear-receptor form. J Biol Chem. 1985;260:418–27.

Meijsing SH. Mechanisms of glucocorticoid-regulated gene transcription. Adv Exp Med Biol. 2015;872:59–81.

Metivier R, Penot G, Flouriot G, Pakdel F. Synergism between ERalpha transactivation function 1 (AF-1) and AF-2 mediated by steroid receptor coactivator protein-1: requirement for the AF-1 alpha-helical core and for a direct interaction between the N- and C-terminal domains. Mol Endocrinol. 2001;15:1953–70.

Meyer ME, Gronemeyer H, Turcotte B, Bocquel MT, Tasset D, Chambon P. Steroid hormone receptors compete for factors that mediate their enhancer function. Cell. 1989;57:433–42.

Michalek RD, Gerriets VA, Nichols AG, Inoue M, Kazmin D, Chang C-Y, Dwyer MA, Nelson ER, Pollizzi KN, Ilkayeva O, Giguere V, Zuercher WJ, Powell JD, Shinohara ML, McDonnell DP, Rathmell JC. Estrogen-related receptor-α is a metabolic regulator of effector T-cell activation and differentiation. Proc Natl Acad Sci. 2011;108:18348–53.

Migliaccio A, Castoria G, Auricchio F. Analysis of androgen receptor rapid actions in cellular signaling pathways: receptor/Src association. Methods Mol Biol. 2011;776:361–70.

Mikkonen L, Pihlajamaa P, Sahu B, Zhang F-P, Jänne OA. Androgen receptor and androgen-dependent gene expression in lung. Mol Cell Endocrinol. 2010;317:14–24.

Mizutani T, Kawabe S, Ishikane S, Imamichi Y, Umezawa A, Miyamoto K. Identification of novel steroidogenic factor 1 (SF-1)-target genes and components of the SF-1 nuclear complex. Mol Cell Endocrinol. 2015;408:133–7.

Mohan HM, Aherne CM, Rogers AC, Baird AW, Winter DC, Murphy EP. Molecular pathways: the role of nr4a orphan nuclear receptors in cancer. Clin Cancer Res. 2012;18:3223–8.

Monroe DG, Secreto FJ, Subramaniam M, Getz BJ, Khosla S, Spelsberg TC. Estrogen receptor {alpha} and {beta} heterodimers exert unique effects on estrogen- and tamoxifen-dependent gene expression in human U2OS osteosarcoma cells. Mol Endocrinol. 2005;19:1555–68.

Moriarty K, Kim KH, Bender JR. Estrogen receptor-mediated rapid signaling. Endocrinology. 2006;147:5557–63.

Morrill GA, Kostellow AB, Gupta RK. Transmembrane helices in "classical" nuclear reproductive steroid receptors: a perspective. Nucl Recept Signal. 2015;13, e003.

Mosselman S, Polman J, Dijkrms R. ERb: identification and characterization of a novel human estrogen receptor. FEBS Lett. 1996;392:49–53.

Mullican SE, DiSpirito JR, Lazar MA. The orphan nuclear receptors at their 25-year reunion. J Mol Endocrinol. 2013;51:T115–40.

Musatov S, Chen W, Pfaff DW, Mobbs CV, Yang X-J, Clegg DJ, Kaplitt MG, Ogawa S. Silencing of estrogen receptor {alpha} in the ventromedial nucleus of hypothalamus leads to metabolic syndrome. Proc Natl Acad Sci U S A. 2007;104:2501–6.

Muscatelli F, Strom TM, Walker AP, Zanaria E, Recan D, Meindl A, Bardoni B, Guioli S, Zehetner G, Rabl W, Schwara HP, Kaplan J-C, Camerino G, Meitinger T, Monaco AP. Mutations in the DAX-1 gene give rise to both X-linked adrenal hypoplasia congenita and hypogonadotropic hypogonadism. Nature. 1994;372:672–6.

Nakajima Y, Yamada M, Taguchi R, Shibusawa N, Ozawa A, Tomaru T, Hashimoto K, Saito T, Tsuchiya T, Okada S, Satoh T, Mori M. NR4A1 (Nur77) mediates thyrotropin-releasing hormone-induced stimulation of transcription of the thyrotropin beta gene: analysis of TRH knockout mice. PLoS One. 2012;7, e40437.

Nardulli AM, Greene GL, BW OM, Katzenellenbogen BS. Regulation of progesterone receptor messenger ribonucleic acid and protein levels in MCF-7 cells by estradiol: analysis of estrogen's effect on progesterone receptor synthesis and degradation. Endocrinology. 1988;122:935–44.

Nardulli AM, Greene GL, Shapiro DJ. Human estrogen receptor bound to an estrogen response element bends DNA. Mol Endocrinol. 1993;7:331–40.

O'Malley BW. The steroid receptor superfamily: more excitement predicted for the future. Mol Endocrinol. 1990;4:363–9.

O'Malley BW, Malovannaya A, Qin J. Minireview: nuclear receptor and coregulator proteomics – 2012 and beyond. Mol Endocrinol. 2012;26:1646–50.

Ogawa S, Inoue S, Watanabe T, Hiroi H, Orimao A. The complete primary structure of human estrogen receptor beta (hER beta) and its heterodimerization with ER alpha in vivo and in vitro. Biochem Biophys Res Commun. 1998;243:122–6.

Ohlsson C, Hellberg N, Parini P, Vidal O, Bohlooly M, Rudling M, Lindberg MK, Warner M, Angelin B, Gustafsson JA. Obesity and disturbed lipoprotein profile in estrogen receptor-alpha-deficient male mice. Biochem Biophys Res Commun. 2000;278:640–5.

Okret S, Dong Y, Bronnegard M, Gustafsson JA. Regulation of glucocorticoid receptor expression. Biochimie. 1991;73:51–9.

Okulicz WC, Evans RW, Leavitt WW. Progesterone regulation of the occupied form of nuclear estrogen receptor. Science. 1981;213:1503–5.

Okun JG, Conway S, Schmidt KV, Schumacher J, Wang X, de Guia R, Zota A, Klement J, Seibert O, Peters A, Maida A, Herzig S, Rose AJ. Molecular regulation of urea cycle function by the liver glucocorticoid receptor. Mol Metab. 2015;4:732–40.

Otte K, Kranz H, Kober I, Thompson P, Hoefer M, Haubold B, Remmel B, Voss H, Kaiser C, Albers M, Cheruvallath Z, Jackson D, Casari G, Koegl M, Paabo S, Mous J, Kremoser C, Deuschle U. Identification of farnesoid X receptor beta as a novel mammalian nuclear receptor sensing lanosterol. Mol Cell Biol. 2003;23:864–72.

Paakinaho V, Kaikkonen S, Makkonen H, Benes V, Palvimo JJ. SUMOylation regulates the chromatin occupancy and anti-proliferative gene programs of glucocorticoid receptor. Nucleic Acids Res. 2014;42:1575–92.

Paech K, Webb P, Kuiper GG, Nilsson S, Gustafsson J, Kushner PJ, Scanlan TS. Differential ligand activation of estrogen receptors ERalpha and ERbeta at AP1 sites. Science. 1997;277:1508–10.

Palstra RJ, Grosveld F. Transcription factor binding at enhancers: shaping a genomic regulatory landscape in flux. Front Genet. 2012;3:195.

Pappas TC, Gametchu B, Watson CS. Membrane estrogen receptors identified by multiple antibody labeling and impeded-ligand binding. FASEB J. 1995;9:404–10.

Parks DJ, Blanchard SG, Bledsoe RK, Chandra G, Consler TG, Kliewer SA, Stimmel JB, Willson TM, Zavacki AM, Moore DD, Lehmann JM. Bile acids: natural ligands for an orphan nuclear receptor [see comments]. Science. 1999;284:1365–8.

Patel SR, Skafar DF. Modulation of nuclear receptor activity by the F domain. Mol Cell Endocrinol. 2015. doi:10.1016/j.mce.2015.07.009.

Pawlak M, Lefebvre P, Staels B. Molecular mechanism of PPARalpha action and its impact on lipid metabolism, inflammation and fibrosis in non-alcoholic fatty liver disease. J Hepatol. 2015;62:720–33.

Pedram A, Razandi M, Levin ER. Nature of functional estrogen receptors at the plasma membrane. Mol Endocrinol. 2006;20:1996–2009.

Pedram A, Razandi M, Sainson RCA, Kim JK, Hughes CC, Levin ER. A conserved mechanism for steroid receptor translocation to the plasma membrane. J Biol Chem. 2007;282:22278–88.

Peluso JJ, Pru JK. Non-canonical progesterone signaling in granulosa cell function. Reproduction. 2014;147:R169–78.

Peluso JJ, DeCerbo J, Lodde V. Evidence for a genomic mechanism of action for progesterone receptor membrane component-1. Steroids. 2012;77:1007–12.

Perrot-Applanat M, Groyer-Picard MT, Logeat F, Milgrom E. Ultrastructural localization of the progesterone receptor by an immunogold method: effect of hormone administration. J Cell Biol. 1986;102:1191–9.

Petz LN, Nardulli AM, Kim J, Horwitz KB, Freedman LP, Shapiro DJ. DNA bending is induced by binding of the glucocorticoid receptor DNA binding domain and progesterone receptors to their response element. J Steroid Biochem Mol Biol. 1997;60:31–41.

Picard D, Kumar V, Chambon P, Yamamoto KR. Signal transduction by steroid hormones: nuclear localization is differentially regulated in estrogen and glucocorticoid receptors. Cell Regul. 1990;1:291–9.

Pietras RJ, Marquez-Garban DC. Membrane-associated estrogen receptor signaling pathways in human cancers. Clin Cancer Res. 2007;13:4672–6.

Porter W, Saville B, Hoivik D, Safe S. Functional synergy between the transcription factor Sp1 and the estrogen receptor. Mol Endocrinol. 1997;11:1569–80.

Porto CS, Lazari MF, Abreu LC, Bardin CW, Gunsalus GL. Receptors for androgen-binding proteins: internalization and intracellular signalling. J Steroid Biochem Mol Biol. 1995;53:561–5.

Powell E, Xu W. Intermolecular interactions identify ligand-selective activity of estrogen receptor alpha/beta dimers. Proc Natl Acad Sci. 2008;105:19012–7.

Pratt WB, Toft DO. Steroid receptor interactions with heat shock protein and immunophilin chaperones. Endocr Rev. 1997;18:306–60.

Prendergast P, Pan Z, Edwards DP. Progesterone receptor-induced bending of its target DNA: distinct effects of the A and B receptor forms. Mol Endocrinol. 1996;10:393–407.

Prossnitz ER, Barton M. Estrogen biology: new insights into GPER function and clinical opportunities. Mol Cell Endocrinol. 2014;389:71–83.

Querol Cano L, Lavery DN, Bevan CL. Mini-review: foldosome regulation of androgen receptor action in prostate cancer. Mol Cell Endocrinol. 2013;369:52–62.

Rajbhandari P, Finn G, Solodin NM, Singarapu KK, Sahu SC, Markley JL, Kadunc KJ, Ellison-Zelski SJ, Kariagina A, Haslam SZ, Lu KP, Alarid ET. Regulation of estrogen receptor α N-terminus conformation and function by peptidyl prolyl isomerase Pin1. Mol Cell Biol. 2012;32:445–57.

Rana K, Davey RA, Zajac JD. Human androgen deficiency: insights gained from androgen receptor knockout mouse models. Asian J Androl. 2014;16:169–77.

Ratman D, Vanden Berghe W, Dejager L, Libert C, Tavernier J, Beck IM, De Bosscher K. How glucocorticoid receptors modulate the activity of other transcription factors: a scope beyond tethering. Mol Cell Endocrinol. 2013;380:41–54.

Razandi M, Pedram A, Greene GL, Levin ER. Cell membrane and nuclear estrogen receptors (ERs) originate from a single transcript: studies of ERα and ERβ expressed in Chinese hamster ovary cells. Mol Endocrinol. 1999;13:307–19.

Razandi M, Pedram A, Park ST, Levin ER. Proximal events in signaling by plasma membrane estrogen receptors. J Biol Chem. 2003;278:2701–12.
Rechoum Y, Rovito D, Iacopetta D, Barone I, Ando S, Weigel NL, O'Malley BW, Brown PH, Fuqua SA. AR collaborates with ERalpha in aromatase inhibitor-resistant breast cancer. Breast Cancer Res Treat. 2014;147:473–85.
Renaud J-P, Rochel N, Ruff M, Vivat V, Chambon P, Gronemeyer H, Moras D. Crystal structure of the RAR-γ ligand-binding domain bound to all-trans retinoic acid. Nature. 1995;378:681–9.
Revelli A, Massobrio M, Tesarik J. Nongenomic actions of steroid hormones in reproductive tissues. Endocrine Rev. 1998;19:3–17.
Riggins RB, Mazzotta MM, Maniya OZ, Clarke R. Orphan nuclear receptors in breast cancer pathogenesis and therapeutic response. Endocr Relat Cancer. 2010;17:R213–31.
Rishi AK, Gerald TM, Shao ZM, Li XS, Baumann RG, Dawson MI, Fontana JA. Regulation of the human retinoic acid receptor alpha gene in the estrogen receptor negative human breast carcinoma cell lines SKBR-3 and MDA-MB-435. Cancer Res. 1996;56:5246–52.
Rodgers JT, Lerin C, Haas W, Gygi SP, Spiegelman BM, Puigserver P. Nutrient control of glucose homeostasis through a complex of PGC-1[alpha] and SIRT1. Nature. 2005;434:113–8.
Rogerson FM, Fuller PJ. Interdomain interactions in the mineralocorticoid receptor. Mol Cell Endocrinol. 2003;200:45–55.
Romanoski CE, Glass CK, Stunnenberg HG, Wilson L, Almouzni G. Epigenomics: roadmap for regulation. Nature. 2015;518:314–6.
Rose AJ, Herzig S. Metabolic control through glucocorticoid hormones: an update. Mol Cell Endocrinol. 2013;380:65–78.
Rosenfeld MG, Glass CK. Coregulator codes of transcriptional regulation by nuclear receptors. J Biol Chem. 2001;276:36865–8.
Rosenfeld MG, Lunyak VV, Glass CK. Sensors and signals: a coactivator/corepressor/epigenetic code for integrating signal-dependent programs of transcriptional response. Genes Dev. 2006;20:1405–28.
Rosner W, Hryb DJ, Khan MS, Nakhla AM, Romas NA. Sex hormone-binding globulin: anatomy and physiology of a new regulatory system. J Steroid Biochem Mol Biol. 1991;40:813–20.
Ruh MF, Chrivia JC, Cox LK, Ruh TS. The interaction of the estrogen receptor with mononucleosomes. Mol Cell Endocrinol. 2004;214:71–9.
Sabbah M, Ricousse SL, Redeuilh G, Baulieu EE. Estrogen receptor-induced bending of the Xenopus vitellogenin A2 gene hormone response element. Biochem Biophys Res Commun. 1992;185:944–52.
Safe S, Kim K. Non-classical genomic estrogen receptor (ER)/specificity protein and ER/activating protein-1 signaling pathways. J Mol Endocrinol. 2008;41:263–75.
Safe S, Jin UH, Hedrick E, Reeder A, Lee SO. Minireview: role of orphan nuclear receptors in cancer and potential as drug targets. Mol Endocrinol. 2014;28:157–72.
Safe S, Jin U-H, Morpurgo B, Abudayyeh A, Singh M, Tjalkens RB. Nuclear receptor 4A (NR4A) family – orphans no more. J Steroid Biochem Mol Biol. 2016;157:48–60.
Safer JD, Cohen RN, Hollenberg AN, Wondisford FE. Defective release of corepressor by hinge mutants of the thyroid hormone receptor found in patients with resistance to thyroid hormone. J Biol Chem. 1998;273:30175–82.
Sauer S. Ligands for the nuclear peroxisome proliferator-activated receptor gamma. Trends Pharmacol Sci. 2015;36:688–704.
Sauer F, Tjian R. Mechanisms of transcriptional activation: differences and similarities between yeast, Drosophila, and man. Curr Opin Genet Dev. 1997;7:176–81.
Scafoglio C, Ambrosino C, Cicatiello L, Altucci L, Ardovino M, Bontempo P, Medici N, Molinari AM, Nebbioso A, Facchiano A, Calogero RA, Elkon R, Menini N, Ponzone R, Biglia N, Sismondi P, De Bortoli M, Weisz A. Comparative gene expression profiling reveals partially overlapping but distinct genomic actions of different antiestrogens in human breast cancer cells. J Cell Biochem. 2006;98:1163–84.

Scarpin KM, Graham JD, Mote PA, Clarke CL. Progesterone action in human tissues: regulation by progesterone receptor (PR) isoform expression, nuclear positioning and coregulator expression. Nucl Recept Signal. 2009;7, e009.

Scherrer LC, Pratt WB. Association of the transformed glucocorticoid receptor with a cytoskeletal protein complex. J Steroid Biochem Mol Biol. 1992;41:719–21.

Schorderet DF, Escher P. NR2E3 mutations in enhanced S-cone sensitivity syndrome (ESCS), Goldmann-Favre syndrome (GFS), clumped pigmentary retinal degeneration (CPRD), and retinitis pigmentosa (RP). Hum Mutat. 2009;30:1475–85.

Schweizer MT, Yu EY. Persistent androgen receptor addiction in castration-resistant prostate cancer. J Hematol Oncol. 2015;8:128.

Seielstad DA, Carlson KE, Kushner PJ, Greene GL, Katzenellenbogen JA. Analysis of the structural core of the human estrogen receptor ligand binding domain by selective proteolysis/mass spectrometric analysis. Biochemistry (Mosc). 1995;34:12605–15.

Sentis S, Le Romancer M, Bianchin C, Rostan M-C, Corbo L. Sumoylation of the estrogen receptor {alpha} hinge region regulates its transcriptional activity. Mol Endocrinol. 2005;19:2671–84.

Seol W, Choi HS, Moore DD. An orphan nuclear hormone receptor that lacks a DNA binding domain and heterodimerizes with other receptors. Science. 1996;272:1336–9.

Seol W, Chung M, Moore DD. Novel receptor interaction and repression domains in the orphan receptor SHP. Mol Cell Biol. 1997;17:7126–31.

Shang Y, Hu X, DiRenzo J, Lazar MA, Brown M. Cofactor dynamics and sufficiency in estrogen receptor-regulated transcription. Cell. 2000;103:843–52.

Shao X, Wang M, Wei X, Deng S, Fu N, Peng Q, Jiang Y, Ye L, Lin Y. Peroxisome proliferator-activated receptor-gamma: master regulator of adipogenesis and obesity. Curr Stem Cell Res Ther. 2015. doi:10.1159/000438585.

Shibata H, Spencer TE, Onate SA, Jenster G, Tsai SY, Tsai MJ, O'Malley BW. Role of co-activators and co-repressors in the mechanism of steroid/thyroid receptor action. Recent Prog Horm Res. 1997;52:141–64.

Shulemovich K, Dimaculangan DD, Katz D, Lazar MA. DNA bending by thyroid hormone receptor: influence of half-site spacing and RXR. Nucleic Acids Res. 1995;23:811–8.

Simpkins JW, Yang S-H, Sarkar SN, Pearce V. Estrogen actions on mitochondria – physiological and pathological implications. Mol Cell Endocrinol. 2008;290:51–9.

Singh M, Su C, Ng S. Non-genomic mechanisms of progesterone action in the brain. Front Neurosci. 2013;7:159.

Sionov RV, Cohen O, Kfir S, Zilberman Y, Yefenof E. Role of mitochondrial glucocorticoid receptor in glucocorticoid-induced apoptosis. J Exp Med. 2006;203:189–201.

Smith CL, O'Malley BW. Coregulator function: a key to understanding tissue specificity of selective receptor modulators. Endocr Rev. 2004;25:45–71.

Solt LA, Burris TP. Action of RORs and their ligands in (patho)physiology. Trends Endocrinol Metab. 2012;23:619–27.

Song I-H, Buttgereit F. Non-genomic glucocorticoid effects to provide the basis for new drug developments. Mol Cell Endocrinol. 2006;246:142–6.

Song RX, Barnes CJ, Zhang Z, Bao Y, Kumar R, Santen RJ. The role of Shc and insulin-like growth factor 1 receptor in mediating the translocation of estrogen receptor {alpha} to the plasma membrane. Proc Natl Acad Sci U S A. 2004;101:2076–81.

Spencer TE, Jenster G, Burcin MM, Allis CD, Zhou J, Mizzen CA, McKenna NJ, Onate SA, Tsai S, Tsai MJ, O'Malley BW. Steroid receptor coactivator-1 is a histone acetyltransferase. Nature. 1997;389:194–8.

Stashi E, York B, O'Malley BW. Steroid receptor coactivators: servants and masters for control of systems metabolism. Trends Endocrinol Metab. 2014;25:337–47.

Stedronsky K, Telgmann R, Tillmann G, Walther N, Ivell R. The affinity and activity of the multiple hormone response element in the proximal promoter of the human oxytocin gene. J Neuroendocrinol. 2002;14:472–85.

Stein S, Schoonjans K. Molecular basis for the regulation of the nuclear receptor LRH-1. Curr Opin Cell Biol. 2015;33:26–34.

Stender JD, Kim K, Charn TH, Komm B, Chang KCN, Kraus WL, Benner C, Glass CK, Katzenellenbogen BS. Genome-wide analysis of estrogen receptor {alpha} DNA binding and tethering mechanisms identifies Runx1 as a Novel tethering factor in receptor-mediated transcriptional activation. Mol Cell Biol. 2010;30:3943–55.

Stenoien DL, Patel K, Mancini MG, Dutertre M, Smith CL, O'Malley BW, Mancini MA. FRAP reveals that mobility of oestrogen receptor-alpha is ligand- and proteasome-dependent. Nat Cell Biol. 2001;3:15–23.

Sternglanz R. Histone acetylation: a gateway to transcriptional activation. Trends Biochem Sci. 1996;21:357–8.

Stoica GE, Franke TF, Wellstein A, Czubayko F, List HJ, Reiter R, Morgan E, Martin MB, Stoica A. Estradiol rapidly activates Akt via the ErbB2 signaling pathway. Mol Endocrinol. 2003;17:818–30.

Stoner M, Wormke M, Saville B, Samudio I, Qin C, Abdelrahim M, Safe S. Estrogen regulation of vascular endothelial growth factor gene expression in ZR-75 breast cancer cells through interaction of estrogen receptor alpha and SP proteins. Oncogene. 2004;23:1052–63.

Stunnenberg HG. Mechanisms of transactivation by retinoic acid receptors. Bioessays. 1993;15:309–15.

Subramaniam N, Cairns W, Okret S. Studies on the mechanism of glucocorticoid-mediated repression from a negative glucocorticoid response element from the bovine prolactin gene. DNA Cell Biol. 1997;16:153–63.

Suntharalingham JP, Buonocore F, Duncan AJ, Achermann JC. DAX-1 (NR0B1) and steroidogenic factor-1 (SF-1, NR5A1) in human disease. Best Pract Res Clin Endocrinol Metab. 2015;29:607–19.

Surjit M, Ganti KP, Mukherji A, Ye T, Hua G, Metzger D, Li M, Chambon P. Widespread negative response elements mediate direct repression by agonist- liganded glucocorticoid receptor. Cell. 2011;145:224–41.

Swanson HI, Wada T, Xie W, Renga B, Zampella A, Distrutti E, Fiorucci S, Kong B, Thomas AM, Guo GL, Narayanan R, Yepuru M, Dalton JT, Chiang JY. Role of nuclear receptors in lipid dysfunction and obesity-related diseases. Drug Metab Dispos. 2013;41:1–11.

Syms AJ, Norris JS, Panko WB, Smith RG. Mechanism of androgen-receptor augmentation. Analysis of receptor synthesis and degradation by the density-shift technique. J Biol Chem. 1985;260:455–61.

Tadepally HD, Burger G, Aubry M. Evolution of C2H2-zinc finger genes and subfamilies in mammals: species-specific duplication and loss of clusters, genes and effector domains. BMC Evol Biol. 2008;8:176.

Talabér G, Jondal M, Okret S. Extra-adrenal glucocorticoid synthesis: immune regulation and aspects on local organ homeostasis. Mol Cell Endocrinol. 2013;380:89–98.

Tan MH, Zhou XE, Soon FF, Li X, Li J, Yong EL, Melcher K, Xu HE. The crystal structure of the orphan nuclear receptor NR2E3/PNR ligand binding domain reveals a dimeric auto-repressed conformation. PLoS One. 2013;8, e74359.

Tang Y, Getzenberg RH, Vietmeier BN, Stallcup MR, Eggert M, Renkawitz R, DeFranco DB. The DNA-binding and tau2 transactivation domains of the rat glucocorticoid receptor constitute a nuclear matrix-targeting signal. Mol Endocrinol. 1998;12:1420–31.

Tan-Wong SM, French JD, Proudfoot NJ, Brown MA. Dynamic interactions between the promoter and terminator regions of the mammalian BRCA1 gene. Proc Natl Acad Sci. 2008;105:5160–5.

Taraborrelli S. Physiology, production and action of progesterone. Acta Obstet Gynecol Scand. 2015;94:8–16.

Teng Y, Radde BN, Litchfield LM, Ivanova MM, Prough RA, Clark BJ, Doll MA, Hein DW, Klinge CM. Dehydroepiandrosterone activation of G-protein-coupled estrogen receptor rapidly stimulates , microRNA-21 transcription in human hepatocellular carcinoma cells. J Biol Chem. 2015;290:15799–811.

Tesarik J, Mendoza C. Direct non-genomic effects of follicular steroids on maturing human oocytes: oestrogen versus androgen antagonism. Hum Reprod Update. 1997;3:95–100.
Theodorou V, Stark R, Menon S, Carroll JS. GATA3 acts upstream of FOXA1 in mediating ESR1 binding by shaping enhancer accessibility. Genome Res. 2013;23:12–22.
Thomas P. Characteristics of membrane progestin receptor alpha (mPR[alpha]) and progesterone membrane receptor component 1 (PGMRC1) and their roles in mediating rapid progestin actions. Front Neuroendocrinol. 2008;29:292–312.
Thomas C, Gustafsson J-Å. The different roles of ER subtypes in cancer biology and therapy. Nat Rev Cancer. 2011;11:597–608.
Thomas P, Pang Y, Zhu Y, Detweiler C, Doughty K. Multiple rapid progestin actions and progestin membrane receptor subtypes in fish. Steroids. 2004;69:567–73.
Thompson EB. Steroid hormones. Membrane transporters of steroid hormones. Curr Biol. 1995;5:730–2.
Thornton JW. Evolution of vertebrate steroid receptors from an ancestral estrogen receptor by ligand exploitation and serial genome expansions. Proc Natl Acad Sci U S A. 2001;98:5671–6.
Thornton JW, Need E, Crews D. Resurrecting the ancestral steroid receptor: ancient origin of estrogen signaling. Science. 2003;301:1714–7.
Toran-Allerand CD. Minireview: a plethora of estrogen receptors in the brain: where will it end? Endocrinology. 2004;145:1069–74.
Traina TA. Results from a phase 2 study of enzalutamide (ENZA), an androgen receptor (AR) inhibitor, in advanced AR+ triple-negative breast cancer (TNBC). In 2015 ASSCO Annual meeting, Vol. 33. J Clin Oncol. 2015.
Tzukerman M, Zhang XK, Pfahl M. Inhibition of estrogen receptor activity by the tumor promoter 12-O- tetradeconylphorbol-13-acetate: a molecular analysis. Mol Endocrinol. 1991;5:1983–92.
Umesono K, Murakami KK, Thompson CC, Evans RM. Direct repeats as selective response elements for thyroid hormone, retinoic acid, and vitamin D_3 receptors. Cell. 1991;65:1255–66.
Valley CC, Solodin NM, Powers GL, Ellison SJ, Alarid ET. Temporal variation in estrogen receptor-{alpha} protein turnover in the presence of estrogen. J Mol Endocrinol. 2008;40:23–34.
Vaquerizas JM, Kummerfeld SK, Teichmann SA, Luscombe NM. A census of human transcription factors: function, expression and evolution. Nat Rev Genet. 2009;10:252–63.
Viengchareun S, Le Menuet D, Martinerie L, Munier M, Pascual-Le Tallec L, Lombes M. The mineralocorticoid receptor: insights into its molecular and (patho)physiological biology. Nucl Recept Signal. 2007;5, e012.
Vinas R, Watson CS. Bisphenol S disrupts estradiol-induced nongenomic signaling in a rat pituitary cell line: effects on cell functions. Environ Health Perspect. 2013;121:352–8.
Wagner RL, Apriletti JW, McGrath ME, West BL, Baxter JD, Fletterick RJ. A structural role for hormone in the thyroid hormone receptor. A structural role for hormone in the thyroid hormone receptor. Nature. 1995;378:690–7.
Walesky C, Apte U. Role of hepatocyte nuclear factor 4alpha (HNF4alpha) in cell proliferation and cancer. Gene Expr. 2015;16:101–8.
Waltering KK, Urbanucci A, Visakorpi T. Androgen receptor (AR) aberrations in castration-resistant prostate cancer. Mol Cell Endocrinol. 2012;360:38–43.
Wang Q, Cooney AJ. Revisiting the role of GCNF in embryonic development. Semin Cell Dev Biol. 2013;24:679–86.
Wang T, Xiong JQ. The orphan nuclear receptor TLX/NR2E1 in neural stem cells and diseases. Neurosci Bull. 2016;32:108–14.
Wang Z-Y, Yin L. Estrogen receptor alpha-36 (ER-α36): a new player in human breast cancer. Mol Cell Endocrinol. 2015. doi:10.1016/j.mce.2015.04.017.
Wang Y, Fischle W, Cheung W, Jacobs S, Khorasanizadeh S, Allis CD. Beyond the double helix: writing and reading the histone code. Novartis Found Symp. 2004;259:3–17. discussion 17-21, 163-9.

Watson CS, Lange CA. Steadying the boat: integrating mechanisms of membrane and nuclear-steroid-receptor signalling. EMBO Rep. 2005;6:116–9.

Watson CS, Pappas TC, Gametchu B. The other estrogen receptor in the plasma membrane: implications for the actions of environmental estrogens. Environ Health Perspect. 1995;103 Suppl 7:41–50.

Watson CS, Campbell CH, Gametchu B. The dynamic and elusive membrane estrogen receptor-alpha. Steroids. 2002;67:429–37.

Watson CS, Bulayeva NN, Wozniak AL, Finnerty CC. Signaling from the membrane via membrane estrogen receptor-[alpha]: estrogens, xenoestrogens, and phytoestrogens. Steroids. 2005;70:364–71.

Watson CS, Jeng Y-J, Kochukov MY. Nongenomic signaling pathways of estrogen toxicity. Toxicol Sci. 2010;115:1–11.

Watson CS, Jeng Y-J, Hu G, Wozniak A, Bulayeva N, Guptarak J. Estrogen- and xenoestrogen-induced ERK signaling in pituitary tumor cells involves estrogen receptor-α interactions with G protein-αi and caveolin I. Steroids. 2012;77:424–32.

Webb P, Lopez GN, Uht RM, Kushner PJ. Tamoxifen activation of the estrogen receptor/AP-1 pathway. Mol Endocrinol. 1995;9:443–56.

Weiser MJ, Foradori CD, Handa RJ. Estrogen receptor beta in the brain: from form to function. Brain Res Rev. 2008;57:309–20.

Welboren W-J, Sweep FCGJ, Span PN, Stunnenberg HG. Genomic actions of estrogen receptor {alpha}: what are the targets and how are they regulated? Endocr Relat Cancer. 2009a;16:1073–89.

Welboren W-J, van Driel MA, Janssen-Megens EM, van Heeringen SJ, Sweep FCGJ, Span PN, Stunnenberg HG. ChIP-Seq of ER[alpha] and RNA polymerase II defines genes differentially responding to ligands. EMBO J. 2009b;28:1418. advanced online publication.

Westphal U. Steroid-protein interactions II. Monogr Endocrinol. 1986;27:1–603.

Willson TM, Moore JT. Genomics versus orphan nuclear receptors – a half-time report. Mol Endocrinol. 2002;16:1135–44.

Willson TM, Brown PJ, Sternbach DD, Henke BR. The PPARs: from orphan receptors to drug discovery. J Med Chem. 2000;43:527–50.

Wong M, Ramayya MS, Chrousos GP, Driggers PH, Parker KL. Cloning and sequence analysis of the human gene encoding steroidogenic factor 1. J Mol Endocrinol. 1996;17:139–47.

Wu C-T, Altuwaijri S, Ricke WA, Huang S-P, Yeh S, Zhang C, Niu Y, Tsai M-Y, Chang C. Increased prostate cell proliferation and loss of cell differentiation in mice lacking prostate epithelial androgen receptor. Proc Natl Acad Sci. 2007;104:12679–84.

Wu Q, Chambliss K, Lee W-R, Yuhanna IS, Mineo C, Shaul PW. Point mutations in the ERα Gαi binding domain segregate nonnuclear from nuclear receptor function. Mol Endocrinol. 2013;27:2–11.

Xue K, Liu J-y, Murphy BD, Tsang BK. Orphan nuclear receptor NR4A1 is a negative regulator of DHT-induced rat preantral follicular growth. Mol Endocrinol. 2012;26:2004–15.

Yamagata K. Chapter sixteen – roles of HNF1α and HNF4α in pancreatic β-Cells: lessons from a monogenic form of diabetes (MODY. In: Gerald L, editor. Vitamins and hormones, vol. 95. New York: Academic; 2014. p. 407–23.

Yang L, Guerrero J, Hong H, DeFranco DB, Stallcup MR. Interaction of the tau2 transcriptional activation domain of glucocorticoid receptor with a novel steroid receptor coactivator, Hic-5, which localizes to both focal adhesions and the nuclear matrix. Mol Biol Cell. 2000;11:2007–18.

Yeh S, Tsai M-Y, Xu Q, Mu X-M, Lardy H, Huang K-E, Lin H, Yeh S-D, Altuwaijri S, Zhou X, Xing L, Boyce BF, Hung M-C, Zhang S, Gan L, Chang C. Generation and characterization of androgen receptor knockout (ARKO) mice: an in vivo model for the study of androgen functions in selective tissues. Proc Natl Acad Sci. 2002;99:13498–503.

Yi P, Wang Z, Feng Q, Pintilie GD, Foulds CE, Lanz RB, Ludtke SJ, Schmid MF, Chiu W, O'Malley BW. Structure of a biologically active estrogen receptor-coactivator complex on DNA. Mol Cell. 2015;57:1047–58.

Yin L, Wu N, Lazar MA. Nuclear receptor Rev-erbalpha: a heme receptor that coordinates circadian rhythm and metabolism. Nucl Recept Signal. 2010;8, e001.

York B, O'Malley BW. Steroid receptor coactivator (SRC) family: masters of systems biology. J Biol Chem. 2010;285:38743–50.

Yoshinaga SK, Peterson CL, Herskowitz I, Yamamoto KR. Roles of SWI1, SWI2, and SWI3 proteins for transcriptional enhancement by steroid receptors. Science. 1992;258:1598–604.

Young MJ, Rickard AJ. Mineralocorticoid receptors in the heart: lessons from cell-selective transgenic animals. J Endocrinol. 2015;224:R1–13.

Zarif JC, Lamb LE, Schulz VV, Nollet EA, Miranti CK. Androgen receptor non-nuclear regulation of prostate cancer cell invasion mediated by Src and matriptase. Oncotarget. 2015;6:6862–76.

Zboray L, Pluciennik A, Curtis D, Liu Y, Berman-Booty LD, Orr C, Kesler CT, Berger T, Gioeli D, Paschal BM, Merry DE. Preventing the androgen receptor N/C interaction delays disease onset in a mouse model of SBMA. Cell Rep. 2015;13:2312–23.

Zhang Y, Dufau ML. EAR2 and EAR3/COUP-TFI regulate transcription of the rat LH receptor. Mol Endocrinol. 2001;15:1891–905.

Zhang J, Lazar MA. The mechanism of action of thyroid hormones. Annu Rev Physiol. 2000;62:439–66.

Zhang Y, Wang L. Nuclear receptor small heterodimer partner in apoptosis signaling and liver cancer. Cancers (Basel). 2011;3:198–212.

Zhang G, Zhang L, Duff GW. A negative regulatory region containing a glucocorticosteroid response element (nGRE) in the human interleukin-1beta gene. DNA Cell Biol. 1997;16:145–52.

Zhang X, Tanaka K, Yan J, Li J, Peng D, Jiang Y, Yang Z, Barton MC, Wen H, Shi X. Regulation of estrogen receptor α by histone methyltransferase SMYD2-mediated protein methylation. Proc Natl Acad Sci. 2013;110:17284–9.

Zhang L, Fang C, Xu X, Li A, Cai Q, Long X. Androgen receptor, EGFR, and BRCA1 as biomarkers in triple-negative breast cancer: a meta-analysis. Biomed Res Int. 2015;2015:357485.

Zhao Y, Bruemmer D. NR4A orphan nuclear receptors: transcriptional regulators of gene expression in metabolism and vascular biology. Arterioscler Thromb Vasc Biol. 2010;30:1535–41.

Zhao C, Dahlman-Wright K, Gustafsson J-Å. Estrogen signaling via estrogen receptor β. J Biol Chem. 2010;285:39575–9.

Zhou W, Slingerland JM. Links between oestrogen receptor activation and proteolysis: relevance to hormone-regulated cancer therapy. Nat Rev Cancer. 2014;14:26–38.

Zhou G, Cummings R, Li Y, Mitra S, Wilkinson HA, Elbrecht A, Hermes JD, Schaeffer JM, Smith RG, Moller DE. Nuclear receptors have distinct affinities for coactivators: characterization by fluorescence resonance energy transfer. Mol Endocrinol. 1998;12:1594–604.

Zhu Y, Rice CD, Pang Y, Pace M, Thomas P. Cloning, expression, and characterization of a membrane progestin receptor and evidence it is an intermediary in meiotic maturation of fish oocytes. Proc Natl Acad Sci U S A. 2003a;100:2231–6.

Zhu Y, Rice CD, Pang Y, Pace M, Thomas P. From the cover: cloning, expression, and characterization of a membrane progestin receptor and evidence it is an intermediary in meiotic maturation of fish oocytes. Proc Natl Acad Sci U S A. 2003b;100:2231–6.

Thyroid Hormone Nuclear Receptors and Molecular Actions

9

Molecular Actions of TRs

Xuguang Zhu and Sheue-yann Cheng

Abstract

The thyroid hormone 3,3′,5-triiodo-L-thyronine (T3) is essential for normal growth, differentiation, and development and maintains metabolic homeostasis. The genomic actions of T3 are mediated by thyroid hormone nuclear receptors (TRs). Two TR genes, located on two different chromosomes, encode three major T3-binding TR isoforms: α1, β1, and β2. TR isoforms are differentially expressed in different target tissues and are developmentally regulated. The transcriptional activity of TR is dictated by types of thyroid hormone response elements on T3 target genes, and is modulated by T3-dependent interaction with nuclear coregulatory proteins, e.g., nuclear corepressors and coactivators. Recent genome-wide analysis shows that T3-induced TR recruitment to chromatin is associated with chromatin remodeling and activated gene transcription. Further, unliganded TR engagement with repressive complexes on chromatin is, similar to activating receptor complexes, a highly dynamic process. Our understanding of the biology and molecular actions of TR was further enhanced by studying human diseases due to mutations of TR isoforms. Lessons learned from mouse models of such human diseases have further advanced our understanding of the diverse and complex genomic actions of TRs.

Keywords

Thyroid hormone receptors • Resistance to thyroid hormone • Hypothyroidism genomic actions • Tumorigenesis • Genetically engineered mouse model • Thyroid cancer

X. Zhu
Laboratory of Molecular Biology, Center for Cancer Research, National Cancer Institute, National Institutes of Health, Bethesda, MD, USA

S.-y. Cheng (✉)
Laboratory of Molecular Biology, National Cancer Institute, Bethesda, MD, USA
e-mail: chengs@mail.nih.gov

A. Belfiore, D. LeRoith (eds.), *Principles of Endocrinology and Hormone Action*, Endocrinology, https://doi.org/10.1007/978-3-319-44675-2_10

Contents

Introduction

The cloning of cDNAs encoding thyroid hormone nuclear receptors (TRs) in the late 1980s has made it possible to characterize their molecular properties and to study directly how TRs regulate the transcriptional activities of T3 target genes (Sap et al. 1986; Weinberger et al. 1986). Two genes, *THRA* and *THRB*, located on chromosomes 17 and 3, respectively, encode three thyroid hormone (T3)-binding TR isoforms. Similar to other members of the nuclear receptor family, TRs consist of domain structures with the highly homologous DNA-binding domain C and T3-binding domain D/E, but with distinct amino A/B domains (Fig. 1a). Early studies on the regulation of the transcription activity of TR concentrated on the identification of thyroid hormone response elements and heterodimeric partners (e.g., such as the retinoid X receptor, RXR) on a gene-by-gene basis. The discoveries of corepressors (e.g., NCOR1, NCOR2) (Chen and Evans 1995; Horlein et al. 1995) and coactivators (e.g., SRC1) (Onate et al. 1995) led to the bimodal switch model to account for the transcription activation of TRs. In the absence of T3, TR complexed with RXR recruits corepressors such as NCOR1 to repress gene transcription. Binding of T3 releases corepressors to allow the liganded TR-RXR to recruit coactivators such as SRC1 to activate gene transcription (Fig. 1b; Xu et al. 1999). Indeed, the ligand binding domain (LBD) of TR assumes a different conformation from that of the unliganded LBD (Apriletti et al. 1998). A hydrophobic cleft on the LBD that binds to nuclear coactivators for ligand-dependent transcription was mapped (Feng et al. 1998).

Recent studies on the transcription regulation of TR have moved beyond the gene-by-gene approach. Technological advances resulted in the modification and expansion of the classical canonical TR signaling pathway. Chromatin immunoprecipitation sequencing (ChIP-seq) allows identification of TR binding sites genome-wide. Digital genome footprinting from DNase-seq genome-wide uncovered new details about the landscape in the interaction of TR with chromatin. The use of

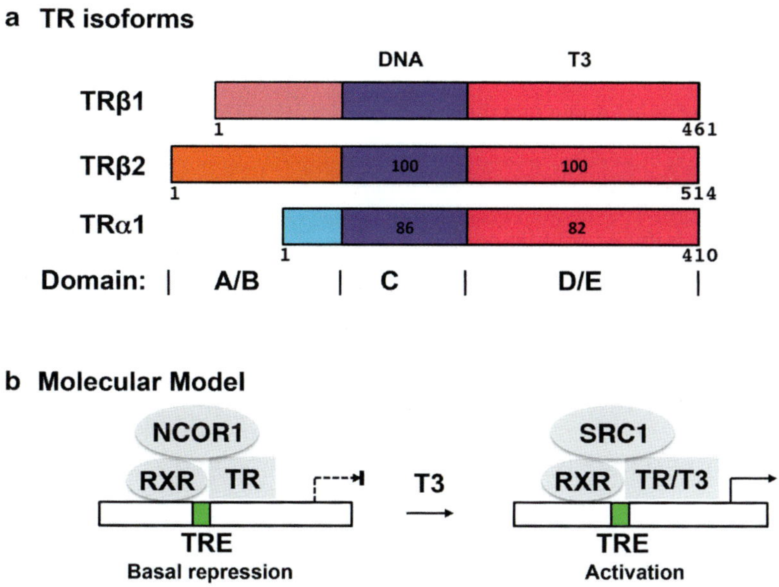

Fig. 1 **(a) Schematic representation of TR isoforms. (b) A simplified model of gene regulation by thyroid hormone T3**. In the absence of T3, a corepressor is bound to the RXR-TR heterodimer at the positive TRE, thereby actively repressing target gene expression. When T3 binds to the TR dimer, the corepressor is released and coactivators are recruited, resulting in activation of gene transcription

mouse models to study human diseases caused by mutations of TRs revealed previously unattainable molecular insights into the pathogenesis of human diseases. This chapter will first briefly review the classical views of TR actions, but with more focus on highlighting recent advances in the understanding of the genomic actions of thyroid hormone and its receptors.

Multilevel Transcription Regulation in TR Signaling

Thyroid Hormone Response Elements

Following the cloning of cDNA of TR isoforms, a flurry of activity ensued to identify the specific cis-elements on the promoters of T3 target genes. Shortly thereafter, the consensus sequence of the six nucleotides (A/G)GGT(C/A/G)A emerged as the thyroid hormone elements (TREs). TREs are composed of two half-site binding motifs with different orientations that can be arranged as an everted repeat with six nucleotides in between the two half-sites, a direct repeat with four nucleotide spacing (DR4), or an inverted repeat as palindromic TRE (Pal) with no spacing between two half binding sites.

Different types of TREs mediate the TR transcription of T3 target genes. For example, the rat growth hormone gene has Pal TRE in its promoter, whereas DR4 motif mediates the TR transcription response on the promoter of the malic enzyme gene. However, it is known that the binding of TR with TREs is TR subtype-, TRE-, and T3-dependent. The strength in the binding of TR to TREs could also be influenced by the neighboring sequences near the TREs. Moreover, it was also found that through DNA looping, two half-sites may not need to be immediately in the near vicinity. As will be discussed below, the interaction of TRE with TR is modulated by an array of nuclear receptor coregulators. Thus, while identification of binding motifs of TR in the promoter of an unknown gene is an indication, functional characterization would be needed for the validation of the binding motifs in the mediation of TR transcription.

Tissue-Dependent Distribution and Isoform-Selective Functions of TR

TR isoforms express at different levels in target tissues during development and in adults. Analysis of mRNA expression in mice showed that *Thra1* mRNA is predominantly expressed in the heart, brain, and bone, whereas the *Thrb1* mRNA is predominantly expressed in the skeletal muscle, kidney, liver, and thyroid. The expression of *Thrb2* mRNA was detected in the hypothalamus, pituitary, retina, and cochlea. Less is known about the expression patterns of *THRA1*, *THRB1*, and *THRB2* mRNA in human target tissues. However, in view of the functional conservation of TRs between the mouse and the human, it is reasonable to expect that the distribution patterns of TR isoform in human tissues could be similar to mice.

The tissue-dependent distribution of TR isoforms raises several important questions in the understanding of transcription activity of TR. What are the biological cues to dictate the TR isoform expression during different stages of development? Do TR isoforms have isoform-specific functions such that the genes needed at certain stages of development will turn on the expression of one TR isoform to activate or suppress? Alternatively, do TR isoforms serve a redundant role to ensure T3 actions are achieved to maintain the genomic integrity? The question of whether TR has isoform-selective or redundant functions has been assessed using TR isoform knockout mice. Analysis of the phenotypes of mice with deletion of the *Thra* gene, the *Thrb* gene, or both the *Thra* and *Thrb* genes indicated that TR isoforms have selective and also overlapping functions to mediate the genomic actions of T3 (Forrest and Vennstrom 2000). Whether TR isoforms exhibit isoform-specific functions was further addressed by using genome-wide analysis (Chatonnet et al. 2013). Analysis of gene expression patterns in neural cells stably expressing TRα1 or TRβ1 showed that a substantial fraction of the T3 target genes preferentially interact with one or the other TR isoform. Genome-wide chromatin occupancy studies demonstrated that the cistromes for TRα1 or TRβ1 are distinct when they function in the identical cellular context (Chatonnet et al. 2013). However, it is intriguing that the receptor-selective regulation of T3 target genes did not result from receptor-selective chromatin occupancy of their promoter regions. Nonetheless, overall, these studies suggested that in addition to the tissue-dependent expression of TR isoforms, TR isoform-selective actions could contribute to the diverse functions of TR.

Modulation of TR Transcription by Nuclear Coregulatory Proteins and Chromatin Remodeling

The groundbreaking discovery of nuclear receptor corepressors (Chen and Evans 1995; Horlein et al. 1995) and the first nuclear receptor coactivator, SRC1 (Onate et al. 1995), opened an exciting new area of studies in the transcription regulation of TR. Shortly after these reports, many additional corepressors (e.g., histone deacetylase family) and coactivators (e.g., SRC family members) and their associated proteins in large complexes were identified (e.g., NCOR/SMRT complex, Sin 3 complex) (Li et al. 2000; Perissi et al. 2010). The identification of corepressors and coactivators led to a simple two-step model as shown in Fig. 1b. The TRE-bound unliganded TR/RXR heterodimer recruits NCOR1 and associated nuclear proteins in a complex, resulting in transcription repression. Binding of T3 leads to conformation change in TR that releases NCOR1 to allow recruitment of coactivators (e.g., SRC1) and associated proteins in the coactivator complex, leading to transcription activation. The corepressor complex and the coactivator complex, each containing series of different enzymatic activities, affect chromatin remodeling and modifications of the histone tails, thereby mediating transcription repression or activation. Thus, the ligand binding is the key event that leads to a switch between two transcription states.

However, this bimodal switch model has been revised by recent genome ChIP-seq studies (Grontved et al. 2015). Analysis of TR binding sites in the mouse liver shows considerable T3- dependent TR recruitment to the genome and de novo remodeling of chromatin. Moreover, in contrast to the classical bimodal switch model in which TR was viewed as a repressor constitutively bound to chromatin in the absence of T3, little evidence of TR footprints from genome-wide DNase-seq hypersensitivity (DHS) analysis was found. Genome-wide DHS analysis also failed to detect footprints of T3-bound TR. These findings suggested that the interaction of TR with chromatin is not static as previously thought, but rather highly dynamic, and, further, that TR can increase accessibility of chromatin in a ligand-dependent manner (Grontved et al. 2015).

TR binding sites genome-wide have also been analyzed in neural cells stably expressing TRα1 or TRβ1 (Chatonnet et al. 2013), in HepG2 cells stably expressing TRβ1 (Ayers et al. 2014), and in the mouse liver expressing biotinylated TRβ1 (Ramadoss et al. 2014). Together with the cistrome identified for the endogenous TRβ1 in the mouse liver (Grontved et al. 2015), these genome-wide analyses showed that the number of T3 binding sites, avidity of TR binding to the sites, and selectivity in target gene binding varied depending on the cellular context. However, two common themes emerged from these studies. One is that DR4 TRE is the preferred TR binding element over other types of TREs. The other is that TR binding sites are not limited to proximal promoter regions but are distributed in the exons, the introns, and the intergenic regions. While genome-wide studies have uncovered a wealth of information previously unattainable to advance our understanding of TR actions in vivo, the findings from these studies also raised additional questions. The genome-wide DHS supported the dynamic interaction of TR with the chromatin; however, the driving force in the dynamic exchange between the repressive and activated states of TR would need to be understood. The molecular nature of enhancers on the chromatin and how they undergo changes from TR-mediated repression to activation would need to be elucidated. Moreover, the key issue of chromatin accessibility would need to be better defined. These exemplary questions and others need to be clarified in future studies.

TR Mutations and Human Diseases

Our understanding of the biology and genomic actions of TR is advanced by understanding the molecular basis of diseases due to mutations of *THR* genes. Mutations of the *THRB* gene or *THRA* genes reduce sensitivity to T3 in target tissues; thus, the disease is known as resistance to thyroid hormone (RTH). However, the resistance phenotypic manifestations in patients caused by TRβ1 mutants or TRα1 mutants are different. To make the distinction, RTH caused by TRβ1 mutations or TRα1 mutations is now referred to as RTHβ or RTHα, respectively.

Resistance to Thyroid Hormone Caused by Mutations of the THRB Gene (RTHβ)

RTHβ was first reported by Refetoff in 1967; however, only after the cloning of TRβ1 cDNA was it possible to establish unequivocally that mutations of the *THRB* gene cause RTHβ. At present, more than 1000 families with 3000 individuals have been reported (Dumitrescu and Refetoff 2013). Except for four patients with two mutated *THRB* alleles, most RTHβ patients are heterozygous mutations exhibiting the characteristic hallmark of elevated serum thyroid hormone accompanied by nonsuppressible TSH. Other common clinical features are goiter, hyperactive behavior, learning disabilities, developmental delay, and sinus tachycardia (Dumitrescu and Refetoff 2013). While clinical manifestations vary from one patient to another, the symptoms are mediated by the dominant negative actions of TRβ mutants.

Understanding the molecular mechanisms by which TRβ mutants act in vivo was facilitated by the genetically engineered mouse models. Two mutant mice with targeted mutations in the *Thrb* gene have been generated, one with a frameshift mutation TRβPV ($Thrb^{PV}$ mouse, Fig. 2a) (Kaneshige et al. 2000) and the other a Δ337T mutation ($Thrb^{\Delta 337T}$ mouse) (Hashimoto et al. 2001). Both TRβPV and TRβΔ337T have lost T3 binding and transcription activity. Both mice display the

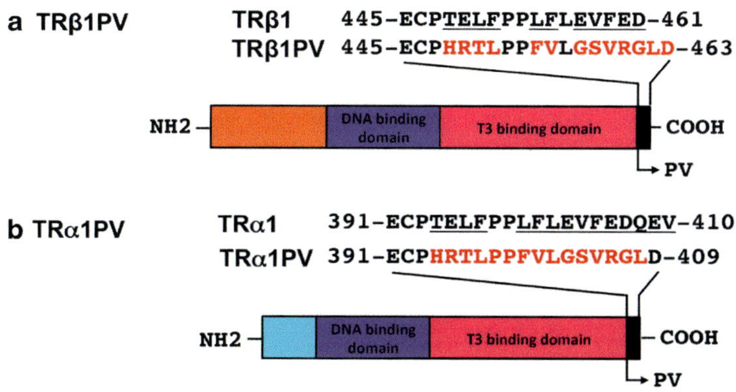

Fig. 2 Schematic comparison of TRβ1, TRβ1PV (a), TRα1, and TRα1PV (b). The TRβ1PV and TRα1PV mutants have frameshift mutations in the carboxyl-terminal amino acid sequences of TRβ1 and TRα1. TRβ1PV and TRα1PV have completely lost T3 binding activity and transcription capacity. The carboxyl-terminal amino acid sequences of the TRβ1, TRβ1PV, TRα1, and TRα1PV mutants are shown

hallmark of dysregulation of the pituitary-thyroid axis; however, TRβPV exerted a stronger effect on the pituitary-thyroid axis so that the *Thrb*^{PV} mouse had higher thyroid hormone and TSH levels than did the *Thrb*$^{\Delta 337T}$mouse.

The availability of the *Thrb*^{PV} mouse allowed the elucidation of the molecular basis underlying variable manifestations of patients with RTHβ. It was puzzling that the clinical manifestations varied between families with different mutations, between families with the same mutation, and also between members of the same family with identical mutations. The role of SRC1 in the variable phenotypic expression of RTHβ was examined by crossing *Thrb*^{PV} mice with SRC1-deficient mice. Lack of SRC1 in *Thrb*^{PV} mice attenuates the extent of RTHβ in a target tissue-dependent manner and alters abnormal expression patterns of known T3 target genes in tissues (Kamiya et al. 2003), indicating the modulating role of SRC1 in RTHβ. The tissue dependency of SRC1 could therefore contribute to the variable manifestations of patients with RTHβ. In addition, characterization of the RTHβ phenotypes of the progeny from the cross of *Thrb*^{PV} mice with mice deficient in TRα1 showed that the lack of TRα1 intensifies the manifestations of RTHβ in *Thrb*^{PV} mice. The tissue-dependent expression of TRα1 can therefore lead to variable manifestations of RTHβ symptoms in different tissues (Suzuki and Cheng 2003). While the studies so far have identified only two modulators that can account for the variable clinical manifestations of RTHβ in patients, the *Thrb*^{PV} mouse can be used for identification of other modulators mediating variable clinical phenotypes.

Genetic analyses indicate that almost all RTHβ patients are heterozygous for the mutant *THRB* allele, a finding consistent with the autosomal dominant pattern of inheritance. Biochemical and genetic analyses show that TRβ1 mutants mediate the pathogenesis of RTHβ via dominant negative actions. The *Thrb*^{PV} mouse facilitated the elucidation of the molecular mechanisms by which TRβ1 mutants act to cause RTHβ phenotypes. Early studies demonstrated that in the target tissue, the liver,

TRβ1PV competes with TRβ1 or TRα1 for binding to TRE and for heterodimerization with RXRs (Zhang et al. 2002). Such competition leads to repression of the positively T3-regulated target genes – S14, malic enzyme, and deiodinase – in the liver of *Thrb*^{PV} mice. These studies demonstrated that one of the molecular mechanisms by which TRβ1 mutants exert their dominant negative activity in vivo is through competition with wild-type TRs for binding to TRE and for heterodimerization with RXRs (Zhang et al. 2002). Recently, the regulatory role of NCOR1 in the dominant negative action of TRβPV was examined in progeny from the cross of *Thrb*^{PV} mice with mutant mice expressing a mutated NCOR1 (NCOR1ΔID, *Thrb*^{PV}/*Ncor1*$^{\Delta ID}$ mice) that cannot interact with TR or TRβPV (Fozzatti et al. 2011). Remarkably, the expression of NCOR1DID in *Thrb*^{PV} mice significantly corrected the abnormally elevated TSH and thyroid hormone levels. Furthermore, thyroid hyperplasia, weight loss, and other hallmarks of RTH were also partially reverted in mice expressing NCOR1ΔID. This study provided the in vivo evidence to show that the aberrant recruitment of NCOR1 by TRβ mutants leads to clinical RTHβ in humans (Fozzatti et al. 2011). Importantly, these findings raised the possibility that therapies aimed at the TR-NCOR1 interaction or its downstream actions could be tested as potential targets in treating RTHβ.

The effects of TRβ mutants on neurological development have been evaluated in the *Thrb*$^{\Delta 337T}$ mouse (Hashimoto et al. 2001). While the major TR isoform is TRα1 in the brain, *Thrb*$^{\Delta 337T}$ mice exhibit severe abnormalities in cerebellar development and function, along with learning defects, suggesting that TRβΔ337T could interfere with the transcription activity of TRα1 via dominant negative action. Moreover, biochemical data also showed that T3 failed to induce dissociation of NCOR1 and SMRT from TRβΔ337T, suggesting that NCOR1 bound to TRβ mutants could also mediate the pathogenesis of neuro-abnormalities. Thus it is possible that strategies to block the interaction of NCOR1 with TRβ mutants could lead to improvement in neuronal dysfunction mediated by TRβ mutants.

Resistance to Thyroid Hormone Caused by Mutations of the THRA Gene (RTHα)

In view of the fact that mutations of the *THRB* gene were shown to cause RTHβ, and given the extensive sequence homology in the functional domains of TRα1 and TRβ1 and their similar in vitro functional characteristics, it was intriguing that no mutation of *THRA* gene had ever been found in RTHβ patients. To sort out whether mutations of the *THRA* gene could be embryonic lethal, inconsequential, or not associated with abnormalities of RTHβ, a mutant mouse targeting the same PV mutated sequence at the C-terminus of the *Thra* gene at the corresponding position as in TRβ1PV was created by homologous recombination (*Thra1*^{PV} mice, Fig. 2b) (Kaneshige et al. 2001). In contrast to *Thrb*$^{PV/+}$ mice, *Thra1*$^{PV/+}$ mice did not exhibit the characteristic hallmark of RTHβ of the pituitary-thyroid axis dysregulation, i.e., elevated thyroid hormone accompanied by nonsuppressible TSH. *Thra1*^{PV} mice are not embryonic lethal but do have decreased fertility and reduced survival. *Thra1*$^{PV/PV}$

neonates die shortly after birth. *Thra1*$^{PV/+}$ mice exhibit severe growth retardation and delayed bone development. The abnormal gene expression patterns in the liver and the pituitary are distinct between *Thra1*$^{PV/+}$ mice (Kaneshige et al. 2001) and *Thrb*$^{PV/+}$ mice (Kaneshige et al. 2000). These distinct phenotypes exhibited by *Thra1*$^{PV/+}$ and *Thrb*$^{PV+}$ mice indicated for the first time that the in vivo functions of TR mutants are clearly isoform-dependent and explained why mutations of the *THRA* gene had never been found in RTHβ patients. However, whether the distinct phenotypes mediated by TR isoform mutants held true in human disease was not known until the patients with mutations of the *THRA* gene were discovered 12 years later after the making of the *Thra1*^{PV} mouse.

Through the use of whole-exome capture and high-throughput sequencing of a DNA sample from a 6-year-old girl exhibiting growth retardation and delayed bone maturation, a mutated TRα1 (E403X) was identified (Bochukova et al. 2012). In the same year, two other patients with another C-terminal truncation mutation were identified in the *THRA* gene (TRα1F397fs406X) (van Mullem et al. 2012). Since then, at least 24 patients with mutations in the *THRA* gene have been reported (Demir et al. 2016). These patients are heterozygous in the mutations of one allele of the *THRA* gene. These patients exhibit classical features of hypothyroidism with growth retardation, delayed mental and bone development, and constipation but with elevated serum T3 and normal TSH (van Mullem et al. 2013). Thus the clinical presentations clearly are not a result of low thyroid hormone but reflect the resistance of target tissues due to the dominant negative actions of TRα1 (RTHα). Moreover, phenotypic expression of patients with TRα1 mutations differ from those observed in patients with TRβ1 mutations, thereby validating the observations in *Thra1*$^{PV/+}$ mice and *Thrb*$^{PV/+}$ mice in that the molecular actions of mutant TR isoforms are distinct to mediate different diseases.

TRα1PV expressed in *Thra1*$^{PV/+}$ mice has a truncated mutated sequence similar to that in two patients reported by van Mullem et al. (2012). *Thra1*$^{PV/+}$ mice faithfully reproduce the hypothyroid phenotypes of patients. The molecular mechanisms by which TRα1PV acts to mediate the dominant negative actions were assessed in the progeny from the cross of *Thra1*$^{PV/+}$ mice with mutant mice expressing NCOR1ΔID (*Thra1*$^{PV/+}$*Ncor1*$^{\Delta ID}$ mice) (Fozzatti et al. 2013a). The severe retarded growth, infertility, and delayed bone development are partially reverted in *Thra1*$^{PV/+}$ mice expressing NCOR1ΔID. The impaired adipogenesis is partially corrected by derepression of peroxisome proliferator-activated receptor γ (*Pparγ*) and CCAAT/enhancer-binding protein α gene (*C/ebpα*) because of the inability of TRαlPV to recruit NCOR1ΔID to form a repressor complex. These studies showed that NCOR1 is a critical regulator of the dominant negative activity of TRα1 mutants in the pathogenesis of hypothyroidism caused by mutations of the *THRA* gene (Fozzatti et al. 2013a).

TRα1PV-NCOR1 complex also recruits histone deacetylase to form a large corepressor complex. The findings that NCOR1 regulates the in vivo dominant negative action of TRα1 mutants suggested that inhibition of deacetylation could improve the hypothyroidism in *Thra1*$^{PV/+}$ mice (Kim et al. 2014a). Indeed, treatment of *Thra1*$^{PV/+}$ mice with a histone deacetylase (HDAC) inhibitor, suberoylanilide hydroxamic acid (SAHA, vorinostat), significantly ameliorates the impaired growth and bone development and the adipogenesis of *Thra1*$^{PV/+}$ mice. In addition, SAHA reverts the impaired adipogenesis by derepressing the expression of the two master regulators of adipogenesis, *C/Ebpα* and *Pparγ*, as well as other adipogenic genes at both the mRNA and protein levels (Kim et al. 2014a). Thus, chromatin histone deacetylation confers in vivo aberrant actions of TRα1 mutants, and HDAC inhibitors are clearly beneficial for hypothyroidism and could be therapeutics for treatment of hypothyroidism caused by TRα1 mutants.

That *Thra1*$^{PV/+}$ mice also could be used as a preclinical mouse model is further demonstrated by the study reported by Bassett et al (Bassett et al. 2014). Affected children with mutations of the *THRA* gene exhibit a consistently severe skeletal dysplasia. It was not clear whether long-term T4 treatment would be beneficial or detrimental. To clarify this issue, *Thra1*$^{PV/+}$ mice were treated with T4 and the adult skeleton was characterized. Although T4 treatment suppresses TSH secretion, it has no effect on skeletal maturation, linear growth, or bone mineralization, thus demonstrating profound tissue resistance to T4. Despite this resistance to T4 effects, prolonged T4 treatment abnormally increases bone stiffness and strength, suggesting the potential for detrimental consequences in the long term. These findings further support the idea that TRα1 has an essential role in the developing and adult skeleton (Bassett et al. 2014). The findings from studying of *Thra1*$^{PV/+}$ mice are valuable in the consideration of using long-term T4 treatment for patients with mutations of the *THRA* gene.

Before the discovery of patients with mutations of the *THRA* gene, in addition to the *Thra1*^{PV} mouse, two other mutant mice with targeted mutations in the *Thra* gene were also created to understand the functions of TRα1 mutants in vivo. The *Thra1*$^{P398H/+}$ mouse exhibited slightly different thyroid function tests than *Thra1*$^{PV/+}$ mice in that TSH, T3, and T4 are all slightly elevated. However, in contrast to *Thra1*$^{PV/+}$ mice which are lean with impaired adipogenesis, *Thra1*$^{P398H/+}$ mice display increased body fat, elevated serum leptin levels, and impairment in catecholamine-stimulated lipolysis (Liu et al. 2003). Another mutant mouse, expressing TRα1R383C (*Thra1*$^{R384C/+}$ mice), similar to *Thra1*$^{PV/+}$ mice, displays severe developmental and growth retardation with only slightly reduced serum thyroxine levels. Similar to *Thra1*$^{PV/PV}$ mice, homozygous *Thra1*$^{R384C/R384C}$ mice survived embryonic development, but neonatal mice cannot survive to adulthood. The *Thra1*^{R384C} mice exhibit several distinct neurological abnormalities with extreme anxiety, reduced recognition memory, and locomotor dysfunction. Interestingly, elevated T4 levels in heterozygotes overcome some defects (Liu et al. 2003; Venero et al. 2005). The reversal of some abnormalities by T4 in *Thra1*$^{R384C/+}$ mice could result from the loss of 90% the ligand binding affinity for TRα1R383C. This is in contrast to TRα1PV for which the ligand binding activity is totally lost. In cell-based studies, high levels of thyroid hormone cannot reverse the loss of transcriptional activity of TRα1PV. In vivo, prolonged T4 treatment of adult *Thra1*$^{PV/+}$ mice failed to correct the bone abnormalities (Bassett et al. 2014).

Clearly, there are some common, but also distinct phenotypic manifestations among *Thra1*$^{PV/+}$, *Thra1*$^{P398H/+}$, and *Thra1*$^{R384C/+}$ mice. The molecular basis of the phenotypic differences has yet to be fully elucidated. The phenotypic differences could reflect the type of mutations, location of the mutation sites, the extent of the loss of ligand binding activity caused by mutations, and how the TRα1 mutants differentially interact with the corepressor complexes. Certainly there are other possibilities that have yet to be explored. However, it would be important to elucidate how these different mutations impact the different phenotypic expression. Currently, only 24 patients with TRα1 mutations have been reported. However, more additional patients could be discovered with distinct clinical presentations as variable as those seen for the three mouse models. Thus, what will be learned from these three mouse models could help in understanding the diversity in the clinical manifestations in patients.

Thyroid Hormone Nuclear Receptors and Cancer

In the past decades, a significant advance has been made in the understanding of TR actions in maintaining normal cellular homeostasis and functions. However, the roles of TR in human cancers are less understood. That TR is critical in regulating cell proliferation and differentiation would predict that aberrant actions of TR could lead to abnormality in cellular functions. Indeed, V-ERBA is a mutated TRα1, which acts in neoplasia by blocking erythroid differentiation and by altering the growth properties of fibroblasts. *V-erb*A is one of the two oncogenes of the avian erythroblastosis virus (AEV), an acute chicken retrovirus that induces lethal erythroleukemia and sarcoma in vivo. While the *v-erb*B locus alone is sufficient to induce erythroleukemia and sarcoma independent of the *v-erb*A gene, the *v-erb*A by itself is not capable of independently causing transformation in either erythroid cells or fibroblasts. V-ERBA functions as a transcription repressor by dominant negative interference with the transcription activity of its normal cellular homologue, c-ERBA (TRα1). That v-ERBA oncoprotein can promote neoplasia in mammals through its dominant negative activity was demonstrated by the development of hepatocellular carcinoma in mice expressing v-ERBA (Barlow et al. 1994). These observations support the idea that TR could play a role in cancer. However, how mutated TRα1 could be directly involved in other human cancers has not been well studied, and so the following section will focus on the role of TRβ1 in human cancers.

The Tumor Suppressor Role of Thyroid Hormone Receptor-β

Association studies indicating the loss of the *THRB* gene by deletion of chromosome 3p were reported in several malignancies including head and neck, renal cell, uterine cervical, lung, melanoma, breast, ovarian, and testicular tumors (Kim and Cheng 2013). Silencing in the expression of the *THRB* gene by promoter hypermethylation and decreased expression of the *THRB* gene has been reported in human cancers including lung, breast, and thyroid carcinoma (Joseph et al. 2007; Ling et al. 2010;

Iwasaki et al. 2010). A recent study demonstrated that abnormally expressed microRNAs could directly target *THRB* to repress its expression in papillary thyroid cancer (Jazdzewski et al. 2011). These findings suggested that TRβ might function as a tumor suppressor in human cancers.

Recent studies have provided direct evidence to demonstrate that TRβt could function as a tumor suppressor in human cancers. Examination of promoter methylation and the expression of the *THRB* gene in tissue specimens from patients with differentiated thyroid carcinoma (DTC) showed a positive correlation between the extent of promoter hypermethylation of the *THRB* gene and the progression of DTC. When human thyroid cancer cell lines in which the *THRB* gene was silenced by hypermethylation were treated with demethylation agents such as 5′aza-CdR and zebularine, the expression of the *THRB* gene was reactivated concurrently with inhibition of cancer cell proliferation, migration, and tumor growth in a xenograft model. Re-expression of the *THRB* gene in thyroid cancer cell lines inhibited cell proliferation and migration through suppressing the activation of the β-catenin signaling pathway. These results unequivocally demonstrated that TRβt can function as a tumor suppressor in human thyroid cancer (Kim et al. 2013). Another study elucidated the mechanisms by which that TRβt could act as a tumor suppressor (Kim et al. 2014b). The *THRB* gene was stably expressed in human follicular thyroid cancer cell lines (FTC-133 and FTC-236 cells). How the expressed TRβt affected cancer cell proliferation, migration, and tumor growth was evaluated in cell-based studies and xenograft models. Expression of TRβt reduced cancer cell proliferation and impeded the migration of tumor cells through inhibition of the AKT-mTOR-p70 S6K pathway. Importantly, new vessel formation was significantly suppressed in tumors via downregulation of vascular endothelial growth factor in FTC cells expressing TRβt (Kim et al. 2014b). These studies not only identified the signaling pathways suppressed by the expressed TRβt in human thyroid cancer cells but also raised the possibility that TRβt could be considered as a potential therapeutic target for thyroid cancer.

That TRβt could function as a tumor suppressor in breast cancer was evaluated in human MCF-7 cells stably expressing the *THRB* gene (Park et al. 2013). Cell-based studies indicate that the estrogen (E2)-dependent growth of MCF-7 cells was inhibited by the expression of TRβt in the presence of the thyroid hormone. In a xenograft mouse model, TRβt suppressed E2-dependent tumor growth of MCF-7 cells. Molecular analysis showed that TRβ1 acted to activate apoptosis and decrease proliferation of tumor cells via downregulation of the JAK-STAT-cyclin D pathways (Park et al. 2013). This in vivo evidence shows that TRβ1 could act as a tumor suppressor in breast tumorigenesis. However, it is notable that TRβ1 functions as a tumor suppressor via different signaling pathways in breast and thyroid cancers (Kim et al. 2014b; Park et al. 2013).

Besides human thyroid cancer cells and breast MCF-7 cancer cells, TRβ1 was also shown to be a tumor suppressor in hepatocarcinoma SK-hep1 cells and breast cancer MDA-MB-468 cells (Martinez-Iglesias et al. 2009). Expression of TRβ1 induces partial mesenchymal-to-epithelial cell transition and inhibits invasiveness, extravasation, and metastasis formation in mice. Cell-based studies demonstrated that TRβ1 abolishes anchorage-independent growth and migration, and it blocks responses to epidermal growth factor, insulin-like growth factor 1, and transforming growth factor β. In addition, TRβ1 suppresses the activated extracellular signal-regulated kinase and phosphatidylinositol 3-kinase signaling pathways to decrease cell proliferation and invasiveness (Martinez-Iglesias et al. 2009). The tumor suppressor role of TRβ1 was demonstrated in neuroblastoma cells. Treatment of cells with T3 inhibits ras-induced cell proliferation, blocks induction of cyclin D1 expression, and suppresses tumor development in nude mice (Garcia-Silva and Aranda 2004). These studies clearly show that TRβ1 can act as a tumor suppressor in many types of cancer cells, and its mechanisms of action depend on cellular context.

Some compelling evidence to support the tumor suppressor role of TRs came from in vivo studies using genetically engineered mice in which both the *Thrb* and *Thra* genes were deleted ($Thral^{-/-}/Thrb^{-/-}$ mice) (Zhu et al. 2010). Remarkably, as $Thral^{-/-}/Thrb^{-/-}$ mice age, they spontaneously develop follicular thyroid cancer with the pathological progression of hyperplasia, capsular invasion, vascular invasion, anaplasia, and metastasis, similar to human thyroid cancer (Zhu et al. 2010). Detailed molecular analysis revealed that known tumor promoters such as the pituitary tumor-transforming gene (*Pttg*) were activated and tumor suppressors such as *Pparγ* and *TP-53* were suppressed during carcinogenesis. In addition, consistent with the human cancer, AKT-mTOR-p70 signaling and vascular growth factor and its receptor were activated to facilitate tumor progression. Thus, loss of normal tumor suppressor functions in both TRβ1 and TRαl promotes tumor development and metastasis. However, the impact of such loss of tumor suppressor functions in other cancers has not been evaluated.

The Oncogenic Actions of TRβ Mutants

That TRb1 could act as a tumor suppressor and its reduced or silenced expression promotes cancer progression predicted that mutated TRβ1 could act as an oncogene. This prediction was borne out by the discovery that the $Thrb^{PV/PV}$ mouse spontaneously develops follicular thyroid cancer (Suzuki et al. 2002). Subsequently, other mouse models of thyroid cancer were also developed to understand the oncogenic actions of TRβ1 mutants in vivo.

Mouse Models of Thyroid Cancer

(a) *The* $Thrb^{PV/PV}$ *mouse*: The pathological progression and frequency of capsular invasion (Fig. 3a), vascular invasion (Fig. 3b), anaplasia (Fig. 3c), and metastasis (Fig. 3d) of thyroid cancer of $Thrb^{PV/PV}$ mice are similar to human follicular thyroid cancer. Extensive characterization of the altered signaling pathways during thyroid carcinogenesis of the $Thrb^{PV/PV}$ mouse identified the activation of tumor promoters such as cyclin D1, β-catenin, phosphatidylinositol 3-kinase (PI3K), protein kinase B (AKT), the steroid receptor coactivator-3, and PTTG and the repression of tumor suppressors such as PPARγ. These altered signaling pathways during thyroid carcinogenesis of $Thrb^{PV/PV}$ mice are consistent with

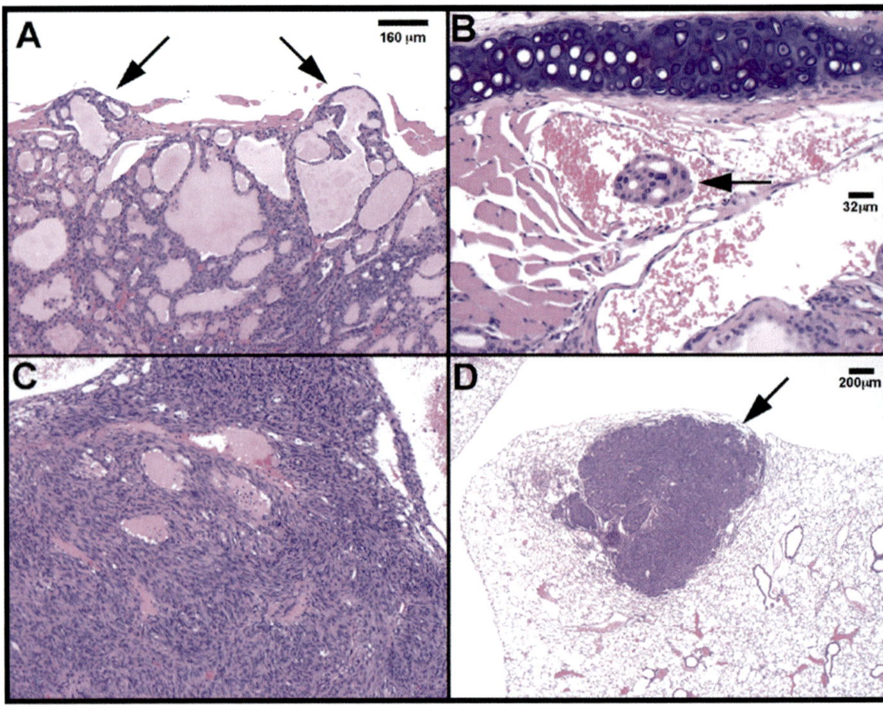

Fig. 3 *Thrb*$^{PV/PV}$ mice spontaneously develop metastatic follicular thyroid carcinoma with pathological progression similar to what is observed in human cancer. Representative features of thyroid carcinogenesis in *Thrb*$^{PV/PV}$ mice: (**a**) capsular invasion in the thyroid; (**b**) vascular invasion in the thyroid; (**c**) anaplasia; and (**d**) metastatic thyroid carcinoma lesions in the lung

the changes reported for the carcinogenesis in the human thyroid. When *Thrb*$^{PV/PV}$ mice were treated with inhibitors of PI3K or an agonist to activate the tumor-suppressing activity of PPARγ, the tumor progression was delayed and metastasis was blocked (Kato et al. 2006; Furuya et al. 2007), further validating the contributions of these two altered signaling pathways in thyroid carcinogenesis.

Subsequently, several mouse models were developed by additional genetic modification of *Thrb*$^{PV/PV}$ mice to gain further insights in the oncogenic actions of TRβ1PV in thyroid carcinogenesis. These mouse models are briefly described below.

(b) *The Thrb*$^{PV/-}$*mouse*: The finding that mutation of one allele of the *Thrb* gene is not sufficient to induce thyroid cancer prompted studies of addressing the question whether the presence of one allele of TR mutation in the absence of the other allele is sufficient to induce thyroid cancer. A *Thrb*$^{PV/-}$mouse was created by crossing heterozygous *Thrb*$^{PV/+}$ mice with *Thrb*$^{+/-}$mice (Kato et al. 2004). Remarkably, mice with one mutated *Thrb* allele together with deletion of the other allele developed thyroid carcinoma with a pathological progression that is similar to that found in *Thrb*$^{PV/PV}$ mice (Kato et al. 2004). These results support the notion that the remaining wild-type *Thrb* allele in heterozygous *Thrb*$^{PV/+}$ mice could act as tumor suppressor to ameliorate the oncogenic activity of TRβ1PV. In *Thrb*$^{PV/-}$mice, the loss of the wild-type *Thrb* allele allows the full expression of oncogenic actions of TRβ1PV to mediate thyroid carcinogenesis.

(c) *The Thrb*$^{PV/PV}$*/Pten*$^{\pm/\sim}$ *mouse*: Inactivation and silencing of phosphatase and tensin homologue deleted from the chromosome 10 (*PTEN*) gene have been observed in follicular thyroid carcinoma. During carcinogenesis, PTEN functions as a tumor suppressor by attenuating the PI3K-AKT signaling pathway critical for cancer development and growth. *Thrb*$^{PV/PV}$*/Pten*$^{+/\sim}$ mice with haploinsufficiency of the *Pten* gene were generated to assess the impact of the PTEN loss in thyroid carcinogenesis (Guigon et al. 2009). PTEN deficiency promoted the progression of thyroid tumor with increased metastatic spread to the lung and resulted in significantly reduced survival. AKT signaling was further aberrantly activated in thyroid tumors in *Thrb*$^{PV/PV}$*/Pten*$^{+/-}$ mice as evidenced by increased activity of the downstream mammalian target of rapamycin (mTOR)-p70S6K signaling and decreased activity of the forkhead family member FOXO3a. Increased cyclin D1 was accompanied by decreased apoptosis as shown by increased nuclear factor-kappaB (NF-kappaB) and decreased caspase-3 activity in thyroid tumors. These results clearly indicated the PI3K-AKT signaling is a driver in thyroid carcinogenesis, and the loss of the *Pten* gene is a critical regulator in thyroid carcinogenesis.

(d) *The Thrb*$^{PV/PV}$*/Pttg*$^{-/-}$ *mouse*: The pituitary tumor-transforming gene (PTTG) is a human securin protein and has a central role in maintaining sister chromatid cohesiveness during mitosis. The roles of PTTG as a transcription factor and in DNA repair suggest that it could also contribute to tumorigenesis. Elucidation of PTTG's role in tumorigenesis has been advanced through study of PTTG knockout mice. While under- and overexpression of PTTG may adversely affect chromosomal stability, PTTG1 knockout mice (*Pttg*$^{/-}$ mice) are viable and fertile. However, when *Pttg*$^{-/-}$ mice were crossed with the *Rb*$^{+/-}$ mouse that develops pituitary tumors, the *Rb*$^{+/-}$*/Pttg*$^{-/-}$ mice had decreased incidence of pituitary tumor development compared to *Rb*$^{+/-}$ mice (Chesnokova et al. 2005). These studies suggest that PTTG1 is a proto-oncogene in the pituitary and deletion of PTTG1 may delay or prevent tumor development. PTTG has also been associated with thyroid cancer through promotion of genetic instability. To define the role of PTTG1 in follicular thyroid cancer, the *Pttg* gene was deleted in *Thrb*$^{PV/PV}$ mice (Kim et al. 2007). Histological examination documented no difference in follicular thyroid cancer occurrence between *Thrb*$^{PV/PV}$ mice and *Thrb*$^{PV/PV}$*/Pttg*$^{-/-}$ mice which indicates that PTTG removal does not prevent the initiation of follicular thyroid cancer. However, *Thrb*$^{PV/PV}$ *Pttg*$^{-/-}$ mice had a significant decrease in vascular invasion and less development of lung metastasis as they progressively aged. Tumor cell proliferation was decreased via decreased protein levels of phosphorylated Rb and an elevation of the CDK inhibitor p21 in *Thrb*$^{PV/PV}$ *Pttg*$^{-/-}$ mice (Kim et al. 2007). These findings indicate that PTTG1 could affect thyroid carcinogenesis. How PTTG1 could impact thyroid carcinogenesis was elucidated by Ying et al (Ying et al. 2006) which showed that the stability of PTTG1 was increased by physical association with TRβ1PV. The accumulated PTTG1 impeded mitotic progression in cells expressing TRβ1PV, thus contributing to thyroid carcinogenesis (Ying et al. 2006).

(e) *The* $Thrb^{PV/PV}Ncor1^{\Delta ID/\Delta ID}$ *mouse*: Studies have indicated that the dominant negative activity of TRβ1PV in mediating RTHβ is regulated by NCOR1 (Fozzatti et al. 2011).

$Thrb^{PV/PV}/Ncor1^{\Delta ID/\Delta ID}$ mice were generated to examine the oncogenic actions of TRβ1PV in thyroid carcinogenesis of the corepressor complex (Fozzatti et al. 2013b). The lack of association of TRβ1PV with NCOR1ΔID in $Thrb^{PV/PV}/Ncor1^{\Delta ID/\Delta ID}$ mice led to suppression of thyroid tumor growth, delayed tumor progression, and prolonged survival. Molecular analysis demonstrated that increased expression of CDK inhibitor 1 ($p21^{waf1/cip1}$, *Cdkn1A*) inhibited tumor cell proliferation and the elevated expression of proapoptotic BCL-associated X (Bax) promoted apoptosis. The expression of *Cdkn1A* and *Bax* genes is directly regulated by p53. In the thyroid tumor of $Thrb^{PV/PV}$ mice, p53 was recruited to the p53-binding site on the proximal promoter of the *Cdkn1A* and the *Bax* genes to associate with TRb1PV-NCOR1-histone deacetylase-3 (HDAC-3) complexes, leading to repression of the *Cdkn1A* gene as well as the *Bax* gene. In the thyroid tumor of $Thrb^{PV/PV}/Ncor1^{\Delta ID/\Delta ID}$ mice, p53 associated with TRβ1PV cannot be recruited to the corepressor complex, resulting in the derepression of these two genes to suppress cancer progression. Thus, NCOR1 can not only modulate RTHβ but also regulate the carcinogenesis of the thyroid.

(f) *The* $Thrb^{PV/PV}Kras^{G12D}$ *mouse*: To understand how a *RAS* mutated gene can impact thyroid carcinogenesis, a mouse model was created targeting the $Kras^{G12D}$ mutation to thyroid epithelial cells of $Thrb^{PV/PV}$ mice (Zhu et al. 2014a). The expression of the $Kras^{G12D}$ mutated gene in the thyroid dramatically changed the tumor phenotype of $Thrb^{PV/PV}$ mice. In addition to more extensive hyperplasia (Fig. 4a) and development of capsular and vascular invasion at an earlier age (Fig. 4b), a higher frequency of occurrence and an earlier appearance of anaplastic foci (Fig. 4c, d) were detected in $Thrb^{PV/PV}/Kras^{G12D}$ mice than $Thrb^{PV/PV}$ mice. Moreover, an increased frequency of occurrence of lung (Fig. 4e) and heart metastasis (Fig. 4f) was also found in $Thrb^{PV/PV}/Kras^{G12D}$ mice. These double mutant mice display markedly reduced survival. Further analysis of the anaplastic foci indicated the complete loss of differentiation with loss of normal thyroid follicular morphology and with reduced expression of the differentiation marker, the transcription factor paired box gene 8 (PAX8). These aggressive phenotypic cancer characteristics mimic those of anaplastic thyroid cancer. Within the anaplastic foci, the loss of PAX8 expression was accompanied by concomitant upregulation of c-MYC (hereafter referred to as MYC). Upregulated MYC contributes to the initiation of undifferentiated thyroid cancer, in part, via enhancing TRβ1PV-mediated repression of the *Pax8* expression. cDNA microarray analyses comparing global gene expression profiles of thyroid tumor lesions of $Thrb^{PV/PV}$ and $Thrb^{PV/PV}Kras^{G12D}$ mice identified 14 upstream

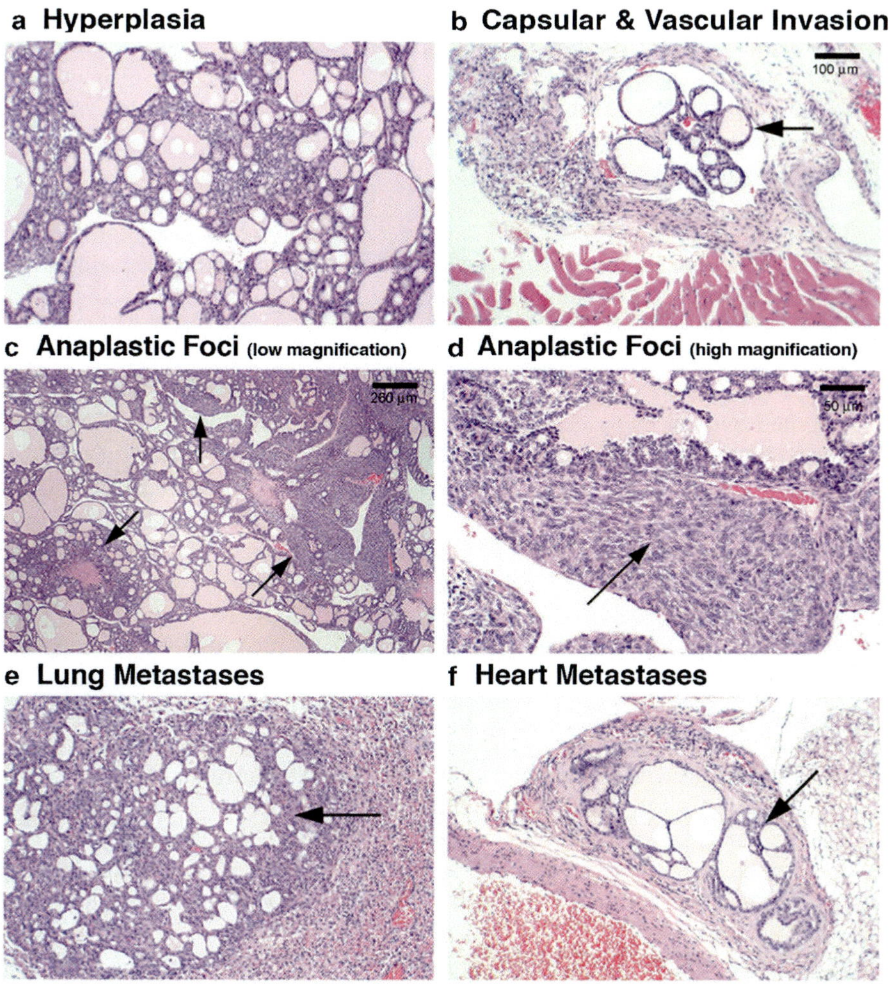

Fig. 4 Histopathologic features of anaplastic thyroid carcinoma in $Thrb^{PV/PV}Kras^{G12D}$ mice. Panels show (**a**) hyperplasia, (**b**) capsular invasion and vascular invasion, (**c**) anaplastic foci at low magnification and (**d**) anaplastic foci at high magnification, (**e**) microscopic lung metastases, and (**f**) heart metastases in $Thrb^{PV/PV}/Kras^{G12D}$ mice at 2–5 months of age

regulators that functioned as key effectors in growth factor-induced signaling to promote thyroid tumor growth of $Thrb^{PV/PV}/Kras^{G12D}$ mice. Further analysis identified integrins as key upstream regulators to stimulate ERBB2-mediated downstream signaling in thyroid tumors of $Thrb^{PV/PV}Kras^{G12D}$ mice.

Additional studies uncovered integrin-activated ERBB2 signaling as one of the mechanisms in synergy between TRβPV and KRASG12D signaling to promote aggressive tumor growth in undifferentiated thyroid cancer (Zhu et al. 2014a, b).

Molecular Mechanisms of Oncogenic Actions of TRβ Mutants

Studies in the mouse models of thyroid cancer (see section "Mouse Models of Thyroid Cancer") have provided insights of molecular mechanisms of oncogenic actions of TRβ mutants and uncovered complex signaling pathways critical in thyroid carcinogenesis. Lessons learned from the mouse models of thyroid cancer are summarized below.

(a) *Oncogenic actions of TRβ mutants via direct protein-protein interaction with key cellular regulators*. Aberrant activation of PI3K-AKT signaling is a major driver in the carcinogenesis of human thyroid (Xing 2010). This abnormal activation of PI3K-AKT signaling is reproduced in the $Thrb^{PV/PV}$ mouse, the $Thrb^{PV/-}$ mouse, and the $Thrb^{PV/PV}/Pten^{+/-}$ mouse. These observations indicate a common molecular mechanism by which TRβ1PV activates PI3K-AKT signaling. Accordingly, the mechanisms by which TRβ1PV acted to increase PI3K activity were ascertained (Furuya et al. 2006). Co-immunoprecipitation assays and confocal microscopy showed that TRβ1PV complexed with the p85α subunit of PI3K to activate the enzymatic activity of PI3K. The sequestering of TRβ1PV by p85α in both the nuclear and extranuclear compartments allowed TRβ1PV to activate various PI3K downstream signaling cascades. Studies also showed that TRβ1PV competes with NCOR1 to interact with p85 (Furuya et al. 2007). The NCOR1 protein level is lower in the thyroid of $Thrb^{PV/PV}$ mice, thereby favoring the physical interaction of TRβ1PV with p85 to overactivate PI3K activity, leading to increased cell proliferation, motility, and migration, and to inhibit apoptosis in thyroid tumor cells (Furuya et al. 2007).

Via direct protein-protein interaction, TRβ1PV also acted to alter the stability of the pituitary tumor-transforming gene (*PTTG*). PTTG is a mammalian securin that is a critical mitotic checkpoint protein involved in maintaining sister chromatid cohesiveness before entering anaphase. The search for genes underlying the chromosomal aberrations in $Thrb^{PV/PV}$ mice by cDNA microarray led to the discovery that *Pttg* mRNA levels were significantly increased in thyroid cancer (Ying et al. 2003a). In addition, cellular PTTG protein levels were markedly increased in the primary lesions of thyroid as well as lung metastasis of $Thrb^{PV/PV}$ mice (Ying et al. 2006). Subsequently, studies elucidated that TRβ1PV physically interacts with PTTG, but because it does not bind T3, it does not interact with SRC-3/PA28 to activate PTTG degradation. The absence of degradation leads to PTTG accumulation and inhibition of mitotic progression (Ying et al. 2006). In $Thrb^{PV/PV}/Pttg^{-/-}$ mice as compared with $Thrb^{PV/PV}$ mice, there was a consistent decrease in thyroid cell proliferation. The thyroids of $Thrb^{PV/PV}/Pttg^{-/-}$ mice were significantly smaller, and the occurrence of metastasis spread to the lung was less frequent (Kim et al. 2007). Altogether, these data indicate that abnormal accumulation of PTTG via direct interaction with TRβ1PV in the thyroids of $Thrb^{PV/PV}$ mice contributes to thyroid carcinogenesis by affecting cell cycle progression and inducing genetic instability.

TRβ1PV also found to physically interact with β-catenin, a central mediator of the Wnt signaling pathway, that is critical for a variety of cellular processes including cell proliferation, cell apoptosis, and cell migration. In thyroid tumors of *Thrb*$^{PV/PV}$ mice, the cellular abundance of β-catenin was aberrantly highly elevated. Elucidation of the underlying mechanism of the elevated β -catenin showed that TRβ1PV strongly interacts with β-catenin. The loss of T3-binding activity in TRβ1PV inhibits the release of β-catenin from TRβ1PV-β-catenin complexes in the presence of T3, thereby preventing β-catenin degradation via proteasome pathways. The absence of β-catenin degradation leads to β-catenin accumulation, resulting in constitutive activation of its oncogenic signaling to promote thyroid carcinogenesis (Guigon et al. 2008).

The discovery that TRβ1PV physically interacts with integrins α5 and β1, c-Src (hereafter referred to as Src), and focal adhesion kinase (FAK) in the integrin-regulated FAK-Src signaling pathway greatly increased our understanding of how TRβ1PV drives invasion and metastasis in *Thrb*$^{PV/PV}$ mice, the *Thrb*$^{PV/-}$ mouse, and the *Thrb*$^{PV/PV}$/*Pten*$^{+/-}$ mouse. Interactions of integrin receptors and basement membrane/extracellular membrane components with subsequent degradation of extracellular membrane by matrix metalloproteinases (MMPs) promote cancer cell invasion through the membrane barriers. Activated by their ligands, integrin receptors undergo conformational changes to activate intracellular signaling molecules such as Src and FAK. Overactivation of Src and its downstream effector, FAK, is associated with invasive potential in thyroid cancer. In thyroid tumors of *Thrb*$^{PV/PV}$ mice, increased protein abundance of integrins α5, αV, β1, and β3 and their ligand fibronectin were detected (Lu et al. 2010). TRβtPV was found to directly interact with integrins α5 and β1 to activate the Src kinase pathway by increasing phosphorylation, resulting in activation of FAK by increasing phosphorylation on several tyrosine sites (Lu et al. 2010). In addition, TRβtPV also physically interacts with FAK to form large PV-integrin-FAK-PI3K complexes. Subsequent activation of downstream signaling of p38 mitogen-activated protein kinase (MAPK) via increased phosphorylation cascades stimulates the expression of MMP-9 at the mRNA and protein levels. The activation of Src-FAK signaling is known to remodel the actin cytoskeleton in cancer cells critical for aberrant cell migration and invasion. It is known that β-actin in association with erzin links the cytoskeletal structure and the plasma membrane. The protein abundance of both β-actin and erzin was increased to affect cell cytoskeletal structure in thyroid tumors. Thus, formation of TRβtPV complexes with proteins such as integrins, β-actin, as well as erzin is a novel mechanism by which TRβtPV could change cytoskeletal organization to promote cell migration and invasion.

The activation of integrin-Src-FAK signaling by complexing with TRβtPV led to the hypothesis that inhibition of Src activity in the *Thrb*$^{PV/PV}$/*Pten*$^{+/-}$mouse would block cell invasion and metastasis. This hypothesis was tested by treating *Thrb*$^{PV/PV}$/*Pten*$^{+/-}$mice with a Src-specific inhibitor, SKI-606. Remarkably, inhibition of Src activity ameliorated the aberrant activation of Src and its downstream targets and markedly inhibited the growth of thyroid tumor, thereby prolonging the survival of treated mice. Importantly, SKI-606 dramatically prevented dedifferentiation, vascular invasion, and lung metastasis of thyroid cancer cells. These responses were meditated by downregulation of mitogen-activated protein kinase pathways and inhibition of the epithelial-mesenchymal transition. Thus the aberrant activation of Src via physical interaction with TRβtPV could be blocked by specific inhibitors (Kim et al. 2012).

(b) *Oncogenic actions of TRB mutants via transcription regulation.* PPARγ is a member of the nuclear receptor superfamily, acting as a ligand-dependent transcription factor. It was proposed to be a tumor suppressor in human thyroid follicular cancer (Kroll et al. 2000). In $Thrb^{PV/PV}$ mice, the *Pparγ* mRNA, as well as the PPARγ protein level, is markedly decreased. In lung metastases, the PPARγ protein level was not detectable (Ying et al. 2003b). Elucidation of the underlying molecular mechanism regarding how TRβ1PV suppresses the expression of the *Pparγ* gene showed that TRβ1PV cross talks with PPARγ signaling and represses the ligand-dependent transcription activity of PPARγ (Kato et al. 2006). TRβ1PV either competes with PPARγ for binding to the peroxisome proliferator-responsive element (PPRE) as homodimers or forms heterodimers with PPARγ, thereby repressing the transcription activity of PPARγ. The PPRE-bound TRβ1PV recruits NCOR1 to the promoters of PPARγ target genes to block the recruitment of the coactivators to the PPRE-bound PV-PPARγ complexes. In the thyroid tumors of $Thrb^{PV/PV}$ mice, signaling of PPARγ downstream tumor suppressor target genes was reduced as a result of the repression of transcriptional activity of PPARγ as well as reduced PPARγ expression, to promote thyroid cancer progression (Ying et al. 2003b). In other studies, the role of PPARγ as a tumor suppressor was examined in a mouse model in which the oncogenic *Pax8-Pparγ* (*PPFP*) gene was targeted to the thyroid with deficiency of the *Pten* gene (Dobson et al. 2011). The mice with both the expression of *PPFP* and deficiency of the *Pten* gene developed metastatic thyroid cancer. Furthermore, treatment of the mice with the PPARγ agonist pioglitazone decreased thyroid growth and prevented metastatic disease, thus supporting the critical role of PPARγ in thyroid carcinogenesis (Dobson et al. 2011) and further highlighting the important mode of TRbPV oncogenic action in transcription regulation via cross talking with PPARγ.

In addition to cross talk with other transcription factors, TRβ1PV can also exert its oncogenic actions via transcription regulation. The genomic expression profiles of laser capture microdissected thyroid tumor lesions of $Thrb^{PV/PV}$ mice, and hyperplastic thyroid cells of PTU-treated wild-type mice were compared (Lu et al. 2011). Analyses of the gene expression data indicated that the expression of 150 genes were significantly altered between $Thrb^{PV/PV}$ and PTU-treated wild-type mice (87 genes had higher expression and 63 genes had lower expression in $Thrb^{PV/PV}$ mice than in PTU-treated wild-type mice). Thirty-six percent of genes with altered expression function as key regulators in metastasis. The remaining genes were involved in various cellular processes including metabolism, intracellular trafficking, transcriptional regulation, post-transcriptional modification, and cell-cell/extracellular matrix signaling. While these altered profiles in the primary lesions of $Thrb^{PV/PV}$ mice could be caused by both primary and secondary effects, it is reasonable to assume that TRβ1PV might exert its oncogenic effects via transcription regulation. In addition, the global gene expression studies have uncovered novel genes responsible for the metastatic spread of follicular thyroid cancer. The gene expression profile also indicated that the metastatic process of thyroid cancer requires effective collaboration among genes with diverse cellular functions (Lu et al. 2011).

How TRβ1PV collaborates with KRASG12D in the thyroid of $Thrb^{PV/PV}/Kras^{G12D}$ mice to induce aggressive dedifferentiated thyroid cancer was also examined at the transcription level by global gene expression profiling (Zhu et al. 2014b). Comparison analysis of the array data between $Thrb^{PV/PV}/Kras^{G12D}$ mice and $Thrb^{PV/PV}$ mice showed that 311 genes were differentially expressed. Of those 311 genes, 150 were upregulated and 161 were downregulated. Comparison between $Thrb^{PV/PV}/Kras^{G12D}$ mice and $Kras^{G12D}$ mice displayed 2,492 genes; among them 1436 genes were upregulated and 1056 were downregulated. Comparison between $Thrb^{PV/PV}$ mice and $Kras^{G12D}$ mice identified 1952 differentially expressed genes of which 1143 were upregulated and 809 were downregulated. No thyroid cancer was detected in $Kras^{G12D}$ mice (Zhu et al. 2014a) and only differentiated follicular thyroid cancer was observed in $Thrb^{PV/PV}$ mice. Further analyses of microarray data identified 14 upstream regulators that were significantly altered in thyroid tumors of $Thrb^{PV/PV}$ mice and $Thrb^{PV/PV}/Kras^{G12D}$ mice. Most of these genes with altered expression function as key regulators in growth factor-induced signaling. Q/PCR analysis validated the array data by showing that integrins were elevated to act as upstream activators to stimulate ERBB2-mediated downstream signaling in thyroid tumors of $Thrb^{PV/PV}/Kras^{G12D}$ mice. Thus, the integrin-activated ERBB2 signaling is one of the mechanisms in synergy between TRβPV and KRASG12D signaling via transcription regulation that promotes aggressive tumor growth in undifferentiated thyroid cancer (Zhu et al. 2014a, b).

Summary and Conclusions

The bimodal switch model (Fig. 1b) has been used to understand the functions of thyroid hormone in gene transcription via study gene-by-gene. Recent technological advances make it possible to concurrently examine the details of gene regulation for each individual gene in different cell types. Genome-wide studies have provided important new insights into how TR interacts with thyroid hormone response elements, transcription enhancers, and other regulatory proteins in the genome. Such studies have significantly advanced our understanding of TR actions in that the interaction of TR with chromatin is not static but is a dynamic process. As genome-wide studies have continued to expand to include more target tissues and with different hormonal conditions, more valuable insights into the genomic actions of thyroid hormone, having broader scope and greater depth, are foreseeable in the near future.

Studies in mouse models further advance our understanding of thyroid hormone receptors in human diseases. Mutations of the *THRB* gene were first identified in RTHβ, and since then significant progress has been made in the understanding of the molecular actions of TRβ mutants in RTHβ. Discovery of patients with mutations of the *THRA* gene has clearly demonstrated that the actions of TR mutants are TR isoform-dependent because the pathological manifestations of RTHα and RTHβ patients are distinct. Additional mutations of the *THRA* gene will certainly continue to be discovered to understand RTHα. Beyond RTH, mutated TRs have been shown to play critical roles in the development and progression of cancer via direct protein-protein interaction as well as transcription regulation. Although most studies have focused on thyroid cancer, the link of TR mutations to other cancers such as breast cancer and renal cancer has also been established (Martinez-Iglesias et al. 2009; Szymanski et al. 2016). The studies on the roles of TRs in diseases may provide new insights into how to better treat the patients with mutations of *THR* genes. Understanding of the functions and biology of mutant TRs will facilitate the study of functions and mechanisms of action of other mutated receptors in the nuclear receptor family.

Cross-References

- ▶ Endocrine Functions of Bone
- ▶ Molecular Mechanisms of Thyroid Hormone Synthesis and Secretion
- ▶ Nongenomic Actions of Thyroid Hormones
- ▶ Steroid Hormones: Synthesis, Secretion, and Transport
- ▶ Synthesis, Secretion, and Transport of Peptide Hormones
- ▶ Targeting of Steroid Hormone Receptor Function in Breast and Prostate Cancer
- ▶ The Endocrine System
- ▶ The Parathyroids
- ▶ The Thyroid

References

Apriletti JW, et al. Molecular and structural biology of thyroid hormone receptors. Clin Exp Pharmacol Physiol Suppl. 1998;25:S2–11.

Ayers S, et al. Genome-wide binding patterns of thyroid hormone receptor beta. PLoS One. 2014;9 (2), e81186.

Barlow C, Meister B, Lardelli M, Lendahl U, Vennstrom B. Thyroid abnormalities and hepatocellular carcinoma in mice transgenic for v-erbA. EMBO J. 1994;13(18):4241–50.

Bassett JH, et al. Thyroid hormone receptor alpha mutation causes a severe and thyroxine-resistant skeletal dysplasia in female mice. Endocrinology. 2014;155(9):3699–712.

Bochukova E, et al. A mutation in the thyroid hormone receptor alpha gene. N Engl J Med. 2012;366(3):243–9.

Chatonnet F, Guyot R, Benoit G, Flamant F. Genome-wide analysis of thyroid hormone receptors shared and specific functions in neural cells. Proc Natl Acad Sci U S A. 2013;110(8):E766–75.

Chen JD, Evans RM. A transcriptional co-repressor that interacts with nuclear hormone receptors. Nature. 1995;377(6548):454–7.

Chesnokova V, Kovacs K, Castro AV, Zonis S, Melmed S. Pituitary hypoplasia in Pttg−/− mice is protective for Rb+/− pituitary tumorigenesis. Mol Endocrinol. 2005;19(9):2371–9.

Demir K, et al. Diverse genotypes and phenotypes of three novel thyroid hormone receptor-alpha mutations. J Clin Endocrinol Metab. 2016;101(8):2945–54.
Dobson ME, et al. Pioglitazone induces a proadipogenic antitumor response in mice with PAX8-PPARgamma fusion protein thyroid carcinoma. Endocrinology. 2011;152(11):4455–65.
Dumitrescu AM, Refetoff S. The syndromes of reduced sensitivity to thyroid hormone. Biochim Biophys Acta. 2013;1830(7):3987–4003.
Feng W, et al. Hormone-dependent coactivator binding to a hydrophobic cleft on nuclear receptors. Science. 1998;280(5370):1747–9.
Forrest D, Vennstrom B. Functions of thyroid hormone receptors in mice. Thyroid. 2000;10 (1):41–52.
Fozzatti L, et al. Resistance to thyroid hormone is modulated in vivo by the nuclear receptor corepressor (NCOR1). Proc Natl Acad Sci U S A. 2011;108(42):17462–7.
Fozzatti L, et al. Nuclear receptor corepressor (NCOR1) regulates in vivo actions of a mutated thyroid hormone receptor alpha. Proc Natl Acad Sci U S A. 2013a;110(19):7850–5.
Fozzatti L, Park JW, Zhao L, Willingham MC, Cheng SY. Oncogenic actions of the Nuclear Receptor Corepressor (NCOR1) in a mouse model of thyroid cancer. PLoS One. 2013b;8(6), e67954.
Furuya F, Hanover JA, Cheng SY. Activation of phosphatidylinositol 3-kinase signaling by a mutant thyroid hormone beta receptor. Proc Natl Acad Sci U S A. 2006;103(6):1780–5.
Furuya F, Lu C, Willingham MC, Cheng SY. Inhibition of phosphatidylinositol 3-kinase delays tumor progression and blocks metastatic spread in a mouse model of thyroid cancer. Carcinogenesis. 2007;28(12):2451–8.
Garcia-Silva S, Aranda A. The thyroid hormone receptor is a suppressor of ras-mediated transcription, proliferation, and transformation. Mol Cell Biol. 2004;24(17):7514–23.
Grontved L, et al. Transcriptional activation by the thyroid hormone receptor through ligand-dependent receptor recruitment and chromatin remodelling. Nat Commun. 2015;6:7048.
Guigon CJ, Zhao L, Lu C, Willingham MC, Cheng SY. Regulation of beta-catenin by a novel nongenomic action of thyroid hormone beta receptor. Mol Cell Biol. 2008;28(14):4598–608.
Guigon CJ, Zhao L, Willingham MC, Cheng SY. PTEN deficiency accelerates tumour progression in a mouse model of thyroid cancer. Oncogene. 2009;28(4):509–17.
Hashimoto K, et al. An unliganded thyroid hormone receptor causes severe neurological dysfunction. Proc Natl Acad Sci U S A. 2001;98(7):3998–4003.
Horlein AJ, et al. Ligand-independent repression by the thyroid hormone receptor mediated by a nuclear receptor co-repressor. Nature. 1995;377(6548):397–404.
Iwasaki Y, et al. Epigenetic inactivation of the thyroid hormone receptor beta1 gene at 3p24.2 in lung cancer. Ann Surg Oncol. 2010;17(8):2222–8.
Jazdzewski K, et al. Thyroid hormone receptor beta (THRB) is a major target gene for microRNAs deregulated in papillary thyroid carcinoma (PTC). J Clin Endocrinol Metab. 2011;96(3):E546–53.
Joseph B, Ji M, Liu D, Hou P, Xing M. Lack of mutations in the thyroid hormone receptor (TR) alpha and beta genes but frequent hypermethylation of the TRbeta gene in differentiated thyroid tumors. J Clin Endocrinol Metab. 2007;92(12):4766–70.
Kamiya Y, et al. Modulation by steroid receptor coactivator-1 of target- tissue responsiveness in resistance to thyroid hormone. Endocrinology. 2003;144(9):4144–53.
Kaneshige M, et al. Mice with a targeted mutation in the thyroid hormone beta receptor gene exhibit impaired growth and resistance to thyroid hormone. Proc Natl Acad Sci U S A. 2000;97 (24):13209–14.
Kaneshige M, et al. A targeted dominant negative mutation of the thyroid hormone alpha 1 receptor causes increased mortality, infertility, and dwarfism in mice. Proc Natl Acad Sci U S A. 2001;98 (26):15095–100.
Kato Y, Ying H, Willingham MC, Cheng SY. A tumor suppressor role for thyroid hormone beta receptor in a mouse model of thyroid carcinogenesis. Endocrinology. 2004;145(10):4430–8.
Kato Y, et al. PPARgamma insufficiency promotes follicular thyroid carcinogenesis via activation of the nuclear factor-kappaB signaling pathway. Oncogene. 2006;25(19):2736–47.

Kim WG, Cheng SY. Thyroid hormone receptors and cancer. Biochim Biophys Acta. 2013;1830 (7):3928–36.

Kim CS, Ying H, Willingham MC, Cheng SY. The pituitary tumor-transforming gene promotes angiogenesis in a mouse model of follicular thyroid cancer. Carcinogenesis. 2007;28(5):932–9.

Kim WG, et al. SKI-606, an Src inhibitor, reduces tumor growth, invasion, and distant metastasis in a mouse model of thyroid cancer. Clin Cancer Res. 2012;18(5):1281–90.

Kim WG, et al. Reactivation of the silenced thyroid hormone receptor beta gene expression delays thyroid tumor progression. Endocrinology. 2013;154(1):25–35.

Kim DW, Park JW, Willingham MC, Cheng SY. A histone deacetylase inhibitor improves hypothyroidism caused by a TRalpha1 mutant. Hum Mol Genet. 2014a;23(10):2651–64.

Kim WG, Zhao L, Kim DW, Willingham MC, Cheng SY. Inhibition of tumorigenesis by the thyroid hormone receptor beta in xenograft models. Thyroid. 2014b;24(2):260–9.

Kroll TG, et al. PAX8-PPARgamma1 fusion oncogene in human thyroid carcinoma [corrected]. Science. 2000;289(5483):1357–60.

Li J, et al. Both corepressor proteins SMRT and N-CoR exist in large protein complexes containing HDAC3. EMBO J. 2000;19(16):4342–50.

Ling Y, et al. Aberrant methylation of the THRB gene in tissue and plasma of breast cancer patients. Cancer Genet Cytogenet. 2010;196(2):140–5.

Liu YY, Schultz JJ, Brent GA. A thyroid hormone receptor alpha gene mutation (P398H) is associated with visceral adiposity and impaired catecholamine-stimulated lipolysis in mice. J Biol Chem. 2003;278(40):38913–20.

Lu C, Zhao L, Ying H, Willingham MC, Cheng SY. Growth activation alone is not sufficient to cause metastatic thyroid cancer in a mouse model of follicular thyroid carcinoma. Endocrinology. 2010;151(4):1929–39.

Lu C, Mishra A, Zhu YJ, Meltzer P, Cheng SY. Genomic profiling of genes contributing to metastasis in a mouse model of thyroid follicular carcinoma. Am J Cancer Res. 2011;1(1):1–13.

Martinez-Iglesias O, et al. Thyroid hormone receptor beta1 acts as a potent suppressor of tumor invasiveness and metastasis. Cancer Res. 2009;69(2):501–9.

Onate SA, Tsai SY, Tsai MJ, O'Malley BW. Sequence and characterization of a coactivator for the steroid hormone receptor superfamily. Science. 1995;270(5240):1354–7.

Park JW, Zhao L, Cheng SY. Inhibition of estrogen-dependent tumorigenesis by the thyroid hormone receptor beta in xenograft models. Am J Cancer Res. 2013;3(3):302–11.

Perissi V, Jepsen K, Glass CK, Rosenfeld MG. Deconstructing repression: evolving models of co-repressor action. Nat Rev Genet. 2010;11(2):109–23.

Ramadoss P, et al. Novel mechanism of positive versus negative regulation by thyroid hormone receptor beta1 (TRbeta1) identified by genome-wide profiling of binding sites in mouse liver. J Biol Chem. 2014;289(3):1313–28.

Sap J, et al. The c-erb-A protein is a high-affinity receptor for thyroid hormone. Nature. 1986;324 (6098):635–40.

Suzuki H, Cheng SY. Compensatory role of thyroid hormone receptor (TR) alpha 1 in resistance to thyroid hormone: study in mice with a targeted mutation in the TR beta gene and deficient in TR alpha 1. Mol Endocrinol. 2003;17(8):1647–55.

Suzuki H, Willingham MC, Cheng SY. Mice with a mutation in the thyroid hormone receptor beta gene spontaneously develop thyroid carcinoma: a mouse model of thyroid carcinogenesis. Thyroid. 2002;12(11):963–9.

Szymanski L, Matak D, Bartnik E, Szczylik C, Czarnecka AM. Thyroid hormones as renal cell cancer regulators. J Signal Transduct. 2016;2016:1362407.

van Mullem A, et al. Clinical phenotype and mutant TRalpha1. N Engl J Med. 2012;366 (15):1451–3.

van Mullem AA, et al. Clinical phenotype of a new type of thyroid hormone resistance caused by a mutation of the TRalpha1 receptor: consequences of LT4 treatment. J Clin Endocrinol Metab. 2013;98(7):3029–38.

Venero C, et al. Anxiety, memory impairment, and locomotor dysfunction caused by a mutant thyroid hormone receptor alpha1 can be ameliorated by T3 treatment. Genes Dev. 2005;19 (18):2152–63.

Weinberger C, et al. The c-erb-A gene encodes a thyroid hormone receptor. Nature. 1986;324 (6098):641–6.

Xing M. Genetic alterations in the phosphatidylinositol-3 kinase/Akt pathway in thyroid cancer. Thyroid. 2010;20(7):697–706.

Xu L, Glass CK, Rosenfeld MG. Coactivator and corepressor complexes in nuclear receptor function. Curr Opin Genet Dev. 1999;9(2):140–7.

Ying H, et al. Alterations in genomic profiles during tumor progression in a mouse model of follicular thyroid carcinoma. Carcinogenesis. 2003a;24(9):1467–79.

Ying H, et al. Mutant thyroid hormone receptor beta represses the expression and transcriptional activity of peroxisome proliferator-activated receptor gamma during thyroid carcinogenesis. Cancer Res. 2003b;63(17):5274–80.

Ying H, et al. Aberrant accumulation of PTTG1 induced by a mutated thyroid hormone beta receptor inhibits mitotic progression. J Clin Invest. 2006;116(11):2972–84.

Zhang XY, et al. Differential expression of thyroid hormone receptor isoforms dictates the dominant negative activity of mutant beta receptor. Mol Endocrinol. 2002;16(9):2077–92.

Zhu XG, Zhao L, Willingham MC, Cheng SY. Thyroid hormone receptors are tumor suppressors in a mouse model of metastatic follicular thyroid carcinoma. Oncogene. 2010;29(13):1909–19.

Zhu X, Zhao L, Park JW, Willingham MC, Cheng SY. Synergistic signaling of KRAS and thyroid hormone receptor beta mutants promotes undifferentiated thyroid cancer through MYC up-regulation. Neoplasia. 2014a;16(9):757–69.

Zhu X, Zhu YJ, Kim DW, Meltzer P, Cheng SY. Activation of integrin- ERBB2 signaling in undifferentiated thyroid cancer. Am J Cancer Res. 2014b;4(6):776–88.

Nongenomic Actions of Thyroid Hormones

10

Sandra Incerpi, Paul J. Davis, Jens Z. Pedersen, and Antonia Lanni

Abstract

Nongenomic actions of thyroid hormone do not require a direct interaction of 3,5,3′-triiodo-L-thyronine (T_3) with the transcriptionally active nuclear receptors TRα and TRβ. A rapid response time is a characteristic of many nongenomic actions; the onset of the majority of these effects is within minutes because the action is independent of gene expression and protein synthesis. While only T_3 is able to generate a genomic response, the different nongenomic effects may be activated by either T_3 or T_4 or by other iodothyronine derivatives such as T_2. In the last decade, the discovery of a large number of nongenomic actions of thyroid hormones has increasingly attracted the interest of researchers, and different specific binding sites or receptors for these hormones/messengers have now been described in several cellular compartments, including the external surface of the plasma membrane. The function of nongenomic effects of these hormones has mainly been considered to relate to homeostasis, such as actions on plasma membrane ion transporters or maintenance of the cytoskeleton, but recent evidence supports the existence of crosstalk between nongenomic and genomic

S. Incerpi (✉)
Department of Sciences, University Roma Tre, Rome, Italy
e-mail: sandra.incerpi@uniroma3.it

P.J. Davis
Pharmaceutical Research Institute, Albany College of Pharmacy and Health Sciences, and Albany Medical College, Albany, NY, USA
e-mail: pdavis.ordwayst@gmail.com

J.Z. Pedersen
Department of Biology, University of Rome Tor Vergata, Rome, Italy
e-mail: j.z.pedersen@gmail.com

A. Lanni
Department of Environmental, Biological, Pharmaceutical Sciences and Technologies, Second University of Naples, Caserta, Italy
e-mail: antonia.lanni@unina2.it

A. Belfiore, D. LeRoith (eds.), *Principles of Endocrinology and Hormone Action*, Endocrinology, https://doi.org/10.1007/978-3-319-44675-2_32

effects of the hormone. Further examination of such crosstalk may reveal hitherto unappreciated mechanisms underlying global illnesses, such as cardiovascular diseases, inflammatory and immune diseases, and mechanisms of tumor cell function. Indeed, these new aspects have already improved our understanding of the contributions of nongenomic thyroid hormone actions to the regulation of cancer-related angiogenesis and to cancer cell survival pathways. In the present report, we provide a concise overview of the main observations that define the nongenomic actions of thyroid hormones and give a description of the state of the art.

Keywords
Thyroid hormones • Nongenomic actions • Extranuclear receptors • Nuclear receptors • Integrin αvβ3 • Mitochondrial receptors • Signal transduction • Membrane transport • Immune system • Growth factors

Contents

Introduction

"Thyroid hormone" is conventionally defined as two compounds, L-thyroxine (T_4) and 3,5,3′-triiodo-L-thyronine (T_3), which are well known from standard textbooks and from routine clinical laboratory blood testing. T_3 acts through binding to nuclear thyroid hormone receptors (TRs) TRα and TRβ, which are protein transcription factors modulating the expression of many different genes. T_3 and T_4 also produce nongenomic effects that do not depend upon a primary interaction of hormone and TRs. The thyroid hormone family also includes several T_4- and T_3-derived metabolites, which are able to induce distinct biological effects of their own.

Our understanding of the mechanism of action of thyroid hormones began with the studies of Tata and coworkers who showed that the cell nucleus was the principal target of the hormone (Tata et al. 1962; Tata 1963). These authors found that

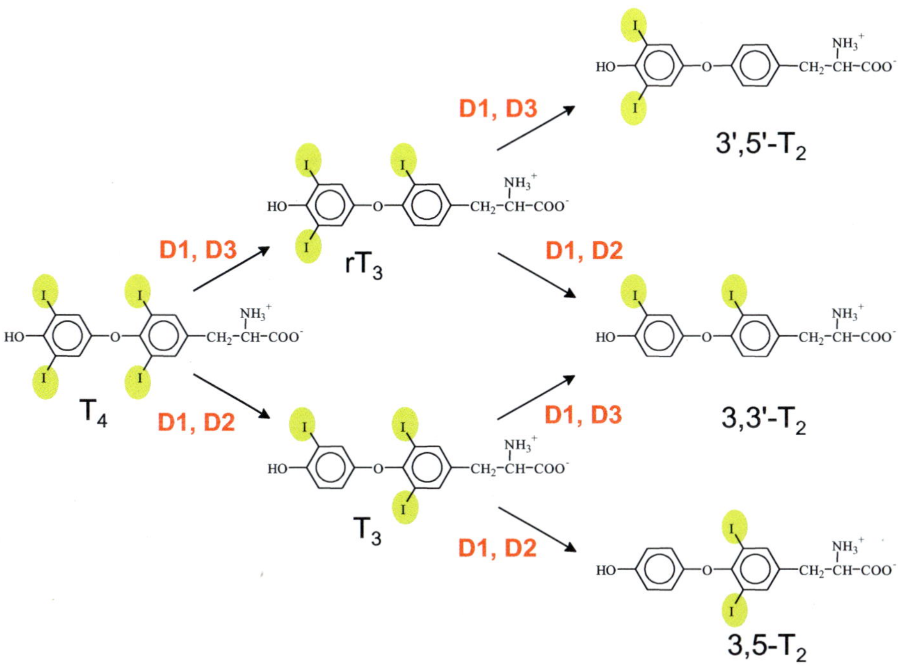

Fig. 1 Structures of the thyroid hormones and their principal metabolites. From the two main thyroid hormones T_4 and T_3 several other iodothyronine metabolites can be formed through the stepwise removal of the iodides through the catalytic activity of different deiodinase enzymes. The non-specific deiodinase D1 can remove iodide from both of the rings, whereas D2 only acts on the outer ring and D3 only on the inner ring. The isomer 3,3′,5-T_3 is the normal thyroid hormone that activates the nuclear receptors, while the form 3,3′,5′-T_3 is known as reverse-T_3 and produces several nongenomic effects. Of the three T_2 isomers only 3,5-T_2 at present appears to be of physiological importance as documented by a significant number of studies on its various biological actions, but the precise role of this iodothyronine is still not established. The same is true for other thyroid metabolites such as tetrac and triac. Finally it should be mentioned that also a 3-iodothyronamine compound with only one iodide remaining is known to produce different nongenomic effects (Piehl et al. 2011)

administration of T_3 to rats induced an increase in basal metabolic rates, but injecting T_3 in combination with actinomycin D (an inhibitor of transcription) completely abolished the stimulatory effect of T_3. Such observations led to the identification of specific nuclear binding sites or receptors for T_3 that initially were found in rat liver and kidney, and later in a variety of other tissues and cells (Lazar 2003; Oppenheimer et al. 1972, 1987). Eventually they were characterized as a family of nuclear receptors. Another step forward in the field of thyroid hormone action was the discovery of the deiodinases, which are involved in the peripheral metabolism of iodothyronines. These enzymes regulate the local and systemic availability of T_3 – the form of thyroid hormone principally active in the nucleus – and of other partially iodinated thyronines (Fig. 1). Today it is generally accepted that the majority of thyroid hormone effects are exerted by T_3 via the nuclear receptors, but it is also clear that not all the actions known involve the nuclear pathway and that iodothyronines other than T_3 also produce important biological responses (Moreno et al. 2008).

The Dawn of Nongenomic Effects

The discovery of the nongenomic effects of thyroid hormones dates to the late 1970s and the beginning of the 1980s. Injections of low doses of T_3 into thyroidectomized animals increased mitochondrial ATP production within minutes, accompanied by an increase in oxygen consumption. The stimulation was not abolished by inhibitors of protein synthesis, thus excluding the nuclear pathway (Sterling et al. 1978, 1980). Among the first reports of the existence of specific extranuclear targets were the nongenomic effects on the erythrocyte plasma membrane Na^+/K^+-ATPase activity, where high-affinity binding sites for triiodothyronine were found in rat erythrocyte membranes (Botta et al. 1983). One aspect that it is important to take into account in such studies is the structure–activity relationship, which can add value to the specificity of the nongenomic effects observed. In this case competition experiments involving the use of different analogs of T_3 showed a high affinity for L-T_3, whereas L-T_4, D-T_3, triiodothyroacetic acid (the deaminated analog of T_3), and reverse-T_3 had much lower affinity, suggesting a site specific for L-T_3. At that time it was not understood that it was the binding of the hormone that actually led to a nongenomic physiological response. However, in other studies a good correlation was found between the binding of T_3 to membranes and various "biological effects," such as changes in the Hill coefficient of membrane-bound acetylcholinesterase.

It was then discovered that T_3 also could affect protein phosphorylation in different tissues in less than 1 h, clearly implicating nongenomic actions. In the same years, other such "extranuclear" effects, as they were called originally (de Mendoza et al. 1978), were reported for various membrane transport systems and enzyme activities such as Ca^{2+}-ATPase, acetylcholinesterase, Na^+/K^+-ATPase, and glucose transport (de Mendoza et al. 1978; Galo et al. 1981; Davis and Blas 1981; Davis et al. 1983; Segal and Ingbar 1979, 1989). Later a nongenomic effect was also reported to involve the capability of T_4 to convert soluble actin to the fibrous form, affecting the cytoskeleton and type II iodothyronine 5′-deiodinase function (Siegrist-Kaiser et al. 1990), and from that study onward, several reports considered T_4 as the principal form of thyroid hormone involved in the nongenomic effects of thyroid hormones that we discuss here.

The Plasma Membrane, Transport Systems, and Channels

One of the main targets of thyroid hormones is the cardiovascular system. In this system the modulation of membrane transport systems such as the calcium pump and the Na^+/K^+-ATPase has a precise physiological relevance. Several genes are positively regulated by thyroid hormone in cardiomyocytes, in particular the α-myosin heavy chain; sarcoplasmic reticulum Ca^{2+}-ATPase; voltage-dependent potassium channels Kv 1.5, Kv 4.2, and Kv 4.3; the Na^+/K^+-ATPase; ryanodine receptors; the L-type calcium channel; and β-adrenergic receptors. Negatively regulated are β-myosin heavy chain, the Na^+/Ca^{2+} exchanger, phospholamban, and certain isoforms of adenylate cyclase (Farias et al. 2006). The physiological result of these activities is that T_3 increases the heart rate, speed, and force of systolic contraction, shortens the duration of diastolic relaxation, enhances vascular tone, and lowers plasma membrane lipid levels. The improved myocardial contractility and increased speed of diastolic relaxation induced by T_3 may be related to specific alterations in the level of the mRNA for Ca^{2+}-ATPase, resulting in an increased number of pump units. The major effects of T_3 are mediated by the nuclear receptors, and the degree of expression of the TR isoforms can affect cardiac function in a differential way, but the activities of the Ca^{2+}-ATPases of myocardial sarcolemma and sarcoplasmic reticulum can also be activated nongenomically. Both effects contribute to a reduction of sarcoplasmic (heart cytoplasmic) calcium content and improve myocardial relaxation and diastolic function, resulting in a cardioprotective effect (Farias et al. 2006). An interesting note is that the transport systems and other activities modulated by genomic mechanisms via the nuclear TR receptors also are the targets of nongenomic actions, and this is one of the first pieces of evidence for the existence of crosstalk between genomic and nongenomic pathways. Studies on rabbit heart ventricle by the patch clamp technique have shown that the opening of Na^+ channels is increased by T_3 at nanomolar concentrations in less than 1 minute. This effect has been confirmed by several later studies. The duration of the action potential in hypothyroid rat cardiomyocytes was significantly longer than in euthyroid cells, but treatment of the myocytes with T_3 (100 nM) shortened the duration of the potential, and the response was significant after only 5 min. This nongenomic action of T_3 in hypothyroid animals was ascribed to a modulation on the voltage-dependent potassium channel, the main contributor to repolarization. The effect was not observed in cells of euthyroid animals, unless the current was inhibited by pharmacological means (Ojamaa et al. 1996; Incerpi et al. 2011).

Also the functioning of potassium channels, such as the inward rectifier K^+ channel of the guinea pig ventriculum, is increased by T_3 (1 nM to μM) in 5 to 15 min after hormone addition, reaching a maximum at 25 min. This current is a determinant of the duration of the action potential (Sakaguki et al. 1996). In pituitary cells in culture, T_3 was found to stimulate the ether-à-go-go-related potassium channels rapidly through a mechanism that required the activation of phosphatidylinositol 3-kinase (PI3K) and was clearly nongenomic (Storey et al. 2002).

Very low plasma concentrations of free T_3 have been reported in patients after open heart surgery, but administration of the hormone has been able to restore normal levels within 1 h. In these cases T_3 may act as an inotropic agent capable of increasing cardiac output and reducing systemic vascular resistance (Novitzky et al. 1989a, b). A series of experiments have demonstrated acute effects of T_3 on myocyte contractile function. This effect was apparently not mediated solely through binding to the adrenergic receptor, but also appeared to reflect T_3-induced cAMP generation in the myocytes. In contrast, T_3 alone did not directly affect myocyte Na^+, K^+-ATPase activity, and it had no rapid effects on L-type Ca^{2+} channels or the intracellular Ca^{2+} levels (Walker et al. 1995). In vascular smooth muscle cells, both T_3 and T_4 rapidly induced coronary vasodilation (within seconds), and this mechanism was found to be independent of nitric oxide production (Ojamaa et al. 1996). It is likely that the effect is mediated by specific ion channels through kinase activation.

A stimulatory effect of physiological levels of thyroid hormones on the Na^+/H^+ exchanger, a transporter and housekeeping modulator of intracellular cell volume and pH, has been shown in rat skeletal muscle in culture (Incerpi et al. 1999; D'Arezzo et al. 2004). The effect appears to help cell recovery from an acid load after muscle contraction, and it was shown to be due to mobilization of intracellular calcium and activation of protein kinase C and mitogen-activated protein kinase (MAPK). That study was not extended to the heart muscle cells, but it has been shown that inhibition of the exchanger in myocardiocytes improved cardiomyocyte survival in the course of ischemia.

Another example of nongenomic activity of nuclear receptors is the T_3-dependent activation of PI3K. In human endothelial cells, the activation is achieved through direct interaction of nuclear receptor with the p85 subunit of PI3K, leading to phosphorylation and activation of Akt and endothelial nitric oxide synthase (Hiroi et al. 2006). In rat pituitary cells, the binding of T_3 to TRβ2 leads to activation of PI3K; consequent production of phosphatidylinositol 3,4,5-triphosphate and Rac regulates activity of KCHN2 channels, which are voltage-dependent potassium channels regulating the firing in electrically excitable cells (Storey et al 2006). The nuclear thyroid hormone receptor TRβ1 has also been shown to rapidly activate Akt in pancreatic β cells (Verga Falzacappa et al. 2007). An important contribution to the nongenomic effects of thyroid hormones has come from studies on mutant thyroid hormone receptors isolated from patients with thyroid hormone resistance (Refetoff et al. 2014). In particular the PV mutation (due to an insertion at codon-448 of the TRβ) leads to a mutant form in which T_3 binding and transcriptional function are lost. The TRβPV mouse exhibits thyroid hormone resistance and with time develops thyroid carcinoma. The mutant mouse displays higher PI3K activity than the wild type; this may be due to a physical interaction of the PV protein with the p85 regulatory subunit of PI3K, leading to cell growth and proliferation, as well as to cell migration, invasion and inhibition of apoptosis (Furuya et al. 2009). Furthermore, unliganded TRβ is known to associate with the nuclear receptor corepressor (NCoR), and this interaction modulates TRβ activity.

Nongenomic effects of thyroid hormones have also been studied in vivo in rat striated muscle (Irrcher et al. 2008). A single injection of T_3 gave rise to the selective activation of kinases in skeletal muscle, including p38 and AMP-activated protein kinase (AMPK), but not ERK1/2. p38 MAPKs are a family of kinases activated by environmental stress, cytokines, and the production of reactive oxygen species, an important component of signaling in muscle contraction. AMPK is a serine/threonine kinase and a nutritional sensor that responds to changes in AMP/ATP levels. The contractile activity of the muscle leads to mitochondrial biogenesis and to activation of transcription factors such as Nrf1, PPAR-γ, and PGC-1α. The latter is a nuclear-encoded transcriptional coactivator that plays a role in glucose metabolism, mitochondrial biogenesis, muscle fiber differentiation, and adaptive thermogenesis. PGC-1α is also a strong coactivator of TRβ and this may play a role in mitochondrial biogenesis (Irrcher et al. 2008).

Thyroid hormones are very important for the normal development and differentiation of the cells of the central nervous system (CNS) (Koibuchi and Chin 2000). Deficiency of thyroid hormones during the perinatal period may result in mental and physical retardation, leading to what in humans is called cretinism. Both genomic and nongenomic actions of thyroid hormones have been described for the central nervous system. In astrocytes T_4 is converted to T_3 by a 5′-deiodinase, and T_3 is then transferred to neurons where it binds to nuclear receptors to regulate gene expression. Both thyroid hormone T_4 and reverse T_3, but not T_3 itself, can modulate processes such as actin polymerization and the extracellular arrangement of laminin, an extracellular matrix protein which plays a primary role in nerve cell migration during the morphogenesis of the CNS, via interactions between components of the cytoskeleton and integrins (Farwell and Dubord-Tomasetti 1999). The cytoskeleton is an important element in the intracellular transport of organelles and vesicles. Cytoskeletal microfilaments are involved in intracellular transport of membrane proteins such as type II iodothyronine deiodinase. T_4 increases cytoskeletal actin turnover and the action of T_4 is inhibited by chemical disruption of microfilaments. The brain is particularly dependent upon the activity of type II deiodinase to generate T_3 from circulating T_4. In fact, T_4 promotes deiodinase inactivation by a mechanism that does not involve the nuclear receptor, but is strictly related to neuronal F-actin content. Both T_4 and reverse T_3, but not T_3, nongenomically increase cell F-actin content in parallel with an increase in the turnover of type II deiodinase, but the synthesis of the deiodinase is not altered (Siegrist-Kaiser et al. 1990; Farwell et al. 2005, 2006).

Experimental hypothyroidism has been widely used to study the roles of thyroid hormones in adult brain and in brain development. Experimental hypothyroidism has been achieved by thyroidectomy of pregnant female animals or induced by administration of an antithyroid drug, such as 6-propyl-2-thiouracil, and the biochemical and morphological results were evaluated in fetuses and newborns (Ahmed et al. 2012; Zamoner and Pessoa-Pureur 2011). The brain components primarily affected under these experimental conditions are the neurotransmitter system, the expression and activities of plasma membrane ion transport systems (Na^+/H^+-exchanger, Na^+/K^+-ATPase, and Ca^{2+}-ATPase), and the neuronal cytoskeleton. The same systems can also be modulated by nongenomic mechanisms of the hormone, as shown by many reports, some of which are discussed here (Davis and Blas 1981; Davis et al. 1983; Incerpi et al. 1999; D'Arezzo et al. 2004; Farwell et al. 2005; Lei et al. 2008; Scapin et al. 2009, 2010; Lei and Ingbar 2011). For a more detailed analysis, the reader is referred to the review by Ahmed et al. (2013).

Direct binding of T_3 to the ionotropic $GABA_A$ receptor was shown to result in a concentration-dependent biphasic modulation of chloride current in synaptoneurosomes (Martin et al. 1996). Local administration in vivo of T_4 rapidly inhibited fast excitatory postsynaptic potentials in the dentate gyrus of the hippocampus and consequent stimulation of the perforant pathway. This effect was particularly significant in hypothyroid rats. A similar response was found in isolated hippocampal slices. The perforant pathway together with the mossy fibers and Schaffer collaterals represents a circuit of long-term potentiation and is one of the components of long-term memory. Nongenomic actions of thyroid hormones lead to rapid changes in neuronal excitability in the hippocampus in adult euthyroid rats, depending on the relative levels of T_3 and T_4 (Caria et al. 2009). The ionotropic receptors of glutamate, the main excitatory neurotransmitter of CNS, are also affected by thyroid hormones by nongenomic mechanisms in different experimental systems (Puia 2011; Losi et al. 2008; Cao et al. 2011). Thyroid hormones also modulate activities of the AMPA receptor and kainate ionotropic channels as well as the ionotropic receptor for GABA, the main inhibitory neurotransmitter of the CNS. This regulation occurs in different ways, for example, through the levels of glutamate, through the synthesis and degradation of GABA, and through its release and reuptake by neurons. The majority of these effects are mediated by transcriptional mechanisms, but evidence also exists for a direct nongenomic action of thyroid hormones on ionotropic GABA receptors. In cultured hippocampal neurons, T_3 and T_4 in the micromolar concentration range decrease $GABA_A$-evoked currents (Puia 2011) by a noncompetitive nongenomic mechanism (Chapell et al. 1998; Martin et al. 2004) that perhaps involves direct interaction of the hormones with the $GABA_A$ receptor (Puia and Losi 2011).

Nongenomic Effects of Thyroid Hormones on the Immune Response

The immune system provides other examples of crosstalk between genomic and nongenomic mechanisms of thyroid hormones. In general hyperthyroidism enhances the immune response. This is indicated in terms of antibody production, immune cell migration, lymphocyte proliferation, and reactive oxygen species production, and it is associated with decreased proinflammatory marker release, antioxidant enzyme production, and increased immune functions (De Vito et al. 2011, 2012). Hypothyroidism often gives rise to the opposite effects for some of these parameters, decreasing the immune response, antibody production, cell migration, and lymphocyte proliferation (Barreiro Arcos et al. 2011). Of interest here is that thyroid hormones modulate immune function also by nongenomic mechanism; in fact, they are able to potentiate the antiviral state induced by IFN-γ on HLA-DR expression in CV-1 fibroblasts and HeLa cells; these cells are particularly useful in studies on nongenomic effects because they are devoid of the nuclear receptors. The signal transduction mechanism includes the downstream activation of the MEK-MAPK signaling pathway, that in turn activates signal transducer and activator of transcription (STAT1α), which normally is activated by proinflammatory cytokines. Tetraiodothyroacetic acid (tetrac), a product of thyroid hormone metabolism, was able to inhibit the effect of thyroid hormones, and membrane-impermeant T_4-agarose mimicked this effect, confirming that the hormone acts at the plasma membrane by a nongenomic mechanism (Lin et al. 1999). Nongenomic effects of thyroid hormones have been found in microglia, the immune cells of the nervous system, mainly in processes such as cell migration, membrane ruffling, and phagocytosis. Membrane transport systems are modulated also by different mechanisms, and these effects may be important for a proper neural activity, while their impairment may at least in part contribute to psychiatric symptoms (Noda 2015).

Iodothyronines and Mitochondria

Energy balance is an important aspect of physiological homeostatic mechanisms and is determined by the relation between energy intake and energy expenditure, and the latter is an important factor in the maintenance of energy homeostasis. Energy expenditure is evaluated by measuring heat production (and indirectly by measuring the oxygen consumption), hence the use of the terms thermogenesis or calorigenesis. Thyroid hormones stimulate this well-known effect, and several hypotheses have been put forward to try to explain the mechanisms underlying this effect, but the molecular details remain incompletely understood. One of the oldest and most intriguing hypotheses was proposed several decades ago and was called the "uncoupling hypothesis." It suggested that thyroid hormone stimulates oxygen consumption in a way that does not result in the synthesis of ATP. In other words, the hormone stimulates the metabolic rate by directly uncoupling, at the mitochondrial level, the electron transport chain from ATP synthesis. This hypothesis was later questioned but never completely abandoned, and it still continues to be investigated using new approaches. The principal reasons for the abandonment of the uncoupling hypothesis were as follows: (i) the concentration of hormone administered in vivo or added to isolated mitochondria was several hundred or thousand times higher compared to the physiological range, and possibly the quantities used induced a toxic effect; (ii) analogs of thyroid hormone considered inactive were as effective as T_4 or T_3; and (iii) the effects in vivo were very rapid in onset, in contrast to the long latent period normally preceding the physiological response to thyroid hormone (for a recent review see Lanni et al. 2016).

Because of the previously cited action of T_3 on energy metabolism and because of the known physiological roles of mitochondria, these organelles continue to be the target of most studies on the calorigenic effects of thyroid hormones. Interest in a possible mitochondrial pathway of action of T_3 caused investigators to seek a specific receptor for the hormone in these organelles. Specific, high-affinity binding sites for T_3 in mitochondria were first reported by Sterling and Milch (1975), and later the existence of these sites was confirmed by others (Goglia et al. 1981). Despite such evidence, the physiological significance of the direct effects and the presence of mitochondrial receptors were initially viewed with some skepticism. However, the possible existence of a mitochondrial receptor for T_3 has received support from more recent work, in partial agreement with the data reported originally. Morel and coworkers (1996) showed by quantitative electron microscopic autoradiography that after injection of radiolabeled T_3, specific binding was evident in several cellular sites, including mitochondria. Wrutniak et al. (1995) identified two T_3-binding proteins from rat liver mitochondrial extracts; one called p43 (43 kDa) was located in the matrix and the other, p28 (28 kDa), in the inner membrane. Both of these proteins are shortened forms of TRα1. The p43 contained domains for intact DNA binding, ligand binding, and ligand-dependent activation domain AF-2, but was largely devoid of the N-terminal activation domain AF-1. The same group overexpressed a truncated 43 kDa c-erbAK1 protein in CV1 cells and then demonstrated by cyto-immunofluorescence that this truncated TRK protein was specifically imported into mitochondria. They also showed that p43 bound to TRE-like sequences on the mitochondrial genome – in the D-loop region, which contains the promoters of the mitochondrial genome – and stimulated transcription in the presence of thyroid hormones in a ligand-dependent manner (Casas et al. 1999, 2009). In transgenic mice, overexpression of p43 in muscle stimulated mitochondrial respiration and increased body temperature (see review by Wrutniak-Cabello et al. 2001). Little is known about the function of mitochondrial p28, but this protein has recently been shown to have a high affinity for T_3 ($K_A = 3.3 \times 10^{10}$ M^{-1}) and to be directed to mitochondria in response to T_3 (Pessemesse et al. 2014).

Several recent reports have indicated that iodothyronines other than T_3 may have important biological effects (Lanni et al. 2005; Senese et al. 2014). In particular, 3,5-diiodo-L-thyronine (T_2) attracted interest because of its effects on energy metabolism and on mitochondria. The first study showing an interaction of a diiodothyronine with mitochondria was published in 1981 (Goglia et al. 1981). Some years later T_2 at very low (pM) concentrations was shown to induce rapid stimulation of oxygen consumption in perfused rat livers. A similar effect was exerted by T_3, but this was largely abolished by the addition of an inhibitor of D1 deiodinase, while the effect of T_2 was not (Horst et al. 1989). Several reports from various laboratories have since confirmed that acute or chronic administration of T_2 to rats results in significant changes in energy metabolism. Some of these studies (Lanni et al. 1996; Moreno et al. 1997) were intended to show whether T_2, when injected into rats, could mimic the effects of T_3 reported by Tata in the early 1960s (Tata et al. 1962; Tata 1963). Using acute injection of T_3 and T_2 into hypothyroid rats, it was found that T_2 had a more rapid effect on the resting metabolic rate than T_3, and in addition, while the effect of T_3 was abolished by the addition of actinomycin D, the effect of T_2 was not. These observations appeared to exclude the involvement of the nuclear pathway in the effect exerted by T_2. Further details about the actions of T_2 can be found in recent reviews (Coppola et al. 2014; Gnocchi et al. 2015, 2016).

The effect of T_2 on resting metabolic rates continues to attract attention (Table 1). By using the "top-down elasticity analysis," it has been possible to show that T_2 stimulated the reduction of cytochrome *c* in the respiratory chain, as well as its oxidation by cytochrome *c* oxidase. These effects are obtained within 1 hour after the injection of 3,5-T_2 (Lombardi et al. 1998) and clearly show a direct interaction of T_2 with the respiratory chain. Observations in vitro showing stimulation by T_2 of complex IV of the respiratory chain confirm an apparently direct interaction at the respiratory chain level and indicate the complex IV as the possible site of interaction (Goglia et al. 1999). It has also been shown that 3,5-T_2 can bind specifically to

Table 1 Biological activities enhanced by the thyroid hormone metabolite 3,5-T_2

Process or activity	Reference
Oxygen consumption in perfused rat liver	Horst et al. (1989)
Ca^{2+} uptake by mitochondria	Hummerich and Soboll (1989)
Rate of oxygen consumption by blood mononuclear cells	Kvetny (1992)
Rate of oxygen consumption by rat liver	Lanni et al. (1992, 1993) and O'Reilly and Murphy (1992)
α-Glycerophosphate dehydrogenase activity	Lombardi et al. (2000) and Cavallo et al. (2016)
Respiratory chain activity	Lombardi et al. (1998)
Cytochrome *c* oxidase activity	Arnold et al. (1998), Goglia et al. (1994), Grasselli et al. (2016), and Lanni et al. (1993, 1994)
β-Oxidation rate	Cimmino et al. (1996) and Lombardi et al. (2009)

subunit Va of the cytochrome *c* oxidase, and in doing so, it abolishes the allosteric inhibition of respiration induced by ATP. Thus, subunit Va appears to be the mitochondrial site of action of T_2 (Arnold et al. 1998). The stimulatory effects exerted by T_2 on resting metabolic rates suggested its application to reduce body fat accumulation and overweight, avoiding the deleterious side effect experienced with the use of T_3 for this purpose. This might turn out to be an effective strategy (Padron et al. 2014); in fact, T_2 prevents high fat-diet-induced insulin resistance in rats (Moreno et al. 2011; de Lange et al. 2011).

Other studies have shown an antidepressant-like effect of T_2 in rats and that T_2 can be effective against renal damage in the nephropathy of streptozotocin-induced diabetes in rats (Markova et al. 2013; Shang et al. 2013). This has not yet been adequately studied clinically (Antonelli et al. 2011), and there may be deleterious side effects with long-term administration of T_2, for example, on the cardiovascular system (Jonas et al. 2015).

Our understanding of the physiological and pathophysiological roles of T_2 would benefit from the development and standardization of new methods for analytical measurement of T_2. A recent method consists of a competitive chemiluminescence immunoassay, based on the use of a selected mouse monoclonal anti-T_2 antibody with very low cross-reactivity to structurally related thyroid hormones and thyronamines (Lehmphul et al. 2014). Liquid chromatography–tandem mass spectrometry techniques have also been applied to this measurement (Rathmann et al. 2015). However, intrinsic instrumental limits still restrain the application of such approaches as routine tools.

Integrin αvβ3

Integrins are a family of plasma membrane-spanning heterodimeric protein receptors formed by the noncovalent association of various α and β monomers. They are very important for cell–cell interactions and for cellular interactions with extracellular matrix proteins. All integrins have large extracellular domain for the binding to extracellular matrix proteins and to other proteins of the plasma membrane, such as vascular growth factor receptors. The integrins also contain a transmembrane domain and a short cytoplasmic domain that interacts with the actin of the cytoskeleton and with other proteins involved in signal transduction pathways (Hynes 1992). The different integrins can be assembled from 18 different α subunits and at least 8 β subunits (in mammals), giving rise to at least 24 αβ heterodimers. The interactions of these integrins modulate cell functions such as differentiation, proliferation, cell migration, tumor invasiveness, metastasis, gene expression, and cell survival (De Vito et al. 2012). Integrins also contribute to angiogenesis, wound healing, and tissue differentiation and stability (Giancotti and Ruoslahti 1999). Dysregulation of integrins is found in the pathogenesis of many diseases (e.g., autoimmune diseases, cardiovascular diseases, osteoporosis), and their overexpression has been reported for several types of tumors (Inaba et al. 2004). A common feature of several integrins is a binding site recognizing the tripeptide sequence Arg-Gly-Asp (RGD). It is known that for bone resorption, osteoclasts must first adhere to the bone matrix, and this effect is mediated by the interaction of the osteoclastic vitronectin receptor with the RGD sequence present in several bone matrix proteins (Clover et al. 1992; Nesbitt et al. 1993). In 2002 it was reported that a vitronectin receptor antagonist, SB 273005, inhibited thyroxine-induced bone resorption in aged rats (Hoffman et al. 2002); this finding is now understood to reflect a primary interaction between integrin αvβ3 and thyroid hormone. Some years later it was discovered that a specific thyroid hormone receptor site exists on αvβ3 integrin (Bergh et al. 2005). Crystallographic data and mathematical modeling of the interaction of thyroid hormone molecules with integrin αvβ3 have shown that a hormone binding site is located in close proximity to the RGD sequence recognition site and that there is no structural homology of this receptor with the nuclear binding sites of thyroid hormones (Incerpi 2005).

The receptor site for thyroid hormone on the αvβ3 integrin is known to contain two domains for the binding of thyroid hormones: T_3 binds to the S1 site and activates Src kinase, which then activates PI3K and the consequent downstream signaling that leads to translocation of TRα resident in the cytoplasm into the cell nucleus and to the activation of the HIF-1α gene. These effects are inhibited by the RGD tripeptide and by tetrac, which can be used as a probe for participation of the αvβ3 integrin in cell actions of thyroid hormones. Both T_3 and T_4 are able to bind to the second integrin thyroid hormone receptor domain, S2, with T_4 being more efficient than T_3. Binding of T_4 to S2 causes activation of ERK1/2, leading to translocation of cytosolic TRβ to nucleus and, importantly, to tumor cell proliferation. This effect of T_4 is inhibited by PD98059, an inhibitor of the MAPK pathway. The RGD peptide does not inhibit the actions of T_4 at this site, but it does block effects of supraphysiological concentrations of T_3 here. Tetrac inhibits actions of both T_4 and T_3 at S2 (Lin et al. 2009b).

Recently a new signaling pathway has been found that involves protein kinase D1 (PKD1), previously called protein kinase Cμ, a conserved serine/threonine protein kinase that promotes integrin αvβ3 recycling and mediates class IIa histone deacetylase (HDAC) phosphorylation; therefore it gives rise to posttranslational modifications of nuclear proteins. PKD1 can be activated by T_4 interaction with the thyroid hormone receptor site on integrin αvβ3, and it activates human umbilical vein endothelial cell angiogenesis through a pathway involving αvβ3/PKD/HDAC5 and upregulation of basic fibroblasts growth factor (bFGF) (Liu et al. 2014). The control of MAPK and phospholipase C activities at the plasma membrane level by thyroid hormones, or by the metabolite 3,5-T_2, contributes to the nongenomic modulation of transport activities reported in the previous paragraphs, such as the Ca^{2+}-ATPase, Na^+/K^+-ATPase, Na^+/H^+-exchanger, the glucose and amino acid transport, and Na^+- and K^+-channels (Incerpi et al. 2002; Scapin et al. 2009).

Crosstalk exists between thyroid hormones and certain growth factors, because some of the latter can use integrin αvβ3 as a coreceptor. Stimulation of glucose uptake by IGF-1 in myoblasts from rat skeletal muscle was inhibited by T_4, and pretreatment with αvβ3 inhibitors such as RGD peptides or tetrac prevented the effect of the hormone (Incerpi et al. 2014). A similar result was reported for the amino acid uptake in Sertoli cells, which was stimulated by T_4 and inhibited by RGD and tetrac, implicating αvβ3 in the function (Zanatta et al. 2013). Also the action of growth factors TGF and EGF was found to be modified by the αvβ3-mediated crosstalk with T_4, but interestingly not in the same way: T_4 potentiated the effect of EGF on cell proliferation, but inhibited the effect in cells treated with TGFα (Shih et al. 2004). This result is particularly interesting because these two growth factors are known to share the same cell surface receptor.

The interaction of thyroid hormone with a receptor on αvβ3 appears to be conserved in evolution. In fact T_4, but not T_3, regulates the sodium channel activity in zebra fish spinal cord mechanosensory neurons (Rohon Beard cells). T_4 enhanced the abundance and the activity of the channel by about 40%, both in the short term and in the long term, and the acute application of T_4 increased the activity of the channel within 5 min. The action of T_4 on the sodium current was reduced by inhibitors of the αvβ3 integrin such as the αvβ3-antibody LM609 and tetrac. The signaling mediated by the integrin involves phosphorylation, and the inhibition of p38 or the presence of phosphatases prevented the effect of T_4 on the sodium current (Yonkers and Ribera 2011).

Particularly interesting is the role of integrins and cadherins in the dental bud, the precursor of the tooth, since it is well known that mesenchymal stem cells are important for tissue repair and regeneration. New deposits of mesenchymal stem cells are found in the dental bud, and osteogenic stimulation upregulates the integrin and cadherins, including integrin αvβ3 (Di Benedetto et al. 2015). It therefore seems possible that thyroid hormones might have a role in this process too.

Thyroid Hormones in Tumor Cell Proliferation and Angiogenesis

Integrin αvβ3 is present in substantial amounts in the plasma membrane of many tumor cells, in dividing endothelial cells, and in osteoclasts. T_4 at physiological levels and T_3 (although only at supraphysiological concentrations) modulate several pathophysiological cell functions through the integrin αvβ3, including tumor cell proliferation. As specified above, the thyroid hormone receptor on integrin αvβ3 is not related to the nuclear receptor, in terms of structure or function. Despite this lack of receptor similarities, the hormone binding site on the integrin may influence the activity and the trafficking of the nuclear receptors for T_3 and estrogen from the cytoplasm to the nucleus, as well as their posttranslational modifications such as phosphorylation, methylation, acetylation, and sumoylation. These modifications extend the duration of nongenomically initiated actions, for example, on the expression of genes subject to regulation by TRs or estrogen receptors (Davis et al. 2013a). As described above, the actions of T_4 and T_3 through αvβ3 initiate the downstream intracellular signaling involved in angiogenesis and angiogenesis-related activities, such as the transcription of vascular growth factor genes and modulation of the activity of vascular growth factor receptors (Lin et al. 2015). The thyroid hormone receptor on integrin αvβ3 also plays a role in brain neocortex expansion and development (Stenzel et al. 2014). Pharmacologic or immunologic inhibition of thyroid hormone action through integrin αvβ3 significantly decreases the angiogenic activity of the hormone in the chick chorioallantoic membrane assay. The application of this particular integrin αvβ3-dependent model may enable the development of innovative approaches to study antiangiogenesis in oncology (Davis et al. 2015d).

At physiological concentrations T_4 induces αvβ3-mediated tumor cell proliferation, whereas physiological levels of T_3 do not stimulate tumor cell division (Davis et al. 2016). Clinical induction of the euthyroid hypothyroxinemia state – by pharmacologically interrupting the production of T_4 in thyroid gland, but maintaining the euthyroid state with exogenous T_3 – prolonged the survival of patients with advanced cancers, who had exhausted conventional chemotherapeutic options (Hercbergs et al. 2015). This encouraging observational study still requires confirmation. The thyroid hormone metabolite tetrac, as well as its nanoformulation, acts at the hormone receptor site on αvβ3 to block binding of T_4 (and, less efficiently, of T_3). Tetrac acts as an antitumor compound through this mechanism, but it has also been shown in preclinical studies to have other important anticancer properties independently of T_4 and T_3. These include nongenomically initiated disruption of tumor cell division, induction of apoptosis, and effects on tumor cell chemosensitivity. Studies on tetrac emphasize the overlapping effects of thyroid hormone analogs on both nongenomic and genomic mechanisms. It should be mentioned that tetrac and its formulations do not affect the proliferation of nonmalignant immortalized primate cells (Davis et al. 2015a, 2016).

Thyroid hormone acting through the integrin increases the expression of the hypoxic-inducible factor-1α (HIF-1α) gene by a PI3K-dependent mechanism (Lin et al. 2015). This effect is subject to inhibition by tetrac, and targeting this effect via the integrin is a strategy to influence tumor cell proliferation and tumor-relevant angiogenesis (Cayrol et al. 2015; Davis et al. 2016). Hypoxia is a reduction in tissue oxygen content, an important parameter for the molecular mechanisms promoting tumor growth. Hypoxia is also related to resistance to chemotherapy and radiotherapy, and to poor survival rates. Successful inhibition by tetrac of the action of thyroid hormones through the integrin pathway has been demonstrated in PC-12 pheochromocytoma cells, both differentiated and undifferentiated, and in mesenchymal stem cells in a cell-conditioned environment (Barbakadze et al. 2014; Schmohl et al. 2015).

The first demonstrations that integrin αvβ3 was essential to the proangiogenic actions of T_3 and T_4 at 10^{-8}–10^{-7} M concentrations were obtained in the chick chorioallantoic membrane model and in a tridimensional endothelial sprouting assay. These hormone concentrations gave physiologic levels of free T_4 in the buffer system used (Bergh et al. 2005). Thyroid hormones had the same angiogenic efficacy as VEGF and bFGF in these model systems. GC-1, an analog of T_4 developed as a specific TRβ1 agonist, as well as diiodothyropropionic acid (DITPA), was also very effective proangiogenically, and the action of both analogs was blocked by tetrac (Mousa et al. 2005).

Thyroid Hormone and Normal Granulocytes and Platelets

Nonmalignant cells may also express sufficient αvβ3 to exhibit nongenomic hormonal effects. This is the case with high turnover of hematologic cells, such as granulocytes and megakaryocytes. Phagocytosis of bacteria by white blood cells may be stimulated by thyroid hormone via αvβ3 (Chen et al. 2012), and platelet aggregation and ATP release are stimulated nongenomically by T_4 (Mousa et al. 2010). The latter was demonstrated in vitro, but thromboembolism occurs in clinical hyperthyroidism (Grine et al. 2013; Min et al. 2014; Elbers et al. 2014; Horacek et al. 2015) and may reflect hormone action on platelets. That there is a distinction between the functions, and perhaps also the structure, of the thyroid hormone receptor on αvβ3 in certain nonmalignant tissues is clear, for example, GC-1 and DITPA are proangiogenic like T_4, but neither GC-1 nor DITPA induces platelet aggregation (Mousa et al. 2010).

Integrin αvβ3 and Gene Expression

Gene expression is modulated by thyroid hormones in many cases via integrin αvβ3 at the plasma membrane; the genes identified so far are listed in Table 2. This has been seen particularly in the capability of tetrac to inhibit tumor cell growth and induce apoptosis (Davis et al. 2016). RNA microarray studies have shown that the treatment of tumor cells with tetrac or its nanoformulation downregulates pro-survival pathway gene expression and upregulates pro-apoptotic gene transcription. The ultimate hormonal effect is genomic, but the action is initiated nongenomically at the plasma membrane integrin αvβ3. The desirable anticancer actions of tetrac include downregulation of the genes *XIAP* (X-linked inhibitor of apoptosis) and *MCL1* (myeloid cell leukemia 1) and upregulation of *CASP2* (caspase 2), *CBY1* (catenin inhibitor chibby homolog 1), and *THBS1* (anti-angiogenic thrombospondin 1). The epidermal growth factor receptor gene *EGFR* is downregulated very efficiently by nanoparticulate tetrac, whereas unmodified tetrac fails to affect expression of this gene. The effect on *EGFR* expression is particularly important since the gene product is a principal factor in tumor cell growth; therefore an efficient way to target this gene through tetrac may have clinical implications

Table 2 Genes modulated by thyroid hormones through integrin αvβ3. Increased expression (↑), decreased expression (↓)

Gene expression	Reference
FGF2 ↑	Shih et al. (2004)
HIF1A ↑	Lin et al. (2009b)
PTGS2 ↑	Davis et al. (2016)
THRA ↑	Lin et al. (2009a)
THRB ↑	Lin et al. (2013)
ESR1 ↑	Lin et al. (2009b)
MMP9 ↑	Davis et al. (2016)
APAF1 ↓	Davis et al. (2016)
CASP3 ↓	Davis et al. (2016)
INOS ↑	Barreiro Arcos et al. (2011)
SREBP1 ↑	Gnoni et al. (2012)
CX3CL1 ↑	Davis et al. (2016)
PCNA ↑	Hsieh et al. (2016)

(Glinskii et al. 2009). In contrast to such actions of the different tetrac formulations, T_4 is anti-apoptotic (Lin et al. 2015) and, as indicated above, proangiogenic (Davis et al. 2015d; Mousa et al. 2014). Thus thyroid hormones support cancer cell proliferation and tumor vascularization, whereas tetrac, and the more efficient nanotetrac, inhibits these processes.

Integrin αvβ3 binds specific extracellular matrix proteins, and in addition to thyroid hormone, it also binds small molecules such as dihydrotestosterone (Lin et al. 2009a) and resveratrol (Lin et al. 2006), which initiate actions that are also cancer relevant. The integrin may also contain a cell surface estrogen receptor (Davis et al. 2013b). Although all of these small molecule receptors appear to be proximal to the RGD recognition site on αvβ3, there is very little interaction among these sites from the standpoint of binding or function.

P-Glycoprotein (also known as P-gp, MDR1, and ABCB1) is a plasma membrane pump that extrudes a number of anticancer agents and other potentially toxic substances from the cell. It is an important component of cancer cell chemoresistance. The gene for P-glycoprotein and the activity of the protein are both subject to stimulation by thyroid hormone (Davis et al. 2015b), but it is not yet known whether αvβ3 is involved in the contributions of the hormone to affect the quantity and function of P-glycoprotein in the membrane.

Integrin Monomer αv and Thyroid Hormones

Integrin αvβ3 is internalized by cells treated with thyroid hormone (Lin et al. 2013). However, this is not a mechanism of cell uptake of thyroid hormone. The αv monomer is trafficked to the nucleus in T_4-exposed tumor cells where it functions as a coactivator protein that is phosphorylated and binds to the promoter regions of several genes, such as *ESR1* (estrogen receptor α), *HIF1A*, (HIF-1α), *PTGS2* (cyclooxygenase-2), and *THRA* (thyroid hormone receptor TRα1). Estrogen receptor α is well known to be involved in the activity of cancers of the breast, ovary, and lung, and cyclooxygenase-2 is involved in the induction of apoptosis by several drugs. HIF-1α is a pro-survival factor that stimulates angiogenesis and cellular conversion to anaerobic metabolism. The recycling of integrin αvβ3 involves the PI3K/Akt pathway (Roberts et al. 2004), but the internalization process in response to thyroid hormone is incompletely understood at the molecular level. It is remarkable that a cell surface protein capable, when stimulated by a specific ligand, of inducing downstream specific gene expression has a monomeric component with intranuclear transcriptional function. The function of the β3 monomer within the cell is unknown; the protein does not enter the nucleus in hormone-exposed cells (Lin et al. 2013).

Additional Receptor Proteins for Nongenomic Effects of Thyroid Hormones

In the course of the years, the separation between genomic and nongenomic effects of thyroid hormones has become mixed up, and it is now recognized that nuclear genomic effect may also start at the plasma membrane level. It has been known for years that the nuclear thyroid hormone receptor TRβ1 may reside either in the nucleus or in the cytosol, and that there are also truncated forms of TRα1 in the cytosol or in the mitochondria. These receptors may shuttle between the plasma membrane, the mitochondria, cytosol, and nucleus (Davis et al. 2015c). In this section we present a brief overview of the variety of receptors able to modulate the nongenomic effects of thyroid hormones, besides the integrin αvβ3.

Only T_3 binds to the nuclear receptors, whereas the other thyroid hormone metabolites and analogs normally are not active at the nuclear level. An examination of their possible binding sites resulted in the discovery of a 16 kDa protein, called the TRΔα1 isoform, which does not bind T_3. This modified nuclear receptor is widely expressed in the brain and is believed to be a possible candidate for the binding to T_4 in the cytosol. Another truncated and transcriptionally incompetent form of TRα1, that binds to the plasma membrane and is subject to palmitoylation, has recently been described by Kalyanaraman et al. (2014). When liganded to thyroid hormone, this interesting receptor nongenomically induces an increase in calcium ion levels, nitric oxide, and cyclic guanosine monophosphate that lead to proliferation of bone cells in particular. This protein may be an important regulator of proliferation in nonmalignant cells exposed to thyroid hormone. Another truncated TRα isoform is localized in lipid rafts, and its downstream signaling involves ERK1/2 and PI3K. A TRβ mutant binds to the regulatory subunit of PI3K in the absence of the ligand. There seems to be a plethora of signaling pathways from different TR receptor isoforms to ERK and PI3K, and NOS may be achieved by such isoforms but also by integrin αvβ3 (Shih et al. 2001; Chen et al. 2012). Also the trafficking of the TRα and TRβ receptors can be regulated by integrin αvβ3, and this appears to be pivotal in the control of cell response to hormones. Furthermore truncated variants of TRα1 may also be found in mitochondria, such as the p43 and p28 proteins mentioned above.

In endothelial cells TRα1 may associate with the p85α subunit of PI3K, activating Akt and eNOS (Hiroi et al. 2006). When thyroid hormone T_3 is bound to TRβ1, it interacts in the cytosol with the p85 subunit of PI3K, leading to the activation of HIF-1α and its target genes related to glucose uptake and metabolism; the latter include glucose transporter-1 (*SLC2A1*) and platelet phosphofructokinase (*PFKP*) (Moeller et al. 2006). Another nuclear receptor isoform, TRβ1, supports postnatal development of pyramidal neurons by a nongenomic mechanism (Martin et al. 2014; Davis et al. 2015b). It is interesting to observe that new nongenomic mechanisms and responses are being discovered practically every year, and it is a general feeling among researchers in the field that we still only know fragments of the complete picture. After more than 30 years, we are still very far from understanding the physiological role and importance of the nongenomic effects of thyroid hormones.

Summary

Nongenomic actions of thyroid hormones do not require direct activation of the nuclear receptors TRα and TRβ, but instead depend on hormone binding to various extranuclear receptors or binding sites. Only thyroid hormone T_3 can produce a genomic response, but the different nongenomic effects may be activated by T_3, T_4, or other iodothyronine derivatives such as T_2. The nongenomic actions are typically observed within minutes, because they are independent of gene expression and protein synthesis. In the last ten years many nongenomic actions have been discovered and characterized, and binding sites have been identified in several cellular compartments and on the external surface of the plasma membrane. Recent results confirm the existence of crosstalk between nongenomic and genomic effects of thyroid hormones, suggesting a hitherto unknown mechanism that could be involved in cardiovascular, inflammatory and immune diseases, and in the mechanisms of cancer-related angiogenesis.

Conclusions

The nongenomic effects of thyroid hormones have been widely studied for almost four decades. The physiologic and pathophysiologic consequences of these effects are increasingly well defined, and some of these nongenomic functions are candidates to become new pharmacologic targets. Thyroid hormones contribute to the basic functioning of the cell, such as membrane transport systems, basal metabolic rates, and cell proliferation, but they are also involved in more specialized cell functions as shown by their effects on actin polymerization in the central nervous system and their nongenomic action on deiodinase activity. Among the specific responses to thyroid hormone that are nongenomic in mechanism are (1) immune system responses by potentiation of the IFN-γ antiviral effect, cell migration, activation of STAT-1α, and nitric oxide production; (2) ion channel modulation in excitable tissues, leading to potentiation of cardiac contraction and fast relaxation in heart tissue, and vasodilation in vascular tissue; (3) ion channel modulation in nerve cells and muscle cells, leading to physiological responses such as altered firing activity and the expansion of progenitor cells in the development of the cerebral cortex; and (4) cancer cell proliferation and cell survival pathway regulation and modulation of cancer-relevant angiogenesis. Nongenomic effects and genomic effects of thyroid hormones overlap or engage in crosstalk, particularly in the setting of cancer. Improving our understanding of these nongenomic effects may lead to the development of new therapeutic tools for a variety of diseases.

Cross-References

► Molecular Mechanisms of Thyroid Hormone Synthesis and Secretion
► Targeting of Steroid Hormone Receptor Function in Breast and Prostate Cancer
► The Thyroid
► Thyroid Hormone Nuclear Receptors and Molecular Actions

References

Ahmed OM, Ahmed RG, El-Gareib AW, El-Bakry AM, Abd El-Tawab SM. Effects of experimentally induced maternal hypothyroidism and hyperthyroidism on the development of rat offspring: II–The developmental pattern of neurons in relation to oxidative stress and antioxidant defense system. Int J Dev Neurosci. 2012;30(6):517–37.

Ahmed RG, Davis PJ, Davis FB, De Vito P, Farias RN, Luly P, et al. Nongenomic actions of thyroid hormones. From basic research to clinical applications. An update. Immune Endocr Metab Agents Med Chem. 2013;13:45–69.

Antonelli A, Fallahi P, Ferrari SM, Di Domenicantonio A, Moreno M, Lanni A, Goglia F. 3,5-diiodo-L-thyronine increases resting metabolic rate and reduces body weight without undesirable side effects. J Biol Regul Homeost Agents. 2011;25(4):655–60.

Arnold S, Goglia F, Kadenbach B. 3,5-Diiodothyronine binds to subunit Va of cytochrome-*c* oxidase and abolishes the allosteric inhibition of respiration by ATP. Eur J Biochem. 1998;252(2):325–30.

Barbakadze T, Natsvlishvili N, Mikeladze D. Thyroid hormones differentially regulate phosphorylation of ERK and Akt via integrin αvβ3 receptor in undifferentiated and differentiated PC-12 cells. Cell Biochem Funct. 2014;32(3):282–6.

Barreiro Arcos ML, Sterle HA, Paulazo MA, Valli E, Klecha AJ, Isse B, et al. Cooperative nongenomic and genomic actions on thyroid hormone mediated-modulation of T cell proliferation involve up-regulation of thyroid hormone receptor and inducible nitric oxide synthase expression. J Cell Physiol. 2011;226(12):3208–18.

Bergh JJ, Lin HY, Lansing L, Mohamed SN, Davis FB, Mousa S, Davis PJ. Integrin αvβ3 contains a cell surface receptor site for thyroid hormone that is linked to activation of mitogen-activated protein kinase and induction of angiogenesis. Endocrinology. 2005;146(7):2864–71.

Botta JA, de Mendoza D, Morero RD, Farías RN. High affinity L-triiodothyronine binding sites on washed rat erythrocyte membranes. J Biol Chem. 1983;258(11):6690–2.

Cao JH, Pan J, Lin H-Y, Davis FB, Zhou M, Davis PJ. L-Thyroxine attenuates pyramidal neuron excitability in rat acute prefrontal cortex slices. Immun Endocr Metab Agents Med Chem. 2011;11:152–6.

Caria MA, Dratman MB, Kow LM, Mameli O, Pavlides C. Thyroid hormone action: nongenomic modulation of neuronal excitability in the hippocampus. J Neuroendocrinol. 2009;21 (2):98–107.

Casas F, Rochard P, Rodier A, Cassar-Malek I, Marchal-Victorion S, Wiesner RJ, et al. A variant form of the nuclear triiodothyronine receptor c-Erb?1 plays a direct role in regulation of mitochondrial RNA synthesis. Mol Cell Biol. 1999;19(12):7913–24.

Casas F, Pessemesse L, Grandemange S, Seyer P, Baris O, Gueguen N, et al. Overexpression of the mitochondrial T3 receptor induces skeletal muscle atrophy during aging. PLoS ONE. 2009;4(5), e5631.

Cavallo A, Taurino F, Damiano F, Siculella L, Sardanelli AM, Gnoni A. Acute administration of 3,5-diiodo-L-thyronine to hypothyroid rats stimulates bioenergetic parameters in liver mitochondria. J Bioenerg Biomembr. 2016;48(5):521–529.

Cayrol F, Díaz Flaqué MC, Fernando T, Yang SN, Sterle HA, Bolontrade M, et al. Integrin αvβ3 acting as membrane receptor for thyroid hormones mediates angiogenesis in malignant T cells. Blood. 2015;125(5):841–51.

Chapell R, Martin J, Machu TK, Leidenheimer NJ. Direct channel-gating and modulatory effects of triiodothyronine on recombinant $GABA_A$ receptors. Eur J Pharmacol. 1998;349(1):115–21.

Chen Y, Sjölinder M, Wang X, Altenbacher G, Hagner M, Berglund P, et al. Thyroid hormone enhances nitric oxide-mediated bacterial clearance and promotes survival after meningococcal infection. PLoS ONE. 2012;7(7), e41445.

Cimmino M, Mion F, Goglia F, Minaire Y, Géloën A. Demonstration of in vivo metabolic effects of 3,5-di-iodothyronine. J Endocrinol. 1996;149(2):319–25.

Clover J, Dodds RA, Gowen M. Integrin subunit expression by human osteoblasts and osteoclasts in situ and in culture. J Cell Sci. 1992;103(Pt 1):267–71.

Coppola M, Glinni D, Moreno M, Cioffi F, Silvestri E, Goglia F. Thyroid hormone analogues and derivatives: actions in fatty liver. World J Hepatol. 2014;6(3):114–29.

D'Arezzo S, Incerpi S, Davis FB, Acconcia F, Marino M, Farias RN, et al. Rapid nongenomic effects of 3,5,3′-triiodo-L-thyronine on the intracellular pH of L-6 myoblasts are mediated by intracellular calcium mobilization and kinase pathways. Endocrinology. 2004;145(12):5694–703.

Davis PJ, Blas SD. In vitro stimulation of human red blood cell Ca^{2+}-ATPase by thyroid hormone. Biochem Biophys Res Commun. 1981;99(4):1073–80.

Davis FB, Cody V, Davis PJ, Borzynski LJ, Blas SD. Stimulation by thyroid hormone analogues of red blood cell Ca^{2+}-ATPase activity in vitro. Correlations between hormone structure and biological activity in a human cell system. J Biol Chem. 1983;258(20):12373–7.

Davis PJ, Lin HY, Tang HY, Davis FB, Mousa SA. Adjunctive input to the nuclear thyroid hormone receptor from the cell surface receptor for the hormone. Thyroid. 2013a;23(12):1503–9.

Davis PJ, Mousa SA, Cody V, Tang HY, Lin HY. Small molecule hormone or hormone-like ligands of integrin αVβ3: implications for cancer cell behavior. Horm Cancer. 2013b;4(6):335–42.

Davis PJ, Glinsky GV, Lin HY, Leith JT, Hercbergs A, Tang HY, et al. Cancer cell gene expression modulated from plasma membrane integrin αvβ3 by thyroid hormone and nanoparticulate tetrac. Front Endocrinol (Lausanne). 2015a;5:240.

Davis PJ, Incerpi S, Lin HY, Tang HY, Sudha T, Mousa SA. Thyroid hormone and P-glycoprotein in tumor cells. Biomed Res Int. 2015b;2015:168427.

Davis PJ, Leonard JL, Lin H-Y, Incerpi S, Luidens MK, Tang HY, et al. Receptor proteins for nongenomic actions of thyroid hormones. Immun Endocr Metab Agents Med Chem. 2015c;15:94–7.

Davis PJ, Sudha T, Lin HY, Mousa SA. Thyroid hormone, hormone analogs, and angiogenesis. Compr Physiol. 2015d;6(1):353–62.

Davis PJ, Goglia F, Leonard JL. Nongenomic action of thyroid hormone. Nat Rev Endo. 2016;12 (2):111–21.

de Lange P, Cioffi F, Senese R, Moreno M, Lombardi A, Silvestri E, et al. Nonthyrotoxic prevention of diet-induced insulin resistance by 3,5-diiodo-L-thyronine in rats. Diabetes. 2011;60(11):2730–9.

de Mendoza D, Moreno H, Farías RN. Membrane cooperative enzymes. High molecular specificity for blocking action of thyroxine on triiodothyronine effect in rat erythrocyte and *Escherichia coli* systems. J Biol Chem. 1978;253(17):6255–9.

De Vito P, Incerpi S, Pedersen JZ, Luly P, Davis FB, Davis PJ. Thyroid hormones as modulators of immune activities at the cellular level. Thyroid. 2011;21(8):879–90.

De Vito P, Balducci V, Leone S, Percario Z, Mangino G, Davis PJ, et al. Nongenomic effects of thyroid hormones on the immune system cells: new targets, old players. Steroids. 2012;77 (10):988–95.

Di Benedetto A, Brunetti G, Posa F, Ballini A, Grassi FR, Colaianni G, et al. Osteogenic differentiation of mesenchymal stem cells from dental bud: role of integrins and cadherins. Stem Cell Res. 2015;15(3):618–28.

Elbers LP, van Zaane B, Gerdes VE, Coutinho JM, Bisschop PH, Fliers E. Venous thromboembolism in overt hyperthyroidism – a direct association with clinical implications? Neth J Med. 2014;72(4):242–4.

Farias RN, Fiore AM, Pedersen JZ, Incerpi S. Nongenomic actions of thyroid hormones: focus on membrane transport systems. Immun Endocr Metab Agents Med Chem. 2006;6:6241–54.

Farwell A, Dubord-Tomasetti SA. Thyroid hormone regulates the extracellular organization of laminin on astrocytes. Endocrinology. 1999;140:5014–21.

Farwell AP, Dubord-Tomasetti SA, Pietrzykowski AZ, Stachelek SJ, Leonard JL. Regulation of cerebellar neuronal migration and neurite outgrowth by thyroxine and 3,3′,5′-triiodothyronine. Brain Res Dev Brain Res. 2005;154(1):121–35.

Farwell AP, Dubord-Tomasetti SA, Pietrzykowsky AZ, Leonard JL. Dynamic nongenomic actions of thyroid hormone in the developing rat brain. Endocrinology. 2006;147:2567–74.

Furuya F, Lu C, Guigon CJ, Cheng SY. Nongenomic activation of phosphatidylinositol 3-kinase signaling by thyroid hormone receptors. Steroids. 2009;74(7):628–34.

Galo MG, Uñates LE, Farías RN. Effect of membrane fatty acid composition on the action of thyroid hormones on (Ca^{2+} + Mg^{2+})-adenosine triphosphatase from rat erythrocyte. J Biol Chem. 1981;256(14):7113–4.

Giancotti FG, Ruoslahti E. Integrin signaling. Science. 1999;285(5430):1028–32.

Glinskii AB, Glinsky GV, Lin HY, Tang HY, Sun M, Davis FB, et al. Modification of survival pathway gene expression in human breast cancer cells by tetraiodothyroacetic acid (tetrac). Cell Cycle. 2009;8(21):3562–70.

Gnocchi D, Alisi A, Bruscalupi G. Thyroid hormones and their metabolites: biological roles and association with non-alcoholic fatty liver disease. Immun Endocr Metab Agents Med Chem. 2015;15:43–59.

Gnocchi D, Steffensen KR, Bruscalupi G, Parini P. Emerging role of thyroid hormone metabolites. Acta Physiol (Oxf). 2016;217(3):184–216.

Gnoni GV, Rochira A, Leone A, Damiano F, Marsigliante S, Siculella L. 3,5,3′-Triiodo-L-thyronine induces SREBP-1 expression by non-genomic actions in human HEP G2 cells. J Cell Physiol. 2012;227(6):2388–97.

Goglia F, Torresani J, Bugli P, Barletta A, Liverini G. In vitro binding of triiodothyronine to rat liver mitochondria. Pflugers Arch. 1981;390(2):120–4.

Goglia F, Lanni A, Barth J, Kadenbach B. Interaction of diiodothyronines with isolated cytochrome c oxidase. FEBS Lett. 1994;346(2–3):295–8.

Goglia F, Moreno M, Lanni A. Action of thyroid hormones at the cellular level: the mitochondrial target. FEBS Lett. 1999;452(3):115–20.

Grasselli E, Voci A, Demori I, Vecchione G, Compalati AD, Gallo G, et al. Triglyceride mobilization from lipid droplets sustains the anti-steatotic action of iodothyronines in cultured rat hepatocytes. Front Physiol. 2016;6:418.

Grine S, Charfi N, Kamoun M, Mnif F, Naceur BB, Rekik N, et al. Hyperthyroidism: a rare cause of pulmonary embolism: report of two cases. Indian J Endocrinol Metab. 2013;17(6):1104–7.

Hercbergs A, Johnson RE, Ashur-Fabian O, Garfield DH, Davis PJ. Medically induced euthyroid hypothyroxinemia may extend survival in compassionate need cancer patients: an observational study. Oncologist. 2015;20(1):72–6.

Hiroi Y, Kim HH, Ying H, Furuya F, Huang Z, Simoncini T, et al. Rapid nongenomic actions of thyroid hormone. Proc Natl Acad Sci U S A. 2006;103(38):14104–9.

Hoffman SJ, Vasko-Moser J, Miller WH, Lark MW, Gowen M, Stroup G. Rapid inhibition of thyroxine-induced bone resorption in the rat by an orally active vitronectin receptor antagonist. J Pharmacol Exp Ther. 2002;302(1):205–11.

Horacek J, Maly J, Svilias I, Smolej L, Cepkova J, Vizda J, et al. Prothrombotic changes due to an increase in thyroid hormone levels. Eur J Endocrinol. 2015;172(5):537–42.

Horst C, Rokos H, Seitz HJ. Rapid stimulation of hepatic oxygen consumption by 3,5-di-iodo-L-thyronine. Biochem J. 1989;261:945–50.

Hsieh M, Wang LM, Changou CA, Chin YT, Yang YS, Lai HY, et al. Crosstalk between integrin αvβ3 and ERα contributes to thyroid hormone-induced proliferation of ovarian cancer cells. Oncotarget. 2016. doi:10.18632/oncotarget.10757. Epub ahead of print.

Hummerich H, Soboll S. Rapid stimulation of calcium uptake into rat liver by L-tri-iodothyronine. Biochem J. 1989;258(2):363–7.

Hynes RO. Integrins: versatility, modulation, and signaling in cell adhesion. Cell. 1992;69 (1):11–25.

Inaba M. Secondary osteoporosis: thyrotoxicosis, rheumatoid arthritis, and diabetes mellitus. J Bone Miner Metab. 2004;22(4):287–92.

Incerpi S. Thyroid hormones: rapid reply by surface delivery only. Endocrinology. 2005;146 (7):2861–3.

Incerpi S, Luly P, De Vito P, Farias RN. Short-term effects of thyroid hormones on the Na/H antiport in L-6 myoblasts: high molecular specificity for 3,3′,5-triiodo-L-thyronine. Endocrinology. 1999;140(2):683–9.

Incerpi S, De Vito P, Luly P, Spagnuolo S, Leoni S. Short-term effects of thyroid hormones and 3,5-diiodothyronine on membrane transport systems in chick embryo hepatocytes. Endocrinology. 2002;143(5):1660–8.

Incerpi S, De Vito P, Pedersen JZ, Luly P. Extranuclear effects of thyroid hormones in skeletal muscle. Immun Endo Metab Agents Med Chem. 2011;11:188–98.

Incerpi S, Hsieh MT, Lin HY, Cheng GY, De Vito P, Fiore AM, et al. Thyroid hormone inhibition in L6 myoblasts of IGF-I-mediated glucose uptake and proliferation: new roles for integrin αvβ3. Am J Physiol Cell Physiol. 2014;307(2):C150–61.

Irrcher I, Walkinshaw DR, Sheehan TE, Hood DA. Thyroid hormone (T_3) rapidly activates p38 and AMPK in skeletal muscle in vivo. J Appl Physiol. 2008;104(1):178–85.

Jonas W, Lietzow J, Wohlgemuth F, Hoefig CS, Wiedmer P, Schweizer U, et al. 3,5-Diiodo-L-thyronine (3,5-T_2) exerts thyromimetic effects on hypothalamus-pituitary-thyroid axis, body composition, and energy metabolism in male diet-induced obese mice. Endocrinology. 2015;156(1):389–99.

Kalyanaraman H, Schwappacher R, Joshua J, Zhuang S, Scott BT, Klos M, et al. Nongenomic thyroid hormone signaling occurs through a plasma membrane-localized receptor. Sci Signal. 2014;7(326):ra48.

Koibuchi N, Chin WW. Thyroid hormone action and brain development. Trends Endocrinol Metab. 2000;11(4):123–8.

Kvetny J. 3,5-T2 stimulates oxygen consumption, but not glucose uptake in human mononuclear blood cells. Horm Metab Res. 1992;24(7):322–5.

Lanni A, Moreno M, Cioffi M, Goglia F. Effect of 3,3′-diiodothyronine and 3,5-diiodothyronine on rat liver oxidative capacity. Mol Cell Endocrinol. 1992;86(3):143–8.

Lanni A, Moreno M, Cioffi M, Goglia F. Effect of 3,3′-di-iodothyronine and 3,5-di-iodothyronine on rat liver mitochondria. J Endocrinol. 1993;136(1):59–64.

Lanni A, Moreno M, Lombardi A, Goglia F. Rapid stimulation in vitro of rat liver cytochrome oxidase activity by 3,5-diiodo-L-thyronine and by 3,3′-diiodo-L-thyronine. Mol Cell Endocrinol. 1994;99(1):89–94.

Lanni A, Moreno M, Lombardi A, Goglia F. Calorigenic effect of diiodothyronines in the rat. J Physiol. 1996;494:831–7.

Lanni A, Moreno M, Lombardi A, de Lange P, Silvestri E, Ragni M, et al. 3,5-diiodo-L-thyronine powerfully reduces adiposity in rats by increasing the burning of fats. FASEB J. 2005;19 (11):1552–4.

Lanni A, Moreno M, Goglia F. Mitochondrial Actions of Thyroid Hormone. Compr Physiol. 2016;6 (4):1591–1607.

Lazar MA. Nuclear receptor corepressors. Nucl Recept Signal. 2003;1, e001.

Lehmphul I, Brabant G, Wallaschofski H, Ruchala M, Strasburger CJ, Köhrle J, et al. Detection of 3,5-diiodothyronine in sera of patients with altered thyroid status using a new monoclonal antibody-based chemiluminescence immunoassay. Thyroid. 2014;24(9):1350–60.

Lei J, Ingbar DH. Src kinase integrates PI_3K/Akt and MAPK/ERK1/2 pathways in T_3-induced Na-K-ATPase activity in adult rat alveolar cells. Am J Physiol Lung Cell Mol Physiol. 2011;301(5): L765–71.

Lei J, Mariash CN, Bhargava M, Wattenberg EV, Ingbar DH. T_3 increases Na-K-ATPase activity via a MAPK/ERK1/2-dependent pathway in rat adult alveolar epithelial cells. Am J Physiol Lung Cell Mol Physiol. 2008;294(4):L749–54.

Lin HY, Davis FB, Gordinier JK, Martino LJ, Davis PJ. Thyroid hormone induces activation of mitogen-activated protein kinase in cultured cells. Am J Physiol. 1999;276(5 Pt 1):C1014–24.

Lin HY, Lansing L, Merillon JM, Davis FB, Tang HY, Shih A, et al. Integrin αVβ3 contains a receptor site for resveratrol. FASEB J. 2006;20(10):1742–4.

Lin HY, Sun M, Lin C, Tang HY, London D, Shih A, et al. Androgen-induced human breast cancer cell proliferation is mediated by discrete mechanisms in estrogen receptor-α-positive and -negative breast cancer cells. J Steroid Biochem Mol Biol. 2009a;113(3–5):182–8.

Lin HY, Sun M, Tang HY, Lin C, Luidens MK, Mousa SA, et al. L-Thyroxine vs. 3,5,3′-triiodo-L-thyronine and cell proliferation: activation of mitogen-activated protein kinase and phosphatidylinositol 3-kinase. Am J Physiol Cell Physiol. 2009b;296:C980–91.

Lin HY, Su YF, Hsieh MT, Lin S, Meng R, London D, et al. Nuclear monomeric integrin αv in cancer cells is a coactivator regulated by thyroid hormone. FASEB J. 2013;27(8):3209–16.

Lin HY, Glinsky GV, Mousa SA, Davis PJ. Thyroid hormone and anti-apoptosis in tumor cells. Oncotarget. 2015;6(17):14735–43.

Liu X, Zheng N, Shi YN, Yuan J, Li L. Thyroid hormone induced angiogenesis through the integrin αvβ3/protein kinase D/histone deacetylase 5 signaling pathway. J Mol Endocrinol. 2014;52 (3):245–54.

Lombardi A, Lanni A, Moreno M, Brand MD, Goglia F. Effect of 3,5-di-iodo-L-thyronine on the mitochondrial energy-transduction apparatus. Biochem J. 1998;330(Pt 1):521–6.

Lombardi A, Beneduce L, Moreno M, Diano S, Colantuoni V, Ursini MV, et al. 3,5-diiodo-L-thyronine regulates glucose-6-phosphate dehydrogenase activity in the rat. Endocrinology. 2000;141(5):1729–34.

Lombardi A, de Lange P, Silvestri E, Busiello RA, Lanni A, Goglia F, et al. 3,5-Diiodo-L-thyronine rapidly enhances mitochondrial fatty acid oxidation rate and thermogenesis in rat skeletal muscle: AMP-activated protein kinase involvement. Am J Physiol Endocrinol Metab. 2009;296(3):E497–502.

Losi G, Garzon G, Puia G. Nongenomic regulation of glutamatergic neurotransmission in hippocampus by thyroid hormones. Neuroscience. 2008;151(1):155–63.

Markova N, Chernopiatko A, Schroeter CA, Malin D, Kubatiev A, Bachurin S, et al. Hippocampal gene expression of deiodinases 2 and 3 and effects of 3,5-diiodo-L-thyronine T2 in mouse depression paradigms. Biomed Res Int. 2013;2013:565218.

Martin JV, Williams DB, Fitzgerald RM, Im HK, Vonvoigtlander PF. Thyroid hormonal modulation of the binding and activity of the $GABA_A$ receptor complex of brain. Neuroscience. 1996;73 (3):705–13.
Martin JV, Padron JM, Newman MA, Chapell R, Leidenheimer NJ, Burke LA. Inhibition of the activity of the native γ-aminobutyric $acid_A$ receptor by metabolites of thyroid hormones: correlations with molecular modeling studies. Brain Res. 2004;1004(1–2):98–107.
Martin NP, Marron Fernandez de Velasco E, Mizuno F, Scappini EL, Gloss B, Erxleben C, et al. A rapid cytoplasmic mechanism for PI3 kinase regulation by the nuclear thyroid hormone receptor, TR*β*, and genetic evidence for its role in the maturation of mouse hippocampal synapses in vivo. Endocrinology. 2014;155(9):3713–24.
Min T, Benjamin S, Cozma L. Thromboembolic complications of thyroid storm. Endocrinol Diabet Metab Case Rep. 2014;2014:130060.
Moeller LC, Cao X, Dumitrescu AM, Seo H, Refetoff S. Thyroid hormone mediated changes in gene expression can be initiated by cytosolic action of the thyroid hormone receptor β through the phosphatidylinositol 3-kinase pathway. Nucl Recept Signal. 2006;4, e020.
Morel G, Ricard-Blum S, Ardail D. Kinetics of internalization and subcellular binding sites for T_3 in mouse liver. Biol Cell. 1996;86(2–3):167–74.
Moreno M, Lanni A, Lombardi A, Goglia F. How the thyroid controls metabolism in the rat: different roles for triiodothyronine and diiodothyronines. J Physiol. 1997;505(2):529–38.
Moreno M, de Lange P, Lombardi A, Silvestri E, Lanni A, Goglia F. Metabolic effects of thyroid hormone derivatives. Thyroid. 2008;18:239–53.
Moreno M, Silvestri E, De Matteis R, de Lange P, Lombardi A, Glinni D, et al. 3,5-Diiodo-L-thyronine prevents high-fat-diet-induced insulin resistance in rat skeletal muscle through metabolic and structural adaptations. FASEB J. 2011;25(10):3312–24.
Mousa SA, O'Connor LJ, Bergh JJ, Davis FB, Scanlan TS, Davis PJ. The proangiogenic action of thyroid hormone analogue GC-1 is initiated at an integrin. J Cardiovasc Pharmacol. 2005;46 (3):356–60.
Mousa SS, Davis FB, Davis PJ, Mousa SA. Human platelet aggregation and degranulation is induced in vitro by L-thyroxine, but not by 3,5,3′-triiodo-L-thyronine or diiodothyropropionic acid (DITPA). Clin Appl Thromb Hemost. 2010;16(3):288–93.
Mousa SA, Lin HY, Tang HY, Hercbergs A, Luidens MK, Davis PJ. Modulation of angiogenesis by thyroid hormone and hormone analogues: implications for cancer management. Angiogenesis. 2014;17(3):463–9.
Nesbitt S, Nesbit A, Helfrich M, Horton M. Biochemical characterization of human osteoclast integrins. Osteoclasts express αvβ3, α2β1, and αvβ1 integrins. J Biol Chem. 1993;268 (22):16737–45.
Noda M. Possible role of glial cells in the relationship between thyroid dysfunction and mental disorders. Front Cell Neurosci. 2015;9:194.
Novitzky D, Cooper DK, Barton CI, Greer A, Chaffin J, Grim J, et al. Triiodothyronine as an inotropic agent after open heart surgery. J Thorac Cardiovasc Surg. 1989a;98(5Pt 2):972–7. discussion 977–8.
Novitzky D, Cooper DK, Swanepoel A. Inotropic effect of triiodothyronine (T_3) in low cardiac output following cardioplegic arrest and cardiopulmonary bypass: an initial experience in patients undergoing open heart surgery. Eur J Cardiothorac Surg. 1989b;3(2):140–5.
Ojamaa K, Klemperer JD, Klein I. Acute effects of thyroid hormone on vascular smooth muscle. Thyroid. 1996;6(5):505–12.
Oppenheimer JH, Koerner D, Schwartz HL, Surks MI. Specific nuclear triiodothyronine binding sites in rat liver and kidney. J Clin Endocrinol Metab. 1972;35:330–3.
Oppenheimer JH, Schwartz HL, Mariash CN, Kinlaw WB, Wong NCW, Freake HC. Advances in our understanding of thyroid hormone action at the cellular level. Endocr Rev. 1987;8:288–308.
O'Reilly I, Murphy MP. Studies on the rapid stimulation of mitochondrial respiration by thyroid hormones. Acta Endocrinol (Copenhagen). 1992;127(6):542–6.

Padron AS, Neto RA, Pantaleão TU, de Souza dos Santos MC, Araujo RL, de Andrade BM, et al. Administration of 3,5-diiodothyronine (3,5-T2) causes central hypothyroidism and stimulates thyroid-sensitive tissues. J Endocrinol. 2014;221(3):415–27.

Pessemesse L, Lepourry L, Bouton K, Levin J, Cabello G, Wrutniak-Cabello C, et al. p28, a truncated form of TRα1 regulates mitochondrial physiology. FEBS Lett. 2014;588(21):4037–43.

Piehl S, Hoefig CS, Scanlan TS, Köhrle J. Thyronamines – past, present, and future. Endocr Rev. 2011;32(1):64–80.

Puia G. Non genomic modulation of ligand gated ionotropic receptors by thyroid hormones. Immun Endocr Metab Agents Med Chem. 2011;11:179–87.

Puia G, Losi G. Thyroid hormones modulate $GABA_A$ receptor-mediated currents in hippocampal neurons. Neuropharmacology. 2011;60(7–8):1254–61.

Rathmann D, Rijntjes E, Lietzow J, Köhrle J. Quantitative analysis of thyroid hormone metabolites in cell culture samples using LC-MS/MS. Eur Thyroid J. 2015;4 Suppl 1:51–8.

Refetoff S, Bassett JH, Beck-Peccoz P, Bernal J, Brent G, Chatterjee K, et al. Classification and proposed nomenclature for inherited defects of thyroid hormone action, cell transport, and metabolism. J Clin Endocrinol Metab. 2014;99(3):768–70.

Roberts MS, Woods AJ, Dale TC, Van Der Sluijs P, Norman JC. Protein kinase B/Akt acts via glycogen synthase kinase 3 to regulate recycling of αvβ3 and α5β1 integrins. Mol Cell Biol. 2004;24(4):1505–15.

Sakaguchi Y, Cui G, Sen L. Acute effects of thyroid hormone on inward rectifier potassium channel currents in guinea pig ventricular myocytes. Endocrinology. 1996;137(11):4744–51.

Scapin S, Leoni S, Spagnuolo S, Fiore AM, Incerpi S. Short-term effects of thyroid hormones on Na^+-K^+-ATPase activity of chick embryo hepatocytes during development: focus on signal transduction. Am J Physiol Cell Physiol. 2009;296(1):C4–12.

Scapin S, Leoni S, Spagnuolo S, Gnocchi D, De Vito P, Luly P, et al. Short-term effects of thyroid hormones during development: focus on signal transduction. Steroids. 2010;75(8–9):576–84.

Schmohl KA, Müller AM, Wechselberger A, Rühland S, Salb N, Schwenk N, et al. Thyroid hormones and tetrac: new regulators of tumour stroma formation via integrin αvβ3. Endocr Relat Cancer. 2015;22(6):941–52.

Segal J, Ingbar SH. Stimulation by triiodothyronine of the in vitro uptake of sugars by rat thymocytes. J Clin Invest. 1979;63(3):507–15.

Segal J, Ingbar SH. Evidence that an increase in cytoplasmic calcium is the initiating event in certain plasma membrane-mediated responses to 3,5,3′-triiodothyronine in rat thymocytes. Endocrinology. 1989;124(4):1949–55.

Senese R, Cioffi F, de Lange P, Goglia F, Lanni A. Thyroid: biological actions of 'nonclassical' thyroid hormones. J Endocrinol. 2014;221:R1–12.

Shang G, Gao P, Zhao Z, Chen Q, Jiang T, Zhang N, et al. 3,5-Diiodo-L-thyronine ameliorates diabetic nephropathy in streptozotocin-induced diabetic rats. Biochim Biophys Acta. 2013;1832(5):674–84.

Shih A, Lin HY, Davis FB, Davis PJ. Thyroid hormone promotes serine phosphorylation of p53 by mitogen-activated protein kinase. Biochemistry. 2001;40(9):2870–8.

Shih A, Zhang S, Cao HJ, Tang HY, Davis FB, Davis PJ, et al. Disparate effects of thyroid hormone on actions of epidermal growth factor and transforming growth factor-α are mediated by 3′,5′-cyclic adenosine 5′-monophosphate-dependent protein kinase II. Endocrinology. 2004;145(4):1708–17.

Siegrist-Kaiser CA, Juge-Aubry C, Tranter MP, Ekenbarger DM, Leonard JL. Thyroxine–dependent modulation of actin polymerization in cultured astrocytes: a novel, extranuclear action of thyroid hormone. J Biol Chem. 1990;265:5296–02.

Stenzel D, Wilsch-Bräuninger M, Wong FK, Heuer H, Huttner WB. Integrin αvβ3 and thyroid hormones promote expansion of progenitors in embryonic neocortex. Development. 2014;141(4):795–806.

Sterling K, Milch PO. Thyroid hormone binding by a component of mitochondrial membrane. Proc Natl Acad Sci U S A. 1975;72(8):3225–9.

Sterling K, Lazarus JH, Milch PO, Sakurada T, Brenner MA. Mitochondrial thyroid hormone receptor: localization and physiological significance. Science. 1978;201(4361):1126–9.

Sterling K, Brenner MA, Sakurada T. Rapid effect of triiodothyronine on the mitochondrial pathway in rat liver in vivo. Science. 1980;210(4467):340–2.

Storey NM, O'Bryan JP, Armstrong DL. Rac and Rho mediate opposing hormonal regulation of the ether-a-go-go-related potassium channel. Curr Biol. 2002;12(1):27–33.

Storey NM, Gentile S, Ullah H, Russo A, Muessel M, Erxleben C, et al. Rapid signaling at the plasma membrane by a nuclear receptor for thyroid hormone. Proc Natl Acad Sci U S A. 2006;103(13):5197–201.

Tata JR. Inhibition of the biological action of thyroid hormones by actinomycin D and puromycin. Nature. 1963;197:1167–8.

Tata JR, Ernster L, Lindberg O. Control of basal metabolic rate by thyroid hormones and cellular function. Nature. 1962;193:1058–60.

Verga Falzacappa C, Petrucci E, Patriarca V, Michienzi S, Stigliano A, Brunetti E, et al. Thyroid hormone receptor TRβ1 mediates Akt activation by T3 in pancreatic β cells. J Mol Endocrinol. 2007;38(1–2):221–33.

Walker JD, Crawford Jr FA, Mukherjee R, Spinale FG. The direct effects of 3,5,3′-triiodo-L-thyronine (T_3) on myocyte contractile processes. Insights into mechanisms of action. J Thorac Cardiovasc Surg. 1995;110(5):1369–79. discussion 1379–80.

Wrutniak C, Cassar-Malek I, Marchal S, Rascle A, Heusser S, Keller JM, et al. A 43-kDa protein related to c-Erb A α1 is located in the mitochondrial matrix of rat liver. J Biol Chem. 1995;270:16347–54.

Wrutniak-Cabello C, Casas F, Cabello G. Thyroid hormone action in mitochondria. J Mol Endocrinol. 2001;26:67–77.

Yonkers MA, Ribera AB. Nongenomic thyroxine regulation of voltage-gated sodium current during embryonic development. Immun Endo Metab Agents Med Chem. 2011;11(3):157–64.

Zamoner A, Pessoa-Pureur R. Nongenomic actions of thyroid hormones: every why has a wherefore. Immun Endocr Metab Agents Med Chem. 2011;11(3):165–78.

Zanatta AP, Zanatta L, Gonçalves R, Zamoner A, Silva FR. Integrin participates in the effect of thyroxine on plasma membrane in immature rat testis. Biochim Biophys Acta. 2013;1830(3):2629–37.

Part IV

The Classical Endocrine System and Endocrine Glands

The Hypothalamus–Pituitary Axis

11

Linda Johnston Rohrbasser, Hussain Alsaffar, and Joanne Blair

Abstract

The hypothalamic pituitary axis is an intricate pathway with a central role in maintaining homeostasis by integrating complex physiological and endocrine inputs, and neuronal and hormonal output. Disorders of the pathway result in profound disturbance in blood pressure, thirst and electrolyte balance, body temperature, appetite and energy metabolism, reproduction, circadian rhythms and sleep, and the emergency response to stress. Untreated, abnormalities of the axis are incompatible with life.

In this chapter we discuss the embryology, anatomy and physiology of the axis. The function of the hypothalamus as the primary regulator of neuroendocrine system is described, examining the neurological and endocrine responses that maintain physiological set points in response to neurological, chemical, and hormonal inputs. The physiology of the endocrine function of the pituitary is discussed, drawing on examples of developmental abnormalities in man to illustrate the clinical consequences of deficiencies in this pathway.

Keywords

Hypothalamus • Pituitary • Homeostasis • Neuroendocrine

Contents

L.J. Rohrbasser
Paediatric Endocrinology and Diabetes Practice, Starnberg, Germany

H. Alsaffar • J. Blair (✉)
Department of Paediatric Endocrinology, Alder Hey Children's Hospital, Liverpool, UK
e-mail: jo.blair@alderhey.nhs.uk

A. Belfiore, D. LeRoith (eds.), *Principles of Endocrinology and Hormone Action*, Endocrinology, https://doi.org/10.1007/978-3-319-44675-2_12

The neuroendocrine system plays a critical role in homeostatic regulation, which is essential for survival and reproduction. Homeostasis is the process by which a steady state is achieved in physiological functions, primarily, heart rate and blood pressure, thirst and electrolyte balance, body temperature, appetite and energy metabolism, reproduction, circadian rhythms and sleep, and the emergency response to stress.

Hypothalamus

The hypothalamus is the integrator of the neuroendocrine system monitoring neurological, chemical, and hormonal inputs, comparing these to physiological set points (electrolyte and fluid balance, body temperature, blood pressure, and body weight) and responding both neurologically and through hormone secretion to restore homeostasis (Fig. 1). This involves the complex integration of positive and negative feedback loops and synaptic inputs from other brain areas and from the autonomic nervous system. Hypothalamic neuropeptides are also secreted in regions of the brain out with the hypothalamus where they modulate and coordinate behavior to complement their hormonal actions. The hypothalamic hormones include thyrotropin-releasing hormone, gonadotropin-releasing hormone, growth hormone-releasing hormone, somatostatin, corticotrophin-releasing hormone, dopamine, oxytocin, and AVP. The set points remain stable from day to day through homeostasis, the coordinated integration of the classic neuroendocrine pathways with the autonomic and central nervous systems.

Embryology

Three weeks following conception, the cells of the developing embryo have organized in to three sheets: ectoderm, mesoderm, and endoderm. The ectoderm, the most exterior or distal layer, gives rise to epidermal skin cells and neuroectoderm,

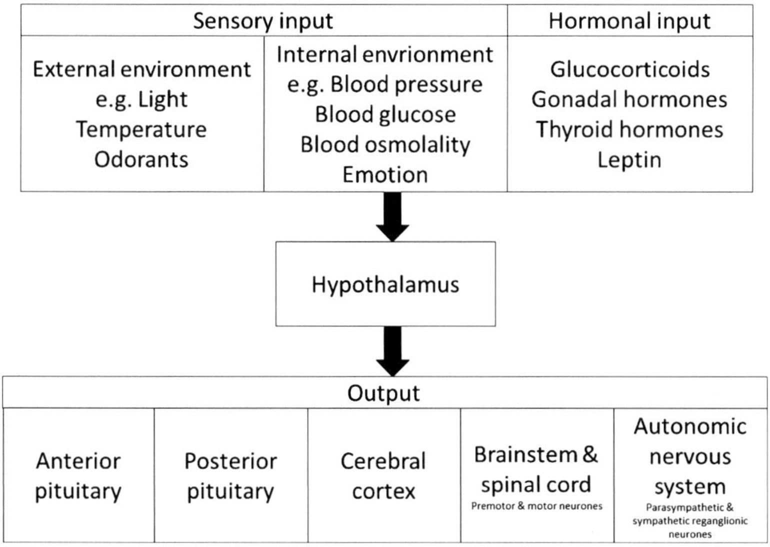

Fig. 1 Simplified overview of hypothalamic integration and coordination

which in turn produces the neural tube and neural crest. Vesicles develop at the cranial end of the neural tube. At the end of fourth week, as the vesicles grow, the neural tube undergoes flexion to form three vesicles: the prosencephalon (future forebrain), mesencephalon (future midbrain), and rhombencephalon (future hindbrain).

In the fifth week, the three vesicles become five, with the forebrain and hindbrain both splitting into two, forming the telencephalon and diencephalon from the forebrain and the metencephalon and the myelencephalon from the hindbrain. Historically, the optic cup and stalk, pituitary gland, thalamus, hypothalamus, and pineal body were thought to arise from the diencephalon. The more recently proposed "prosomere model" (Puelles 2009), the segmental structural model based on gene expression in the mouse, suggests that the hypothalamus is derived from the secondary prosencephalon; ventral aspects of the two or three rostral (anterior) segments of the neural tube and the dorsal derivatives of which form the telencephalon (Freeman 2003; Puelles 2001; Alvarez-Bolado 2015) (Fig. 2).

Anatomy

The hypothalamus constitutes less than 1% of brain volume and weighs approximately 5 g. It is a highly conserved region of the brain whose destruction is not compatible with life. The hypothalamus is a bilateral structure like the cerebral hemispheres, unlike the pituitary. It extends from the optic chiasm and anterior

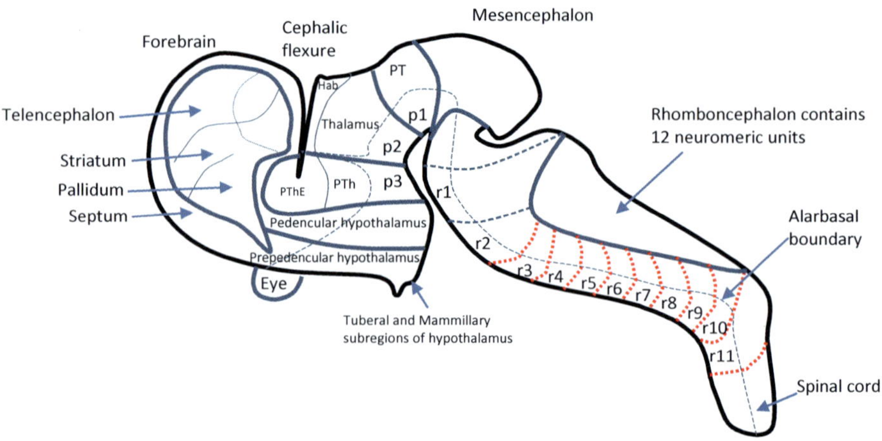

Fig. 2 The scheme shows all longitudinal components, but the floor and roof plates are not represented. The caudal forebrain or diencephalon consists of three prosomeres (p1–p3) whose alar regions include the pretectum (PT), the thalamus and habenula (Th–hab), and the prethalamus and prethalamic eminence (PTh, PThE) (Modified from the prosomeric model of Puelles and Rubenstein (2003))

commissure to the posterior margins of the mammillary bodies and from the thalamus laterally to form the floor and part of the lateral wall of the third ventricle. The regional structures of the hypothalamus are defined by nuclei with distinct functions (Figs. 3, and 4 and Table 1).

The hypothalamic floor projects down to continue as the median eminence, then the infundibulum, and ultimately the posterior pituitary (neurohypophysis). Hormones released from the median eminence reach the anterior pituitary via the hypophysial portal system.

The floor of hypothalamus between the infundibulum and mammillary bodies is known as the tuberal area and contains most of the cell bodies of the small neurons containing hypothalamic-releasing hormones.

Functional Aspects of Hypothalamic Function

Neurosecretory cells are neurons that do not terminate in classical synapses but secrete their neurotransmitters/hormones direct into the bloodstream. In the hypothalamic region, these have been classified as "magnocellular," large cells with high synthetic activity located in the supraoptic and paraventricular regions, and "parvocellular," small neurons in the paraventricular nucleus and rostrally in adjacent parts of the septal region. Magnocellular neurosecretory cells synthesize and secrete oxytocin and AVP. Parvocellular neurosecretory cells release factors at the median eminence into the hypophysial portal blood system to regulate pituitary

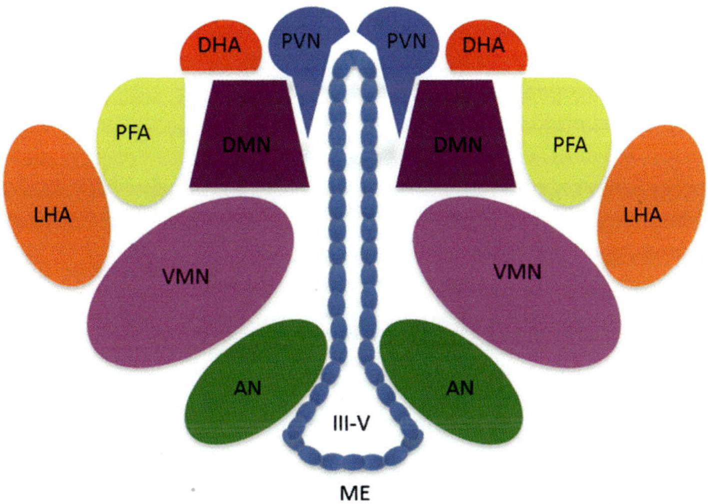

Fig. 3 Schematic coronal view of hypothalamic nuclei location around the third ventricle (III-V). *III-V* third ventricle, *ME* median eminence, *AN* arcuate nucleus, *VMN* ventromedial nucleus, *DMN* dorsomedial nucleus, *PVN* periventricular nucleus, *DHA* dorsal hypothalamic area, *PFA* perifornical area, *LHA* lateral hypothalamic area, *SCN* suprachiasmatic nucleus, *SON* supraoptic nucleus, *POA* preoptic area, *MB* mammillary bodies, *AHN* anterior hypothalamic nuclei, *PHN* posterior hypothalamic nuclei

Fig. 4 Schematic sagittal view of the hypothalamic nuclei. *III-V* third ventricle, *ME* median eminence, *AN* arcuate nucleus, *VMN* ventromedial nucleus, *DMN* dorsomedial nucleus, *PVN* periventricular nucleus, *DHA* dorsal hypothalamic area, *PFA* perifornical area, *LHA* lateral hypothalamic area, *SCN* suprachiasmatic nucleus, *SON* supraoptic nucleus, *POA* preoptic area, *MB* mammillary bodies, *AHN* anterior hypothalamic nuclei, *PHN* posterior hypothalamic nuclei

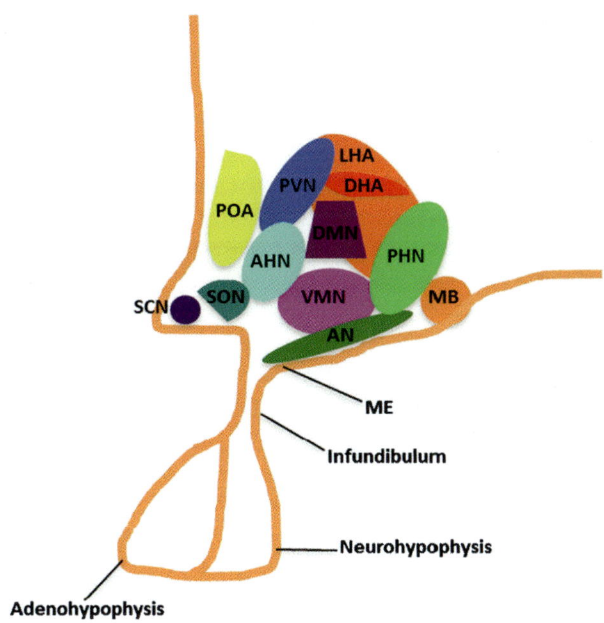

Table 1 A summary of the hypothalamic nuclei and their functions

Nucleus	Output	Functions
Paraventricular	Autonomic system	Fluid balance
	TRH	Milk letdown
	CRH	Parturition
	Oxytocin, vasopressin	Autonomic
	Somatostatin	Ant pit control
Preoptic	LHRH	Lateral anterior thermoregulation
		Sexual behavior
Anterior	Thermoregulation, panting, sweating	Lateral anterior thermoregulation
	Thyrotropin inhibition	Sexual behavior
Suprachiasmatic (SCN)	Projections to hypothalamic nuclei	Major pacemaker
Supraoptic	Vasopressin	Fluid balance
	Oxytocin	Milk letdown
		Parturition
Dorsomedial		Emotion (rage)
		BP, heart rate
		GI stimulation
Ventromedial	Satiety	Appetite
	Neuroendo control	Body weight
		Insulin regulation
Arcuate	ANS, caudal brainstem, parts of cortex, and limbic system	Control of anterior pituitary
	GHRH (neuroendocrine neurons)	Energy balance
	Dopamine	Prolactin inhibition
Posterior	Increase BP	Thermoregulation
	Pupillary dilation	
	Shivering	
	Vasopressin release	
Mammillary	Memory	Emotion, short-term memory
Tuberomammillary		Arousal, feeding, and energy balance
		Learning, memory, sleep
Lateral complex	Orexin	Arousal, appetite
	Melanin-concentrating hormone	Feeding, mood, sleep/wake cycle

function. Their hormones in turn control the secretion, and often synthesis, of hormones from five classic cell types in the anterior pituitary. These cells receive multiple neuronal inputs and integrate these in their subsequent neurosecretory response. While the anterior pituitary releases hormones in response to the stimulatory or inhibitory hypothalamic hormones, these are in turn influenced by neurological input from several regions of the brain.

The hypophysial portal system is a rich complex of blood vessels from the base of the hypothalamus, draining into a mesh of capillaries and ultimately the pituitary sinusoids. They create a great increase in vascular surface area and are also fenestrated, further facilitating the diffusion of hypothalamic factors to the anterior pituitary.

Another major input to neuroendocrine homeostatic regulation through the hypothalamus is the autonomic nervous system. Additionally direct innervation of glands, including the adrenals, pancreas, and pineal and salivary glands, influences the regulation of their exocrine and endocrine functions. The pancreas receives both sympathetic and parasympathetic inputs whose interplay exquisitely influences glucose homeostasis through insulin and glucagon secretion.

The hypothalamus, as part of the brain, is protected from peripheral humoral and chemical signals through the blood–brain barrier. However for homeostatic control, key regions of the brain must receive sensory information from the bloodstream including hormone levels, electrolytes, and glucose as well as potential toxins. The circumventricular organs (CVOs) are regions that allow the passage of peripheral cues into key neuronal cell groups, facilitating homeostasis. The CVOs lie along the third and fourth ventricles in the midline and include the subfornical organ (SFO), the organum vasculosum of the lamina terminalis (OVLT), the median eminence, and the neurohypophysis. In these CVO regions, there is a rich blood supply with fenestrated capillaries that allow relatively free diffusion of proteins and peptide hormones. Several of the CVOs have major projections to hypothalamic nuclei that play a role in homeostasis.

Circadian Rhythms

Circadian rhythms refer to the daily fluctuations that occur in hormone secretion, body temperature, and sleep/wake cycle. The main hypothalamic nucleus involved is the suprachiasmatic nucleus (SCN), the body's master clock. SCN neurons have intrinsic rhythmical discharge activity with a 25 h cycle in the absence of light input. Light-stimulated input from the retinohypothalamic tract entrains the SCN neuronal rhythm to a 24 h cycle. The SCN has output projections into multiple hypothalamic nuclei controlling the circadian rhythm of several specific functions including thermoregulation, glucocorticoid secretion, sleep, arousal, and feeding.

Light-stimulated activation of the SCN results in increased input to the paraventricular nucleus which stimulates sympathetic pathways which inhibit the secretion of melatonin from the pineal gland. Thus darkness and the subsequent loss of sympathetic inhibitory signals allow increased melatonin secretion.

Disorders of circadian rhythm can manifest themselves as sleep disorders, for example, phase shifting or jet lag, delayed sleep phase syndrome often seen in teenagers, or advanced sleep phase syndrome seen in the elderly. Disorders of circadian rhythm often, but not always, affect the blind. The retinohypothalamic tract is not a visual tract and can thus be normal in the blind or defective in those with normal vision.

Sleep allows energy conservation through reduced organic and physical activities and thus influences energy homeostasis. During wakefulness activities lead to hunger which promotes feeding. Chronic circadian rhythm disruption influences sleep, the immune system, appetite, and energy balance (Markwald 2013).

The SCN functionally connects hypothalamic sleeping to feeding centers. The SCN efferent projections target the subparaventricular zone (SPZ) with axons also extending to the dorsomedial nuclei (DMN). Lesions in the ventral SPZ have demonstrated its key regulation of rhythmicity in sleep, feeding, and activity. The DMN sends efferents to the sleep regulation center in the ventrolateral preoptic area, the PVN (corticotrophin-releasing hormone, CRH) neurons and signals to autonomic nervous system, and the lateral hypothalamus (orexin- and melanin-concentrating hormone). The DMN also receive inputs from the arcuate nucleus (appetite and energy expenditure regulation). The ventromedial hypothalamus expresses brain-derived neurotrophic factor (BDNF) under regulation of the melanocortin 4 receptor (MC4R). BDNF regulates sleep onset and hedonic food intake (Faraguna et al. 2008).

In humans a diurnal variation in temperature has been observed depending on the periods of rest and activity, with core temperature lowest between 23 and 3 h during sleep and peaking during the day between 10 and 18 h.

Energy Homeostasis

The obesity epidemic has been the stimulus to much research in energy homeostasis. Imbalance between food intake and energy expenditure causes weight gain and metabolic dysfunction with significant morbidity and mortality in energy excess, whereas in starvation, energy must be conserved for essential organs, e.g., the brain, and diverted from nonessential functions, e.g., reproduction.

The central melanocortin system in the hypothalamus integrates peripheral signals and regulates peripheral organ functions. Arcuate nucleus pro-opiomelanocortin (POMC)-expressing neurons and neuropeptide Y (NPY) and agouti-related peptide (AgRP) co-expressing neurons interact with melanocortin 4 receptor (MC4R)-expressing neurons in the paraventricular nucleus. POMC neurons stimulate MC4R and induce reduced food intake and increased energy expenditure (anorexigenic effect), while NPY–AgRP neurons are orexigenic, antagonizing POMC action and inducing increased food intake and reduced energy expenditure.

In POMC knockout mice and patients with POMC gene mutations, early-onset obesity is observed (Krude 1998; Yaswen et al. 1999). In contrast NPY and AgRP mutations have no significant effect on food intake or body weight (Qian et al. 2002).

The POMC gene protein precursor generates a number of bioactive peptides (ACTH, α-, β-, and γ-melanocyte-stimulating hormone (MSH), β-endorphin)

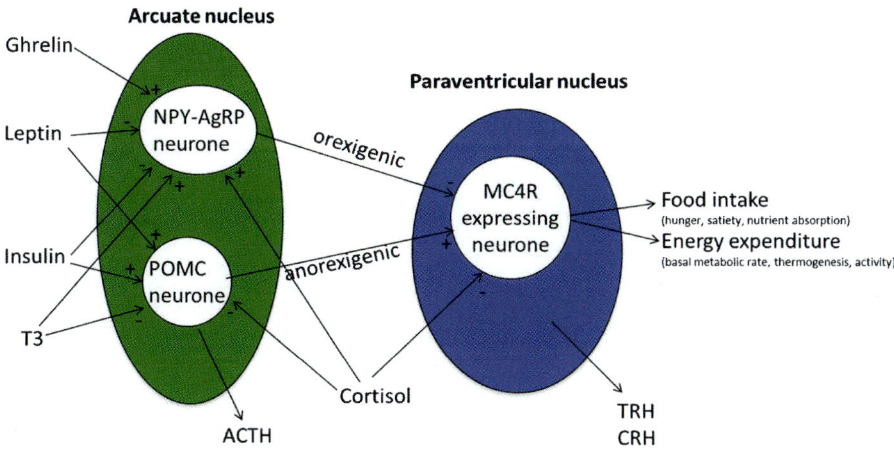

Fig. 5 Schematic overview of hormonal regulation of energy homeostasis

through posttranslational modifications. Alpha MSH mediates its anorexigenic and AgRP its orexigenic effects through binding and activation of MCRs. The MC3R is expressed in the POMC neurons of the arcuate nucleus, and MC4R are expressed in several regions of the central nervous system (CNS) including the hypothalamic paraventricular nucleus. MC3R and MC4R mice mutations are associated with reduced energy expenditure and MC4R mutations also with hyperphagia. Human MC4R mutations have been reported in nonsyndromic obesity (Vaisse et al. 1998).

The melanocortin system is in turn influenced by many peripheral signals including leptin, ghrelin, insulin, glucocorticoids, and thyroid hormones. These hormones feed information into the melanocortin system regarding the metabolic status of the organism (Fig. 5).

Leptin is anorexigenic and produced by white adipose tissue in amounts proportional to the body fat mass. While leptin has several receptors, only the long form with extracellular and cytoplasmic domains mediates the effect of leptin. Leptin or leptin receptor deficiency is associated with a morbid obese phenotype with hyperphagia, hyperglycemia, hyperlipidemia, and reduced energy expenditure (Montague et al. 1997; Clément et al. 1998). In mice neuron-specific Ob-R deficiency was associated with obesity, while hepatocyte-specific deficiency was not, showing that the direct effect of leptin on the CNS is key to exerting its metabolic effects. Leptin has been shown to activate POMC neurons and suppress activation of NPY–AgRP neurons.

Insulin, secreted from pancreatic β islet cells, stimulates glucose uptake in peripheral organs promoting weight gain. However, in the CNS, insulin receptors are widely expressed, and insulin's actions are anorexigenic. Brain-specific insulin receptor-deficient mice have a phenotype of obesity with hyperphagia (Brüning et al. 2000). Studies in L1 mice (reduced insulin receptor in the arcuate nucleus) suggest that insulin receptor activation in POMC neurons positively regulates hepatic glucose production and energy expenditure, while insulin signaling in AgRP neurons has the opposite effect. Insulin and leptin appear to have similar effects on glucose homeostasis but opposing effects on body weight (Williams et al. 2010).

Ghrelin is secreted from endocrine stomach cells when the stomach is empty. It exerts its orexigenic effects through activation of the growth hormone secretagogue receptor (GHSR). GHSR is strongly expressed in the hypothalamus, predominantly in the NPY–AgRP neurons of the arcuate nucleus, ghrelin's main site of action in the CNS. Ghrelin's inhibition of POMC action is probably mediated through the activation of NPY–AgRp neurons. Indeed its effect is abolished in NPY–AgRP double knockout mice (Chen et al.). Ghrelin also increases enzymatic degradation of α-MSH to further enhance its orexigenic effects (Kwon Jeong et al. 2013). Ghrelin resistance develops in obese overfed mice but not in ob/ob mice suggesting leptin plays a role in this resistance. CNS administration of leptin to ob/ob mice induced ghrelin resistance confirming this hypothesis (Wang et al. 2013).

Thyroid hormones affect both food intake and energy expenditure. Hyperthyroidism induces hyperphagia by T_3 stimulation of NPY and inhibition of POMC neurons in the arcuate nucleus (Ishii et al. 2003). Starvation leads to increased T_4 to T_3 conversion in the hypothalamus. T_3 regulates uncoupling protein 2 activity which mediates ghrelin action on the NPY–AgRp neurons to increase feeding behavior (Vella et al. 2011).

Glucocorticoid excess in Cushing's syndrome is associated with rapid weight gain, hypertension, hyperglycemia, and insulin resistance, whereas hypocortisolism in Addison's disease or after adrenalectomy is associated with weight loss, reduced appetite, and hypoglycemia. ACTH produced by POMC cells stimulates adrenal glucocorticoid production. However POMC also has direct central effects (Smart et al. 2006). In adrenalectomized mice, there are changes in the synaptic organization of arcuate POMC neurons and enhanced central effects of leptin.

There are many additional influences on appetite – glucose, fatty acid, and amino acids also function as signal molecules of peripheral energy homeostasis. These components have differential effects by altering the activity levels of different components of the system.

Glucose is the primary energy source of the brain, and hypothalamic glucose-sensing neurons are present in several hypothalamic nuclei, suggesting that nutrient status can influence many other systems (Routh et al. 2012). Brain glucose levels are lower than blood glucose levels, and there are distinct diffusion barriers (e.g., circumventricular organs) allowing movement of glucose from the periphery to the CNS and also between brain regions. Controlled by glial cells capable of glucose sensing, this diffusion is regionally differentially regulated and influenced by nutritional status.

Glucose-excited neurons have been found among GnRH neurons of the anterior hypothalamus, the preautonomic neurons in the paraventricular hypothalamus, and the melanin-concentrating hormone neurons in the lateral hypothalamus. Glucose sensing through activation of the KATP channel as in the beta pancreatic cell has been described but not for all regions.

Glucose-inhibited neurons are also found in many hypothalamic regions, e.g., ventromedial nucleus, arcuate nucleus, paraventricular nucleus, dorsolateral nucleus, and the lateral hypothalamus. While nitric oxide signaling is responsible for glucose sensing in some glucose-inhibited neurons, the exact mechanism is not understood in many regions, including the arcuate NPY–AgRP neurons.

There is a sensitive mechanism for providing the brain with a constant supply of glucose, and glucose-sensing neurons detect hypoglycemia and play a role in the initiation of the counter-regulatory response to hypoglycemia. During fasting, reduced leptin and ghrelin levels lead directly and indirectly to activation of NPY–AgRP and orexigenic glucose inhibitory neurons. This is associated with increased food intake, gluconeogenesis, and ketogenesis in order to maintain a supply of energy to the brain. Additionally, glucose-sensing neurons may divert energy away from competing systems or allow such functions, e.g., reproduction, only when glucose levels are adequate.

The hypothalamus is the main integrator of inputs and responses in the control of appetite and energy expenditure. It is a complex process involving the input of several endocrine, chemical, and neurological signals, coordinated predominantly by the melanocortin system into an endocrine and neurological response to maintain body weight. However there is much research still needed to understand the exact details of the control of energy homeostasis.

The homeostatic control of energy intake and expenditure is tightly controlled by the hypothalamus. Signals from the "hedonic" corticolimbic pathways are also integrated but can override the homeostatic system increasing desire to consume palatable foods despite satiety. Environmental changes with increased availability of energy-rich foods, increased portion size, and reduced physical activity due to more sedentary jobs further facilitate the development of obesity through "hedonic" overriding the homeostatic controls (Lenard and Berthoud 2008).

Water and Electrolyte Balance

The balance of water and electrolyte intake must be carefully balanced with water and electrolyte loss in order to maintain a stable total body fluid volume and osmolality. Osmoreceptors in the anterior hypothalamus and circumventricular organs detect changes in plasma osmolality. Projections from these regions then activate both stimulatory and inhibitory neurons connecting with the supraoptic and paraventricular nuclei. So, if osmolality increases, then AVP, which is produced in the supraoptic nucleus and magnocellular neurons in the paraventricular nucleus, is released from the posterior pituitary gland into the circulation. In the nephron, AVP promotes water reabsorption to correct the increased osmolality.

Non-osmotic stimuli from baroreceptors influence the same hypothalamic nuclei via the medulla and nucleus tractus solitarius. In addition to AVP released from the posterior pituitary, there are AVP-secreting neurons stretching from the PVN and SCN to the brainstem and spinal cord where they influence the sympathetic nervous system.

Thirst regulates water intake and involves neural and hormonal input. Activation of the hypothalamic thirst center occurs when the mouth is dry and when osmolality increases. Decreased blood volume results in release of renin from the kidney and subsequent activation of the angiotensin II which directly stimulates the hypothalamic thirst center too.

Renin-stimulated aldosterone production results in increased nephron reabsorption of sodium with secretion of potassium. In addition to AVP action, this makes sure that the volume and osmolality are restored. Activation of the sympathetic nervous system also causes vasoconstriction of the afferent arteriole and reduced nephron perfusion resulting in a fall in urine output.

Blood Pressure and Heart Rate

Blood pressure homeostasis primarily involves the interplay between sympathetic and parasympathetic autonomic nervous systems but is also influenced by the neuroendocrine factors (e.g., CRF, GH, angiotensin II, AVP). Changes in hypothalamic nuclei output can result in a rise or reduction of blood pressure by altering sympathetic nervous activity. These nuclei are closely interconnected and receive afferent input from the midbrain, medulla, and chemo- and baroreceptors in the heart, aorta, carotids, and kidneys with efferent outputs to spinal sympathetic preganglionic neurons which control the sympathetic ganglia and adrenal medulla.

The hypothalamic regions particularly involved in blood pressure homeostasis lie along the third ventricle and also include the circumventricular organs (SFO and OVLT) which allow the input of peripheral chemical signals, including sodium ion concentration. The paraventricular, arcuate, medial preoptic, and supraoptic are primarily involved, but there are many projections to, and input from, other hypothalamic nuclei including the SCN which influences the circadian rhythm of heart rate and blood pressure related to sleep. The dorsomedial nucleus has direct and indirect connections to the autonomic nervous system.

The arterial baroreceptors autonomic reflexes respond rapidly to changes in blood pressure and alter heart rate through changed sympathetic tone. Low-pressure baroreceptors in the large veins and right atrium influence blood volume through autonomic stimulation of the neuroendocrine system. A drop in blood pressure will also stimulate retention of salt and water and increase thirst. A wide range of neurotransmitters and hormones play a role in this process including GABA, natriuretic peptides, angiotensin II, AVP, nitric oxide, serotonin, NPY, opioids, bradykinins, thyrotropin-releasing hormone (TRH), and corticotropin-releasing hormone (CRH). Their individual roles and complex peripheral and central interactions are out with the scope of the chapter. A few examples are discussed below.

The angiotensin pathways from the lamina terminalis to the PVN, supraoptic nucleus, and rostral ventrolateral medulla are activated by circulating angiotensin II, CSF sodium ion concentration, and possibly aldosterone. Activation leads to increased sympathetic output largely by reducing GABA and raising glutamate release in fast synaptic transmission pathways.

High dietary salt is detected in the circumventricular organs of the brain when CSF sodium ion concentration rises. This in turn promotes endogenous ouabain release from the adrenal gland which leads to a sustained increase in angiotensin II. The latter is a much slower pathway, but these two neuromodulatory paths allow the CNS to shift gears rapidly and cause sustained sympathetic hyperactivity in an efficient manner (Blaustein et al. 2012; Hamlyn et al. 2014).

Temperature

Body temperature is tightly regulated as excursions from this range result in detrimental changes to cellular function, e.g., reduced enzyme efficiency and altered membrane diffusion, which in turn have significant impact on energy availability. While recovery from low temperatures in hibernating mammals is usual, smaller increases in brain temperature are incompatible with life. Small increases in temperature can occur in the febrile response to endogenous pyrogens released during infections. This is supposed to improve host defense and reduce pathogen viability. Thus temperature homeostasis is essential for survival and plays a role in defense against pathogens.

Information on temperature is provided by cutaneous thermal receptors through sensory nerves to the spinal dorsal horn neurons and to the lateral parabrachial nucleus in the pons. Body core structures including the brain, spinal cord, and abdomen transmit temperature information through the splanchnic and vagal nerve afferents. At the level of the hypothalamus, this information is integrated in the preoptic and anterior areas. The preoptic area has been shown to respond to both increases and decreases in temperature and integrates these sensory inputs to generate signals aimed at restoring normal body temperature. Signals from the dorsomedial hypothalamus to the rostral ventromedial medulla complete the pathway to the sympathetic nervous system. The effectors in thermoregulation under sympathetic nerve control include cutaneous circulation (vasoconstriction or vasodilation); thermogenesis from brown adipose tissue, skeletal muscle (shivering), or the heart (increased heart rate); and evaporative loss (e.g., sweating, panting) (Morrison and Nakamura 2011).

Pituitary

The anterior pituitary gland plays a critical role in homeostasis by integrating complex peripheral signals from the hypothalamus and other peripheral organs, intrapituitary signals, and external stimuli to regulate release of anterior pituitary hormones into the peripheral circulation.

The classical feedback mechanisms of the hypothalamic pituitary axis and its target organs were described many years ago. In more recent years, our understanding of the role of intrapituitary regulators of pituitary cell growth, apoptosis, hormone secretion, and hormone release has expanded rapidly, to give finer detail of the complex mechanisms underlying the release of anterior pituitary hormones.

Embryology

The pituitary gland is similar in all vertebrates and has been studied extensively in the mouse (Fig. 2) (Kelberman and Dattani 2007; Alatzoglou et al. 2009). The anterior and intermediate lobes arise from oral ectoderm, while the posterior pituitary is derived from neural ectoderm.

During the third week of gestation, an outpocketing of oral ectoderm, the hypophysial diverticulum, appears in front of the buccopharyngeal membrane, preceded by localized thickening of the ectoderm (pituitary placode). This placode is located ventrally in the midline of the anterior neural ridge and in the continuity with the future hypothalamo–infundibular region, which is located posteriorly in the rostral part of the neural plate (Alatzoglou et al. 2009). The hypophysial diverticulum forms Rathke's pouch which, in time, will become the anterior lobe of the pituitary. During week 5 of gestation, the neuroectoderm from the diencephalon extends to form the infundibulum (neurohypophysial diverticulum) which grows downward developing into the posterior lobe. The hypophysial diverticulum and the infundibulum grow toward one another, and by the second month, the hypophysial diverticulum is isolated from its ectodermal origin in the oral cavity and lies close to the infundibulum.

Hesx1 is the first transcription factor to be expressed in the developing pituitary, and normal function is required for the development of Rathke's pouch and other midline structures. Abnormalities in this gene are reported in children with pituitary hypoplasia, ectopic posterior pituitaries, optic nerve hypoplasia, and loss of pituitary function (Kelberman et al. 2009). These features may present together as septo-optic dysplasia, in which the corpus callosum is also affected.

The expression of Pitx1 and Pitx2 is evident in the early stages of pituitary embryogenesis and persists during pituitary cell differentiation. Mutations of the Pitx2 gene are associated with Axenfeld–Rieger syndrome. Affected patients have abnormalities of the anterior segment of the eye, dental hypoplasia, a protuberant umbilicus, and abnormalities of the brain. Pituitary involvement is suggested by the presence of a small sella turcica in some patients.

The SOXB1 group of transcription factors, Sox2 and Sox3, are expressed throughout the developing brain and in high levels in the infundibulum and developing hypothalamus. Mutations of the SOX2 gene are associated with anophthalmia, optic nerve hypoplasia, and pituitary hypoplasia and with gonadotropin deficiency and genital abnormalities in boys and growth hormone deficiency. Abnormalities of forebrain structures, including hypoplasia of the corpus callosum, hypothalamic hamartoma, and hippocampal malformations, are also reported.

The SOX3 gene is located on the X chromosome, and the phenotype of SOX3 mutations is inherited in an X-linked manner. Affected boys have learning difficulties and variable pituitary failure, in which GH deficiency is constant and other pituitary hormones may be involved. Imaging studies demonstrate pituitary and infundibular hypoplasia, ectopic posterior pituitary, and hypoplasia of the corpus callosum.

Lhx3 and Lhx4 are essential for normal pituitary development, the role of Lhx3 being primarily in the regulation of cell differentiation and maturation and Lhx4, cell proliferation. Abnormalities of the LHX3 and LHX4 genes have been associated with hypopituitarism, pituitary hypoplasia, and abnormalities of the spine (Kelberman et al. 2009).

The differentiation and proliferation of pituitary stem cells into five distinct hormone-producing cell types are regulated by a spatial and temporal distribution of key transcription factors and signaling pathways. The wingless (WNT) and the sonic hedgehog pathways are important for the regulation of cell proliferation, while bone morphogenetic protein (BMP) and fibroblast growth factor (Fgf) are important in regulating cell proliferation and migration.

Within the ventral ectoderm of Rathke's pouch, a ventral-to-dorsal gradient of BMP 2 and, in the opposite direction, a gradient of Fgf 8 are established. In this way, overlapping sets of transcription factors are synthesized in different

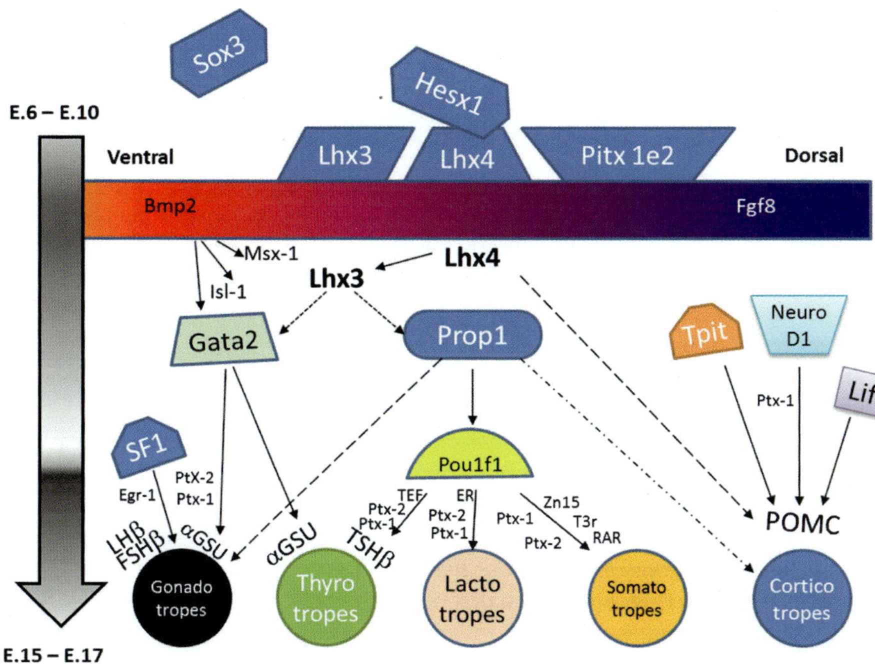

Fig. 6 Activation of pituitary transcription factors. In response to the BMP2–FGF8 ventral–dorsal gradient. *Solid arrows* indicate the activation of expression, *dotted arrows* indicate an unknown role in the activation of expression, *dashed arrows* indicate an undefined role, and *dash–dot arrows* indicate an action of an important factor in the maintenance of long-term cell function. *BMP2* bone morphogenetic protein 2, *EGR1* early growth response 1, *ER* estrogen receptor, *FGF8* fibroblast growth factor 8, *GATA2* GATA-binding protein 2, *HESX1* HESX homeobox 1, *ISL1* ISL LIM homeobox 1, *LHX3* LIM homeobox 3, *LHX4* LIM homeobox 4, *LIF* leukemia inhibitory factor, *MSX1* MSH homeobox 1, *NeuroD1* neurogenic differentiation 1, *PIT1* POU class 1 homeobox 1, *PITX1* paired-like homeodomain 1, *PITX2* paired-like homeodomain 2, *POMC* pro-opiomelanocortin, *PROP1* prophet of Pit-1, *RAR* retinoic acid receptor, *SF1* steroidogenic factor 10, *T3r* thyroid hormone nuclear receptor, *TEF* thyrotroph embryonic factor, *TPIT* T-box19, *Zn15* zinc finger protein Zn15 (Adapted from de Moraes et al (2012)

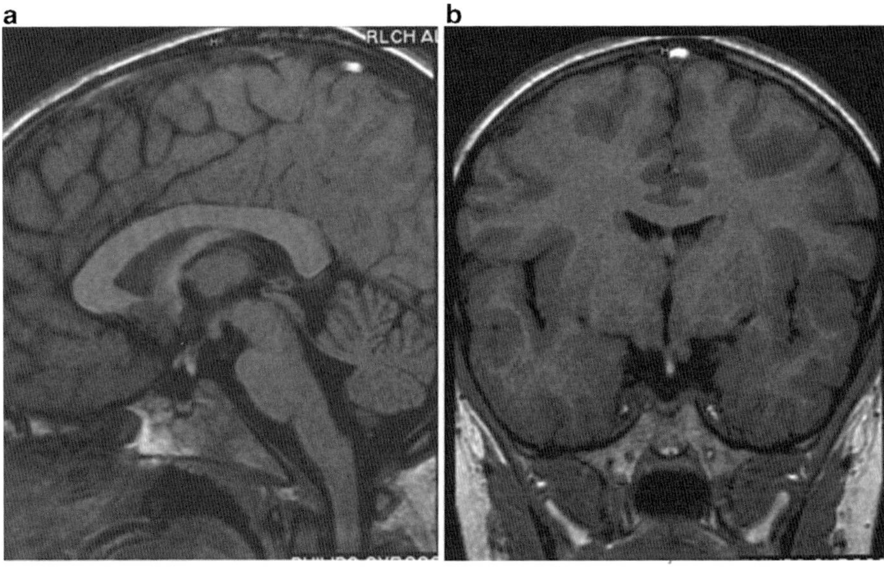

Fig. 7 Pituitary stalk interruption syndrome (PSIS). (**a**) Sagittal and (**b**) coronal T1-weighted MR images show that the posterior lobe of the pituitary is in an ectopic location, the pituitary stalk is absent, and the anterior lobe of the pituitary is hypoplastic (Images courtesy of Dr Laurence Abernethy, Alder Hey Children's NHS Foundation Trust, Liverpool)

populations of cells, dependent upon their location along the dorsal–ventral axis. A simplified cartoon illustrating key transcription factors in the regulation of pituitary cell differentiation is given in Fig. 6.

Mutations in pituitary transcription factors have been identified in patients with multiple pituitary hormone deficiencies (MPHD), less commonly, an isolated pituitary hormone deficiency which may be associated with anatomical changes. Pituitary stalk interruption (Fig. 7) has been described in patients with mutations of the HESX1, LHX4, and SOX3 genes (Yang et al. 2013), while the more severe phenotype of septo-optic dysplasia (Fig. 8) has been described in patients with mutations of HESX1.

The clinical phenotype of patients with mutations of pituitary transcription factors is summarized in Table 2.

Anatomy

The pituitary gland, a small pea-sized organ weighing approximately 0.5 g, rests in the sella turcica, a saddle-shaped depression in the body of sphenoid bone. The pituitary lies between optic chiasm, separated by the diaphragma sellae from above and the sphenoid air cells which located below it. The cavernous sinus and its contents are to be found on each side of the pituitary. The pituitary stalk, which connects the median eminence of the hypothalamus to the pituitary gland, passes through an opening in the dura surrounding the brain.

The pituitary comprises of anterior (adenohypophysis) and posterior (neurohypophysis) lobes. The anterior lobe is subdivided into the pars anterior (pars distalis) and the pars intermedia, which may be separated by a cleft that is a remnant of an embryonic pouch. The pars tuberalis is a projection from the pars anterior that extends upward and forward along the anterior and lateral surfaces of the pituitary.

During childhood the upper border of the anterior pituitary is flat on magnetic resonance imaging, and the height of the pituitary is <6 mm. During normal puberty, physiological pituitary hypertrophy is observed, and the upper border may appear convex. These changes are more evident in girls than in boys, with pituitary height reaching 10 mm in girls (Elster et al. 1990) (Figs. 8 and 9).

Blood Supply of the Pituitary

The principal arterial supply of the pituitary gland is from the superior and inferior hypophysial arteries. The superior hypophysial arteries originate from the internal carotid artery shortly after it enters the cranial cavity and then promptly divide into posterior and anterior branches, each of which anastomoses with the corresponding branch from the opposite side to form an arterial ring around the upper pituitary stalk. Trabecular or loral arteries, from the anterior branches, descend along the upper surface of the anterior lobe toward the pituitary stalk and terminate in long stalk arteries. Short stalk arteries, from both the posterior and anterior branches of the superior hypophysial arteries, penetrate the superior aspect of the pituitary stalk to run superiorly or inferiorly.

The inferior hypophysial arteries originate from the meningohypophysial trunks within the cavernous sinuses. They pass along the inferolateral portions

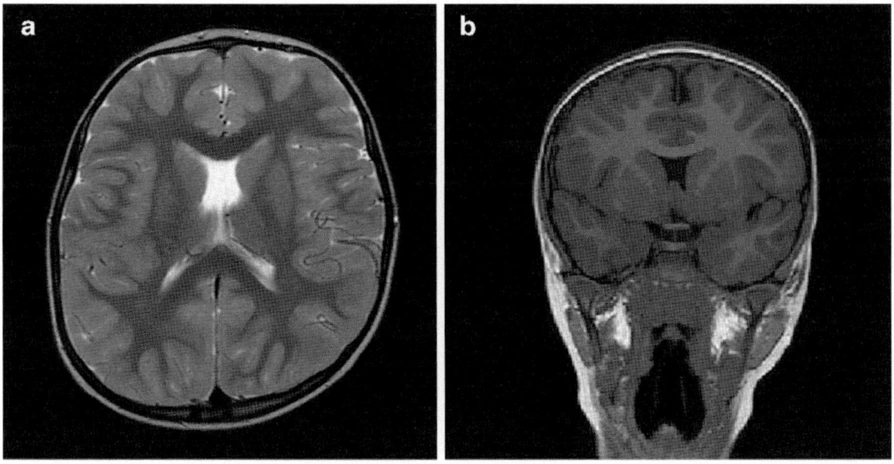

Fig. 8 Septo-optic dysplasia. (**a**) Axial T2-weighted MRI shows the absence of the interventricular septum and an abnormal configuration of the frontal horns of the lateral ventricles. (**b**) Coronal T1-weighted MRI shows absence of the interventricular septum and hypoplasia of the optic chiasm and anterior pituitary (Images courtesy of Dr Laurence Abernethy, Alder Hey Children's NHS Foundation Trust, Liverpool)

Table 2 Mutations in pituitary transcription factors and associated phenotypes

Gene	Key clinical features	Endocrine phenotype
HESX1	Variable, no obvious phenotype–genotype correlation	IGHD or combined with ACTH, TSH, LH, and FSH deficiency
OTX2	Anophthalmia or microphthalmia	CPHD
SOX2	Esophageal atresia, genital abnormalities in males, bilateral anophthalmia, or severe microphthalmia, sensorineural hearing loss, hypothalamic hamartoma	Hypogonadotropic hypogonadism
SOX3	Short male with varying degree of mental retardation, facial anomalies in some patients	IGHD or combined with ACTH, TSH, LH, and FSH deficiency
GLI2	Single nares, single central incisor, postaxial polydactyly, and partial agenesis of the corpus callosum	GH, TSH, PRL, LH, and FSH
LHX3	Short, rigid cervical spine with or without sensorineural deafness	Sparing ACTH in majority, however it has been reported in c.80–32_775 _ 454 del3,088 and p.K50X mutations. Mainly GH, TSH, and gonadotropin deficiency
LHX4	Variable, persistent craniopharyngeal canal and abnormal cerebellar tonsils	IGHD or combined with TSH, ACTH
PROP1	Enlarged pituitary with later involution	GH, TSH, PRL, and gonadotropin deficiency. Evolving ACTH deficiency
POU1F1 (PIT1)	Clinical features of central hypothyroidism at early age	GH, PRL, TSH deficiency
PITX2	Malformation of the anterior segment of the eye, dental hypoplasia, and a protuberant umbilicus	GH deficiency

of the gland and bifurcate into medial and lateral branches that anastomose with their opposite counterparts to form an arterial circle about the posterior lobe. Branches of the inferior hypophysial arteries supply the posterior lobe and lower portion of the stalk, with only a minor contribution to the periphery of the anterior lobe (Fig. 10).

Gomitoli, “balls of thread,” are unique vascular complexes formed from arterial branches of the pituitary stalk and infundibulum. Blood flow through these vessels is regulated by thick smooth muscle sphincters located in short specialized arterioles at the transition from central arteries to capillaries. The periarteriolar capillaries drain into an extensive pampiniform network, the portal system, which envelopes the stalk. The anterior pituitary receives the majority of its blood supply not from arteries but from the portal system which forms a vital link between the hypothalamus and the pituitary gland.

Venous outflow of the pituitary is via collecting vessels that drain into the subhypophysial sinus, cavernous sinus, and superior circular sinus.

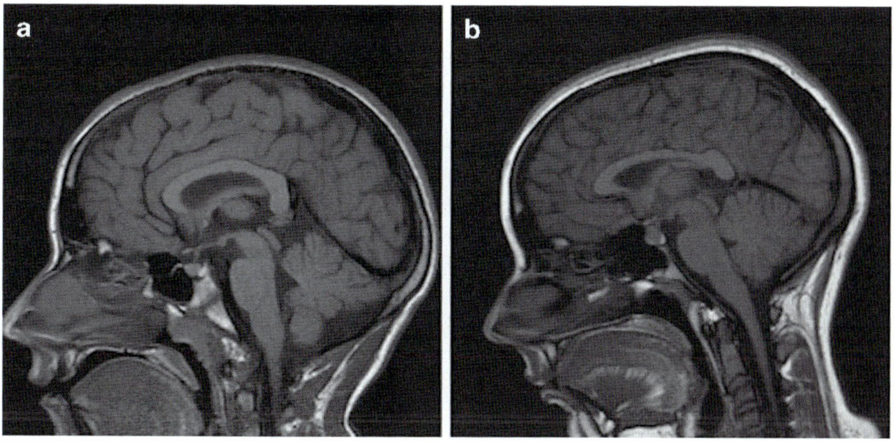

Fig. 9 MRI of pituitary. Sagittal T1-weighted images. (**a**) Normal prepubertal girl. The upper surface of the anterior lobe of the pituitary is flat. (**b**) Normal pubertal girl. The upper surface of the anterior lobe of the pituitary is convex and almost reaches the optic chiasm (Images courtesy of Dr Laurence Abernethy, Alder Hey Children's NHS Foundation Trust, Liverpool)

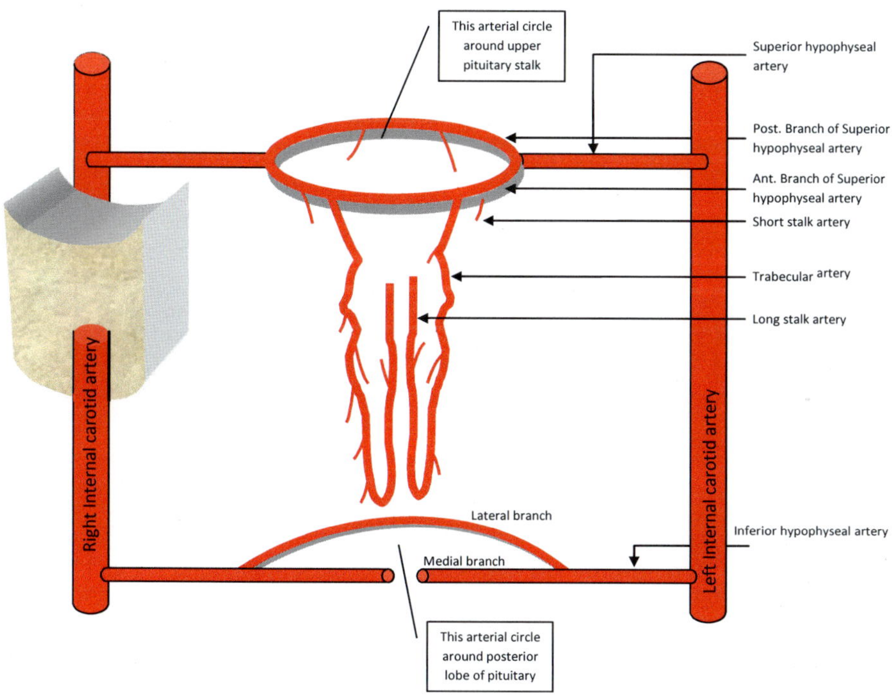

Fig. 10 Blood supply of the pituitary gland

Folliculostellate Cells

Folliculostellate (FS) cells are star-shaped, non-endocrine cells that comprise approximately 5% of the total pituitary cell mass. They form follicles within the pituitary that increase in number and size during aging. FS cells have phagocytic properties, removing cell debris from pituitary cell apoptosis, and a supportive role for other pituitary cells, surrounding them with long cytoplasmic processes.

FS cells have an additional, critical role in coordinating pituitary hormone release, communicating directly with each other through desmosomes and gap junctions and with endocrine cells by gap junctions. They function within a complex network that coordinates FS cell and endocrine cell function and activity over long distances. The rapid communication of secondary messengers through this network is dependent on the density and size of intercellular gap junctions, which may be influenced by hormones, such as glucocorticoids (GC) and sex hormones, and other factors such as leptin, tumor necrosis factor (TNF)-α, and transforming growth factor (TGF)-β3.

Anterior pituitary cells also communicate in a paracrine manner through soluble factors, including growth factors, cytokines, hormones, and peptides, some of which may be produced primarily or exclusively by FS cells. One important example is vascular endothelial growth factor (VEGF-A), which was first identified in the pituitary FS cells in 1989 and has since been recognized as a key regulator of blood vessel and lymph angiogenesis (Ferrara 1989; Gospodarowicz et al. 1989). Two VEGF receptors (VEGFR-1 and VEGFR-2) are expressed in the pituitary, VEGFR-1 located in endocrine cells and VEGFR-2 primarily in endothelial cells (Onofri et al. 2006). VEGF-A may play an important role in the development of the intrapituitary vascular network during embryogenesis, maintenance in postnatal life, and in enabling pituitary plasticity during adult life, for example, by promoting angiogenesis to support the increased lactotroph cell mass during pregnancy and lactation (Turner et al. 2000). VEGF also increases vascular permeability by altering fenestration of endothelial cells. In this way, FS cells may regulate the activity of pituitary gland messengers, by increasing the exchange of soluble factors between the bloodstream and endocrine cells.

Anterior Pituitary Hormones

There are six principle hormones synthesized and secreted by specialized cells of the anterior pituitary: prolactin, thyrotrophin (thyroid-stimulating hormone, TSH), adrenocorticotropin (ACTH), growth hormone (GH), luteinizing hormone (LH), and follicle-stimulating hormone (FSH). Each hormone is regulated by multiple sources of input acting at the level of the pituitary and hypothalamus.

The pituitary hormones regulate their own synthesis and secretion, acting at the level of the pituitary and through log loop feedback, at the level of the pituitary. Within the pituitary, there are multiple ultrashort loop feedback

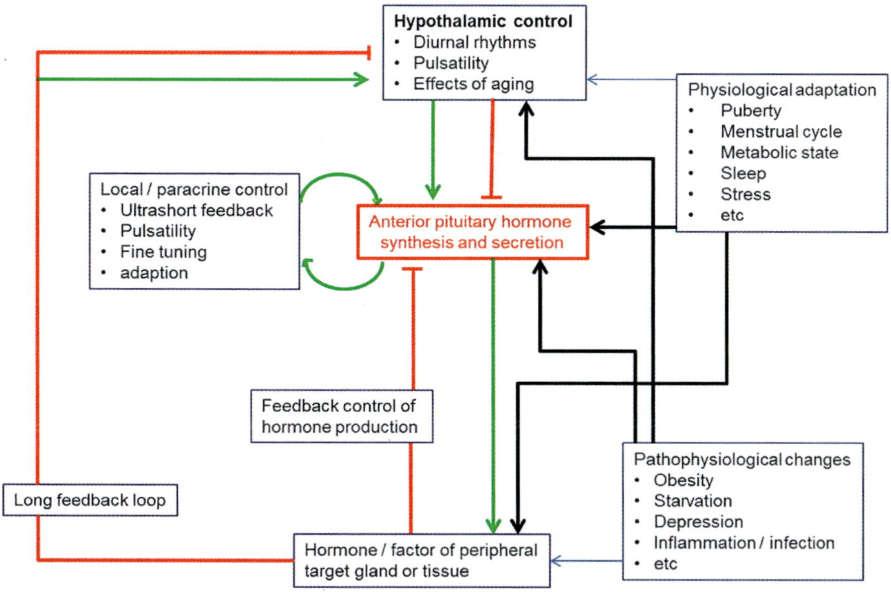

Fig. 11 Principle regulators of anterior pituitary hormone synthesis and release. *Green lines* indicate factors that stimulate hormone secretion, *red lines* factors that inhibit hormone secretion, and *black lines* factors that may either stimulate of inhibit secretion (From Perez-Castro et al. 2012)

pathways that are thought to be important in fine-tuning pituitary hormone release. The activity of the pituitary is also subject to multiple peripheral influences, including nutritional status, temperature, illness, mood, sleep, etc. The general principles of anterior pituitary hormone regulation are illustrated in Fig. 11.

Lactotrophs and Prolactin

Prolactin is secreted from lactotrophs, cells derived from the Pit-1-dependent lineage of pituitary cells, of which there are two types: large polyhedral cells, containing large secretory granules that are found throughout the pituitary, and smaller elongated cells, containing smaller secretory granules that are located in the lateral wings. Together they comprise approximately 15–20% of pituitary functional cell mass. Both cell types hypertrophy during pregnancy and lactation when the pituitary may more than double in size.

Animal studies suggest that lactotrophs are derived from postmitotic somatotrophs (Burrows et al. 1996), and occasional cells (mammosomatotrophs) secrete both prolactin and growth hormone. Lactotrophs have the highest mitotic and apoptotic rate of all pituitary cells.

Prolactin

The prolactin gene is 10 kb in size, comprising five exons and four introns encoding a 199 amino acid polypeptide hormone with three intramolecular disulfide bonds. There are a number of prolactin variants which are the product of alternative splicing of the primary transcript, proteolytic cleavage, and other posttranslational modifications of the amino acid chain (Sinha 1995). The most abundant form of prolactin, monomeric (23 kDa), is also the most potent variant. Other variants include dimeric (48–56 KDa) and polymeric (>100 KDa) prolactin. An abundance of polymeric prolactin ("macroprolactinemia") is rarely associated with the clinical manifestations of prolactin excess.

Prolactin is secreted in a pulsatile manner, with 4–14 pulses in 24 h, each lasts approximately an hour. There is a diurnal pattern of hormone release: Peaks of greatest amplitude are secreted overnight, with a temporal relationship with REM sleep, and those of lowest amplitude are secreted during the morning (Sassin et al. 1972). Prolactin pulses are more frequent and of higher amplitude in females than in males and decline with age in both genders.

Regulation of Prolactin Secretion

Prolactin secretion is stimulated by thyroid hormone-releasing hormone, which preferentially increases the secretion of monomeric prolactin. Other factors that stimulate prolactin secretion include fibroblast and epidermal growth factors, vasoactive intestinal polypeptide (VIP), and hypothalamic prolactin-releasing hormone, which binds to a specific receptor.

The dominant action of estrogen on lactotrophs is to increase prolactin gene transcription and secretion; however it is also recognized that estrogen also promotes both lactotroph proliferation and apoptosis. There is some evidence that these contrary actions of estrogen are mediated through different receptors, apoptosis being medicated by membrane bound receptors and cell proliferation by intracellular estrogen receptors (Zárate et al. 2009). Estrogen-induced changes in lactotroph cell growth are mediated through growth factors including TGF-α, TGF-β, epidermal growth factor (EGF), basic fibroblast growth factor (bFGF), IGF-I, IGF-II, interleukin-6, and others. Prolactin levels also increase in response to opiates.

Prolactin secretion is inhibited, primarily, by dopamine synthesized and secreted from the tuberoinfundibular cells and the hypothalamic tuberohypophysial dopaminergic system. It reaches the lactotrophs of the pituitary via the hypothalamic pituitary portal circulation, to bind on specific type 2 dopamine receptors on lactotroph cell membranes. Disruption of the hypothalamic pituitary portal circulation is often associated with an increase in peripheral prolactin concentrations.

Prolactin increases dopamine synthesis by promoting tyrosine hydroxylase activity, thus regulating its own secretion through a classical negative feedback loop. Other inhibitors of prolactin release include endothelin 1 and TGT-β1, which act in a paracrine manner, and calcitonin which maybe of hypothalamic origin.

Prolactin Actions

The prolactin receptor, a member of the cytokine receptor superfamily, is expressed in a wide range of tissues, including the breast, pituitary, liver, adrenal cortex, kidney, prostate, ovary, testes, intestine, epidermis, pancreatic islet cells, myocardium, lung, brain, and lymphocytes. Collectively, human and animal studies have identified more than 300 prolactin actions (Freeman et al. 2000), leading some authors to speculate that prolactin is a prohormone that exerts these diverse actions through a number of prolactin derivatives.

The most important role of prolactin in humans is lactation (milk production), and women with mutations of the prolactin gene do not lactate (Falk 1992). Prolactin is not essential for human breast development, which requires growth hormone, epidermal growth factor, estrogen, parathyroid hormone-related protein, and progesterone.

During the third trimester of pregnancy, prolactin acts in a synergistic manner with estrogen, progesterone, and other breast-derived growth factors, to stimulate the production of colostrum. Following birth, suckling stimulates prolactin release which is essential for the maintenance of lactation, and in the absence of suckling, prolactin levels return to nonpregnant levels approximately 7 days. During lactation, prolactin inhibits GnRH and gonadotropin secretion and therefore acts as a natural contraceptive.

Thyrotrophs and Thyrotrophin

Thyrotrophin, or thyroid-stimulating hormone (TSH), is synthesized and secreted by thyrotrophs, irregularly shaped cells with flattened nuclei that are located in the anterior medial aspects of the pituitary. Thyrotrophs are smaller than the other pituitary cells and comprise approximately 5% of pituitary cell mass.

TSH Structure

TSH, one of four glycoprotein hormones which comprise an α-subunit, covalently bound to a unique β-subunit which confers biological specificity. Other glycoprotein hormones include TSH, LH, FSH, and placental chorionic gonadotropin. The gene encoding the common α-subunit is located on 6p14.3. The gene encoding the TSH β-subunit is located on 1p13.2 and comprises three exons, of which the first is noncoding. The TSH β-subunit is 112 amino acid long.

Thyrostimulin, a heterodimer of two more recently identified glycoprotein subunits, also stimulates the TSH receptor (Nakabayashi et al. 2002). The role of thyrostimulin is a subject of ongoing research, but it appears to have a number of important peripheral actions (Sun et al. 2010; Bassett et al. 2015).

Regulation of TSH Secretion

Like other pituitary hormones, secretion of TSH is pulsatile and shows a diurnal pattern of secretion, with concentrations of TSH being highest in the late evening.

TSH secretion is stimulated by hypothalamic TRH, secreted from the paraventricular nuclei as pro-TRH which contains five copies of the TRH molecule. Peptidase action, followed by cyclization of the glutamine residue to form a pyroglutamyl residue, results in the release of individual TRH molecules which act on G protein-coupled type 1 TRH receptors and induce the inositol phosphate/calcium/protein kinase C signaling pathway to stimulate TSH release.

The TRH neuron has an important role in setting TSH levels in response to external stimuli. In response to cold, adrenergic input increases the set point for TRH inhibition by T_3, allowing thyroid hormone levels to rise, increasing thermogenesis. In response to fasting, stimulation of the pro-opiomelanocortin (POMC) system, which promotes weight loss, and inhibition of the neuropeptide Y/agouti-related peptide system, which promotes weight gain, result in a reduction of TRH expression.

The major inhibitors of TRH and TSH synthesis and secretion are thyroxine (T_4), synthesized in the thyroid gland, and 3,3′,5′-triiodothyronine (T_3), the product of T_4 deiodination. The effects of T_3 are mediated through thyroid hormone receptors (TR), part of the superfamily of nuclear hormone receptors, of which α and β are the major isoforms. TR-α is the principal mediator of T_3 suppression of hypothalamic TRH synthesis and TRH receptor expression. Levels of T_3 are determined by type 2 and type 3 deiodinase, which increase and inactivate T_3, respectively. Type 2 deiodinase is found in the glial cells of the hypothalamus and tanycytes, which line the third ventricle, while type 3 deiodinase is found in the TRH neuron, indicating complex mechanisms of local regulation of TRH secretion.

TSH secretion is regulated within the pituitary by FS cells which express TSH receptors, type 2 deiodinase, and the specific T_3 transporter, monocarboxylate transporter 8. It is proposed that FS cells act in an ultrashort feedback, releasing an inhibitor of TSH secretion, possibly TGF-β2, upon stimulation of FS cell TSH receptors (Pazos-Mour et al. 2003). Type 3 deiodinase and TR are found in thyrotrophs, again indicating a complex local interplay between promoters and inhibitors of hormones regulating thyroid hormone release.

Transporter proteins play an important role in mediating the actions of T_3 in the brain, of which two, organic anion-transporting polypeptide and MOAT8, are the two most important.

Somatostatin inhibits the nocturnal release of TSH acting at the level of the pituitary and possibly through inhibition of TRH secretion and TRH receptor expression. Dopamine also has the effect of inhibiting the nocturnal rise in TSH secretion. TRH and TSH secretion is also inhibited by glucocorticoids and inflammatory cytokines.

Corticotrophs and Adrenocorticotropic Hormone (ACTH)

Corticotrophs are large, irregular cells with prominent neurosecretory granules located around the median pituitary wedge and posteriorly adjacent to the pars nervosa. They are the first endocrine cells of the pituitary to produce hormones,

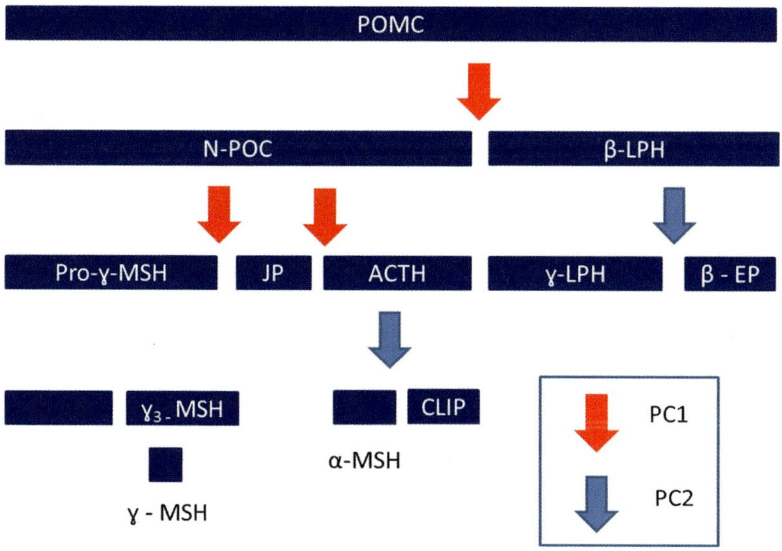

Fig. 12 Processing and cleavage of pro-opiomelanocortin. *ACTH* adrenocorticotropic hormone, *CLIP* corticotropin-like intermediate lobe protein, *EP* endorphin, *JP* joining peptide, *LPH* lipoprotein, *MSH* melanocyte-stimulating hormone, *N-POC* N-terminal POMC fragment (From Clark and Swords 2001)

being active from the eighth week of gestation. They comprise approximately 20% of functional pituitary cell mass and produce the products of the POMC gene, including adrenocorticotropic hormone (ACTH) and opioid and melanotropic peptides. These POMC gene products have a high glycoprotein content, making the corticotroph stain strongly positive for periodic acid–Schiff.

The POMC gene is located on the short arm of chromosome2, 2p23, and consists of three exons: The first encodes a leader sequence and the second the signal initiation sequence and N-terminal portion of the POMC peptide, and the third contains most of the sequence for corticotropic, melanotropic, and opioid peptides. Translation of the gene results in a 266 amino acid preprohormone which undergoes extensive modification and processing including removal of the N-terminal sequence, glycosylation of Thr45, N-linkage of Asn65, and serine phosphorylation (Fig. 12). Cleavage of POMC at pairs of basic residues (lys–lys or lys–arg) by prohormone convertase 1 (PC1) releases N-terminal POMC fragment (N-POC) and β-LPH. Further cleavage of N-POC by PC1 releases pro-γ-MSH, joining peptide and ACTH, and further cleavage of β-LPH by PC2 results in γ-LPH and β-endorphin. ACTH may be further cleaved by PC2 to α-melanocyte-stimulating hormone (α-MSH) and corticotrophin-like intermediate lobe peptide (CLIP).

Products of POMC have a wide range of actions. ACTH binds to the melanocortin receptor type 2 receptor to induce synthesis of adrenal glucocorticoids, androgens, and, to a lesser degree, mineralocorticoids. Stimulation of the melanocortin receptor type 1 on melanocytes by ACTH, β-lipotropin (β-LPH), and γ-LPH induces skin pigmentation. The effects of leptin on appetite suppression are mediated by the melanocortin system via α-MSH, acting at the level of the hypothalamus. Deficiency of POMC results in hyperphagia and weight gain in both mice (Yaswen et al. 1999) and humans (Krude et al. 1998), which can be reversed by infusing α-MSH into the ventricles.

α-MSH also has an important role in the inflammatory response, regulating the activity of antigen-presenting cells and T cells and inhibiting macrophage activity and leukocyte migration.

The hypothalamic pituitary adrenal axis plays a central role in the stress response to pain, hemorrhage, hypovolemia, trauma, psychological stress, infection, inflammation, and hypoglycemia. Upregulation of the axis in response to peripheral and central signals of stress, including vasovagal, catecholamine, and cytokine messengers, results in an increase in glucocorticoid synthesis and release, affecting energy supply, metabolism, cardiovascular function, and immunity.

ACTH Secretion

ACTH is secreted in a pulsatile manner, with pulses of ACTH being followed, approximately 15 min later, by pulses of cortisol. A circadian pattern of ACTH secretion is evident, with maximum levels of ACTH being observed between 06.00 and 09.00, falling to a nadir between 23.00 and 02.00 The circadian rhythm is set by the suprachiasmatic nucleus of the hypothalamus.

Regulation of ACTH

Levels of ACTH are regulated by factors from the hypothalamic, including CRH, dopamine and arginine vasopressin (AVP), within the pituitary by cytokines and growth factors and by glucocorticoids through a negative feedback loop at the level of the hypothalamus and pituitary.

CRH is a 41-amino acid peptide derived from a 196-amino acid prohormone synthesized by neurons in the parvocellular division of the hypothalamic paraventricular nuclei. These neurons also secrete other ACTH secretagogues including AVP, cholecystokinin, and opioid peptides. Hypothalamic CRH secretion is increased by a number of cytokines and neurotransmitters, including acetylcholine, norepinephrine, histamine, serotonin, tumor necrosis factor, oxytocin, vasoactive peptide (VIP), catecholamines, angiotensin II, and interleukins (IL), with the exception of IL2, which appears to act at the level of the pituitary. Secretion is inhibited by gamma-aminobutyric acid.

AVP is synthesized in the supraoptic and periventricular nuclei of the hypothalamus and corticotrophs, where it acts in a paracrine manner. AVP stimulates ACTH release via the V1b receptor. It is a relatively weak stimulant of ACTH but acts synergistically with CRH by increasing the number of corticotrophs responsive to CRH.

In response to CRH binding with the CRH type 1 receptor (CRH-R1), corticotrophs release ACTH stored in secretory vesicles. CRH also activates

POMC gene expression, resulting in a second, slower wave of ACTH release. Subpopulations of corticotroph cells may differ in their CRH-R1 expression, with some subpopulations responding quickly with immediate release of stored ACTH, while others respond more slowly, thus ensuring a sustained ACTH rise during periods of prolonged stress (Mason et al. 2002).

CRH and AVP are thought to be the major mediators of stress-related ACTH release, and physical and psychological stress increases transcription of both secretagogues. Cytokines released from immune cells (TNF-α, IL-1, IL-6), FS cells, and corticotrophs of the pituitary (leukemia inhibitory factor (LIF), IL-6) are also potent stimulators of ACTH secretion during periods of stress (Arzt et al. 1999).

Glucocorticoids inhibit ACTH release at three levels: at the level of the hypothalamus by inhibiting CRH and AVP synthesis, at the level of the pituitary by inhibiting POMC transcription, and by modifying corticotroph response to CRH-R1 and V1b receptor stimulation.

Growth Hormone and Somatotrophs

Somatotrophs

Growth hormone (GH) is synthesized in somatotrophs, cells that comprise approximately 50% of pituitary cell mass and are located in the lateral wings of the pituitary. They are polyhedral in appearance and a small subpopulation (mammosomatotrophs) stain for both GH and prolactin.

The human growth hormone gene is located on the long arm of chromosome 17q22-24. GH is a 191 amino acid single-chain polypeptide hormone consisting of four α-helixes with two disulfide bonds. There are two major isoforms, full length (22 kDa) which accounts for approximately 70% of circulating GH. An alternatively spliced GH (20 kDa), which lacks residues 32–46 and has a slower clearance rate than 22 kDa GH, accounts for a further 15% of pituitary-derived GH. An acetylated 22KDA GH isoform can also be detected, and other isoforms are present in low concentrations (Bauman 2009).

Patterns of Growth Hormone Secretion

From early infancy, growth hormone is secreted in pulses of the greatest frequency and amplitude during sleep with the onset of slow-wave sleep being the trigger for the peaks of the greatest amplitude and frequency (Van Cauter et al. 1998). Between pulses, growth hormone concentrations return to levels below the limits of detection of most laboratory assays.

Growth hormone levels are higher during the neonatal period than in later childhood, and over the first 4 days of life, the magnitude and frequency of growth hormone pulses fall by 50% (Vigneri and Agata 1971). In the first few months of life, there is no relationship between sleep and growth hormone secretion.

Production of GH during childhood ranges from 200 to 600 μg/L per day. During adolescence GH production rises sharply in concert with the increase in sex hormones, to 1,000–1,800 μg/L per day, falling to 200–600 μg/L once again during young adult life and falling progressively during middle and old age (Giustina and Veldhuis 1998).

Regulators of Growth Hormone Secretion

Growth hormone peaks are regulated primarily, by the balance between growth hormone-releasing hormone (GHRH), the principle GH secretagogue which stimulates GH gene transcription and GH release, and somatostatin which is the primary inhibitor of GH secretion. The secretion of these two hormones is under complex and multilayered control by neurotransmitters, neuropeptides, and opiates.

GHRH, of which there are two principal forms, GHRH (1–40) and GHRH (1–44), is derived from a 108 amino acid preprohormone. The C-terminal residues 30–44 may be redundant as full biological activity is retained in their absence. GHRH acts through a seven-transmembrane domain G protein-coupled receptor to stimulate GH synthesis and release and somatotroph proliferation.

Ghrelin, a peptide released primarily from the gastric mucosal cells, is a potent GH secretagogue, acting directly at the level of the pituitary and via hypothalamic GHRH where it binds with the GH secretagogue receptor (Kojima et al. 1999). Other sources of ghrelin include the hypothalamus, and somatotrophs, thyrotrophs, and lactotrophs, where it acts in a paracrine manner. The actions of ghrelin are mediated, at least in part, by GHRH, as transection of the pituitary stalk results in loss of ghrelin-mediated GH suppression.

Clonidine, arginine, exercise, and L-dopa all augment GH secretion via α-adrenergic pathways. In contrast, β-adrenergic pathways inhibit GH secretion. Enkephalins and endorphins increase GH release, as do galanin, neurotensin, VIP, motilin, cholecystokinin, and glucagon.

Sex steroids promote GH secretion, increasing the amplitude of GH pulses. Estrogen promotes GH secretion through the estrogen receptor α, expressed on both GHRH neurons and somatotrophs, but also reduces GH sensitivity, resulting in a fall in IGF-I levels. Testosterone promotes GH secretion, with no loss of GH sensitivity, increasing levels of both GH and IGF-I.

The primary action of leptin, a hormone released from white adipose tissue, is the maintenance of a healthy body fat mass by inhibiting the appetite centers of the brain. Short-term exposure to leptin increases GH release, probably by enhancing GHRH release and inhibiting somatostatin, but prolonged exposure results in a reduction in GHRH sensitivity and lower GH levels. During periods of fasting, GH levels rise. In contrast, GH levels are low in obese subjects.

GH secretion is stimulated for up to 3 h following glucocorticoid exposure, followed by suppression within 12 h of sustained exposure. Thyroid hormones are essential for the maintenance of normal GH levels. In hypothyroid patients, the GH response to stimulation is impaired and recovers after restoration of normal thyroid hormone levels. Sex steroids increase GH levels. In men, testosterone effects are mediated via aromatization to estrogen

Somatostatin is the primary inhibitor of GH secretion. It is also the product of a preprohormone and circulates in two forms: somatostatin-28 and somatostatin-14. Somatostatin has diverse effects within the pituitary and in other organs including the gut, pancreas, and liver. Pituitary actions of somatostatin include inhibition of GH secretion directly and also through inhibition of GHRH release from the hypothalamus. Somatostatin levels rise in response to increases in GHRH, growth hormone, and IGF-I.

Gonadotropins and Gonadotrophs

The gonadotropins LH and FSH are synthesized and released by gonadotrophs, which contribute approximately 10% of the pituitary cell mass and are located throughout the pars distalis and pars tuberalis. They are in intimate contact with lactotrophs, with which they interact in a paracrine manner.

LH and FSH are members of the glycoprotein hormone family, which also includes TSH and placental chorionic gonadotropin. They comprise a common 92 amino acid α-subunit covalently bound to a hormone-specific β-subunit, which varies in size from 110 to 145 amino acids. The gene encoding the common α-subunit is located on chromosome 6 and comprises four exons, of which the first is noncoding. The gene encoding the LH-β-subunit is located on 19q.13.3 and comprises three exons. The FSH β-subunit gene also comprises three exons and is located on 11p.14.1.

Regulators of Gonadotropin Secretion

The major regulators of LH and FSH concentrations are hypothalamic GnRH, which stimulates release, and gonadal factors, including testosterone, estradiol, progesterone, and inhibin, which inhibit release. Auto and paracrine pathways within the pituitary also regulate gonadotropin release and are of particular importance in determining the differential regulation of LH and FSH from the same cell.

During embryogenesis, the migration of GnRH neurons from the medial olfactory placode along the olfactory bulb to the infundibulum, medial basal and the periventricular regions of the hypothalamus, is dependent on a number of factors including anosmin-1 (the product of KAL gene), leukemia inhibitory factor, and fibroblast growth factor receptor 1. Kallmann syndrome, characterized by anosmia and hypogonadotropic hypogonadism, results from defective GnRH neuron migration in patients with mutations of the KAL1 gene (Bick et al. 1992).

GnRH is encoded by two genes. $GNRH_1$ is found in hypothalamic neurons. It encodes a 92 amino acid precursor protein which regulates pituitary release of gonadotropins. The second GnRH gene, $GNRH_2$, is found in the midbrain and encodes a decapeptide that serves as a neurotransmitter rather than a pituitary-releasing factor.

Like other hypothalamic hormones, GnRH is released in a pulsatile manner. This pulsatility is essential for normal activity of the hypothalamic pituitary axis, as continuous exposure of to GnRH results in downregulation of GnRH receptors and desensitization of gonadotrophs.

GnRH binding to its membrane receptor on gonadotrophs stimulates the release of both LH and FSH, and differential regulation of LH and FSH is achieved, in part through changes in GnRH pulse frequency (Dalkin et al. 1989). LH, FSH, and TSH share a common α-subunit, and hormone specificity is conferred from the β-subunit. High-frequency GnRH pulses increase transcription of α- and LH-β-subunits, whereas low-frequency GnRH pulses increase FSH-β gene transcription. Furthermore, animal studies report that GnRH pulses released once an hour favor LH secretion over FSH secretion, while pulses of lower frequency favor FSH secretion.

The frequency of GnRH pulses also influences the half-life and biological activity of gonadotropins. Prior to secretion, terminal sugars are attached to gonadotropin molecules, influencing gonadotropin activity. These sugars include sialic acid, the most important, galactose, n-acetylglucosamine, and mannose. Gonadotropins with sialic acid are protected from degradation and have a longer half-life, while gonadotropins with less sialic acid are able to bind the gonadotropin receptor with greater affinity. Glycosylation is influenced by the frequency of GnRH pulses. In the follicular phase, the frequency of GnRH pulses is slow, favoring glycosylation of FSH and sustained FSH support of developing follicles. Just before the midcycle gonadotropin surge, GnRH pulses are released with higher frequency. Glycosylation is less, favoring the release of more potent gonadotropins with a shorter half-life at the time of ovulation.

GnRH release is regulated, in part, by Kisspeptin, which acts directly on the GnRH neuron to stimulate GnRH release into the portal circulation. Kisspeptin binding with its receptor on gonadotropins has been reported to upregulate LHβ and FSHβ gene expression and to increase LH and FSH secretion. Animal models with inactivating mutations of Kiss1 and the Kiss1 receptor have delayed puberty (Chan et al. 2009), while an activating mutation of the receptor has been reported in a girl with precocious puberty (Teles et al. 2008).

Inhibins are members of the transforming growth factor β family which inhibit FSH secretion. They comprise a common α-subunit and two β-subunits, which confer specificity: βA and βB. Inhibins are produced in gonadal tissue and gonadotrophs and to a lesser degree somatotrophs, thyrotrophs, and FS cells. In males, inhibin B is released in response to FSH stimulation. In females inhibin A is released from dominant ovarian follicles and corpora lutea in the late follicular and luteal phase of the menstrual cycle, whereas inhibin B levels rise during the late luteal and early follicular phase.

Activins comprise two β-subunits, of which two have been most extensively studied: activin A (βA, βA) and activin B (βB, βB). In contrast to the action of inhibin, activins stimulate FSH release. Inhibins compete with activins for type II activin receptors, thereby modulating activin effects on FSH secretion. The relative production of inhibins and activins may depend on the relative availability of intracellular α- and β-subunits: In the presence of a surplus of α-subunit, the production of inhibin may be favored over activin, whereas the contrary would be true in the presence of a surplus of β-subunits. This raises the possibility that the regulation of FSH release is mediated, in part, by the relative production of α- and β-subunits.

Follistatin is a monomeric peptide that is synthesized and released from gonadal cells and intrapituitary endocrine and FS cells. Follistatin binds activin with high affinity, preventing it from binding to its receptor and thereby blocking the effect of activin on FSH secretion.

Sex steroids (testosterone, estradiol, and progesterone) act at the level of the hypothalamus to slow the pulsatile release of GnRH into the portal circulation. The GnRH neuron lacks steroid hormone receptors, so these actions of sex steroids on GnRH release must be mediated through another pathway or messenger. Sex steroids also inhibit gonadotropin release, acting directly at the level of the pituitary to reduce LH and FSH release and to reduce the sensitivity of gonadotrophs to GnRH stimulation.

In the female, during the follicular phase of the menstrual cycle, estrogen switches from a negative to a positive feedback effect, resulting in the gonadotropin surge. This switch is dependent on the maintenance of critical estrogen concentration for a critical period of time, which is associated with an increase in GnRH receptors and increased GnRH responsiveness.

Menstrual Cycle

The menstrual cycle starts with the onset of menstrual bleeding, when ovaries contain multiple small follicles and estrogen concentrations are low. Pulses of LH are relatively fast, and FSH levels are higher than at other times of the cycle, stimulating the development of ovarian follicles. As follicles develop, estrogen levels rise, increasing the negative feedback effect on GnRH and gonadotropin release.

In response to the rise in estrogen, the frequency of LH pulses falls, until estrogen levels are maintained at an adequate level to induce the switch from a negative to a positive feedback effect. As gonadotropin levels rise, the follicular wall dissolves, and the matured ovum is released into the fallopian tube. Progesterone is released in high concentrations, slowing LH pulses. If fertilization does not occur, progesterone levels fall after 14 days, and LH and FSH levels rise once again. The fall in progesterone also results in the shedding of the endometrium and the start of a new menstrual cycle.

Conclusion

The activity of the hypothalamic pituitary axis is exquisitely regulated, integrating messages from within the pituitary, the hypothalamus, peripheral tissues and organs, and the external environment, to ensure hormone levels that support physiological and homeostatic processes, critical to health and well-being. It is an awe-inspiring example of the complexity, elegance, and sophistication of the endocrine system, and no doubt, there is still much for us to learn.

Cross-References

- ▶ Ovarian Physiology
- ▶ The Adrenal Glands
- ▶ The Endocrine Pancreas
- ▶ The Endocrine Regulation of Blood Pressure
- ▶ The Endocrine Regulation of Energy and Body Weight
- ▶ The Endocrinology of Puberty
- ▶ The Physiology of the Testis
- ▶ The Thyroid

References

Alatzoglou KS, Kelberman D, Dattani MT. The role of SOX proteins in normal pituitary development. J Endocrinol. 2009;200(3):245–58. 1479-6805.

Alvarez-Bolado G, Grinevich V, Puelles L. Editorial: development of the hypothalamus. Front Neuroanat. 2015;9:83. doi:10.3389/fnana.2015.00083.

Arzt E, Pereda MP, Castro CP, Pagotto U, Renner U, Stalla GK. Pathophysiological role of the cytokine network in the anterior pituitary gland. Front Neuroendocrinol. 1999;20(1):71–95.

Bassett JH, van der Spek A, Logan JG, Gogakos A, Bagchi-Chakraborty J, Murphy E, van Zeijl C, Down J, Croucher PI, Boyde A, Boelen A, Williams GR. Thyrostimulin regulates osteoblastic bone formation during early skeletal development. Endocrinology. 2015;156(9):3098–113.

Baumann GP. Growth hormone isoforms. Growth Horm IGF Res. 2009;19(4):333–40.

Bick D, Franco B, Sherins RJ, Heye B, Pike L, Crawford J, Maddalena A, Incerti B, Pragliola A, Meitinger T, Ballabio A. Brief report: intragenic deletion of the KALIG-1 gene in Kallmann's syndrome. N Engl J Med. 1992;326:1752–5.

Blaustein MP, Leenen FH, Chen L, Golovina VA, Hamlyn JM, Pallone TL, Van Huysse JW, Zhang J, Wier WG. How NaCl raises blood pressure: a new paradigm for the pathogenesis of salt-dependent hypertension. Am J Physiol Heart Circ Physiol. 2012;302(5):H1031–49.

Brüning JC, Gautam D, Burks DJ, Gillette J, Schubert M, Orban PC, Klein R, Krone W, Müller-Wieland D, Kahn CR. Role of brain insulin receptor in control of body weight and reproduction. Science. 2000;289(5487):2122–5.

Burrows HL, Birkmeier TS, Seasholtz AF, Camper SA. Targeted ablation of cells in the pituitary primordia of transgenic mice. Mol Endocrinol. 1996;10(11):1467–77.

Chan YM, Broder-Fingert S, et al. Kisspeptin/Gpr54-independent gonadotrophin-releasing hormone activity in Kiss1 and Gpr54 mutant mice. J Neuroendocrinol. 2009;21(12):1015–23.

Chen HY, Trumbauer ME, Chen AS, Weingarth DT, Adams JR, Frazier EG, Shen Z, Marsh DJ, Feighner SD, Guan XM, Ye Z, Nargund RP, Smith RG, Van der Ploeg LH, Howard AD, MacNeil DJ, Qian S. Orexigenic action of peripheral ghrelin is mediated by neuropeptide Y and agouti-related protein. Endocrinology. 2004;145(6):2607–12.

Clark AJL, Swords FM. Molecular biology of corticoroph function. In: Rappaport R, Anselm S, editors. Hypothalamic-pituitary development. Basel: Karger; 2001.

Clément K, Vaisse C, Lahlou N, Cabrol S, Pelloux V, Cassuto D, Gourmelen M, Dina C, Chambaz J, Lacorte JM, Basdevant A, Bougnères P, Lebouc Y, Froguel P, Guy-Grand B. A mutation in the human leptin receptor gene causes obesity and pituitary dysfunction. Nature. 1998;392(6674):398–401.

Dalkin AC, Haisenlender DJ, et al. The frequency of gonadotropin-releasing-hormone stimulation differentially regulates gonadotropin subunit messenger ribonucleic acid expression. Endocrinology. 1989;125(2):917–23.

de Moraes DC, Vaisman M, Conceição FL, Ortiga-Carvalho TM. Pituitary development: a complex, temporal regulated process dependent on specific transcriptional factors. J Endocrinol. 2012;215(2):239–45. doi:10.1530/JOE-12-0229. Epub 2012 Aug 7.

Elster AD, Chen MY, Williams 3rd DW, Key LL. Pituitary gland: MR imaging of physiologic hypertrophy in adolescence. Radiology. 1990;174(3 Pt 1):681–5.

Falk RJ. Isolated prolactin deficiency: a case report. Fertil Steril. 1992;58(5):1060–2.

Faraguna U, Vyazovskiy VV, Nelson AB, Tononi G, Cirelli C. A causal role for brain-derived neurotrophic factor in the homeostatic regulation of sleep. J Neurosci. 2008;28(15):4088–95.

Ferran, et al. Molecular codes defining rostrocaudal domains in the embryonic mouse hypothalamus. Front Neuroanat. 2015;9:46.

Ferrara N, Henzel WJ. Pituitary follicular cells secrete a novel heparin-binding growth factor specific for vascular endothelial cells. 1989. Biochem Biophys Res Commun. 2012;425 (3):540–7.

Freeman J. The anatomy and embryology of the hypothalamus in relation to hypothalamic hamartomas. Epileptic Disord. 2003;5:177–86.

Freeman ME, Kanyicska B, Lerant A, Nagy G. Prolactin: structure, function, and regulation of secretion. Physiol Rev. 2000;80(4):1523–631.

Giustina A, Veldhuis JD. Pathophysiology of the neuroregulation of growth hormone secretion in experimental animals and the human. Endocr Rev. 1998;19(6):717–97.

Gospodarowicz D, Abraham JA, Schilling J. Isolation and characterization of a vascular endothelial cell mitogen produced by pituitary-derived folliculo stellate cells. Proc Natl Acad Sci U S A. 1989;86(19):7311–5.

Hamlyn JM, Linde CI, Gao J, Huang BS, Golovina VA, Blaustein MP, Leenen FH. Neuroendocrine humoral and vascular components in the pressor pathway for brain angiotensin II: a new axis in long term blood pressure control. PLoS One. 2014;9(9):e108916.

Ishii S, Kamegai J, Tamura H, Shimizu T, Sugihara H, Oikawa S. Hypothalamic neuropeptide Y/Y1 receptor pathway activated by a reduction in circulating leptin, but not by an increase in circulating ghrelin, contributes to hyperphagia associated with triiodothyronine-induced thyrotoxicosis. Neuroendocrinology. 2003;78(6):321–30.

Kelberman D, Dattani MT. Hypothalamic and pituitary development: novel insights into the aetiology. Eur J Endocrinol/Eur Fed Endocr Soc. 2007;157 Suppl 1:S3. 0804-4643 (August 2007).

Kelberman D, Rizzoti K, Lovell-Badge R, Robinson IC, Dattani M. Genetic regulation of pituitary gland development in human and mouse. Endocr Rev. 2009;30(7):790–829.

Kojima M, Hosoda H, Date Y, Nakazato M, Matsuo H, Kangawa K. Ghrelin is a growth-hormone-releasing acylated peptide from stomach. Nature. 1999;402(6762):656–60.

Krude H, Biebermann H, Luck W, Horn R, Brabant G, Grüters A. Severe early-onset obesity, adrenal insufficiency and red hair pigmentation caused by POMC mutations in humans. Nat Genet. 1998;19(2):155–7.

Kwon Jeong J, Dae Kim J, Diano S. Ghrelin regulates hypothalamic prolyl carboxypeptidase expression in mice. Mol Metab. 2013;2(1):23–30.

Lenard NR, Berthoud HR. Central and peripheral regulation of food intake and physical activity: pathways and genes. Obesity (Silver Spring). 2008;16 Suppl 3:S11–22.

Markwald RR, Melanson EL, Smith MR, Higgins J, Perreault L, Eckel RH, Wright Jr KP. Impact of insufficient sleep on total daily energy expenditure, food intake, and weight gain. Proc Natl Acad Sci U S A. 2013;110(14):5695–700.

Mason D, Hassan A, Chacko S, Thompson P. Acute and chronic regulation of pituitary receptors for vasopressin and corticotropin releasing hormone. Arch Physiol Biochem. 2002;110 (1–2):74–89.

Montague CT, Farooqi IS, Whitehead JP, Soos MA, Rau H, Wareham NJ, Sewter CP, Digby JE, Mohammed SN, Hurst JA, Cheetham CH, Earley AR, Barnett AH, Prins JB, O'Rahilly S. Congenital leptin deficiency is associated with severe early-onset obesity in humans. Nature. 1997;387(6636):903–8.

Morrison SF, Nakamura K. Central neural pathways for thermoregulation. Front Biosci (Landmark Ed). 2011;16:74–104.
Nakabayashi K, Matsumi H, Bhalla A, Bae J, Mosselman S, Hsu SY, Hsueh AJ. Thyrostimulin, a heterodimer of two new human glycoprotein hormone subunits, activates the thyroid-stimulating hormone receptor. J Clin Invest. 2002;109(11):1445–52.
Onofri C, Theodoropoulou M, Losa M, Uhl E, Lange M, Arzt E, Stalla GK, Renner U. Localization of vascular endothelial growth factor (VEGF) receptors in normal and adenomatous pituitaries: detection of a non-endothelial function of VEGF in pituitary tumours. J Endocrinol. 2006;191 (1):249–61.
Pazos-Mour, Otiga-Carvalho TM, Gasper de Moura E. The autocrine/paracrine regulation of thyrotropin secretion. Thyroid. 2003;13:167–75.
Perez-Castro C, Renner U, Haedo MR, Stalla GK, Arzt E. Cellular and molecular specificity of pituitary gland physiology. Physiol Rev. 2012;92(1):1–38.
Puelles L. Brain segmentation and forebrain development in amniotes. Brain Res Bull. 2001;55 (6):695–710.
Puelles L. Forebrain development: prosomere model. Murcia: University of Murcia; 2009. Elsevier Ltd.
Puelles L, Rubenstein JL. Forebrain gene expression domains and the evolving prosomeric model. Trends Neurosci. 2003;26(9):469–76.
Qian S, Chen H, Weingarth D, Trumbauer ME, Novi DE, Guan X, Yu H, Shen Z, Feng Y, Frazier E, Chen A, Camacho RE, Shearman LP, Gopal-Truter S, MacNeil DJ, Van der Ploeg LH, Marsh DJ. Neither agouti-related protein nor neuropeptide Y is critically required for the regulation of energy homeostasis in mice. Mol Cell Biol. 2002;22(14):5027–35.
Routh VH, Donovan CM, Ritter S. 2. Hypoglycemia detection. Transl Endocrinol Metab. 2012;3 (4):47–87.
Sassin JF, Frantz AG, Weitzman ED, Kapen S. Human prolactin: 24-hour pattern with increased release during sleep. Science. 1972;177(4055):1205–7.
Sinha YN. Structural variants of prolactin: occurrence and physiological significance. Endocr Rev. 1995;16(3):354–69.
Smart JL, Tolle V, Low MJ. Glucocorticoids exacerbate obesity and insulin resistance in neuron-specific proopiomelanocortin-deficient mice. J Clin Invest. 2006;116(2):495–505.
Sun SC, Hsu PJ, Wu FJ, Li SH, Lu CH, Luo CW. Thyrostimulin, but not thyroid-stimulating hormone (TSH), acts as a paracrine regulator to activate the TSH receptor in mammalian ovary. J Biol Chem. 2010;285(6):3758–65.
Teles MG, Bianco SD, et al. A GPR54-activating mutation in a patient with central precocious puberty. N Engl J Med. 2008;7:709–15.
Turner HE, Nagy Z, Gatter KC, Esiri MM, Harris AL, Wass JA. Angiogenesis in pituitary adenomas and the normal pituitary gland. J Clin Endocrinol Metab. 2000;85(3):1159–62.
Vaisse C, Clement K, Guy-Grand B, Froguel P. A frameshift mutation in human MC4R is associated with a dominant form of obesity. Nat Genet. 1998;20(2):113–4.
Van Cauter E, Plat L, Copinschi G. Interrelations between sleep and the somatotropic axis. Sleep. 1998;21(6):553–66.
Vella KR, Ramadoss P, Lam FS, Harris JC, Ye FD, Same PD, O'Neill NF, Maratos-Flier E, Hollenberg AN. NPY and MC4R signaling regulate thyroid hormone levels during fasting through both central and peripheral pathways. Cell Metab. 2011;14(6):780–90.
Vigneri R, D'Agata R. Growth hormone release during the first year of life in relation to sleep-wake periods. J Clin Endocrinol Metab. 1971;33(3):561–3.
Wang Q, Liu C, Uchida A, Chuang JC, Walker A, Liu T, Osborne-Lawrence S, Mason BL, Mosher C, Berglund ED, Elmquist JK, Zigman JM. Arcuate AgRP neurons mediate orexigenic and glucoregulatory actions of ghrelin. Mol Metab. 2013;3(1):64–72.
Williams KW, Margatho LO, Lee CE, Choi M, Lee S, Scott MM, Elias CF, Elmquist JK. Segregation of acute leptin and insulin effects in distinct populations of arcuate proopiomelanocortin neurons. J Neurosci. 2010;30(7):2472–9.

Yang Y, Guo QH, Wang BA, Dou JT, Lv ZH, Ba JM, Lu JM, Pan CY, Mu YM. Pituitary stalk interruption syndrome in 58 Chinese patients: clinical features and genetic analysis. Clin Endocrinol (Oxf). 2013;79(1):86–92.

Yaswen L, Diehl N, Brennan MB, Hochgeschwender U. Obesity in the mouse model of pro-opiomelanocortin deficiency responds to peripheral melanocortin. Nat Med. 1999;5(9):1066–70.

Zárate S, Jaita G, Zaldivar V, Radl DB, Eijo G, Ferraris J, Pisera D, Seilicovich A. Estrogens exert a rapid apoptotic action in anterior pituitary cells. Am J Physiol Endocrinol Metab. 2009;296(4): E664–71.

The Posterior Pituitary

12

Joseph G. Verbalis

Abstract

The posterior pituitary is comprised of the end terminals of specialized hypothalamic neurons called neurohypophyseal neurons. The two hormones of the posterior pituitary, arginine vasopressin (AVP) and oxytocin (OT), are synthesized in the cell bodies of the neurohypophyseal neurons. The pre-prohormones are cleaved from the signal peptide in the endoplasmic reticulum, and the prohormones, provasopressin and pro-oxytocin, are packaged along with processing enzymes into neurosecretory granules. The neurosecretory granules are transported out of the perikaryon of the neurohypophyseal neurons via microtubules down the long axons that form the supraopticohypophyseal tract to terminate in axon terminals in the posterior pituitary. The entire unit including the magnocellular neurons in the SON and PVN, the supraopticohypophyseal tract, and the axon terminals in the posterior pituitary is called the neurohypophysis. The primary physiologic action of AVP is its function as a water-retaining hormone via activation of vasopressin V2 receptors in the principal cells of the kidney collecting duct. Disorders of AVP synthesis or secretion can lead to excessive water excretion (diabetes insipidus) or inappropriate water retention (syndrome of inappropriate antidiuretic hormone secretion). The primary physiologic action of OT is its function to stimulate milk secretion during suckling via activation of OT receptors in the breast with subsequent contraction of myoepithelial cells around the breast alveoli and ductules to eject milk. Disorders of OT synthesis or secretion can lead to inability to eject breast milk postpartum,

J.G. Verbalis (✉)
Division of Endocrinology and Metabolism, Georgetown University School of Medicine, Washington, DC, USA
e-mail: verbalis@georgetown.edu

A. Belfiore, D. LeRoith (eds.), *Principles of Endocrinology and Hormone Action*, Endocrinology, https://doi.org/10.1007/978-3-319-44675-2_13

though clinical cases have not been described in humans. Both AVP and OT are also synthesized in parvocellular hypothalamic neurons that project within the brain and regulate a variety of central nervous system functions, not all of which have been characterized.

Keywords
Neurohypophysis • Osmolality • Oxytocin • Vasopressin • Water homeostasis

Contents

Neurohypophysis, Anatomy and Hormones

The hormones of the posterior pituitary, arginine vasopressin (AVP) and oxytocin (OT), are synthesized in specialized neurons in the hypothalamus, the neurohypophyseal neurons. These are neurons that are specialized for synthesis and secretion of each hormone and are notable for their large size, hence their designation as *magnocellular* neurons (Sofroniew et al. 1981). In the hypothalamus, the neurohypophyseal magnocellular neurons are clustered in the paired paraventricular (PVN) and supraoptic (SON) nuclei (Fig. 1). AVP and OT are also synthesized in *parvocellular* (i.e., small-cell) neurons of the PVN, and AVP (but not OT) is also synthesized in the suprachiasmatic nucleus (Swanson and Sawchenko 1980). Transcription of AVP and OT mRNA and translation of the AVP and OT prohormones occur entirely in the cell bodies of the neurohypophyseal neurons. The

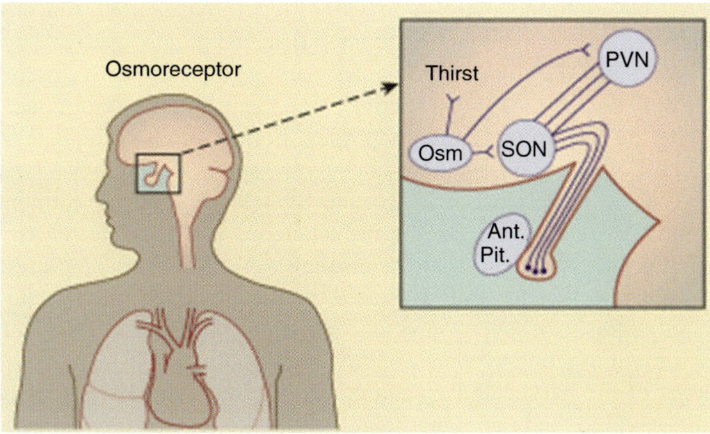

Fig. 1. Sagittal view of the head demonstrating the position of the neurohypophysis. The magnocellular neurons are clustered in two paraventricular nuclei (*PVN*) and two supraoptic nuclei (*SON*). Only one nucleus of each pair is illustrated. The supraoptic nuclei are located lateral to the edge of the optic chiasm, whereas the paraventricular nuclei are central along the wall of the third ventricle. The axons of the four nuclei combine to form the supraopticohypophyseal tract as they course through the pituitary stalk to their storage terminals in the posterior pituitary. The osmostat (*Osm*) is located in the hypothalamus anterior to the third ventricle, whereas the thirst center (*Thirst*) is distributed across different brain areas. *Ant. Pit.* anterior pituitary (From Verbalis (2016a))

pre-prohormones are cleaved from the signal peptide in the endoplasmic reticulum, and the prohormones, provasopressin and pro-oxytocin, are packaged along with processing enzymes into neurosecretory granules. The neurosecretory granules are transported out of the perikaryon of the neurohypophyseal neurons via microtubules down the long axons that form the supraopticohypophyseal tract to terminate in axon terminals in the posterior pituitary. The entire unit including the magnocellular neurons in the SON and PVN, the supraopticohypophyseal tract, and the axon terminals in the posterior pituitary is called the *neurohypophysis*.

During transport, the processing enzymes cleave provasopressin into AVP (9 amino acids), vasopressin-neurophysin (95 amino acids), and vasopressin glycopeptide, also called copeptin (39 amino acids). Pro-oxytocin is similarly cleaved to OT (which differs from vasopressin by only two of nine amino acids) and oxytocin-neurophysin, but there is no glycopeptide contained in pro-oxytocin. Within the neurosecretory granules, neurophysins form neurophysin-hormone complexes that stabilize the hormones. Stimulatory (e.g., cholinergic and angiotensin) neurotransmitter terminals and inhibitory (e.g., γ-aminobutyric acid, noradrenergic, and atrial natriuretic peptide [ANP]) neurotransmitter terminals control the release of AVP through the activity of synaptic contacts on the cell bodies. Physiologic release of AVP or OT into the general circulation occurs at the posterior pituitary, where, in response to an action potential, intracellular calcium is increased and causes the neurosecretory granules to fuse with the axon membrane thereby releasing the entire contents of the granule via exocytosis into the pericapillary space. Once released, each hormone has no further association with its respective neurophysin, and each of the peptide products can be independently detected in the general circulation. Although AVP and OT comprise only small parts of their respective prohormones, they are the only known biologically active components of the prohormones. Factors that stimulate the release of neurohypophyseal hormones also stimulate their synthesis; however, whereas release is instantaneous, synthesis requires a longer time. Because synthesis is delayed, maintenance of a large store of hormone in the posterior pituitary is essential for the instantaneous and massive release of each hormone that is necessary with acute hemorrhage (AVP) or during parturition (OT). In most species, sufficient AVP is stored in the posterior pituitary to support maximum antidiuresis for several days and to maintain baseline levels of antidiuresis for weeks without ongoing synthesis of new hormone.

The axons of the parvocellular neurons of the paraventricular nuclei project to different areas within the brain rather than to the posterior pituitary. Some terminate in the median eminence of the basal hypothalamus, where, similar to other hypothalamic releasing factors, the hormones are secreted into the portal capillary system and where AVP serves as one of the regulators of secretion of adrenocorticotropic hormone. Other neurons project to the limbic system, the brainstem, and the spinal cord, where AVP and OT serve neurotransmitter and neuromodulatory roles. Still other axons secrete hormones into the cerebrospinal fluid of the third ventricle, the function of which is unknown.

Vasopressin, Regulation and Functions

Regulation of Osmolality

The primary physiologic action of AVP is its function as a water-retaining hormone. The central sensing system (osmostat) for control of release of vasopressin is anatomically discrete, located in a small area of the hypothalamus just anterior to the third ventricle that also includes the circumventricular organs, the organum vasculosum of the lamina terminalis (OVLT), and the subfornical organ (SFO) (see Fig. 1). The osmostat controls release of AVP to cause water retention and also stimulates thirst to cause water repletion. Osmotic regulation of AVP secretion and osmotic regulation of thirst are usually tightly coupled, but experimental lesions and some pathologic situations in humans demonstrate that each can be regulated independently. The primary extracellular osmolyte to which the osmoreceptor responds is sodium. Under normal physiologic conditions, glucose and urea readily traverse neuron cell membranes and do not stimulate release of AVP. Although basal osmolality in normal subjects lies between 280 and 295 mOsm/kg H_2O, for each individual extracellular fluid (ECF) osmolality is maintained within narrow ranges. Increases in plasma osmolality as little as 1% will stimulate the osmoreceptors to release AVP. Basal plasma levels of AVP are generally 0.5–2 pg/mL, which are sufficient to maintain urine osmolality above plasma osmolality and urine volume in the range of 2–3 L/day. When AVP levels are suppressed below 0.5 pg/ml, maximum urine osmolality decreases to less than 100 mOsm/kg H_2O and a free water diuresis ensues to levels approaching 800–1000 ml/h (18–24 L/d). Increases in plasma osmolality cause a linear increase in plasma AVP and a corresponding linear increase in urine osmolality. At a plasma osmolality of approximately 295 mOsm/kg H_2O, urine osmolality is maximally concentrated to 1000–1200 mOsm/kg H_2O. Thus, the entire physiologic range of urine osmolality is accomplished by relatively small changes in plasma AVP in the range of 0–5 pg/mL (Fig. 2).

To maintain fluid balance, water must be not just conserved but consumed as well to replace insensible water losses and obligate urine output. Most studies have indicated that thirst is not stimulated until a somewhat higher plasma osmolality (5–10 mOsm/kg H_2O) than the threshold for release of AVP. During the course of a normal day, most humans obtain sufficient water from habitual fluid intake and catabolism of food to maintain plasma osmolality below the threshold required to activate thirst. Therefore, under normal physiological conditions, water balance (and hence plasma osmolality) is regulated more by secretion of AVP than by true thirst.

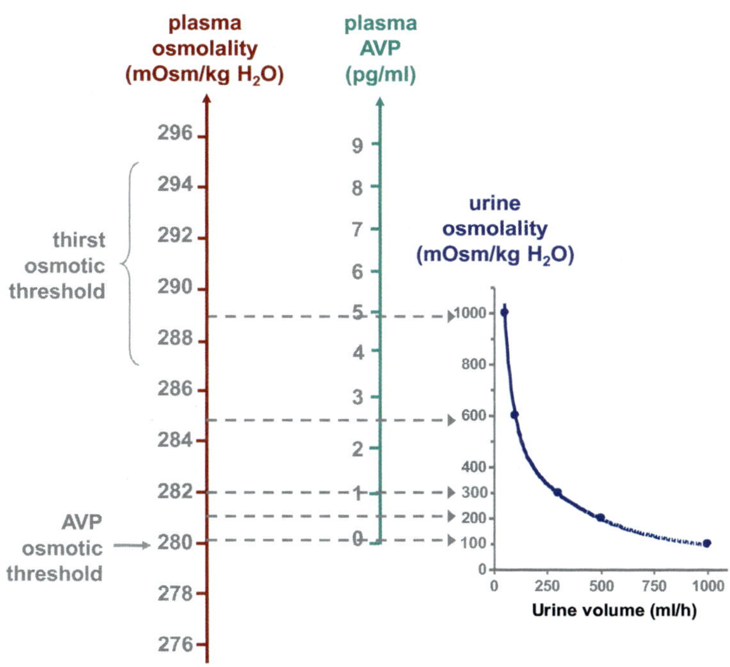

Fig. 2. Relationship of plasma osmolality, plasma AVP concentrations, urine osmolality, and urine volume in humans. Note that the osmotic threshold for AVP secretion defines the point at which urine concentration begins to increase, but the osmotic threshold for thirst is significantly higher and approximates the point at which maximal urine concentration has already been achieved. Note also that, because of the inverse relation between urine osmolality and urine volume, changes in plasma AVP concentrations have much larger effects on urine volume at low plasma AVP concentrations than at high plasma AVP concentrations (Adapted from Robinson (1985))

However, with more severe degrees of dehydration thirst is essential to restore body water deficits.

AVP acts on V2, or antidiuretic, receptors in the collecting duct cells of the kidney to cause water retention, or antidiuresis. AVP V2 receptors are G protein-coupled receptors that activate adenylyl cyclase with subsequent increased intracellular cyclic AMP levels upon ligand activation of the receptor. The increased cAMP initiates the movement of aquaporin-2 water channels from the cytoplasm to the apical (luminal) membrane of the collecting duct cells. Once inserted into the apical membrane, these channels allow facilitated rapid transport of water from the collecting duct lumen into the cell along osmotic gradients. The water then exits the cell through the basolateral membrane and into the kidney medullary circulation via aquaporin-3 and aquaporin-4 water channels, which are constitutively present in the basolateral membrane. This entire process is termed antidiuresis. In the absence of AVP, the aquaporin-2 channels are re-internalized from the apical membrane into subapical vesicles. This prevents active reabsorption of water from the collecting duct lumen, resulting in diuresis. In addition to this rapid "shuttling" of the aquaporin-2 channels to regulate water reabsorption on a minute-to-minute basis, AVP also acts via V2 receptors to regulate long-term stores of aquaporin-2; that is, increased AVP stimulates aquaporin-2 synthesis and the absence of AVP results in decreased aquaporin-2 synthesis. The hypertonic medullary interstitium determines the maximum concentration of the final urine, which is isotonic with the inner medulla of the kidney under conditions of maximal antidiuresis.

Blood Pressure and Blood Volume Regulation

In contrast to the osmoregulatory system, volume regulation is anatomically more diffuse. High-pressure baroreceptors are located in the aorta and carotid sinus, and low-pressure baroreceptors are located in the right and left atria. Stimuli for pressure and volume receptors are carried via the glossopharyngeal (ninth) and vagal (tenth) cranial nerves to the nucleus tractus solitarius in the brainstem. Subsequent secondary and tertiary projections converge on the magnocellular neurons, where they provide inhibitory as well as excitatory inputs. Decreases in blood pressure or vascular volume stimulate AVP release, whereas situations that increase blood volume or left atrial pressure (e.g., negative-pressure breathing) decrease secretion of AVP. The release of AVP in response to changes in volume or pressure is less sensitive than the release in response to osmoreceptors, and generally a 10–15% reduction in blood volume or pressure is needed to stimulate release of AVP. However, once arterial pressure falls below this threshold, the stimulated response is exponential, and plasma levels of AVP are achieved that are markedly greater than those achieved by osmotic stimulation. Other nonosmotic stimuli such as nausea and intestinal traction probably act through similar nonosmotic neural pathways to release AVP. The pressor effects of AVP are mediated through AVP V1a receptors located on vascular smooth muscle. For both AVP V1a and V1b receptors, the cellular mechanism of action of AVP is to increase intracellular calcium rather than to stimulate adenylate cyclase. In intact animals, the pressor activity of relatively is weak because of compensatory vasodilatory systems that act to modulate all vasopressor effects. The relatively insensitive regulation of AVP secretion by changes in volume and pressure and the modest role of AVP to regulate blood pressure are consistent with the notion that regulation of body sodium homeostasis via the renin-angiotensin-aldosterone system (RAAS) is more important for control of ECF and blood volume than is regulation of water homeostasis. However, the action of AVP to regulate blood pressure can become prominent when other blood pressure regulatory systems are deficient (e.g., autonomic neuropathy or RAAS blockade), or in states of pathological vasodilatation (e.g., liver cirrhosis, septic shock).

Adrenocorticotropic Hormone Regulation

AVP in the parvocellular neurons whose axons terminate in the median eminence is released into the pituitary portal capillaries and carried to the anterior pituitary. Anterior pituitary corticotrophs are stimulated via AVP V1b receptors to release adrenocorticotropic hormone (ACTH). Although the major regulator of ACTH secretion is corticotropin-releasing hormone (CRH), because AVP and CRH activate different signal transduction systems in the corticotrophs, each hormone has synergistic effects on the actions of the other to release ACTH.

Interactions of Osmotic and Volume Regulation

The AVP system has evolved to optimize mammalian drinking behavior. Under normal conditions, water is consumed as available in the absence of stimulated thirst and AVP secretion regulates renal water excretion to maintain plasma osmolality; this allows extensive geographic movement without thirst, which would produce time-consuming and potentially dangerous water-seeking behavior. But thirst still serves as a backup if dehydration becomes excessive despite stimulated AVP secretion to cause maximal antidiuresis. Similarly, because the blood pressure/volume regulation of AVP is less sensitive, modest changes in pressure or volume, which are exacerbated by upright posture, do not interfere with regulation of osmolality. But the pressor effects of high AVP levels still serve as a backup if volume depletion or hypotension become excessive. Usually, the physiologic regulation of osmolality and pressure/volume are synergistic. Dehydration causes an increase in plasma osmolality and a decrease in blood volume, both of which stimulate release of AVP. Excess administration of fluid causes both a decrease in plasma osmolality and an expansion of blood volume, both of which inhibit AVP secretion. However, other pathologic situations can result in opposing signals to AVP secretion, for example, hyponatremia resulting from diuretic use with a decreased extracellular fluid volume, or from cardiac failure or cirrhosis with a decreased effective arterial blood volume. In these situations, AVP secretion represents a balance between the excitatory and inhibitory inputs provided by the osmotic and volume/pressure stimuli.

In addition, other factors can modulate the osmotic release and action of AVP. With volume expansion, natriuretic factors such as atrial natriuretic peptide (ANP) and brain natriuretic peptide (BNP) are released from atrial myocytes and act at the kidney to induce natriuresis. ANP is also synthesized in the hypothalamus, where it may act to decrease AVP secretion. During pregnancy, there is a decrease of plasma osmolality by approximately 10 mOsm/kg H_2O as a result of a resetting of the osmostat, in which AVP increases and decreases appropriately around the lower plasma osmolality; the osmostat for thirst is reset in parallel. Data suggests that this effect may be mediated, in part, by the placental hormone relaxin. Abnormalities in water and electrolyte balance are very common in elderly humans. This is in part due to age-related changes in body volume (as much as a 50% decrease in total body water above age 75) and renal function. However, elderly humans also have a decreased sense of thirst; although there is a normal or even increased ability to secrete AVP with age, there is a decreased ability to achieve either maximum urine concentration to retain water, and maximum dilution of urine to excrete water. Consequently, elderly patients are particularly prone to hyper- or hyponatremia with diseases that affect water balance, or from the drugs used as therapy for these diseases.

Oxytocin, Regulation and Functions

OT is also synthesized in the magnocellular neurons of the neurohypophysis, and only differs in structure from AVP by two of nine amino acids. OT has similar concentrations in the posterior pituitary of both men and women, but to date a physiologic function for oxytocin has been described only in women. While prolactin is the main hormone necessary for milk production, OT is essential for milk secretion. Suckling stimulates tactile receptors in the nipple, producing an afferent signal to the hypothalamus that causes release of OT from the posterior pituitary. OT binds to OT receptors (OTR) in the breast and induces contraction myoepithelial cells around the alveoli and ductules to eject milk. OT also participates in parturition, though this action is more complex and is variable among species. In all species, there is interaction of OT with gonadal steroid hormones, prostaglandins, and relaxin. Additionally, upregulation of the uterine receptors for OT dramatically increases the response to OT at the end of pregnancy. The interaction of these various hormones in a cross-stimulation feed-forward cascade to support parturition is important to ensure survival of the species, so it is understandable that during parturition, lack of any single hormone (including OT) is generally not sufficient to inhibit delivery. The greatest release of OT occurs with, not before, delivery of the infant, probably secondary to stretching of the vaginal wall. This "Fergusson reflex" may aid delivery of subsequent fetuses in animals with multiple births; in humans, OT release may be more important to induce uterine contraction to inhibit blood loss after delivery than to initiate parturition.

No pathological syndromes of either increased or decreased secretion of OT have yet been defined. Women with diabetes insipidus secondary to traumatic damage of the magnocellular neurons often have normal pregnancy and delivery and can breastfeed their infants, but it may be that in these cases OT neurons survive better than AVP neurons. In animal studies, administration of OT to males increases sperm transport, but this function has not been documented in humans. Although only a single receptor for OT has been identified, similar to the receptors for AVP, the receptors for OT in the breast and in the myometrium are independently regulated. Because of the structural similarity between AVP and OT, at high plasma levels, OT can activate AVP receptors and AVP can activate OT receptors. One example of this is that administration of OT to induce labor can stimulate AVP V2 receptors of the kidney and cause water retention and hyponatremia if excess fluids are administered simultaneously.

Although peripheral effects of OT have only been described in females, similar to AVP, parvocellular OT neurons in the paraventricular nuclei project to multiple different areas within the brain where OT serves as a neurotransmitter and neuromodulator. Evidence in animals has strongly implicated brain OT in the production of maternal behaviors in females and in affiliative, that is, affection and bonding, behaviors in both sexes. These may prove to be of equal or greater importance than the peripheral actions of this hormone.

Disorders of Posterior Pituitary Function

Disorders of posterior pituitary function can result in body fluid and electrolyte disorders, which are among the most commonly encountered problems in the practice of clinical medicine. This is in large part because many different disease states can potentially disrupt the finely balanced mechanisms that control the intake and output of water and solute. Since body water is the primary determinant of the osmolality of the ECF, disorders of the posterior pituitary can be broadly divided into disorders of insufficient AVP, or AVP effect, and disorders of excess AVP, or AVP effect. The former often leads to hyperosmolality, where there is a deficiency of body water relative to body solute, and the latter often leads to hypoosmolality, where there is an excess of body water relative to body solute. Because sodium is the main constituent of plasma osmolality, these disorders are typically characterized by hypernatremia and hyponatremia, respectively.

Disorders of Deficient AVP or AVP Effect: Hyperosmolality and Hypernatremia

Hyperosmolality indicates a deficiency of water relative to solute in the ECF. Because water moves freely between the ICF and ECF, this also indicates a deficiency of total body water relative to total body solute. Although hypernatremia can be caused by an excess of body sodium, the vast majority of cases are due to losses of body water in excess of body solutes, caused by either insufficient water intake or excessive water excretion. Consequently, most of the disorders causing hyperosmolality are those associated with inadequate water intake and/or deficient pituitary AVP secretion. Although hyperosmolality from inadequate water intake is seen frequently in clinical practice, this is usually not due to an underlying defect in thirst but rather results from a generalized incapacity to obtain and/or ingest fluids, often stemming from a depressed sensorium.

Etiologies and Diagnosis

Evaluation of the patient's ECF volume status is important as a guide to fluid replacement therapy, but is not as useful for differential diagnosis since most hyperosmolar patients will manifest some degree of hypovolemia. Rather, assessment of urinary concentrating ability provides the most useful data with regard to the type of disorder present. Using this approach, disorders of hyperosmolality can be categorized as those in which renal water conservation mechanisms are intact but are unable to compensate for inadequately replaced losses of hypotonic fluids from other sources, or those in which renal concentrating defects are a contributing factor to the deficiency of body water (Verbalis 2012).

Diabetes Insipidus *Diabetes insipidus (DI)* can result from either inadequate AVP secretion (*central or neurogenic DI*) or inadequate renal response to AVP (*nephrogenic DI*). Central DI is caused by a variety of acquired or congenital anatomic lesions that disrupt the neurohypophysis, including pituitary surgery, tumors, trauma, hemorrhage, thrombosis, infarction, or granulomatous disease (Robertson 1995), as well as less commonly by genetic mutations of the AVP gene (Babey et al. 2011). Severe nephrogenic DI is most commonly congenital due to defects in the gene for the AVP V2R (X-linked recessive pattern of inheritance) or in the gene for the AQP2 water channel (autosomal recessive pattern of inheritance) (Fujiwara and Bichet 2005), but relief of chronic urinary obstruction or therapy with drugs such as lithium can cause an acquired form sufficient to warrant treatment. Acquired nephrogenic DI can result from hypokalemia or hypercalcemia, but the mild concentrating defect generally does not by itself cause hypertonicity and responds to correction of the underlying disorder (Khanna 2006). Regardless of the etiology of the DI, the end result is a water diuresis due to an inability to concentrate urine appropriately.

Because patients with DI do not have impaired urine Na^+ conservation, the ECF volume is generally not markedly decreased and regulatory mechanisms for maintenance of osmotic homeostasis are primarily activated: stimulation of thirst and pituitary AVP secretion (to whatever degree the neurohypophysis is still able to secrete AVP). In cases where AVP secretion is totally absent (complete DI), patients are dependent entirely on water intake for maintenance of water balance. However, in cases where some residual capacity to secrete AVP remains (partial DI), plasma osmolality can eventually reach levels that allow moderate degrees of urinary concentration. Although untreated DI can lead to both hyperosmolality and volume depletion, until the water losses become severe, volume depletion is minimized by osmotic shifts of water from the ICF into the more osmotically concentrated ECF (Robinson and Verbalis 2011).

Osmoreceptor Dysfunction The primary osmoreceptors that control AVP secretion and thirst are located in the anterior hypothalamus, and lesions of this region in animals cause hyperosmolality through a combination of impaired thirst and osmotically stimulated AVP secretion (Johnson and Buggy 1978). Initial reports in humans described this syndrome as "essential hypernatremia," and subsequent studies used the term *adipsic hypernatremia* in recognition of the profound thirst deficits found in most of the patients. All of these syndromes are now grouped together as *disorders of osmoreceptor function* (Baylis and Thompson 1988). Most of the cases reported to date have represented various degrees of osmoreceptor destruction associated with different brain lesions (Baylis and Thompson 2001). In contrast to lesions causing central DI, these lesions usually occur more rostrally in the hypothalamus. For all cases of osmoreceptor dysfunction, it is important to remember that afferent pathways from the brainstem to the hypothalamus generally remain intact; therefore, these patients will usually have normal AVP and renal concentrating responses to baroreceptor-mediated stimuli such as hypovolemia and hypotension.

Differential Diagnosis

Distinguishing between central and nephrogenic DI in a patient who is already hyperosmolar entails simply evaluating the response to a trial of AVP or desmopressin. Administration of AVP (5 units SC) or, preferably, the selective AVP V2R agonist desmopressin (2 μg SC or IV) should cause a significant increase in urine osmolality within 1–2 h after injection in patients with central DI, indicating insufficient endogenous AVP secretion. An absent or suboptimal response suggests renal resistance to AVP effects and, therefore, nephrogenic DI. Although conceptually simple, interpretational difficulties often arise because the water diuresis produced by AVP deficiency causes a downregulation of AQP2 synthesis along with a washout of the renal medullary concentrating gradient, such that increases in urine osmolality in response to administered AVP or desmopressin are not as great as would be expected (see Interpretation of urine concentration after AVP/desmopressin, Table 1).

Because patients with DI generally have an intact thirst mechanism, such patients often do not present with hyperosmolality, but rather have normal plasma osmolality and serum sodium levels with polyuria and polydipsia (Robertson 1995). In these cases, a fluid deprivation test should be performed in order to raise the serum osmolality and confirm the diagnosis of DI (see Table 1 for the procedure and interpretation of a fluid deprivation test).

When a diagnosis of central DI is made, magnetic resonance imaging (MRI) of the hypothalamus and neurohypophyseal tract is mandatory to rule out a neoplasm or granulomatous disease as an etiology. In individuals with a normal posterior

Table 1 Fluid deprivation test for the diagnosis of diabetes insipidus (*DI*)

Procedure
1. Initiation of the deprivation period depends on the severity of the DI; in routine cases, the patient should be made NPO after dinner, whereas in cases with more severe polyuria and polydipsia, this may be too long a period without fluids and the water deprivation should be begun early on the morning (e.g., 6 a.m.) of the test
2. Obtain plasma and urine osmolality, serum electrolytes, and a plasma AVP level at the start of the test
3. Measure urine volume and osmolality hourly or with each voided urine.
4. Stop the test when body weight decreases by ≥3%, the patient develops orthostatic blood pressure changes, the urine osmolality reaches a plateau (i.e., <10% change over two or three consecutive measurements), or the serum $[Na^+]$ > 145 mmol/L
5. Obtain plasma and urine osmolality, serum electrolytes, and a plasma AVP level at the end of the test, when the plasma osmolality is elevated, preferably >300 mOsm/kg H_2O
6. If the serum $[Na^+]$ < 146 mmol/L or the plasma osmolality <300 mOsm/kg H_2O when the test is stopped, then consider a short infusion of hypertonic saline (3% NaCl at a rate of 0.1 ml/kg/min for 1–2 h) to reach these endpoints
7. If hypertonic saline infusion is not required to achieve hyperosmolality, administer AVP (5 U) or DDAVP (1 μg) SC and continue following urine osmolality and volume for an additional 2 h
Interpretation
1. An unequivocal urine concentration after AVP/DDAVP (>50% increase) indicates central DI (CDI) and an unequivocal absence of urine concentration (<10%) strongly suggests nephrogenic DI (NDI) or primary polydipsia (PP)
2. Differentiating between NDI and PP, as well as for cases in which the increase in urine osmolality after AVP/DDAVP administration is more equivocal (e.g., 10–50%), is best done using the relation between plasma AVP levels and plasma osmolality obtained at the end of the dehydration period and/or hypertonic saline infusion and the relation between plasma AVP levels and urine osmolality under basal conditions

pituitary, the presence of pituitary "bright spot" (i.e., a hyperintense signal in the absence of contrast administration, representing the AVP-containing neurosecretory granules) is usually seen on T1-weighted noncontrast sagittal images. Conversely, in patients with central DI, the bright spot is usually absent. However, this test is not definitive, since the pituitary bright spot decreases with age and with disorders that cause dehydration, and it can be present in up to 5% of patients with DI due to the presence of pituitary oxytocin, which also leads to a hyperintense signal on T1-weighted imaging (Robinson and Verbalis 2011).

Evaluation of anterior pituitary function should be performed in all patients with central DI, especially if glucocorticoid administration and/or replacement unmasks underlying DI. Adrenal insufficiency can cause hypersecretion of AVP, which may be due in part to reductions in systemic blood pressure and cardiac output caused by cortisol deficiency, thereby stimulating pituitary AVP release. Cortisol deficiency is also known to cause increased AVP release from the median eminence into the pituitary portal circulation in an attempt to increase ACTH secretion via effects at pituitary V1bR on corticotrophs, which may also contribute to increased systemic AVP levels (Oelkers 1989).

The recent development of a commercial assay for the C-terminal glycoprotein of the AVP prohormone, copeptin, offers the possibility of a more stable and easier to measure marker of AVP secretion in response to induced dehydration and hypertonicity. Copeptin is secreted from the posterior pituitary in equimolar amounts as AVP, but is not degraded proteolytically as rapidly as AVP; in addition, its larger size renders measurement by two-site immunoassays possible, in contrast to AVP, which is too small for use of this technique (Morgenthaler et al. 2008). However, the clinical use of copeptin levels as a surrogate marker of AVP secretion during fluid deprivation tests will require standardization of normal and abnormal responses relative to plasma AVP levels.

Clinical Manifestations

The characteristic clinical symptoms of DI are the polyuria and polydipsia that result from the underlying impairment of urinary concentrating mechanisms, which have already been covered in the previous section discussing pathophysiology of specific types of DI. Interestingly, patients with DI typically describe a craving for cold water, which appears to quench their thirst better. Patients with CDI also typically describe a precipitous onset of their polyuria and polydipsia, which simply reflects the fact that urinary concentration can be maintained fairly well until the number of AVP-producing neurons in the hypothalamus decreases to 10–15% of normal, after which plasma AVP levels decrease to the range where urine output increases dramatically (Heinbecker and White 1941).

However, patients with DI, and particularly those with osmoreceptor dysfunction syndromes, can also present with varying degrees of hyperosmolality and dehydration depending on their overall hydration status. It is therefore important to be aware of the clinical manifestations of hyperosmolality as well. These can be divided into the signs and symptoms produced by dehydration, which are largely cardiovascular, and those caused by the hyperosmolality itself, which are predominantly neurological and reflect brain dehydration as a result of osmotic water shifts out of the central nervous system (Verbalis 2012). Cardiovascular manifestations of hypertonic dehydration include hypotension, azotemia, acute tubular necrosis secondary to renal hypoperfusion or rhabdomyolysis, and shock. Neurological manifestations range from nonspecific symptoms such as irritability and cognitive dysfunction to more severe manifestations of *hypertonic encephalopathy* such as disorientation, decreased level of consciousness, obtundation, chorea, seizures, coma, focal neurological deficits, subarachnoid hemorrhage, and cerebral infarction. The severity of symptoms can be roughly correlated with the degree of hyperosmolality, but individual variability is marked and for any single patient the level of serum [Na^+] at which symptoms will appear cannot be accurately predicted.

Similar to hypoosmolar syndromes, the length of time over which hyperosmolality develops can markedly affect the clinical symptomatology. Rapid development of severe hyperosmolality is frequently associated with marked neurological symptoms, whereas gradual development over several days or weeks generally causes milder symptoms. In this case, the brain counteracts osmotic shrinkage by increasing intracellular content of solutes. These include electrolytes such as potassium and a variety of *organic osmolytes*, which previously had been called *idiogenic osmoles*; for the most part these are the same organic osmolytes that are lost from the brain during adaptation to hypoosmolality (Gullans and Verbalis 1993). The net effect of this process is to protect the brain against excessive shrinkage during sustained hyperosmolality. However, once the brain has adapted by increasing its solute content, rapid correction of the hyperosmolality can produce brain edema, since it takes a finite time (24–48 h in animal studies) to dissipate the accumulated solutes, and until this process has been completed the brain will accumulate excess water as plasma osmolality is normalized (Verbalis 2010). This effect is most often seen in dehydrated pediatric patients who can develop seizures with rapid rehydration, but it has been described only rarely in adults.

General Principles of Therapy

The general goals of treatment of all hyperosmolar disorders are (1) correction of preexisting water deficits and (2) reduction in ongoing excessive urinary water losses. The specific therapy required varies with the clinical situation. Awake ambulatory patients with diabetes insipidus and normal thirst have little body water deficit but benefit from relief of the polyuria and polydipsia that disrupt normal activities. In contrast, comatose patients with or without diabetes insipidus are unable to drink in response to thirst, and in these patients progressive hypertonicity may be life-threatening. The established water deficit may be estimated using the following formula (Robinson and Verbalis 1997):

$$\text{Water deficit} = 0.6 \times \text{premorbid weight} \times [1 - 140/\text{serum } [\text{Na}^+] \text{ (mmol/L)}]$$

This formula is dependent on several assumptions (total body water is approximately 60% of body weight, no body solute is lost as hypertonicity developed, and the premorbid [Na^+] is 140 mmol/L), but nonetheless provides a valid estimate of the approximate total body water deficit. To reduce the risk of central nervous system injury from protracted exposure to severe hypertonicity, the serum osmolality should be lowered to the range of 330 mOsm/kg H_2O within the first 24 h of therapy. As noted previously, because the organic osmolytes accumulated in the brain during chronic hyperosmolality cannot be immediately dissipated, further correction to a normal osmolality should be spread over the subsequent 1–3 days to avoid producing cerebral edema during treatment, particularly in pediatric patients (Adrogue and Madias 2000a).

It should be remembered that formulae which estimate body water deficits do not take ongoing water losses into account. Consequently, frequent serum electrolyte determinations must be made, and the administration rate of oral water or intravenous 5% dextrose in water should be adjusted accordingly. For example, the estimated water deficit of a 70 kg patient whose serum [Na^+] is 160 mmol/L would be 5.25 l. In such an individual, administration of water at a rate > 200 ml per hour would be required simply to correct the established deficit over 24 h, but additional fluid would be needed to keep up with any ongoing losses in a patient with diabetes insipidus until a response to treatment has occurred.

Treatment of Central DI

A variety of antidiuretic agents have been used to treat central diabetes insipidus, but desmopressin is the treatment of choice for this disorder. Desmopressin was synthesized as a selective antagonist of AVP V2R, and it is particularly useful therapeutically because it has a much longer half-life than AVP and is devoid of the pressor activity of AVP at vascular V1aR (Robinson 1976). Desmopressin is generally administered intranasally (5–20 μg every 8–24 h), but can be given parenterally in acute situations (1–2 μg IV, IM and SC). For both the intranasal and parenteral preparations, increasing the administered dose generally has the effect of prolonging the duration of antidiuresis rather than increasing its magnitude; consequently, altering the dose can be useful to reduce the required frequency of administration. Synthetic AVP (Pitressin) can also be used to treat central DI, but its use is limited by a much shorter half-life necessitating more frequent dosing or a continuous infusion, and the production of pressor effects due to vasoconstriction.

Treatment of Nephrogenic DI

Nephrogenic diabetes insipidus is more difficult to treat since the kidney is resistant to all AVP-type agents. Limited responses can sometimes be achieved using thiazide diuretics (any drug of the thiazide class may be used with equal potential for benefit). Thiazides cause natriuresis by blocking sodium absorption in the cortical diluting site; when combined with dietary sodium restriction a modest hypovolemia results, which stimulates isotonic proximal tubular solute reabsorption and diminishes solute delivery to the distal parts of the nephron. Together, these effects diminish free water clearance independently of actions of AVP, thereby decreasing the polyuria of patients with nephrogenic DI (Sands and Bichet 2006). Monitoring for hypokalemia is necessary and K^+ supplementation is occasionally required. Care must be exercised when treating patients taking lithium with diuretics, since the induced contraction of plasma volume may increase lithium concentrations by increasing proximal tubular absorption and worsen potential toxic effects of the therapy (Grunfeld and Rossier 2009). Because prostaglandins increase renal medullary blood flow and diminish medullary solute concentration, effects that modestly decrease the interstitial gradient for water reabsorption, drugs that block renal prostaglandin synthesis (e.g., nonsteroidal anti-inflammatory agents) can increase non-AVP-mediated water reabsorption and impair urinary dilution, thereby reducing free water clearance and urine output. Although these agents are somewhat effective in central diabetes insipidus, their main usefulness is as adjunctive therapy in nephrogenic diabetes insipidus, in which more direct antidiuretic therapies are limited.

Disorders of Excess AVP or AVP Effect: Hypoosmolality and Hyponatremia

Hypoosmolality indicates excess water relative to solute in the ECF; because water moves freely between the ECF and the intracellular fluid (ICF), this also indicates an excess of total body water relative to total body solute. Imbalances between body water and solute can be generated either by *depletion* of body solute more than body water, or by *dilution* of body solute from increases in body water more than body solute. This is an oversimplification of complex physiology, and most hypoosmolar states include components of both solute depletion and water retention. Nonetheless, this general concept has proven to be useful because it provides a simple framework for understanding the basic etiologies of hypoosmolar disorders.

Differential Diagnosis

Definitive identification of the etiology of hypoosmolality is not always possible at the time of presentation, but categorization according to the patient's ECF volume status represents the first step in ascertaining the underlying cause of the disorder (Verbalis 2012).

Decreased ECF Volume (Hypovolemia) Clinically detectable hypovolemia indicates some degree of solute depletion. Even isotonic or hypotonic fluid losses can cause hypoosmolality if water or hypotonic fluids are subsequently ingested or infused. A low urine sodium concentration (U_{Na}) suggests a nonrenal cause of solute depletion, whereas a high U_{Na} suggests renal causes of solute depletion. Diuretic use is the most common cause of hypovolemic hypoosmolality. Most etiologies of solute losses causing hypovolemic hypoosmolality will be clinically apparent, although some salt-wasting nephropathies and mineralocorticoid deficiency may be difficult to diagnose during early phases of these diseases.

Normal ECF Volume (Euvolemia) Virtually any disorder causing hypoosmolality can present with a volume status that appears normal by standard methods of clinical evaluation. Because clinical assessment of volume status is not very sensitive, the presence of normal or low blood urea nitrogen and uric acid concentrations are helpful laboratory correlates of relatively normal ECF volume. In these cases, a low U_{Na} (<30 mmol/L) suggests depletional hypoosmolality secondary to ECF losses with subsequent volume replacement by water or other hypotonic fluids. Such patients may appear euvolemic by the usual clinical parameters used to assess hydration status. A high U_{Na} ($\geq$30 mmol/L) generally indicates a dilutional hypoosmolality such as the syndrome of inappropriate antidiuretic hormone secretion (SIADH), the most common cause of euvolemic hypoosmolality. The clinical criteria necessary to diagnose SIADH remain as initially defined by Bartter and Schwartz in 1967 (Bartter and Schwartz 1967). Many different disorders are associated with SIADH, which can be divided into four major etiologic groups: tumors, CNS disorders, drug effects, and pulmonary diseases.

Increased ECF Volume (Hypervolemia) Clinically detectable hypervolemia indicates whole body sodium excess, and hypoosmolality in these patients suggests a relatively decreased intravascular volume and/or pressure leading to water retention as a result of elevated plasma AVP levels and decreased distal delivery of glomerular filtrate to the kidneys. Such patients usually have a low U_{Na} because of secondary hyperaldosteronism, but under certain conditions the U_{Na} may be elevated (e.g., diuretic therapy). Hyponatremia generally does not occur until relatively advanced stages of congestive heart failure, cirrhosis, or the nephrotic syndrome, by which time diagnosis is usually not difficult. Renal failure can also cause retention of both sodium and water.

Clinical Manifestations

The clinical manifestations of hyponatremia are largely neurological, and primarily reflect brain edema resulting from osmotic water shifts into the brain (Verbalis 2010). These range from nonspecific symptoms such as headache and confusion, to more severe manifestations such as decreased sensorium, coma, seizures, and death. Significant central nervous system (CNS) symptoms generally do not occur until the serum sodium concentration ([Na^+]) falls below 125 mmol/L, and the severity of symptoms can be roughly correlated with the degree of hypoosmolality. Individual variability is marked, and for any patient the level of serum [Na^+] at which symptoms will appear cannot be accurately predicted. Several factors other than the severity of the hypoosmolality also affect the degree of neurological dysfunction. The most important is the time course over which hypoosmolality develops. Rapid development of severe hypoosmolality frequently causes marked neurological symptoms, whereas gradual development over several days or weeks is often associated with relatively mild symptomatology despite profound degrees of hypoosmolality. This is because the brain counteracts osmotic swelling by extruding extracellular and intracellular solutes, including potassium and a variety of small organic molecules (amino acids, polyols, and methylamines) called *organic osmolytes* (Gullans and Verbalis 1993). Since this is a time-dependent process, rapid development of hypoosmolality can result in brain edema before this adaptation occurs, but with slower development of the same degree of hypoosmolality brain cells can lose solute sufficiently rapidly to prevent cell swelling, brain edema, and neurological dysfunction (Verbalis 2010). Underlying neurological disease also affects the level of hypoosmolality at which CNS symptoms appear; moderate hypoosmolality is of little concern in an otherwise healthy patient, but can cause morbidity in a patient with an underlying seizure disorder. Nonneurological metabolic disorders (hypoxia, hypercapnia, acidosis, hypercalcemia, etc.) similarly can affect the level of osmolality at which CNS symptoms occur.

General Principles of Therapy

Correction of hyponatremia is associated with markedly improved neurological outcomes in patients with severely symptomatic hyponatremia. In a retrospective review of patients who presented with severe neurological symptoms and serum $[Na^+] < 125$ mmol/L, prompt therapy with isotonic or hypertonic saline resulted in a correction in the range of 20 mmol/L over several days and neurological recovery in almost all cases. In contrast, in patients who were treated with fluid restriction alone, there was very little correction over the study period (<5 mmol/L over 72 h), and the neurological outcomes were much worse, with most of these patients either dying or entering a persistently vegetative state (Ayus 1986). Consequently, based on this and many similar retrospective analyses, prompt therapy to rapidly increase the serum $[Na^+]$ represents the standard of care for treatment of patients presenting with severe life-threatening symptoms of hyponatremia.

Chronic hyponatremia is much less symptomatic as a result of the process of brain volume regulation. Because of this adaptation process, chronic hyponatremia is arguably a condition that clinicians feel they may not need to be as concerned about, which has been reinforced by the common usage of the descriptor *asymptomatic hyponatremia* for many such patients. However, it is clear that many such patients very often do have neurological symptoms, even if milder and more subtle in nature, including headaches, nausea, mood disturbances, depression, difficulty concentrating, slowed reaction times, unstable gait, increased falls, confusion, and disorientation (Renneboog et al. 2006). Consequently, all patients with hyponatremia who manifest any neurological symptoms that could possibly be related to the hyponatremia should be considered as potential candidates for treatment of the hyponatremia, regardless of the chronicity of the hyponatremia or the level of serum $[Na^+]$.

Currently Available Therapies for Treatment of Hyponatremia

Conventional management strategies for hyponatremia range from saline infusion and fluid restriction to pharmacologic measure to adjust fluid balance. Consideration of treatment options should always include an evaluation of the benefits as well as the potential toxicities of any therapy, and must be individualized for each patient (Verbalis et al. 2007; Verbalis 2013). It should always be remembered that sometimes simply stopping treatment with an agent that is associated with hyponatremia is sufficient to reverse a low serum $[Na^+]$.

Isotonic Saline The treatment of choice for depletional hyponatremia (i.e., hypovolemic hyponatremia) is isotonic saline ($[Na^+] = 154$ mmol/L) to restore ECF volume and ensure adequate organ perfusion. This initial therapy is appropriate for patients who either have clinical signs of hypovolemia, or in whom a spot U_{Na} is <30 mmol/L. However, this therapy is ineffective for dilutional hyponatremias such as SIADH (Schwartz et al. 1957), and continued inappropriate administration of isotonic saline to a euvolemic patient may worsen their hyponatremia (Steele et al. 1997), and/or cause fluid overload.

Hypertonic Saline Acute hyponatremia presenting with severe neurological symptoms is life-threatening, and should be treated promptly with hypertonic solutions, typically 3% NaCl ($[Na^+] = 513$ mmol/L), as this represents the most reliable method to quickly raise the serum $[Na^+]$. A continuous infusion of hypertonic NaCl is usually utilized in inpatient settings. Various formulae have been suggested for calculating the initial rate of infusion of hypertonic solutions (Adrogue and Madias 2000b), but until now there has been no consensus regarding optimal infusion rates of 3% NaCl. One of the simplest methods to estimate an initial 3% NaCl infusion rate utilizes the following relationship (Verbalis et al. 2007; Verbalis 2013):

$$\begin{aligned}&\text{Patient's weight (kg) x desired correction rate } (\text{mEq/L/h})\\&\quad = \text{infusion rate of 3\% NaCl } (\text{mL/h})\end{aligned}$$

Depending on individual hospital policies, the administration of hypertonic solutions may require special considerations (e.g., placement in the ICU, sign-off by a consultant).

An alternative option for more emergent situations is administration of a 100 mL bolus of 3% NaCl, repeated 1–2 times every 30 min if there is no clinical improvement, which has been recommended by a consensus conference organized to develop guidelines for prevention and treatment of exercise-induced hyponatremia, an acute and potentially lethal condition (Hew-Butler et al. 2008). Injecting this amount of hypertonic saline intravenously raises the serum $[Na^+]$ by an average of 2–4 mmol/L, which is well below the recommended maximal daily rate of change of 10–12 mmol/24 h or 18 mmol/48 h (Sterns et al. 1994). Because the brain can only accommodate an average increase of approximately 7–8% in brain volume before herniation occurs, quickly increasing the serum $[Na^+]$ by as little as 2–4 mmol/L in acute hyponatremia can effectively reduce brain swelling and intracranial pressure (Battison et al. 2005).

Many physicians are hesitant to use hypertonic saline in patients with chronic hyponatremia, because it can cause an overly rapid correction of serum sodium levels that can lead to the *osmotic demyelination syndrome* (ODS) (Sterns et al. 1986). Nonetheless, this remains the treatment of choice for patients with severe neurological symptoms, even when the time course of the hyponatremia is nonacute or unknown.

Fluid Restriction For patients with chronic hyponatremia, fluid restriction has been the most popular and most widely accepted treatment. When SIADH is present, fluids should generally be limited to 500–1000 mL/24 h. Because fluid restriction increases the serum [Na^+] largely by under-replacing the excretion of fluid by the kidneys, some have advocated an initial restriction to 500 ml less than the 24-h urine output (Robertson 2006). When instituting a fluid restriction, it is important for the nursing staff and the patient to understand that this includes *all* fluids that are consumed, not just water. Generally, the water content of ingested food is not included in the restriction because this is balanced by insensible water losses (perspiration, exhaled air, feces, etc.), but caution should be exercised with foods that have high fluid concentrations (such as fruits and soups). Restricting fluid intake can be effective when properly applied and managed in selected patients, but serum [Na^+] are increased only slowly (1–2 mmol/L/d) even with severe restriction (Schwartz et al. 1957). In addition, this therapy is often poorly tolerated because of an associated increase in thirst leading to poor compliance with long-term therapy. However, it is economically favorable, and some patients do respond well to this option.

Fluid restriction should not be used with hypovolemic patients, and is particularly difficult to maintain in patients with very elevated urine osmolalities secondary to high AVP levels; in general, if the sum of urine Na^+ and K^+ exceeds the serum [Na^+], most patients will not respond to a fluid restriction since a negative electrolyte-free water clearance will be difficult to achieve (Berl 2008; Decaux 2009; Furst et al. 2000). In addition, fluid restriction is not practical for some patients, particularly patients in intensive care settings who often require administration of significant volumes of fluids as part of their therapies.

Demeclocycline Demeclocycline, a tetracycline antibiotic, inhibits adenylyl cyclase activation after AVP binds to the V2R in the kidney, and thus targets the underlying pathophysiology of SIADH. This therapy is typically used when patients find severe fluid restriction unacceptable and the underlying disorder cannot be corrected. However, demeclocycline is not approved by the US Food and Drug Administration (FDA) or the European Medicines Agency (EMA) to treat hyponatremia, and can cause nephrotoxicity in patients with heart failure and cirrhosis, although this is usually reversible (Singer and Rotenberg 1973).

Mineralocorticoids Administration of mineralocorticoids, such as fludrocortisone, has been shown to be useful in a small number of elderly patients (Ishikawa et al. 1996). However, the initial studies of SIADH did not show it to be of benefit in patients with SIADH, and it carries the risk of fluid overload and hypertension. Consequently, it is rarely used as primary therapy for hyponatremia.

Urea Administration of urea has been successfully used to treat hyponatremia because it induces osmotic diuresis and augments free water excretion. Effective doses of urea for treatment of hyponatremia are 30–90 g daily in divided doses (Decaux and Genette 1981). Unfortunately, its use is limited because there is no US Pharmacopeia (USP) formulation for urea, it is not currently approved by any regulatory agency for treatment of hyponatremia, and there are limited data to support its long-term use. Furthermore, urea is associated with poor palatability leading to patient compliance problems. However, patients with feeding tubes may be excellent candidates for urea therapy since palatability is not a concern, and the use of fluid restriction may be difficult in some patients with high obligate intake of fluids as part of their nutritional and medication therapy. Although mild azotemia can occur with urea therapy, this rarely reaches clinically significant levels.

Furosemide and NaCl The use of furosemide (20–40 mg/day) coupled with a high salt intake (200 mmol/day), which represents an extension of the treatment of acute symptomatic hyponatremia to the chronic management of euvolemic hyponatremia, has also been reported to be successful in selected cases (Decaux et al. 1981). However, the long-term efficacy and safety of this approach is unknown.

Arginine Vasopressin Receptor (AVPR) Antagonists Clinicians have used all of the above conventional therapies for hyponatremia over the past decades. However, conventional therapies for hyponatremia, although effective in specific circumstances, are suboptimal for many different reasons, including variable efficacy, slow responses, intolerable side effects, and serious toxicities. But perhaps the most striking deficiency of most conventional therapies is that, with the exception of demeclocycline, these therapies do not directly target the underlying cause of most all dilutional hyponatremias, namely inappropriately elevated plasma AVP levels. A new class of pharmacological agents, *vasopressin receptor antagonists*, also called *vaptans,* which directly block AVP-mediated receptor activation has recently been developed for clinical use (Greenberg and Verbalis 2006; Thibonnier et al. 2001).

Conivaptan and tolvaptan are competitive receptor antagonists of the AVP V2R and have been approved by the FDA for the treatment of euvolemic and hypervolemic hyponatremia and by the EMA for treatment of hyponatremia caused by SIADH. These agents compete with AVP/ADH for binding at its site of action in the kidney, thereby blocking the antidiuresis caused by elevated AVP levels and directly attacking the underlying pathophysiology of dilutional hyponatremia. AVPR antagonists produce electrolyte free water excretion (called *aquaresis*) without affecting renal sodium and potassium excretion (Ohnishi et al. 1993). The overall result is a reduction in body water without natriuresis, which leads to an increase in the serum [Na^+]. One of the major benefits of this class of drugs is that serum [Na^+] is significantly increased by an average of 4–8 mmol/L within 24–48 h (Schrier et al. 2006; Zeltser et al. 2007), which is considerably faster than the effects of fluid restriction that can take many days. Also, compliance has not been shown to be problem for vaptans, whereas this is a major problem with attempted long-term use of fluid restriction.

Conivaptan is FDA-approved for euvolemic and hypervolemic hyponatremia in hospitalized patients. It is available only as an intravenous preparation and is given as a 20 mg loading dose over 30 min, followed by a continuous infusion of 20 or 40 mg (Li-Ng and Verbalis 2010). Generally, the 20 mg continuous infusion is used for the first 24 h to gauge the initial response. If the correction of serum [Na^+] is felt to be inadequate (e.g., <5 mmol/L), then the infusion rate can be increased to 40 mg/d. Therapy is limited to a maximum duration of 4 days because of drug-interaction effects with other agents metabolized by the CYP3A4 hepatic isoenzyme. Importantly, for conivaptan and all other vaptans, it is critical that the serum [Na^+] concentration is measured frequently during the active phase of correction of the hyponatremia (a minimum of every 6–8 h for conivaptan, but more frequently in patients with risk factors for development of osmotic demyelination, such as severely low serum [Na^+], malnutrition, alcoholism, and hypokalemia (Verbalis et al. 2007). If the correction approaches 12 mmol/L in the first 24 h, the infusion should be stopped and the patient monitored on a fluid restriction. If the correction exceeds 12 mmol/L, consideration should be given to administering sufficient water, either orally or as intravenous D_5W to bring the overall correction below 12 mEq/L. The maximum correction limit should be reduced to 8 mEq/L over the first 24 h in patients with risk factors for development of osmotic demyelination mentioned previously. The most common adverse effects include injection-site reactions, which are generally mild and usually do not lead to treatment discontinuation, headache, thirst, and hypokalemia (Zeltser et al. 2007).

Tolvaptan, an oral AVPR antagonist, is FDA-approved for treatment of dilutional hyponatremias. In contrast to conivaptan, oral administration allows it to be used for both short- and long-term treatment of hyponatremia (Schrier et al. 2006). Similar to conivaptan, tolvaptan treatment must be initiated in the hospital so that the rate of correction can be monitored carefully. Patients with a serum [Na^+] < 125 mmol/L are eligible for therapy with tolvaptan as primary therapy; if the serum [Na^+] is ≥125 mmol/L, tolvaptan therapy is only indicated if the patient has symptoms that could be attributable to the hyponatremia and the patient is resistant to attempts at fluid restriction (Otsuka Pharmaceutical Co and Tokyo 2009). The starting dose of tolvaptan is 15 mg on the first day, and the dose can be titrated to 30 mg and 60 mg at 24 h. intervals if the serum [Na^+] remains <135 mEq/L or the increase in serum [Na^+] has been ≤5 mmol/L in the previous 24 h. As with conivaptan, it is essential that the serum [Na^+] concentration is measured frequently during the active phase of correction of the hyponatremia (a minimum of every 6–8 h, but more frequently in patients with risk factors for development of osmotic demyelination). Limits for safe correction of hyponatremia and methods to compensate for overly rapid corrections are the same as described previously for conivaptan. One additional factor that helps to avoid overly rapid correction with tolvaptan is the recommendation that fluid restriction not be used during the active phase of correction, thereby allowing the patient's thirst to compensate for an overly vigorous aquaresis. Common side effects include dry mouth, thirst, increased urinary frequency, dizziness, nausea, and orthostatic hypotension, which were relatively similar between placebo and tolvaptan groups in clinical trials (Otsuka Pharmaceutical Co and Tokyo 2009; Schrier et al. 2006).

Because inducing increased renal fluid excretion via either a diuresis or an aquaresis can cause or worsen hypotension in patients with hypovolemic hyponatremia, vaptans are contraindicated in this patient population (Verbalis et al. 2007). However, clinically significant hypotension was not observed in either the conivaptan or tolvaptan clinical trials in euvolemic and hypervolemic hyponatremic patients. Although vaptans are not contraindicated with decreased renal function, these agents generally will not be effective if the serum creatinine is >3.0 mg/dl. By virtue of their solubility properties, the vaptans are readily absorbed through the gastrointestinal tract and therefore likely cross the blood–brain barrier as well, but alterations of central nervous system (CNS) functions have not been observed to date with clinical use of vaptans. This may be due to the fact that most of the CNS effects of AVP have been attributed to V1aR, with no evidence to support the presence or biological function of V2R in the CNS (Thibonnier et al. 1998); however, such effects have not been reported even with clinical use of conivaptan, a combined V1aR/V2R antagonist. Therefore, until more directed and sensitive studies are done to assess potential CNS effects of AVP receptor antagonists, it must be concluded that such effects are absent, or minimal.

Hyponatremia Treatment Guidelines

Although various authors have published recommendations for the treatment of hyponatremia (Adrogue and Madias 2000b; Ellison and Berl 2007; Spasovski et al. 2014; Sterns et al. 2009; Verbalis et al. 2007; Verbalis 2009), no standardized treatment algorithms have yet been widely accepted. A synthesis of existing expert recommendations for treatment of hyponatremia is illustrated in Fig. 3. This algorithm is based primarily on the symptomatology of hyponatremic patients, rather than the serum [Na^+] or on the chronicity of the hyponatremia, the latter of which is often difficult to ascertain.

A careful neurological history and assessment should always be done to identify potential causes for the patient's symptoms other than hyponatremia, although it will not always be possible to exclude an additive contribution from the hyponatremia to an underlying neurological condition. In this algorithm, patients are divided into three groups based on their presenting symptoms: ***severe symptoms*** (seizures, coma, respiratory arrest, obtundation, and vomiting; these symptoms usually imply a more acute onset or worsening of hyponatremia requiring immediate active treatment); ***moderate symptoms*** (nausea, confusion, disorientation, and altered mental status; these symptoms may be either chronic or acute, but allow time to elaborate a more deliberate approach to treatment); ***mild symptoms*** (headache, irritability, inability to concentrate, altered mood, and depression, or a virtual absence of discernible symptoms; these symptoms usually indicate that the patient may have chronic or slowly evolving hyponatremia). (Verbalis 2012)

Patients with severe symptoms should be treated with hypertonic saline as first-line therapy, followed by fluid restriction with or without AVPR antagonist therapy. Patients with moderate symptoms will benefit from a regimen of vaptan therapy or limited hypertonic saline administration, followed by fluid restriction or long-term vaptan therapy. Although moderate neurological symptoms can indicate that a patient is in an early stage of acute hyponatremia, they more often indicate a chronically hyponatremic state with sufficient brain volume adaptation to prevent

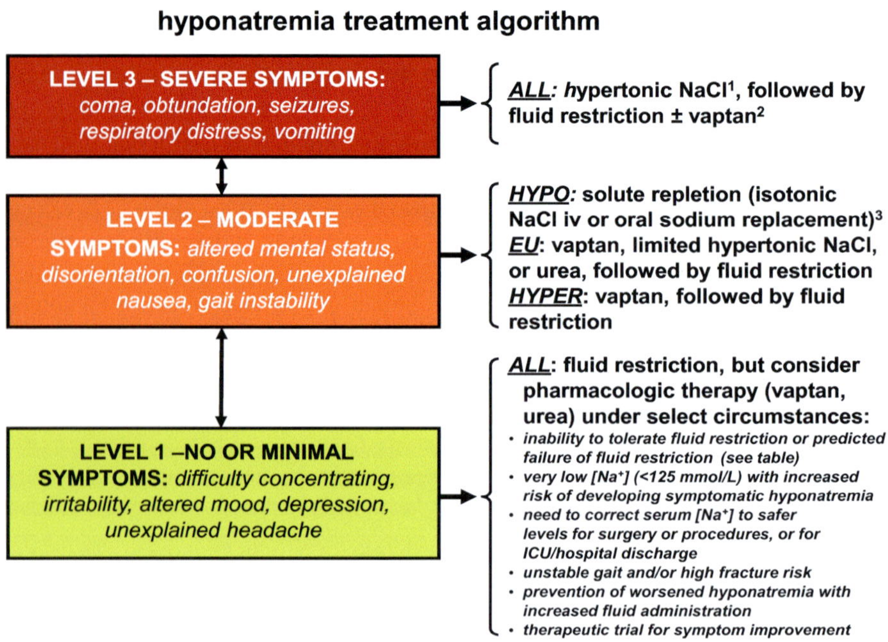

Fig. 3. Algorithm for treatment of patients with euvolemic hyponatremia based on their presenting symptoms. The *arrows* between the symptom boxes indicate movement of patients between different symptom levels. *HYPO* hypovolemic hyponatremia, *EU* euvolemic hyponatremia, *HYPER* hypervolemic hyponatremia, *ALL* all types of hypotonic hyponatremia. [1]some authors recommend simultaneous treatment with desmopressin to limit speed of correction; [2]no active therapy should be started within 24 h of hypertonic saline to decrease the chance of overly rapid correction of [Na^+] and risk of ODS; [3]with isotonic NaCl infusion, serum [Na^+] must be followed closely to prevent overly rapid correction and risk of ODS due to secondary water diuresis (From Verbalis (2016b))

marked symptomatology from cerebral edema. Regardless, close monitoring of these patients in a hospital setting is warranted until the symptoms improve or stabilize. Patients with no or minimal symptoms should be managed initially with fluid restriction, although treatment with vaptans may be appropriate for a wide range of specific clinical conditions, foremost of which is a failure to improve the serum [Na^+] despite reasonable attempts at fluid restriction.

A special case is when spontaneous correction of hyponatremia occurs at an undesirably rapid rate as a result of the onset of a water diuresis. This can occur following cessation of desmopressin therapy in a patient who has become hyponatremic, replacement of glucocorticoids in a patient with adrenal insufficiency, replacement of solutes in a patient with diuretic-induced hyponatremia, or spontaneous resolution of transient SIADH. Brain damage from ODS can clearly ensue in this setting if the preceding period of hyponatremia has been of sufficient duration (usually $\geq$48 h) to allow brain volume regulation to occur. If the previously discussed correction parameters have been exceeded and the correction is proceeding more rapidly than planned (usually because of continued excretion of hypotonic urine), the pathological events leading to demyelination can be reversed by administration of hypotonic fluids and desmopressin. Efficacy of this approach is suggested both from animal studies (Soupart et al. 1994) as well as case reports in humans (Goldszmidt and Iliescu 2000; Sterns et al. 2009), even when patients are overtly symptomatic (Oya et al. 2001).

Although this algorithm is based on presenting symptoms at the time of initial evaluation, it should be remembered that in some cases patients initially exhibit more moderate symptoms because they are in the early stages of hyponatremia. In addition, some patients with minimal symptoms are prone to develop more symptomatic hyponatremia during periods of increased fluid ingestion. In support of this, approximately 70% of 31 patients presenting to a university hospital with symptomatic hyponatremia and a mean serum [Na^+] of 119 mmol/L had preexisting “asymptomatic” hyponatremia as the most common risk factor identified (Bissram et al. 2007). Consequently, therapy of hyponatremia should also be considered to prevent progression from lower to higher levels of symptomatic hyponatremia, particularly in patients with a past history of repeated presentations for symptomatic hyponatremia.

Monitoring the Serum [Na^+] in Hyponatremic Patients

The frequency of serum [Na^+] monitoring is dependent on both the severity of the hyponatremia and the therapy chosen. In all hyponatremic patients neurological symptomatology should be carefully assessed very early in the diagnostic evaluation to assess the symptomatic severity of the hyponatremia and to determine whether the patient requires more urgent therapy. All patients undergoing active treatment with hypertonic saline for symptomatic hyponatremia should have frequent monitoring of serum [Na^+] and ECF volume status (every 2–4 h) to ensure that the serum [Na^+] does not exceeded the recommended levels during the active phase of correction (Verbalis et al. 2007), since overly rapid correction of serum sodium can cause damage to the myelin sheath of nerve cells, resulting in ODS (Sterns et al. 1986). Patients treated with vaptans for mild to moderate symptoms should have serum [Na^+] monitored every 6–8 h during the active phase of correction, which will generally be the first 24–48 h of therapy. Active treatment with hypertonic saline or vaptans should be stopped when the patient’s symptoms are no longer present, a safe serum [Na^+] (usually >120 mmol/L) has been achieved, or the rate of correction has reached 12 mmol/L within 24 h or 18 mmol/L within 48 h (Sterns et al. 1994; Verbalis et al. 2007). Importantly, ODS has not yet been reported either in clinical trials or with therapeutic use of any vaptan as monotherapy to date. In patients with a stable level of serum [Na^+] treated with fluid restriction or therapies other than hypertonic saline, measurement of serum [Na^+] daily is generally sufficient, since levels will not change that quickly in the absence of active therapy or large changes in fluid intake or administration.

Long-Term Treatment of Chronic Hyponatremia

Some patients will benefit from continued treatment of hyponatremia following discharge from the hospital. In many cases, this will consist of a continued fluid restriction. However, as discussed previously, long-term compliance with this therapy is poor due to the increased thirst that occurs with more severe degrees of fluid restriction. Thus, for selected patients who have responded to tolvaptan in the hospital, consideration should be given to continuing the treatment as an outpatient after discharge. In patients with established chronic hyponatremia, tolvaptan has shown to be effective at maintaining a normal [Na^+] for as long as 3 years of continued daily therapy (Berl et al. 2010). However, many patients with inpatient hyponatremia have a transient form of SIADH without need for long-term therapy. Selection of which patients with inpatient hyponatremia are candidates for long-term therapy should be based on the etiology of the SIADH. In all cases, consideration should be given to a trial of stopping the drug 2–4 weeks following discharge to see if hyponatremia is still present. A reasonable period of tolvaptan cessation to evaluate the presence of continued SIADH is 7 days, since this period was sufficient for demonstration of a recurrence of hyponatremia in the tolvaptan SALT trials (Berl et al. 2010; Schrier et al. 2006). Serum [Na^+] should be monitored every 2–3 days following cessation of tolvaptan so that the drug can be resumed as quickly as possible in those patients with recurrent hyponatremia, since the longer the patient is hyponatremic the greater the risk of subsequent ODS with overly rapid correction of the low serum [Na^+].

References

Adrogue HJ, Madias NE. Hypernatremia. N Engl J Med. 2000a;342(20):1493–9. Available from: PM:10816188.

Adrogue HJ, Madias NE. Hyponatremia. N Engl J Med. 2000b;342(21):1581–9. Available from: PM:0010824078.

Ayus JC. Diuretic-induced hyponatremia [editorial]. Arch Intern Med. 1986;146(7):1295–6. Available from: PM:0003718124.

Babey M, Kopp P, Robertson GL. Familial forms of diabetes insipidus: clinical and molecular characteristics. Nat Rev Endocrinol. 2011;7(12):701–14. Available from: PM:21727914.

Bartter FC, Schwartz WB. The syndrome of inappropriate secretion of antidiuretic hormone. Am J Med. 1967;42:790–806.

Battison C, Andrews PJ, Graham C, Petty T. Randomized, controlled trial on the effect of a 20% mannitol solution and a 7.5% saline/6% dextran solution on increased intracranial pressure after brain injury. Crit Care Med. 2005;33(1):196–202. Available from: PM:15644669.

Baylis PH, Thompson CJ. Osmoregulation of vasopressin secretion and thirst in health and disease. Clin Endocrinol (Oxf). 1988;29(5):549–76. Available from: PM:3075528.

Baylis PH, Thompson CJ. Diabetes insipidus and hyperosmolar syndromes. In: Becker KL, editor. Principles and practice of endocrinology and metabolism. 3rd ed. Philadelphia: Lippincott Williams & Wilkins; 2001. p. 285–93.

Berl T. Impact of solute intake on urine flow and water excretion. J Am Soc Nephrol. 2008;19(6):1076–8. Available from: PM:18337482.

Berl T, Quittnat-Pelletier F, Verbalis JG, Schrier RW, Bichet DG, Ouyang J, Czerwiec FS. Oral tolvaptan is safe and effective in chronic hyponatremia. J Am Soc Nephrol. 2010;21(4):705–12. Available from: PM:20185637.

Bissram M, Scott FD, Liu L, Rosner MH. Risk factors for symptomatic hyponatraemia: the role of pre-existing asymptomatic hyponatraemia. Intern Med J. 2007;37(3):149–55. Available from: PM:17316332.

Decaux G. The syndrome of inappropriate secretion of antidiuretic hormone (SIADH). Semin Nephrol. 2009;29(3):239–56. Available from: PM:19523572.

Decaux G, Genette F. Urea for long-term treatment of syndrome of inappropriate secretion of antidiuretic hormone. Br Med J – Clin Res. 1981;283:1081–3.

Decaux G, Waterlot Y, Genette F, Mockel J. Treatment of the syndrome of inappropriate secretion of antidiuretic hormone with furosemide. N Engl J Med. 1981;304:329–30.

Ellison DH, Berl T. Clinical practice. The syndrome of inappropriate antidiuresis. N Engl J Med. 2007;356(20):2064–72. Available from: PM:17507705.

Fujiwara TM, Bichet DG. Molecular biology of hereditary diabetes insipidus. J Am Soc Nephrol. 2005;16:2836. Available from: PM:16093448.

Furst H, Hallows KR, Post J, Chen S, Kotzker W, Goldfarb S, Ziyadeh FN, Neilson EG. The urine/plasma electrolyte ratio: a predictive guide to water restriction. Am J Med Sci. 2000;319(4):240–4. Available from: PM:0010768609.

Goldszmidt MA, Iliescu EA. DDAVP to prevent rapid correction in hyponatremia. Clin Nephrol. 2000;53(3):226–9. Available from: PM:0010749304.

Greenberg A, Verbalis JG. Vasopressin receptor antagonists. Kidney Int. 2006;69(12):2124–30. Available from: PM:16672911.

Grunfeld JP, Rossier BC. Lithium nephrotoxicity revisited. Nat Rev Nephrol. 2009;5(5):270–6. Available from: PM:19384328.

Gullans SR, Verbalis JG. Control of brain volume during hyperosmolar and hypoosmolar conditions. Annu Rev Med. 1993;44:289–301.

Heinbecker P, White HL. Hypothalamico-hypophyseal system and its relation to water balance in the dog. Am J Physiol. 1941;133:582–93.

Hew-Butler T, Ayus JC, Kipps C, Maughan RJ, Mettler S, Meeuwisse WH, Page AJ, Reid SA, Rehrer NJ, Roberts WO, Rogers IR, Rosner MH, Siegel AJ, Speedy DB, Stuempfle KJ, Verbalis JG, Weschler LB, Wharam P. Statement of the second international exercise-associated hyponatremia consensus development conference, New Zealand, 2007. Clin J Sport Med. 2008;18(2):111–21. Available from: PM:18332684.

Ishikawa S, Fujita N, Fujisawa G, Tsuboi Y, Sakuma N, Okada K, Saito T. Involvement of arginine vasopressin and renal sodium handling in pathogenesis of hyponatremia in elderly patients. Endocr J. 1996;43(1):101–8.

Johnson AK, Buggy J. Periventricular preoptic-hypothalamus is vital for thirst and normal water economy. Am J Physiol. 1978;234(3):R122–9. Available from: PM:629368.

Khanna A. Acquired nephrogenic diabetes insipidus. Semin Nephrol. 2006;26(3):244–8. Available from: PM:16713497.

Li-Ng M, Verbalis JG. Conivaptan: evidence supporting its therapeutic use in hyponatremia. Core Evid. 2010;4:83–92. Available from: PM:20694067.

Morgenthaler NG, Struck J, Jochberger S, Dunser MW. Copeptin: clinical use of a new biomarker. Trends Endocrinol Metab. 2008;19(2):43–9. Available from: PM:18291667.

Oelkers W. Hyponatremia and inappropriate secretion of vasopressin (antidiuretic hormone) in patients with hypopituitarism. N Engl J Med. 1989;321:492–6.

Ohnishi A, Orita Y, Okahara R, Fujihara H, Inoue T, Yamamura Y, Yabuuchi Y, Tanaka T. Potent aquaretic agent. A novel nonpeptide selective vasopressin 2 antagonist (OPC-31260) in men. J Clin Invest. 1993;92(6):2653–9. Available from: PM:8254021.

Oya S, Tsutsumi K, Ueki K, Kirino T. Reinduction of hyponatremia to treat central pontine myelinolysis. Neurology. 2001;57(10):1931–2. Available from: PM:11723299.

Renneboog B, Musch W, Vandemergel X, Manto MU, Decaux G. Mild chronic hyponatremia is associated with falls, unsteadiness, and attention deficits. Am J Med. 2006;119(1):71. Available from: PM:16431193.
Robertson GL. Diabetes insipidus. Endocrinol Metab Clin North Am. 1995;24(3):549–72. Available from: PM:0008575409.
Robertson GL. Regulation of arginine vasopressin in the syndrome of inappropriate antidiuresis. Am J Med. 2006;119(7 Suppl 1):S36–42. Available from: PM:16843083.
Robinson AG. DDAVP in the treatment of central diabetes insipidus. N Engl J Med. 1976;294 (10):507–11. Available from: PM:1250255.
Robinson AG. Disorders of antidiuretic hormone secretion. J Clin Endocrinol Metab. 1985;14:55–88.
Robinson AG, Verbalis JG. Diabetes insipidus. Curr Ther Endocrinol Metab. 1997;6:1–7.
Robinson AG, Verbalis JG. Posterior pituitary. In: Melmed S, et al., editors. Williams textbook of endocrinology. 12th ed. Philadelphia: W.B. Saunders; 2011. p. 291–323.
Sands JM, Bichet DG. Nephrogenic diabetes insipidus. Ann Intern Med. 2006;144(3):186–94. Available from: PM:16461963.
SAMSCA (tolvaptan) Prescribing Information. Otsuka America Pharmaceutical, Inc., Princeton, N.J. 07US14L-0919A, Rev. 02,2014.
Schrier RW, Gross P, Gheorghiade M, Berl T, Verbalis JG, Czerwiec FS, Orlandi C. Tolvaptan, a selective oral vasopressin V2-receptor antagonist, for hyponatremia. N Engl J Med. 2006;355 (20):2099–112. Available from: PM:17105757.
Schwartz WB, Bennett S, Curelop S, Bartter FC. A syndrome of renal sodium loss and hyponatremia probably resulting from inappropriate secretion of antidiuretic hormone. Am J Med. 1957;23:529–42.
Singer I, Rotenberg D. Demeclocycline-induced nephrogenic diabetes insipidus. In-vivo and in-vitro studies. Ann Intern Med. 1973;79(5):679–83. Available from: PM:4356453.
Sofroniew MV, Weindl A, Schrell U, Wetzstein R. Immunohistochemistry of vasopressin, oxytocin and neurophysin in the hypothalamus and extrahypothalamic regions of the human and primate brain. Acta Histochem Suppl. 1981;24:79–95. Available from: PM:6785843.
Soupart A, Penninckx R, Crenier L, Stenuit A, Perier O, Decaux G. Prevention of brain demyelination in rats after excessive correction of chronic hyponatremia by serum sodium lowering. Kidney Int. 1994;45:193–200.
Spasovski G, Vanholder R, Allolio B, Annane D, Ball S, Bichet D, Decaux G, Fenske W, Hoorn EJ, Ichai C, Joannidis M, Soupart A, Zietse R, Haller M, van der Veer S, Van BW, Nagler E. Clinical practice guideline on diagnosis and treatment of hyponatraemia. Nephrol Dial Transplant. 2014;29:i1. Available from: PM:24569496.
Steele A, Gowrishankar M, Abrahamson S, Mazer CD, Feldman RD, Halperin ML. Postoperative hyponatremia despite near-isotonic saline infusion: a phenomenon of desalination [see comments]. Ann Intern Med. 1997;126(1):20–5.
Sterns RH, Riggs JE, Schochet Jr SS. Osmotic demyelination syndrome following correction of hyponatremia. N Engl J Med. 1986;314:1535–42.
Sterns RH, Cappuccio JD, Silver SM, Cohen EP. Neurologic sequelae after treatment of severe hyponatremia: a multicenter perspective. J Am Soc Nephrol. 1994;4:1522–30.
Sterns RH, Nigwekar SU, Hix JK. The treatment of hyponatremia. Semin Nephrol. 2009;29 (3):282–99. Available from: PM:19523575.
Swanson LW, Sawchenko PE. Paraventricular nucleus: a site for the integration of neuroendocrine and autonomic mechanisms. Neuroendocrinology. 1980;31(6):410–7. Available from: PM:6109264.
Thibonnier M, Conarty DM, Preston JA, Wilkins PL, Berti-Mattera LN, Mattera R. Molecular pharmacology of human vasopressin receptors. Adv Exp Med Biol. 1998;449:251–76. Available from: PM:10026814.

Thibonnier M, Coles P, Thibonnier A, Shoham M. The basic and clinical pharmacology of nonpeptide vasopressin receptor antagonists. Annu Rev Pharmacol Toxicol. 2001;41:175–202. Available from: PM:11264455.

Verbalis JG. Hyponatremia and hypo-osmolar disorders. In: Greenberg A, et al., editors. Primer on kidney diseases. 5th ed. Philadelphia: Saunders Elsevier; 2009. p. 52–9.

Verbalis JG. Brain volume regulation in response to changes in osmolality. Neuroscience. 2010;168 (4):862–70. Available from: PM:20417691.

Verbalis JG. Disorders of water balance. In: Taal MW, et al., editors. Brenner & Rector's the kidney. 9th ed. Philadelphia: Elsevier; 2012. p. 540–94.

Verbalis JG. The syndrome of inappropriate antidiuretic hormone secretion and other hypoosmolar disorders. In: Coffmna TM, et al., editors. Schrier's diseases of the kidney. 9th ed. Philadelphia: Lippincott, Williams & Wilkins; 2013. p. 2012–54.

Verbalis JG. Posterior pituitary. In: Goldman L, Ausiello D, editors. Cecil medicine. 25th ed. Philadelphia: Saunders Elsevier; 2016a. p. 1494–9.

Verbalis JG. Disorders of water balance. In: Brenner B, editor. Brenner & Rector's the kidney. 10th ed. Philadelphia: W.B. Saunders Elsevier; 2016b. p. 460–510.

Verbalis JG, Goldsmith SR, Greenberg A, Schrier RW, Sterns RH. Hyponatremia treatment guidelines 2007: expert panel recommendations. Am J Med. 2007;120(11 Suppl 1):S1–21. Available from: PM:17981159.

Zeltser D, Rosansky S, van Rensburg H, Verbalis JG, Smith N. Assessment of the efficacy and safety of intravenous conivaptan in euvolemic and hypervolemic hyponatremia. Am J Nephrol. 2007;27(5):447–57. Available from: PM:17664863.

The Thyroid

13

Trevor E. Angell, Stephen A. Huang, and Erik K. Alexander

Abstract

The thyroid gland is an endocrine organ located in the lower neck that is responsible for the production of thyroid hormone, an iodinated peptide hormone integral to proper physiologic function. The thyroid follicular cell uniquely concentrates iodine and, via the process of organification, incorporates it into thyroid hormone. Thyroid hormone is released from the gland predominantly in the form of thyroxine (T4) and circulates bound to specific plasma proteins that create an available pool of thyroid hormone. Thyroid hormones are metabolism via a system of selenoproteins called iodothyronine deiodinases that can convert thyroxine to more active forms, such as triiodothyronine (T3), or create inactive metabolites. In response to inadequate thyroid hormone, the pituitary gland secretes thyrotropin (TSH) that stimulates thyroid hormone production, which in turn inhibits pituitary TSH release in a classical negative feedback loop. This chapter discusses the synthesis of thyroid hormone and the exquisite mechanisms of regulation and metabolism that govern thyroid status in the body. Particular attention is paid to important physiologic states affecting thyroid status including pregnancy and aging.

Keywords

Thyroid hormone • Metabolism • Transport • Iodine deficiency • Pregnancy • Deiodinase enzymes • Synthesis • Thyroxine • Regulation

T.E. Angell (✉) • E.K. Alexander
The Thyroid Section, Department of Medicine, Brigham and Women's Hospital, Boston, MA, USA

Harvard Medical School, Boston, MA, USA
e-mail: tangell@partners.org; ekalexander@partners.org

S.A. Huang
Thyroid Program of the Division of Endocrinology, Boston Children's Hospital, Boston, MA, USA
e-mail: shuang.2011@gmail.com

A. Belfiore, D. LeRoith (eds.), *Principles of Endocrinology and Hormone Action*, Endocrinology, https://doi.org/10.1007/978-3-319-44675-2_14

Contents

Introduction

The thyroid gland is an endocrine organ in the human body responsible for the production and secretion of thyroid hormone. The two principle thyroid hormones, triiodothyronine (T3) and thyroxine (T4), circulate throughout the body and stimulate receptors found in most cells and organs. Through this process, thyroid hormones play a principle role in controlling cellular metabolism and energy expenditure. The presence of a thyroid gland in all vertebrates confirms its evolutionary importance. Without thyroid hormone, illness will ensue and eventually lead to death.

During embryogenesis, the thyroid develops from a diverticulum of the pharynx and is attached by the thyroglossal duct. The primitive thyroid descends into the lower neck in conjunction with the process of cardiac formation. As this migration occurs, the thyroglossal duct elongates and eventually degenerates. Once fully formed, the thyroid gland is the largest endocrine organ in the human body and weighs approximately 20 g. It is anatomically composed of three sections, a left and right lobe and a connecting isthmus. In some patients, a pyramidal lobe is also identified.

Histologically, the thyroid is composed of follicles of varying size that consist of an outer layer of follicular cells. Inside the follicle, thyroid hormone is stored in a matrix of colloid containing thyroglobulin and other proteins. The follicular cells regulate the production, storage, and secretion of the thyroid hormones, largely in response to serum thyrotropin (TSH) (Collins and Capend 1980). The major substrate for thyroid hormone production is iodine, a necessary nutritional supplement in all human beings. C cells are also found in the thyroid gland, though they do not play a role in thyroid hormone physiology. Rather, C cells regulate the production of a different hormone called calcitonin, relevant to calcium homeostasis.

On physical examination, the thyroid is located in the anterior, lower neck. Anatomically important landmarks include the thyroid cartilage and cricoid cartilage, which are often referred to as the “Adam’s apple” and are readily identifiable in most patients. The thyroid gland is a soft tissue organ that lies just inferior to these cartilaginous structures. With swallowing, the thyroid moves upward, or cephalad. This important maneuver is critical for accurate examination and assessment of the gland. Typically, the thyroid gland is soft, mobile with swallowing, and non-tender to palpation. As patients age, the thyroid examination can become more difficult as the gland frequently descends and is partially substernal. In these scenarios, swallowing will nonetheless allow effective examination of the thyroid in most patients. Thyroid agenesis or dysgenesis occurs in approximately 1 in 3,500 live births (Klett 1997). Newborn screening is now universally performed in nearly all developed countries, as early identification of this process allows for effective treatment and amelioration of harm.

Synthesis of Thyroid Hormone

Iodine is an essential nutrient and necessary for human survival. Iodine is the primary substrate for thyroid hormone formation. Without dietary iodine intake, thyroid hormone cannot be produced. Therefore, adequate intake of this element is critical for health, and the human body has evolved complex means of optimizing its metabolism. Iodine is actively stored in the thyroid gland, where it reaches a concentration that is 20–40 times more than in the plasma (Carrasco 1993). In the follicle, iodine is then made available for the production of both T3 and T4.

Iodine accumulation is an active process that occurs against a concentration gradient. The protein responsible for this process is the sodium-iodine symporter (NIS) (Vilijn and Carrasco 1989). NIS actively transports iodine across the basolateral membrane and into the cytoplasm of the follicular cell. A separate transporter then moves iodide across the apical membrane and into the colloid pool. Regulation of NIS function is primarily through TSH stimulation, though iodide transport and accumulation is also regulated by the concentration of iodide itself. High doses of iodide inhibit the accumulation of further iodine and thus formation of thyroid hormone. This process is known as the Wolff-Chaikoff effect. Interestingly, after a period of days to weeks, an escape from this physiologic effect is frequently observed, during which iodide organification is restored and hormone production once again occurs. Separate from the thyroid gland, the only other tissues in the human body that actively accumulate iodide are the salivary glands, gastric mucosa, and the lactating mammary gland. The latter is felt to be an evolutionary adaptation that allows optimal iodide delivery to the breastfeeding infant during a critical period of neurologic development.

Thyroid hormone synthesis, storage, and secretion are highly regulated steps (Kopp 2005). Once iodide is transported into the follicle, it is oxidized by thyroid peroxidase (TPO). In the follicular lumen, a protein called thyroglobulin serves as a matrix upon which T4 and T3 are built. The TPO enzyme catalyzes the iodination of tyrosyl residues in thyroglobulin. This is referred to as iodination, or organification. The process produces mono-iodinated or di-iodinated tyrosines (MIT and DIT, respectively). Thereafter, MIT and DIT are coupled to produce T4 or T3. Upon stimulation, T4 and T3 are released into the blood stream, where they circulate and exert their effects. The majority of secreted thyroid hormone is T4 (80%), while the remaining minority is T3 (20%). Though T3 is the active form of thyroid hormone, most tissues in the body convert T4 to T3 via a process of deiodination. Thyroglobulin serves as the primary internal reservoir for iodine and its recycling in the human body.

In serum, thyroid hormone is hydrophobic and therefore must be associated with proteins for transport and delivery to tissues and organs throughout the human body (Benvenga et al. 2002). There are three proteins which transport thyroid hormone – thyroxine-binding globulin (TBG), transthyretin, and albumin. Of these, TBG is the major carrier of thyroid hormone. Importantly, the free fraction of T4 in human plasma is only 0.03%, while that of T3 is 0.3%. Thus, the majority of circulating thyroid hormone is inactive, existing in equilibrium between bound and free states, and available for release when needed.

In humans, about 80% of the T3 that is produced each day is created by peripheral deiodination of circulating T4 outside of the thyroid gland itself. This process is catalyzed primarily by the action of type 2 deiodinase. When thyroid hormone enters the cells, it is transported into the nucleus, where it binds to nuclear thyroid hormone receptors. This complex then interacts via a highly complex series of events with thyroid hormone response elements, as well as repressors and corepressors, to activate target genes and transcriptionally regulate thyroid hormone action (Brent 2012).

Metabolism of Thyroid Hormone

While both T4 and T3 can regulate thyroid hormone-responsive genes, T3 binds thyroid hormone nuclear receptors with 12-fold greater affinity and is thus the more active, or potent, thyroid hormone. As mentioned above, most thyroid hormone secreted from the gland is T4 and its conversion to T3 in peripheral tissues provides the vast majority of T3 found in the circulation. For these reasons, T4 can be considered a prohormone that is metabolized into the active T3 ligand.

In humans (and all vertebrates), the major pathway of thyroid hormone metabolism is sequential monodeiodination (removal of an iodine atom), catalyzed by a family of enzymes called the iodothyronine deiodinases (Fig. 1) (Gereben et al. 2008). The removal of an outer (phenolic) ring iodine from T4 activates it into the more biologically potent T3. Conversely, inner (tyrosyl) ring deiodination leads to substrate inactivation, converting T4 and T3 into rT3 and T2, respectively. The deiodinase enzyme family has three members: type 1, type 2, and type 3 deiodinase. Each deiodinase is encoded by a distinct gene and each has a unique pattern of tissue expression and kinetic properties. Type 1 deiodinase (D1) is highly expressed in the liver and kidneys. While it has some weak inner-ring deiodinase activity, its major function in postnatal physiology is as an activator of T4. The susceptibility of D1 to inhibition by propylthiouracil can be exploited in the treatment of hyperthyroidism to reduce D1-mediated T4 to T3 conversion, and this is the rationale for using high-dose propylthiouracil in rare patients with thyroid storm. Type 2 deiodinase (D2) is widely expressed in skeletal muscle tissue. D2 is the primary activator of T4 and the major source of T3 generation in euthyroid patients. In addition, its focal expression

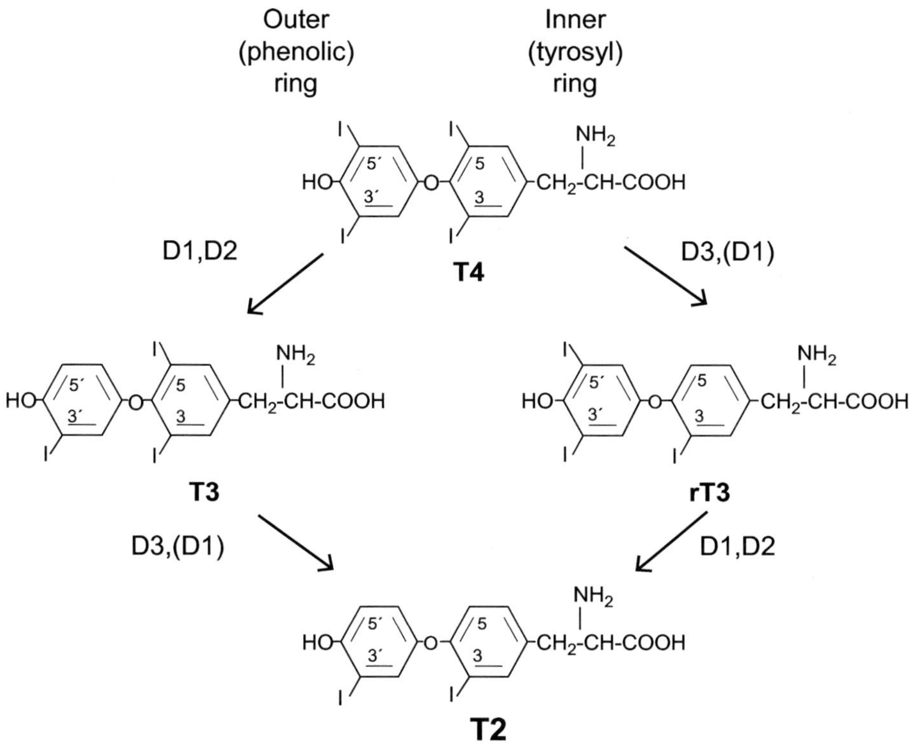

Fig. 1 Metabolism of thyroid hormone by the deiodinase enzyme system. Thyroxine (*T4*) is activated into 3,5,3′-triiodothyronine (*T3*) by phenolic or "outer"-ring deiodination, catalyzed by type 1 (*D1*) and type 2 (*D2*) deiodinase. T4 and T3 are inactivated by tyrosyl or "inner"-ring deiodination, that is, primarily catalyzed type 3 deiodinase (*D3*). rT3 = 3,3′,5′-triiodothyronine. T2 = 3,3′-diiodothyronine

in tissues like the pituitary gland and the brown fat allows the fine control of T3 signaling in processes such as hypothalamic-pituitary-thyroid feedback and adaptive thermogenesis. The expression of type 3 deiodinase (D3) is high in the uteroplacental unit and in embryonic tissues and then falls to lower levels upon birth. D3 is a pure inactivator of thyroid hormones that regulates the transfer of maternal thyroid hormone to the fetus during pregnancy and catalyzes the clearance of circulating thyroid hormone in adults.

Collectively, the dynamic expression of deiodinase enzymes is a potent homeostatic mechanism that works to maintain normal tissue T3 concentrations in the setting of primary thyroid disease. In patients with mild hypothyroidism or iodine deficiency, the upregulation of D2 can maintain serum T3 concentrations in the normal range, even after hyperthyrotropinemia and hypothyroxinemia have developed. Even in patients with complete hypothyroidism, the outer-ring deiodination of levothyroxine (T4) catalyzed by D1 and D2 preserves normal serum T3 concentrations and allows standard monotherapy to be effective (Jonklaas et al. 2014). In thyrotoxic patients, it is D3 that is upregulated and protects the host by accelerating the clearance of circulating thyroid hormones and by reducing local T3 concentrations in sensitive D3-expressing tissues within the central nervous system.

Interestingly, while the major role of deiodination is T3 homeostasis, it is now appreciated that primary changes in deiodination can drive alterations in systemic or local thyroid status. During systemic illness, the downregulation of hepatic D1 and the induction of D3 in injured tissues both contribute to the low T3 syndrome (also called the nonthyroidal illness syndrome) that is commonly observed in hospitalized patients (Boelen et al. 2011). In rare individuals with large deiodinase-expressing tumors, ectopic deiodinase activity can cause either systemic hypothyroidism (as observed in D3-expressing infantile hemangiomas or gastrointestinal stromal tumors) (Maynard et al. 2014) or T3 hyperconversion (as observed in certain D2-expressing follicular carcinomas) (Kim et al. 2003).

In addition to deiodination, the action of secreted thyroid hormone is also regulated by alternative metabolic pathways (thyroid hormone conjugation) (Wu et al. 2005), by thyroid hormone transporters (Visser et al. 2011, 2013; Fu and Dumitrescu 2014), and by nuclear receptors (Visser et al. 2013). The conjugation of thyroid hormone's phenolic hydroxyl group by sulfotransferases or glucuronidases increases inactivation by promoting inner-ring deiodination or biliary excretion, respectively (Gereben et al. 2008). The cellular uptake and efflux of thyroid hormone are highly regulated by tissue-specific transporter proteins, including monocarboxylate transporters (MCT) and organic anion transporter polypeptides (OATP) (Bernal et al. 2015). Intracellular T3 signaling is dependent upon nuclear receptors that are encoded by two distinct genes, *THRA* and *THRB* (Brent 2012), that each expresses tissue-specific T3-binding products. These regulatory pathways have long been studied in cell biology and animal models. In addition, their relevance to human health has been directly demonstrated through the recent discovery of individuals with germline loss-of-function mutations in genes encoding thyroid transporters (*SLC16A2*) or receptors (*THRB* or *THRA*) (Refetoff et al. 2014). Illustrating the ability of these pathways to impact local thyroid hormone status, affected patients manifest pathology including tissue-specific thyroid hormone resistance (including growth failure and abnormal neurodevelopment) despite normal or even elevated serum thyroid hormone concentrations.

Regulation of Thyroid Status

Thyroid status is determined by many factors that combine to govern thyroid hormone availability. Of these, the function and regulation of the hypothalamic-pituitary-thyroid (HPT) axis is the most significant. The thyroid gland also demonstrates important mechanisms of autoregulation with respect of iodine status, which will be discussed below. The HPT axis constitutes a classical negative feedback loop. The main regulator of thyroid function is TSH, which is a glycoprotein consisting of one alpha and one beta subunit released by cells of the anterior pituitary called thyrotrophs. TSH secretion exhibits both pulsatility and diurnal variation, which are affected by physiologic and disease states such as sleep deprivation, depression, and hypothyroidism. Neurons of the hypothalamus produce and release thyrotropin-releasing hormone (TRH), which influences the pattern of TSH secretion. After secretion of TSH by the pituitary thyrotroph, TSH enters the peripheral circulation and, upon reaching the thyroid gland, binds TSH receptors present on the basolateral surface of thyroid follicular cells.

Activation of the TSH receptor initiates complex intercellular signaling involving phospholipase C and cyclic AMP pathways that all serve to augment thyroid function. Under TSH stimulation, there are increased synthesis and activity of NIS, TPO, and Tg and increased cellular trafficking of hormone products, leading to greater iodine uptake, organification, and, ultimately, thyroid hormone secretion. Circulating thyroid hormone in the form of T4 crosses the blood-brain barrier with the assistance of thyroid hormone transport proteins such as MCT. Thyroxine is then converted to biologically active T3 by cells within the central nervous system and acts upon the hypothalamus and pituitary resulting in reductions in TRH and TSH, thus completing the negative feedback loop of the HPT axis (Costa-e-Sousa 2012).

TSH changes approximately tenfold for each unit change in thyroxine (Spencer et al. 1990). This "log-linear" relationship illustrates the exquisite sensitivity of pituitary TSH secretion to changes in peripherally circulating thyroid hormone concentrations. Through this mechanism normal thyroid status is maintained within a narrow physiologic range. Because of this relationship, diseases of thyroid hormone deficiency or excess can be detected through the measurement of abnormal levels of serum TSH even when measured levels of thyroid hormones remain within the reference range. Mild thyroid dysfunction of this kind is referred to a "subclinical" thyroid disease, and while frequently asymptomatic may have adverse effects, particularly on the cardiovascular system.

Since only a slight fraction of T4 and T3 is unbound, or free, in the peripheral circulation, the relative presence of the major thyroid hormone carrier proteins – TBG, transthyretin, and albumin – is an important factor that regulates thyroid status. These carrier proteins function to provide a thyroid hormone reservoir, limit renal losses, and buffer changes in thyroid hormone levels. Conditions altering the plasma binding of thyroid hormones to these carrier proteins may lead to benign abnormalities of circulating thyroid hormone levels or be the source of deleterious changes to thyroid status. The major carrier of thyroid hormone is TBG, a 54 kDa glycoprotein located on the X chromosome (Schussler 2000). TBG undergoes conformational change leading to high- and low-affinity states that modulated the ability to delivery T4 to target tissues (Zhou et al. 2006), and binding of T4 to TBG may be inhibited by some medications including phenytoin and salicylate. Increased levels of serum TBG during normal pregnancy in part account for greater thyroid hormone demand and the clinical need to supplement thyroid hormone in some woman during gestation. Binding-protein conditions leading to altered but benign thyroid hormone levels that do not impact physiologic thyroid status include congenital TBG deficiency, present in ~1/5,000 male newborns, and familial dysalbuminemic hyperthyroxinemia (Ruiz et al. 1982) and should be considered in the clinical evaluation of abnormal thyroid hormone testing.

The regulation of thyroid status is further modulated by inputs from the nervous system, other hormones, and mediators of inflammation, each conveying signals related to nutrition, stress, and overall health of the organism. Increased TSH secretion is exhibited after exposure to cold temperature and in response to increased leptin levels, which are present in the well-fed state. TSH and peripheral thyroid hormone levels are reduced with fasting. TSH secretion is also reduced by mediators of stress or illness, such as during severe infections or inflammation (Chan 2003). Cytokines, IL-1β, TNFα, IL-6, and others, inhibit TSH secretion by the pituitary, as do elevated cortisol levels (Spath-Schwalbe 1996; Blake et al. 1991). In these circumstances, thyroid status may reflect a physiologic response to significant stress or illness that may not be indicative of intrinsic thyroid disease.

The Effects of Iodine on Thyroid Status

Thyroid status is also influenced by the relative presence of inorganic iodine, and the response to iodine deficiency occurs at all levels of the HPT axis in order to maintain the availability of intracellular T3, preserving thyroid hormone action throughout the body. Lower iodine availability itself results in relatively greater production of T3 rather than T4 since the former requires one fewer iodine. As discussed above, detection by the pituitary thyrotrophs of reduced T4 levels results in augmented TSH secretion and subsequent stimulation of thyroidal function that increases iodine uptake and thyroid hormone production. Thyroid enlargement, or goiter, may occur as a result of increased cell division induced by TSH-mediated stimulation. Similar changes to those of iodine deficiency may been seen in conditions during which the thyroid is unable to utilize iodine, such as in Hashimoto's disease or patients with Graves' disease taking thiourea drugs (methimazole or propylthiouracil) that block the activity of the TPO enzyme (Larsen 1975). Additionally, as mentioned above, upregulation of the type 2 deiodinase enzyme in patients with iodine deficiency contributes to the maintenance of normal serum T3 concentrations. These effects result in clinical euthyroidism except when iodine deficiency becomes severe, at which point clinical manifestations of hypothyroidism may emerge. Iodine deficiency remains the leading cause of hypothyroidism worldwide.

The negative effects of iodine deficiency may occur through human life. Miscarriage, congenital anomalies, perinatal and infant mortality, and impaired mental and physical development are all manifestations of iodine deficiency in early life. When iodine deficiency is severe during pregnancy, offspring may suffer from cretinism, a syndrome of severe neuromotor, mental, and physical deficiencies preventable with supplementation of iodine. In adults, iodine deficiency is associated with attenuated mental function, hypothyroidism, goiter, thyroid nodules, autonomously functioning or "toxic" nodular goiters, and a higher incidence of more aggressive forms of thyroid cancer (follicular and anaplastic thyroid carcinomas).

Iodine excess also may adversely affect thyroid status. High doses of iodide inhibit the accumulation of further iodine and the formation of thyroid hormone by direct action on the thyroid gland. This process, known as the Wolff-Chaikoff effect, is a normal physiologic response to iodine excess likely buffering the influence of an iodine load. While not definitively proven, inhibition of thyroid hormone biosynthesis may be mediated by the accumulation of iodinated compounds within the thyroid follicular cell. Resumption of normal organification after approximately 2 days of iodine exposure, so-called escape from the Wolff-Chaikoff effect, is considered to result from reduction in NIS and decreased iodine transport that normalizes intracellular iodine levels and removal of inhibition to thyroid hormone production (Burrow et al. 1994). Failure to escape from the Wolff-Chaikoff effect is observed in patients with underlying thyroid disease, such as chronic lymphocytic thyroiditis (Hashimoto's thyroiditis), in which prolonged hypothyroidism may develop.

The induction or exacerbation of hyperthyroidism due to exposure to iodine excess may also occur and is referred to as the Jod-Basedow phenomenon. Susceptible patients include those with Graves' disease, iodine deficiency, or multinodular goiters harboring autonomously functioning thyroid tissue. Animal studies have demonstrated the development of autoimmune thyroid disease after excess iodine intake in a number of species. This suggestion is supported by the higher prevalence of subclinical hypothyroidism, overt hypothyroidism, and autoimmune thyroid disease in human populations with high iodine intake compared to those with low or normal iodine status.

Age-Related Influence on Thyroid Function

Normal pregnancy is characterized by high maternal-to-fetal gradients of T4 and T3 that are maintained by the expression of type 3 deiodinase and other inactivating enzymes in both the uteroplacental unit and embryonic tissues. Collectively, these enzymes function as a biochemical shield that limits the transfer of maternal thyroid hormone to fetal tissues and permits the local regulation of thyroid hormone signaling by cell-specific activating enzymes and T3 transporters (Dugrillon 1996).

Upon birth, fetal tissues rapidly shift from a profile of thyroid hormone inactivation to one of thyroid hormone activation. Within hours of delivery, the expression of thyroid hormone-inactivating enzymes falls and thyroid hormone activation increases (Bianco et al. 2002). In addition, a robust burst of central stimulation referred to as the neonatal surge increases glandular secretion. This surge is characterized by a rise in serum TSH up to 80 μU/ml, followed by transient elevations in serum T4 and T3 (Fisher and Odell 1969). In full-term infants, the transition to mature thyroid physiology is rapid, and serum thyroid hormone concentrations approximate adult levels by 1 month of age. Premature infants can demonstrate a blunted version of these changes, characterized by a smaller TSH surge and a prolonged depression of serum T4 referred to as the "hypothyroxinemia of prematurity" (Delahunty et al. 2010).

The aging process is accompanied by apparent changes in thyroid function. While most studies have shown no or minimal change in free thyroxine levels with age, circulating free T3 levels decrease, though remain within the reference range with advancing age. TSH concentration has been reported to change with age. Particular interest exists regarding the relationship between aging and elevated TSH concentrations and whether this reflects a physiologic aspect of aging or the existence of thyroid hormone deficiency. Symptoms of hypothyroidism may be difficult to distinguish from physical changes present during normal aging, making the appropriate interpretation of serum TSH measurement an important issue in the care of geriatric patients.

In a population free of any discernible thyroid disease analyzed from the third National Health and Nutrition Examination Survey (NHANES III), 15% of individuals greater than 70 years old had a TSH level above the upper limit of the calculated reference range (Hollowell et al. 2002). One explanation of this finding is that mild, but nevertheless true, thyroid disease is present in these individuals. It has been noted that TSH distribution curves of supposedly healthy individuals contain a rightward skew toward higher TSH concentration that has been attributed to possible unrecognized thyroid disease in the reference population (Baloch et al. 2003). Further assessment of NHANES databases has generated age-specific TSH reference ranges that show a shift toward higher TSH values most apparent in patients over 80 years old compared to those 20–29 years old. Most striking is that when stratified by age, these reference curves lack the right skew in TSH values often reported (Surks and Hollowell 2007). Thus, there exists an age-related rise in TSH that is present in apparently healthy individuals, and this higher TSH concentration in people older than 85 years has been shown by some to predict longevity without associated functional impairment (Gussekloo et al. 2004). The mechanism underlying the observed change in TSH with age remains unclear. Decrease in the biological activity of TSH, changes in diurnal pattern or pulsatility, and polymorphisms in the TSH receptor have all been postulated, but data scrutinizing these hypotheses in population studies are lacking.

Thyroid Physiology in Pregnancy

Pregnancy is a unique physiologic process, during which thyroid hormone production and metabolism are substantially modified from the nonpregnant state. Thyroid hormone is critical for human development, substantially impacting fetal growth, infant development, and neurocognitive ability. While both too much and too little thyroid hormone can impact pregnancy as well as the developing fetus, maternal hypothyroidism may be harmful even when mild to moderate in severity. A classic example of the detrimental effects imparted by maternal hypothyroidism is endemic cretinism. Now thankfully rare, cretinism is the consequence of severe iodine insufficiency during pregnancy and newborn development. Affected offspring suffer profound neurocognitive and developmental impairments, with extremely impaired cognitive ability.

During human pregnancy, the maternal-fetal unit must produce approximately 40% more thyroid hormone to adequately meet the needs of both the mother and developing fetus (Alexander et al. 2004). In a healthy mother, this increase in hormone demand occurs seamlessly through the stimulatory effects of both TSH and pregnancy-derived human chorionic gonadotropin (hCG). As hCG shares homology with serum TSH, both peptides stimulate the gland to produce thyroid hormone, increasing the available pool throughout the body. This process of increasing production is unique to gestation and reverts to prepregnancy status after delivery. Studies of human physiology have demonstrated that the increase in thyroid hormone production begins very early in gestation (~4 to 6 weeks) and then rises linearly through mid-gestation (16–20 weeks). The increase in thyroid hormone demand then plateaus but is sustained for the remainder of pregnancy.

Several studies have documented the harmful effects of maternal hypothyroidism, especially when severe (Haddow et al. 1999; Negro et al. 2010). Such adverse effects include increased risk of miscarriage, as well as direct harmful effects on the cognitive status of the developing fetus. Interestingly, these effects appear to be augmented by the presence of the thyroid peroxidase antibody (TPO Ab) in the maternal circulation. For example, one study demonstrated an increased risk of miscarriage in TPO Ab-negative women when maternal TSH concentrations were elevated greater than 5 mIU/L, but demonstrated similar effects in TPO Ab-positive women when maternal TSH concentrations were elevated greater than 2.5 mIU/L (Liu et al. 2014). The reason for this additional detrimental effect when TPO Ab is elevated is unknown.

Women at highest risk for the harmful effects of hypothyroidism during pregnancy are those suffering from primary thyroid dysfunction. Such women must take exogenous levothyroxine, often because of prior thyroid surgery or radioactive iodine ablation. Other women suffer from autoimmune destruction of the thyroid (Hashimoto's disease) and can produce only a partial amount of endogenous thyroid hormone. All such women do not have the ability to augment further production necessary during pregnancy. In these women, thyroid hormone tests must be performed early in gestation, once pregnancy is confirmed. Thereafter, levothyroxine supplementation should be increased to prevent maternal hypothyroidism during gestation.

Summary

In summary, the above text describes a highly complex, tightly regulated, and evolutionarily preserved system that is necessary for optimal human health. The critical importance of optimal dietary iodine should be stressed. The production, secretion, and action of the thyroid hormones (T4 and T3) provide a means by which the body regulates overall metabolism and cellular function. It is not surprising, therefore, that thyroid physiology demonstrates properties of rapid responsiveness, active storing of necessary substrates (iodine), as well as mechanisms for tight control (the Wolff-Chiakoff effect). Together, this physiologic system has evolved to optimize human health and development. More recent understanding of thyroid physiology during pregnancy further delineates the importance of this endocrine organ and its hormonal effects.

Cross-References

- ▶ Growth Hormones and Aging
- ▶ Molecular Mechanisms of Thyroid Hormone Synthesis and Secretion
- ▶ Steroid Hormones: Synthesis, Secretion, and Transport
- ▶ The Hypothalamus–Pituitary Axis

References

Alexander EK, Marqusee E, Lawrence J, Jarolim P, Fischer GA, Larsen PR. Timing and magnitude of increases in Levothyroxine requirements during pregnancy in women with hypothyroidism. N Eng J Med. 2004;351(3):25–33.

Baloch Z, Carayon P, Conte-Devolx B, Demers LM, Feldt-Rasmussen U, Henry JF, LiVosli VA, Niccoli-Sire P, John R, Ruf J, Smyth PP, Spencer CA, Stockigt JR. Laboratory medicine practice guidelines. Laboratory support for the diagnosis and monitoring of thyroid disease. Thyroid. 2003;13:3–126.

Benvenga S, Lapa D, Trimarchi F. Thyroxine binding to members and nonmembers of the serine protease inhibitor family. J Endocrinol Invest. 2002;25:32–8.

Bernal J, Guadaño-Ferraz A, Morte B. Thyroid hormone transporters-functions and clinical implications. Nat Rev Endocrinol. 2015;11:406–17.

Bianco AC, Salvatore D, Gereben B, Berry MJ, Larsen PR. Biochemistry, cellular and molecular biology, and physiological roles of the iodothyronine selenodeiodinases. Endocr Rev. 2002;23:38–89.

Blake NG, Eckland DJ, Foster OJ, Lightman SL. Inhibition of hypothalamic thyrotropin-releasing hormone messenger ribonucleic acid during food deprivation. Endocrinology. 1991;129:2714–8.

Boelen A, Kwakkel J, Fliers E. Beyond low plasma T3: local thyroid hormone metabolism during inflammation and infection. Endocr Rev. 2011;32:670–93.

Brent GA. Mechanisms of thyroid hormone action. J Clin Invest. 2012;122:3035–43.

Burrow GN, Fisher DA, Larsen PR. Maternal and fetal thyroid function. N Engl J Med. 1994;331:1072–8.

Carrasco N. Iodide transport in the thyroid gland. Biochim Biophys Acta. 1993;1154:65–82.

Chan JL, Heist K, DePaoli AM, Veldhuis JD, Mantzoros CS. The role of falling leptin levels in the neuroendocrine and metabolic adaptation to short-term starvation in healthy men. J Clin Invest. 2003;111:1409–21.

Collins WT, Capend CC. Ultrastructural and functional alterations of the rat thyroid gland produced by polychlorinated biphenyls compared with iodide excess and deficiency, and thyrotropin and thyroxine administration. Virchows Arch. 1980;33:213.

Costa-e-Sousa RH, Hollenberg AN. Minireview: The neural regulation of the hypothalamic-pituitary-thyroid axis. Endocrinology. 2012;153:4128–35.

Delahunty C, Falconer S, Hume R, Jackson L, Midgley P, Mirfield M, Ogston S, Perra O, Simpson J, Watson J, Willatts P, Williams F, SPT Group. Levels of neonatal thyroid hormone in preterm infants and neurodevelopmental outcome at 5 1/2 years: millennium cohort study. J Clin Endocrinol Metab. 2010;95:4898–908.

Dugrillon A. Iodolactones and iodoaldehydes – mediators of iodine in thyroid autoregulation. Exp Clin Endocrinol Diabetes. 1996;104 Suppl 4:41–5.

Fisher DA, Odell WD. Acute release of thyrotropin in the newborn. J Clin Invest. 1969;48:1670–7.

Fu J, Dumitrescu AM. Inherited defects in thyroid hormone cell-membrane transport and metabolism. Best Pract Res Clin Endocrinol Metab. 2014;28:189–201.

Gereben B, Zavacki AM, Ribich S, Kim BW, Huang SA, Simonides WS, Zeöld A, Bianco AC. Cellular and molecular basis of deiodinase-regulated thyroid hormone signaling. Endocr Rev. 2008;29:898–938.

Gussekloo J, van Exel E, de Craen AJ, Meinders AE, Frölich M, Westendorp RG. Thyroid status, disability and cognitive function, and survival in old age. JAMA. 2004;292(21):2591–9.

Haddow JE, Palomaki GE, Allan WC, Williams JR, Knight GJ, Gagnon J, O'Heir CE, Mitchell ML, Hermos RJ, Waisbren SE, Faix JD, Klein RZ. Maternal thyroid deficiency during pregnancy and subsequent neuropsychological development of the child. N Engl J Med. 1999;341:549–55.

Hollowell JG, Staehling NW, Flanders WD, Hannon WH, Gunter EW, Spencer CA, Braverman LE. Serum TSH, T(4), and thyroid antibodies in the United States population (1988 to 1994): National Health and Nutrition Examination Survey (NHANES III). J Clin Endocrinol Metab. 2002;87:489–99.

Jonklaas J, Bianco AC, Bauer AJ, Burman KD, Cappola AR, Celi FS, Cooper DS, Kim BW, Peeters RP, Rosenthal MS, Sawka AM. Guidelines for the treatment of hypothyroidism: prepared by the american thyroid association task force on thyroid hormone replacement. Thyroid. 2014;24:1670–751.

Kim BW, Daniels GH, Harrison BJ, Price A, Harney JW, Larsen PR, Weetman AP. Overexpression of type 2 iodothyronine deiodinase in follicular carcinoma as a cause of low circulating free thyroxine levels. J Clin Endocrinol Metab. 2003;88:594–8.

Klett M. Epidemiology of congenital hypothyroidism. Exp Clin Endocrinol Diabetes. 1997;105 Suppl 4:19–23.

Kopp P. Thyroid hormone synthesis. In: Braverman L, Utiger R, editors. Werner and Ingbar's the thyroid: a fundamental and clinical text. 9th ed. Philadelphia: Lippincott, Williams & Wilkens; 2005. p. 52.

Larsen PR. Thyroidal triiodothyronine and thyroxine in Graves' disease: correlation with pre-surgical treatment, thyroid status, and iodine content. J Clin Endocrinol Metab. 1975;41:1098–104.

Liu H, Shan Z, Li C, Mao J, Xie X, Wang W, Fan C, Wang H, Zhang H, Han C, Wang X, Liu X, Fan Y, Bao S, Teng W. Maternal subclinical hypothyroidism, thyroid autoimmunity, and the risk of miscarriage: a prospective cohort study. Thyroid. 2014;24:1642–9.

Maynard MA, Marino-Enriquez A, Fletcher JA, Dorfman DM, Raut CP, Yassa L, Guo C, Wang Y, Dorfman C, Feldman HA, Frates MC, Song H, Jugo RH, Taguchi T, Hershman JM, Larsen PR, Huang SA. Thyroid hormone inactivation in gastrointestinal stromal tumors. N Engl J Med. 2014;370:1327–34.

Negro R, Schwartz A, Gismondi R, Tinelli A, Mangieri T, Stagnaro-Green A. Universal screening versus case finding for detection and treatment of thyroid hormonal dysfunction during pregnancy. J Clin Endocrinol Metab. 2010;95:1699–707.

Refetoff S, Bassett JH, Beck-Peccoz P, Bernal J, Brent G, Chatterjee K, De Groot LJ, Dumitrescu AM, Jameson JL, Kopp PA, Murata Y, Persani L, Samarut J, Weiss RE, Williams GR, Yen PM. Classification and proposed nomenclature for inherited defects of thyroid hormone action, cell transport, and metabolism. J Clin Endocrinol Metab. 2014;99:768–70.

Ruiz M, Rajatanavin R, Young RA, Taylor C, Brown R, Braverman LE, Ingbar SH. Familial dysalbuminemic hyperthyroxinemia: a syndrome that can be confused with thyrotoxicosis. N Engl J Med. 1982;306:635–9.

Schussler GC. The thyroxine-binding proteins. Thyroid. 2000;10:141–9.

Späth-Schwalbe E, Schrezenmeier H, Bornstein S, Burger K, Porzsolt F, Born J. Endocrine effects of recombinant interleukin 6 in man. Neuroendocrinology. 1996;63:237–43.

Spencer CA, LoPresti JS, Patel A, Guttler RB, Eigen A, Shen D, Gray D, Nicoloff JT. Applications of a new chemiluminometric thyrotropin assay to subnormal measurement. J Clin Endocrinol Metab. 1990;70:453–60.

Surks MI, Hollowell JG. Age-specific distribution of serum thyrotropin and antithyroid antibodies in the US population: implications for the prevalence of subclinical hypothyroidism. J Clin Endocrinol Metab. 2007;92:4575–82.

Vilijn F, Carrasco N. Expression of the thyroid sodium/iodide symporter in Xenopus laevis oocytes. J Biol Chem. 1989;264:11901–3.

Visser WE, Friesema EC, Visser TJ. Minireview: thyroid hormone transporters: the knowns and the unknowns. Mol Endocrinol. 2011;25:1–14.

Visser WE, van Mullem AA, Visser TJ, Peeters RP. Different causes of reduced sensitivity to thyroid hormone: diagnosis and clinical management. Clin Endocrinol (Oxf). 2013;79:595–605.

Wu SY, Green WL, Huang WS, Hays MT, Chopra IJ. Alternate pathways of thyroid hormone metabolism. Thyroid. 2005;15:943–58.

Zhou A, Wei Z, Read RJ, Carrell RW. Structural mechanism for the carriage and release of thyroxine in the blood. Proc Natl Acad Sci U S A. 2006;103:13321–6.

The Parathyroids

14

Christopher S. Kovacs

Abstract

The parathyroids respond to low serum ionized calcium or increased serum phosphorus by releasing parathyroid hormone (PTH); additional parathyroid products include chromogranins and possibly PTH-related protein (PTHrP). In turn PTH has actions in three target organs (the bone, kidney, intestines) to raise serum calcium and lower phosphorus. PTH is also an important regulator of bone turnover, having a biphasic action to either stimulate osteoblast activity and bone formation or osteoclast activity and bone resorption. PTH interacts with other calciotropic and phosphotropic hormones, including that it stimulates production of calcitriol and fibroblast growth factor-23 (FGF23) and is itself inhibited by both hormones. This chapter reviews the embryology, anatomy, and physiology of the parathyroid glands and PTH and the functions that PTH has to regulate mineral ion concentrations and skeletal mass and strength.

Keywords

Parathyroid hormone • Ionized calcium • Calcium • Phosphorus • Inorganic phosphorus • Magnesium • Parathyroid hormone-related protein • Calcitriol • Fibroblast growth factor-23 • Adult • Fetus • Neonate • Familial hypocalciuric hypercalcemia • Autosomal dominant hypocalcemia • Hyperparathyroidism • Hypoparathyroidism • Pseudohypoparathyroidism • Pseudohyperparathyroidism • Parathyromatosis

C.S. Kovacs (✉)
Faculty of Medicine – Endocrinology, Memorial University of Newfoundland, Health Sciences Centre, St. John's, Newfoundland, Canada
e-mail: ckovacs@mun.ca

A. Belfiore, D. LeRoith (eds.), *Principles of Endocrinology and Hormone Action*, Endocrinology, https://doi.org/10.1007/978-3-319-44675-2_15

Contents

Extracellular Calcium Homeostasis

Extracellular calcium is required for innumerable cellular processes, ranging from neurotransmission to hormone release to blood coagulation to muscle contraction. Calcium circulates in several forms, including free or ionized (~50% of total), bound to albumin and other proteins (~40% of total), and complexed to citrate or phosphate (~10% of total). Assay of serum calcium, also called total serum calcium, determines the combined concentration of all three forms without distinguishing their relative contributions. The ionized fraction of calcium in the bloodstream is tightly regulated between 1.10 and 1.30 mmol/L, which is about 10,000 times higher than the concentration of calcium in the intracellular fluid. The protein-bound and complexed fractions are maintained by other processes independent of physiological need for calcium. Alterations in ionized calcium above (hypercalcemia) or below (hypocalcemia) the normal physiological range can lead to significant dysfunction of cells and tissues, specific symptoms and signs, and even acute mortality. In general a reduction in ionized calcium is much less well tolerated than comparable elevations in ionized calcium. Increases or decreases in the bound or complexed fractions of serum calcium are physiologically unimportant unless they also lead to alterations in the ionized calcium. Consequently, the ionized calcium, albumin-corrected serum calcium, and protein-adjusted serum calcium are preferred over the unadjusted serum calcium as indicators of normal or abnormal concentrations of extracellular calcium.

The intracellular calcium concentration is also tightly regulated at low levels in order to serve as a second messenger within the cytosol, separated by cellular membranes from the high extracellular calcium concentration. Intracellular calcium is maintained by calcium entry channels, sodium-calcium exchangers, ATP-dependent calcium pumps, intracellular calcium-binding proteins, and intracellular storage (microsomes, mitochondria, and the Golgi apparatus). Sudden fluxes in calcium that serve as second messenger signals are rapidly terminated by pumping calcium back into the extracellular fluid or causing it to be taken up by intracellular storage sites again. The regulation of intracellular calcium is not directly dependent upon the parathyroids and as such is beyond the scope of this chapter.

Maintaining the ionized calcium concentration in the circulation requires key interactions among the calcium-sensing receptor, parathyroids, kidneys, intestines, and the skeleton (wherein 99% of calcium in the body resides). The calcium-sensing receptor, which is expressed predominantly by the parathyroids, C cells of the thyroid, and renal tubules, specifies the set level of ionized calcium that must be maintained in the circulation. This level of calcium is near the saturation point with phosphorus, such that a small increase in calcium or phosphorus can lead to calcium-phosphate crystals precipitating in the soft tissues, nerves, and the conducting system of the heart. The calcium-sensing receptor acts to inhibit the synthesis and release of parathyroid hormone (PTH) by the parathyroids, stimulate synthesis and release of calcitonin by the C cells of the thyroid, and inhibit the reabsorption of calcium by the kidney tubules independent of PTH.

The parathyroids, by releasing PTH when the inhibiting control of the calcium-sensing receptor is released (such as from a fall in ionized calcium), play a central role in regulating calcium homeostasis. PTH increases serum calcium by stimulating skeletal resorption, reabsorption of calcium by the kidneys, and synthesis of calcitriol (which in turn stimulates intestinal calcium and phosphorus absorption). These actions of PTH would otherwise lead to a simultaneous increase in serum phosphorus, except that PTH has additional actions to increase renal phosphorus excretion (directly and through stimulating release of fibroblast growth factor-23 [FGF23]). This provides a safety valve to allow excess phosphorus that was resorbed from the skeleton and absorbed through the diet to be excreted into the urine.

The key role of the parathyroids is best exemplified by genetic or acquired conditions of aparathyroidism and hypoparathyroidism, in which PTH is either absent or present at very low concentrations. Ionized calcium is low, phosphorus is high, calcitriol is low, intestinal calcium absorption is reduced, the kidneys waste calcium but retain phosphorus, extraskeletal calcium-phosphate crystals may form in basal ganglia and other tissues, and bone turnover is low, leading to inappropriate skeletal retention of calcium. An activating mutation of the calcium-sensing receptor leads to identical results by keeping PTH suppressed to very low levels.

Although PTH plays this central and critical role, normal calcium and phosphorus homeostasis also depends upon other hormones such as calcitriol, estradiol, PTH-related protein (PTHrP), FGF23, etc. For example, if the contribution of calcitriol is absent (from severe vitamin D deficiency, absence of the vitamin D receptor [VDR], or lack of the Cyp27b1 enzyme that synthesizes calcitriol), then intestinal delivery of calcium and phosphorus is reduced and skeletal homeostasis is disrupted despite the presence of PTH. Loss of estradiol leads to increased sensitivity to normal circulating levels of PTH, increased osteoclast activity, increased skeletal resorption, and net bone loss leading to osteoporosis. The many interactions of these calciotropic hormones are beyond the scope of this chapter, but it should be kept in mind that despite its critical role, normal calcium and bone homeostasis requires more than just sufficiency of PTH.

Embryology and Anatomy of the Parathyroids

The parathyroids originate in the endoderm of the third and fourth pharyngeal pouches and migrate during embryogenesis with the thymus and thyroid to their final positions in the neck. The fourth pouch gives rise to a superior pair of parathyroids that often resides posterior to the middle of the thyroid, while the third pouch produces an inferior pair of parathyroids that usually end up at the inferior poles of the thyroid but can have a quite variable final resting position. There are commonly four and occasionally just three parathyroids in humans; however, their friable nature during embryonic development can lead to supernumerary parathyroids in approximately 5–10% of individuals (typically 5 glands, but as many as 12 have been seen). Errant migration can lead to ectopic parathyroids that range from high up in the neck to as low as the diaphragm. Although ectopic parathyroids are most commonly located in the thymus, they can be located in diverse tissues such as the esophagus, larynx, and carotid sheath. More rarely, multiple parathyroid rests can give rise to diffuse, functioning parathyroid tissue throughout the neck, a condition termed parathyromatosis (this condition can also iatrogenically arise from spillage of parathyroid tissue during a neck exploration).

Genetic causes of hypoparathyroidism can include mutations affecting the development of the third and fourth pharyngeal arches (including DiGeorge and other 22q11.2 deletion syndromes), thereby leading not only to absent parathyroids but also thyroid hypoplasia and absence of the thymus. More specific gene deletions (e.g., *GCM2*) can lead to selective loss of the parathyroids, or a null mutation in the *PTH* gene itself can occur.

The parathyroids are typically yellow brown in appearance, 2–5 mm in length and width, 0.5–2 mm in thickness, and 30–55 g in weight. A thin fibrous capsule surrounds a lobulated interior that is largely composed of stromal fat and PTH-producing chief cells, with other cells (oxyphil, clear, and transitional oxyphil) also noted. These other cell types also express PTH and it remains unclear whether their secretory role or function differs from those of chief cells. Clear cells are glycogen rich and more abundant in embryonic and fetal parathyroids. Oxyphil and transitional cells are relatively scarce until they increase significantly in number after birth.

The parathyroids produce immunoreactive PTH beginning at about 10 weeks of gestation. Low circulating levels of PTH (as compared to simultaneous maternal and normal adult values) are usually maintained in the embryonic and fetal circulation, which then normally rise to adult levels during the first 48 h after birth. The fetal parathyroids are evidently kept suppressed by high levels of calcium that are normally present in the fetal circulation and cord blood. The high level of ionized calcium is sufficient to act through the calcium-sensing receptor to suppress the fetal parathyroids. However, the fetal parathyroids are certainly capable of higher levels of PTH production and release. This will occur, for example, in response to severe maternal hypocalcemia. Such compensatory fetal hyperparathyroidism is ultimately detrimental to the fetus because it leads to undermineralization of the skeleton and fractures that may occur in utero, during delivery, or soon after birth.

Parathyroid Hormone

Pth Gene Expression

PTH is located on chromosome 11 and contains three exons and two introns. It is predominantly and abundantly expressed in the chief cells of the parathyroids, but low levels of expression have also been noted in rodent hypothalamus, thymus, and placental trophoblasts. Whether or not equivalent human tissues express PTH has not been determined. Quite rarely PTH has been unequivocally shown to be ectopically produced by certain malignancies.

Synthesis and Processing

The initial *PTH* gene transcript is a 115 amino acid precursor protein called preproPTH. The prepro sequence enables recognition of the immature protein by signal recognition particles, which bind to preproPTH when it emerges from the ribosome and guide it to the endoplasmic reticulum where the pre-sequence is cleaved. In turn the pro sequence is cleaved upon passage through the Golgi apparatus, resulting in mature PTH being packaged into secretory granules. The intact PTH molecule is 84 amino acids in length and has a molecular weight of 9,300.

The secretory granules released by the parathyroids contain other products, including chromogranin A. The chromogranins may represent 50% of the protein output of the parathyroids, but whether these have functional roles is uncertain. Chromogranin expression increases with hypocalcemia and decreases with hypercalcemia, and there is some evidence that chromogranins may inhibit PTH synthesis and release. However, the possible role that non-PTH secretory products of the parathyroids may have on mineral and skeletal homeostasis has not been rigorously studied.

Secretion of PTH

Synthesis and secretion of PTH is mainly controlled by the calcium-sensing receptor, which is a classical seven-transmembrane-spanning, G-protein-coupled receptor whose ligand is primarily calcium. When calcium ions bind to the receptor on parathyroid glands, coupling to G_q leads to activation of phospholipase C, hydrolysis of phospholipid phosphatidylinositol 4,5-bisphosphate, and the generation of the second messengers IP3 and diacylglycerol and a rise in intracellular calcium. This receptor activation ultimately inhibits release of PTH by blocking fusion of storage granules with the plasma membrane and release of their contents (PTH and chromogranins) into the circulation. More prolonged activation of the receptor, such as through chronic hypercalcemia that is not mediated by PTH, leads to reduced *PTH* transcription and translation and reduced parathyroid cell growth.

There is a sigmoidal relationship between PTH and calcium, with the steep part of the curve corresponding to the normal physiological range of ionized calcium (Fig. 1). An ionized calcium concentration that is above the level set by the calcium-sensing receptor will suppress PTH completely. Conversely, reduced binding of calcium to the receptor (such as by a low serum calcium) leads to disinhibition of PTH transcription, translation, and release; the stability of *preproPth* mRNA is also increased. An inactivating mutation of the calcium-sensing receptor shifts the curve to the right, leading to increased PTH and higher ionized calcium, whereas an activating mutation shifts the curve to the left, resulting in low PTH and low ionized calcium. The presence of PTH in storage granules enables rapid release when the ionized calcium falls. In addition to controlling the moment-to-moment release of PTH, the calcium-sensing receptor also has longer-term trophic effects on the relative growth of the parathyroids.

Magnesium is an additional regulator of PTH synthesis and release, although its effects are weaker and more complex. It is also a ligand for the calcium-sensing receptor. High serum magnesium inhibits PTH and can lead to hypocalcemia. Conversely low serum magnesium can acutely stimulate PTH release, whereas chronic hypomagnesemia inhibits PTH release and also blunts PTH action in target cells. Why chronic hypomagnesemia inhibits parathyroid responsiveness and PTH action is not fully understood.

Phosphorus is also a regulator of PTH release with high serum phosphorus leading to increased PTH irrespective of the ionized calcium level. This most commonly occurs in renal failure patients, in whom high serum phosphorus provokes increased PTH, despite the actions of the calcium-sensing receptor to keep PTH in check. How phosphorus is sensed and in turns leads to stimulation of PTH release is unclear. Low phosphorus has inhibitory effects on PTH synthesis and release, thereby clearly establishing that PTH is responsive to the spectrum of high to

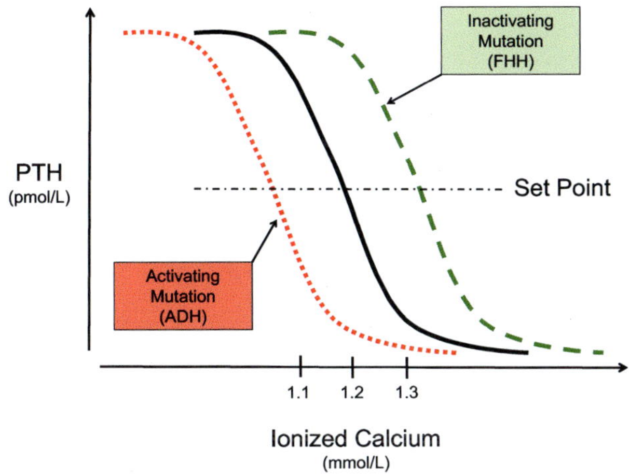

Fig. 1 Sigmoidal relationship between ionized calcium and PTH. Ionized calcium activates the calcium receptor to inhibit PTH, with the greatest responsiveness (represented by the near-vertical slope of the *solid black line*) occurring within the physiological range of 1.10–1.30 mmol/L for ionized calcium. Consequently, a rise in ionized calcium inhibits PTH, while a fall in ionized calcium disinhibits PTH synthesis and release. The set point is the level of ionized calcium that results in 50% of the capacity of the parathyroids to acutely release PTH. An inactivating mutation of the calcium-sensing receptor (such as that occurs in familial hypocalciuric hypercalcemia or FHH) makes the receptor less responsive to a rise in calcium and shifts the set point to the right, resulting in higher than normal ambient concentrations of both ionized calcium and PTH (*green dashed line*). FHH begins causing hypercalcemia in utero and is generally asymptomatic in children and adults. An activating mutation of the calcium-sensing receptor (such as that occurs in autosomal dominant hypocalcemia or ADH) makes the receptor more responsive to low levels of ionized calcium, shifting the set point to the left and resulting in low ionized calcium and PTH concentrations (*red dotted line*). ADH likely causes hypocalcemia beginning in utero and usually results in symptomatic hypocalcemia and tetany in children and adults. It is indistinguishable from hypoparathyroidism except by genetic testing

low phosphorus. FGF23 similarly increases in response to high serum phosphorus, but one of its actions is to suppress PTH transcription and synthesis.

Calcitriol itself will inhibit transcription and synthesis of *PTH*, while independently increasing calcium and phosphorus absorption from the intestines. Analogs of calcitriol have been developed for use in renal failure patients that reduce the synthesis and secretion of PTH, but do not cause the increase in calcium and phosphorus delivery that occurs in response to treatment with calcitriol.

Clearance and Metabolism

Upon its release, PTH has a very short circulating half-life of less than 4 min. In the kidneys and liver, intact PTH is cleaved to produce amino-terminal and carboxy-terminal fragments. C-terminal fragments are cleared by renal filtration and are known to accumulate in renal failure.

PTH Receptors

The biological activity of PTH is almost entirely attributable to actions of the N-terminal molecule on the PTH/PTHrP receptor (also called the type 1 PTH receptor or PTH1R). It is abundantly expressed in osteoblasts and renal tubules. Additional sites of expression include cells within the placenta. The PTH1R is a seven-transmembrane-spanning, G-protein-coupled receptor with a large extracellular domain to which PTH binds. The first six amino acids of PTH are required for activation of PTH1R, while residues between 18 and 34 are responsible for PTH binding to the receptor. Activation of PTH1R in turn activates two G proteins, G_s and G_q. G_s in turn activates adenylyl cyclase, which generates cAMP as the second messenger. G_q couples to phospholipase C, prompting an increase in intracellular calcium and activation of protein kinase C as second messengers.

A second but less well-characterized receptor, which PTH binds to and activates while PTHrP does not, is called the PTH2R. However, its endogenous ligand appears to be TIP39 (tuberoinfundibular peptide of 39 residues) and not PTH. It is expressed within the brain only and may not have any role in calcium and bone homeostasis.

Additional receptors have been proposed for the mid or C-terminal portions of PTH, and there is some evidence from rodents for functions of these molecules. Whether the accumulating C-terminal fragment in renal failure patients contribute to disturbances in calcium and bone metabolism remains uncertain.

Assays

Modern assays measure an "intact" form of the PTH molecule by requiring two antibodies, one that recognizes an amino-terminal sequence and a second antibody that recognizes a mid-molecular sequence. In this way the biologically relevant molecule is detected, while nonfunctional C-terminal and N-terminal fragments should not be detected; PTHrP is also not detected by these assays. With such assays PTH has a normal range of approximately 1.0–6.0 pmol/L. In primary and secondary hyperparathyroidism, the values will be increased, whereas in hypoparathyroidism the values will either be below the lower limit of normal or "inappropriately normal" in the presence of hypocalcemia. When hypercalcemia is not mediated by autonomous parathyroid function, the calcium-sensing receptor should shut off PTH synthesis and release, leading to a very low or undetectable PTH level.

A further refinement in assays resulted after the recognition that an N-terminal truncated form of PTH, which lacks the first six amino acids and is inactive, can represent 50% of the circulating "intact PTH" level in renal failure patients. The N-terminal antibody has been revised in newer assays to capture the first six amino acids, thereby eliminating the possibility of detecting the inactive N-terminal-truncated forms of PTH. These assays are said to detect "bio-intact PTH" as opposed to "intact PTH." They are useful for more accurately determining the magnitude of secondary hyperparathyroidism in renal failure and whether it requires treatment to lower the PTH concentration to maintain bone health. It is unclear that bio-intact PTH assays have any benefit over intact PTH assays in other clinical situations, since the truncated N-terminal forms of intact PTH have only been shown to accumulate in renal failure.

Biological Actions: Adult

PTH has important direct and indirect actions in kidneys, intestines, and the bone, the three dominant organs that contribute to calcium and bone homeostasis in the adult (Fig. 2).

In the kidneys PTH has several direct actions. It stimulates active reabsorption of calcium against an electrochemical gradient in the distal convoluted tubules by activating transient receptor potential vanilloid 5 (TRPV5) and stimulating the expression of the sodium-calcium exchanger NCX1. These actions are independent of the calcium-sensing receptor and calcitonin to affect calcium reabsorption. In the proximal renal tubules, PTH potently inhibits the expression of sodium-phosphate cotransporter subtypes 2a and 2c (NaPi2a and NaPi2c), which leads to renal phosphorus excretion. It also stimulates the excretion of bicarbonate by inhibiting the actions of Na^+-H^+ antiporters; consequently, hyperparathyroidism can lead to a mild hyperchloremic metabolic acidosis. Furthermore, it stimulates the expression and activity of 1α-hydroxylase (Cyp27b1), which converts 25-hydroxyvitamin D into calcitriol, the active or hormonal form of vitamin D. Finally, PTH also increases calcitriol by inhibiting the expression of Cyp24a1, the enzyme that catabolizes calcitriol and 25-hydroxyvitamin D. PTH has indirect actions in the kidney through its ability to stimulate the expression of FGF23, which in turn acts on the kidney tubules to downregulate the expression of NaPi2a and NaPi2c, thereby promoting renal phosphorus excretion. FGF23 also inhibits Cyp27b1, stimulates Cyp24a1, and inhibits PTH, thereby lowering calcitriol, an action that opposes the effect of PTH to increase calcitriol.

The interactions between PTH and FGF23 in the kidney tubules are not well understood. It is evident that both hormones are required, since loss of either PTH or FGF23 results in a similar degree of reduced urinary phosphorus excretion, increased renal expression of NaPi2a and NaPi2c, and hyperphosphatemia. In turn, the resultant hyperphosphatemia leads to extraskeletal calcifications and disturbed mineralization of the bone. It is clear that neither hormone can make up for absence of the other, and so both are required.

PTH has no direct actions in intestinal cells (enterocytes). However, it does have indirect actions, the most dominant of which is that through its stimulation of calcitriol, it causes upregulation of both active and passive absorption of calcium and phosphorus. Another indirect action is through stimulation of FGF23, which then acts to reduce the expression of NaPi2b by enterocytes and lower the serum calcitriol concentration, thereby reducing intestinal phosphorus absorption through two pathways.

PTH has several distinct, time-dependent actions upon bone cells.

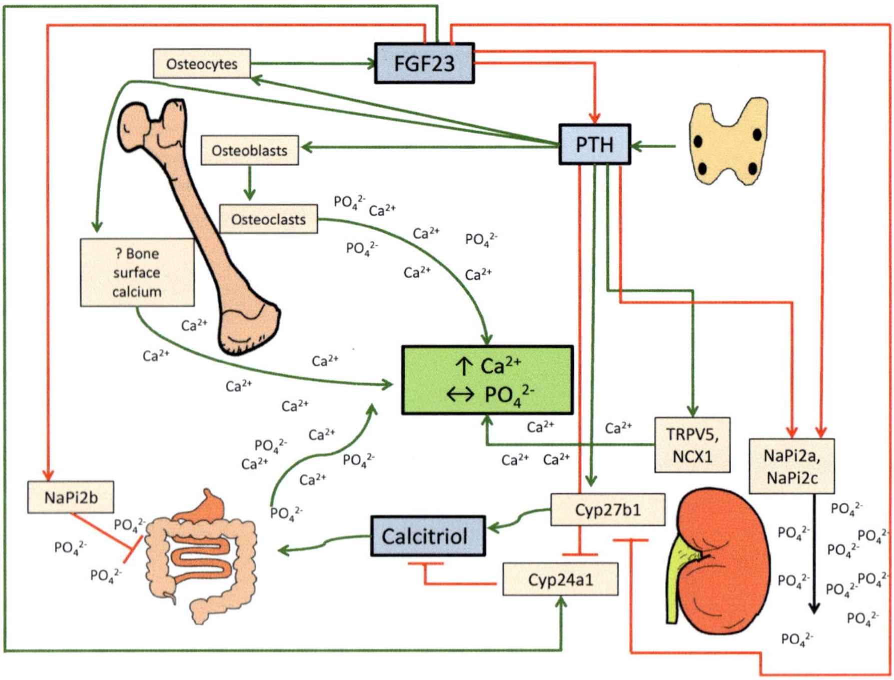

Fig. 2 Central role of PTH in regulating calcium and phosphorus economy and bone mass. The main sites of PTH action are the bone, kidney, and (indirectly) intestines. **Within bone cells**, PTH has three main actions that take progressively more time to be invoked. First, in response to acute hypocalcemia, PTH responds within 1–2 min to liberate calcium from the bone surface via uncertain mechanisms. Second, short and low amplitude pulses of PTH activate the PTH1R to stimulate osteoblasts, resulting in bone formation and incorporation of calcium and phosphorus into bone. Third, prolonged and higher amplitude pulses of PTH also activate osteoblasts, but in turn osteoblasts upregulate release of RANKL to stimulate osteoclast recruitment and activity, thereby resorbing the bone to bring calcium and phosphorus into the circulation. This third action takes hours to be invoked. A fourth action with the bone is that PTH acts on osteocytes to stimulate FGF23 release. **Within kidney tubules**, PTH increases reabsorption of calcium by stimulating TRPV5 and NCX1, increases renal excretion of phosphorus by inhibiting expression of NaP12a and NaPi2c, and increases calcitriol by stimulating Cyp27b1 (which synthesizes calcitriol) and inhibiting Cyp24a1 (which catabolizes calcitriol and 25-hydroxyvitamin D). **Within the intestines**, PTH acts via its stimulation of calcitriol to increase intestinal calcium and phosphorus absorption. These PTH-induced effects bring more calcium into the circulation from all three target organs but also cause an influx in phosphorus from bone and intestines. The potential for phosphorus to rise and cause widespread precipitation of calcium-phosphate crystals is offset by PTH's potent effect to stimulate renal phosphorus excretion. Consequently, the net effect of a rise in PTH in response to acute hypocalcemia is that the ionized calcium increases to normal while serum phosphorus remains relatively stable. The longer-term effects of physiological actions of PTH on the bone are to maintain ionized calcium, phosphorus, and bone mass/strength. Also depicted are that PTH stimulates FGF23, which in turn also stimulates renal phosphorus excretion, lowers calcitriol, and has both direct and indirect actions to lower intestinal phosphorus absorption. Not depicted is that calcitriol stimulates the synthesis and release of FGF23 but inhibits the synthesis and release of PTH, thereby helping to counterbalance some of the actions invoked by a rise in PTH

The most rapid but poorly understood PTH action is its response to acute hypocalcemia, such as that induced by hyperventilation or treatment with EDTA or old citrated blood products, or which can be mimicked by observing the acute hypercalcemic response to a PTH infusion. The rapid recovery from hypocalcemia is preceded by a surge in PTH, requires intact parathyroids, and does not depend upon the kidneys; therefore, it must be due to some action on the bone to liberate calcium (possibly from the surface of the bone). However, this is not the result of osteoclast-mediated bone resorption since this takes hours to be induced. Instead, recent work has suggested that the rapid response to PTH may be the result of its PTH1R-dependent actions on osteocytes, which can respond rapidly to release calcium from their surrounding matrices (a process called osteocytic osteolysis). This fast response to PTH has also been conjectured to proceed via actions on the bone surface such as an outwardly directed calcium pump, proton production and mineral solubility, changes to calcium-binding protein properties, or other actions on bone lining cells.

The second action of PTH is to bind to and activate the PTH1R expressed by preosteoblasts and osteoblasts. This results in increased osteoblast number, recruitment, and activity and reduced osteoblast apoptosis and conceivably could lead to a reduction in the ionized calcium in the circulation. A short pulse of PTH (which can be experimentally mimicked by a subcutaneous daily injection or an intravenous infusion lasting no more than 2 h) has been shown to stimulate these effects in osteoblasts. These short pulses likely mimic the brief pulses in PTH release that will occur physiologically as a consequence of its release being controlled by the calcium-sensing receptor and a phosphorus sensor and its rapid removal from the circulation.

The third but more delayed action of PTH is to stimulate osteoclasts and thereby resorb calcium and phosphorus from the skeleton. Historically this has always been perceived as the dominant effect of PTH, since PTH is considered to be a hormone that raises the blood calcium and hyperparathyroidism (a form of PTH excess) causes increased skeletal resorption and elevates the serum calcium. However, the PTH1R is expressed by osteoblasts and not osteoclasts, and only in the past 15 years has it become clear how PTH indirectly stimulates osteoclasts. Prolonged and higher magnitude pulses of PTH (which can be mimicked by a continuous infusions of PTH) result in osteoblasts upregulating the expression of receptor activator of nuclear factor kappa-B ligand (RANKL), which in turn increases osteoclast formation, recruitment, and activity. The consequence is increased bone resorption, but this takes hours for the effect to be achieved, and that is why this mechanism cannot account for rapid (i.e., within several minutes) recovery from acute hypocalcemia or the rapid hypercalcemic response to a PTH infusion.

The cumulative long-term effect of these diverse actions of PTH is to maintain the ionized calcium and phosphorus concentrations at target levels in the circulation and regulate bone turnover at a rate that enables ongoing repair of microdamage and maintenance of bone mass and strength. By interacting with calcitriol and FGF23, the supply of calcium and phosphorus entering the circulation from the diet is controlled by PTH. Hypoparathyroidism reduces bone turnover, leading to slow skeletal accretion of mineral and microdamage and systemic hypocalcemia. Hyperparathyroidism increases osteoclast activity, resulting in thinned trabeculae, conversion from platelike to weaker rodlike structures within the microarchitecture, and reduced bone strength.

Biological Actions: Fetus

The fetal circulation is characterized by elevated concentrations of ionized calcium and phosphorus and low levels of PTH and calcitriol, as compared to the maternal circulation and normal adult values. Cord blood has long been recognized to have high levels of PTH-like bioactivity despite low circulating levels of intact PTH, and in the past two decades, it has become clear that this is due to the presence of high circulating levels of PTHrP. Fetal mineral metabolism also differs significantly from the adult due to the presence of the placenta, which actively transports calcium, phosphorus, and magnesium from the maternal circulation against concentration and electrochemical gradients. Furthermore, the intestines and kidneys, which are key organs in adult mineral and bone homeostasis, play little or no role in fetal mineral homeostasis. The fetal kidneys do not have the same capability to actively reabsorb calcium or phosphorus that adult kidneys do; moreover, any mineral excreted by the kidneys ends up in the amniotic fluid, from where it can be swallowed and reabsorbed.

The characteristically low levels of PTH in the fetal circulation do not mean that it plays no role in fetal mineral homeostasis. In animal models, fetal parathyroidectomy or genetic deletion of parathyroids, PTH, and PTH1R receptor have each led to significant fetal hypocalcemia and hyperphosphatemia. The skeleton is significantly undermineralized in the absence of PTH, whereas the length and morphology of the developing limbs and spine may be normal. PTH also has a very modest effect to stimulate placental calcium transport that has only be clearly shown in an animal model lacking PTH; placental expression of certain cation transporters is also reduced in the absence of PTH. (PTHrP has a more important role in placental calcium and magnesium transport; see below.) These findings support that the main role of PTH during fetal development is to participate in maintaining the fetal ionized calcium at a high level that facilitates rapid mineralization of the developing skeleton during the third trimester. In the absence of PTH, the ionized calcium falls, delivery of mineral to osteoblasts is reduced, and the skeleton cannot be fully mineralized.

As noted earlier, if severe maternal hypocalcemia is present, such as that caused by maternal hypoparathyroidism or severe maternal vitamin D deficiency, then fetal hyperparathyroidism will result in an effort to maintain the fetal ionized calcium at its normally high level. An unavoidable consequence of fetal hyperparathyroidism is increased resorption of the fetal skeleton, which has been found to cause skeletal fragility and fractures.

The findings in animal models predict that human babies lacking PTH (such as with DiGeorge syndrome) will have reduced calcium and increased phosphorus in cord blood and undermineralized skeletons.

Biological Actions: Neonate

At birth the loss of the placental mineral pump and its associated hormones, combined with the onset of breathing, leads to a sudden 20–30% fall in ionized calcium from the high values of fetal life. By 12–24 h after birth, the ionized calcium is transiently below normal adult values and is accompanied by a rising serum phosphorus. Low ionized calcium and high phosphorus are consistent with a hypoparathyroid state. This is followed by rising intact PTH concentrations that are followed in turn by increased ionized calcium, decreased phosphorus, and increased calcitriol. Initially the neonatal intestines have reduced responsiveness to calcitriol and largely absorb calcium through passive mechanisms that are enhanced by lactose. As the postnatal days pass, upregulation of the vitamin D receptor and expression of calcitriol-dependent factors in the enterocytes herald an increase in the ability to actively absorb calcium. And so each neonate goes through a transient phase of physiological hypoparathyroidism as the parathyroids "wake up" over the first 48 h from the physiological expression that had been experienced during all of fetal life.

Maternal hypercalcemia during pregnancy leads to increased flow of calcium across the placenta and suppression of the fetal parathyroids to a greater degree than normal. In turn this can lead to prolonged parathyroid suppression after birth, thereby increasing the risk of neonatal hypocalcemia, tetany, seizures, and even sudden death. In some cases, the neonatal parathyroid suppression has lasted for months, and in a few cases, it has been permanent. Conversely when significant maternal hypocalcemia during pregnancy leads to compensatory fetal hyperparathyroidism, this relatively autonomous hyperfunction can last for weeks to months after birth and result in neonatal hypercalcemia. These findings underscore that the fetal parathyroids are active and responsive to the fetal blood calcium level and that both high and low calcium levels in utero can have harmful effects that persist in the neonate.

Parathyroid Hormone-Related Protein

PTHLH Gene Expression

PTHrP is encoded by *PTHLH* on the short arm of chromosome 12. It has a complex structure with multiple promoters. The exon/intron organization of *PTHLH* and *PTH* is identical in the prepro sequence regions, highly homologous in regions encoding amino acids 1–13, and similar in regions encoding amino acids 14–34. Beyond those regions, the structures of *PTHLH* and *PTH* have no similarities. The two genes are believed to have derived from a common ancestor through gene duplication.

Unlike the expression of *PTH* that is almost exclusive to the parathyroids, *PTHLH* is expressed in multiple and diverse tissues in the embryo, fetus, and adult.

Synthesis and Processing

Three distinct promoters and alternative splicing of *PTHLH* result in three separate PTHrP isoforms in humans that are identical through their first 139 amino acids: $PTHrP^{1-139}$, $PTHrP^{1-141}$, and $PTHrP^{1-173}$. All three forms of PTHrP share 8 of the first 13 amino acids with PTH and have a similar secondary structure as PTH over amino acids 14–34. These structural similarities enable PTHrP to bind to and activate the PTH1R. There are no similar amino acid sequences or structures between PTHrP and PTH in their mid- or C-terminal regions.

The prepro isoforms of PTHrP have a bipartite nuclear localization signal (NLS) in the mid-region at amino acids 88–91 and 102–106 and a 36-amino acid sequence within the N-terminal that functions as a signal peptide. Posttranslational processing of preproPTHrP generates full-length, N-terminal ($PTHrP^{1-36}$, $PTHrP^{1-86}$, etc.), mid-region, and C-terminal peptides forms of PTHrP. Each of these forms may have distinct receptor(s). The signal peptide directs full-length and N-terminal forms of PTHrP to the secretory pathway. The NLS directs full-length and mid-region PTHrP to the nucleus and nucleolus, wherein PTHrP has intracrine actions.

Full-length PTHrP is essentially a polyhormone or polycytokine with multiple capabilities and actions, depending upon how it is processed, secreted, or internalized.

Secretion of PTHrP

Factors that have been shown to stimulate PTHrP transcription and synthesis include prolactin, placental lactogen, serotonin, estradiol, TGF-B, and EGF. Both high estradiol levels in pregnancy and low estradiol levels during lactation have been shown to stimulate PTHrP production. Within lactating mammary epithelial cells, the act of suckling also increases production of PTHrP.

Although PTH is under control of the calcium-sensing receptor expressed on the parathyroids, PTHrP is not responsive to it. Its secretion during fetal development appears to be autonomous from placenta and other sources, such that it does not increase in response to systemic hypocalcemia or to inactivating mutations of the calcium-sensing receptor (whereas PTH increases in both situations). Conversely during lactation the expression and release of PTHrP are responsive to the calcium-sensing receptor expressed by mammary epithelial cells. Binding of calcium ions to the receptor inhibits the transcription, synthesis, and release of PTHrP, whereas reduced activation of the receptor leads to increased PTHrP expression. There may also be a modest effect of systemic hypocalcemia or low dietary calcium intake that acts through the calcium-sensing receptor in breast tissue to locally stimulate PTHrP production.

Clearance and Metabolism

Like PTH, full-length forms of PTHrP have a half-life of a few minutes in the circulation because of rapid cleavage. The various metabolites of PTHrP may each have different clearance rates. Transcription, translation, and posttranslational processing of PTHrP should lead to equal appearance of N-terminal, mid-region, and C-terminal forms of PTHrP. However, when PTHrP is produced to excess in humoral hypercalcemia of malignancy, the circulating concentrations of the mid-region forms, which begin at amino acid 38, greatly exceed the serum levels of N-terminal and C-terminal PTHrP. This likely results from a slower rate of clearance of the mid-regional forms of PTHrP as compared to N-terminal and C-terminal forms.

PTHrP Receptors

PTHrP binds to and activates PTH1R with similar affinity as PTH. However, three-dimensional crystal structures of PTH^{1-34}, $PTHrP^{1-36}$, and PTH1R predict that PTHrP binds less avidly than PTH to the PTH1R, thereby leading to a shorter duration of binding and signaling. This is in part because the more tightly wound amphipathic helix of PTH^{1-34} facilitates a tighter fit into the hydrophobic pocket of the PTH1R, as compared to the looser fit of the curved and slightly unwound helix of $PTHrP^{1-36}$. In most in vitro assays, the ability of N-terminal PTH and PTHrP to induce signaling has been relatively indistinguishable; however, upregulation of Cyp27b1 to synthesize calcitriol appears to be less marked in the presence of elevated PTHrP (such as from lactation, humoral hypercalcemia of malignancy, or experimental infusions of PTHrP), as compared to the increase in calcitriol that is achieved with similar elevations of PTH.

As noted earlier, PTHrP does not bind to or activate the PTH2R. A PTH3R that is activated by PTHrP but not PTH has been observed in zebra fish but not humans.

There is functional evidence in specific tissues and at various developmental stages, for other unique receptors that recognize N-terminal, mid-molecular, and C-terminal forms of PTHrP. However, to date none of these receptors have been identified or characterized.

Assays

PTHrP appears to be subjected to more rapid metabolism and degradation than PTH, and this renders serum as a problematic source for reliable measurement of PTHrP. Plasma is best collected in chilled tubes containing EDTA and a protease inhibitor such as aprotinin, processed rapidly under refrigerated conditions, and frozen promptly. Even with such rigorous methods of plasma collection, PTHrP begins degrading within 15 min.

Similar to the assays for PTH, a two-antibody system is largely used to detect near full-length PTHrP. These antibodies are highly specific to PTHrP such that they do not cross-react with PTH. However, the most widely used assays measure $PTHrP^{1-86}$, which does not a naturally occurring product based on the predicted cleavage sites of PTHrP. A $PTHrP^{1-86}$ assay will detect all three full-length isoforms, including $PTHrP^{1-130}$, $PTHrP^{1-141}$, or $PTHrP^{1-173}$, but it will not detect $PTHrP^{1-36}$. This is problematic because $PTHrP^{1-36}$ derives from posttranslational processing of all three full-length forms of PTHrP and conceivably may be the most abundant of the biologically active N-terminal forms of PTHrP. A few assays use a two-antibody method to measure $PTHrP^{1-34}$, and these will detect both the N-terminal and full-length forms. In most PTHrP assays, the normal adult range is <1.0 pmol/L, but the sensitivity of the assays is at the same level.

None of these clinically available assays will specifically detect the mid-region ($PTHrP^{38-94}$ and $PTHrP^{38-101}$) or C-terminal ($PTHrP^{107-139}$ and $PTHrP^{141-173}$) forms of PTHrP. The mid-region will be present in any molecule detected by a $PTHrP^{1-86}$ assay, but the C-terminal portions are not necessarily present.

Biological Actions: Adult

PTHrP is normally not detectable in the circulation of adults, and as a result, it is not believed to have a hormonal role in regulating normal mineral homeostasis. Its expression persists in certain tissues, and it has been detected in normal, hyperplastic, and adenomatous parathyroid tissue from humans. Whether it increases together with PTH in patients with hyperparathyroidism has not been determined.

There are two physiological circumstances in which PTHrP rises in the adult circulation and exerts hormonal effects, but in each of these instances, the parathyroids are not the source of PTHrP.

During pregnancy PTHrP rises in the maternal circulation and likely derives from both the placenta and breasts. The increase in PTHrP may contribute to the normal two- to fourfold increase in calcitriol that normally occurs during pregnancy and which occurs despite a fall in PTH to low levels. Individual case reports have revealed that this increase in PTHrP can impact calcium and bone metabolism and lead to maternal hypercalcemia. When due to a placental source, the hypercalcemia and increased PTHrP are followed within hours of delivery by hypocalcemia, undetectable PTHrP, and a surge in PTH. Conversely, when due to PTHrP production by the breasts, the hypercalcemia persists postpartum and may last for weeks to months after weaning.

During lactation the breasts upregulate the expression of PTHrP even more and contribute to accelerated skeletal resorption from which most of the calcium content of milk is derived. This expression contributes to most lactating women experiencing a rise in the ionized or albumin-corrected serum calcium while lactating, during which the PTH concentration often becomes undetectable. The role the breasts play is exemplified by hypoparathyroid women who, while breastfeeding, often normalize mineral homeostasis such that supplemental calcium or calcitriol must be substantially reduced or discontinued in order to avoid the development of severe hypercalcemia. Around the time of weaning, the production of PTHrP by the breasts declines significantly, but the effect of lactation to normalize mineral homeostasis has persisted for over a year after weaning in some women.

Biological Actions: Fetus

In fetal life PTHrP is expressed in a myriad of tissues, and so it has roles in the development of many different tissues, from placenta to mammary buds to alveolar type II cells in the lungs to the skin, cartilage, and bone. It is also present at high levels in the fetal circulation. Whether the circulating form results from release by the fetal parathyroids, the placenta, or both, has not been made clear. With respect to fetal mineral and bone homeostasis, several local and systemic actions of PTHrP have become clear through study of genetically manipulated animal models.

PTHrP is expressed within chondrocytes of the developing endochondral skeleton, where it acts to delay their terminal differentiation into hypertrophic chondrocytes. In the absence of PTHrP, accelerated terminal differentiation occurs, followed by premature resorption of the cartilaginous template, and then the laying down of primary spongiosa by osteoblasts. In certain locations, such as the ribs, absence of PTHrP leads to bone forming where cartilage normally persists in the adult. Shortened long bones result from the accelerated differentiation of chondrocytes.

Conversely, overexpression of PTHrP during fetal life delays terminal differentiation of chondrocytes, resulting in a largely cartilaginous skeleton at term. In such mouse models, the development of normal bone is delayed until after birth, but otherwise proceeds normally.

From its expression in placenta, and possibly the fetal parathyroids, PTHrP stimulates the active transport of calcium and magnesium across the placenta. PTHrP does not affect placental phosphorus transport and nor do PTH or FGF23; the regulators of placental phosphorus transport remain unknown. Absence of PTHrP leads to modest hypocalcemia and hyperphosphatemia, but skeletal mineral content is not reduced due to the competing problem of accelerated skeletal development and mineralization invoked by loss of PTHrP.

While these findings have been established in animal models, there is limited evidence from humans that loss of PTHrP may lead to similar effects. Blomstrand chondrodysplasia is due to loss of the PTH1R, and it causes an embryonically lethal chondrodysplasia that is quite similar to what has been found in *Pth1r* null and *Pthrp* null fetal mice. An autosomal dominant microdeletion in *PTHLH* occurs in brachydactyly type E, a condition characterized by short stature, metacarpals, and metatarsals.

PTHrP is expressed by human placenta, but whether human fetal parathyroids express PTHrP has not been determined. Cord blood reveals high PTHrP concentrations that are up to 15-fold higher than PTH and which correlate with and likely explain the high cord blood calcium.

Biological Actions: Neonate

At some point after birth and before adult life, PTHrP disappears from the circulation and is no longer important for mineral homeostasis until the later time points of pregnancy and lactation. Exactly when PTHrP becomes undetectable has not been determined. The speed of disappearance of PTHrP from the neonatal circulation will depend upon whether the parathyroids are a significant source of it during fetal development. Furthermore, milk contains high concentrations of PTHrP that are 1,000–10,000 times that in the circulation of lactating women or patients with humoral hypercalcemia of malignancy. PTHrP obtained from milk may exert effects within the neonatal intestines or could conceivably be absorbed to systematically affect neonatal mineral and skeletal metabolism. Limited animal data are compatible with PTHrP blunting the accretion of mineral by the neonatal skeleton, and there is also some evidence that PTHrP in milk may be absorbed into the neonatal circulation. The potential role of PTHrP in milk has not been systematically investigated in humans.

Disorders of Parathyroid Function

Hyperparathyroidism

High systemic levels of intact PTH cause increased osteoclast-mediated bone resorption, increased bone turnover, hyperphosphaturia, low or low-normal serum phosphorus, relatively reduced renal calcium excretion (hypercalciuria occurs due to the magnitude of calcium release from bone), increased calcitriol, and potentially hypercalcemia. In primary hyperparathyroidism, autonomous production of PTH by a parathyroid adenoma or hyperplasia of all four glands leads to hypercalcemia. In contrast, in secondary hyperparathyroidism the parathyroids are responding appropriately to an abnormal stimulus (such as hypocalcemia or hyperphosphatemia), and the ionized calcium is not elevated, but will be normal or low.

There is evidence that parathyroid adenomas also produce PTHrP, and so it is conceivable that high circulating levels of PTHrP are contributing to activation of the PTH1R. However, PTHrP levels have not been investigated in patients with primary hyperparathyroidism.

Hypoparathyroidism

In hypoparathyroidism, whether genetic (e.g., DiGeorge syndrome) or acquired (e.g., surgical or autoimmune), the circulating levels of intact PTH are either frankly low, or inappropriately normal but biologically inactive. Low effective PTH levels lead to reduced bone turnover (both osteoclast and osteoblast activity are lowered), reduced urine phosphorus excretion, hyperphosphatemia, renal calcium wasting, low calcitriol, and hypocalcemia.

PTHrP should be normal (i.e., undetectable) in these patients since PTHrP does not respond to systemic hypocalcemia. However, its production upregulates during pregnancy and lactation, and PTHrP will then have systemic effects to normalize mineral and bone metabolism despite hypoparathyroidism.

Pseudohypoparathyroidism

Pseudohypoparathyroidism is characterized by renal but not skeletal resistance to PTH and displays increased circulating levels of PTH together with low urine phosphorus excretion, hyperphosphatemia, renal calcium wasting, low calcitriol, and hypocalcemia. It is due to post-receptor or G protein defects and is not a problem with the receptor itself.

Pseudohyperparathyroidism

Pseudohyperparathyroidism is hypercalcemia induced by physiological excess release of PTHrP from placenta or breasts during pregnancy, or the breasts during lactation. It is characterized by hypercalcemia, high circulating levels of PTHrP, and low to undetectable PTH. When caused by PTHrP released by the placenta, the condition reverses within a few hours after delivery and can result in life-threatening hypocalcemia before the parathyroids recover. When caused by excess release of PTHrP from the breasts, the condition is slower to involute and may persist after weaning. No cases have clearly identified the parathyroids as the culprit source of PTHrP; in fact, some cases have occurred in hypoparathyroid women.

Hypercalcemia of Malignancy

There are two main classifications of disorders leading to hypercalcemia of malignancy. The first category is humoral hypercalcemia of malignancy, in which the skeleton has no or few metastases, but systemic resorption of the skeleton leads to release of calcium and phosphorus more rapidly than it can be excreted. This is most commonly due to excess production of PTHrP by a tumor that may not be located in the bone (e.g., breast, squamous lung tumor, etc.). It is rare for humoral hypercalcemia of malignancy to be caused by PTH, but it can occur with parathyroid carcinoma and even more rarely with tumors that ectopically produce PTH.

The second category is local osteolytic hypercalcemia, in which the skeleton is riddled with metastases and the hypercalcemia is occurring as a consequence of resorption localized to the immediate surroundings of each metastasis. In these situations the tumors are also producing PTHrP to cause localized resorption of the bone, thereby enabling the tumor to erode and invade bone. In such patients, PTHrP does not escape into the circulation in detectable amounts, but is only measurable within and surrounding the metastases.

In both categories of hypercalcemia of malignancy, unless it is the rare case of a PTH-producing tumor, the intact PTH level should be undetectable as a result of the calcium-sensing receptor reacting to the high ionized calcium and shutting down the parathyroids completely.

Summary

The parathyroids play an important, central role in regulating calcium and bone homeostasis, with direct actions in the kidney and bone and indirect actions in the intestines. PTH acts acutely to raise the blood calcium, but over the long term to maintain the ionized calcium and normal skeletal microarchitecture, mineralization, and strength. Without PTH or with excess PTH, mineral and skeletal metabolism is significantly disrupted and cannot be fully compensated for by other calciotropic hormones. On the other hand, it is important to recognize that there are key interactions of PTH with other regulators of calcium and bone metabolism (e.g., calcitriol, FGF23, estradiol, PTHrP) and that loss of any one of these other factors will disrupt normal mineral physiology despite the presence of intact parathyroids and normal PTH signaling.

Cross-References

▶ Endocrine Functions of Bone
▶ G protein-Coupled Receptors
▶ Synthesis, Secretion, and Transport of Peptide Hormones
▶ Targeting of Steroid Hormone Receptor Function in Breast and Prostate Cancer
▶ The Endocrine Control of Human Pregnancy

References

Bilezikian JP, Marcus R, Levine MA, Marcocci C, Silverberg SJ, Potts Jr JT, editors. The parathyroids: basic and clinical concepts. 3rd ed. San Diego: Academic; 2015.

Kovacs CS. Bone development and mineral homeostasis in the fetus and neonate: roles of the calciotropic and phosphotropic hormones. Physiol Rev. 2014;94(4):1143–218.

Kovacs CS. Maternal mineral and bone metabolism during pregnancy, lactation, and post-weaning recovery. Physiol Rev 2016;96:449–547.

Parfitt AM. Misconceptions (3): calcium leaves bone only by resorption and enters only by formation. Bone. 2003;33(3):259–63.

The Adrenal Glands

15

Filippo Ceccato, Carla Scaroni, and Marco Boscaro

Abstract

The adrenal glands (also known as suprarenal glands) are endocrine glands, found above the kidneys, which produce a variety of intracellular hormones.

Steroidogenesis is the complex pathway used to transform cholesterol in steroid hormones. Three main types of steroids are produced by the adrenal cortex: glucocorticoids (cortisol), mineralocorticoids (aldosterone), and sex steroids (mainly androgens). Corticotropin (adrenocorticotropic hormone, ACTH) is the principal hormone stimulating adrenal glucocorticoid biosynthesis and secretion; it is produced in the anterior pituitary and derives from pro-opiomelanocortin (POMC). The most important aspect of pituitary–adrenal axis control is the negative feedback control exerted by cortisol (and so glucocorticoids), inhibiting both POMC gene transcription in the anterior pituitary and CRH mRNA synthesis and secretion in the hypothalamus. Aldosterone, controlled by the renin–angiotensin system, is involved mainly in the cardiovascular homeostasis. Since renin–aldosterone is one of the main regulators of blood pressure, several drugs have been developed to block this system. Both cortisol and aldosterone exert their effects following uptake of free hormone from the circulation and binding to intracellular receptors, termed the glucocorticoid and mineralocorticoid receptors. These are both members of the thyroid/steroid hormone receptor superfamily of transcription factors comprising a C-terminal ligand-binding domain, a central DNA-binding domain interacting with specific DNA sequences on target genes.

The term catecholamine refers to substances that contain catechol and a side chain with an amino group – the catechol nucleus. Adrenomedullary cells are also called chromaffin cells, because cytoplasmic granules stain brown with chromium salts,

F. Ceccato (✉) • C. Scaroni • M. Boscaro
Endocrinology Unit, Department of Medicine DIMED, University-Hospital of Padova, Padova, Italy
e-mail: ceccato.filippo@gmail.com; carla.scaroni@unipd.it; marco.boscaro@unipd.it

A. Belfiore, D. LeRoith (eds.), *Principles of Endocrinology and Hormone Action*, Endocrinology, https://doi.org/10.1007/978-3-319-44675-2_16

due to the oxidation of epinephrine and norepinephrine to melanin. Catecholamines affect many cardiovascular and metabolic processes, including increasing the heart rate, blood pressure, myocardial contractility, and cardiac conduction velocity.

Keywords
Adrenal glands • Physiology • Steroidogenesis • Catecholamine

Contents

Anatomy

The adrenal glands (also known as suprarenal glands) are endocrine glands, found above the kidneys, which produce a variety of intracellular hormones.

Bartolomeo Eustachi, also known by his Latin name of Eustachius, was one of the founders of the science of human anatomy. He was an Italian anatomist, and he first described the adrenal glands in 1500. However, these publications were part of the papal library and did not receive public attention, which was first received with Caspar Bartholin 100 years after. The adrenal glands are named for their location relative to the kidneys. The term "adrenal" comes from *ad* (Latin, "near") and *renes* (Latin, "kidney"). Until the nineteenth century, there was some debate as to whether the glands were indeed suprarenal or part of the kidney, and the suprarenal nature of the glands was not truly accepted; then anatomists clarified the ductless nature of the glands and their only secretory role.

The adrenal glands have a pyramidal structure and are located on both sides of the body in the retroperitoneum, above and slightly medial to the kidneys, or on its posteromedial surface. In humans, the right adrenal gland is pyramidal in shape, whereas the left is semilunar and somewhat larger. The glands are usually yellowish in color and about $5 \times 3 \times 1$ cm in size, and their combined weight is about 7–10 g (in adult, because the newborn adrenal glands are bigger and weigh approximately 20–25% of the total body).

The adrenal glands are surrounded by a fatty capsule and lie within the renal fascia, which also surrounds the kidneys, separated from the kidneys with a wall of connective tissue. The adrenal glands are directly below the diaphragm and are attached to the crura of the diaphragm by the renal fascia.

Each gland has an outer *cortex*, which produces steroid hormones, divided into three zones as summarized in Fig. 1:

- Zona glomerulosa, 15–20%, secreting mineralocorticoids (mainly aldosterone)
- Zona fasciculata, 60–70%, secreting glucocorticoids (mainly cortisol)
- Zona reticularis, 10–15%, secreting androgens (mainly androstenedione) and an inner *medulla*, which produces catecholamines

The vasculature is complex. The adrenal glands have one of the greatest blood supply rates per gram of tissue, divided in three principal arteries that usually supply each adrenal gland:

- The superior suprarenal artery, a branch of the inferior phrenic artery
- The middle suprarenal artery, a direct branch of the abdominal aorta
- The inferior suprarenal artery, a branch of the renal artery

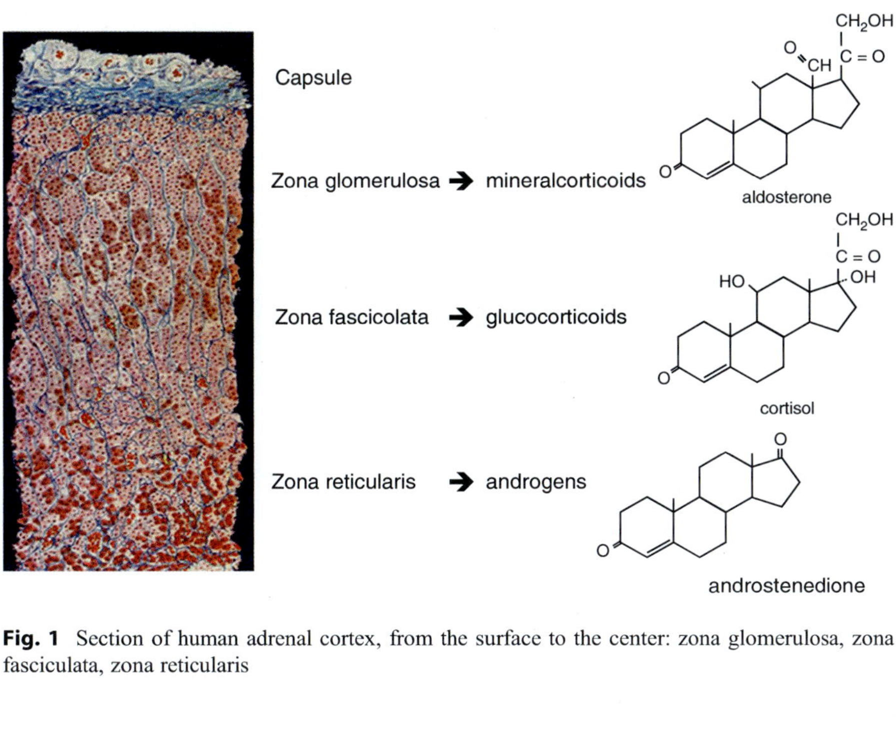

Fig. 1 Section of human adrenal cortex, from the surface to the center: zona glomerulosa, zona fasciculata, zona reticularis

These blood vessels supply a network of small arteries within the capsule of the adrenal glands. Thin strands of the capsule enter the glands, carrying blood to them. In the zona reticularis, a dense sinusoidal plexus is created, which empties into a central vein, the suprarenal veins: the right adrenal vein is short and drains into the inferior vena cava, while the longer left adrenal vein drains into the left renal vein or the left inferior phrenic vein (this anatomical difference is one of the most important issue when a surgeon perform adrenalectomy). The central adrenomedullary vein, in the adrenal medulla, is an unusual type of blood vessel and different from the other veins: the smooth muscle in its tunica media (the middle layer of the vessel) is arranged in conspicuous, longitudinally oriented bundles (Mesiano and Jaffe 1997; Jaffe et al. 1998).

Adrenal Cortex

The adrenal cortex derives from mesenchymal cells attached to the coelomic cavity, adjacent to the urogenital ridge. The fetal adrenal is evident after 2 months and rapidly increases in size: by midgestation it is larger than the kidney. In fetal life, and up to 12 months postpartum, two distinct zones are evident, an inner prominent fetal zone and an outer definitive zone that differentiates into the adult adrenal gland. Postpartum the fetal zone regresses to adult adrenal. The innermost zone, the zona reticularis, is evident after 1 year of life. The differentiation of the adrenal cortex into distinct zones has important functional consequences and is thought to be dependent upon the temporal expression of peculiar transcription factors (Vinson 2016).

Beneath the capsule, the zona glomerulosa comprises approximately 15% of the cortex (depending upon sodium intake); cells are clustered in spherical nests and are small with small nuclei. The zona fasciculata comprises 75% of the cortex (therefore cortisol secretion is higher than aldosterone production); cells are large and lipid laden and form radial cords between the fibrovascular radial networks. The innermost zona reticularis is sharply demarcated from both the zona fasciculata and adrenal medulla; cells here are irregular with little lipid content (Mesiano and Jaffe 1997; Okamoto and Takemori 2000).

Adrenal Medulla

The adrenal medulla occupies the central portion of the adrenal gland and accounts for 10% of the total adrenal gland volume, although there is no clear demarcation between the adrenal cortex and medulla. Some of the plexus arteries penetrate the cortex and supply the medulla, as capillaries do, forming the corticomedullary portal system.

Adrenomedullary cells are also called chromaffin cells, because cytoplasmic granules stain brown with chromium salts, due to the oxidation of epinephrine and norepinephrine to melanin. Chromaffin cells differentiate in the center of the adrenal gland in response to cortisol; some chromaffin cells also migrate to form paraganglia, collections of chromaffin cells on both sides of the aorta. The largest cluster of chromaffin cells outside the adrenal medulla is near the level of the inferior mesenteric artery and is referred to as the organ of Zuckerkandl, which is the major source of catecholamines in the first year of life. The preganglionic sympathetic neurons receive synaptic input from neurons within the pons, medulla, and hypothalamus, providing regulation of sympathetic activity by the brain. Adrenal medulla is innervated via splanchnic nerves through axons from the lower thoracic and lumbar preganglionic neurons.

Human Steroidogenesis and Control

Steroidogenesis

Three main types of steroids are produced by the adrenal cortex:

- Glucocorticoids (cortisol)
- Mineralocorticoids (aldosterone)
- Sex steroids (mainly androgens)

All steroid hormones derived from the cyclopentanoperhydrophenanthrene structure, based upon three cyclohexane rings and a single cyclopentane ring. The carbon atoms are indicated by numbers, and the rings are designated by letters according to standard convention (Fig. 2).

As depicted in Fig. 2, there are four rings in a steroid skeleton and hence there are three fusion points: A/B, B/C, and C/D rings share two carbons each (called fusion center). Every fusion center can either be *cis*- or *trans*-fused. The three-dimensional structures of the major part of natural steroids are *trans-trans-trans*: the structure of a steroid molecule is essential for the binding with the receptor; little modification could increase this affinity.

Fig. 2 Cyclopentanoperhydrophenanthrene structure: three cyclohexane rings (**a–d**) and a single cyclopentane ring (**d**)

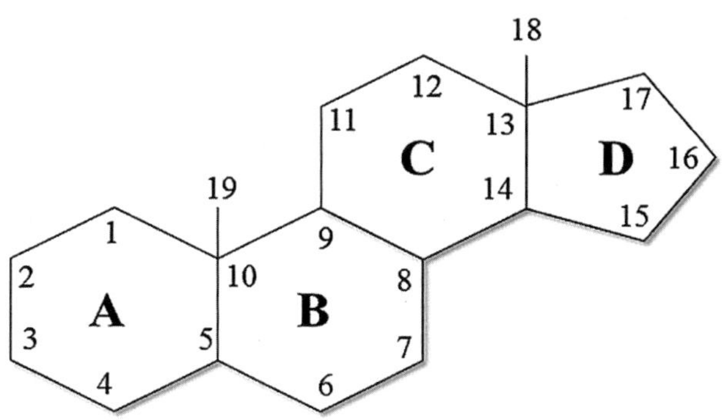

Table 1 IUPAC and trivial names of natural and synthetic steroids (IUPAC 1972)

Trivial name	IUPAC name
Aldosterone	4-Pregnen-11β,21-diol-3,18,20-trione
Androstenedione	4-Androsten-3,17-dione
Cortisol	4-Pregnen-11β,17α,21-triol-3,20-dione
Cortisone	4-Pregnen-17α,21-diol-3,11,20-trione
Dehydroepiandrosterone	5-Androsten-3β-ol-17-one
Deoxycorticosterone	4-Pregnen-21-ol-3,20-dione
Dexamethasone	1,4-Pregnadien-9α-fluoro-16α-methyl-11β,17α,21-triol-3,20-dione
Dihydrotestosterone	5α-Androstan-17β-ol-3-one
Estradiol	1,3,5(10)-Estratrien-3,17β-diol
Fludrocortisone	4-Pregnen-9α-fluoro-11β,17α,21-triol-3,20-dione
17-Hydroxyprogesterone	4-Pregnen-17α-ol-3,20-dione
Methylprednisolone	1,4-Pregnadien-6α-methyl-11β,17α,21-triol-3,20-dione
Prednisolone	1,4-Pregnadien-11β,17α,21-triol-3,20-dione
Prednisone	1,4-Pregnadien-17α,21-diol-3,11,20-trione
Pregnenolone	5-Pregnen-3β-ol-20-one
Progesterone	4-Pregnen-3,20-dione
Testosterone	4-Androsten-17β-ol-3-one
Triamcinolone	1,4-Pregnadien-9α-fluoro-11β,16α,17α,21-tetrol-3,20-dione

Steroid nomenclature is usually defined in two ways: by trivial names (e.g., cortisol, aldosterone), the most used in the scientific literature, or by the chemical structure as defined by the International Union of Pure and Applied Chemistry (Table 1). The number of carbon atoms is also used to separate steroids: estrogens have 18 carbon atoms (C18 steroids) and androgens have 19 carbon atoms (C19), while glucocorticoids/progestogens are C21 steroid derivatives (see Fig. 3).

Cholesterol is the first step of steroid synthesis. The sources of cholesterol are:

- *Dietary cholesterol.* Uptake of LDL (low-density lipoproteins) in adrenal is mediated by LDL receptors; LDL are then internalized via receptor-mediated endocytosis, the resulting vesicles fuse with lysozymes, and free cholesterol is produced following hydrolysis.
- *De novo cholesterol synthesis.* Within the adrenal cortex from acetate (acetyl coenzyme A).

Children with abetalipoproteinemia or defective LDL receptors still have normal basal adrenal steroidogenesis, thanks to de novo cholesterol synthesis in adrenals (which is physiologically used in part, since LDL uptake is easier). Adrenal steroidogenesis is summarized in Fig. 4. The initial hormone-dependent rate-limiting step is the transport of intracellular cholesterol (regardless whether derived from LDL or de novo production) from the outer to inner mitochondrial membrane to create pregnenolone. Steroidogenic acute regulatory protein (StAR) is a 30-κD

Fig. 3 Structure of some endogenous and synthetic steroids

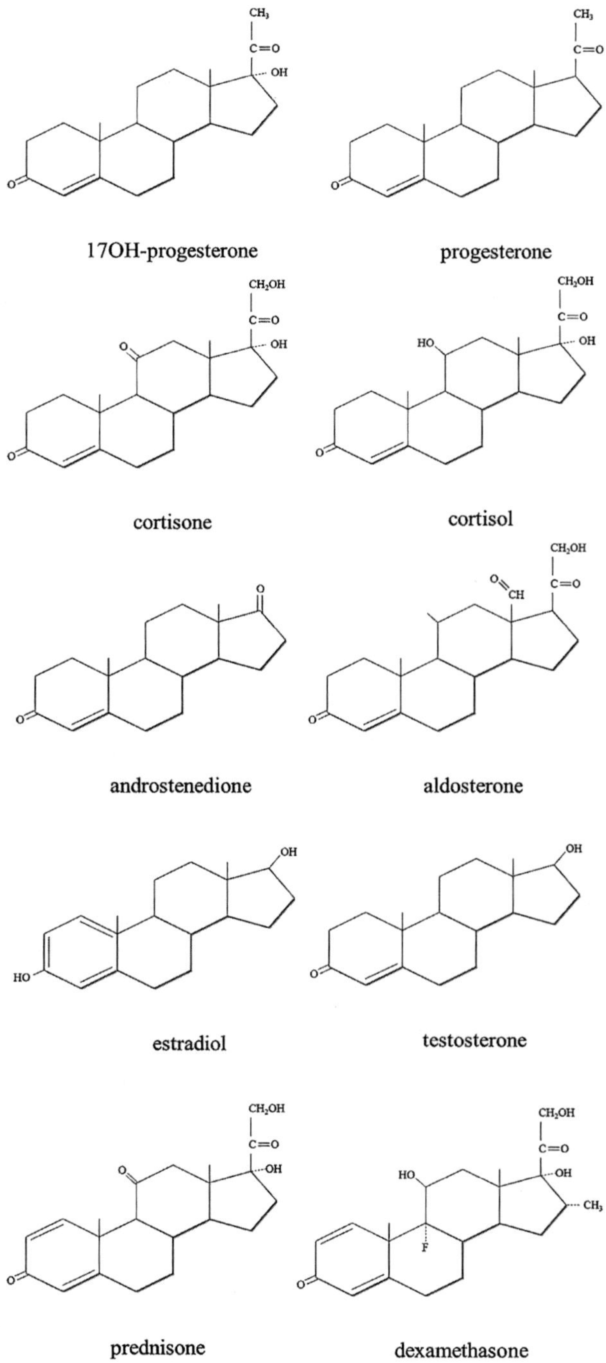

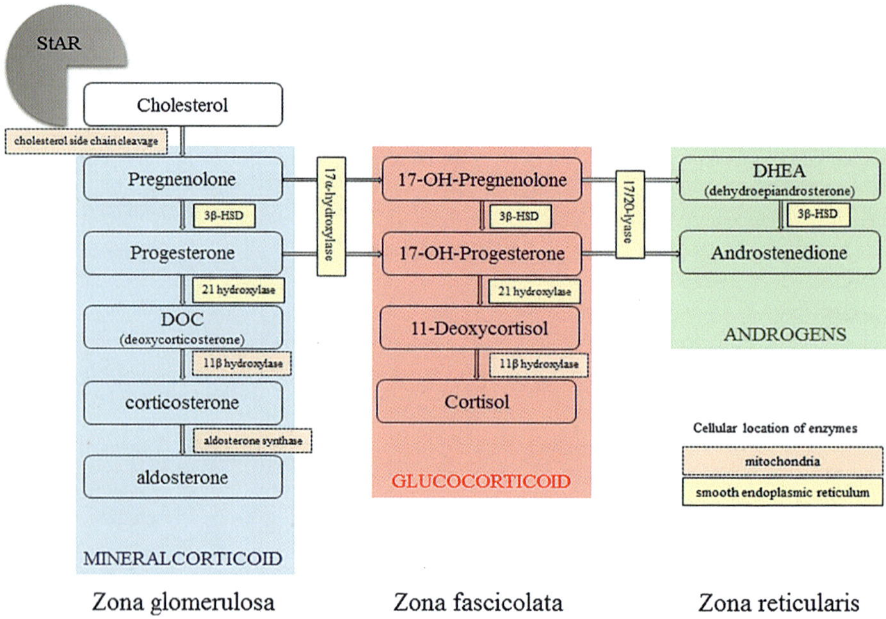

Fig. 4 Adrenal steroidogenesis

protein cytochrome P450 enzyme, called side-chain cleavage. The binding of ACTH to its receptor, in the adrenal cell, mediates an increase in intracellular cAMP (cyclic adenosine monophosphate), providing the first important rate-limiting and controlled step in adrenal steroidogenesis (Midzak and Papadopoulos 2016).

Most enzymes involved in steroid biosynthesis are either cytochrome P450s (CYPs, termed pigment 450 because all absorb light at 450 nm) or hydroxysteroid dehydrogenase (HSD). All enzymes have been cloned and characterized functionally; all enzymes are in general unidirectional, although not absolutely, in normal adrenals, the accumulation of products does not drive flux back to the precursor. All P450-mediated hydroxylations and carbon–carbon bond cleavage reactions are mechanistically and physiologically irreversible. On the other hand, only in in vitro conditions, HSD reactions are mechanistically reversible and can run in either direction under certain conditions. Cholesterol side-chain cleavage enzyme (StAR) and the CYP11B enzymes are localized to the mitochondria and require an electron shuttle system. 17α-Hydroxylase and 21-hydroxylase enzymes are localized in the microsomal/endoplasmic reticulum fraction and require electron transfer from NADPH by the enzyme P450 oxidoreductase (P450-OR). In addition, the 17,20-lyase activity of P450 CYP17 is dependent upon a flavoprotein that functions as an allosteric facilitator of the CYP17 and P450-OR interaction. Mutations in the genes encoding these enzymes result in human disease.

Steroidogenesis is a complex pathway. Briefly, after cholesterol uptake in the mitochondria, it is cleaved by the P450 enzyme cholesterol side-chain cleavage

(StAR) to pregnenolone. In the cytoplasm, pregnenolone is converted to progesterone by the type II isozyme of 3β-hydroxysteroid dehydrogenase by a reaction involving dehydrogenation of the 3-hydroxyl group and isomerization of the double bond at C5. Progesterone is then hydroxylated to 17-OH progesterone through the activity of CYP 17α-hydroxylase. 17-Hydroxylation is an essential prerequisite for glucocorticoid synthesis (especially cortisol), and the zona glomerulosa (which produces mainly mineralocorticoid, aldosterone) does not express 17-hydroxylase. CYP 17α-hydroxylase also possesses 17,20-lyase activity, which results in the production of the C19 adrenal androgens, dehydroepiandrosterone, and androstenedione. In humans, however, 17-OH progesterone is not an efficient substrate for CYP 17α-hydroxylase, and there is negligible conversion of 17-OH progesterone to androstenedione. Adrenal androstenedione secretion is dependent upon the conversion of dehydroepiandrosterone to androstenedione by 3β-HSD – this enzyme will also convert 17-OH pregnenolone to 17-OH progesterone, but the preferred substrate is pregnenolone.

21-Hydroxylase, derived from CYP21A2 gene, performs 21-hydroxylation of progesterone to deoxycorticosterone (in the zona glomerulosa) or 17-OH progesterone to 11-deoxycortisol (in the zona fasciculata). The final step in cortisol biosynthesis takes place in the mitochondria and involves the conversion of 11-deoxycortisol to cortisol by the enzyme CYP11B1, 11β-hydroxylase. In the zona glomerulosa, 11β-hydroxylase may also convert deoxycorticosterone to corticosterone. However, the enzyme CYP11B2 (aldosterone synthase) may also carry out this reaction and, in addition, is required for the conversion of corticosterone to aldosterone via the intermediate 18-OH corticosterone. Thus, CYP11B2 (expressed in the zona glomerulosa, in a typical zonal and functional control of steroidogenesis) can carry out 11β-hydroxylation, 18-hydroxylation, and 18-methyl oxidation to yield the characteristic C11–18 hemi-acetyl structure of aldosterone (Miller 1988; Miller and Auchus 2011).

Human Steroidogenesis in Clinical Practice: Disease and Drugs

Adrenal steroidogenesis inhibitors have been the mainstay of medical treatment for Cushing's syndrome (CS).

- Ketoconazole is an imidazole fungicide that has been used off-label to reduce hypercortisolism because of its effect in considerably inhibiting the activity of cytochrome P450 adrenal steroidogenic enzymes, including 11β-, 17α-, and 18-hydroxylase. Dosages varied from 200 to 1,200 mg/day, and biochemical efficacy was usually achieved with 600–800 mg/day, obtaining overall response rates of 53–88% in CS.
- Metyrapone has been used successfully in some countries for 40 years. It inhibits the conversion of 11-deoxycortisol into cortisol by 11β-hydroxylase (CYP11B1), with a nadir in cortisol levels within 2 h of its administration; CS was controlled in 75% of patients in few weeks using a median dose of 2,000 mg/day in weeks 1–3, which was raised to 2,250 mg/day (range 500–6,000) by week 6. Its side effects depend on the excess of adrenal mineralocorticoids and androgens due to the

CYP11B1 blockade causing hypertension, edema, hypokalemia, and hirsutism in women. LCI699 is an 11β-hydroxylase inhibitor similar to metyrapone, except that it is 100 times more potent.

- Mitotane [1-(2-chlorophenyl)-1-(4-chlorophenyl)-2,2-dichloroethane (o, p′-DDD)] has been used in adrenocortical carcinoma for several years, as an adjuvant therapy, or to reduce cortisol levels in severe form of CS, the specific mechanisms underlying its adrenolytic action (with a direct cytotoxic effect on the adrenal cortex) and anti-steroidogenic effect are not fully understood (Ceccato et al. 2015).

Congenital adrenal hyperplasia (CAH) is a group of autosomal recessive disorders characterized by impaired cortisol synthesis, ranging from 1:10,000 to 1:20,000 births. The most common form of CAH is caused by mutations in CYP21A2, causing 21-hydroxylase deficiency (21OHD). In addition to the salt-wasting (75% of cases) and simple virilizing forms of 21OHD, there is also a mild nonclassic CAH form, which may show variable degrees of postnatal androgen excess and does not lead to severe cortisol insufficiency. Nonclassic forms of CAH are more prevalent, occurring in approximately 0.1–0.2% in the general Caucasian population. In the complete absence of 21-hydroxylase P450c21 activity (the salt-wasting form), inability to convert progesterone to deoxycorticosterone results also in aldosterone deficiency (other than cortisol insufficiency) causing severe hyponatremia, hyperkalemia, and acidosis with concomitant hypotension, shock, cardiovascular collapse, and death in untreated newborns. The goal of 21OHD therapy is to reduce excessive androgen secretion by replacing the deficient hormones (cortisol, and aldosterone if needed).

Another rare disease concerning steroidogenesis enzyme is 3β-hydroxysteroid dehydrogenase (3β-HSD), characterized by a variable glucocorticoid and mineralocorticoid deficiency that may be fatal if not diagnosed early in infancy. In its classic form, genetic females may have clitoromegaly and mild virilization because the fetal adrenal overproduces large amounts of dehydroepiandrosterone, a small portion of which is converted to testosterone via extra-adrenal 3β HSD1. Genetic males also synthesize some androgens by peripheral conversion of adrenal and testicular dehydroepiandrosterone, but the concentrations are insufficient for complete male genital development so that these males have a small phallus and severe hypospadias.

Regulation of Adrenal Steroidogenesis

"Functional Zonation" of the Adrenal Cortex

Glucocorticoids are secreted in relatively high amounts (cortisol 10–20 mg/day) from the zona fasciculata under the control of ACTH. Recently a more precise estimation of endogenous cortisol production rate, believed to be around 9–11 mg/m^2/day (so a normal man with 1.73 m^2 of body area produces 16–19 mg/die that has to be considered during glucocorticoid treatment), has recently led to the dosage of glucocorticoid replacement therapy being reduced. In other words, since there are no defined tools to titrate cortisol therapy in adrenal insufficiency, this estimation and clinical features are essential to avoid cortisol overtreatment and to reduce the risk of mild but chronic glucocorticoid replacement therapies (able to induce osteoporosis, hypertension, diabetes as in Cushing's syndrome).

Mineralocorticoids are secreted in low amounts (aldosterone 100–150 μg/day) from the zona glomerulosa under the principal control of angiotensin II. In "mineralocorticoid-target" tissues, there is relatively "high" concentration of aldosterone than cortisol, since cortisol is metabolized to cortisone (to prevent activation of the mineralocorticoid receptor by cortisol) by the 11β-hydroxysteroid dehydrogenase type 2, expressed in many tissues such as the kidney, colon, salivary glands, and placenta.

As a class, adrenal androgens are the most abundant steroids secreted from the adult adrenal gland (>20 mg/day), but their role is not yet fully understood.

Steroidogenesis is guided through the expression of steroidogenic enzymes in a specific "zonal" manner. The zona glomerulosa cannot synthesize cortisol because it does not express 17α-hydroxylase. In contrast, aldosterone secretion is confined to the outer zona glomerulosa through the restricted expression of CYP11B2 (aldosterone synthase). Although CYP11B1 and CYP11B2 share 95% homology, the 5′ promoter sequences differ and permit regulation of the final steps in glucocorticoid and mineralocorticoid biosynthesis by ACTH and angiotensin II, respectively. In the zona reticularis, high levels of cytochrome b5 confer 17,20-lyase activity upon CYP17 and androgen production. The difference between CYP11B1 and CYP11B2 has recently been used to develop a novel CYP11B2-specific nuclear imaging agent for detection of primary aldosteronism during positron emission tomography, since adrenal vein sampling (the gold standard method for lateralization) is an invasive and technically difficult procedure (Abe et al. 2016).

Dehydroepiandrosterone is sulfated in the zona reticularis by the sulfotransferase to form dehydroepiandrosterone sulfate. In the fetal adrenal, steroidogenesis occurs primarily within the inner fetal zone. Because of a relative lack of 3β-HSD and high sulfotransferase activity, the principal steroidogenic products are DHEA and DHEAS, which are then aromatized by placental trophoblast to estrogens. Thus, the majority of maternal estrogen across pregnancy is, indirectly, fetally derived.

Classical endocrine feedback loops are in place to control the secretion of both hormones – cortisol inhibits the secretion of both corticotropin-releasing factor and ACTH from the hypothalamus and pituitary, respectively, and the aldosterone-induced sodium retention inhibits renal renin secretion.

Pro-opiomelanocortin and ACTH

Corticotropin (adrenocorticotropic hormone, ACTH) is the principal hormone stimulating adrenal glucocorticoid biosynthesis and secretion. ACTH has 39 amino acids and is synthesized within the anterior pituitary as part of a much larger 241 amino acid precursor, pro-opiomelanocortin (POMC). POMC is cleaved in a tissue-specific fashion to yield smaller peptide hormones.

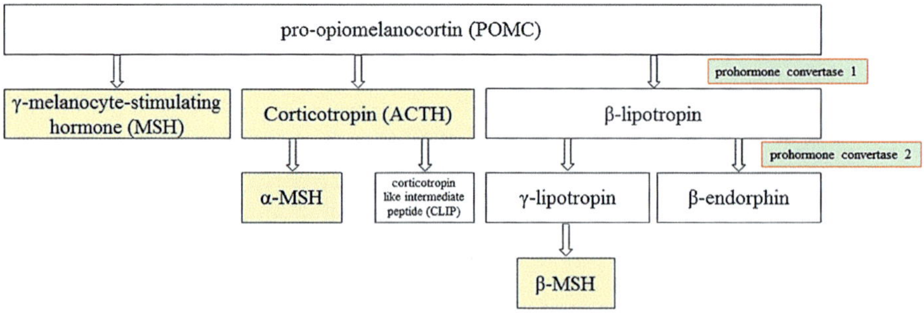

Fig. 5 Synthesis and cleavage of pro-opiomelanocortin within the human anterior pituitary gland

Proprotein convertase 1, also known as prohormone convertase, is an enzyme encoded by the PCSK1 gene. Prohormone convertase 1 cleaves pro-opiomelanocortin and is similar to that involved in the process proinsulin and proglucagon in pancreatic islets. In the anterior pituitary, this results in the secretion of β-lipoprotein (β-LPH) and pro-ACTH, the latter being further cleaved to an N-terminal peptide, joining peptide and ACTH itself (Fig. 5).

The first 24 amino acids of ACTH are common to all species, and synthetic ACTH 1–24 (Synacthen) is available commercially for clinical testing of the hypothalamic–pituitary–adrenal (HPA) axis. Melanocyte-stimulating hormones (a, β, and γ) are also cleaved products from POMC, but the increased pigmentation characteristic of Addison's disease or Nelson's syndrome is thought to arise directly from increased ACTH concentrations binding to the melanocortin-1 receptor rather than the result of high serum α-MSH levels.

POMC is also transcribed in the brain, liver, kidney, gonad, and placenta. In these tissues, POMC mRNA is usually shorter than the pituitary 1,200-bp species due to lack of exons 1 and 2 and the 5′ region of exon 3. As a result, it is probable that these POMC-like peptides are not secreted and are not active (low affinity to ACTH receptor). However, in ectopic ACTH syndrome, additional POMC mRNA species are described, which are longer than normal pituitary 1,200-bp POMC species (typically 1,450 bp) due to the use of alternative promoters in the 5′ region of the gene, explaining the resistance of POMC secretion to glucocorticoid feedback in these neuroendocrine tumors (in pituitary a low dose of glucocorticoid is able to suppress ACTH). The cleavage of POMC is also tissue specific, and, at least in some cases of ectopic ACTH syndrome, it is possible that circulating ACTH precursors, notably pro-ACTH, may cross-react in current ACTH radioimmunoassays (although they are not hormonally active).

POMC expression and processing within neurons in the hypothalamus, specifically the generation of α-MSH that interacts with MCR-4 receptors, appear to be of crucial importance in energy control.

ACTH binds to a G-protein-coupled, melanocortin-2 receptor; signal transduction is cAMP mediated, although both extracellular and intracellular Ca^{2+} play a role. Other factors synergize with or inhibit the effects of ACTH on the adrenal cortex, including angiotensin II, activin, inhibin, and cytokines (TNF-α and leptin). Cell-to-cell communication via gap junctions is also important in mediating the effects of ACTH that are both rapid and chronic; the end result is the stimulation of adrenal steroidogenesis and growth (in ACTH-dependent Cushing's syndrome, it is common to find adrenal hyperplasia during abdominal imaging). Acutely, steroidogenesis is stimulated through a StAR-mediated increase in cholesterol delivery to the CYP11A1 enzyme in the inner mitochondrial membrane. Chronically (within 24–26 h of exposure), ACTH acts to increase the synthesis of all steroidogenic enzymes. ACTH also increases synthesis of the LDL receptors and possibly also HMG-CoA reductase, the rate-limiting step in cholesterol biosynthesis. ACTH increases adrenal weight by inducing both hyperplasia and hypertrophy, and on the contrary, ACTH deficiency causes adrenal atrophy (Chrétien 2016).

Corticotropin-Releasing Hormone and Other Hypothalamic Controls

POMC secretion is controlled by numerous factors, the main of which is corticotropin-releasing hormone (CRH). Additional control is provided through an endogenous circadian rhythm, stress and feedback inhibition by cortisol itself. CRH is a 41 amino acid peptide that is synthesized in neurons within the paraventricular nucleus of the hypothalamus. Ovine CRH differs from human by seven amino acids; it is slightly more potent than human CRH in stimulating ACTH secretion and is therefore used to perform CRH test (used in the differential diagnosis of ACTH-dependent CS). CRH is secreted into the hypophyseal portal blood, where it binds to specific receptors on corticotroph cells; this binding is able to stimulate POMC gene transcription through adenylate cyclase. It is unclear whether hypothalamic CRH contributes in any way to circulating levels; CRH is also synthesized in other tissues, and it is likely that circulating CRH reflects synthesis from testis, gastrointestinal tract, adrenal medulla, and particularly the placenta, where the increased secretion across pregnancy results in a threefold increase in circulating CRH levels. In the circulation, CRH is bound to CRH-binding protein (CRH-BP); levels of CRH-BP also increase during pregnancy so that cortisol secretion is not markedly elevated. CRH is the principal stimulus for ACTH secretion, but AVP is able to potentiate CRH-mediated secretion (Smith and Funder 1988; Lovejoy et al. 2014).

Physical stresses increase ACTH and cortisol secretion, again through central actions mediated via CRH and AVP. Thus, cortisol secretion rises in response to stress events (fever, surgery, burn injury, hypoglycemia, hypotension, exercise, and so on). In all of these cases, this can be viewed as a normal counterregulatory response to the insult. Intriguingly, although acute psychological stress will raise cortisol levels, its secretion rates appear to be normal in patients with chronic anxiety states.

Circadian Rhythm

ACTH, and as a consequence cortisol, is secreted in a pulsatile fashion with a circadian rhythm so that levels are highest on wakening and decline throughout the day, reaching nadir values in the evening (see Fig. 6).

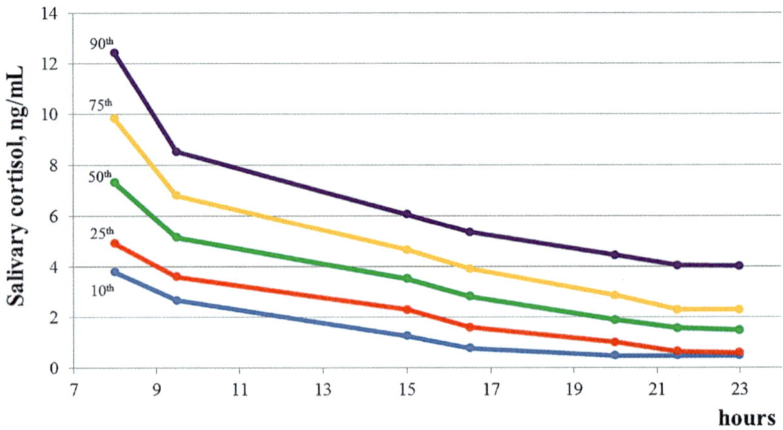

Fig. 6 Figure 1: Percentiles of salivary cortisol (depicting physiological rhythm) in 120 healthy subjects

Moreover, this circadian rhythm is impaired in patients with endogenous Cushing's syndrome, which is characterized by increased night cortisol values that could be easily measured in saliva as salivary cortisol.

ACTH and cortisol are secreted in rather irregular pulses: both pulse frequency and amplitude contribute to connect circulating levels and function in the receptor. Cortisol presents an ultradian periodicity of around 1 h, and it has been speculated that this is an intrinsic part of glucocorticoid signaling.

ACTH pulse frequency is higher in normal adult males compared with females (on average, 18 pulses versus 10 pulses/24 h), and the circadian ACTH rhythm appears to be mediated principally by an increased ACTH pulse amplitude between 05.00 and 09.00 h but also by a reduction in ACTH pulse frequency between 18.00 and 24.00 h. Food ingestion is a further stimulus to ACTH secretion. Circadian rhythm is dependent upon both day–night and sleep–wake patterns and is disrupted by alternating day–night shift working patterns and by long-distance travel across time zones: it may take up to 2 weeks for circadian rhythm to reset to an altered day–night cycle (Gamble et al. 2014).

Negative Feedback

An important aspect of CRH and ACTH secretion is the negative feedback control exerted by cortisol (and so glucocorticoids), inhibiting both POMC gene transcription in the anterior pituitary and CRH mRNA synthesis and secretion in the hypothalamus. This negative feedback effect is dependent upon the dose, potency, half-life, and duration of administration of the glucocorticoid: suppression of the HPA axis by pharmacologic corticosteroids may persist for many months after cessation of therapy. Diagnostically, the lost of feedback mechanism in Addison's disease explains ACTH hypersecretion and undetectable ACTH levels in patients with a cortisol-secreting adrenal adenoma. Feedback inhibition is principally mediated via the glucocorticoid receptor (GR). Moreover, negative feedback is checked in a screening test for Cushing's syndrome diagnosis: in normal subjects, the administration of a supraphysiological dose of glucocorticoid results in suppression of cortisol secretion: 1 mg DST, which explores this normal feedback of the hypothalamic–pituitary–adrenal (HPA) axis, is a simple dynamic test, usually performed in outpatients. A morning serum cortisol <50 nmol/l is sufficient to exclude Cushing's, unless high clinical suspicion.

Mineralocorticoid Secretion: The Renin–Angiotensin–Aldosterone Axis

Aldosterone is secreted from the zona glomerulosa under the control of three principal factors: angiotensin II (the so-called renin–angiotensin–aldosterone system, RAA), potassium, and to a lesser extent ACTH (El Ghorayeb et al. 2016).

The secretion of aldosterone is restricted to the zona glomerulosa because of the zonal-specific expression of aldosterone synthase. Corticosterone and deoxycorticosterone, while synthesized in both the zona fasciculata and glomerulosa, can act as mineralocorticoids, which become significant in some clinical conditions (as congenital adrenal hyperplasia, adrenal-secreting tumors, or therapy with metyrapone, in Cushing's syndrome). Similarly, cortisol can act as a mineralocorticoid in the setting of impaired metabolism to cortisone carried out by the enzyme 11β-hydroxysteroid dehydrogenase; this is important in patients with resistant severe hypertension (i.e., in apparent mineralocorticoid excess, AME), ectopic ACTH syndrome, and renal disease. In AME, a rare autosomal recessive disorder causing severe hypervolemic hypertension and hypokalemic alkalosis (similar to primary hyperaldosteronism), increased levels of tissue cortisol (in mineralocorticoid-target tissue, as the kidney) are able to activate the mineralocorticoid receptor (cortisol and aldosterone share similar affinity to mineralocorticoid receptor), leading to aldosterone-like effects in the kidney. AME differential diagnosis is based upon suppressed plasma renin activity and absence of measurable serum mineralocorticoids (aldosterone) and confirmed with cortisol-to-cortisone ratio (if available). AME responds to glucocorticoid treatment (administered to suppress endogenous cortisol secretion), and hypertension is treated with spironolactone (mineralocorticoid receptor antagonist).

Angiotensin II and potassium stimulate aldosterone secretion principally by increasing the transcription of CYP11B2 through common intracellular signaling pathways, with cAMP, intracellular Ca^{2+}, and activation of calmodulin kinases. The potassium effect is mediated through membrane depolarization and opening of calcium channels.

The effect of ACTH upon aldosterone secretion is modest and differs in time: an acute ACTH bolus (used to test HPA axis and cortisol reserve) will increase aldosterone secretion, principally by stimulating the early pathways of adrenal steroidogenesis but no effect upon CYP11B2 gene transcription. Contrariwise, chronic continual ACTH stimulation has either no effect or an inhibitory effect on aldosterone production, possibly because of receptor downregulation or suppression of angiotensin II-stimulated secretion because of a mineralocorticoid effect of cortisol, DOC, or corticosterone. Dopamine, heparin, and atrial natriuretic peptide inhibit aldosterone secretion.

The separate control of glucocorticoid biosynthesis through the HPA axis and mineralocorticoid synthesis via the RAA system has important clinical consequences. Patients with primary adrenal failure invariably have both cortisol and aldosterone deficiencies, whereas patients with ACTH deficiency due to pituitary disease have only glucocorticoid deficiency; in the latter, aldosterone concentrations are normal because the RAA system is intact (see Fig. 7).

Approximately 50–70% of aldosterone circulates bound to either albumin or weakly to corticosteroid-binding globulin; 30–50% of the total plasma aldosterone is free, with a short half-life of 15–20 min. In the liver, aldosterone is rapidly inactivated to tetrahydroaldosterone. The classic functions of aldosterone are regulation of extracellular volume and control of potassium homeostasis. These effects are mediated by binding of free aldosterone to the mineralocorticoid receptor in the cytosol of epithelial cells, principally in the kidney. Mineralocorticoid receptors have a tissue-specific expression: distal nephron, colon, and hippocampus present the highest concentrations of mineralocorticoid receptors. Aldosterone leads to modification of the apical sodium channel, resulting in increased sodium ion transport across the cell membrane. Glucocorticoids and mineralocorticoids bind equally to the mineralocorticoid receptor. Specificity of action is provided in many tissues by the presence of a glucocorticoid-degrading enzyme, 11β-hydroxysteroid dehydrogenase, which prevents glucocorticoids from interacting with the receptor. Mineralocorticoid "escape" refers to the counterregulatory mechanisms that are manifested after 3–5 days of excessive mineralocorticoid administration.

Renin is an enzyme produced primarily in the juxtaglomerular apparatus of the kidney; it is stored in granules and released in response to specific secretagogues. The protein consists of 340 amino acids; the first 43 are a prosegment cleaved to produce the active enzyme. Renin release is controlled by:

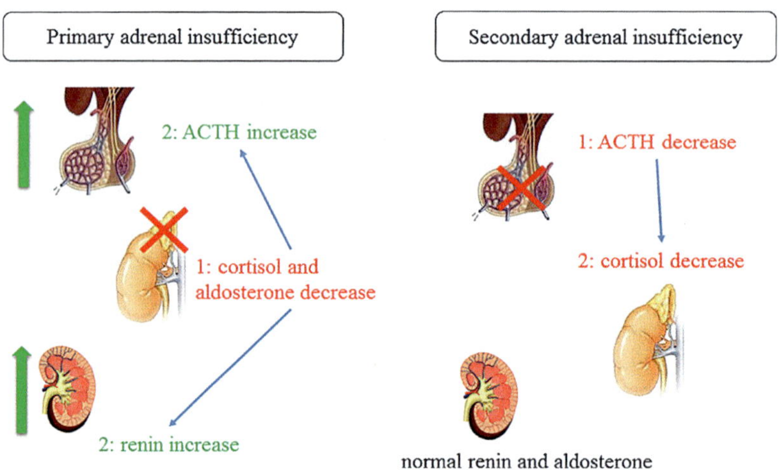

Fig. 7 Difference between primary (adrenal) and secondary adrenal insufficiency

- The macula densa, a specialized group of distal convoluted tubular cells that function as chemoreceptors for monitoring the sodium concentration.
- Juxtaglomerular cells acting as pressure transducers that sense stretch of the afferent arteriolar wall and thus renal perfusion pressure.
- The sympathetic nervous system, which modifies the release of renin, particularly in response to upright posture in humans.
- Potassium: renin release is increased directly by hypokalemia and decreased by hyperkalemia.

Thus, renin release is maximized in conditions of low renal perfusion pressure or low tubular sodium content (e.g., renal artery stenosis, hemorrhage, dehydration). Renin release is suppressed by elevated perfusion pressure at the kidney (i.e., arterial hypertension) and high-sodium diets.

Since renin–aldosterone is one of the main regulators of blood pressure, several drugs have been developed to block this system, as summarized in Fig. 8 (Zaman et al. 2002).

Angiotensinogen, synthesized in the liver, is a substrate for renin and is broken down into the angiotensin peptides. The protein consists of 485 amino acids, 33 of which constitute a presegment that is removed after secretion. The action of renin on angiotensinogen produces angiotensin I. Angiotensin I is composed of the first ten amino acid sequence following the presegment and does not appear to have biologic activity. Angiotensin II, the main form of biologically active angiotensin, is formed by cleavage of the two carboxyl-terminal peptides of angiotensin I by angiotensin-converting enzyme (ACE), localized to cell membranes in the lung and intracellular granules in certain tissues that produce angiotensin II. The half-life in the circulation of angiotensin II is very short (<60 s). Elements of the RAA system are present in the adrenal, the kidneys, the heart, and the brain. For example, the adrenal glomerulosa cells contain the proteins needed to produce and secrete angiotensin II. Other tissues contain one or more components of the renin–angiotensin system and require other cells or circulating components, or both, to generate angiotensin II (De Mello 2016). Angiotensin II functions through the angiotensin receptor to maintain normal extracellular volume and blood pressure by:

- Increasing aldosterone secretion from the zona glomerulosa by increasing transcription of CYP11B2
- Constriction of vascular smooth muscle, thereby increasing blood pressure and reducing renal blood flow
- Release of norepinephrine and epinephrine from the adrenal medulla
- Enhancement of the activity of the sympathetic nervous system by increasing central sympathetic outflow, thereby increasing norepinephrine discharge from sympathetic nerve terminals
- Promotion of the release of vasopressin

In addition to the classic genomic actions mediated by aldosterone binding to cytosolic receptors, mineralocorticoids have acute, nongenomic actions due to activation of an unidentified cell surface receptor. This action involves a

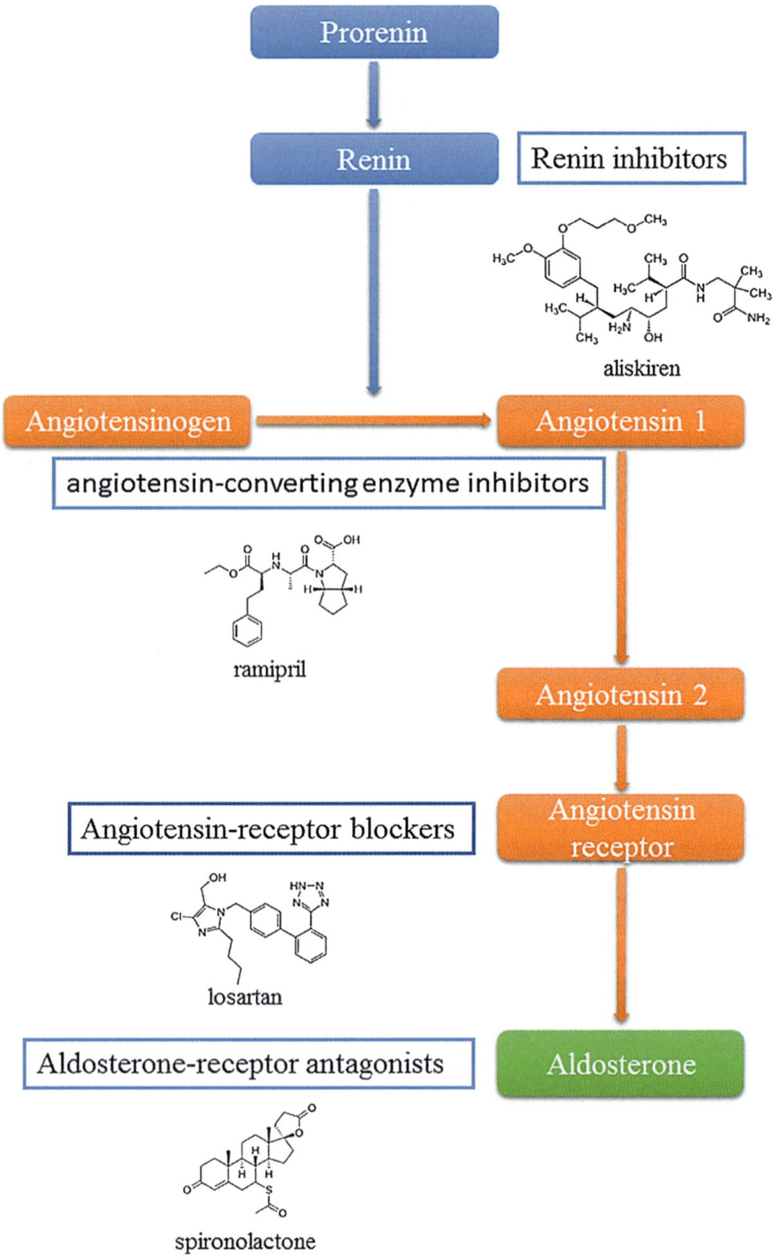

Fig. 8 Pharmacology of the renin–angiotensin–aldosterone system

G-protein signaling pathway and probably a modification of the sodium–hydrogen exchange activity. This effect has been demonstrated in both epithelial and non-epithelial cells.

Aldosterone has additional, nonclassic effects primarily on nonepithelial cells. These actions, although probably genomic and therefore mediated by activation of the cytosolic mineralocorticoid receptor, do not include modification of sodium–potassium balance. Aldosterone-mediated actions include the expression of several collagen genes, growth factors, plasminogen activator inhibitor type 1, or genes mediating inflammation. The resultant actions lead to microangiopathy and fibrosis in various tissues such as the heart, the vasculature, and the kidney. Increased levels of aldosterone are not necessary to cause this damage; an imbalance between the volume or sodium balance state and the level of aldosterone appears to be the critical factor (Gao et al. 2016).

The action of angiotensin II on aldosterone involves a negative feedback loop that also includes extracellular fluid volume. The major function of this feedback loop is to modify sodium homeostasis and, secondarily, to regulate blood pressure. Thus, sodium restriction activates the renin–angiotensin–aldosterone axis. The effects of angiotensin II on both the adrenal cortex and the renal vasculature promote renal sodium conservation. Conversely, with suppression of renin release and suppression of the level of circulating angiotensin, aldosterone secretion is reduced and renal blood flow is increased, thereby promoting sodium loss. The renin–angiotensin–aldosterone loop is very sensitive to dietary sodium intake. Sodium excess enhances the renal and peripheral vasculature responsiveness and reduces the adrenal responsiveness to angiotensin II. Sodium restriction has the opposite effect. Thus, sodium intake modifies target tissue responsiveness to angiotensin II.

Adrenal Androgen Secretion

Adrenal androgens represent an important component (>50%) of circulating androgens in premenopausal females. In males, this contribution is much smaller because of the testicular production of androgens, but adrenal androgen excess even in males may be of clinical significance, mainly in CAH. The adult adrenal secretes approximately 4 mg/day of dehydroepiandrosterone (DHEA), 7–15 mg/day of DHEAS, 1.5 mg of androstenedione, and 0.05 mg/day of testosterone. DHEA is a crucial precursor of human sex steroid biosynthesis and exerts androgenic or estrogenic activity following conversion by the activities of 3β-HSD, a superfamily of β-HSD isozymes and aromatase, expressed in peripheral target tissues, which is of clinical importance in many diseases. Only desulfated DHEA is converted downstream and biologically active.

ACTH stimulates androgen secretion; DHEA (but not DHEAS because of its increased plasma half-life) and androstenedione demonstrate a similar circadian rhythm to cortisol.

Corticosteroid Hormone Actions

Receptors and Gene Transcription

Both cortisol and aldosterone exert their effects following uptake of free hormone from the circulation and binding to intracellular receptors, termed the glucocorticoid (GR) and mineralocorticoid receptors (MR). These are both members of the thyroid/steroid hormone receptor superfamily of transcription factors comprising a C-terminal ligand-binding domain, a central DNA-binding domain interacting with specific DNA sequences on target genes.

Glucocorticoid hormone action has been studied in more depth than mineralocorticoid action. The binding of steroid to the GR in the cytosol results in activation of the steroid-receptor complex involving heat-shock proteins (HSP 90 and HSP 70) that release GR. Following translocation to the nucleus, gene transcription is stimulated or repressed following binding of dimerized GR-ligand complexes to specific DNA sequences in the promoter regions of target genes. This "glucocorticoid-response element" binds with high affinity to two loops of DNA within the DNA-binding domain of the GR, stabilizing the RNA polymerase II complex, in several tissues of the organism, leading to a high number of cortisol-mediated effects (stress, growth, energy intake, inflammation, and so on). In contrast to the diverse actions of glucocorticoids, mineralocorticoids have a more restricted role, principally to stimulate epithelial sodium transport in the distal nephron, distal colon, and salivary glands. This is mediated through the induction of the apical sodium channel through transcriptional regulation. Aldosterone binds to the MR, principally in the cytosol, followed by translocation of the hormone-receptor complex to the nucleus. The MR and GR share considerable homology – 57% in the steroid-binding domain and 94% in the DNA-binding domain. Aldosterone (and the synthetic "mineralocorticoid" fludrocortisone) could bind to the GR and cortisol to the MR (in vitro the MR has the same inherent affinity for aldosterone and cortisol). Specificity upon the MR is conferred through the "pre-receptor" metabolism of cortisol via the enzyme 11β-hydroxysteroid dehydrogenase type 2 (11β-HSD2), which inactivates cortisol and corticosterone to 11-keto metabolites, enabling aldosterone to bind to the MR. The underlying signaling pathways remain to be fully clarified, but the effects are reversible with MR antagonists.

There are several receptor antagonists developed in the last years, commonly used in several adrenal diseases. Mifepristone (RU486) was originally developed as an anti-progesterone drug, and it is currently used in many countries as antiprogestin medication. It has also been found to act as a glucocorticoid receptor antagonist, so it has been proposed in Cushing's syndrome, but its widespread use is limited by the difficulty of judging its effectiveness, because its action prompts a rise in circulating cortisol levels (Ceccato et al. 2015). Mifepristone, administered at doses of up to 1,200 mg daily, improved diabetes, clinical signs, and symptoms, rather than in cortisol levels; since mifepristone could increase ACTH levels and could not control pituitary adenoma, further studies are needed to establish its safety.

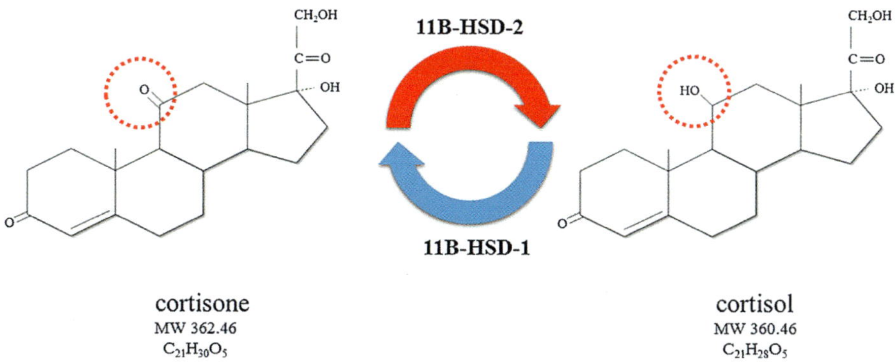

Fig. 9 Cortisol and cortisone, the box highlight the difference among hormones; *MW* molecular weight, *HSD* 11β-hydroxysteroid dehydrogenase

Cortisol-Binding Globulin and Corticosteroid Hormone Metabolism

More than 90% of circulating cortisol is bound to cortisol-binding globulin (CBG), an a_2-globulin with 383 amino acid protein and synthesized in the liver. CBG does not carry synthetic corticosteroids (except prednisolone, which has an affinity for CBG approximately 50% of that of cortisol). Circulating CBG concentrations are approximately 700 nmol/L. Levels are increased by estrogens (be careful in measuring total serum cortisol in pregnancy) and hepatitis and reduced by glucocorticoids, cirrhosis, nephrosis, and hyperthyroidism. The excretion of "free" cortisol through the kidneys is termed urinary free cortisol and represents only 1% of the total cortisol secretion rate.

The circulating half-life of cortisol varies between 70 and 120 min (Hammond 2016).

The interconversion of the 11-hydroxyl (cortisol, termed Kendall's compound F) to the 11-oxo group (cortisone, compound E) through the activity of 11-β-hydroxysteroid dehydrogenase (HSD) types 1 and 2 explains analytical bias in cortisol measurement. There are two methods to measure cortisol: immunoassays (as radioimmunoassay, RIA; enzyme-linked immunosorbent assay, ELISA; automated electro-chemiluminescence immunoassay, ECLIA) and liquid chromatography–tandem mass spectrometry (LC-MS/MS). Antibody-based immunoassays can be affected by cross-reactivity (especially cortisone, whose structure is similar to cortisol, as shown in Fig. 9) and synthetic glucocorticoids. By contrast, structurally based assays such as LC-MS/MS do not pose this problem, allowing the separation of various glucocorticoids and metabolites.

Two distinct 11β-HSD isozymes have been reported, a type 1, NADPH-dependent oxo-reductase expressed principally in the liver, which confers bioactivity upon orally administered cortisone by converting it to cortisol, and a type 2, NAD-dependent dehydrogenase. It is 11β-HSD2, coexpressed with the MR in the kidney, colon, and salivary gland, which inactivates cortisol to cortisone and permits aldosterone to bind to the MR in vivo. If this "enzyme-protective mechanism" is impaired, cortisol is able to act as a mineralocorticoid; this explains some forms of endocrine hypertension (apparent mineralocorticoid excess, liquorice ingestion), and the mineralocorticoid excess state that characterizes the ectopic ACTH syndrome.

Aldosterone is also metabolized in the liver and kidneys. In the liver, it undergoes tetrahydro-reduction and is excreted in the urine as a 3-glucuronide tetrahydroaldosterone derivative. However, glucuronide conjugation at the 18 position occurs directly in the kidney as does 3a and 5α/5b metabolism of the free steroid. Because of the aldehyde group at the C18 position, aldosterone is not metabolized by 11β-HSD2. Hepatic aldosterone clearance is reduced in patients with cirrhosis, ascites, and severe congestive heart failure.

Effects of Glucocorticoids

Carbohydrate, Lipid Metabolism, and Blood Pressure

Glucocorticoids increase blood glucose concentrations through their action on glycogen, protein, and lipid metabolism. In the liver, cortisol stimulates glycogen deposition by increasing glycogen synthase and inhibiting glycogen phosphorylase. Hepatic glucose output increases through the activation of key enzymes involved in gluconeogenesis, principally glucose 6-phosphatase and phosphoenolpyruvate kinase. In peripheral tissues (muscle, fat), cortisol inhibits glucose uptake and utilization. In adipose tissue, lipolysis is activated, resulting in the release of free fatty acids into the circulation. An increase in total circulating cholesterol and triglycerides is observed, but HDL cholesterol levels fall. The resultant effect is to cause insulin resistance and an increase in blood glucose concentrations, at the expense of protein and lipid catabolism.

Glucocorticoids stimulate adipocyte differentiation, promoting adipogenesis through the transcriptional activation of key differentiation genes, including lipoprotein lipase, glycerol-3-phosphate dehydrogenase, and leptin. In the long term, the effects of glucocorticoid excess upon adipose tissue are complex, where the deposition of visceral or central adipose tissue is stimulated, related to the increased expression of both the GR and 11β-HSD1 in visceral rather than in subcutaneous adipose tissue.

Glucocorticoids increase blood pressure by a variety of mechanisms involving actions on the kidney and vasculature. In vascular smooth muscle, they increase sensitivity to pressor agents such as catecholamines and angiotensin II while reducing nitric oxide-mediated endothelial dilatation. Angiotensinogen synthesis is increased by glucocorticoids. In the kidney, depending upon the activity 11β-HSD2, cortisol can act on the distal nephron to cause sodium retention and potassium loss (mediated via the MR). Elsewhere across the nephron, glucocorticoids increase glomerular filtration rate, proximal tubular epithelial sodium transport, and free water clearance. This latter effect involves antagonism of the action of vasopressin and explains the hyponatremia seen in patients with glucocorticoid deficiency (Goodwin 2015).

Skin, Muscle, and Connective Tissue

In addition to inducing insulin resistance in muscle tissue, glucocorticoids also cause catabolic changes in the muscle, skin, and connective tissue. In the skin and connective tissue, glucocorticoids inhibit epidermal cell division and DNA synthesis and reduce collagen synthesis and production. In muscle, glucocorticoids cause atrophy (but not necrosis), and overall muscle protein synthesis is reduced.

Glucocorticoids inhibit osteoblast function, explaining the osteopenia and osteoporosis that characterize glucocorticoid excess. With up to 1% of Western populations taking long-term glucocorticoid therapy, glucocorticoid-induced osteoporosis is becoming a prevalent health concern, affecting 50% of patients treated with corticosteroids for more than 12 months. Cortisol excess could also induce an avascular necrosis (rapid and focal deterioration in bone quality), especially in the femoral head, leading to pain and ultimately collapse of the bone, often requiring hip replacement. It can affect individuals of all ages and may occur with relatively low doses of glucocorticoids (e.g., during corticosteroid replacement therapy for adrenal failure). Recent data implicate glucocorticoid-induced osteocyte apoptosis in the pathogenesis of the condition, and the lack of a direct role for an interrupted blood supply suggests that the term osteonecrosis is preferable to avascular femoral necrosis. However, there is still no explanation for individual susceptibility.

Glucocorticoids also induce negative calcium balance by inhibiting intestinal calcium absorption and increasing renal calcium excretion. Therefore, PTH secretion is usually increased. In children, glucocorticoids suppress growth, but the increases in body mass index are thought to offset a deleterious effect on bone mineral density.

Anti-Inflammatory Actions and the Immune System

Glucocorticoids suppress immunologic responses at many levels. In the peripheral blood, an acute glucocorticoid bolus reduces lymphocyte counts (by redistributing lymphocytes from the intravascular compartment to spleen, lymph nodes, and bone marrow) and eosinophils, while cortisol bolus increases neutrophil counts. The immunologic actions of glucocorticoids involve direct actions on both T and B lymphocytes, which include inhibition of immunoglobulin synthesis and stimulation of lymphocyte apoptosis. Inhibition of cytokine production from lymphocytes is mediated through inhibition of the action of NF-κB. Additional anti-inflammatory effects involve inhibition of monocyte differentiation into macrophages and macrophage phagocytosis and cytotoxic activity. Glucocorticoids reduce the local inflammatory response by preventing the action of histamine and plasminogen activators. Prostaglandin synthesis is impaired through the induction of lipocortins, which inhibit phospholipase A2 activity.

Central Nervous System and Mood

Clinical observations in patients with glucocorticoid excess and deficiency reveal that the brain is an important target tissue for glucocorticoids, with depression, euphoria, psychosis, apathy, and lethargy being important manifestations. Both glucocorticoid and mineralocorticoid receptors are expressed in the brain, including the hippocampus, hypothalamus, cerebellum, and cortex. Glucocorticoids cause neuronal death, especially in the hippocampus, impairing cognitive function and memory and leading to neurodegenerative diseases. Local blockade of cortisol generation by 11β-HSD1 has been shown to improve cognitive function. DHEA has been shown to have neuroprotective effects in the hippocampus region. In the eye, glucocorticoids act to raise intraocular pressure through an increase in aqueous humor production and deposition of matrix within the trabecular meshwork, which inhibits aqueous drainage. Steroid-induced glaucoma appears to have a genetic predisposition, but the underlying mechanisms are unknown.

Growth and Endocrine Glands

Although glucocorticoids stimulate GH gene transcription in vitro, glucocorticoids in excess inhibit linear skeletal growth, probably as a result of catabolic effects on connective tissue, muscle, and bone and through inhibition of the effects of IGF-1. Experiments on mice lacking the GR gene emphasize the role of glucocorticoids in normal fetal development. In particular, glucocorticoids stimulate lung maturation through the synthesis of surfactant proteins, and mice lacking the GR die shortly after birth due to hypoxia from lung atelectasis. Glucocorticoids also stimulate the enzyme phenylethanolamine N-methyltransferase (PNMT), which converts noradrenaline to adrenaline in adrenal medulla and chromaffin tissue. Mice lacking the GR do not develop an adrenal medulla.

Glucocorticoids suppress the thyroid axis, probably through a direct action on TSH secretion. In addition, they inhibit 5′ deiodinase activity mediating the conversion of thyroxine to active triiodothyronine. Glucocorticoids also act centrally to inhibit GnRH pulsatility and LH FSH release.

Therapeutic Corticosteroids

After the first demonstration of anti-inflammatory effect in the 1950s, a series of synthetic corticosteroids have been developed for therapeutic purposes. These are used to treat a diverse variety of human diseases and principally rely on their anti-inflammatory and immunologic actions. The main corticosteroids used in clinical practice, their structure together with their relative glucocorticoid and mineralocorticoid potencies, are listed in Table 2.

Biologic activity of a corticosteroid is dependent upon a 4-3-keto, 11β-hydroxy, 17α,21-trihydroxyl configuration. Conversion of the C11 hydroxyl group to a C11 keto group (cortisol to cortisone) inactivates the steroid. The addition of a 1,2 unsaturated bond to cortisol results in prednisolone, which is four times more potent than cortisol actions. Prednisone is the "cortisone equivalent" of prednisolone and relies upon conversion by 11β-HSD1 in the liver for bioactivity. Potency is further increased by the addition of a 6α-methyl group to prednisolone (methylprednisolone). Fludrocortisone is a synthetic mineralocorticoid having 125-fold greater potency than cortisol in bonding mineralocorticoid receptor and so stimulating sodium reabsorption, achieved through the addition of a 9α-fluoro group to

Table 2 Structures and anti-inflammatory corticoid drugs

		Anti-inflammatory action	Mineralocorticoid action
Cortisol	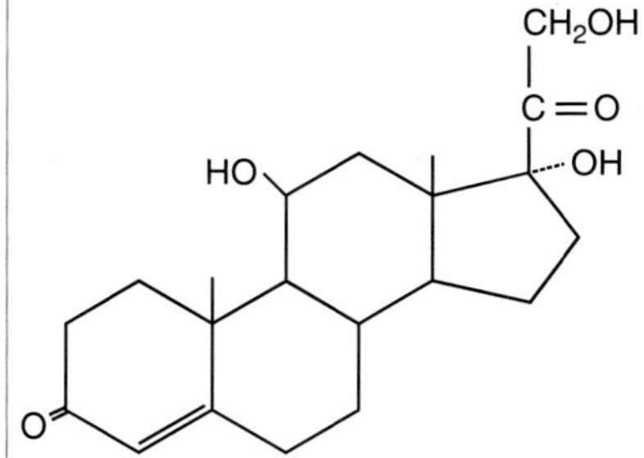 cortisol	1	1
Prednisolone	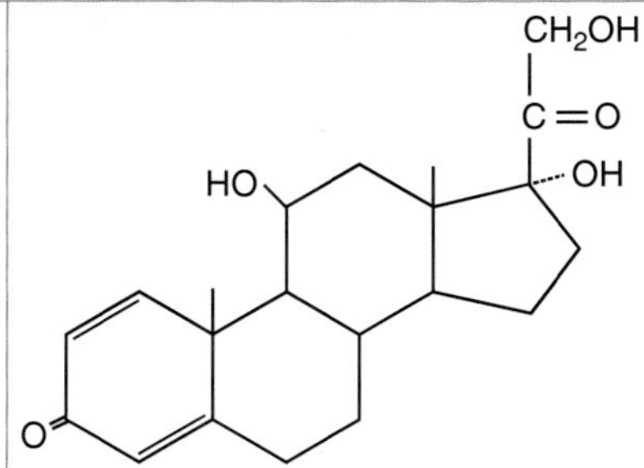 prednisolone	3	0.75

(*continued*)

Table 2 (continued)

		Anti-inflammatory action	Mineralocorticoid action
Methylprednisolone	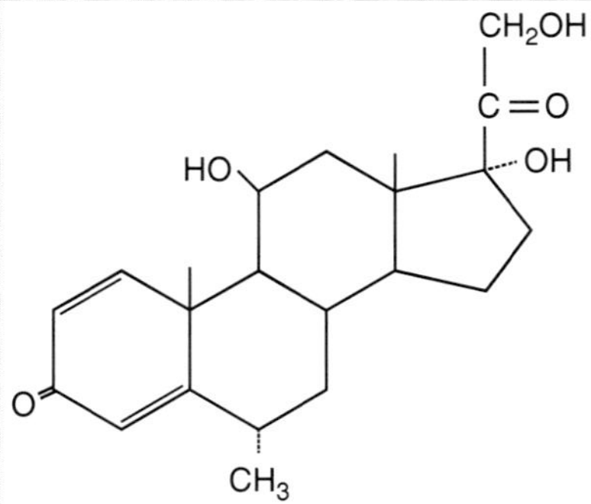 methylprednisolone	6.2	0.5
Fludrocortisone	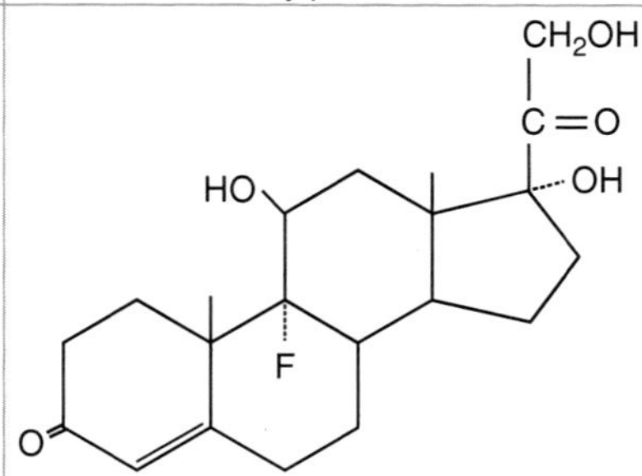 fludrocortisone	12	125

Triamcinolone	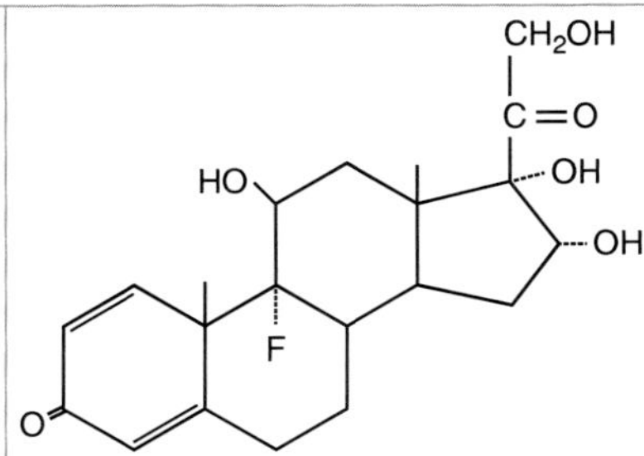 triamcinolone	5	0
Dexamethasone	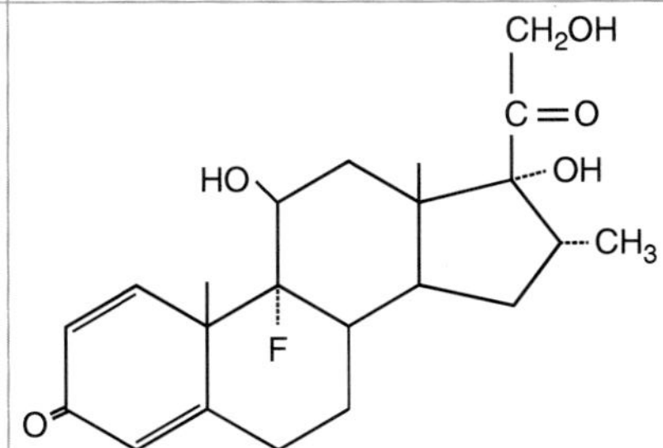 dexamethasone	26	0

(continued)

Table 2 (continued)

		Anti-inflammatory action	Mineralocorticoid action
Betamethasone	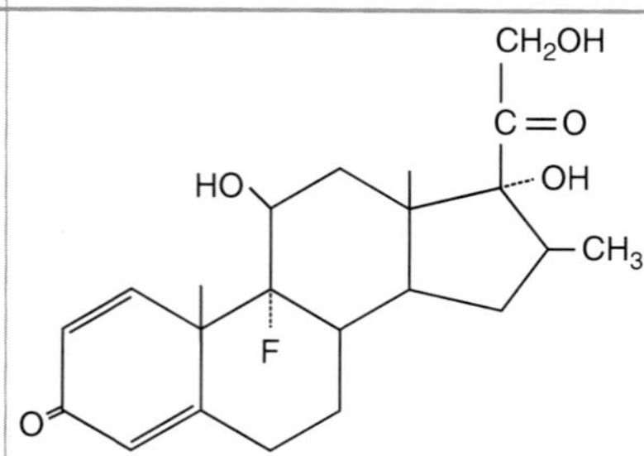 betamethasone	25	0

cortisol, and is used to treat mineralocorticoid deficiency in Addison disease and after bilateral adrenalectomy. Interestingly, fludrocortisone also has glucocorticoid potency (12-fold greater than cortisol), and the addition of a 16α-methyl group and 1,2 saturated bond to fludrocortisone results in dexamethasone, a highly potent glucocorticoid (25-fold that of cortisol) but without significant mineralocorticoid activity. Betamethasone has the same structure of dexamethasone, but with a 16β-methyl group, and is widely used in respiratory and nasal aerosol sprays, and betamethasone is not able to bond to mineralocorticoid receptor (Peacy 1997).

Corticosteroids are given orally, parenterally, and by numerous topical routes (e.g., eyes, skin, nose, inhalation, rectal suppositories). Unlike hydrocortisone, which has a high affinity for CBG, most synthetic steroids have low affinity for this binding protein and circulate as free steroid (~30%) or bound to albumin (up to 70%). Circulating half-lives vary depending upon individual variability and underlying disease, particularly renal and hepatic impairment. Cortisone acetate should not be used parenterally as it requires metabolism by the liver to active cortisol.

Synthetic corticosteroids similarly suppress the function of the HPA axis through a process that is dependent on both dose and duration of treatment. As a result, the sudden cessation of corticosteroid therapy may result in adrenal failure. This may also occur following treatment with high doses of the synthetic progestogen, medroxyprogesterone acetate, which possesses glucocorticoid agonist activity. In patients taking any steroid dose for less than 3–4 weeks, a clinically significant suppression of the HPA axis is rarely a problem, and patients can withdraw from steroids suddenly with no ill effect. The possible exception to this is the patient who receives frequent "short" courses of corticosteroid therapy, for example, patients with recurrent episodes of severe asthma. Conversely, suppression of the HPA axis is invariable in patients taking the equivalent of 15 mg/day or more of prednisolone long term. Recovery from suppression may take 6–9 months. CRH secretion returns to normal, and within a few weeks, ACTH levels begin to increase and indeed rise above normal values until adrenal steroidogenesis recovers. In the interim, and without replacement therapy, patients may experience symptoms of glucocorticoid deficiency, including anorexia, nausea, weight loss, arthralgia, lethargy, skin desquamation, and postural dizziness. To avoid symptoms of glucocorticoid deficiency, steroids should be cautiously withdrawn over a period of months.

Catecholamines

The term catecholamine refers to substances that contain catechol (ortho-dihydroxybenzene) and a side chain with an amino group – the catechol nucleus (Fig. 10).

Dopamine, found in the adrenal medulla and peripheral sympathetic nerves, acts primarily as a neurotransmitter in the central nervous system; epinephrine is synthesized and stored in the adrenal medulla and released into the systemic circulation, whereas norepinephrine is synthesized and stored not only in the adrenal medulla but also in the peripheral sympathetic nerves.

Catecholamines affect many cardiovascular and metabolic processes, including increasing the heart rate, blood pressure, myocardial contractility, and cardiac conduction velocity. Specific receptors mediate the biologic actions. The three types of adrenergic receptors (α, β, DA) and their receptor subtypes have led to an understanding of the physiologic responses to exogenous and endogenous administration of catecholamines. The a_1 subtype is a postsynaptic receptor that mediates vascular and smooth muscle contraction; stimulation causes vasoconstriction and increased blood pressure. The a_2 receptors are located on presynaptic sympathetic nerve endings and, when activated, inhibit release of norepinephrine; stimulation causes suppression in central sympathetic outflow and decreased blood pressure. There are three major β-receptor subtypes:

- β_1 receptor mediates cardiac effects and is more responsive to isoproterenol than to epinephrine or norepinephrine; β_1 receptor stimulation causes positive inotropic and chronotropic effects in the heart, increased renin secretion in the kidney, and lipolysis in adipocytes.
- β_2 receptor mediates bronchial, vascular, and uterine smooth muscle relaxation; stimulation causes bronchodilatation, vasodilatation in skeletal muscle, glycogenolysis, and increased release of norepinephrine from sympathetic nerve terminals.
- β_3 receptor regulates energy expenditure and lipolysis, especially in adipocytes.

Most cells in the body have adrenergic receptors. The pharmacologic development of selective α- and β-adrenergic agonists and antagonists has advanced the pharmacotherapy for various clinical disorders. For example, β_1-antagonists (e.g., atenolol and metoprolol) are considered standard therapies for angina pectoris, hypertension, and cardiac arrhythmias. Administration of β_2-agonists causes bronchial smooth muscle relaxation and is commonly prescribed in inhaled formulations for the treatment of asthma.

Catecholamine Synthesis

Catecholamines are synthesized from tyrosine by a process of hydroxylation and decarboxylation (see Fig. 10). Tyrosine is derived from ingested food or synthesized

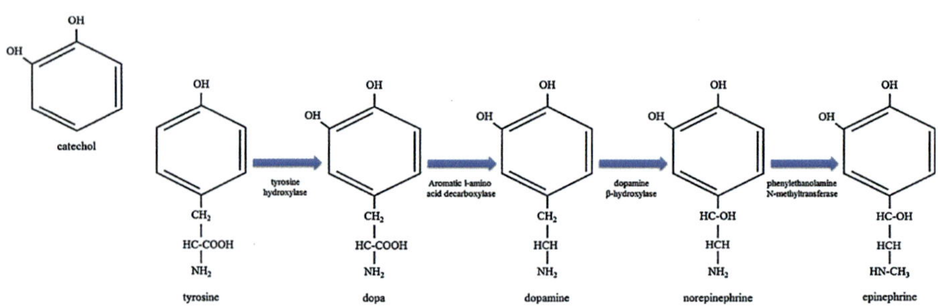

Fig. 10 Biosynthetic pathway for catecholamines

from phenylalanine in the liver, and it enters neurons and chromaffin cells by active transport. Tyrosine is converted to dopa by tyrosine hydroxylase, the first step of synthesis. Increased intracellular levels of catechols downregulate the activity of tyrosine hydroxylase; as catecholamines are released from secretory granules in response to a stimulus, cytoplasmic catecholamines are depleted and the feedback inhibition of tyrosine hydroxylase is released. Transcription of tyrosine hydroxylase is stimulated by glucocorticoids (cortisol also is a cofactor of phenylethanolamine N-methyltransferase PNMT, explaining that epinephrine-secreting pheochromocytomas are almost exclusively localized to the adrenal medulla), cAMP-dependent protein kinases, calcium-/phospholipid-dependent protein kinase, and calcium-/calmodulin-dependent protein kinase. α-Methyl-para-tyrosine (metirosine) is a tyrosine hydroxylase inhibitor that may be used therapeutically in patients with catecholamine-secreting tumors.

Aromatic l-amino acid decarboxylase catalyzes the decarboxylation of dopa to dopamine. Dopamine is actively transported into granulated vesicles to be hydroxylated to norepinephrine by the copper-containing enzyme dopamine β-hydroxylase. These reactions occur not only in chromaffin cells of the adrenal medulla but also in the synaptic vesicle of adrenergic neurons in the central and peripheral nervous system. In the adrenal medulla, norepinephrine is released from the granule into the cytoplasm, where the cytosolic enzyme PNMT converts it to epinephrine. Epinephrine is then transported back into another storage vesicle. The N-methylation reaction by PNMT involves S-adenosylmethionine as the methyl donor as well as oxygen and magnesium. In normal adrenal medullary tissue, approximately 80% of the catecholamine released is epinephrine (Eisenhofer et al. 2004).

Catecholamine Storage and Secretion

Catecholamines, found in the adrenal medulla and sympathetically innervated, are stored in electron-dense granules that also contain ATP, neuropeptides (e.g., adrenomedullin, ACTH, vasoactive intestinal polypeptide), calcium, magnesium, and chromogranins. Uptake into the storage vesicles is facilitated by active transport using vesicular monoamine transporters (VMATs). The VMAT ATP-driven pump maintains a steep electrical gradient. For every monoamine transported, ATP is hydrolyzed and two hydrogen ions are transported from the vesicle into the cytosol. ^{123}I- and ^{131}I-labeled metaiodobenzylguanidine (MIBG) is imported by VMATs into the storage vesicles in the adrenal medulla, which makes ^{123}I-MIBG useful for imaging localization of catecholamine-secreting tumors (Fig. 11) and ^{131}I-MIBG potentially useful in treating malignant catecholamine-secreting tumors (Flatmark et al. 2002; Eisenhofer et al. 2004).

Stressful stimuli (e.g., hypoglycemia, myocardial infarction, anesthesia) are able to trigger catecholamine secretion. Acetylcholine from preganglionic sympathetic fibers stimulates nicotinic cholinergic receptors and causes depolarization of adrenomedullary chromaffin cells, leading to activation of voltage-gated calcium channels, which results in exocytosis of secretory vesicle contents. A calcium-sensing

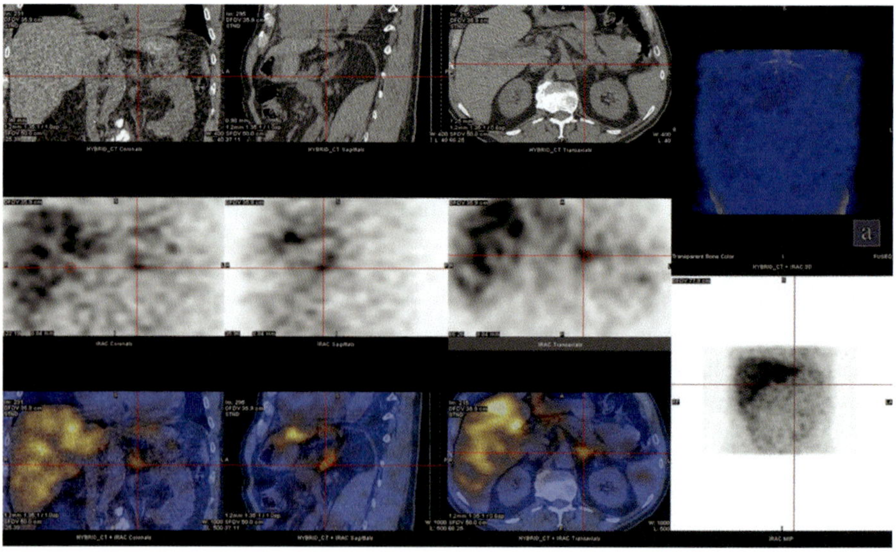

Fig. 11 ^{123}I-MIBG of a pheochromocytoma

receptor appears to be involved in the process of exocytosis. During exocytosis, all the granular contents are released into the extracellular space. Norepinephrine modulates its own release by activating the a_2-receptors on the presynaptic membrane. Stimulation of the presynaptic a_2-receptors inhibits norepinephrine release (the mechanism of action of some antihypertensive medications such as clonidine). Catecholamines are among the shortest-lived signaling molecules in plasma; the initial biologic half-life of circulating catecholamines is between 10 and 100 s; half of the catecholamines circulate in plasma associated with albumin.

Catecholamine Metabolism and Inactivation

Catecholamines are removed from the circulation either by reuptake by sympathetic nerve terminals or by metabolism through two enzyme pathways, followed by sulfate conjugation and renal excretion. Most of the metabolism of catecholamines occurs in the same cell in which they are synthesized. Almost 90% of catecholamines released at sympathetic synapses are taken up locally by the nerve endings (uptake-1). Uptake-1 can be blocked by cocaine, tricyclic antidepressants, and phenothiazines. Most of these catecholamines are metabolized by catechol-O-methyltransferase (COMT).

Although COMT is found primarily outside neural tissue, O-methylation in the adrenal medulla is the predominant source of metanephrine (COMT converts epinephrine to metanephrine) and a major source of normetanephrine (COMT converts norepinephrine to normetanephrine) by methylating the 3-hydroxy group (also in this reaction, S-adenosylmethionine is used as the methyl donor). Metanephrine and

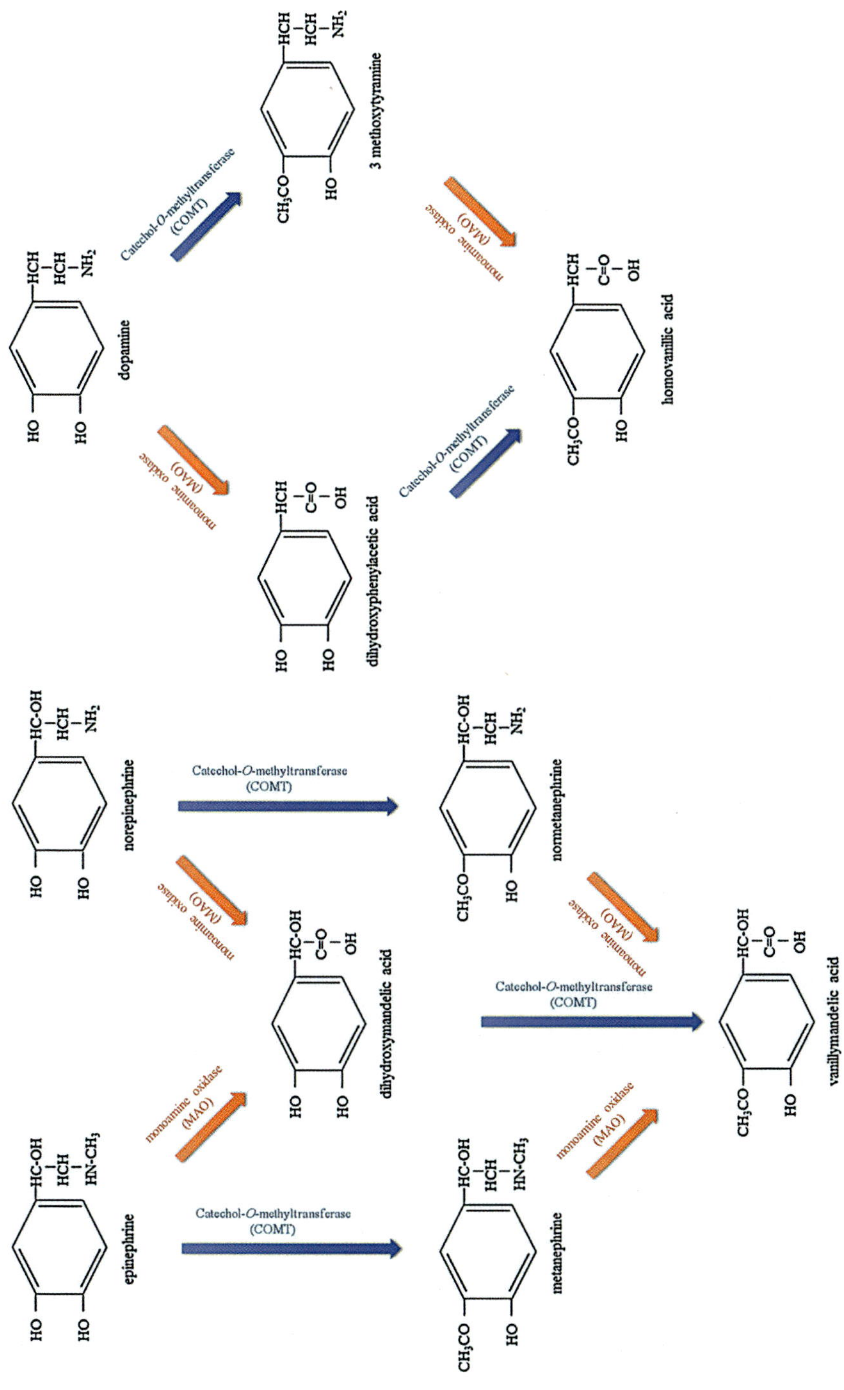

Fig. 12 Catecholamine metabolism

normetanephrine are oxidized by monoamine oxidase (MAO) to vanillylmandelic acid (VMA) by oxidative deamination. MAO may also oxidize epinephrine and norepinephrine to 3,4-dihydroxymandelic acid, which is then converted by COMT to VMA. MAO is located on the outer membrane of mitochondria (Flatmark et al. 2002; Eisenhofer et al. 2004) (Fig. 12).

There is compelling evidence that measurements of plasma free or urinary fractionated metanephrines (especially by mass spectrometry) are superior to other tests of catecholamine excess for diagnosis of pheochromocytoma; the theoretical basis for this is provided by improved understanding of catecholamine metabolism. Metanephrines are produced within adrenal chromaffin cells (or the tumors derived from these cells) by membrane-bound COMT: the lack of this enzyme in sympathetic nerves, the major site of initial norepinephrine metabolism, means that the O-methylated metabolites are relatively specific markers of chromaffin tumors. Most importantly, these metabolites are produced continuously within tumors by a process that is independent of exocytotic release.

Summary

In the present chapter, we have illustrated some general notions regarding adrenal physiology.

Adrenal cortex, through steroidogenesis, produces and secretes glucocorticoids (cortisol), mineralocorticoids (aldosterone) and sex steroids (mainly androgens). The inner part of adrenals, the medulla, secretes catecholamines.

Disclosure Summary *Declaration of interest*: All authors declare that they have no conflicts of interest that might be perceived as influencing the impartiality of the reported research.

Funding: This study did not receive any specific grant from any funding agency in the public, commercial, or not-for-profit sector.

Cross-References

▶ The Endocrine Regulation of Blood Pressure
▶ The Hypothalamus–Pituitary Axis

References

Abe T, Naruse M, Young Jr WF, Kobashi N, Doi Y, Izawa A, Akama K, Okumura Y, Ikenaga M, Kimura H, Saji H, Mukai K, Matsumoto H. A novel CYP11B2-specific imaging agent for detection of unilateral subtypes of primary aldosteronism. J Clin Endocrinol Metab. 2016;101 (3):1008–15.

Ceccato F, Barbot M, Zilio M, Albiger N, Mantero F, Scaroni C. Therapeutic strategies for Cushing's Syndrome: an update. Expert Opin Orphan Drugs. 2015;3(1):45–56. doi:10.1517/21678707.2015.991714.

Chrétien M, Mbikay M. 60 YEARS OF POMC: from the prohormone theory to pro-opiomelanocortin and to proprotein convertases (PCSK1 to PCSK9). J Mol Endocrinol. 2016;56(4):T49–62. doi:10.1530/JME-15-0261.

De Mello WC. Intracellular angiotensin II as a regulator of muscle tone in vascular resistance vessels. Pathophysiological implications. Peptides. 2016;78:87–90. doi:10.1016/j.peptides.2016.02.006.

Eisenhofer G, Kopin IJ, Goldstein DS. Catecholamine metabolism: a contemporary view with implications for physiology and medicine. Pharmacol Rev. 2004;56:331–49.

El Ghorayeb N, Bourdeau I, Lacroix A. Role of ACTH and other hormones in the regulation of aldosterone production in primary aldosteronism. Front Endocrinol (Lausanne). 2016;7:72. doi:10.3389/fendo.2016.00072.

Flatmark T, Almas B, Ziegler MG. Catecholamine metabolism: an update on key biosynthetic enzymes and vesicular monoamine transporters. Ann N Y Acad Sci. 2002;971:69–75.

Gamble KL, Berry R, Frank SJ, Young ME. Circadian clock control of endocrine factors. Nat Rev Endocrinol. 2014;10(8):466–75. doi:10.1038/nrendo.2014.78.

Gao J, Zhang K, Chen J, Wang MH, Wang J, Liu P, Huang H. Roles of aldosterone in vascular calcification: an update. Eur J Pharmacol. 2016;786:186–93. doi:10.1016/j.ejphar.2016.05.030.

Goodwin JE. Glucocorticoids and the cardiovascular system. Adv Exp Med Biol. 2015;872:299–314. doi:10.1007/978-1-4939-2895-8_13.

Hammond GL. Plasma steroid-binding proteins: primary gatekeepers of steroid hormone action. J Endocrinol. 2016;230(1):R13–25. doi:10.1530/JOE-16-0070.

International Union of Pure and Applied Chemistry. Definitive rules for the nomenclature of steroids. Pure Appl Chem. 1972;31:285–322.

Jaffe RB, Mesiano S, Smith R, et al. The regulation and role of fetal adrenal development in human pregnancy. Endocr Res. 1998;24:919–26.

Lovejoy DA, Chang BS, Lovejoy NR, del Castillo J. Molecular evolution of GPCRs: CRH/CRH receptors. J Mol Endocrinol. 2014;52(3):T43–60. doi:10.1530/JME-13-0238.

Mesiano S, Jaffe RB. Developmental and functional biology of the primate fetal adrenal cortex. Endocr Rev. 1997;18:378–404.

Midzak A, Papadopoulos V. Adrenal mitochondria and steroidogenesis: from individual proteins to functional protein assemblies. Front Endocrinol (Lausanne). 2016;7:106. doi:10.3389/fendo.2016.00106.

Miller WL. Molecular biology of steroid hormone synthesis. Endocr Rev. 1988;9:295–318.

Miller WL, Auchus RJ. The molecular biology, biochemistry, and physiology of human steroidogenesis and its disorders. Endocr Rev. 2011;32(1):81–151.

Okamoto M, Takemori H. Differentiation and zonation of the adrenal cortex. Curr Opin Endocrinol Diab. 2000;7:122–7.

Peacy SR. Glucocorticoid replacement therapy: are patients over treated and does it matter? Clin Endocrinol. 1997;46:255–61.

Smith AI, Funder JW. Proopiomelanocortin processing in the pituitary, central nervous system, and peripheral tissues. Endocr Rev. 1988;9:159–79.

Vinson GP. Functional zonation of the adult mammalian adrenal cortex. Front Neurosci. 2016;10:238. doi:10.3389/fnins.2016.00238.

Zaman MA, Oparil S, Calhoun DA. Drugs targeting the renin-angiotensin-aldosterone system. Nat Rev Drug Discov. 2002;1(8):621–36.

The Endocrine Pancreas

16

Salvatore Piro, Francesca Urbano, Franco Folli, Giovanna Finzi, Lorella Marselli, and Piero Marchetti

Abstract

The mammalian pancreas comprises an endocrine compartment, secreting hormones in the bloodstream, and an exocrine part, releasing digestive enzymes into the intestine. This chapter summarizes some of our current understanding of endocrine cells in the mammalian pancreas. These comprise α-cells secreting glucagon, β-cells secreting insulin, δ-cells secreting somatostatin, PP cells secreting pancreatic polypeptide, and ϵ-cells secreting ghrelin. Altogether these cells, organized in islets, and their hormones regulate blood glucose levels, glucose, lipid and protein metabolism, body weight, energy expenditure, food intake, and many other functions in peripheral tissues. Dysfunction or destruction of endocrine islets leads to diabetes mellitus and metabolic alteration of great medical importance.

The main purpose of this chapter is to illustrate the pancreatic islet composition and cell function and the physiological role of the islet hormones. Moreover we aim to discuss the pathophysiology of diseases caused by abnormal secretion or activity of these hormones.

S. Piro (✉) • F. Urbano
Department of Clinical and Experimental Medicine, Division of Internal Medicine, Garibaldi-Nesima Hospital, University of Catania, Catania, Italy
e-mail: piro@unict.it; francescaurbano@hotmail.it

F. Folli
Department of Medicine, Division of Diabetes, University of Texas Health Science Center, San Antonio, TX, USA
e-mail: folli@uthscsa.edu

G. Finzi
Azienda Socio Sanitaria Territoriale Dei Sette Laghi (ASST), Varese, Italy
e-mail: giovanna.finzi@asst-settelaghi.it

L. Marselli • P. Marchetti
Department of Clinical and Experimental Medicine, University of Pisa, Pisa, Italy
e-mail: lorella.marselli@med.unipi.it; piero.marchetti@med.unipi.it

A. Belfiore, D. LeRoith (eds.), *Principles of Endocrinology and Hormone Action*, Endocrinology, https://doi.org/10.1007/978-3-319-44675-2_31

Keywords
Pancreatic islets • Alpha cell • Beta cell • Delta cell • PP cell • Glucagon • Insulin • Somatostatin • Diabetes

Contents

Introduction

The mammalian pancreas comprises an endocrine compartment, secreting hormones into the bloodstream, and an exocrine part, secreting pancreatic digestive juices and enzymes into the duodenum. The endocrine components are grouped in the so-called islets of Langerhans, a small group of cells secreting distinct types of hormones; the exocrine function of the pancreas is involved in digestion, and the associated structures are known as the pancreatic acini (acinar and duct cells) (Kim et al. 2009).

The islets of Langerhans, present in the entire pancreas, show different shapes and sizes, which vary from approximately 30 to 300 μm in diameter (Berclaz et al. 2012). Each islet is composed of approximately 500–3,000 cells, and every cell produces a single hormone type (Fig. 1). Each cell contains granules that act as hormone deposit; granule exocytosis is the mechanism of hormonal release from islet cells. Beta cells are the predominant cell type and are the source of circulating insulin. The other cell types present within the islets are the glucagon-secreting alpha cells, the somatostatin-secreting delta cells, the ghrelin-secreting epsilon cells, and the pancreatic polypeptide (PP)-secreting cells (Rutter et al. 2015). Recently, experiments on the movement of hormonal granules in the islet cells

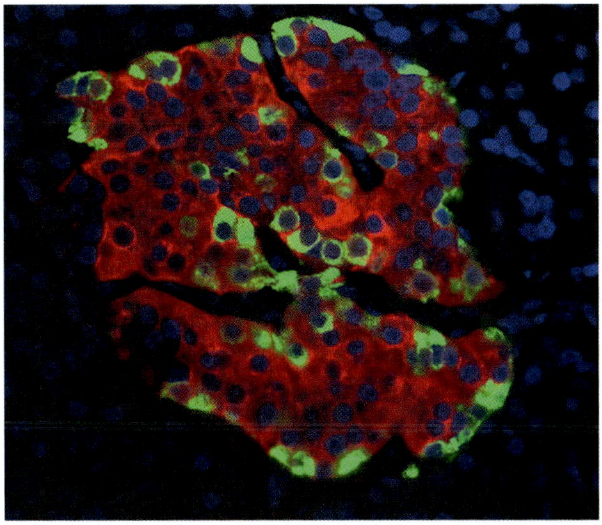

Fig. 1 A representative human pancreatic islet with insulin-containing beta cells in *red* and glucagon-containing alpha cells in *green*

have attracted great interest. Careful application of these approaches may provide evidence of how islet cells work and how intracellular granules are released (Michael et al. 2004, 2007).

Ultrastructural analysis has demonstrated a complex cell-cell interaction inside the islet, involving intricate interactions among the endocrine cells (Williamson et al. 1961; Benninger et al. 2008). This complexity includes contiguity of one cell type with other cells, *cell-to-cell* gap junctions, structural polarization of cells between capillaries, and alignment of complex endothelial cell pores with regions of exocytosis in endocrine cells.

Altogether these cells and their hormones regulate blood glucose levels, glucose, lipid, and protein metabolism in peripheral tissues. Maintenance of glucose homeostasis is essential for life, and the regulation of blood sugar levels is achieved by peptide hormone secretion from the endocrine cells located in the islets of Langerhans. Dysfunction or destruction of endocrine islets leads to diabetes mellitus and metabolic alterations of great medical importance. However, it should not be excluded that in the coming years, new hormones produced within the pancreatic islets could be identified. Such a discovery could lead to new scenarios in diabetes physiology and in the physiopathology of metabolic diseases.

Over the last 100 years, the scientific and clinical point of view on diabetes has centered on beta cells and insulin. The greater presence of beta cells within the islets has generated the syllogism *beta cell = diabetes*. To date it is known that all the hormones produced by the islets contribute to the development of diabetes and metabolic abnormalities. Every cell within the islets represents a single unit, and a single islet could be identified as a micro-organ within the pancreas. Moreover, every single islet, *autonomically* innerved and microperfused, receives an independent circulation from the general blood flow, and the intra-islet flow is essential for the interactions and reciprocal hormonal influences among the different cells within the islet. The anatomical organization of the islets reflects this system of interactions; in particular, it permits insulin β-cell secretion to inhibit α-cell glucagon secretion and somatostatin δ-cell secretion to inhibit both α- and β-cell hormone releases. The knowledge of these secretory dynamics has contributed to the discovery of the islet composition and the difference among different islet sizes and aspects.

Furthermore, notable cytoarchitectural differences among different animal species and human islets have been reported. For example, in rodent islets, the β-cells are located predominately in the central core with α- and δ-cells localized in the periphery forming a mantle (Kim et al. 2009; Jeon et al. 2009). In human and primate islets, the α-cells are not localized in the periphery but are rather dispersed throughout the islet. These different models of organization suggest different roles and functions of the islet cells in different species. The range of islet sizes closely overlaps among humans, primates, rabbits, and mice. However, islet composition varies among species and also within the same species under normal conditions. The effect of these differences on function is still unknown. Some evidence has recently suggested that metabolic alterations could influence islet composition and size, and cell function; certain metabolic conditions, such as diabetes or obesity, could contribute to modify cell identity and islet plasticity during life (Rhodes 2005). Pregnancy and obesity have been reported to be accompanied with cytoarchitectural changes of the islets in terms of increase in beta-cell mass. Overt diabetes is associated with a massive decrease of beta-cell function and number and with a correlated change in islet composition (Cinti et al. 2016).

Other evidence has recently shown that cells within the islets could *trans-differentiate* from one type to another. This evidence (i.e., alpha to beta-cell conversion or *vice versa*) was proposed to be the major mechanism underlying beta-cell regeneration in conditions of extreme beta-cell loss or to be one possible mechanism that contributes to the loss of cell function during diabetes. This property demonstrates an extreme plasticity of the islet, and it may depend on the common embryological origin of these cells (Thorel et al. 2010; Bramswig et al. 2013). Metabolic perturbations or increase of hormonal demand could influence these aspects. In particular, regarding the last topic, an emerging role of alpha cells must be highlighted. Alpha and beta cells could share some differentiating aspects, and certain conditions might determine a transition of one cell type to another.

Furthermore, epigenetic studies have shown that manipulation of rodent histone acetylation signatures can modify embryonic pancreatic differentiation and composition (Bramswig et al. 2013). A better comprehension of these new aspects could be useful for a better understanding of the pathophysiology of diabetes. Although the β-cell is central to these observations, dysfunction in α- or δ-cells can contribute to the disease etiology during diabetes.

In the present chapter, we aim to illustrate some general notions, fundamental in medicine, regarding the pancreatic islet composition and cell function. Moreover, in order to focus on the current knowledge on pancreatic endocrine cells, we will report some salient features that distinguish the cells that make up the islet.

Alpha as the First Cell

The α-cells that co-occupy the islets of Langerhans represent the source of glucagon, the primary glucoregulatory hormone that counteracts the metabolic consequences of excessive insulin action (Cryer 2014; Campbell and Drucker 2015). The history of glucagon begins with that of insulin. In 1921, when F. Banting and C. Best tested their first pancreatic extracts in depancreatized dogs, they observed that insulin-induced hypoglycemia was preceded by a transient hyperglycemia (Gromada et al. 2007). The historical evidence suggesting that elevated glucagon is the glucoregulatory partner of insulin was reviewed in 1975, in the Banting Lecture of the American Diabetes Association (Unger 1976), only 50 years after its discovery; in the same year, Unger and Orci enunciated their "bi-hormonal hypothesis," concerning the central role of the combination of hypoinsulinemia and relative hyperglucagonemia in diabetic hyperglycemia (Unger and Orci 1975). The hormone glucagon has long been dismissed as a minor contributor to metabolic disease, but critical findings during the past few years have moved α-cells and glucagon into the spotlight of scientific discovery. The α-cell and glucagon have gained much attention with the recent recognition of the glucagon-suppressive effect, and related clinical utility in the treatment of type 2 diabetes, of the gut-derived incretin hormone glucagon-like peptide 1 (GLP-1) (able to powerfully stimulate insulin secretion from β-cells) and amylin, co-secreted with insulin from pancreatic β-cells (Hvidberg et al. 1994; Hare et al. 2009). Several other findings over the last few years have contributed to the recognition of islet α-cells and glucagon as key and essential players in energy homeostasis: α-cells appear to act as guardians of β-cells to ensure their health (Campbell and Drucker 2015), α-cells contain a local GLP-1 system that locally produces GLP-1 for paracrine action within the islets (Hope et al. 2004; Marchetti et al. 2012b), α-cells have the capacity to trans-differentiate into insulin-producing β-cells (Gromada et al. 2007; Plamboeck et al. 2013; Bagger et al. 2011), and moreover, impairment of glucagon signaling leads to a marked hyperplasia of α-cell mass that provides an increased supply of α-cells for their trans-differentiation into new β-cells.

Furthermore, recent pharmacologic investigations have focused on the therapeutic potential of targeting the α-cell with glucagon receptor antagonists. This approach could be effective in lowering hyperglycemia in patients with type 2 diabetes (Bagger et al. 2011).

The Pancreatic α-Cell

Pancreatic α-cells were discovered in 1907 as histologically distinct cells from the β-cells of the islets of Langerhans. The α-cells are one of five distinct polypeptide-secreting islet cell types: glucagon-secreting α-cells, insulin-producing β-cells, somatostatin-releasing delta cells, pancreatic polypeptide (PP)-secreting cells, and ghrelin-producing epsilon cells (Wierup et al. 2002, 2004; Lee et al. 2002).

The α-cells, accounting for approximately 20% of islet cells, are in close contact with β-cells. Human islets do not show the anatomical subdivisions of rodent islets where the β-cells are concentrated in the core of the islet, and α- and delta cells are located in the mantle (Cabrera et al. 2006); in humans, non-β-cells are often observed both at the periphery and also, seemingly, at the center of islets scattered throughout the human islet (Cabrera et al. 2006). Anatomical studies have shown that islets are densely vascularized, with at least one arteriole supplying every islet (Murakami and Fujita 1992). This would permit simultaneous exposure of islets to changes in arterial milieu and rate of flow (Moldovan and Brunicardi 2001). The cytoarchitecture of the human islet, where most of the β-cells show associations with other endocrine cells, suggests the existence of a network of intercellular paracrine signaling (Unger and Orci 2010).

The Glucagon Gene

The "glucagon" gene (GCG) encodes an mRNA for a prohormone, proglucagon, that, when translated into protein, gives rise to numerous peptides belonging to the glucagon superfamily of hormones. Despite the significant peptide sequence homology, members of this superfamily exert diverse and sometimes opposing regulatory functions (Kieffer and Habener 1999; Campbell and Drucker 2013). These hormones include glucagon-like peptides 1 and 2 (GLP-1, GLP-2), oxyntomodulin, glicentin, glicentin-related polypeptide (GRPP), and the intervening peptides 1 and 2. These peptides are formed from the proglucagon precursor by selected and tissue-specific enzymatic cleavages.

Proglucagon is expressed in pancreatic α-cells, intestinal L cells, and specific neurons in the central nervous system, and tissue-specific cleavages mediated by particular endopeptidases result in a different profile of proglucagon-derived peptides in these tissues.

Intestinal L cells predominantly express neuroendocrine convertase 1 [also known as prohormone convertase 1, (PC1/3) encoded by proprotein convertase subtilisin/kexin (PCSK-1)], which generates glicentin, oxyntomodulin, glucagon-like peptide 1 (GLP-1), and glucagon-like peptide 2 (GLP-2). By contrast, neuroendocrine convertase 2 (also known as prohormone convertase 2, PC2) is expressed in α-cells and liberates glucagon and the major proglucagon fragment, which contains unprocessed GLP-1 and GLP-2 (Campbell and Drucker 2015). The spectrum of proglucagon-derived peptides (PGDPs) produced by post-translational proteolysis of proglucagon differs among different tissues and is determined by the metabolic environment. There is evidence that glucagon was also found in enteroendocrine gut cells (Grimelius et al. 1976; Sasaki et al. 1975; Stanojevic and Habener 2015), and under such conditions of β-cell injuries, α-cell hyperplasia, and diabetes, α-cells are able to turn on the expression of PC1/3 and produce GLP-1 in addition to glucagon.

Glucagon Physiology and Hormone Secretion

Glucagon is secreted in response to hypoglycemia, with a robust secretory response that is triggered when levels of glucose decline below a key threshold, which differs slightly between different species (Cryer et al. 2003; Cryer 2013). The "intra-islet" hypothesis regarding glucagon secretion, first published in 1972 (Hope et al. 2004; Samols et al. 1988), indicates that a decrease in arterial glucose causes β-cell secretion decrease, whereby a tonic α-cell inhibition by insulin is diminished and glucagon secretion increases (Hope et al. 2004; Samols et al. 1988; Raju and Cryer 2005). Therefore, insulin and plasma glucose are considered strong regulators of the non-diabetic α-cell (Hare et al. 2009; Vilsboll et al. 2002; Knop et al. 2007a, b). Glucagon secretion also rises in response to adrenergic stimulation and to some regulatory peptides as well as following increases in circulating levels of amino acids and fatty acids (Gromada et al. 2007). The important role of multiple β-cell-derived secretory products, including insulin, zinc, and γ-aminobutyric acid (GABA), in the suppression of glucagon secretion is widely recognized (Gromada et al. 2007) and might account for the failure of insulin alone to completely suppress glucagon secretion under conditions of impaired or lost β-cell function (Campbell and Drucker 2015).

Moreover, the peptide produced by delta cells, somatostatin, potently inhibits glucagon secretion (Luft et al. 1978; Sakurai et al. 1974), and the human α-cell expresses several of the five somatostatin receptor subtypes (Ludvigsen et al. 2004; Portela-Gomes et al. 2000). Furthermore, also the central nervous system (CNS) represents an important sensor of glucose levels in the body and drives neural signals that augment glucagon secretion during hypoglycemia. Multiple regions and nuclei within the CNS contribute to the stimulation of glucagon secretion when glucose levels fall via increased parasympathetic input (Lamy et al. 2014). In addition, glucagon secretion is also influenced by the gut hormones GLP-1 and GIP (glucose-dependent insulinotropic polypeptide) (Nauck et al. 1993; Creutzfeldt et al. 1996).

Although glucose levels, free fatty acids, or amino acids primarily control glucagon release directly or indirectly through β-cells and δ-cells, the same metabolites could affect α-cell functionality. Inhibitory or stimulatory substances may reach the α-cell via the microcirculation and/or interstitial fluid (Charollais et al. 2000; Kleinman et al. 1995). In addition to all external factors, glucagon itself works as an extracellular messenger. It exerts a positive autocrine feedback that stimulates secretion in both isolated rat and mouse α-cells by an increase in exocytosis associated with a rise in cAMP levels (Ma et al. 2005).

Ion Channels and Regulation of Electrical Activity in the α-Cell

Similar to insulin secretion from β-cells, glucagon secretion from α-cells is regulated by electrical communication between various ion channels. Pancreatic α-cells are, indeed, equipped with a specific set of channels that generate action potentials. There are at least four different types of K^+-selective channels: the ATP-sensitive K^+ channel (K^+_{ATP} channel), the delayed K^+ channel (K_{Dr} channel), a G protein-gated K^+ channel activated by somatostatin (K_I channel), and a transient K^+ channel (A channel). Four types of voltage-gated Ca^{++} channel (T, N, R, and L type), a Na^+ channel, and $GABA_A$ receptor chloride channels have been observed (Gromada et al. 2007).

The K^+_{ATP} channel is considered to be the primary channel and the main regulatory component of glucagon secretion (MacDonald et al. 2007) (Fig. 2). It plays a central role in many tissues by coupling cell metabolism to electrical activity. Glucose metabolism in α-cells is mediated by the activity of glucokinase and the glucose transporter 1 (GLUT 1), a lower capacity isoform than GLUT 2, expressed in β-cells (Heimberg et al. 1995, 1996; Tu et al. 1999). Studies on isolated α-cells have shown that, unlike β-cells, they produce spontaneous action potentials in the absence of glucose (Franklin et al. 2005; Gromada et al. 1997, 2001a, 2004; Rorsman et al. 1989; Yoshimoto et al. 1999; Bokvist et al. 1999; Rorsman and Hellman 1988). Under resting conditions, the tonic activity of the K^+_{ATP} channels maintains a negative membrane potential at around -60 mV. Glucose metabolism produces a concentration-dependent inhibition of the channels, which is mediated by changes in the intracellular concentrations of ATP and ADP. The resulting increase in the ATP-to-ADP ratio leads to closure of K^+_{ATP} channels and membrane depolarization. This in turn activates voltage-dependent

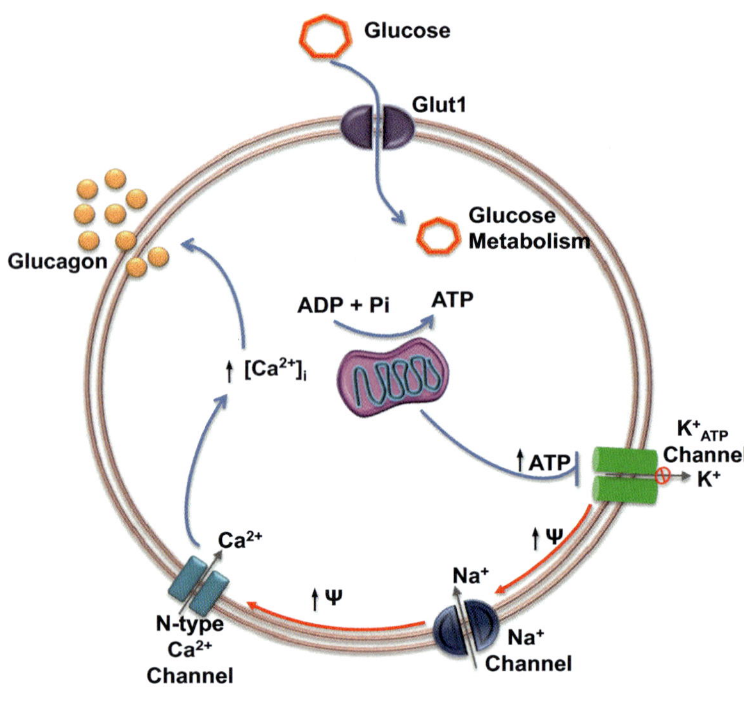

Fig. 2 Model for glucose-dependent regulation of glucagon secretion in rat alpha cells

Na^+- and L- and N-type Ca^{++} channels responsible for action potential generation, Ca^{++} influx, elevation of the intracellular Ca^{++} concentration, and stimulation of glucagon secretion (Gromada et al. 1997; Gopel et al. 2000). Sulfonylureas are able to bind to the SUR moiety of the K^+_{ATP} channel. The sulfonylurea-induced closure of the K^+_{ATP} channels initiates the same series of events in the α-cell as glucose or pyruvate.

Hormone Physiological Action

Several lines of defense protect the organism against hypoglycemia and its potential damaging effects, especially in the brain, which depends on a continuous supply of glucose, its principal metabolic fuel. Among all these protection systems, glucagon plays a central role in the response to hypoglycemia and also opposes insulin effects (Quesada et al. 2008). Therefore, it is conceivable that the structure and function of glucagon have been strictly preserved in the process of evolution. Following secretion into the portal circulation, glucagon targets its primary site of action, the liver. The actions of glucagon in the liver are complex. They involve binding to the glucagon receptor, a G protein-coupled receptor (gcgr), member of the class II G protein-coupled receptor subfamily (Jelinek et al. 1993), located in the plasma membrane, which results in amplification of signal transduction cascades and regulation of transcription factors. Gcgr primarily acts through activation of adenylate cyclase and subsequent increase in intracellular cyclic AMP (cAMP) concentrations. Specifically, receptor-binding activates G protein-mediated signal transduction (Gsα and Gq), and Gsα activates adenylate cyclase resulting in increasing cAMP and thereby protein kinase A (PKA) activity. Gq activation leads to an increase in intracellular Ca^{++} through activation of phospholipase C (Jiang and Zhang 2003). The glucagon receptor in the liver is highly selective for glucagon, but it exhibits a modest affinity for glucagon-like peptides (Hjorth et al. 1994). In hepatocytes, receptor activation ultimately leads to increased hepatic glucose production by enhancing both glycogenolysis and gluconeogenesis along with inhibition of glycogenesis and glycolysis (Gromada et al. 2007; Consoli et al. 1989; Gastaldelli et al. 2004; Lefebvre 2002). In this way glucagon action ensures an appropriate glucose supply to the body and brain. Thus, in healthy individuals, the balance of glucagon suppression and stimulation critically contributes to preserve normoglycemia. Glucagon can also stimulate the uptake of amino acids for gluconeogenesis in the liver. Indeed, subjects with hyperglucagonemia can develop plasma hypoaminoacidemia, especially of amino acids involved in gluconeogenesis, such as alanine, glycine, and proline (Cynober 2002). In addition to the liver, Gcgr is expressed in other tissues, including the adipose tissue, pancreas, gastrointestinal tract, heart, brain, and kidney, suggesting a broader physiological role beyond glucose and nutrient homeostasis (Christensen et al. 2011) (Fig. 3). In islet cells, the elevation of cAMP by glucagon has been reported to stimulate insulin and glucagon secretion from β- and α-cells, respectively (Ma et al. 2005; Huypens et al. 2000), by

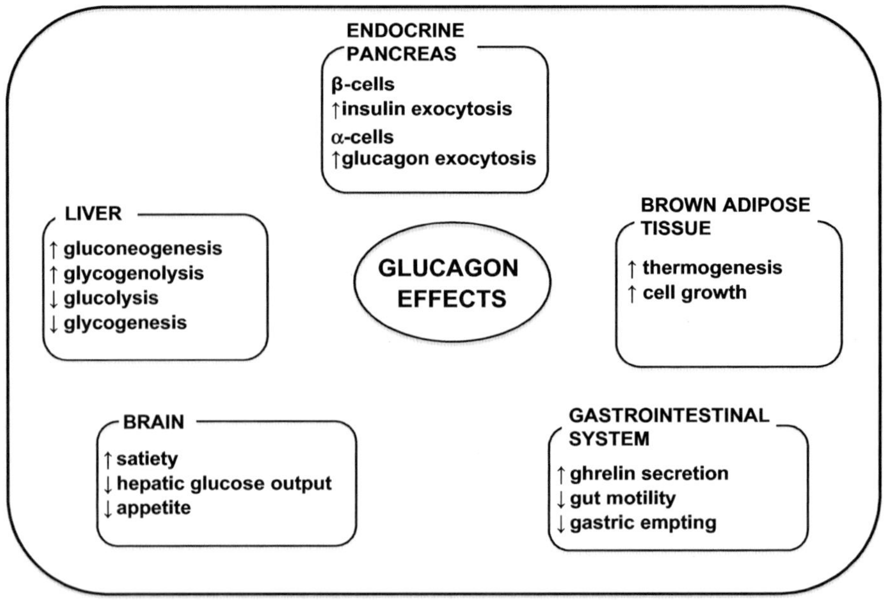

Fig. 3 Schematic representation of glucagon effects on various target tissues

PKA-dependent and PKA-independent mechanisms. Upregulation of cAMP activates cAMP-regulated guanine nucleotide exchange factors (cAMPGEFs/Epac), which modulate intracellular Ca^{++} ion mobilization, enhancing exocytosis (Ma et al. 2005; Holz et al. 2006).

Role of Glucagon in Hyperglycemia

As already reported, 40 years ago, Unger and Orci (1975) proposed the "bi-hormonal hypothesis" to explain the pathophysiology of diabetes (Unger and Orci 1975). According to this hypothesis, this metabolic disease is the result of an insulin deficiency or resistance along with an absolute or relative excess of glucagon (hyperglucagonemia), which can cause a higher rate of hepatic glucose production than glucose utilization, favoring hyperglycemia (Quesada et al. 2008). In recent years a glucagon-centered view of diabetes mellitus has reemerged, and it is supported by the requirement for glucagon in the development of hyperglycemia in preclinical models of type 1 diabetes mellitus (T1DM), type 2 diabetes mellitus (T2DM), and insulin deficiency (Campbell and Drucker 2013; Unger and Cherrington 2012). In particular the diabetic α-cell suffers from resistance to the glucagon-suppressive effects normally exerted by glucose and insulin (Dunning et al. 2005). Exogenous insulin is not effective as a negative feedback for hepatic glucose output, while glucagon potentiates glucose mobilization from the liver, thus contributing to hyperglycemia. Moreover in diabetic patients, the lack of suppression of glucagon release in hyperglycemic conditions is impaired, which would contribute further to postprandial hyperglycemia in both type 1 and type 2 diabetes. Recent investigations, using *in vitro* model, have furthermore indicated that also the long-term exposure to free fatty acids (in particular palmitate) restrains the insulin inhibitory effect on glucagon secretion leading to an inappropriate hormone release (Piro et al. 2010). These results suggest that hyperglucagonemia during diabetes might be a consequence of metabolic disorders (i.e., lipotoxicity) rather than a cause of diabetes and, for these reason, could be prevented.

Interestingly, it has been recently reported that a model of mice in absolute absence of glucagon receptors ($Gcgr^{-/-}$) is not hyperglycemic and shows normal glucose tolerance, even after complete destruction of β-cells (Lee et al. 2011). Moreover, restoration of hepatic Gcgr expression led to activation of gluconeogenesis and the rapid reappearance of hyperglycemia (Lee et al. 2012). Suppression of glucagon release with somatostatin in dogs that had been subjected to chemical destruction of their β-cells and in insulin-deprived humans with T1DM suppressed hyperglucagonemia and alleviated hyperglycemia (Dobbs et al. 1975). These experiments provide the first concrete evidence that glucagon might play an essential pathogenic role in the hyperglycemia during insulin deficiency state.

The Second Type of Cell: The Beta Cell

The pancreatic beta cells are unique endocrine cells that produce, store, and secrete insulin, the hormone that maintains circulating glucose concentrations within a narrow physiologic range, despite wide fluctuations in energy intake and expenditure. They also release additional proteins and small molecules, such as C-peptide, amylin, zinc, ATP, and GABA. Beta cells were first described more than one century ago and their morphology, ultrastructure, function, turnover, and molecular features investigated in depth afterward; this was mainly due to their key role in the pathophysiology of diabetes. They have an average diameter of 10 μm, contain approximately 20 pg insulin *per* cell, and are the predominant cell type in the pancreatic islets (50–80% of all islet endocrine cells). In the human pancreas, beta-cell mass varies from 0.6 to 2.1 g, and the amount of insulin in the gland has been reported to range from 50 to 250 μg/g (Berclaz et al. 2012; Masini et al. 2012). In a normal adult, beta cells may release approximately 30–70 U of insulin per day (mainly depending on body weight), 50% of which is secreted under basal conditions and the remaining amount in response to meals. The secretion of insulin is regulated by a complex interplay between nutrients, hormones, and neuronal signals, which allows the supply of insulin in quantity, dynamics, and flexibility matching the minute-by-minute needs of the body. In this chapter we will describe some key features of human pancreatic beta cells, focusing on insulin production and the cellular as well as molecular mechanism regulating the secretion of this hormone and also including the case of type 2 diabetes.

Gene Expression and Biosynthesis of Insulin

The insulin gene in humans is located on the short arm of chromosome 11, at position 15.5, from base pair 2,159,779 to base pair 2,161,209 and contains three exons and two introns. The beta-cell insulin gene transcriptional control is conferred by *cis*-acting regulatory DNA sequences that bind beta cell restricted as well as ubiquitous transcription factors. Specifically, the insulin gene is regulated at a DNA promoter region located approximately 340 base pairs upstream of the transcription initiation site. Beta cell-enriched proteins regulating insulin gene transcription include insulin promoter factor 1 (PDX1) and MAF bZIP transcription factor A (MAFA), whereas mechanisms not restricted to beta cells involve transcription factors responsive to specific signaling pathways (Ca^{++} signaling in particular) as well as several kinases and phosphatases (such as ERK and calcineurin) (Marchetti et al. 2012a). These factors also mediate the regulation of insulin gene expression induced by glucose. For instance, increased glucose concentrations determine phosphorylation of PDX1 by a number of different kinases [(including phosphatidylinositol-4,5-bisphosphate 3-kinase (PI3K) and mitogen-activated protein kinases (MAPK)], followed by the translocation of PDX1 to the nucleus. In addition, glucose stabilizes preproinsulin mRNA, the half-life of which increases more than twofold (from about 30 to 70 h). Several other factors modulate insulin gene expression, including a few hormones. GLP-1 upregulates the expression of insulin by potentiating the action of glucose on PDX1 and through other mechanisms, such as direct activation of cAMP response elements (CRE) and nuclear factor of activated T cells (NFAT); conversely, somatostatin and leptin reduce insulin gene expression by a number of different mechanisms, which in some cases also include decreased mRNA stability.

The product of insulin gene transcription is preproinsulin mRNA, which leads to the synthesis of a single polypeptide chain insulin precursor (Brezar et al. 2011). During translation of preproinsulin mRNA to preproinsulin protein, the emerging signal sequence of preproinsulin is bound to the membrane of the rough endoplasmic reticulum (RER), and preproinsulin enters the RER lumen. There, a specific peptidase cleaves the signal sequence, resulting in the formation of the nascent proinsulin molecule. Proinsulin then undergoes folding and formation of disulfide bonds between the A and B chains catalyzed by RER disulfide isomerase activity. The newly synthesized proinsulin is then transported from the RER to the cis-Golgi apparatus within transport vesicles in an ATP-dependent process. This is followed by trafficking through the stacks of the medial- and trans-Golgi apparatus to reach the clathrin-coated regions of the trans-Golgi network, which is the site of secretory granules biogenesis (Masini et al. 2012; Hou et al. 2009). In the immature secretory granule compartment, conversion begins of proinsulin to insulin and C-peptide by the action of two Ca^{++}-dependent endopeptidases (PC2 and PC1/3) and a Ni^{++}-dependent exopeptidase (CPH). Besides proinsulin conversion, maturation of the insulin granules involves loss of clathrin and progressive acidification (to reach a pH of 5.0–5.5), which is necessary for proinsulin conversion and insulin crystallization. In fact, within the mature granule and in the presence of high Zn^{++} concentrations,

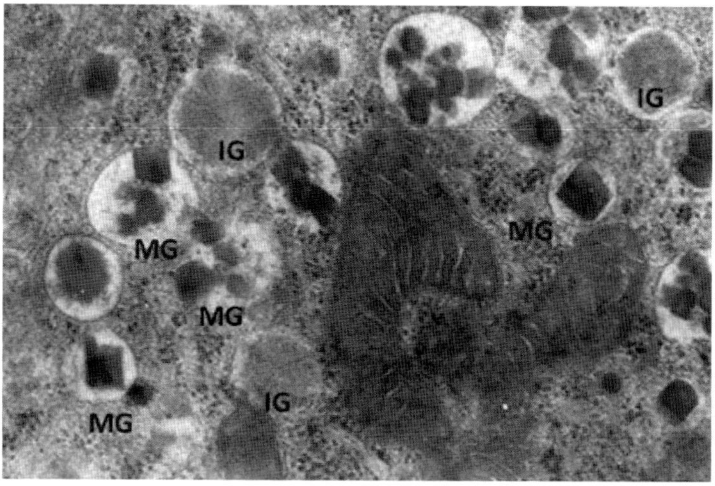

Fig. 4 Electron microscopy image of a human beta cell showing immature insulin granules (*IG*), with a less electron-dense structure, and mature insulin granules (*MG*), with a dense core (insulin crystals) and a white halo

insulin associates to form hexamers, a process that is coordinated by the histidine residue at position 10 of the insulin B chain. As a result, the dense core of the secretory granule observed by electron microscopy (Masini et al. 2012) is considered to be an insulin crystal (Fig. 4). Since C-peptide does not co-crystallize with insulin, this protein is assumed to be present in the clear halo of the granule (Fig. 4). Once formed, beta-cell granules are retained until exocytosis occurs, and insulin is released into the circulation (see below).

The Mechanisms of Glucose-Induced Insulin Secretion

Insulin secretion is a dynamic and finely controlled process, regulated in a feedback system, to maintain physiological plasma glucose concentrations in a relatively narrow range. In the fasting state, insulin controls glucose production by the liver and limits the release of free fatty acids from adipocytes; in this condition, the glucose produced by hepatocytes is mostly used by the brain, whose uptake of the hexose is insulin independent. After a meal, glucose enters the circulation through the portal system, with signals originating from the intestine able to amplify the release of insulin; the hormone is secreted in large amounts and promotes glucose uptake by peripheral tissues (mostly muscle) and the liver (which also curbs glucose production); at the level of the adipocytes, insulin stimulates glucose uptake and inhibits the release of free fatty acids.

The main physiological regulators of insulin secretion are listed in Table 1. Among them, glucose is predominant and exerts its effects through complex mechanisms that over the years have been described by models of stimulus-secretion

Table 1 Main physiological regulators of insulin secretion

Stimulators	Inhibitors
Nutrients	
Glucose	
Amino acids	
Free fatty acids (>C12)	
Ketones	
Hormones	**Hormones**
GLP-1	Somatostatin
GIP	Ghrelin
CCK	
Glucagon	
VIP	
Gastrin	
Secretin	
PACAP	
Neurotransmitters	**Neurotransmitters**
Acetylcholine	Adrenaline (α2 receptors)
Adrenaline (β2 receptors)	Noradrenaline (α2 receptors)
	NPY

coupling (Juhl and Hutton 2004). Glucose is both a trigger and an amplifier of the release of insulin. It is transported into the cytoplasm of the beta cell through facilitated glucose transport, mainly mediated by glucose transporter 2 (GLUT2) in rodents and GLUT1 in humans. Glucose is then rapidly phosphorylated by glucokinase (hexokinase IV, a high-*Km* isoform of hexokinase) in the glycolytic pathway (Fig. 5). The formation of glucose-6-phosphate occurs without allosteric inhibition of the product. Therefore, glucokinase determines the rate of glycolysis and is considered the molecular glucose sensor for insulin secretion in the beta cell. The end product of the glycolytic cascade is the three-carbon molecule, pyruvate. In principle, pyruvate could be used for either aerobic or anaerobic respiration. Since in the beta cell the expression of lactate dehydrogenase (the enzyme that converts pyruvate to lactate) is very low, under normal conditions pyruvate rapidly enters the mitochondrion to undergo oxidation.

In the mitochondrion, pyruvate is converted to acetyl CoA by the enzyme pyruvate kinase, to then react with oxaloacetate to produce citrate, a metabolite of the tricarboxylic acid (TCA) cycle. The activation of TCA leads to the production of reducing equivalents in the form of NADH and $FADH_2$, which will be used for the generation of ATP in the electron transport chain. There, NADH and $FADH_2$ act as donors of electrons, which move through a series of complexes (complex I, NADH-ubiquinone reductase; complex II, succinate dehydrogenase; complex III, ubiquinol-cytochrome c reductase; complex IV, cytochrome c oxidase), where redox reactions occur. The terminal electron acceptor is O_2. These reactions are coupled with the production of a proton gradient across the inner mitochondrial membrane. The resulting transmembrane proton gradient is used by the ATP synthase complex to

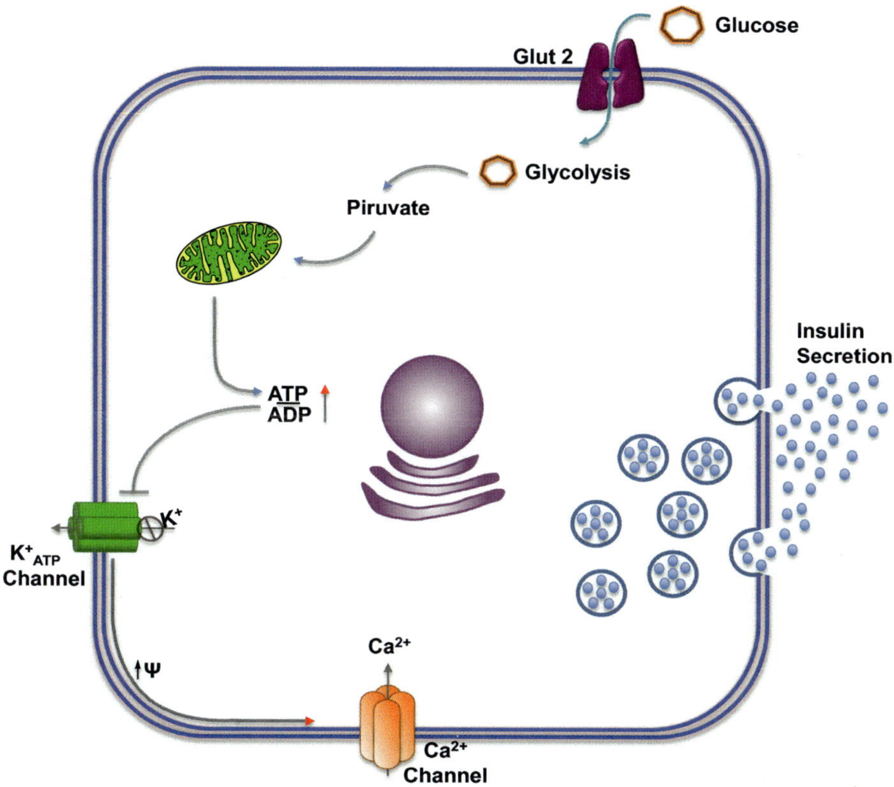

Fig. 5 Model for glucose-dependent stimulation of insulin secretion by beta cells of the pancreas

produce ATP via oxidative phosphorylation. The ATP synthesized in this way is finally translocated to the cytosol by the adenine nucleotide translocator (ANT).

The rise in cytosolic ATP concentrations causes the closure of the K^{+}_{ATP} channels, reduction of the K^{+} conductance, and depolarization of the plasma membrane of the beta cell. Therefore, the K^{+}_{ATP} channels couple the metabolic state of the beta cell to the electrical activity. These channels are tetramers of a complex of two proteins, a high-affinity sulfonylurea receptor (SUR1) and an inwardly rectifying K^{+} channel (Kir6.2). Each channel is composed of four outer subunits of SUR1, which mediate the opening property of Mg^{++} ADP and confer the sensitivity to pharmacological agents such as sulfonylureas and diazoxide, which, respectively, close and open the channel; the inner pore of the channels is formed by four subunits of Kir6.2 to which ATP binds (Fig. 6). Once the threshold potential induced by membrane depolarization is reached, voltage-dependent Ca^{++} channels (mainly of the L type) open, allowing the influx of Ca^{++}. In turn, this induces a rapid depolarization to a plateau potential on which bursts of Ca^{++} potentials appear. This is followed by oscillations of membrane potentials and rhythmic openings of the channels and influx of the ion. The influx of the extracellular Ca^{++} to the beta-cell cytosol allows

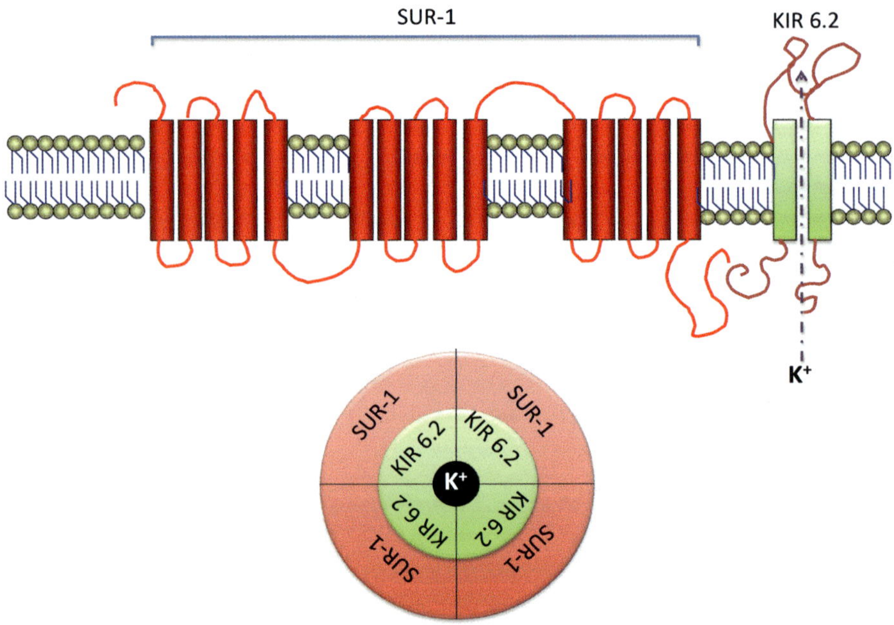

Fig. 6 Model for SUR-1/Kir6.2 channel. The *upper* part of the figure shows the channel into the membrane; the *lower* part shows the complex of two proteins of SUR-1 and Kir 6.2 forming a tetramer. SUR-1 isoform is expressed mainly in beta cells and in the brain, SUR-2 isoform in the cardiac and in skeletal muscle, and SUR 2B in the smooth muscle

mobilization of the insulin granules and their exocytosis. The signals regulating the transport of insulin secretory granules to the plasma membrane of the beta cells and the mechanisms involved in insulin exocytosis show analogies to the processes observed with synaptic vesicle exocytosis in neurons. Transport of insulin granules is likely mediated by the interaction of the granules with cytosolic microtubules and microfilaments, which is triggered by different intracellular secondary signals, including an increase in cytosolic Ca^{++}. Docking of the granules to the plasma membrane and subsequent fusion are believed to depend on the interaction of proteins on the granules (v-SNAREs, such as the synaptobrevin family) with cognate members of proteins located on the membrane (t-SNAREs, such as syntaxin and SNAP-25) (Fig. 7). Granules that are not used for exocytosis are degraded through a mechanism termed crinophagy, i.e., an autophagic process involving fusion with lysosomes. The mechanisms linking Ca^{++} to these last events are still relatively unknown; however, a major role is probably played by Ca^{++}-calmodulin protein kinase II, which is associated with the secretory granules and is involved in the mobilization of the insulin granules from the Golgi apparatus to the exocytotic sites.

In summary, therefore, the triggering pathway model through which glucose induces insulin secretion involves the entry of glucose into the beta cells via facilitated transport (which is not rate limiting, allowing rapid balance between extra- and intracellular

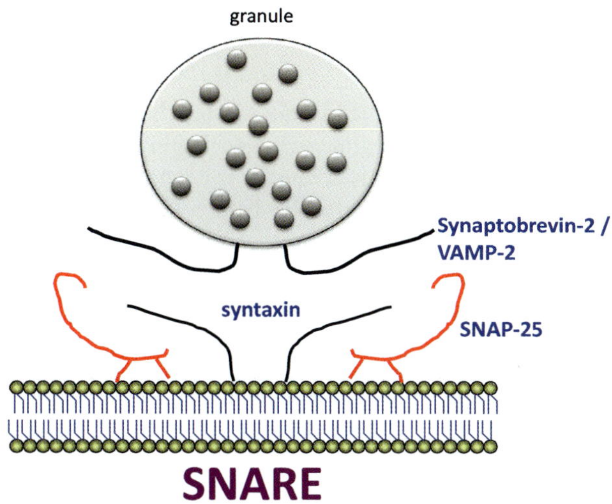

Fig. 7 Representation of docking granules to the plasma membrane in beta cell

glucose concentrations), followed by glucose metabolism by glycolysis. The tight coupling of glycolysis and mitochondrial activity leads to quick changes in the cytosolic ATP/ADP ratio, which in turn regulate the function of the K^{+}_{ATP} channels. These latter transduce biochemical signals into biophysical events, with their closure (due to increased ATP/ADP ratio) determining depolarization of the plasma membrane, opening of voltage-dependent Ca^{++} channels, and increasing Ca^{++} influx. Finally, Ca^{++} activates effector mechanisms leading to the exocytosis of the insulin granules.

As mentioned above, glucose also possesses the capacity of amplifying insulin release, meaning that glucose metabolism produces signals that do not further increase cytosolic Ca^{++} concentrations but promotes Ca^{++}-mediated exocytosis of insulin granules (Henquin 2011). This has been demonstrated by studies using pharmacological blocking of the K^{+}_{ATP} channels or clamping Ca^{++} concentrations at elevated levels. At such experimental conditions, glucose increased insulin secretion with negligible effects on the already high Ca^{++} concentrations (Henquin 2011). The mechanisms responsible of the amplifying pathway are still unsettled, but events mediated by ATP at steps distal to the increase of Ca^{++} levels and/or metabolites produced in the mitochondrion may play a role.

The Role of Compounds Other Than Glucose

As listed in Table 1, several other compounds can affect the beta-cell insulin secretory function. Amino acids, either alone or in combination, regulate the release of insulin by both metabolic and/or biophysical mechanisms (Newsholme et al. 2014). They may have triggering actions but more frequently amplify insulin release. Leucine alone, for instance, can weakly increase insulin secretion in the absence of glucose, but it is much more potent in the presence of glutamine that, alone, is not effective (Anello et al. 2004). Leucine and, more markedly, its combination with glutamine exert both triggering and amplifying effects on insulin release. Biochemically, leucine is metabolized to produce acetyl CoA, which is used in the TCA cycle. Glutamine is transformed in glutamate which, in the presence of leucine, is further metabolized to α-ketoglutarate, also fueling the TCA cycle. The two amino acids, therefore, act at steps involving the mitochondrion. Another amino acid, arginine, is, instead, poorly metabolized by beta cells. Arginine depolarizes the plasma membrane due to its transport into the cell in a positively charged form. This depolarization activates the voltage-dependent Ca^{++} channels to allow Ca^{++} entry and the successive steps leading to exocytosis of insulin granules.

Free fatty acids represent metabolic substrates for the beta cells and can regulate the secretory function of these cells by modulating the oxidation of fuel molecules in the mitochondria (Henquin 2011). More recently, it has become clear that they are able to exert signaling functions by binding to some G protein-coupled receptors (GPRs) that are expressed on the surface of beta cells (GPR40 in particular but also GPR119 and GPR120) (Morgan and Dhayal 2009) and mediate, at least in part, the acute insulin secretagogue effects of free fatty acids. Activation of the receptors induces the production of inositol trisphosphate (IP3) and diacylglycerol (DAG). In turn, IP3 triggers the release of Ca^{++} from the endoplasmic reticulum, and DAG activates protein kinase C (PKC) to amplify the effects of glucose metabolism on insulin secretion. It has been shown that palmitate and stearate can slightly increase basal insulin secretion in the presence of low (3 mmol/l) glucose concentrations and that the rank of potency of fatty acids to potentiate glucose-induced insulin secretion (at 10–15 mmol/l) is palmitate > myristate > stearate approximately = oleate > linoleate approximately = linolenate (Warnotte et al. 1999).

The beta-cell GPR system is also involved in the regulation of insulin secretion by neurotransmitters and several hormones (Table 1). In particular, the role of the incretin hormone GLP-1 has been extensively studied, also in view of its potential as a target for type 2 diabetes therapy (Drucker and Nauck 2006). GLP-1 is released from enteroendocrine L cells in response to nutrient ingestion and potentiate insulin release in a glucose concentration-dependent manner. Its mechanisms of action on the beta cell are complex but seem to be mediated by activation of adenylate cyclase and also the production of IP3 and DAG (this latter is similar to the case of free fatty acids). Adenylate cyclase activation leads to increased cyclic adenosine monophosphate (cAMP) production. In turn, cAMP activates protein kinase A (PKA)-dependent and independent mechanisms that mainly through the action of Epac2 and the phosphorylation activity of PKA on several substrates influence insulin granule kinetics and ion channel activity (Doyle and Egan 2007).

Beta Cells in Human Type 2 Diabetes

Diabetes mellitus is a heterogeneous disease, consisting of four main types: (a) type 1 diabetes, due to autoimmune beta-cell destruction, usually leading to absolute insulin deficiency; (b) type 2 diabetes, due to a progressive loss of insulin secretion on the background of insulin resistance; (c) gestational diabetes, which is diagnosed in the second or third trimester of pregnancy; and (d) specific types of diabetes due to other causes, e.g., monogenic diabetes syndromes, diseases of the exocrine pancreas, drug- or chemical-induced diabetes, and others (American Diabetes A. 2016). Since type 2 diabetes is by far the most common form of diabetes (85–90% of all cases) and given the key role of beta-cell failure in its onset and progression (Halban et al. 2010), much work has been done to understand the condition of beta cells in this type of diabetes, mainly focusing on beta-cell loss and functional incompetence.

Although quantification of beta cells in the human pancreas is a difficult task, morphometric analyses have been performed by several authors to assess beta-cell mass (when the weight of pancreas specimens was available), volume (usually assuming that the islets are spherical), and/or area (insulin-positive proportions in the islets or the pancreatic tissue) (Marchetti et al. 2012a). The amount of beta cells has been usually reported to be significantly lower in the pancreata of patients with type 2 diabetes (30–40% reduction on average). Interestingly, however, work performed by the use of light and electron microscopy suggests that the loss of beta cells in this type of diabetes, as assessed by insulin staining, may be overestimated because of degranulation or other changes in the beta-cell phenotype (dedifferentiation is an example) (Cinti et al. 2016).

The reasons why there is a reduced amount of beta cells in type 2 diabetes are still a matter of debate. It is likely that in this condition more beta cells die because of a form of programmed cell death called apoptosis (characterized by marked nuclear chromatin condensation and additional morphological characteristics) (Fig. 8), possibly due to increased stress of the RER (Marchetti et al. 2007; Eizirik et al. 2008) on the basis of the interplay between genetic and environmental factors (Butler et al. 2007). This is probably associated with defects of beta-cell regeneration. The latter may essentially occur by replication (proliferation) of existing cells, neogenesis from precursors, or trans-differentiation of existing mature cells. It has been generally observed, by the use of indirect morphological methods, that regeneration events in

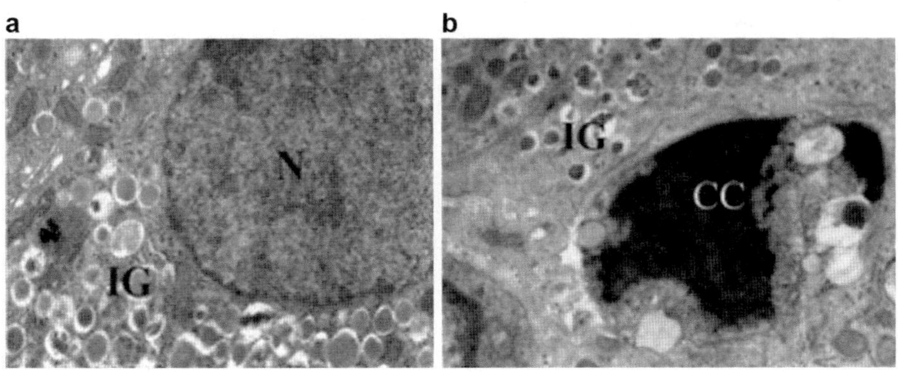

Fig. 8 Electron microscopy of a normal beta cell (*left panel*) and a beta cell with signs of apoptosis (*right panel*). *IG* insulin granules, *CC* chromatin condensation in the nucleus

human type 2 diabetes occur at similar very low rates as in the nondiabetic condition, not compensating for the loss of beta cells described above (Butler et al. 2007). Currently, however, the insulin-secretory defects of beta cells are considered more important than the reduced beta-cell amount in the pathophysiology of type 2 diabetes. As a matter of fact, there are several quantitative and qualitative alterations of insulin release in type 2 diabetes (Ferrannini 1998; Kahn et al. 2014). Commonly found abnormalities include reduced or absent first phase insulin secretion to intravenous glucose, delayed or blunted responses to mixed meal ingestion, and, with time, reduced second phase release and diminished responses to non-glucose stimuli. Qualitative defects are mainly represented, besides changes of early phase insulin secretion, by alterations of oscillatory patterns and increased proinsulin release. As mentioned above, insulin is secreted in pulses and oscillations. The pulses take place every 8–10 min in normal individuals and are superimposed on much longer oscillations. The higher-frequency pulses appear to be intrinsically controlled by the islets themselves, whereas the lower-frequency oscillations may be regulated by signaling from outside the islets. In type 2 diabetes patients, the pulsed pattern has been reported to be disrupted, although the mechanisms involved are unclear. Increased proinsulin/insulin ratio has also been reported in type 2 diabetes. Within beta-cell secretory granules, under normal conditions, proinsulin is mostly cleaved into insulin and C-peptide, leaving around 2% of the intact or incompletely cleaved proinsulin precursor molecules. In patients with type 2 diabetes, the proportion of proinsulin molecules is increased four- to fivefold when compared with that of normal individuals, indicating less efficient conversion of proinsulin to insulin.

In conclusion, pancreatic beta cells are unique endocrine cells with extraordinarily sophisticated architectural, biological, and molecular features. Their key role is the production and secretion of insulin in a tightly regulated manner, to maintain circulating glucose concentrations in the physiological range. Although the large amount of information available on the processes modulating insulin release, shedding light on additional mechanisms governing the health of the beta cells will contribute to better understand the cause of diabetes and conceive strategies for its prevention, better treatment, and, hopefully, cure.

The Third Cell: The Delta Cell and Somatostatin

The presence of a third cell type in the islets of Langerhans of a variety of species was originally described by Felice Caramia (Caramia et al. 1965; Merlini and Caramia 1965; Munger et al. 1965; Caramia 1963). In 1975, for the first time, the presence of immunoreactive somatostatin-containing cells that were scattered throughout the islets of Langerhans was demonstrated by Maurice Dubois in a variety of species ranging from humans to sheep, thus confirming the existence of this third cell type, as originally described by Felice Caramia (Dubois 1975).

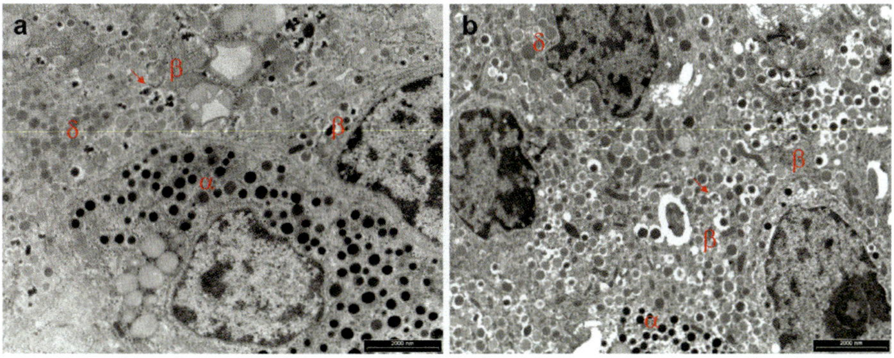

Fig. 9 Islets of Langerhans of man (**a**) and baboon (**b**) pancreas: β-cell granules are heterogeneous, showing dense cores which become crystalline when the granules mature (*arrows*); α-cell granules are characterized by a dense, osmophilic core surrounded by a less dense eccentric halo; and δ-cell granules are round, homogeneous, and of low electron density

Somatostatin-secreting δ-cells are the third most common cell type in the islets of Langerhans, where they constitute from 8% to 12% of the total cells there (Fig. 9). The same studies also demonstrated that insulin-containing β-cells range from ~50% to 60%, and glucagon-containing α-cells range from ~10% to 20% in adult human and nonhuman primates' islets of Langerhans (Rufener et al. 1975; Dubois et al. 1975; Rahier et al. 1983b). Interestingly, the cellular composition of human and nonhuman primates' islets is not dramatically different from rodent islets in terms of relative abundance of cell type, with the relative abundance decreasing progressively from β–α–δ-PP-ghrelin (~70% to 15% to 10% to 4% to 1%, respectively) cells. However, while in rodents (mice and rats) β-cells are present in the center of the islet, with α- and δ-cells constituting a crown around them, in adult human and nonhuman primate islets (baboon and monkey), β-cells, α-cells, and δ-cells are found scattered throughout the islets of Langerhans, most of them aligned along blood vessels with no particular arrangements, suggesting that the islet microcirculation is not a key determinant in the order of paracrine interaction of different cell types, differently from the rodents' islets of Langerhans (Cabrera et al. 2006; Rahier et al. 1980, 1981; Guardado-Mendoza et al. 2009, 2015; Quinn et al. 2012; Folli et al. 2011; Di Cairano et al. 2016). It is also interesting to note that while in the mouse's islets of Langerhans ~70% of β-cells display only homotypic association (i.e., juxtaposition between same cell type), in human islets ~30% show this kind of association. In human and nonhuman primates' islets, the majority of contacts, ~70%, are heterotypic contacts (i.e., juxtaposition between different cell types) (Bosco et al. 2010). These data imply that human and nonhuman primate islets have a distinct physiology from rodent islets, consistent with the striking morphological differences between primates (human and nonhuman) and rodents (mice and rats).

Somatostatin

Somatostatin was originally described as a substance that inhibited the release of growth hormone (GH) from pituitary glands (Burgus et al. 1973; Brazeau et al. 1973). Subsequently, this hormone was also found in islets of Langerhans' extracts and was described as capable to inhibit insulin secretion (Koerker et al. 1974; Hellman and Lernmark 1969). Somatostatin was sequenced in 1973 by the group of Guillemin (Burgus et al. 1973; Brazeau et al. 1973). There are two major forms of somatostatin, somatostatin-14 and somatostatin-28, which are derived from the same gene, by differential cleavage of the prohormone by prohormone-converting enzymes, furin, PC1, and PC2 (prohormone convertase) (Galanopoulou et al. 1993). In the central nervous system including the hypothalamus, somatostatin-14 is the predominant form, where it inhibits not only GH release but also TSH and PRL release. Somatostatin-28 is the predominant form in the gastrointestinal tract. The genes encoding somatostatin in humans, rodents, and fish display very strong sequence homology (Reichlin 1983a, b; Shen and Rutter 1984; Morel et al. 1984; Montminy et al. 1984, 1986a, b).

Somatostatin is a powerful inhibitor of glucagon as well as insulin secretion in mammals, either through the islet microcirculation and/or direct paracrine-juxtacrine mechanisms and possibly the mechanisms by which somatostatin acts in rodents are quite different when compared to primates (human and nonhuman), given the different cytoarchitecture of the islets of Langerhans in the two genera (Walker et al. 2011; Watts et al. 2016; Pipeleers et al. 1985a, b; Hauge-Evans et al. 2009; Malaisse 2014).

Somatostatin release in the islets of Langerhans is stimulated by hyperglycemia, by arginine, and by sulfonylurea, tolbutamide (Cheng-Xue et al. 2013).

There are five different somatostatin receptors (SSTR1, SSTR2, SSTR3, SSTR4, and SSTR5) (Patel and Srikant 1994, 1997). α-Cells express predominantly the SSTR2, while β-cells express prevalently the SSTR1 and SSTR5 receptors (Strowski et al. 2000). A number of mechanisms were described by which somatostatin leads to inhibition of glucagon secretion in α-cell. Somatostatin can activate G protein-coupled K^+ channels in α-cells, thus causing plasma membrane hyperpolarization and inhibition of electrical activity (Gromada et al. 2001a; Yoshimoto et al. 1999). Furthermore, the effect of somatostatin to inhibit α-cell exocytosis depends on the activity of a pertussis toxin-sensitive G protein (Gi2) as well as calcineurin (Gromada et al. 2001b). Studies employing knockout (KO) mice for SSTR2 and somatostatin receptor agonists and antagonists have shown that somatostatin inhibits glucagon release primarily through the SSTR2 receptor, while insulin secretion is inhibited primarily through SSTR5 (Cheng-Xue et al. 2013; Wang et al. 2005a, b). These data are also reinforced by studies on SST (somatostatin)-KO mice. These mice were phenotypically normal and exhibited increased insulin as well as glucagon secretion, in response to physiological stimuli. Glucose also suppressed glucagon secretion from control, but not SST-KO islets. These data support the concept that δ-cell somatostatin acts as a paracrine-inhibitory signal to inhibit insulin and glucagon secretion, also in response to nutrients, such as glucose and which may also

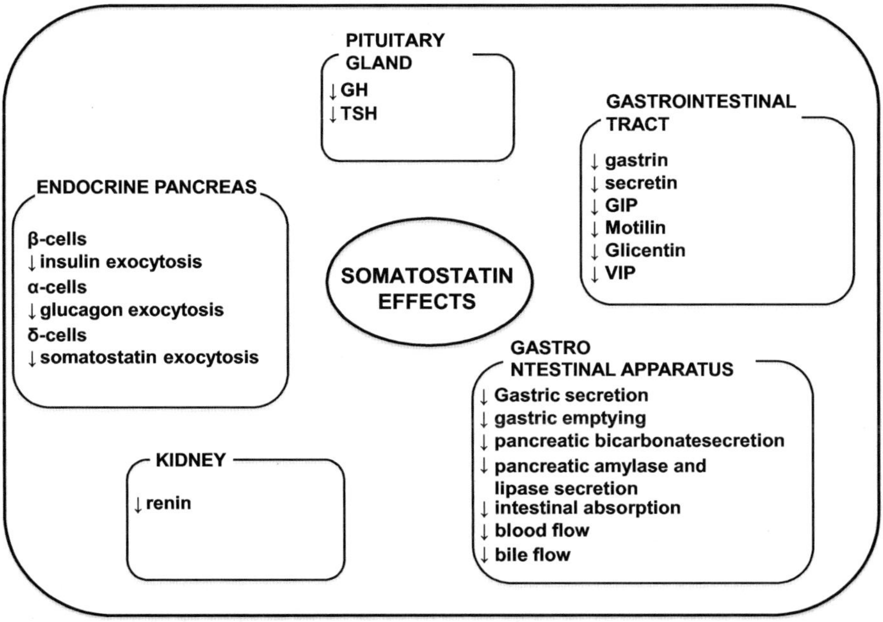

Fig. 10 Schematic representation of somatostatin effects on various target tissues

prime the islets of Langerhans' response to cholinergic activation (Hauge-Evans et al. 2009; Rorsman and Braun 2013). The main biological effects of somatostatin on various target tissues are summarized in Fig. 10.

Ion Channels and Regulation of Electrical Activity in the δ-Cell

The physiology of the human delta cells has recently been studied in detail by the laboratory of Matthias Braun and Peter Rorsman (Braun et al. 2009). Somatostatin secretion from human δ-cells is stimulated by glucose and tolbutamide and inhibited by diazoxide. δ-Cells display sporadic electrical activity, which is increased by tolbutamide, but not by glucose. Interestingly, somatostatin cells have a tolbutamide-insensitive/Ba2+ -sensitive inwardly rectifying K^+ current as well as two voltage-gated K^+ currents, one sensitive to tetraethylammonium/stromatoxin (delayed rectifying, Kv2.1/2.2) and 4-aminopyridine (A current). Voltage-gated tetrodotoxin (TTX)-sensitive Na^+ currents contributed to the action upstroke, with no effect on somatostatin release. D-cells are also equipped with Ca^{++} channels, which can be blocked by isradipine (L-type channels), ω-agatoxin (P/Q-type channels), and NNC 55-0396 (T-type channels). The blockade of any of these channels affects the δ-cell electrical activity and eliminates glucose-stimulated somatostatin release. Exocytosis is regulated by Ca^{++} influx through P/Q-type Ca^{++} channels. Glucose stimulation of somatostatin secretion involves both K^+ ATP channel-dependent and K^+ ATP channel-independent mechanisms.

The PP Cells

Although glucagon-secreting α-cells, insulin-secreting β-cells, and somatostatin-secreting δ-cells are predominant, other cell types are present in pancreatic islets; these other cells could play a role in intra-islet coordination and thus in the control of glucose homeostasis. However, our knowledge about these other cells is extremely limited.

The pancreatic polypeptide (PP)-secreting cells, also known as F cells, represent the fourth cell population within the islets. PP cells produce pancreatic polypeptide (PP), a 36 amino acid peptide, present in secretory granules bounded by a membrane. These cells were first identified in an avian pancreas and later in murine and mammalian pancreas (Kimmel et al. 1975; Larsson et al. 1975). They are located with other non-beta cells toward the periphery of rodent islets; in human islets they are present close to the capillaries. The size and the distribution of the PP cells in the pancreas are very heterogeneous, but the head of the pancreas shows the highest concentration (Rahier et al. 1983a; Stefan et al. 1982; Wang et al. 2013a, b). PP hormone regulates gastric emptying, intestinal motor activity, and glucagon secretion; thus PP is an important element of the islet-gut-brain axis. Recent evidence suggests a role of PP cells in the context of GLP-1 and GIP actions in islets; in particular, GIP could act on PP cells to control glucagon secretion (Chia et al. 2014).

Other Cell Types

In the last few years, epsilon cells or ghrelin-positive cells have received much attention. The hormone ghrelin is an endocrine peptide that has been identified in gastric oxyntic glands and that induces growth hormone secretion in the pituitary gland. Moreover, this hormone is expressed in many tissues such as the stomach, placenta, testis, pituitary gland, and thyroid. Although a number of studies have reported ghrelin expression in the developing pancreas, the location of ghrelin-immunoreactive cells in the adult pancreas remains controversial. Some authors report ghrelin expressed in epsilon cells, as a distinct cell type present in islets, and some other authors found ghrelin co-expressed with other hormones. Recently Raghay et al. demonstrated that ghrelin immunoreactivity co-localizes with glucagon in the human islet, whereas ghrelin is expressed in insulin-secreting cells in the rat pancreas, as confirmed by double immunofluorescence and in situ hybridization (Raghay et al. 2013). Following this point of view, epsilon cells could represent some constitutive cells in islets and could contribute to maintaining the architecture of the organ. Understanding how diabetes-related disorders could influence islet structure, cell identity and intra-islet cellular communication could clarify how non-β-cells contribute to the control of islet function and composition. Diabetes results not only from dysfunction of one or more of the hormone-expressing cells but also from changes to the islet architecture and a breakdown in the communication between the endocrine cells of the pancreatic islet (Foulis et al. 1991; Foulis and Stewart 1984).

Summary and Conclusions

In the present chapter, we have illustrated some general notions regarding the pancreatic islet composition and cell function. We have reported that every cell within the islet represents a single unit, and a single islet could be identified as a micro-organ in the pancreas. Moreover, we have illustrated that reduction of beta-cell mass is fundamental for the pathogenesis of both type 1 and type 2 diabetes and that non-beta cells are essential to islet architecture. We need to know more about cell physiology and physiopathology of islet cells. Understanding how diabetes-related disorders influence islet structure and intra-islet cellular metabolic abnormalities could clarify how every cell present in the islet contributes to the control of islet function. Therefore, therapeutic strategies should aim to target all cell types in islets and both cellular function and islet architecture to help restore glucose homeostasis in diabetes. These issues are among the highest priorities in the field of diabetes and metabolic diseases in humans.

Cross-References

► Synthesis, Secretion, and Transport of Peptide Hormones
► Principles of Endocrine Diseases
► The Endocrine System

References

American Diabetes Association. Classification and diagnosis of diabetes. Diabetes Care. 2016;39 Suppl 1:S13–22.

Anello M, Spampinato D, Piro S, Purrello F, Rabuazzo AM. Glucosamine-induced alterations of mitochondrial function in pancreatic beta-cells: possible role of protein glycosylation. Am J Physiol Endocrinol Metab. 2004;287(4):E602–8.

Bagger JI, Knop FK, Holst JJ, Vilsboll T. Glucagon antagonism as a potential therapeutic target in type 2 diabetes. Diabetes Obes Metab. 2011;13(11):965–71.

Benninger RK, Zhang M, Head WS, Satin LS, Piston DW. Gap junction coupling and calcium waves in the pancreatic islet. Biophys J. 2008;95(11):5048–61. Pubmed Central PMCID: 2586567.

Berclaz C, Goulley J, Villiger M, Pache C, Bouwens A, Martin-Williams E, et al. Diabetes imaging-quantitative assessment of islets of Langerhans distribution in murine pancreas using extended-focus optical coherence microscopy. Biomed Opt Express. 2012;3(6):1365–80. Pubmed Central PMCID: 3370976.

Bokvist K, Olsen HL, Hoy M, Gotfredsen CF, Holmes WF, Buschard K, et al. Characterisation of sulphonylurea and ATP-regulated K+ channels in rat pancreatic A-cells. Pflugers Arch – Eur J Physiol. 1999;438(4):428–36.

Bosco D, Armanet M, Morel P, Niclauss N, Sgroi A, Muller YD, et al. Unique arrangement of alpha- and beta-cells in human islets of Langerhans. Diabetes. 2010;59(5):1202–10. Pubmed Central PMCID: 2857900.

Bramswig NC, Everett LJ, Schug J, Dorrell C, Liu C, Luo Y, et al. Epigenomic plasticity enables human pancreatic alpha to beta cell reprogramming. J Clin Invest. 2013;123(3):1275–84. Pubmed Central PMCID: 3582140.

Braun M, Ramracheya R, Amisten S, Bengtsson M, Moritoh Y, Zhang Q, et al. Somatostatin release, electrical activity, membrane currents and exocytosis in human pancreatic delta cells. Diabetologia. 2009;52(8):1566–78.

Brazeau P, Vale W, Burgus R, Ling N, Butcher M, Rivier J, et al. Hypothalamic polypeptide that inhibits the secretion of immunoreactive pituitary growth hormone. Science. 1973;179 (4068):77–9.

Brezar V, Carel JC, Boitard C, Mallone R. Beyond the hormone: insulin as an autoimmune target in type 1 diabetes. Endocr Rev. 2011;32(5):623–69.

Burgus R, Ling N, Butcher M, Guillemin R. Primary structure of somatostatin, a hypothalamic peptide that inhibits the secretion of pituitary growth hormone. Proc Natl Acad Sci U S A. 1973;70(3):684–8. Pubmed Central PMCID: 433335.

Butler PC, Meier JJ, Butler AE, Bhushan A. The replication of beta cells in normal physiology, in disease and for therapy. Nat Clin Pract Endocrinol Metab. 2007;3(11):758–68.

Cabrera O, Berman DM, Kenyon NS, Ricordi C, Berggren PO, Caicedo A. The unique cytoarchitecture of human pancreatic islets has implications for islet cell function. Proc Natl Acad Sci U S A. 2006;103(7):2334–9. Pubmed Central PMCID: 1413730.

Campbell JE, Drucker DJ. Pharmacology, physiology, and mechanisms of incretin hormone action. Cell Metab. 2013;17(6):819–37.

Campbell JE, Drucker DJ. Islet alpha cells and glucagon – critical regulators of energy homeostasis. Nat Rev Endocrinol. 2015;11(6):329–38.

Caramia F. Electron microscopic description of a third cell type in the islets of the rat pancreas. Am J Anat. 1963;112:53–64.

Caramia F, Munger BL, Lacy PE. The ultrastructural basis for the identification of cell types in the pancreatic islets. I. Guinea pig. Z Zellforsch Mikrosk Anat. 1965;67(4):533–46.

Charollais A, Gjinovci A, Huarte J, Bauquis J, Nadal A, Martin F, et al. Junctional communication of pancreatic beta cells contributes to the control of insulin secretion and glucose tolerance. J Clin Invest. 2000;106(2):235–43. Pubmed Central PMCID: 314309.

Cheng-Xue R, Gomez-Ruiz A, Antoine N, Noel LA, Chae HY, Ravier MA, et al. Tolbutamide controls glucagon release from mouse islets differently than glucose: involvement of K(ATP) channels from both alpha-cells and delta-cells. Diabetes. 2013;62(5):1612–22. Pubmed Central PMCID: 3636641.

Chia CW, Odetunde JO, Kim W, Carlson OD, Ferrucci L, Egan JM. GIP contributes to islet trihormonal abnormalities in type 2 diabetes. J Clin Endocrinol Metab. 2014;99(7):2477–85. Pubmed Central PMCID: 4079310.

Christensen M, Bagger JI, Vilsboll T, Knop FK. The alpha-cell as target for type 2 diabetes therapy. Rev Diabet Stud: RDS. 2011;8(3):369–81. Pubmed Central PMCID: 3280671.

Cinti F, Bouchi R, Kim-Muller JY, Ohmura Y, Sandoval PR, Masini M, et al. Evidence of beta-cell dedifferentiation in human type 2 diabetes. J Clin Endocrinol Metab. 2016;101(3):1044–54.

Consoli A, Nurjhan N, Capani F, Gerich J. Predominant role of gluconeogenesis in increased hepatic glucose production in NIDDM. Diabetes. 1989;38(5):550–7.

Creutzfeldt WO, Kleine N, Willms B, Orskov C, Holst JJ, Nauck MA. Glucagonostatic actions and reduction of fasting hyperglycemia by exogenous glucagon-like peptide I(7-36) amide in type I diabetic patients. Diabetes Care. 1996;19(6):580–6.

Cryer PE. Mechanisms of hypoglycemia-associated autonomic failure in diabetes. N Engl J Med. 2013;369(4):362–72.

Cryer PE. Glycemic goals in diabetes: trade-off between glycemic control and iatrogenic hypoglycemia. Diabetes. 2014;63(7):2188–95.

Cryer PE, Davis SN, Shamoon H. Hypoglycemia in diabetes. Diabetes Care. 2003;26(6):1902–12.

Cynober LA. Plasma amino acid levels with a note on membrane transport: characteristics, regulation, and metabolic significance. Nutrition. 2002;18(9):761–6.

Di Cairano ES, Moretti S, Marciani P, Sacchi VF, Castagna M, Davalli A, et al. Neurotransmitters and neuropeptides: new players in the control of Islet of Langerhans' cell mass and function. J Cell Physiol. 2016;231:756–67.

Dobbs R, Sakurai H, Sasaki H, Faloona G, Valverde I, Baetens D, et al. Glucagon: role in the hyperglycemia of diabetes mellitus. Science. 1975;187(4176):544–7.

Doyle ME, Egan JM. Mechanisms of action of glucagon-like peptide 1 in the pancreas. Pharmacol Ther. 2007;113(3):546–93. Pubmed Central PMCID: 1934514.

Drucker DJ, Nauck MA. The incretin system: glucagon-like peptide-1 receptor agonists and dipeptidyl peptidase-4 inhibitors in type 2 diabetes. Lancet. 2006;368(9548):1696–705.

Dubois MP. Immunoreactive somatostatin is present in discrete cells of the endocrine pancreas. Proc Natl Acad Sci U S A. 1975;72(4):1340–3. Pubmed Central PMCID: 432529.

Dubois PM, Paulin C, Assan R, Dubois MP. Evidence for immunoreactive somatostatin in the endocrine cells of human foetal pancreas. Nature. 1975;256(5520):731–2.

Dunning BE, Foley JE, Ahren B. Alpha cell function in health and disease: influence of glucagon-like peptide-1. Diabetologia. 2005;48(9):1700–13.

Eizirik DL, Cardozo AK, Cnop M. The role for endoplasmic reticulum stress in diabetes mellitus. Endocr Rev. 2008;29(1):42–61.

Ferrannini E. Insulin resistance versus insulin deficiency in non-insulin-dependent diabetes mellitus: problems and prospects. Endocr Rev. 1998;19(4):477–90.

Folli F, Okada T, Perego C, Gunton J, Liew CW, Akiyama M, et al. Altered insulin receptor signalling and beta-cell cycle dynamics in type 2 diabetes mellitus. PLoS One. 2011;6(11): e28050. Pubmed Central PMCID: 3227614.

Foulis AK, Stewart JA. The pancreas in recent-onset type 1 (insulin-dependent) diabetes mellitus: insulin content of islets, insulitis and associated changes in the exocrine acinar tissue. Diabetologia. 1984;26(6):456–61.

Foulis AK, McGill M, Farquharson MA. Insulitis in type 1 (insulin-dependent) diabetes mellitus in man – macrophages, lymphocytes, and interferon-gamma containing cells. J Pathol. 1991;165 (2):97–103.

Franklin I, Gromada J, Gjinovci A, Theander S, Wollheim CB. Beta-cell secretory products activate alpha-cell ATP-dependent potassium channels to inhibit glucagon release. Diabetes. 2005;54 (6):1808–15.

Galanopoulou AS, Kent G, Rabbani SN, Seidah NG, Patel YC. Heterologous processing of prosomatostatin in constitutive and regulated secretory pathways. Putative role of the endoproteases furin, PC1, and PC2. J Biol Chem. 1993;268(8):6041–9.

Gastaldelli A, Miyazaki Y, Pettiti M, Buzzigoli E, Mahankali S, Ferrannini E, et al. Separate contribution of diabetes, total fat mass, and fat topography to glucose production, gluconeogenesis, and glycogenolysis. J Clin Endocrinol Metab. 2004;89(8):3914–21.

Gopel SO, Kanno T, Barg S, Weng XG, Gromada J, Rorsman P. Regulation of glucagon release in mouse-cells by KATP channels and inactivation of TTX-sensitive Na+ channels. J Physiol. 2000;528(Pt 3):509–20. Pubmed Central PMCID: 2270147.

Grimelius L, Capella C, Buffa R, Polak JM, Pearse AG, Solcia E. Cytochemical and ultrastructural differentiation of enteroglucagon and pancreatic-type glucagon cells of the gastrointestinal tract. Virchows Arch B Cell Pathol. 1976;20(3):217–28.

Gromada J, Bokvist K, Ding WG, Barg S, Buschard K, Renstrom E, et al. Adrenaline stimulates glucagon secretion in pancreatic A-cells by increasing the Ca2+ current and the number of granules close to the L-type Ca2+ channels. J Gen Physiol. 1997;110(3):217–28. Pubmed Central PMCID: 2229364.

Gromada J, Hoy M, Olsen HL, Gotfredsen CF, Buschard K, Rorsman P, et al. Gi2 proteins couple somatostatin receptors to low-conductance K+ channels in rat pancreatic alpha-cells. Pflugers Arch – Eur J Physiol. 2001a;442(1):19–26.

Gromada J, Hoy M, Buschard K, Salehi A, Rorsman P. Somatostatin inhibits exocytosis in rat pancreatic alpha-cells by G(i2)-dependent activation of calcineurin and depriming of secretory granules. J Physiol. 2001b;535(Pt 2):519–32. Pubmed Central PMCID: 2278803.

Gromada J, Ma X, Hoy M, Bokvist K, Salehi A, Berggren PO, et al. ATP-sensitive K+ channel-dependent regulation of glucagon release and electrical activity by glucose in wild-type and SUR1-/-mouse alpha-cells. Diabetes. 2004;53 Suppl 3:S181–9.

Gromada J, Franklin I, Wollheim CB. Alpha-cells of the endocrine pancreas: 35 years of research but the enigma remains. Endocr Rev. 2007;28(1):84–116.

Guardado Mendoza R, Perego C, Finzi G, La Rosa S, Capella C, Jimenez-Ceja LM, et al. Delta cell death in the islet of Langerhans and the progression from normal glucose tolerance to type 2 diabetes in non-human primates (baboon, Papio hamadryas). Diabetologia. 2015;58(8):1814–26.

Guardado-Mendoza R, Davalli AM, Chavez AO, Hubbard GB, Dick EJ, Majluf-Cruz A, et al. Pancreatic islet amyloidosis, beta-cell apoptosis, and alpha-cell proliferation are determinants of islet remodeling in type-2 diabetic baboons. Proc Natl Acad Sci U S A. 2009;106(33):13992–7. Pubmed Central PMCID: 2729008.

Halban PA, German MS, Kahn SE, Weir GC. Current status of islet cell replacement and regeneration therapy. J Clin Endocrinol Metab. 2010;95(3):1034–43. Pubmed Central PMCID: 2841538.

Hare KJ, Knop FK, Asmar M, Madsbad S, Deacon CF, Holst JJ, et al. Preserved inhibitory potency of GLP-1 on glucagon secretion in type 2 diabetes mellitus. J Clin Endocrinol Metab. 2009;94 (12):4679–87.

Hauge-Evans AC, King AJ, Carmignac D, Richardson CC, Robinson IC, Low MJ, et al. Somatostatin secreted by islet delta-cells fulfills multiple roles as a paracrine regulator of islet function. Diabetes. 2009;58(2):403–11. Pubmed Central PMCID: 2628614.

Heimberg H, De Vos A, Pipeleers D, Thorens B, Schuit F. Differences in glucose transporter gene expression between rat pancreatic alpha- and beta-cells are correlated to differences in glucose transport but not in glucose utilization. J Biol Chem. 1995;270(15):8971–5.

Heimberg H, De Vos A, Moens K, Quartier E, Bouwens L, Pipeleers D, et al. The glucose sensor protein glucokinase is expressed in glucagon-producing alpha-cells. Proc Natl Acad Sci U S A. 1996;93(14):7036–41. Pubmed Central PMCID: 38931.

Hellman B, Lernmark A. Inhibition of the in vitro secretion of insulin by an extract of pancreatic alpha-1 cells. Endocrinology. 1969;84(6):1484–8.

Henquin JC. The dual control of insulin secretion by glucose involves triggering and amplifying pathways in beta-cells. Diabetes Res Clin Pract. 2011;93 Suppl 1:S27–31.

Hjorth SA, Adelhorst K, Pedersen BB, Kirk O, Schwartz TW. Glucagon and glucagon-like peptide 1: selective receptor recognition via distinct peptide epitopes. J Biol Chem. 1994;269 (48):30121–4.

Holz GG, Kang G, Harbeck M, Roe MW, Chepurny OG. Cell physiology of cAMP sensor Epac. J Physiol. 2006;577(Pt 1):5–15. Pubmed Central PMCID: 2000694.

Hope KM, Tran PO, Zhou H, Oseid E, Leroy E, Robertson RP. Regulation of alpha-cell function by the beta-cell in isolated human and rat islets deprived of glucose: the "switch-off" hypothesis. Diabetes. 2004;53(6):1488–95.

Hou JC, Min L, Pessin JE. Insulin granule biogenesis, trafficking and exocytosis. Vitam Horm. 2009;80:473–506. Pubmed Central PMCID: 4324607.

Huypens P, Ling Z, Pipeleers D, Schuit F. Glucagon receptors on human islet cells contribute to glucose competence of insulin release. Diabetologia. 2000;43(8):1012–9.

Hvidberg A, Nielsen MT, Hilsted J, Orskov C, Holst JJ. Effect of glucagon-like peptide-1 (proglucagon 78-107amide) on hepatic glucose production in healthy man. Metab Clin Exp. 1994;43(1):104–8.

Jelinek LJ, Lok S, Rosenberg GB, Smith RA, Grant FJ, Biggs S, et al. Expression cloning and signaling properties of the rat glucagon receptor. Science. 1993;259(5101):1614–6.

Jeon J, Correa-Medina M, Ricordi C, Edlund H, Diez JA. Endocrine cell clustering during human pancreas development. J Histochem Cytochem: Off J Histochem Soc. 2009;57(9):811–24. Pubmed Central PMCID: 2728126.

Jiang G, Zhang BB. Glucagon and regulation of glucose metabolism. Am J Physiol Endocrinol Metab. 2003;284(4):E671–8.

Juhl K, Hutton J. Stimulus-secretion coupling in the pancreatic beta-cell. Adv Exp Med Biol. 2004;552:66–90.

Kahn SE, Cooper ME, Del Prato S. Pathophysiology and treatment of type 2 diabetes: perspectives on the past, present, and future. Lancet. 2014;383(9922):1068–83. Pubmed Central PMCID: 4226760.

Kieffer TJ, Habener JF. The glucagon-like peptides. Endocr Rev. 1999;20(6):876–913.

Kim A, Miller K, Jo J, Kilimnik G, Wojcik P, Hara M. Islet architecture: a comparative study. Islets. 2009;1(2):129–36. Pubmed Central PMCID: 2894473.

Kimmel JR, Hayden LJ, Pollock HG. Isolation and characterization of a new pancreatic polypeptide hormone. J Biol Chem. 1975;250(24):9369–76.

Kleinman R, Gingerich R, Ohning G, Wong H, Olthoff K, Walsh J, et al. The influence of somatostatin on glucagon and pancreatic polypeptide secretion in the isolated perfused human pancreas. Int J Pancreatol: Off J Int Assoc Pancreatol. 1995;18(1):51–7.

Knop FK, Vilsboll T, Madsbad S, Holst JJ, Krarup T. Inappropriate suppression of glucagon during OGTT but not during isoglycaemic i.v. glucose infusion contributes to the reduced incretin effect in type 2 diabetes mellitus. Diabetologia. 2007a;50(4):797–805.

Knop FK, Vilsboll T, Hojberg PV, Larsen S, Madsbad S, Volund A, et al. Reduced incretin effect in type 2 diabetes: cause or consequence of the diabetic state? Diabetes. 2007b;56(8):1951–9.

Koerker DJ, Ruch W, Chideckel E, Palmer J, Goodner CJ, Ensinck J, et al. Somatostatin: hypothalamic inhibitor of the endocrine pancreas. Science. 1974;184(4135):482–4.

Lamy CM, Sanno H, Labouebe G, Picard A, Magnan C, Chatton JY, et al. Hypoglycemia-activated GLUT2 neurons of the nucleus tractus solitarius stimulate vagal activity and glucagon secretion. Cell Metab. 2014;19(3):527–38.

Larsson LI, Sundler F, Hakanson R. Immunohistochemical localization of human pancreatic polypeptide (HPP) to a population of islet cells. Cell Tissue Res. 1975;156(2):167–71.

Lee HM, Wang G, Englander EW, Kojima M, Greeley Jr GH. Ghrelin, a new gastrointestinal endocrine peptide that stimulates insulin secretion: enteric distribution, ontogeny, influence of endocrine, and dietary manipulations. Endocrinology. 2002;143(1):185–90.

Lee Y, Wang MY, Du XQ, Charron MJ, Unger RH. Glucagon receptor knockout prevents insulin-deficient type 1 diabetes in mice. Diabetes. 2011;60(2):391–7. Pubmed Central PMCID: 3028337.

Lee Y, Berglund ED, Wang MY, Fu X, Yu X, Charron MJ, et al. Metabolic manifestations of insulin deficiency do not occur without glucagon action. Proc Natl Acad Sci U S A. 2012;109 (37):14972–6. Pubmed Central PMCID: 3443167.

Lefebvre PJ. The intriguing diversity of the glucagon gene products. Curr Diab Rep. 2002;2 (3):201–2.

Ludvigsen E, Olsson R, Stridsberg M, Janson ET, Sandler S. Expression and distribution of somatostatin receptor subtypes in the pancreatic islets of mice and rats. J Histochem Cytochem: Off J Histochem Soc. 2004;52(3):391–400.

Luft R, Efendic S, Hokfelt T. Somatostatin – both hormone and neurotransmitter? Diabetologia. 1978;14(1):1–13.

Ma X, Zhang Y, Gromada J, Sewing S, Berggren PO, Buschard K, et al. Glucagon stimulates exocytosis in mouse and rat pancreatic alpha-cells by binding to glucagon receptors. Mol Endocrinol. 2005;19(1):198–212.

MacDonald PE, De Marinis YZ, Ramracheya R, Salehi A, Ma X, Johnson PR, et al. A K ATP channel-dependent pathway within alpha cells regulates glucagon release from both rodent and human islets of Langerhans. PLoS Biol. 2007;5(6):e143. Pubmed Central PMCID: 1868042.

Malaisse WJ. Paracrine control of glucagon release by somatostatin (Review). Int J Mol Med. 2014;33(3):491–8.

Marchetti P, Bugliani M, Lupi R, Marselli L, Masini M, Boggi U, et al. The endoplasmic reticulum in pancreatic beta cells of type 2 diabetes patients. Diabetologia. 2007;50(12):2486–94.

Marchetti P, Lupi R, Bugliani M, Kirkpatrick CL, Sebastiani G, Grieco FA, et al. A local glucagon-like peptide 1 (GLP-1) system in human pancreatic islets. Diabetologia. 2012a;55(12):3262–72.

Marchetti P, Bugliani M, Boggi U, Masini M, Marselli L. The pancreatic beta cells in human type 2 diabetes. Adv Exp Med Biol. 2012b;771:288–309.

Masini M, Marselli L, Bugliani M, Martino L, Masiello P, Marchetti P, et al. Ultrastructural morphometric analysis of insulin secretory granules in human type 2 diabetes. Acta Diabetol. 2012;49 Suppl 1:S247–52.

Merlini D, Caramia F. Effect of dehydroascorbic acid on the islets of Langerhans of the rat pancreas. J Cell Biol. 1965;26(1):245–61. Pubmed Central PMCID: 2106693.

Michael DJ, Geng X, Cawley NX, Loh YP, Rhodes CJ, Drain P, et al. Fluorescent cargo proteins in pancreatic beta-cells: design determines secretion kinetics at exocytosis. Biophys J. 2004;87(6): L03–5. Pubmed Central PMCID: 1304941.

Michael DJ, Xiong W, Geng X, Drain P, Chow RH. Human insulin vesicle dynamics during pulsatile secretion. Diabetes. 2007;56(5):1277–88.

Moldovan S, Brunicardi FC. Endocrine pancreas: summary of observations generated by surgical fellows. World J Surg. 2001;25(4):468–73.

Montminy MR, Goodman RH, Horovitch SJ, Habener JF. Primary structure of the gene encoding rat preprosomatostatin. Proc Natl Acad Sci U S A. 1984;81(11):3337–40. Pubmed Central PMCID: 345502.

Montminy MR, Sevarino KA, Wagner JA, Mandel G, Goodman RH. Identification of a cyclic-AMP-responsive element within the rat somatostatin gene. Proc Natl Acad Sci U S A. 1986a;83 (18):6682–6. Pubmed Central PMCID: 386573.

Montminy MR, Low MJ, Tapia-Arancibia L, Reichlin S, Mandel G, Goodman RH. Cyclic AMP regulates somatostatin mRNA accumulation in primary diencephalic cultures and in transfected fibroblast cells. J Neurosci Off J Soc Neurosci. 1986b;6(4):1171–6.

Morel A, Gluschankof P, Gomez S, Fafeur V, Cohen P. Characterization of a somatostatin-28 containing the (Tyr-7, Gly-10) derivative of somatostatin-14: a terminal active product of prosomatostatin II processing in anglerfish pancreatic islets. Proc Natl Acad Sci U S A. 1984;81(22):7003–6. Pubmed Central PMCID: 392064.

Morgan NG, Dhayal S. G-protein coupled receptors mediating long chain fatty acid signalling in the pancreatic beta-cell. Biochem Pharmacol. 2009;78(12):1419–27.

Munger BL, Caramia F, Lacy PE. The ultrastructural basis for the identification of cell types in the pancreatic islets. II. Rabbit, dog and opossum. Z Zellforsch Mikrosk Anat. 1965;67(6):776–98.

Murakami T, Fujita T. Microcirculation of the rat pancreas, with special reference to the insulo-acinar portal and insulo-venous drainage systems: a further scanning electron microscope study of corrosion casts. Arch Histol Cytol. 1992;55(5):453–76.

Nauck MA, Kleine N, Orskov C, Holst JJ, Willms B, Creutzfeldt W. Normalization of fasting hyperglycaemia by exogenous glucagon-like peptide 1 (7-36 amide) in type 2 (non-insulin-dependent) diabetic patients. Diabetologia. 1993;36(8):741–4.

Newsholme P, Cruzat V, Arfuso F, Keane K. Nutrient regulation of insulin secretion and action. J Endocrinol. 2014;221(3):R105–20.

Patel YC, Srikant CB. Subtype selectivity of peptide analogs for all five cloned human somatostatin receptors (hsstr 1–5). Endocrinology. 1994;135(6):2814–7.

Patel YC, Srikant CB. Somatostatin receptors. Trends Endocrinol Metab: TEM. 1997;8 (10):398–405.

Pipeleers DG, Schuit FC, in't Veld PA, Maes E, Hooghe-Peters EL, Van de Winkel M, et al. Interplay of nutrients and hormones in the regulation of insulin release. Endocrinology. 1985a;117(3):824–33.

Pipeleers DG, in't Veld PA, Van de Winkel M, Maes E, Schuit FC, Gepts W. A new in vitro model for the study of pancreatic A and B cells. Endocrinology. 1985b;117(3):806–16.

Piro S, Maniscalchi ET, Monello A, Pandini G, Mascali LG, Rabuazzo AM, et al. Palmitate affects insulin receptor phosphorylation and intracellular insulin signal in a pancreatic alpha-cell line. Endocrinology. 2010;151(9):4197–206.

Plamboeck A, Veedfald S, Deacon CF, Hartmann B, Wettergren A, Svendsen LB, et al. The effect of exogenous GLP-1 on food intake is lost in male truncally vagotomized subjects with pyloroplasty. Am J Physiol Gastrointest Liver Physiol. 2013;304(12):G1117–27.
Portela-Gomes GM, Stridsberg M, Grimelius L, Oberg K, Janson ET. Expression of the five different somatostatin receptor subtypes in endocrine cells of the pancreas. Appl Immunohistochem Mol Morphol: AIMM Off Publ Soc Appl Immunohistochem. 2000;8 (2):126–32.
Quesada I, Tuduri E, Ripoll C, Nadal A. Physiology of the pancreatic alpha-cell and glucagon secretion: role in glucose homeostasis and diabetes. J Endocrinol. 2008;199(1):5–19.
Quinn AR, Blanco CL, Perego C, Finzi G, La Rosa S, Capella C, et al. The ontogeny of the endocrine pancreas in the fetal/newborn baboon. J Endocrinol. 2012;214(3):289–99. Pubmed Central PMCID: 3686495.
Raghay K, Gallego R, Scoazec JY, Garcia-Caballero T, Morel G. Different ghrelin localisation in adult human and rat endocrine pancreas. Cell Tissue Res. 2013;352(3):487–94.
Rahier J, Wallon J, Henquin JC. Abundance of somatostatin cells in the human neonatal pancreas. Diabetologia. 1980;18(3):251–4.
Rahier J, Wallon J, Henquin JC. Cell populations in the endocrine pancreas of human neonates and infants. Diabetologia. 1981;20(5):540–6.
Rahier J, Goebbels RM, Henquin JC. Cellular composition of the human diabetic pancreas. Diabetologia. 1983a;24(5):366–71.
Rahier J, Wallon J, Loozen S, Lefevre A, Gepts W, Haot J. The pancreatic polypeptide cells in the human pancreas: the effects of age and diabetes. J Clin Endocrinol Metab. 1983b;56(3):441–4.
Raju B, Cryer PE. Loss of the decrement in intraislet insulin plausibly explains loss of the glucagon response to hypoglycemia in insulin-deficient diabetes: documentation of the intraislet insulin hypothesis in humans. Diabetes. 2005;54(3):757–64.
Reichlin S. Somatostatin. N Engl J Med. 1983a;309(24):1495–501.
Reichlin S. Somatostatin (second of two parts). N Engl J Med. 1983b;309(25):1556–63.
Rhodes CJ. Type 2 diabetes-a matter of beta-cell life and death? Science. 2005;307(5708):380–4.
Rorsman P, Braun M. Regulation of insulin secretion in human pancreatic islets. Annu Rev Physiol. 2013;75:155–79.
Rorsman P, Hellman B. Voltage-activated currents in guinea pig pancreatic alpha 2 cells. Evidence for Ca2+-dependent action potentials. J Gen Physiol. 1988;91(2):223–42. Pubmed Central PMCID: 2216127.
Rorsman P, Berggren PO, Bokvist K, Ericson H, Mohler H, Ostenson CG, et al. Glucose-inhibition of glucagon secretion involves activation of GABA-receptor chloride channels. Nature. 1989;341(6239):233–6.
Rufener C, Dubois MP, Malaisse Lagae F, Oric L. Immuno-fluorescent reactivity to anti-somatostatin in the gastro-intestinal mucosa of the dog. Diabetologia. 1975;11(4):321–4.
Rutter GA, Pullen TJ, Hodson DJ, Martinez-Sanchez A. Pancreatic beta-cell identity, glucose sensing and the control of insulin secretion. Biochem J. 2015;466(2):203–18.
Sakurai H, Dobbs R, Unger RH. Somatostatin-induced changes in insulin and glucagon secretion in normal and diabetic dogs. J Clin Invest. 1974;54(6):1395–402. Pubmed Central PMCID: 301694.
Samols E, Stagner JI, Ewart RB, Marks V. The order of islet microvascular cellular perfusion is B——A——D in the perfused rat pancreas. J Clin Invest. 1988;82(1):350–3. Pubmed Central PMCID: 303515.
Sasaki H, Rubalcava B, Baetens D, Blazquez E, Srikant CB, Orci L, et al. Identification of glucagon in the gastrointestinal tract. J Clin Invest. 1975;56(1):135–45. Pubmed Central PMCID: 436564.
Shen LP, Rutter WJ. Sequence of the human somatostatin I gene. Science. 1984;224(4645):168–71.
Stanojevic V, Habener JF. Evolving function and potential of pancreatic alpha cells. Best Pract Res Clin Endocrinol Metab. 2015;29(6):859–71. Pubmed Central PMCID: 4690008.

Stefan Y, Grasso S, Perrelet A, Orci L. The pancreatic polypeptide-rich lobe of the human pancreas: definitive identification of its derivation from the ventral pancreatic primordium. Diabetologia . 1982;23(2):141–2.

Strowski MZ, Parmar RM, Blake AD, Schaeffer JM. Somatostatin inhibits insulin and glucagon secretion via two receptors subtypes: an in vitro study of pancreatic islets from somatostatin receptor 2 knockout mice. Endocrinology. 2000;141(1):111–7.

Thorel F, Nepote V, Avril I, Kohno K, Desgraz R, Chera S, et al. Conversion of adult pancreatic alpha-cells to beta-cells after extreme beta-cell loss. Nature. 2010;464(7292):1149–54. Pubmed Central PMCID: 2877635.

Tu J, Tuch BE, Si Z. Expression and regulation of glucokinase in rat islet beta- and alpha-cells during development. Endocrinology. 1999;140(8):3762–6.

Unger RH. The banting memorial lecture 1975. Diabetes and the alpha cell. Diabetes. 1976;25 (2):136–51.

Unger RH, Cherrington AD. Glucagonocentric restructuring of diabetes: a pathophysiologic and therapeutic makeover. J Clin Invest. 2012;122(1):4–12. Pubmed Central PMCID: 3248306.

Unger RH, Orci L. The essential role of glucagon in the pathogenesis of diabetes mellitus. Lancet. 1975;1(7897):14–6.

Unger RH, Orci L. Paracrinology of islets and the paracrinopathy of diabetes. Proc Natl Acad Sci U S A. 2010;107(37):16009–12. Pubmed Central PMCID: 2941311.

Vilsboll T, Krarup T, Madsbad S, Holst JJ. Defective amplification of the late phase insulin response to glucose by GIP in obese type II diabetic patients. Diabetologia. 2002;45(8):1111–9.

Walker JN, Ramracheya R, Zhang Q, Johnson PR, Braun M, Rorsman P. Regulation of glucagon secretion by glucose: paracrine, intrinsic or both? Diabetes Obes Metab. 2011;13 Suppl 1:95–105.

Wang XP, Norman M, Yang J, Liu SH, Magnusson J, DeMayo FJ, et al. The effect of global SSTR5 gene ablation on the endocrine pancreas and glucose regulation in aging mice. J Surg Res. 2005a;129(1):64–72.

Wang XP, Yang J, Norman MA, Magnusson J, DeMayo FJ, Brunicardi FC. SSTR5 ablation in islet results in alterations in glucose homeostasis in mice. FEBS Lett. 2005b;579(14):3107–14.

Wang X, Zielinski MC, Misawa R, Wen P, Wang TY, Wang CZ, et al. Quantitative analysis of pancreatic polypeptide cell distribution in the human pancreas. PLoS One. 2013a;8(1):e55501. Pubmed Central PMCID: 3561199.

Wang X, Misawa R, Zielinski MC, Cowen P, Jo J, Periwal V, et al. Regional differences in islet distribution in the human pancreas – preferential beta-cell loss in the head region in patients with type 2 diabetes. PLoS One. 2013b;8(6):e67454. Pubmed Central PMCID: 3691162.

Warnotte C, Nenquin M, Henquin JC. Unbound rather than total concentration and saturation rather than unsaturation determine the potency of fatty acids on insulin secretion. Mol Cell Endocrinol. 1999;153(1–2):147–53.

Watts M, Ha J, Kimchi O, Sherman A. Paracrine regulation of glucagon secretion: the beta-alpha-delta model. Am J Physiol Endocrinol Metab. 2016;310:E597–611.

Wierup N, Svensson H, Mulder H, Sundler F. The ghrelin cell: a novel developmentally regulated islet cell in the human pancreas. Regul Pept. 2002;107(1–3):63–9.

Wierup N, Yang S, McEvilly RJ, Mulder H, Sundler F. Ghrelin is expressed in a novel endocrine cell type in developing rat islets and inhibits insulin secretion from INS-1 (832/13) cells. J Histochem Cytochem: Off J Histochem Soc. 2004;52(3):301–10.

Williamson JR, Lacy PE, Grisham JW. Ultrastructural changes in islets of the rat produced by tolbutamide. Diabetes. 1961;10:460–9.

Yoshimoto Y, Fukuyama Y, Horio Y, Inanobe A, Gotoh M, Kurachi Y. Somatostatin induces hyperpolarization in pancreatic islet alpha cells by activating a G protein-gated K+ channel. FEBS Lett. 1999;444(2–3):265–9.

The Physiology of the Testis

17

Alessandro Ilacqua, Davide Francomano, and Antonio Aversa

Abstract

The testis is the most important organ for reproductive and sexual function. Male fetal sexual differentiation of the genitalia is driven by Leydig cell-secreted androgens and Sertoli cell (SC)-secreted anti-Müllerian hormone. The hormone insulin-like factor 3 (INSL3) is produced by testicular Leydig cells (LCs) depending on the state of LC differentiation and is stimulated by the long-term trophic effects of luteinizing hormone (see section "Testicular Descent"). INSL3 is, along with the other major Leydig cell hormone testosterone (Te), essential for testicular descent, which in humans should be completed before birth. The absence of androgen receptor expression in SCs underlies a physiological stage of androgen insensitivity within the male gonad in the fetal and early postnatal periods. From fetal life to adulthood, the testis evolves through maturational phases showing specific morphologic and functional features in its different compartments. The seminiferous cords contain Sertoli and germ cells, surrounded by peritubular cells, and the interstitial tissue contains LCs and connective tissue. During infancy and childhood, LCs regress and Te secretion declines dramatically. SCs remain immature and spermatogenesis is arrested at the premeiotic stage. At puberty, LCs differentiate again, and Te concentration increases and provokes SC maturation and germ cells undergo meiosis,

A. Ilacqua
Free Lance, Rome, Italy
e-mail: alessandro_ilacqua@alice.it

D. Francomano
Department Experimental Medicine, Sapienza University of Rome, Rome, Italy
e-mail: davide.francomano@uniroma1.it

A. Aversa (✉)
Department of Experimental and Clinical Medicine, Magna Graecia University of Catanzaro, Catanzaro, CZ, Italy
e-mail: aversa@unicz.it

A. Belfiore, D. LeRoith (eds.), *Principles of Endocrinology and Hormone Action*, Endocrinology, https://doi.org/10.1007/978-3-319-44675-2_17

the hallmark of adult spermatogenesis driving to sperm production (see section "Interstitial Compartment"). During adulthood androgen receptors became expressed and spermatogenesis occurs, while in aging, despite that sperm cell production remains partially affected, the secretion rate of Te declines depending on the presence of comorbidities and drugs affecting its production by LC (see section "Aging").

Keywords
Leydig cell • Sertoli cell • Testosterone • Sperm cell

Contents

Functional Organization of the Testis

The *male reproductive system* (Fig. 1) is essential for the maintenance of the species through two essential functions: *gametogenesis and sexual function*. The testes produce the male gametes and the male sexual hormones (*androgens*). The term *spermatogenesis* describes and includes all the processes involved in the production of gametes, whereas *steroidogenesis* refers to the enzymatic reactions leading to the production of male steroid hormones. Spermatogenesis and steroidogenesis take place in two compartments morphologically and functionally distinguishable from

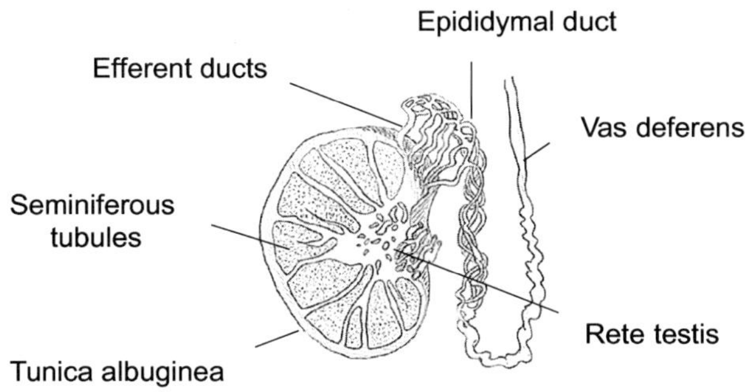

Fig. 1 Essentials of anatomy of the Testis

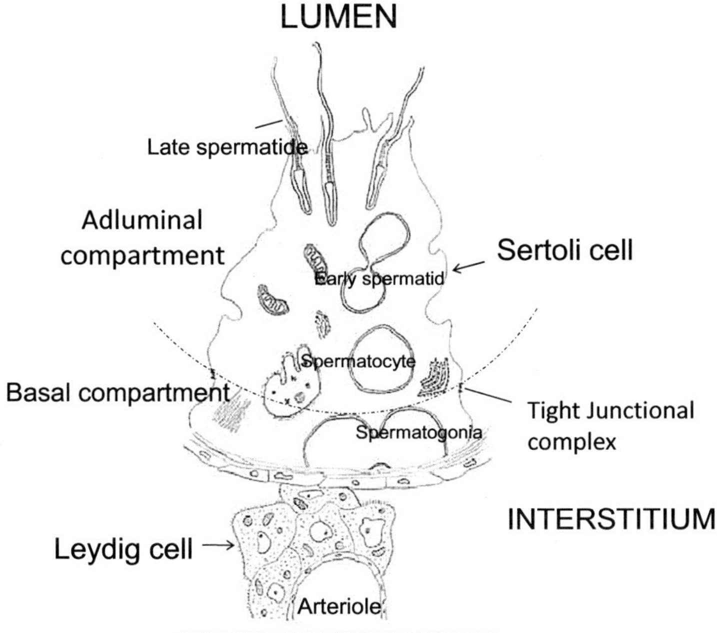

Fig. 2 The Testis

each other. These are the tubular compartment, consisting of the seminiferous tubules and the interstitial compartment between the seminiferous tubules (Fig. 2). Although anatomically separate, both compartments are closely connected with each other. The integrity of both compartments is necessary for quantitative and qualitative production of sperm cells. The function of the testis and thereby also the function of its compartments are regulated by the hypothalamus and the pituitary gland (endocrine regulation). These endocrine effects are mediated and modulated at the testicular level by local control mechanisms (*paracrine and autocrine factors*) (Basciani et al. 2010).

Interstitial Compartment

The most important cells of this compartment are the Leydig cells (LCs). These cells are the source of testicular testosterone (Te) and of insulin-like factor 3 (INSL3). Aside from LCs, the interstitial compartment also contains immune cells, blood and lymph vessels, nerves, fibroblasts, and loose connective tissue. In experimental animals, this compartment comprises about 2.6% of the total testicular volume. In the human testis, the interstitial compartment represents about 12–15% of the total testicular volume, 10–20% of which is occupied by LCs and it counts approximately 200×10^6 cells. LCs produce and secrete the most important male sexual hormone, that is, testosterone. From the developmental, morphological, and functional viewpoint, different types of LCs can be distinguished: stem cells, progenitor committed stem cell, fetal differentiated cells in the fetus, and adult differentiated cells (Ge and Hardy 2007). Fetal LCs become neonatal LCs at birth and degenerate thereafter or regress into immature LCs (Prince 2007). Fetal LCs produce Te. Immature LCs that mainly produce androstane-3-α,17-β-diol instead of T have also been described.

Adult LCs are rich in smooth endoplasmic reticulum and mitochondria with tubular cristae. Other important cytoplasmic components are lipofuscin granules, the final product of endocytosis and lysosomal degradation, and lipid droplets in which the preliminary stages of Te synthesis take place and special formations, called Reinke's crystals, are often found in the adult LCs. These are probably subunits of globular proteins whose functional meaning is not known. The proliferation rate of the LCs in the adult testis is rather low and is influenced by LH. The ontogeny of LCs is not entirely clear and mesonephros, neural crest, and coelomic sources have been involved. In the adult testis, LCs develop from perivascular and peritubular mesenchymal-like cells, and the differentiation of these cells into LCs is induced by LH but also by growth and differentiation factors derived from Sertoli cell (SC).

Tubular Compartment

Spermatogenesis takes place in the tubular compartment. This compartment represents about 60–80% of the total testicular volume. It contains the germ cells and two different types of somatic cells, the peritubular cells and the SC. The testis is divided by septa of connective tissue into about 250–300 lobules, each one containing one to three highly convoluted seminiferous tubules. Overall, the human testis contains about 600 seminiferous tubules. The length of individual seminiferous tubules is about 30–80 cm. Considering an average number of about 600 seminiferous tubules per testis and an average length of the tubuli seminiferi of about 60 cm each, the total length of the tubuli seminiferi is about 360 m per testis, i.e., 720 m of seminiferous epithelium per man. The seminiferous tubules are covered by a lamina propria, which consists of a basal membrane, a layer of collagen, and the peritubular cells (myofibroblasts). These cells are stratified around the tubulus and form concentrical layers that are separated by collagen layers. These characteristics differentiate the human testicle from the majority of the other mammals, whose seminiferous tubules are surrounded only by two to four layers of myofibroblasts. Mature sperm cells are transported toward the exit of the seminiferous tubules by spontaneous contraction of myofibroblast, and several regulators of cell contractions are reported, e.g., oxytocin, oxytocin-like substances, prostaglandins, androgenic steroids, and endothelins. Peritubular contractility is mediated by endothelin and this effect is modulated by the relaxant peptide adrenomedullin produced by SCs. Androgens may regulate contractility of peritubular cells toward their action on contractility-related genes, e.g., endothelin-1 and endothelin receptors A and B, adrenomedullin receptor, and vasopressin receptor 1a (Zhang et al. 2006). In adulthood testis, SCs are somatic cells, mitotically inactive, located within the germinal epithelium, on the basal membrane, extend to the lumen of the tubulus seminiferous, and, in a broad sense, can be considered as the supporting structure of the germinal epithelium; then they are responsible for final testicular volume and sperm production in the adult. The SC has several distinct functions that facilitate the maturation of the germ cells. First, it provides a physical scaffold upon which the germ cells develop and migrate toward the lumen of the tubule. Second, the SCs form the blood−testis barrier with specialized tight junctions that exist between these cells. Third, SCs create the focused microenvironment essential for germ cell maturation. These distinctive functions also encompass phagocytosis, fluid secretion, and production of a variety of molecules. Through the production and secretion of 90% of tubular fluid, SCs create and maintain the patency of the tubulus lumen. Special structural elements of the blood-testis barrier prevent reabsorption of the secreted fluid, resulting in pressurized compartment that maintains the patency of the lumen. The tubular fluid contains a higher concentration of potassium ions and a lower concentration of sodium ions. Other constituents are bicarbonate, magnesium and chloride ions, inositol, glucose, carnitine, glycerophosphorylcholine, amino acids, and several proteins. Therefore, the germ cells are immersed in a fluid of unique composition. The basolateral aspect of neighboring SCs comprises membrane specializations forming a band sealing the cells to each other and obliterating the intracellular space (occluding tight junctions). Through the blood–testis barrier, the seminiferous epithelium is divided into two regions, which are anatomically and functionally completely different from each other. Early germ cells (preleptotene, zygotene) are located in the basal region and the later stages of maturing germ cells in the adluminal region. During their development, germ cells are displaced from the basal to the adluminal compartment. This is accomplished by a synchronized dissolution and reassembly of the tight junctions above and below the migrating germ cells. Two important functions are postulated for the blood–testis barrier: the physical isolation of haploid and thereby antigenic germ cells to prevent recognition by the immune system (prevention of autoimmune orchitis) and the preparation of a special milieu for the meiotic process and sperm development. Along the cell body, extending over the entire height of the germinal epithelium, all morphological and physiological differentiation and maturation of the germinal cell up to the mature sperm cell take place.

Germ Cells (See Hormonal Regulation of Spermatogenesis)

Hormonal Control of Testicular Function

The endocrine regulation of testicular function, i.e., the production of sperm and of androgens is well investigated. Understanding the hormonal interactions has important clinical consequences, presented in the following paragraphs. Figure 3 offers an overview of the hormonal regulation of testicular function and physiological Te actions in different target organs.

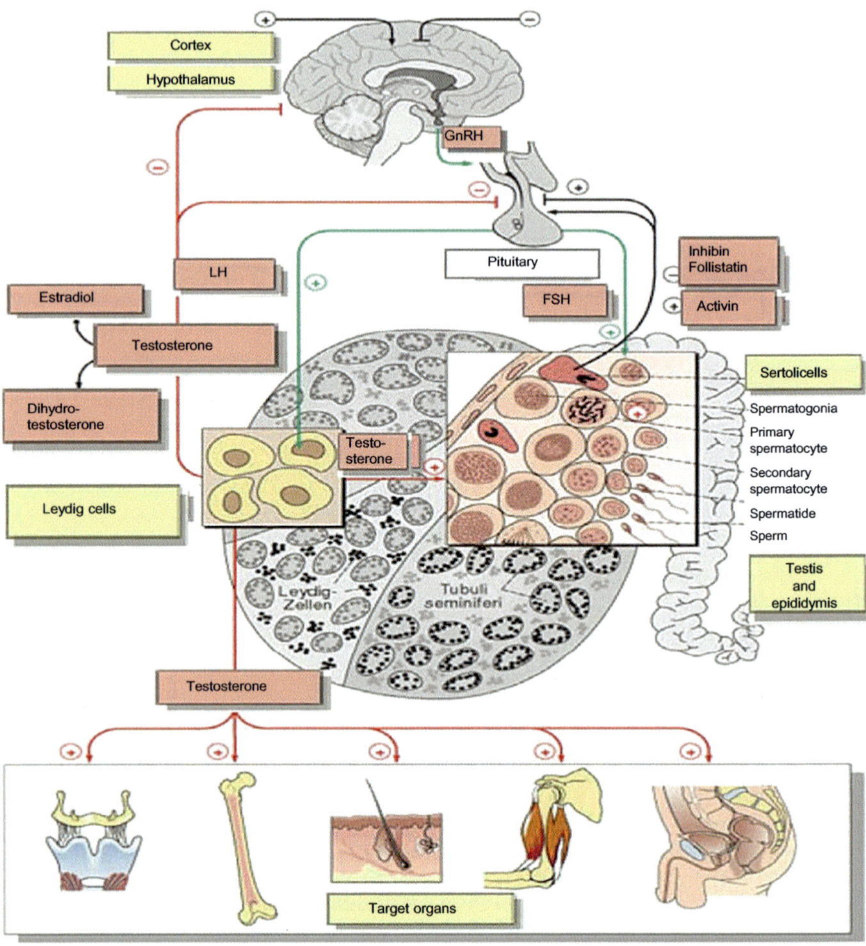

Fig. 3 Hormonal regulation of the testicular function and effects of androgens

Functional Organization of the Hypothalamic–Pituitary System

The *gonadotropins luteinizing hormone* (*LH*) *and follicle-stimulating hormone* (*FSH*) are produced and secreted by the gonadotropic cells of the anterior pituitary. Their designation is derived from the function exerted in females. In males, they control steroidogenesis and gametogenesis in the testis. Pituitary gonadotropins are the central structure controlling gonadal function and, in turn, are regulated by the hypothalamic *gonadotropin-releasing hormone* (*GnRH*). Since GnRH secretion is pulsatile, gonadotropin release also occurs in discrete peaks, more evident in the case of LH, due to its shorter half-life in circulation compared to FSH. In turn, GnRH secretion depends on the activation of the GPR54 receptor, located on the surface of the GnRH neurons and stimulated by the peptide kisspeptin (Fig. 4). The pituitary function is also under the control of gonadal steroids and peptides that influence its activity both directly and through the hypothalamus. Due to their very strict anatomical and functional connection, the hypothalamus and pituitary gland have to be considered as a unique functional unit. The hypothalamus is the rostral extension of the brain stem reticular formation. It contains the cellular bodies of neurons that project their axon terminals toward the median eminence (ME), a specialized region located at the floor of the third ventricle from which the pituitary stalk originates. The hypothalamus is classically subdivided into three longitudinal zones: periventricular, medial, and lateral, the latter functioning as the connecting area between limbic and brain stem regions, whereas the former two contain most of the nuclei controlling neuroendocrine and visceral functions. The ME is the ventral bulge of the hypothalamus and is the site where the axon terminals of the neurosecretory neurons make contact with the capillary plexus, giving rise to the hypophyseal portal circulation. The nerve terminals form buttons on the capillaries and release the neurohormones into the portal blood by diffusion through the basal membrane. The ME is outside the blood–brain barrier and thereby freely accessible to the regulatory influences of hormones and substances present in the systemic circulation and mediating the release of neurohormones in portal blood. The superior hypophyseal arteries provide the blood supply of the ME. The long portal hypophyseal vessels originate from the confluence of capillary loops, which supply the

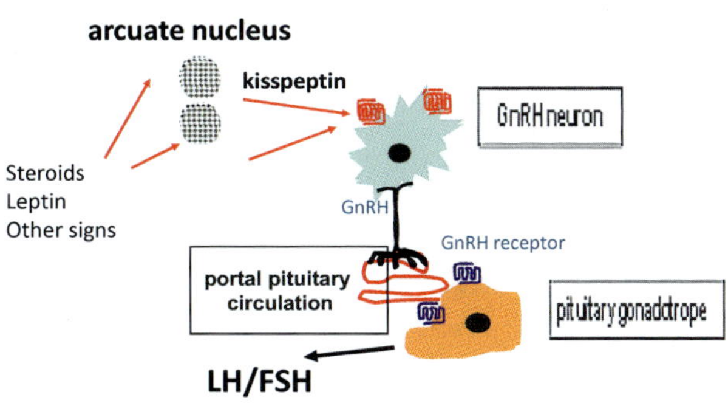

Fig. 4 Current model of regulation of gonadotropin secretion. Role of Kisspeptin

anterior pituitary gland with the highest blood flow of any organ in the body. In humans, the perikarya of neurons stained positive for GnRH are especially found in the ventral part of the mediobasal hypothalamus, between the third ventricle and the ME, scattered throughout the periventricular infundibular region.

The pituitary gland lies in the sella turcica, beneath the hypothalamus and optic chiasm, covered with the sellar diaphragm. Thus, pituitary tumors can result in visual impairment by exerting pressure on the optical nerves. Gonadotropic cells are localized in the anterior pituitary, the most ventral part of the gland, of ectodermic origin from Rathke's pouch. The anterior pituitary consists of the anterior lobe (or pars distalis, the anatomically and functionally most important part), the pars intermedia, and pars tuberalis. The pars distalis is of pivotal importance for pituitary function. Gonadotropin-producing cells constitute approximately 15% of the adenohypophyseal cell population, are scattered in the posteromedial portion of the pars distalis, and are basophilic and PAS positive. Although the secretion of LH and FSH can be partially dissociated under certain circumstances, the same cell type is believed to secrete both gonadotropins. About 80% of the gonadotropic cells in men contain both LH and FSH. The cells have a very well-developed rough endoplasmic reticulum and a large Golgi complex and are rich in secretory granules. In normal men, the pituitary contains approximately 700 IU of LH and 200 IU of FSH. Following gonadectomy or in primary hypogonadism, the cells become vacuolated and large (castration cells). Finally, pituitary gonadotrophs are often found in close connection with prolactin cells, suggesting a paracrine interaction between the two cell types.

The Kisspeptin–GPR54 System

GnRH secretion is under the control of the kisspeptin–GPR54 system. Kisspeptin is the product of the *KISS1* gene, located on chromosome 1q32.1. The name of the *KISS1* gene derives from the chocolate "kisses" of Hershey, Pennsylvania, the city in which the gene was identified. *KISS1* was originally described as a human tumor suppressor gene for its ability to inhibit the growth of melanoma and breast cancer metastasis. Later on, it was shown that kisspeptin (also known as metastin) is the natural ligand of the orphan receptor GPR54 and has an important role in initiating GnRH secretion at puberty. The product of the *KISS1* gene is a 145-amino-acid peptide, which is cleaved into a 54-amino-acid peptide known as kisspeptin-54. Shorter peptides, sharing a common C-terminal, RF-amidated motif with kisspeptin-54, are probably degradation products. Kisspeptin-expressing neurons are located in the *anteroventral periventricular nucleus* (*AVPV*), *periventricular nucleus*, *anterodorsal preoptic nucleus*, and *arcuate nucleus* (*ARC*). Outside the nervous system, the *KISS1* gene is expressed in the placenta, testis, pancreas, liver, and intestine (Popa et al. 2008a). When injected icv or iv to rodents and primates, kisspeptin stimulates LH secretion, an effect mediated by the interaction with its receptor, GPR54, an orphan G protein-coupled receptor, located on the surface of the GnRH-secreting neurons. The *GPR54* gene is located on chromosome 19p13.3. It was discovered that loss-of-function mutations of *GPR54* in the human cause failure to progress through puberty and hypogonadotropic hypogonadism (De Roux et al. 2003). Therefore, the kisspeptin–GPR54 system is essential to initiate gonadotropin secretion at puberty and to maintain normal androgenization in adulthood. In fact, kisspeptin neurons located in ARC and AVPV send projections to the medial preoptic area, a region rich in GnRH cell bodies, providing the anatomical evidence of a direct relationship between kisspeptin fibers and GnRH neurons which, in turn, express *GPR54*. The indispensable role of the kisppeptin–GPR54 system for gonadotropin secretion is proven also by the hypogonadotropic hypogonadal phenotype of mice bearing targeted null mutations of the *kiss1* or *gpr54* gene (Seminara et al. 2003; d'Anglemont de Tassigny et al. 2007) (Fig. 4). GPR54 signals through a Gq type of G protein. Experimentally, kisspeptin stimulates phosphatidylinositol (PI) turnover, calcium mobilization, and arachidonic acid release in GPR54-expressing cells and induces phosphorylation of mitogen-activated protein kinases (MAPK). Continuous infusion of kisspeptin results in rapid increase in LH secretion after 2 h, followed by a decrease to the basal levels by 12 h of infusion due to desensitization of GPR54, since GnRH is still able to elicit LH secretion under these conditions. This suggests that endogenous, pulsatile kisspeptin release is physiologically responsible for pulsatile GnRH and LH secretion.

Kisspeptin is sensitive to steroid levels within the circulation and is the mediator of the negative and positive feedback regulation of gonadotropin secretion. In fact, although androgens, estrogens, and progesterone suppress gonadotropin secretion through androgen receptor (AR)-, estrogen receptor (ER)-α-, and progesterone receptor (PR)-dependent mechanisms, respectively, none of these sex steroids affect GnRH secretion by direct action on GnRH neurons. On the contrary, kisspeptin neurons in the ARC are direct targets of sex steroids in all species and should be viewed as the site of the negative feedback control of GnRH production. In addition, kisspeptin produced by the AVPV, a sexually dimorphic nucleus rich in steroid-sensitive neurons in the female, mediates the positive feedback effects of estrogen on GnRH secretion (Popa et al. 2008b). Finally, kisspeptin neurons seem to be involved in the regulation of the reproductive axis by metabolic signals sensing the energy balance of the organism, e.g., leptin. Reproductive hormones are inhibited during starvation, and kisspeptin mediates some of leptin's effects on reproduction. According to the current model, leptin and perhaps other adiposity and satiety factors stimulate *KISS1* expression, which results in stimulation of GnRH release. When levels of adiposity and satiety factors decrease or when such factors are not detected, the expression of *KISS1* (and presumably its secretion) decreases, thus reducing excitatory input to GnRH neurons (Chou 2014).

GnRH

Structure of GnRH

Two forms of GnRH, termed GnRH-I (or GnRH) and GnRH-II, encoded by separate genes have been identified, and they are structurally very similar but show a significantly different tissue distribution and regulation of gene expression

(Cheng and Leung 2005). GnRH-I, the peptide involved in gonadotropin regulation, is a decapeptide produced in the GnRH neurons of the hypothalamus. They originate from olfactory neurons and during embryonic development migrate toward the basal forebrain along branches of the terminal and vomeronasal nerves, across the nasal septum. This event is regulated by a number of factors that influence the migration of different portions of the GnRH neuronal population at different steps along the route and the formation of the olfactory bulb (Tobet and Schwarting 2006). The importance of such factors is demonstrated by mutations in the respective coding gene in patients with Kallmann syndrome (KS). In about 10% of patients with KS and anosmia due to a hypoplasia of the bulbus olfactorius, mutations or deletions of the KAL1 gene on the X chromosome were detected. This gene was first implicated in KS and encodes for anosmin-1 which is produced in the bulbus and in other tissues and which is transiently expressed as an extracellular matrix and basal membrane protein during organogenesis and interacts with heparan sulfate. Other genes implicated in GnRH neuron migration and KS are those encoding the fibroblast growth factor receptor 1 (*FGFR1*) and its ligand fibroblast growth factor 8 (*FGF8*), as well as prokineticin 2 (*PK2*) and its receptor (*PKR2*) (Kim et al. 2008).

In primates, the main locations of GnRH neurons are the mediobasal hypothalamus and the ARC, but they are found also in the anterior hypothalamus, preoptic area, septum, and other parts of the forebrain. GnRH neurons are synaptically connected with terminals stained positive for pro-opiomelanocortin-related peptides and enzymes involved in the metabolism of catecholamines and gamma-aminobutyric acid (GABA). Furthermore, GnRH-positive neurons of the ARC are connected to neuropeptide Y (NPY) neurons in the preoptical area and in the eminentia mediana. All these substances are known to influence GnRH secretion. The gene encoding GnRH is localized at the chromosomal site 8p21-p11.2. GnRH is produced by successive cleavage stages from a longer precursor, called prepro-GnRH, transported along the axons to the ME and there released into portal blood. In the precursor with a length of 92 amino acids, GnRH is preceded by a signal peptide consisting of 24 amino acids and followed by a stretch of 56 amino acids forming the GnRH-associated peptide (GAP). Prepro-GnRH is processed in the rough endoplasmic reticulum and in the Golgi complex, the first step being the removal of the signal peptide and the cyclization of the aminoterminal Gln residue to pyroGlu. At the junction between GnRH and GAP, a Gly-Lys-Arg sequence provides a processing signal important for the cleavage of GAP and C-terminal amidation of the last Pro residue. Mature GnRH is therefore a single chain decapeptide cyclized at the N terminus and amidated at the C terminus and assumes a folded conformation as the result of a ß-II type bend involving the central Tyr-Gly-Leu-Arg residues that brings the N- and C termini in close proximity (Millar et al. 2008). GnRH has a very short half-life (<10 min) and is mostly retained and degraded in the pituitary gland immediately after secretion by several peptidase systems. As the generation of synthetic analogs of GnRH has shown, the amino acids in position 6–10 are important for *high-affinity* binding of the neuropeptide, whereas positions 1–3 are critical for *biological activity* and positions 5–6 and 9–10 are involved in *enzymatic degradation*. The discovery of the amino acid sequence of GnRH permitted the design of GnRH analogs exerting agonistic or antagonistic action relative to the endogenous GnRH.

Secretion of GnRH

GnRH is released into the portal blood in discrete pulses (Fig. 5). The frequency of GnRH pulses and the amplitude of its secretory episodes determine the quality of LH and FSH secretion from the pituitary gland. GnRH is the sole releasing factor for both gonadotropins, but modulating its frequency results in preferential release of LH or FSH (Hayes and Crowley 1998). The pulsatile nature of GnRH secretion is partly an intrinsic characteristic of the GnRH neurons, since isolated immortalized GnRH neurons have a spontaneous pulsatile secretory activity in vitro. However, in vivo GnRH is under the control of the kisspeptin/GPR54 system, which mediates the effects of the peripheral steroids on GnRH secretion and is involved in the control of GnRH pulsatility. The pulse generator is under the continuous tonic inhibition of peripheral steroids and, e.g., gonadectomy results in an immediate increase of frequency and amplitude of gonadotropin secretion. Thus, in the *absence*

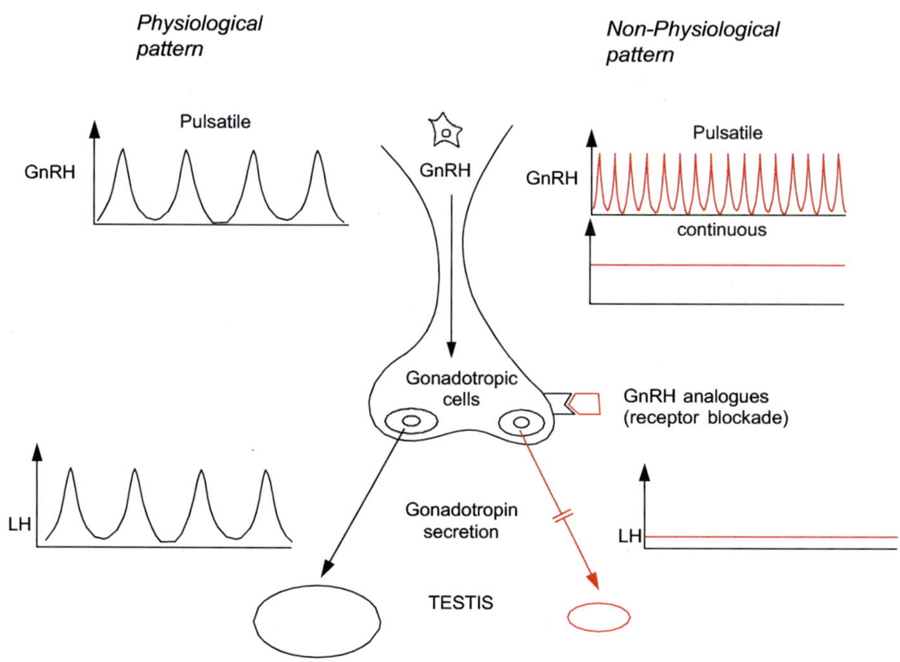

Fig. 5 Importance of the pulsatile pattern of GnRH secretion for gonadotropin secretion and testicular function

of steroids, the pulse generator becomes *free-running* (Lopez et al. 1998). In humans, *the major hormone controlling GnRH secretion is testosterone* (*Te*), which inhibits gonadotropin secretion via negative feedback both at the hypothalamic and pituitary level. Te can act as such or after metabolism to DHT or estradiol. The effects of Te and its metabolites vary depending on the experimental model, but in general, we can assume that both Te and DHT act mainly at the hypothalamic level by decreasing the frequency of GnRH pulsatility, whereas estrogens suppress gonadotropin secretion by reducing the amplitude of their peaks at the pituitary level. Progesterone inhibits gonadotropin release at least in part via ARC dopaminergic and NPY neurons. The negative feedback action of androgens and progestins is most important for the development of a male fertility control regimen. Among the neurotransmitters and neuromodulators that might influence GnRH secretion, the noradrenergic system and NPY show stimulatory activity, whereas interleukin-1, dopaminergic, serotoninergic and GABAergic systems are inhibitory. Opioid peptides seem to modulate the negative feedback of gonadal steroids. Finally, also leptin has been shown to stimulate gonadotropin secretion, as well.

Mechanism of GnRH Action

GnRH acts through interaction with a specific G-coupled receptors linked by the typical seven-membrane domain structure. With 328 amino acids, it is the smallest G protein-coupled receptor known up to now and possesses a rather short extracellular domain. The intracellular C terminus is practically absent, and the signal transduction is probably carried out by the intracytoplasmic loops connecting the seven membrane-spanning segments, especially the third one which is unusually long. The receptor contains two glycosylation sites, projecting into the extracellular space, of uncertain function. The conformation of the binding site is unknown. The gene encoding the human GnRH receptor includes three exons separated by two introns. The 5′ flanking region contains multiple TATA transcription initiation sites and several cis-acting regulatory sequences, which confer responsiveness to cAMP, glucocorticoids, progesterone, thyroxin, PEA-3, AP-1, AP-2, and Pit-1-sensitive sequences. The GnRH receptor is specifically expressed in the gonadotropic cells within the pituitary. An orphan receptor, the steroidogenic factor-1 (SF-1), is involved in the expression of human GnRH. Transcription factors such as SF-1, Pit-1, and Pro-Pit-1 are generally needed for the development and maturation of the hypothalamic–hypophyseal–gonadal axis. SF-1-deficient mice and patients bearing a mutation in the Pro-Pit-1 gene exhibit pronounced alterations of gonadotropin secretion. Recently, a second GnRH receptor gene has been identified in nonhuman primates (type II GnRH receptor) which is structurally and functionally distinct from the classical, type I receptor. The GnRH type II receptor, however, is not functional in humans and many other species and its role is yet unknown. Both GnRH-I and GnRH-II were shown to signal through the GnRH type I receptor (ligand-selective signaling). While GnRH-I regulates gonadotropins, GnRH-II appears to be a neuromodulator and stimulates sexual behavior. Following GnRH receptor interaction, a hormone-receptor complex is formed. This results in the interaction with Gq protein, hydrolysis of PI, and production of diacylglycerol and inositol trisphosphate, which leads to calcium mobilization from the intracellular stores and influx of extracellular calcium into the cell. Diacylglycerol and calcium then activate protein kinase C (PKC), inducing protein phosphorylation and further activation of calcium channels. The increase in intracellular calcium results in prompt gonadotropin release by exocytosis and, with time, more sustained gonadotropin synthesis and secretion. Thereafter, the hormone-receptor complex is internalized by endocytosis and undergoes degradation in lysosomes. GnRH is capable of modulating number and activity of its own receptors, and the effects depend on the secretory pattern and dose of neurohormone. The receptor expression is higher when GnRH is given in a pulsatile manner, and the withdrawal of GnRH during the interpulse intervals leads to increase of GnRH-binding sites just before the next pulse occurs (self priming). Conversely, continuous exposure to GnRH results in an initial rise in response followed by desensitization. This property of the GnRH receptor is exploited in therapy with GnRH agonists that, owing to their prolonged and sustained stimulatory activity, cause slow receptor desensitization and decrease of gonadotropin secretion. The molecular mechanism of receptor desensitization is not completely understood. Owing to the lack of an intracellular domain, GnRH agonists cannot induce phosphorylation and rapid desensitization of the receptor (Kim et al. 2008).

Gonadotropins

Structure of Gonadotropins

LH and FSH are glycoprotein hormones secreted by the pituitary gland that control development, maturation, and function of the gonads. Like the related thyroid-stimulating hormone (TSH) and human chorionic gonadotropin (hCG), they consist of two polypeptide chains, α and β, bearing carbohydrate moieties N-linked to asparagine (Asn) residues. The α-subunit is common to all members of the glycoprotein hormone family, whereas the β-subunit, although structurally very similar, differs in each hormone and confers specificity of action.

Separate but structurally related genes, localized on different chromosomes, encode for the subunits. The gene encoding for the α-subunit is composed of four exons and three introns, whereas the β genes consist of three exons separated by two introns. The FSH-β gene is located on chromosome 11 and differs from the other glycoprotein hormone β-subunit genes in possessing a rather long 3′ untranslated region probably involved in RNA stability. The LH-β gene belongs to an extraordinary complex cluster of genes also including at least seven nonallelic hCGβ-like genes arranged in tandem on chromosome 19. The regulation of gene expression of LH and FSH has been extensively studied in experimental animals, especially rodents, and involves a complex interplay between hypothalamic GnRH and gonadal steroids and peptides acting at the hypothalamic and pituitary level (Burger et al. 2004). The common α-subunit contains two glycosylation sites, at position 52 and 78. The glycosylation sites of FSH-β are 7 and 24, whereas LH is glycosylated only at position 30. In mammals the α-subunit is also produced by the placenta, and conversely, the pituitary gland has been shown to contain and secrete trace amounts of hCG. α- and β-subunits are non-covalently linked, and the probable tertiary structure of pituitary gonadotropins can be approximated and deduced by analogy with its cognate hCG, whose crystal structure has been resolved. LH and hCGβ subunits are structurally very similar and, in fact, LH and hCG act on the same receptor. A peculiar feature of hCGβ is a carboxyl-terminal extension containing four O-linked sugar residues that remarkably reduces the rate of metabolism and increases the half-life of the hormone. This peculiarity of hCGß has been recently exploited for the production of a synthetic gonadotropin hybrid containing a similar C-terminal extension in the β-subunit, which resulted in a conspicuous increase of the gonadotropin half-life. The oligosaccharide structure consists of a central mannose core, bound to an Asn residue through two residues of N-acetylglucosamine, and terminal extensions of tetrasaccharide branches, bi- or tri-antennary, terminating with sialic acid (FSH) or sulfate (LH) residues. These carbohydrate structures can be more or less extended in length and are rich in sugar terminals, constituting the molecular basis of the gonadotropin heterogeneity evident after chromatographic separation. Having a different terminal glycosylation, LH and FSH also have a different half-life. LH is rich in N-acetylglucosamine sulfate and is quickly removed from the circulation after interaction with specific liver receptors that recognize sulfate terminals. This rapid removal of sulfate LH from the blood results in rapid clearance of a relevant amount of the LH discharged in each secretory episode and "amplifies" the pulsatile features of LH in circulation. Conversely, FSH is predominantly sialylated and thereby protected from immediate capture and metabolism within the liver. As a result, LH and FSH half-lives are about 20 min and 2 h, respectively. Therefore, although both gonadotropins are secreted simultaneously from the pituitary gland following a GnRH pulse, LH appears to be highly pulsatile and FSH much less so (Moyle and Campbell 1995). Glycosylation is fundamental for gonadotropin secretion and bioactivity and strongly influences the half-life in circulation and in vivo biopotency. It is well known that gonadotropin activity depends on glycosylation, which is not critical for receptor binding but is important for receptor activation. Furthermore, isoforms completely devoid of carbohydrates cannot be secreted by the producing cells and behave as competitive antagonists of the wild type. Polymorphic variants of the FSH-β gene exist as well and are associated with serum FSH levels in men (Grigorova et al. 2008). Such a variant was found to be associated with a significant reduction in free Te and testes volume, but, on the contrary, in an increase of semen volume, sex hormone-binding globulin, serum Te, and estradiol.

Secretion of Gonadotropins

After the synthetic process is completed, LH and FSH are stored in different secretion granules, ready to be released upon stimulation with GnRH. A portion of molecules, however, is not stored in secretory granules, i.e., does not enter the regulated pathway of secretion and is, instead, constitutively secreted. FSH especially follows the latter route. Storage in separate granules and the natural propensity to follow one of the two secretory pathways are the main reasons why the same GnRH stimulus can, under certain conditions, preferentially release one of the two gonadotropins. Low GnRH pulse frequency causes preferential release of FSH probably due to differential expression of the FSH receptor (Ferris and Shupnik 2006).

LH and FSH are measurable in the pituitary gland as early as the 10th week of gestation and during the 12th week in peripheral blood. In fetal life and in infancy, FSH is predominant over LH and the FSH/LH ratio is higher in females than in males. The relative abundance of the two gonadotropins undergoes changes during development. Te drives the initial phase of testicular migration and the development of male external genitalia. The fetal testicle already produces Te during the 10th week of gestation, under the stimulation of fetal LH and maternal hCG. The role of maternal hCG in this crucial phase of gonadal development is suggested by the fact that a mutation of the LH β chain leading to a biologically inactive gonadotropin is associated with normal sexual differentiation. Conversely, inactivating mutations of the LH receptor produce a clinical syndrome resembling complete androgen insensitivity, with a phenotype of female external genitalia (Huhtaniemi et al. 1999; Themmen et al. 1998).

During infancy gonadotropins in serum are very low. The pulsatile secretion of gonadotropins becomes evident at the time of puberty, when LH and FSH pulses in serum are detected first during nighttime and then progressively also during the day. Before puberty, gonadotropin levels are very low and GnRH secretion appears to be extremely limited, even in the presence of negligible steroid production by the gonads. High sensitivity of the hypothalamus to negative steroid feedback is believed to suppress GnRH production before puberty, but certainly other factors such as body mass, leptin, and signals from the central nervous system are important to maintain the hypothalamic–pituitary–gonadal axis silent before the programmed time.

The steroid regulation of gonadotropin gene expression, synthesis, and secretion is rather complex and shows many facets depending on the experimental model. In general, however, it is currently accepted that gonadal steroids exert their negative control on gonadotropins mainly at the hypothalamic level, depressing the release of GnRH most probably via the kisspeptin/GPR54 system. The steroid effect at the pituitary level is more complex, but there is considerable evidence that estrogens inhibit GnRH-stimulated gonadotropin synthesis and secretion at this level. Te is the main testicular product suppressing FSH and LH secretion in men. FSH secretion is, obviously, also under the control of some other factor(s) related to the efficiency of spermatogenesis, since oligozoospermia is often accompanied by selective increase of serum FSH in the presence of normal Te levels. The mutual relationship between FSH and inhibin secretion in man is well established: a pronounced inverse correlation was found between serum concentrations of inhibin B and serum levels of FSH, testis size, and sperm numbers. Clearly, inhibin B is the physiologically relevant form of inhibin in men. It appears at present that the serum levels of inhibin B directly reflect the integrity of the germinal epithelium and of the Sertoli cells (Boepple et al. 2008).

Mechanism of Action of Gonadotropins

LH and FSH exert their function via *specific receptors*. The gonadotropin receptors also belong to the family of the G protein-coupled receptors and are characterized by a very large extracellular domain to which the hormone binds, specifically, the usual membrane-spanning domain including seven hydrophobic segments connected to each other through three extracellular and three intracellular tracts and an intracellular carboxyl-terminal domain (Simoni and Casarini 2014).

The genes for LH and FSH receptors are localized on chromosome 2 and consist of 11 and 10 exons, respectively. The last exon encodes a small portion of the extracellular domain, the entire transmembrane domain, and the intracellular C terminus. The extracellular domain contains the high-affinity hormone-binding site and is rich in leucine repeats. The 5′-flanking region of the two genes contains no conventional promoter and has multiple transcriptions start sites. In addition, the human LH receptor was recently shown to contain a cryptic exon (denominated exon 6A) which plays a very important role in the intracellular processing of the mature receptor protein and can be mutated in rare cases of LH resistance. Several alternatively spliced transcripts of LH and FSH receptors have been described, lacking one or more exons, but presently it is not known whether these RNA isoforms are translated into proteins of any physiological function. Single nucleotide polymorphisms give rise to allelic variants with different biological activity in vitro and/or in vivo.

The mature receptor proteins are glycosylated at several points, a process that does not seem to be involved in receptor activation and signal transduction but probably necessary for receptor folding and transport to the cell membrane. Recently, the partially deglycosylated complex of human FSH bound to the extracellular hormone-binding domain of its receptor was crystallized, showing that binding specificity is mediated by key interaction sites involving both the common α- and hormone-specific β-subunits. On binding, FSH undergoes a concerted conformational change that affects protruding loops implicated in receptor activation. The FSH–FSHR complexes form dimers in the crystal important for transmembrane signal transduction resulting in activation of the G protein, cAMP production, and activation of PKA. Gonadotropins act mainly through stimulation of intracellular cAMP. More recently it has been shown that LH and FSH can also induce an increase of calcium influx in target cells, but the physiological importance of this mechanism is still unknown. cAMP remains, therefore, the main signal transducer and calcium could possibly act as a signal amplification or modulating mechanism. Following the hormone-receptor interaction, there is an increase in cAMP concentrations and subsequent activation of PKs which, in turn, phosphorylate existing proteins such as enzymes, structural and transport proteins, and transcriptional activators. Activating and inactivating mutations of the gonadotropin receptors have been identified. Recent human data suggest that gonadotropins may act as cell survival factors for spermatogonia rather than as stimulators of cell proliferation, permitting differentiation of Ap spermatogonia into B-type spermatogonia (Simoni and Casarini 2014; Piersma et al. 2007).

Endocrine Regulation and Relative Importance of LH and FSH for Spermatogenesis

Spermatogenesis starts with the division of stem cells and ends with the formation of mature sperm. The various germ cells are arranged in typical cellular associations within the seminiferous tubules known as spermatogenic stages, and the entire spermatogenic process can be divided into four phases and requires 16 days for the development and differentiaton of an Ap spermatogonium into a mature sperm:

1. Mitotic proliferation and differentiation of diploid germ cells (spermatogonia) (spermatogoniogenesis)
2. Meiotic division of tetraploid germ cells (spermatocytes) resulting in haploid germ cells (spermatids)
3. Transformation of spermatids into testicular sperm (spermiogenesis)
4. Release of sperm from the germinal epithelium into the tubular lumen (spermiation).

It must be pointed out, however, that a recent review recommends 74 days by including time for spermatogonial renewal (Amann 2008).

The gamete development through several stages (from spermatogenesis to spermiation) is regulated by the brain, e.g., the hypothalamus and pituitary via GnRH and gonadotropins. Importantly, the hypothalamic–hypophyseal circuit is subject to negative feedback regulation mediated by testicular factors. Te inhibits the secretion of LH and FSH. For FSH, the protein hormone inhibin B plays an important role.

For the interpretation of hormonal regulation and hormonal effects on spermatogenesis, the following terminology should be remembered:

1. Initiation: First complete cycle of spermatogenesis during puberty.
2. Maintenance: Hormonal requirements of intact spermatogenesis in the adult.
3. Reinitiation: Hormonal requirements for the restimulation of gametogenesis after transitory interruption.
4. Qualitatively normal spermatogenesis: All germ cells are present although in subnormal numbers.
5. Quantitatively normal spermatogenesis: All germ cells are present in normal numbers.

Considerable efforts were undertaken to unravel the relative importance of LH/Te and FSH for qualitative and quantitative initiation, maintenance, and reinitiation of spermatogenesis (Fig. 6). It is generally assumed that either Te or FSH alone is able

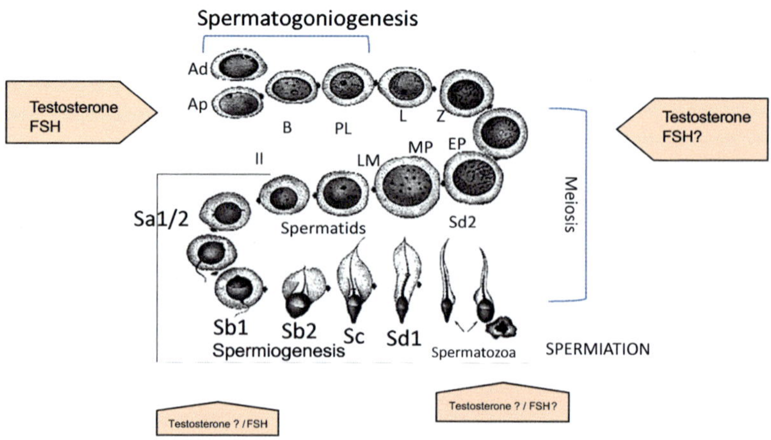

Ad = A-dark spermatogonium (testicular stem cells, divides rarely), Ap = A-pale spermatogonium (self-renewing and progenitor cell for spermatogenesis), B = B spermatogonium, Pl = preleptotene spermatocytes, L = leptotene spermatocytes, EP = early pachytene spermatocytes, MP = mid pachytene spermatocytes, LP = late pachytene spermatocytes, II = 2nd meiotic division, RB = residual body, Sa1–Sd2 = developmental stages of spermatid maturation

Fig. 6 Sites of action of testosterone and FSH on the spermatogenic process in primates

to initiate, maintain, and reinitiate spermatogenesis but only to a qualitative extent. In order to achieve quantitative effects on germ cell production and sperm numbers, at least under physiological conditions, both LH and FSH activities are needed (Weinbauer et al. 2004).

These assertions are based upon controlled studies in nonhuman primate models and volunteers and on studies in patient populations and case reports. The latter has provided interesting information but can also confound interpretation of findings owing to the variable endocrine and medical history of the patients. Complete spermatogenesis is seen in the vicinity of Te-producing LC tumors and in patients with activating mutations of the LH receptor, suggesting that pharmacologically high local Te concentrations induce sperm formation. The aim of treatment is to obtain sufficiently high intratesticular Te concentrations, which are crucial. This is normally pursued clinically by giving hCG, which contains high LH activity, together with FSH. On the other hand, patients bearing a defective FSH-β subunit, presented with azoospermia. One of these patients was normally virilized, suggesting the need of FSH for complete initiation of spermatogenesis in man (Lindstedt et al. 1998); conversely, patients with selective LH deficiency can have complete spermatogenesis, indicating the ability of FSH to initiate the entire male germ cell development cascade.

Exogenous provision of supranormal doses of Te or of gestagenic compounds suppresses gonadotropin secretion through the negative feedback mechanism and leads to a drastic decrease of sperm numbers in the ejaculate. In primates it is essential that complete suppression of FSH secretion be achieved despite inhibition of LH secretion. In the latter study, albeit LH bioactivity had been completely eliminated, a slight and transient rebound of FSH secretion provoked an escape of spermatogenic suppression. In gonadotropin-suppressed men, either FSH or LH maintained spermatogenesis. The importance of FSH is also evident from a hypophysectomized patient in whom an activating mutation of the FSH receptor coexisted with normal spermatogenesis in the absence of LH. Conversely, inactivating mutations of FSH action do not necessarily lead to a complete block of spermatogenesis. Although either hormone on its own has the potential to elicit the entire spermatogenic process, this is not always the case in patients receiving androgen/hCG therapies. In case of failure of hCG, however, the addition of FSH has been shown to permit completion of spermatogenesis in hypogonadotropic men with azoospermia. Finally, in primates, both gonadotropins are necessary for spermatogenesis. The biological meaning of this dual regulation system is not clear yet. From a clinical viewpoint it is concluded that the synergistic action of LH/Te and FSH is necessary for the initiation, maintenance and also for reinitiation of normal spermatogenesis (Tobet and Schwarting 2006). The regulation of testicular function is primarily controlled by central structures, but the complexity of the testicular cell types and architecture also mandates a variety of *local control* and regulatory mechanisms. The categories of local interactions and communication can be classified as *paracrine, autocrine, and intracrine*. In addition, the interplay between the different testicular compartments is also subsumed under local interactions. It is evident that the endocrine mechanisms play the central role in the regulation of testicular function and factors produced locally are important for the modulation of hormone activity and local factors could thus be seen as mediators of hormone action and intra-/intercellular communication. Moreover, it can be reasonably assumed that other still unidentified protein factors mediate the communication between interstitial and tubular compartments, between SC and germ cells and between germ cells (Weinbauer and Wessels 1999). Growth factors bind to surface receptors and induce cell-specific differentiation events via specific signal transduction cascades. Among those factors participating in the local regulation of spermatogenesis are transforming growth factor (TGF)-α and TGF-β, inhibin and activin, nerve growth factor (NGF), insulin-like growth factor I (IGF-I), fibroblast growth factor (FGF), and epidermal growth factor (EGF) (Laron and Klinger 1998).

Insulin-Like Factor 3 (INSL3)

INSL3 is a member of the relaxin-like peptide family, and it is emerging as a key factor in the regulation of a variety of developmental processes related to reproduction (Foresta et al. 2004). The binding of the hormone to its specific receptor LGR8 (also known as leucine-rich repeat-containing G protein-coupled receptor) activates adenylate cyclase and cAMP production through Gs proteins, although alternative mechanisms have been proposed (Kumagai et al. 2002). INSL3 is expressed in pre- and postnatal LC of the testis. The major known endocrine role of INSL3 is related to the regulation of the transabdominal phase of testicular descent by action on the gubernaculum. As a consequence, *Insl3* and *Rxfp2* knockout mice have bilateral cryptorchid testes, and mutations in the *INSL3* and *RXFP2* genes have been associated with testis maldescent also in humans (Ferlin et al. 2003). In addition to the

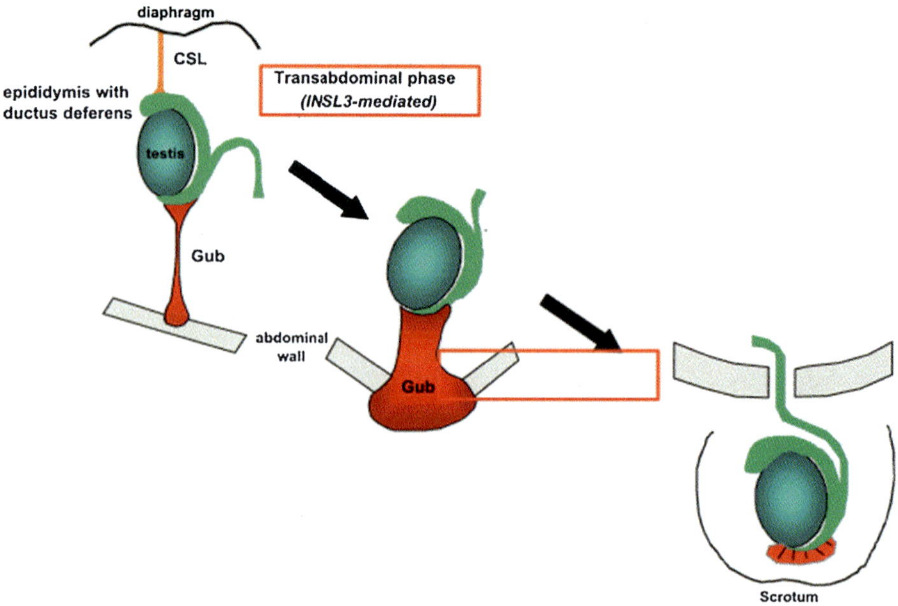

Fig. 7 Hormonal control of testicular descent

prenatal role for INSL3, further possible endocrine and paracrine actions in adult males have recently gained particular attention based on several observations. First, in adults, INSL3 is produced constitutively but in a differentiation-dependent manner by the LC under the effect of luteinizing hormone (LH), and substantial circulating INSL3 levels are present in adult men. Reduced plasma concentrations are seen in situations of undifferentiated or altered LC status (such as hypogonadism), and INSL3 has been suggested to be even more sensitive than Te to impaired LC function (Ferlin et al. 2006). Second, RXFP2 is expressed in many tissues besides the gubernaculum, including the kidney, skeletal muscle, thyroid, pituitary gland, brain, and bone marrow, and paracrine roles for INSL3 have been suggested in the testis, ovary, thyroid, and mammary gland (Fig. 7).

Steroid Hormones

Te is the main secretory product of the testis, along with 5α-dihydrotestosterone (DHT), androsterone, androstenedione, 17-hydroxyprogesterone (17-OH-Pg), progesterone (Pg), and pregnenolone. The role of androsterone, 17-OH-Pg, and Pg in the testis is unknown, but progesterone receptors have been found in some peritubular cells and on spermatozoa. For Te, a classic endocrine factor, compelling evidence is available as a pivotal local regulator of spermatogenesis. Rodent data demonstrated that selective elimination of LC, interruption of testicular Te transport, and specific SC androgen receptor knockout models provoked profound alterations of germ cell maturation (Takaimya et al. 1998). Selective peritubular cell androgen receptor knockout mice exhibited specific SC and peritubular cell defects. Spermatogenesis was present in boys with Te-producing LC tumors but only in seminiferous tubules adjacent to the tumor and not in tumor-free areas. Similarly, activating mutations of the LH receptor prematurely induced qualitatively normal spermatogenesis.

In fertile men, testicular Te concentrations exceed that of SHBG/ABP by about 200-fold, indicating a substantial surplus of Te in the testis. Testicular Te concentrations are >80-fold higher than those in plasma (Coviello et al. 2005). Te is metabolized to DHT by testicular 5α-reductase activity and to estradiol by testicular aromatase activity. To what extent these metabolic activities are essential for spermatogenesis besides Te itself is not entirely clear.

Although it is established beyond doubt that Te is an essential local regulator of spermatogenesis, it has been surprisingly difficult to demonstrate a clear-cut relationship between testicular Te concentrations and germ cell production. In *nonhuman primates*, no correlation between testicular androgen levels and germ cell production/spermatozoa number was observed. Similarly, contraceptive studies in volunteers failed to demonstrate a correlation between intratesticular steroids and germ cell numbers (Matthiesson et al. 2005b). In the nonhuman primate, Te induces the formation of smooth muscle actin in the peritubular cells during prepubertal testicular maturation. Peritubular cells express the androgen receptor. Te effect is significantly reinforced by FSH. Since FSHR are found only in SC, it follows that FSH influences androgen action indirectly through factors arising in the SC. This indicates that as an endocrine factor, FSH can also induce the formation of physiologically relevant, locally acting factors in the primate testis. Interestingly, recombinant FSH stimulates Te production in men (Levalle et al. 1998) and in patients with selective FSH deficiency, lending further support to the importance of local interactions between SCs, LCs, and peritubular cells in connection with the actions of androgens and gonadotropins (Lofrano-Porto et al. 2008).

Testicular Descent

The incidence of positional anomalies of the testis is over 3% and ranges among the most common congenital defects. These defects are associated with spermatogenic disturbances such as fewer spermatogonial stem cells at birth compared with normal boys and increased risk of testicular tumor development. Testicular descent is multifactorial with two distinct phases. The first is descending phase from the lower kidney pole to the pelvic cavity (*transabdominal phase of descent*) controlled by the swelling of the gubernaculum. The shortening of the gubernacular cord and the outgrowth of the gubernacular bulb controlled by the genitofemoral nerve are independent of androgens. The gubernaculum deposits extracellular matrix, rich in glycosaminoglycans and hyaluronic acid, and forms a cone-like structure at the caudal end of the gonad, anchoring the developing testis close to the inguinal region during fetal growth. In the second phase, the descent into the scrotum (*inguino-*

scrotal phase of descent) is controlled by androgen action. In the 26th gestational week, the gubernaculum begins to grow through the inguinal canal and reaches the scrotum by gestational week 35, pulling the testis in its path before the gubernaculum shrinks to a fibrous remnant. The intra-abdominal pressure and the shrinkage of the gubernaculum may force the testis through the inguinal canal. At birth, the testes reach at the bottom of the scrotum, and in 97% of boys, testicular descent is completed within another 12 weeks (Fig. 7). The physiological and endocrine mechanisms that govern testicular descent are not known in detail. INSL3 is a potential regulator of testicular descent as suggested by the fact that in gene knockout mice, maldescended testes remain located in the abdominal cavity. INSL3 produced by the LC together with androgen induces the gubernaculum growth and is therefore needed in the early phase, and knockout mice for INSL3 gene have their testes high in the abdominal cavity. *Estrogens or environmental endocrine disruptors* have also been suspected to induce a downregulated INSL3 expression and thus disturb testicular descent. Genetic analysis in men revealed several functionally deleterious mutations in both INSL3 and its receptor GREAT/LGR8 gene (Boepple et al. 2008).

Vascularization, Temperature, and Regulation of Spermatogenesis

Vascularization of the testis has two main roles: transport and mobilization of endocrine factors and metabolites, as well as regulation of testicular temperature. The arterial supply of the testicular parenchyma follows the lobular division of the seminiferous tubules. Each lobule is supplied by one artery from which segmental arteries, supplying blood to the lateral regions of the lobuli. Segmental arteries and capillaries become branched between the LC and finally give rise to the venous system.

In men, testicular temperature is about 3–4 °C below core body temperature and about 1.5–2.5 °C above the temperature of scrotal skin. For the maintenance of a physiologically lower temperature, the testis relies on two *thermoregulatory systems*. Heat can be transferred to the external environment through the scrotal skin, as the scrotal skin is very thin, possesses hardly any subcutaneous fat tissue, and has a very large surface.

The second regulatory system is the pampiniform plexus. In this system, the convoluted testicular artery is surrounded by several veins coiling around the artery several times. Arterial blood arriving at the testis is thereby cooled down by the surrounding venous blood. The usual explanation for the pampiniform plexus here is to efficiently maintain the optimal temperature, which is below body temperature. Recently, a new theory has been put forward hypothesizing that the process of spermatogenesis results in a large amount of heat, which has to be regulated. Testes are located in the scrotum in order to maintain lower body temperatures. Some mammals' testes remain functional inside the body, e.g., elephants, but these animals lack sweat glands and are closely related to aquatic ancestors which have to compensate for the chilling effects of the heat-conducting environment, namely, water. Human scrotal skin is devoid of subcutaneous fat and the presence of high sweat gland density enables heat transmission. Upon exposure to cold temperatures, the scrotal surface is minimized by contraction for preventing temperature loss, and cremaster muscles retract the testes closer to the abdomen for temperature maintenance.

Testicular Androgens

In men, *testosterone* is by far the most important and abundant androgen in blood. More than 95% of the existing androgens derive from the testis, which synthesizes about 6–7 mg Te per day. Apart the testes, the remaining contribution to androgen production derives mainly from the adrenals. The site of androgen production in the testis is the LC. Both synthesis and secretion are under regulation of pituitary LH and local factors. The starting point for androgen synthesis is cholesterol and adult LCs have additional requirements for cholesterol, because it is the essential precursor for all steroid hormones. LH as the central regulatory factor controls both steroidogenesis and LC cholesterol homeostasis in vivo. Cholesterol can either be incorporated by the cell through receptor-mediated endocytosis from low-density lipoproteins (LDL) or can be synthesized de novo within the LCs starting from acetyl coenzyme A (Sriraman et al. 2005). The conversion of cholesterol to Te goes through five different enzymatic steps in which the side chain of cholesterol is shortened through oxidation from 27-C to 19-C (Fig. 8). Te is the main secretory product of the testis, along with DHT, androsterone, androstenedione, 17-OHPg, Pg, and pregnenolone. The transformation of Te into DHT takes place principally into the target organs. Androstenedione is important as a precursor for the production of extratesticular estrogens. Biologically active estradiol can be produced as a result of extratesticular aromatization of androstenedione to estrone that is subsequently reduced to estradiol in peripheral tissues. Only a very small portion of the Te produced is stored in the testis, and the androgen is mainly secreted in the blood.

Te concentrations in the testicular lymphatic circulation and in the venous blood are very similar, but there are essential differences in the flow rate and velocity of both systems. Therefore, transport of Te in the general blood circulation occurs mainly through the spermatic vein. Androgens diffuse into interstitial fluid and then enter testicular capillaries or enter capillaries directly from LC that is in direct contact with the testicular microvasculature. The mechanism for Te transport from the LC into the blood or lymphatics is not completely known. Probably lipophilic steroids distributed within cells or small cell groups are released through passive diffusion.

Testosterone and Blood Transport

SHBG concentration in men is about one third to one half of the concentration found in women. During transport in plasma, Te is mainly bound to albumin or *to sex hormone-binding globulin* (*SHBG*), which is produced by *hepatocytes*. A protein,

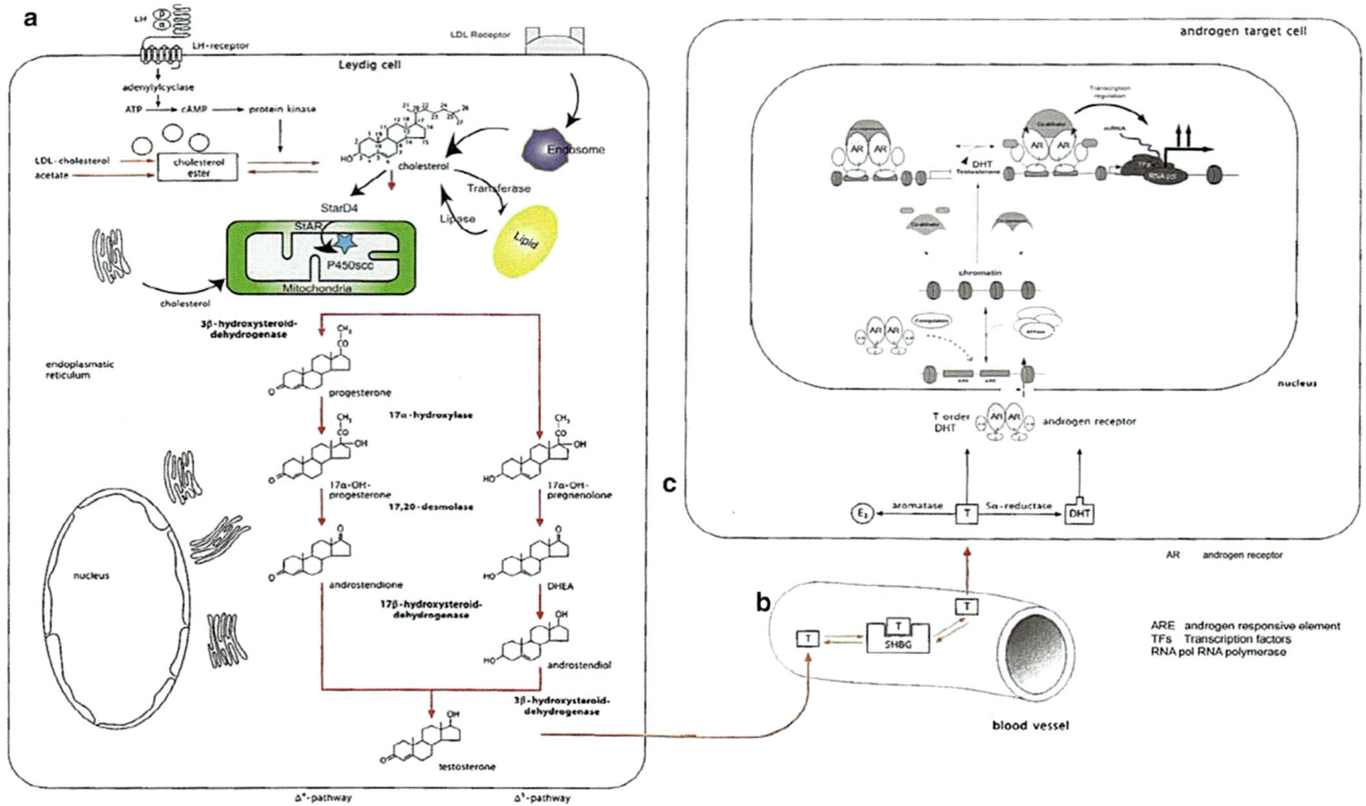

Fig. 8 Biosynthesis of androgen

the *androgen-binding protein* (*ABP*), with similar steroid-binding characteristics is produced in the testis. SHBG is an α-globulin consisting of different protein subunits. In rats it is expressed in SC and is secreted preferentially into the seminiferous tubules and migrates into the caput epididymis where it is internalized by epithelial cells that regulate androgen-dependent mechanisms of sperm maturation. Testicular SHBG isoforms are found in sperm and released from these during the capacitation reaction. Plasma SHBG is about 95 kDa in molecular weight, 30% of which is represented by carbohydrate, and possesses one androgen-binding site per molecule. Human testicular SHBG transcripts are expressed in the germ cells and contain an alternative exon 1 sequence, appearing to encode an SHBG isoform that is 4–5 kDa smaller than plasma SHBG. Te-binding capacity is also much lower compared to the plasma SHBG. In normal men, only 2% of total Te circulates freely in the blood, while 44% is bound to SHBG and 54% to albumin. The binding affinity of Te to albumin is about 100 times lower compared to SHBG. However, since albumin concentration is much higher than that of SHBG, the binding capacity of both proteins for Te is about the same. The ratio of Te bound to SHBG over free SHBG is proportional to SHBG concentration. A direct measurement of free Te is impractical in routine practice, so that several equations are used to estimate the free Te concentration in serum (Selva et al. 2005). The main dissociation of Te from binding proteins takes place in capillaries. The interaction of binding proteins with the endothelial glycocalyx leads to a structural modification of the hormonal binding site and thereby to a change in affinity. As a result Te is set free and can diffuse freely into the target cell. SHBG not only binds Te but also estradiol. The type of binding is influenced by the different SHBG isoforms, but generally Te binds threefold higher than estradiol to SHBG. Its concentration in serum is under hormonal regulation and primarily regulated through opposing actions of sex steroids on hepatocytes, estrogen stimulation, and androgen inhibiting it. Other hormones such as thyroid hormones are also potent stimulators of SHBG production. In normal, healthy men with an intact hypothalamic–pituitary–testicular axis, an increase in plasma concentrations of SHBG leads to an acute decrease of free Te and simultaneous stimulation of Te synthesis, persisting until achievement of normal concentrations. SHBG concentrations can be elevated in hypogonadal men (Rolf 1997).

Extratesticular Metabolism of Testosterone

Te is a precursor of two important hormones: through 5α-reduction, as it gives rise to the highly biologically (three- to sixfold compared to Te) active hormone 5*a*-dihydrotestosterone (DHT), and through aromatization to estradiol. The half-life of Te in plasma is only about 12 min. Reduction of Te to DHT occurs in the endoplasmic reticulum through the enzyme 5α-reductase which is located in cellular microsomes. Both Te and DHT bind to the same intracellular androgen receptor to regulate gene expression in the target tissue. Although they interact with the same androgen receptor, Te and DHT produce distinct biological responses and the molecular mechanisms are still under debate. Two isoforms of 5α-reductase could be identified in humans by NADPH-dependent enzymes reducing the double bond at the four to five positions in C-19 as well as C-21 steroids. The gene for 5α-reductase type I is located on chromosome 5 encoding for a protein with 259 amino acids, while the gene for the 5α-reductase type II is on chromosome 2 encoding for a shorter protein with 254 amino acids. The two isoforms are very similar to each other, but show different biochemical properties. One works optimally at an alkaline pH, the other at acidic pH. Also, the tissue distribution of the two forms is different. Type I 5α-reductase has been localized in the non-genital skin, liver, brain, prostate, ovary, and testis, while type II is mainly active in classical androgen-dependent tissues, such as the epididymis, genital skin, seminal vesicle, testis, and prostate but also in the liver, uterus, breast, hair follicles, and placenta. At the cellular level, DHT sustains differentiation and growth and is particularly important for normal sexual development and virilization in men. It also affects the muscle mass and the deepening of the voice. Overall, Te effects result from influences of the hormone itself and of its metabolites estradiol and DHT. Changes in the property of type II 5α-reductase due to mutation can result in *c*omplete *a*ndrogen *i*nsensitivity *s*yndrome (CAIS) or *p*artial *a*ndrogen *i*nsensitivity *s*yndrome (PAIS) (Imperato-McGinley and Zhu 2002). In human tissues five aldo-keto reductase isoforms (AKR) exist with varying reductase activity on the 3-, 17-, and 20-ketosteroid position with isoform (AKR1C2) predominately converting 5α-DHT to 3α-diol. The inactivated metabolites are excreted in the urine (Penning et al. 2000). Some androgen metabolites are excreted in free form; others are glucuronated by the liver before excretion. The 17-glucuronidation of the DHT to metabolite androstane-3α,17β-diol is directly correlated with increasing of the risk factors for metabolic syndrome (total fat mass, its distribution, intrahepatic fat, disturbed lipid profile, insulin resistance, and diabetes) (Vandenput et al. 2007).

Mechanism of Androgen Action

Te dissociates from SHBG at the target organ and diffuses into the cells. The conversion of Te into DHT is organ dependent. The first step in androgen action is binding to the androgen receptor, which belongs to the family of steroid hormone receptors. The mechanism through which the androgen receptor and other nuclear receptors act as transcriptional factors has a general mechanism in which they bind to their ligand in the cytosol thus inducing conformational changes, loss of chaperones, dimerization, and nuclear translocation. Into the nucleus both (ligand and nuclear receptor) bind to specific sequences of genomic DNA and induce stimulation of RNA synthesis. Chromatin remodeling such as modification of histones plays a role in gene transcription, and many nuclear receptor-interacting co-regulators perform significant roles in gene transcription. Currently 48 nuclear receptors have been identified in humans. These receptors share substantial functions and are thought to have evolved from a single ancestral gene. Orphan nuclear receptors have also been found for which no ligand has yet been identified. Members of this receptor family possess an N-terminal domain, a DNA-binding domain, a hinge region, and a hormone-binding domain (Kato et al. 2011).

Steroid receptors show high homology with the corresponding DNA-binding and ligand-binding domains in the mineralocorticoid, glucocorticoid, and progesterone receptors. In contrast, at *the N-terminal domain*, little similarity with these receptors remains. The nuclear receptors are subdivided into *two subfamilies* depending on their ligand partners' forming *homodimers* such as the androgen receptor and other steroid receptors; another subfamily forms *heterodimers* with only one ligand, such as the thyroid hormone receptor. An important characteristic of the N-terminal domain of the androgen receptor is the presence of *short tandem repeats* (*STRs*) *CAG* coding for polymorphic polyglutamine, TGG repeats coding for polyproline, and GGC repeats for polyglycine. In normal men, about 17–29 glutamine repeats and 13–17 glycine repeats are present. Alleles of small GGC size have been associated with esophageal cancer, while in patients with Kennedy disease, a disease with degenerating motoneurons, up to 72 such glutamine repeats are present. Furthermore, in the androgen receptor, long CAG and GGC alleles are associated with decreased transactivation function and have been associated with cancers in women. In the androgen receptor, a low-size CAG (<19 repeats) and GGC (<15 repeats) alleles result in higher receptor activity and have been associated with earlier age of onset and a higher grade and more advanced stage of prostate cancer at the time of diagnosis (Francomano et al. 2013a; Tirabassi et al. 2015).

The number of glutamine repeats of the androgen receptor has been associated with azoospermia or oligozoospermia, but no clear association was found. The mentioned subtle differences in the number of repeats, e.g., CAG or TGG and GGC of AR gene, have also been tested for spermatogenic effects. In spite of many efforts to demonstrate that the number of CAG triplets influences the transcriptional activity of the androgen receptor, no clear relationship to disturbances of spermatogenesis has been found in a wide variety of human ethnics. Some oligozoospermic and azoospermic men bearing mutations in the ligand-binding domain have also been identified. Androgen receptor defects such as deletions or inactivating mutations can profoundly alter receptor function. The resulting phenotype is highly variable ranging from poor virilization to testicular feminilization. Inactivating mutations of the androgen receptor gene in a 46 XY male with testes resulted in a female phenotype owing to the complete lack of all androgen activity. However, there is no uterus and only a partially formed vagina, and during puberty pubic and axillary hair is scant or absent. This syndrome of complete androgen insensitivity (AIS) was earlier called testicular feminization. Similar clinical consequences are also typical for mutations which severely damage the function of the androgen receptor, such as those in the DNA-binding or androgen-binding domain. Partial AIS (PAIS) is due to mutations in the androgen receptor gene and over 800 mutations have been reported (http://www.androgendb.mcgill.ca). Furthermore, mutations which involve co-activators or co-repressors can also lead to PAIS of different severity. Moreover, mutations in the N-terminal domain of the androgen receptor, which can lead to elimination of the androgen receptor function, play a minor role in male idiopathic infertility (Zuccarello et al. 2008).

Biological Actions of Androgens

In primates, the androgen receptor can be found not only in the classical androgen-dependent organs, such as the muscles, prostate, seminal vesicles, epididymis, and testes, but also in almost every tissue, e.g., the hypothalamus, pituitary, kidney, spleen, heart, and salivary glands. Hence, Te exerts a variety of actions on many body targets. In the testis, the androgen receptor is expressed in SCs, peritubular cells, and LCs, while the germ cells seem not to express it. Studies in cell-specific androgen receptor knockout mice demonstrated that the SCs require androgen for the maintenance of complete spermatogenesis and that spermatocyte and spermatid development depends on androgens. The peritubular myoid cells maintain their cell contractility, ensuring normal spermatogenesis and sperm output. A functional androgen receptor in LCs is essential to maintain spermatogenesis and Te production and is required for normal male fertility (Xu et al. 2007). Androgens are important in every phase of human life. During the embryonal stage, Te determines the differentiation of the sexual organs and, during puberty, the further development toward the adult male phenotype, which is then maintained along with important anabolic functions. DHT is the main androgen acting on the epididymis, vas deferens, seminal vesicles, and prostate, originating from Te through 5α-reductase. These tissues are particularly dependent on continuous androgen action. In addition, Te aromatization to estrogens plays an important role in prostate growth. Estrogen concentrations in prostate stromal tissue are clearly increased in case of benign prostatic hyperplasia (BPH). Estrogens, acting in synergy with androgens and the estrogen receptor ß, are required to regulate the proliferative and antiproliferative changes that occur during normal prostate development and differentiation. In the epididymis, the seminal vesicles, and the vas deferens, a lack of Te can result in regression of the secretory epithelia, eventually leading to aspermia (ejaculation failure). The androgen effects in these organs are mediated through Te, DHT, and estradiol.

Both Te and DHT are necessary for normal penis growth, which is positively correlated with the increasing Te concentrations during puberty. The masculinization of Wolffian ducts is primarily caused by Te, whereas the transformation of the external genitalia, urethra, and prostate is primarily due to DHT. However, androgen receptors are no longer expressed in the penis of adult men, and any androgen deficiency after puberty results in only minor decrease of penis size. Similarly, Te administration to adults is not capable of increasing penis size. Te is the main androgen present in *muscles*, which have very low 5α-reductase activity. Skeletal muscles are capable of converting circulating dehydroepiandrosterone (DHEA) to Te and estrogen. Te has direct anabolic effects both on smooth and striated muscles with an increase of muscular mass and hypertrophy of the fibers. In modern sports these effects have led to an abuse of these steroids to increase the muscle mass in both sexes, and loss of Te can lead to muscular atrophy. Also, androgens influence the neuromuscular system (NM) throughout genomic and non-genomic pathways. The genomic pathways are mainly involved in long-term effects of Te on muscle structure and function, whereas the non-genomic pathways are responsible for rapid effects of Te on NM metabolisms and functions and, probably, only as an integrated step also on muscle structure. Even if scarce data exist in humans, probably, steroids influence the nervous component of NM system (e.g., motor behavior, neuronal activity, intracellular signaling) mainly through non-genomic mechanisms (i.e., voltage-dependent K+ currents, Ca2+ channels, neurotransmitters, etc.). Te replacement treatment would reduce excitability of the NM system, and it would favor a predominant recruitment of slow-twitch motor units (Felici et al. 2016). Both *androgens and estrogens* induce an increase of bone density by stimulating mineralization, while the lack of these steroids results in osteoporosis. The *skeleton* develops distinctly in males and females, particularly at the periosteal surface. Sex differences in skeletal morphology and physiology occur at or around puberty, with little effect of gonadal steroids prior to puberty. At the beginning of puberty, the increase in linear growth of bones is directly correlated with increasing Te concentrations. It is known that gender differences, particularly with respect to "bone quality" and architecture (i.e., predominantly bone width), are modulated by the balance of the sex steroids estrogen and androgen. At the end of puberty, depending on the presence of Te, epiphyseal closure occurs, an event that can be consistently delayed in the presence of low Te concentrations. Low Te is associated with increased risk of fracture, particularly with hip and nonvertebral fractures. It is clear now that the androgen action on bone metabolism is mediated through estradiol (Valimaki et al. 2004).

The effects of androgens on the skin and dependent organs vary in the different cutaneous districts and are mediated by Te and, probably, DHT. Depending on Te, the growth of *sebaceous glands* can be stimulated, and sebum production in the face, upper part of the back, and in the skin of the chest can be induced. Te contributes to the development of acne vulgaris, while estrogens can diminish sebum concentration. The effects of DHT and Te on the hair are influenced by the androgen sensitivity of the hair follicle. While axillary hair and the lower part of pubic hair start growing even in the presence of low androgen concentrations, much higher androgen levels are necessary for the growth of the beard, upper part of the pubic hair, and chest hair. The hairline is determined both by genetic factors and individual distribution of the androgen receptor and depends on the androgen milieu. High 5α-reductase activity has been observed in bald men, while in patients with 5α-reductase deficiency or hypogonadism, there is no regression of the hair line. Since the growth of the scalp hair is related to increased 5α-reductase activity, increased activity of this enzyme with consequences for hair loss could be an expression of the precocious aging of the hair follicles. Androgens stimulate hair follicles to alter hair color and size via the hair growth cycle and seem to reduce alopecia (Randall et al. 2008).

During puberty, there is a Te-dependent growth of the length of the *larynx* of about 1 cm. This size increase, together with the length and mass of the vocal cords, leads to a lowering of vocal register. A deep voice is directly related to androgens so that a lower register can also be induced in women by Te treatment. The depth of voice in a man is correlated with the duration of the pubertal phase after which the androgen receptors are lost. Once reached, register remains unchanged and no modification of the voice can be obtained after puberty in hypogonadal patients. The gender-specific change of the vocal register is correlated with the degree of mineralization in human thyroid cartilage. Few chondrocytes near the mineralization front are positive for the androgen receptor and also for alkaline phosphatase, suggesting an involvement in androgen-mediated thyroid cartilage mineralization (Claassen et al. 2006).

The influence of androgens on the hematopoietic system is twice. Through the androgen-dependent, receptor-mediated erythropoietin synthesis, there is robust stimulation of erythrocyte production. Androgens also directly affect the hematopoietic stem cells and lead to increased synthesis of hemoglobin. These effects can also be demonstrated in vitro on the granulopoietic and thrombopoietic stem cells, although the role of androgens in this field is still unclear.

In the central nervous system (CNS), Te can be either aromatized to E2 or reduced to DHT. The individual activities of the different enzymes and distribution of receptors are not homogeneous in the CNS, but rather vary according to the brain region. Recent data show that neural stem/progenitor cells (NSPCs) from the sub-ventricular zone of male and female mice respond to principal sex hormones; therefore circulating estradiol and Te could be prime mediators of sexually dimorphic NSPC regulation (Ransome and Boon 2015). During the intrauterine period, a boy's brain develops in the male direction induced by Te and in a girl in the female direction through its absence. The gender identity, the sexual orientation, and other CNS-controlled behaviors are programmed at this early period of development. Androgens are also important for other male characteristics such as aggressive behavior, initiative, and concentration capacities. A connection with spatial orientation and mathematical and composition skills is still under discussion. There is a close relationship between androgen milieu and normal corporeal and spiritual performance and activity as well as good general mood and self-confidence. The frequency and presence of sexual fantasies, morning erections, frequency of masturbation or copulation, and sexual activity are related to blood Te concentrations in the normal-to-subnormal range. Conversely, androgen deficiency is often accompanied by loss of interest, lethargy, depressive mood, loss of libido, and sexual inactivity. Furthermore in the adult, Te in the brain is neuroprotective and may influence motor neuron regeneration in adulthood (Zitzmann 2006). Reduced Te level is associated with depressive disorders and depends upon the androgen receptor genotype. The role of Te in the CNS is still poorly understood, but evidence suggests that Te could be helpful in the treatment of cognitive diseases, including dementia. Te appears to activate a distributed cortical network and addition of Te may improve spatial cognition in younger and older hypogonadal men (Isidori et al. 2015).

Te plays a key role in *erectile function* through coordinating and facilitating such processes by androgen receptors localized within vascular endothelium and smooth muscle cells. Thus, arterial functions may be directly subject to T influence, and most likely, two independent pathways of T-induced effects within the vessel wall can be assumed (i.e., genomic and non-genomic) (Fig. 9). Androgen sensitivity could be also modulated by a functional polymorphism of the AR that influences the strength of the genomic signal transduced from its interaction with an androgen as a bound ligand. One such functional AR polymorphism is the exon 1 triplet CAG

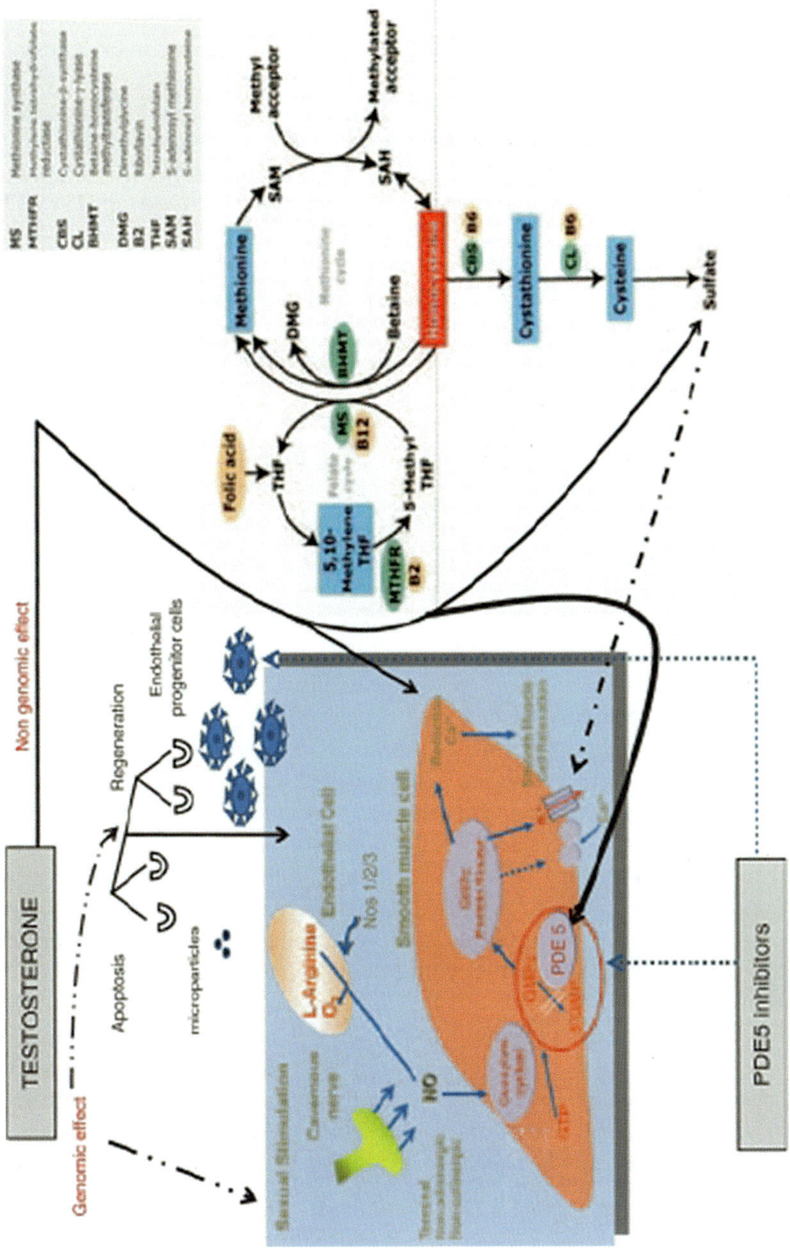

Fig. 9 Genomic and non genomic effects of testosterone on penile endothelial function

(polyglutamine) whereby the repeat length is inversely correlated with androgen sensitivity. Thus, T may directly control the expression and activity of type 5 phosphodiesterases (PDE5) in human corpus cavernosum through the existence of a single androgen-responsive element identified in human PDE5A gene promoter (Francomano et al. 2013b). The effects of androgens on penile tissues in experimental models demonstrated that androgen deprivation induces:

1. Smooth muscle cell degeneration (apoptosis) and adipose tissue deposition with associated fibrosis of corpus cavernosum
2. Reduction in the expression of nitric oxide synthase (eNOS and nNOS) and decrease of arterial
3. Inflow and increase of venous outflow in the corpus cavernosum
4. Enhanced response to mediators of vasoconstriction and smooth muscle contraction such as a-adrenergic agents
5. Decrease of NO-mediated smooth muscle relaxation during sexual stimuli
6. Downregulation of expression of PDE5

Preclinical investigations provided evidence that PDE5i are less effective in androgen-deficient animals and that the re-administration of androgen facilitates PDE5i action, and this was confirmed in humans (Aversa et al. 2015).

Cross Talk Between Testis, Bone Marrow, and Pancreas

Emerging data suggest that bone mass, energy metabolism, and reproduction may be coordinately regulated. Adiponectin has been proposed as a major player with its strong association with impaired glucose tolerance, independently of adiposity. Adiponectin and glucose homeostasis are both regulated by osteocalcin (OSCA), an osteoblast hormone linked to vitamin D metabolism (Lee et al. 2007). Also, the recent animal studies by Oury et al. revealed that the bone is a positive regulator of male fertility and that this action may be mediated through OSCA, via its binding to a specific G-coupled receptor, GPRC6A, present on Leydig cells that favors Te biosynthesis. OSCA-deficient mice show a decrease in testicular, epididymal, and seminal vesicles weights and sperm count, and Leydig cell maturation appears to be halted in the absence of OSCA (Oury et al. 2011). OSCA-stimulated Te biosynthesis is positively regulated by insulin signaling in osteoblasts which in turn stimulates the bioactivation of OSCA. In a feedback loop control, undercarboxylated active OSCA then stimulates insulin secretion by the cells of the pancreatic islets, promotes insulin sensitivity in peripheral organs, and favors Te biosynthesis in Leydig cells of the testis.

Te in turn favors bone growth, maintenance, and maturation (Francomano et al. 2013a). Human data shows an association between visceral fat mass, insulin sensitivity, OSCA, and T levels in humans, which significantly correlate with skeletal health. In this view, OSCA results as an important marker of metabolic and gonadal functionality, other than its well-established function as a marker of bone remodeling (Migliaccio et al. 2013).

Aging

In aging men stochastic damage leads to gradual impairment of the hypothalamic–pituitary–testicular axis, which is manifested as an age-related decrease of total, free, and bioavailable Te. Primary testicular changes, including decreased numbers of LCs, increased deposits of lipofuscin, and disrupted steroidogenesis, reduce Te synthesis and its reserve capacities. Age-associated increases in SHBG serum levels further aggravate decreases in bio-Te and free Te compared to total Te. Although decreased, testicular functional reserve capacity is generally sufficient for adequate GnRH/LH feed-forward signals, which should result in fully compensatory Te secretion. However, inadequate amplitude of GnRH and LH synchronous pulses due to lower numbers and insufficient synchronization of hypothalamic neurons with aging lower testicular Te output and availability. Thus, mild secondary hypogonadism of the hypothalamic–pituitary unit in elderly men results in the inability to compensate for mostly mild primary testicular hypogonadism/hypoandrogenism. This secondary hypogonadism is observed, although there may be reduced Te feedback inhibition, maintained LH secretory capacity of gonadotropins, increased LH metabolic half-life, and increased efficacy of suboptimal effective GnRH pulses. Men >80 years exhibit increasing LH levels, which may also occur in middle-aged men due to the loss of elevated opioid tone (Kaufman and Vermeulen 2005). Te deficiency (TD) is now the preferred terminology by many experts over the traditional term, hypogonadism or late-onset hypogonadism, due to its greater specificity. Whereas hypogonadism refers to inadequate function of the testicles with regard to both Te and sperm production, TD refers only to inadequate Te production. As the large majority of affected men with TD are older and unconcerned with their fertility, the term TD is more appropriate. The Massachusetts Male Aging Study (MMAS) investigated the relationships between age-related transitions in Te and health or lifestyle changes and reported that a 4–5 kg/m2 increase in BMI had a comparable negative impact on Te as 10 years of aging (Travison et al. 2007). MMAS also reported that weight gain was associated with subsequently lower levels of Te than remaining nonobese. In obese diabetic patients, interventional weight loss regimes resulted in increased Te. However, it is not known whether "unsupervised" weight loss in the general population would have a similar impact on Te (Camacho et al. 2013). The diagnosis of TD requires the presence of characteristic symptoms and/or signs together with confirmatory blood tests demonstrating low Te levels (Table 1). It is important to note that individuals with low Te levels may not have any symptoms or signs, and there is no good evidence at this point in time that these men deserve treatment. Conversely, men with suggestive symptoms but with entirely normal Te levels are not considered candidates for treatment.

The clinical diagnosis of TD requires double confirmation via demonstration of low Te levels. The most frequently used test is total Te, and most professional societies and experts recommend this test as their primary biochemical determinant. However, it is critical to note that there is no universally accepted biochemical definition of T deficiency. This is reflected by the different Te thresholds suggested by different society guidelines and expert groups, as well (Table 2). TD is an

Table 1 Sign and symptoms of testosterone deficiency

Sexual symptoms	Non-sexual symptoms	Signs
Low sexual desire (libido)	Decreased energy, vitality, well-being and motivation	Enlarged waist
Erectile dysfunction	Depressed mood, dysthymia, feeling sad or blue	Obesity (increased BMI)
Infrequent morning/nocturnal erection	Poor concentration and memory	Anemia
Difficulty achieving orgasm	Increased sleepiness, fatigue	Reduced testis and prostate volumes
Diminished intensity of the experience of orgasm	Diminished physical or work performance	Reduced muscle bulk and strength
Diminished sexual genital sensation	Hot flushes, sweats	Gynecomastia
	Impaired cognition (“brain fog”)	Reduced beard growth and body hair
		Low bone mineral density

Table 2 Proposed cut-offs for plasma testosterone by different scientific societies

	Total T	Free T (calculated or EqD)
US Endocrine Society 2010 (Boepple et al. 2008; Penning et al. 2000)	<300 ng/dL (<10.4 nmol/L)	<50–90 pg/mL
EAA, ISA, ISSAM 2009 (Vandenput et al. 2007)	<3 50 ng/dL (12.1 nmol/L)	<65 pg/mL (<225 pmol/L)
EAU 2012 Kato et al. (2011)	<3 50 ng/dL (12.1 nmol/L)	< 84 pg/mL (<243 pmol/L)
		80–100 pg/mL
Some experts (Francomano et al. 2013; Tirabassi et al. 2015)	<400 ng/dL (13.9 nmol/L)	1.5 ng/dL (by RIA)

important clinical condition that affects men of all ages. The treatment with Te provides symptom relief for many affected men and improves general health parameters. There is thus great value for the practicing clinician to be aware of the condition and to diagnose and treat it at any age, when present (Aversa and Morgentaler 2015).

Cross-References

▶ Growth Hormones and Aging

References

Amann RP. The cycle of the seminiferous epithelium: a need to revisit? J Androl. 2008;29:469–87.

Aversa A, Morgentaler A. The practical management of testosterone deficiency in men. Nat Rev Urol. 2015;12:641–50.

Aversa A, Francomano D, Lenzi A. Does testosterone supplementation increase PDE5-inhibitor responses in difficult-to-treat erectile dysfunction patients? Expert Opin Pharmacother. 2015;16:625–8.

Basciani S, Mariani S, Spera G, Gnessi L. Role of platelet-derived growth factors in the testis. Endocr Rev. 2010;31:916–39.

Boepple PA, Hayes FJ, Dwyer AA, et al. Relative roles of inhibin B and sex steroids in the negative feedback regulation of follicle-stimulating hormone in men across the full spectrum of seminiferous epithelium function. J Clin Endocrinol Metab. 2008;93:1809–14.

Burger LL, Haisenleder DJ, Dalkin AC, Marshall JC. Regulation of gonadotropin subunit gene transcription. J Mol Endocrinol. 2004;33:559–84.

Camacho EM, Huhtaniemi IT, O'Neill TW, et al. Age-associated changes in hypothalamic–pituitary–testicular function in middle-aged and older men are modified by weight change and lifestyle factors: longitudinal results from the European Male Ageing Study. Eur J Endocrinol. 2013;168:445–55.

Cheng CK, Leung PC. Molecular biology of gonadotropin- releasing hormone (GnRH)-I, GnRH-II, and their receptors in humans. Endocr Rev. 2005;26:283–306.

Chou SH. 20 years of leptin: role of leptin in human reproductive disorders. J Endocrinol. 2014;223: T49–62.

Claassen H, Monig H, Sel S, et al. Androgen receptors and gender-specific distribution of alkaline phosphatase in human thyroid cartilage. Histochem Cell Biol. 2006;126:381–8.

Coviello AD, Matsumoto AM, Bremner WJ, et al. Low-dose human chorionic gonadotropin maintains intratesticular testosterone in normal men with testosterone-induced gonadotropin suppression. J Clin Endocrinol Metab. 2005;90:2595–602.

d'Anglemont de Tassigny X, Fagg LA, et al. Hypogonadotropic hypogonadism in mice lacking a functional Kiss1 gene. Proc Natl Acad Sci U S A. 2007;104:10714–9.

De Roux N, Genin E, Carel JC, et al. Hypogonadotropic hypogonadism due to loss of function of the KiSS1-derived peptide receptor GPR54. Proc Natl Acad Sci U S A. 2003;100:10972–6.

Felici F, Ilenia B, Sgrò P, et al. Acute severe male hypotestosteronemia affects central motor command in humans. J Electrom Kines. 2016. doi:10.1016/j.jelekin.2015.12.004.

Ferlin A, Simonato M, Bartoloni L. The INSL3-LGR8/ GREAT ligand-receptor pair in human cryptorchidism. J Clin Endocrinol Metab. 2003;88:4273–9.

Ferlin A, Garolla A, Rigon F, et al. Changes in serum Insulin-like factor 3 (INSL3) during normal male puberty. J Clin Endocrinol Metab. 2006;91:3426–31.

Ferris HA, Shupnik MA. Mechanisms for pulsatile regulation of the gonadotropin subunit genes by GNRH1. Biol Reprod. 2006;74:993–8.

Foresta C, Bettella A, Vinanzi C, et al. Insulin like factor 3: a novel circulating hormone of testis origin in humans. J Clin Endocrinol Metab. 2004;89:5952–8.

Francomano D, Greco EA, Lenzi A, Aversa A. CAG repeat testing of androgen receptor polymorphism: is this necessary for the best clinical management of hypogonadism? J Sex Med. 2013;10:2373–81.

Ge R, Hardy MP. Regulation of Leydig cells during pubertal development. In: Payne AH, Hardy MP, editors. The Leydig cell in health and disease. Totowa: Humana Press; 2007. p. 55–70.

Grigorova M, Punab M, Ausmees K, Laan M. FSHB promoter polymorphism within evolutionary conserved element is associated with serum FSH level in men. Hum Reprod. 2008;23:2160–6.

Hayes FJ, Crowley Jr WF. Gonadotropin pulsations across development. Horm Res. 1998;49:163–8.

Huhtaniemi I, Jiang M, Nilsson C, Petterson K. Mutations and polymorphisms in gonadotropin genes. Mol Cell Endocrinol. 1999;151:89–94.

Imperato-McGinley J, Zhu YS. Androgens and male physiology the syndrome of 5α-reductase-2 deficiency. Mol Cell Endocrinol. 2002;198(1–2):51–9.

Isidori AM, Balercia G, Calogero AE. Outcomes of androgen replacement therapy in adult male hypogonadism: recommendations from the Italian society of endocrinology. J Endocrinol Invest. 2015;38:103–12.

Kato S, Yokoyama A, Fujiki R. Nuclear receptor coregulators merge transcriptional coregulation with epigenetic regulation. Trends Biochem Sci. 2011;36:272–81.

Kaufman JM, Vermeulen A. The decline of androgen levels in elderly men and its clinical and therapeutic implications. Endocr Rev. 2005;26:833–76.

Kim SH, Hu Y, Cadman S, Bouloux P. Diversity in fibroblast growth factor receptor 1 regulation: learning from the investigation of kallmann syndrome. J Neuroendocrinol. 2008;20: 141–63.

Kumagai J, Hsu SY, Matsumi H, et al. INSL3/Leydig insulin-like peptide activates the LGR8 receptor important in testis descent. J Biol Chem. 2002;277:31283–6.

Laron Z, Klinger B. Effect of insulin-like growth factor on serum androgens and testicular and penile size in males with Laron syndrome (primary growth hormone resistance). Eur J Endocrinol. 1998;138:176–80.

Lee NK, Sowa H, Hinoi E, et al. Endocrine regulation of energy metabolism by the skeleton. Cell. 2007;130:456–69.

Levalle O, Zylbersztein C, Aszpis S, et al. Recombinant human follicle-stimulating hormone administration increases testosterone production in men, possibly by a sertoli cell-secreted non steroid factor. J Clin Endocrinol Metab. 1998;83:3973–6.

Lindstedt G, Nystrom E, Matthews C, et al. Follitropin (FSH) deficiency in an infertile male due to FSHβ gene mutation. Clin Chem Lab Med. 1998;36:663–5.

Lofrano-Porto A, Casulari LA, Nascimento PP, et al. Effects of follicle-stimulating hormone and human chorionic gonadotropin on gonadal steroidogenesis in two sibling with a follicle-stimulating hormone β-subunit mutation. Fertil Steril. 2008;90:1169–74.

Lopez FJ, Merchenthaler IJ, Moretto M, Negro-Vilar A. Modulating mechanisms of neuroendocrine cell activity: the LHRH pulse generator. Cell Mol Neurobiol. 1998;18:125–46.

Matthiesson KL, Stanton PG, O'Donnell L, et al. Effects of testosterone and levonorgestrel combined with a 5α-reductase inhibitor or gonadotropin-releasing hormone antagonist on spermatogenesis and intratesticular steroid levels in normal men. J Clin Endocrinol Metab. 2005;90:5647–55.

Migliaccio S, Francomano D, Bruzziches R, et al. Trunk fat negatively influences skeletal and testicular functions in obese men: clinical implications for the aging male. Int J Endocrinol. 2013. doi:10.1155/2013/182753.Epub2013.

Millar RP, Pawson AJ, Morgan K, et al. Diversity of actions of GnRHs mediated by ligand-induced selective signaling. Front Neuroendocrinol. 2008;29:17–35.

Moyle WR, Campbell RK. Gonadotropins. In: DeGroot JL, Besser M, Burger HG, Jameson LJ, Loriaux DL, Marshall JC, Odell WD, Potts jr JT, Rubenstein AH, editors. Endocrinology. Philadelphia/London: Saunders; 1995. p. 230–41.

Oury F, Sumara G, Sumara O, et al. Endocrine regulation of male fertility by the skeleton. Cell. 2011;144:796–809.

Penning TM, Burczynski ME, Jez JM, et al. Human 3alpha- hydroxysteroid dehydrogenase isoforms of the aldoketo reductase superfamily: functional plasticity and tissue distribution reveals roles in the inactivation and formation of male and female sex hormones. Biochem J. 2000;351:67–77.

Piersma D, Verhoef-Post M, Berns EM, Themmen AP. LH receptor gene mutations and polymorphisms: an overview. Mol Cell Endocrinol. 2007;260–262:282–A286.

Popa SM, Clifton DK, Steiner RA. The role of kisspeptins and GPR54 in the neuroendocrine regulation of reproduction. Annu Rev Physiol. 2008a;70:213–38.

Popa SM, Clifton DK, Steiner RA. The role of kisspeptins and GPR54 in the neuroendocrine regulation of reproduction. Ann Rev Physiol. 2008b;70:213–38.

Prince FP. The human Leydig cell: functional morphology and developmental history. In: Hardy MP, Payne AH, editors. The Leydig cell in health and disease. Totowa: Humana Press; 2007. p. 71–90.

Randall VA, Jenner TJ, Hibberts NA, et al. Stem cell factor/c-Kit signalling in normal and androgenetic alopecia hair follicles. J Endocrinol. 2008;197:11–23.

Ransome M, Boon WC. Testosterone-induced adult neurosphere growth is mediated by sexually-dimorphic aromatase expression. Front Cell Neurosci. 2015;9:253.

Rolf C, Nieschlag E "Senescence". Da "Andrology – Male reproductive health and dysfunction" Cap. 1997;21:397–407.

Selva DM, Bassas L, Munell F, et al. Human sperm sex hormone-binding globulin isoform: characterization and measurement by time-resolved fluorescence immunoassay. J Clin Endocrinol Metab. 2005;90:6275–82.

Seminara SB, Messager S, Chatzidaki EE, et al. The GPR54 gene as a regulator of puberty. N Engl J Med. 2003;349:1614–27.

Simoni M, Casarini L. Mechanisms in endocrinology: genetics of FSH action: a 2014-and-beyond view. Eur J Endocrinol. 2014;170(3):R91–107.

Sriraman V, Anbalagan M, Rao AJ. Hormonal regulation of Leydig cell proliferation and differentiation in rodent testis: a dynamic interplay between gonadotrophins and testicular factors. Reprod BioMed Online. 2005;11:507–18.

Takaimya K, Yamamoto A, Furukawa K, et al. Complex gangliosides are essential in spermatogenesis of mice: possible roles in the transport of testosterone. Proc Natl Acad Sci U S A. 1998;95:12147–52.

Themmen AP, Martens JW, Brunner HG. Activating and inactivating mutations in LH receptor. Mol Cell Endocrinol. 1998;145:137–42.

Tirabassi G, Cignarelli A, Perrini S, et al. Influence of CAG repeat polymorphism on the targets of testosterone action. Int J Endocrinol. 2015;2015:298107.

Tobet SA, Schwarting GA. Recent progress in gonadotropin-releasing hormone neuronal migration. Endocrinology. 2006;147:1159–65.

Travison TG, Araujo AB, Kupelian V, et al. The relative contributions of aging, health, and lifestyle factors to serum testosterone decline in men. J Clin Endocrinol Metab. 2007;92:549–55.

Valimaki VV, Alfthan H, Ivaska KK, et al. Serum estradiol, testosterone, and sex hormone-binding globulin as regulators of peak bone mass and bone turnover rate in young Finnish men. J Clin Endocrinol Metab. 2004;89:3785–9.

Vandenput L, Mellstrom D, Lorentzon M, et al. Androgens and glucuronidated androgen metabolites are associated with metabolic risk factors in men. J Clin Endocrinol Metab. 2007;92:4130–7.

Weinbauer GF, Wessels J. Paracrine control of spermatogenesis. Andrologia. 1999;31:249–62.

Weinbauer GF, Niehaus M, Nieschlag E. The role of testosterone in spermatogenesis. Testosterone: action, deficiency, substitution. Cambridge: Cambridge University Press; 2004. p. 173–206.

Xu Q, Lin HY, Yeh SD, Yu IC, et al. Infertility with defective spermatogenesis and steroidogenesis in male mice lacking androgen receptor in Leydig cells. Endocrine. 2007;32:96–106.

Zhang C, Yeh S, Chen YT, et al. Oligozoospermia with normal fertility in male mice lacking the androgen receptor in testis peritubular myoid cells. Proc Natl Acad Sci U S A. 2006;103:17718–23.

Zitzmann M. Testosterone and the brain. Aging Male. 2006;9:195–9.

Zuccarello D, Ferlin A, Vinanzi C, et al. Detailed functional studies on androgen receptor mild mutations demonstrate their association with male infertility. Clin Endocrinol (Oxf). 2008;68:580–8.

Ovarian Physiology 18

M. O. Verhoeven and C. B. Lambalk

Abstract

This chapter discusses ovarian processes starting in uterine life and subsequently across the following phases: from birth until puberty, the pubertal period itself, then from post puberty until menopause, and finally during menopause and the postmenopausal phase. The ovary has three important functions: first, oocyte and follicle formation and storage; second, oocyte and follicle development resulting in ovulation; and third, reproductive hormone production. The hormone production is inseparable from follicular development. The various processes are described in each of the different phases of life.

Keywords

Androgens • Anti-Müllerian hormone (AMH) • Estrogens • Oocyte • Follicle • Follicle development • Follicle-stimulating hormone (FSH) • Gonadotrophins • Inhibin • Luteinizing hormone (LH) • Ovarian physiology • Ovary • Progesterone

Contents

M.O. Verhoeven (✉) • C.B. Lambalk
Department of Obstetrics and gynecology, VU Medical Center Amsterdam, Amsterdam, The Netherlands
e-mail: m.verhoeven@vumc.nl; cb.lambalk@vumc.nl

A. Belfiore, D. LeRoith (eds.), *Principles of Endocrinology and Hormone Action*, Endocrinology, https://doi.org/10.1007/978-3-319-44675-2_18

Forming the Gonads (Fetal Life)

During intrauterine life the ovary is formed from the gonadal (genital) ridges. The primordial germ cells originating from the yolk sac invade the gonadal ridges from week 6 of development. This journey is performed by amoeboid movement along the dorsal mesentery of the hindgut arriving at the primitive gonads at the beginning of the fifth week and invading them by the sixth week. Different genes and proteins play an important role in this process. If the primordial germ cells fail to reach their goal, the gonads will not develop. When arrived in the gonadal ridges, the primordial germ cells differentiate into oogonia and start to proliferate. The process of mitosis, meiosis, and apoptosis determine the amount of oogonia. By the sixth to seventh week, the number of oogonia is approximately 10,000 with the highest number around 20 weeks of gestation of approximately six to seven million. At this point, the process of apoptosis of oogonia will be dominant, and the amount will fall to 700,000–1,000,000 at birth.

The oogonia enter the prophase of first meiosis forming the primary oocytes. This process starts at 8th–13th weeks/at about 15 weeks of fetal life. Retinoic acid produced in the fetal ovary and mesonephros plays a role in this process protecting the oogonia against programmed apoptosis. Oogonia that did not enter the prophase of the first meiosis after 7 months of gestation undergo apoptosis. The surface epithelial cells proliferate and invade the mesenchyme surrounding the primary oocyte with a single layer forming primordial granulosa cells (also called follicular cells). The primary oocyte and granulosa cells develop a close interaction by gap junctions through which intensive signaling between these cells can take place. The granulosa cells prevent the primary oocytes from continuing the process of first meiosis until the follicle enters ovulation. Then ovulation will disrupt gap junctions allowing the oocyte to enter the final stage of the first meiosis. The primary oocyte and single layer granulosa cells together form the primordial follicle.

The follicles formed in the fetal stage can show abnormalities which are not found after birth anymore. The granulosa surrounding the oocyte can configure tails instead of a regular circle (Peters et al. 1978). Follicles can contain more than one oocyte and the theca layer can be hyper- or hypotrophic. It seems that the follicle selection is targeting to keep the most healthy follicles in the resting pool since these abnormalities are not seen after birth.

Gonadotrophin-releasing hormone (GnRH) is present in the hypothalamus at 9 weeks of gestation, and its storage increases until approximately 20 weeks. Also the concentrations of luteinizing hormone (LH) and follicle-stimulating hormone (FSH) in the pituitary increase during fetal life and stabilize from 20 weeks onward being detectable from the third month of gestational age and reaching a maximum level around fifth to seventh month of gestation. Thereafter, circulatory LH and FSH plasma serum concentrations decrease until lower levels around term. LH and FSH do not influence mitosis of the oogonia or the progression of the oocyte until the diplotene stage of the meiosis and formation of primordial follicles in fetal life (Baker and Scrimgeour 1980).

Prepubertal Silence (Birth Until Puberty)

In this phase of life, the decline of the follicle pool continues. During this phase, there is a continuous development of follicles until the pre-antral stage (1 mm, no formation of lumen). Some follicles may develop slightly further, but in the end, all maturing follicles become atretic (Anderson et al. 2014).

Compared to pubertal ovaries, prepubertal ovaries contain a higher proportion of abnormal nongrowing follicles characterized by indistinct germinal vesicle membrane and absent nucleolus. It is possible that these follicles will be recruited to grow but ending eventually in apoptosis since these abnormalities are not seen in adult ovaries (Anderson et al. 2014).

Immediately after birth, an active GnRH system is triggering pulsatile pituitary LH and FSH secretion causing a mini puberty in the neonate. This pulsatile LH and FSH secretion lasts longer in girls than in boys. But after some time, GnRH secretion reduces and the period of prepubertal silence follows. Consequently, LH and FSH levels in prepubertal girls are extremely low (Fig. 1) (Apter et al. 1989). This is why follicle development at this age will not complete beyond the antral follicle stage. In cord blood taken immediately after birth, high concentrations of estradiol and estriol are found. Estradiol concentrations decrease rapidly after birth. Both estradiol and estriol originate from mother or placenta and not from ovaries of the newborn infant self (Kuijper et al. 2013). During the mini puberty, larger follicles are found then after prepubertal silencing (Kuiri-Hanninen et al. 2013; Kuiri-Hanninen et al. 2011). This mini puberty goes together with a transient increase in anti-Müllerian hormone (AMH), inhibin B, and estrogen concentrations (Andersen et al. 2010; Hagen et al. 2010; Kuiri-Hanninen et al. 2011). Each of these hormones will be in more detail discussed later.

The prepubertal period is characterized by a very low FSH tone which is not necessary for the initial follicular recruitment which does take place prepubertally (Durlinger et al. 2001; Kumar et al. 1997). It has been shown that these early stage developing follicles from the primary until early antral stage in an FSH absent surrounding show more abnormalities (Halpin et al. 1986; McGee et al. 1997) explaining why more oocyte abnormalities are seen in fetal and prepubertal stage compared with later life phases.

AMH concentrations are stably low in an individual prepubertal girl, but prior to the onset of puberty until the onset of puberty, a subtle rise in AMH is observed

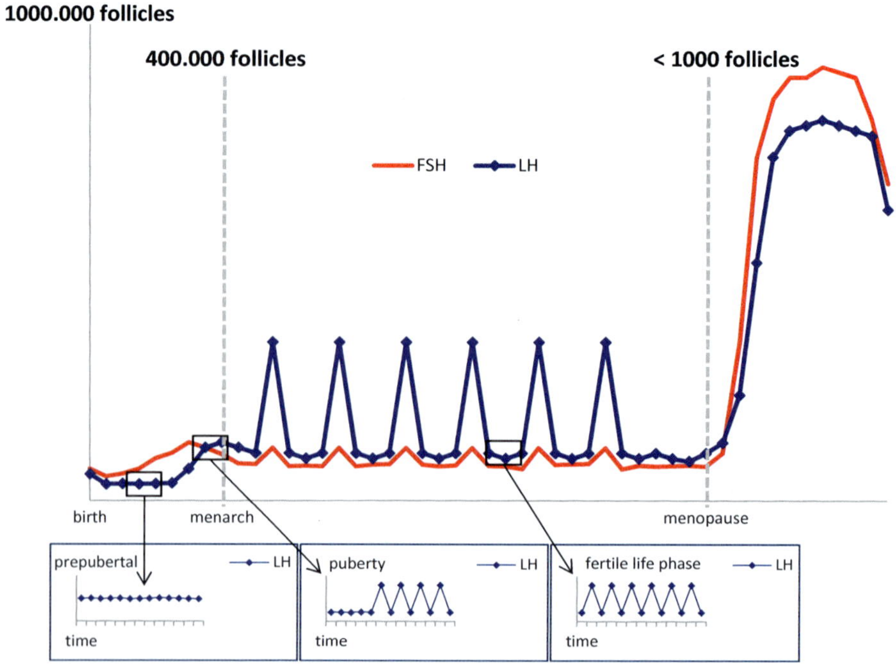

Fig. 1 Schematic graph of gonadotrophins throughout life. Graphical representation of concentrations of follicle stimulating hormone (*FSH*) and luteinizing hormone (*LH*), throughout the life of a women (After Naftolin et al. 1974)

and followed by a small decline after the onset of puberty (Hagen et al. 2012a, b; Lashen et al. 2013). Inhibin B and estrogen concentrations are low in prepubertal girls as well.

During childhood the ovary becomes larger and heavier by growing of the stroma and of the amount of larger antral follicles. It should be noted that the process of follicle maturation until the antral stage is already present in older children. However, these follicles become atretic at any time during the various developmental phases. The presence of large antral follicles increases with age, but they never reach the preovulatory stage yet.

Starting to Work (Puberty)

The definition of puberty is the period during which physical changes appear resulting in being able to procreate. The onset of puberty is independent from the gonads. However, they play an important role in endocrinal changes during puberty resulting in physical changes. Two systems are responsible for the endocrinal changes; first the hypothalamic, pituitary, and gonadal axis and second the adrenal gland (adrenarche).

Puberty starts with an increase in pulsatile GnRH release by the hypothalamus both elevated in pulse frequency and amplitude. The pituitary is stimulated by GnRH and is becoming more sensitive for it resulting in increasing concentrations of LH, FSH, and finally estradiol (Apter et al. 1989; Dickerman et al. 1976). This results first in a nocturnal LH pulse release and secretion of FSH (Fig. 1) followed by increased estrogen concentrations in the early morning. This elevation in estrogen concentration is responsible for the start of breast development (thelarche).

After puberty the development of the antral follicles until the preovulatory phase occurs in monthly cohorts controlled by gonadotrophins. The follicles can continue to develop to Graafian preovulatory size and are able to ovulate, thereby releasing the oocyte with conversion of remaining follicle structure into the corpus luteum that starts to produce progesterone in large quantities. With no fertilization and pregnancy, the endometrium breaks down, and the menstruation will take place.

The first vaginal bleeding a girl experiences is referred to as menarche. The first year after menarche, 55% of the cycles are anovulatory, and the bloodshed is more the result of imbalanced estrogenic endometrial stimulation (Fraser and Baird 1972). This is the result of the immature collaboration of the hypothalamus, pituitary, and ovaries with as a consequence an absent positive feedback response to estrogens which is necessary to induce ovulation (Fraser Michie et al. 1973; Sizonenko 1978; Winter and Faiman 1973).

Less follicles in pubertal ovaries will be morphologically and functionally abnormal than in the prepubertal ovary (Anderson et al. 2014). The maturing follicles produce androgens, estrogens, and after ovulation progesterone. As already mentioned briefly, these endocrinological changes will be responsible for initiating physical changes during puberty development. Estrogens among others cause further growth of the labia minora, increase the size of the uterus, and control thelarche. Androgens are among others responsible for pubarche, body odor, and acne. Progesterone is responsible for among others coloring of the areola of the mamma and mamma development. Despite the fact that adrenarche precedes puberty, thelarche but not pubarche is usually the first sign of the start of puberty in girls (Mouritsen et al. 2013).

The adrenarche is the start of the production of the androgen dehydroepiandrosterone sulfate (DHEAS) and androstenedione in the reticular zone of the adrenal gland. This process starts several years before puberty but is closely linked in timing to the onset of puberty. However, both processes take place independently from each other. In the absence of adrenarche, puberty starts on a normal age, and patients with gonadal deficiency will develop a normal adrenarche. The adrenergic androgen production is supported by ovarian androgen production during and after puberty.

Fertile Life Phase (Menarche Until Menopause)

Follicles are the functional units of the ovary and are responsible for hormone production and the development and potential release of fertile oocytes. At the onset of puberty, 400,000 follicles are left, and only 400–500 follicles will end in ovulation which is less than 1%. The various developmental phases of follicles are illustrated in Fig. 2. At any time frame, the ovary consists of follicles in various developmental phases. The dominant follicle develops each cycle and is not present in the beginning of the cycle and after ovulation. The functional corpus luteum is only present in the luteal phase. The various types of follicles present in the ovary are the primordial follicle (resting follicle), the primary follicle (pre-antral follicle), the secondary follicle (pre-antral follicle), the tertiary follicle (the nondominant small antral follicle), the dominant tertiary follicle (large antral follicle), and finally the mature tertiary follicle (Graafian follicle) (Fig. 2). After ovulation, the remains of the follicle are composed by granulosa and theca cells developing into corpus luteum.

It seems that the process of follicle development is designed to allow the healthiest oocyte to develop to the final stage ending in ovulation. By communication with its environment via paracrine signaling, the oocyte doing this most effectively survives. The earlier follicle phases are controlled by paracrine and autocrine regulation mechanisms. Both inhibiting and activating pathways are suggested to play a role in this early follicular development. The late follicle developmental phases are controlled by an endocrine system with a dominant role of the gonadotrophins. However, FSH is also associated with follicular development in pre-antral follicles: earlier pre-antral follicles are gonadotrophin sensitive but not dependent, while the late antral/preovulatory follicles are gonadotrophin dependent. Early follicle development improves in the presence of FSH but is also present in absent FSH conditions, whereas under these circumstances, late follicle development will not take place (Arendsen de Wolff-Exalto 1982; Durlinger et al. 2001; Halpin et al. 1986; Kumar et al. 1997; McGee et al. 1997). This phenomenon is also referred to as earlier follicle development being FSH sensitive (can do without FSH) and late follicle development being FSH dependent (cannot do without FSH) (Dewailly et al. 2016).

Primordial Follicle Activation

The resting phase is the primordial follicle which consist of an oocyte and flattened granulocytes (Fig. 2). While the primordial follicle is usually referred to as the resting phase of the follicle, it has been demonstrated that the oocyte in these follicles is metabolically active and transcribes genes responsible for follicle growth (Gallardo et al. 2007). This suggests that there are inhibiting factors preventing the oocyte from further maturing and keeping the follicle in a dormant phase. What factors initiate primordial follicles to develop into the growing pool remains largely unclear. Some factors are identified that play a role in this activation such as Kit ligand, neurotrophins, vascular endothelial growth factor, BMP 4, BMP 7, leukemia inhibitory factor, basic fibroblast growth factor, and keratinocyte growth factor. It seems that there is an overkill of factors present that could activate primordial follicles but being actively attenuated. What the physiological proportions between the various factors is for optimal selection of a certain amount of healthy primordial follicles is still not completely elucidated. It is also unclear why certain primordial

	Timing of presence	Hormonal product	Follicle diameter (oocyte diameter)	Configuration
primordial germ cells	Fetal			
oogonia	Fetal		(32 μm)	
primordial follicle	fetal, pre-menarche, fertile phase, postmenopausal		35 μm (32 μm)	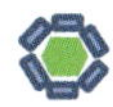
paracrine and autocrine regulated phase FSH sensitive			**primordial → primary follicle: 150 days primary → secundary follicle: 120 days**	
primary or pre-antral stage follicle	fetal, pre-menarche, fertile phase, postmenopausal	AMH	46 μm (32 μm)	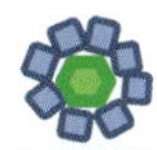
secondary, or pre-antral follicle	fetal, pre-menarche, fertile phase, postmenopausal	AMH androgens estrogens progesterone	60-120 μm (80 μm)	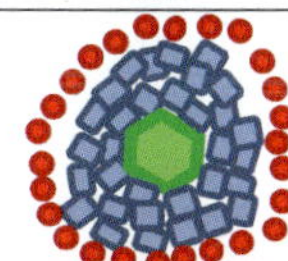
gonadotrophin dependent (cyclic) FSH dependent			**secondary → tertiary follicle: 80 days dominance sellection: 10 days**	
tertiary or antral follicle dominance selection	fetal, pre-menarche, fertile phase, postmenopausal	inhibin B androgens estrogens progesterone	2-10 mm (80 μm)	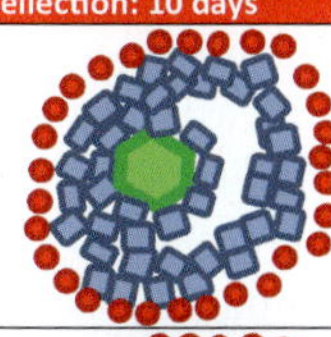
tertiary or antral follicle, dominant follicle	fetal, pre-menarche, fertile phase, postmenopausal	inhibin B androgens estrogens progesterone	10-17 mm (80 μm)	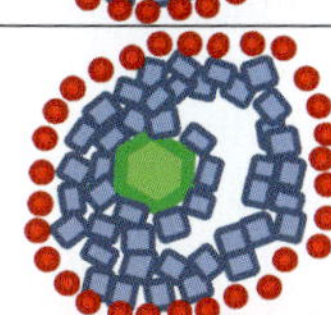
gonadotrophin dependent (cyclic) LH regulated phase			**dominant → Graafian follicle: 14 days**	
mature tertiary or Graafian follicle	fertile phase	inhibin A androgens estrogens progesterone	18-25 mm (80 μm)	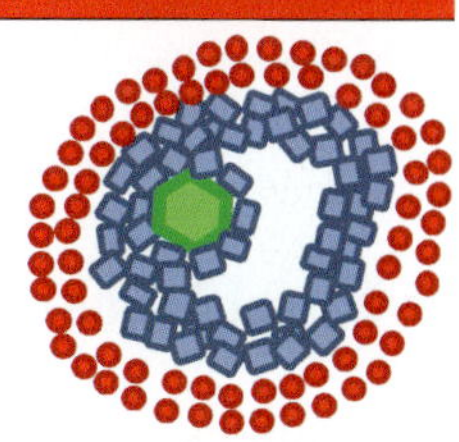
corpus luteum	fertile phase	inhibin A androgens estrogens progesterone		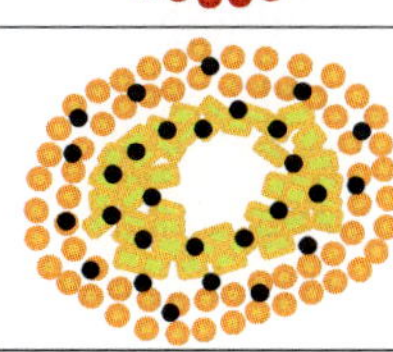

= oocyte, = zona pellucida, = flattened granulosa cell, = cubical granulosa cell, = theca cell, = luteinized granulosa cell, = luteinized theca cell, ● = T-lymphocyte / macrophages.

Fig. 2 Follicular development

follicles are selected over others. There are three pathways identified as important in the recruiting of primordial follicles into the growing pool.

The first pathway being activated by the earlier mentioned different factors starts with the tyrosine kinase receptor (RTK) (Adhikari and Liu 2009). RTK is a cell surface receptor with an extracellular, a transmembrane, and an intracellular domain. When activated a cascade of downstream processes takes place regulating numerous cellular processes. Some of the earlier mentioned activation factors like, for example, Kit ligand, is able to activate RTK with the consequence that the inhibition of the primordial follicle development is broken and the dormant follicle becomes activated (Tarnawa et al. 2013). In mice deficient of one of the factors in the RTK cascades results in enlarged follicle recruitment resulting in immature ovarian insufficiency (Castrillon et al. 2003; Reddy et al. 2008).

The second pathway important for primordial follicle dormancy is suppression of rapamycin (mTOR) that regulates cell growth and proliferation. Both RTK and mTOR pathways are important for preserving the fertile life phase in women by inhibiting follicle activation (Adhikari and Liu 2010). Besides the role in primordial follicles, mTOR plays an important role in granulosa cell growth in antral follicles (Huang et al. 2013).

The third pathway important for attenuation in follicle development is the Hippo signaling pathway. This pathway plays an important role in organ size and management of tumor growth when disrupted (Halder and Johnson 2011; Hergovich and Hemmings 2012; Zhao et al. 2011). It contains a growth-inhibiting action when active. Tissue damage will interrupt the Hippo signaling pathway resulting in tissue proliferation. Both ovarian drilling and transplanted ovarian cortex fragments are followed by follicle growth (Donnez et al. 2011; Farquhar et al. 2012). In both situations, the ovarian tissue is damaged. Moreover, in human ovaries, important genes of the Hippo pathway are found to be expressed in follicles at different developmental phases suggesting a role in follicular development (Hsueh et al. 2015; Kawamura et al. 2013). It is suggested that ovulation disrupts the ovarian surface and therefore interrupts the Hippo signaling pathway allowing follicles to develop further (Hsueh et al. 2015).

The Pre-antral Primary and Secondary Follicle

When the primordial follicle is recruited into the growing pool, the granulosa cells start to change. They will form one cuboid layer granulosa cells (early primary follicle). The granulosa cells proliferate resulting in a mature primary follicle with a stratified layer of granulosa cells and a zona pellucida surrounding the oocyte (Fig. 2). They start to produce substances for the zona pellucida together with the oocyte. The maturing phase from primordial follicle to mature primary follicle takes 150 days. From primary to secondary follicle, the granulosa cell layers increase, and theca cell layers are formed around the granulosa cell layers and the follicle matures. Theca cells are found around follicles with two or more granulosa cell layers (Young and McNeilly 2010). The change from primary to secondary phase takes 120 days. From primordial follicle until secondary follicle takes in total nine menstrual cycles. The fate of a follicle is determined by endocrine, paracrine, and autocrine factors. Despite the fact that several follicles share the same morphological appearance, their hormonal activity and development could be completely different determining their fate. While many follicles start to ripe in a growing pool, in physiological circumstances, most follicles will end in atresia/apoptosis (Gougeon and Testart 1986).

The various genes expressed in follicles in the apparently same developmental phase may explain the variation in developmental course and life span of follicles in one growing cohort (Gougeon 1996). It is suggested that larger follicles use the Hippo signaling pathway to suppress maturation of neighboring follicles of less advantageous stages. It should be noted that during ovulation, the epithelial surface of the ovary is disrupted, and the Hippo signaling pathway is interrupted allowing follicles of lower developmental stage to develop further (Hsueh et al. 2015).

In the pre-antral phase, cell layers are formed around the granulosa cells, the theca interna, and the theca externa. LH stimulates theca cell differentiation and androgens production by theca cells (Figs. 3 and 4). The close connection between the theca cells and granulosa cells facilitates collaboration of these two cell groups. Androgens are transferred to the granulosa cells where they are converted into estrogens by aromatase under the influence of FSH. This typical two cell principle interplay is graphically shown in Figs. 3 and 4. This means that follicles without a theca layer are not able to produce estrogens. Follicles are able to grow in an LH-deprived condition, while no estrogens are produced in the absence of its precursor androgens not being synthesized in the theca cells.

The Antral Tertiary and Preovulatory (Graafian)Follicle

The period after puberty is characterized by cyclic activity governed by pituitary gonadotrophin stimulation and ovarian hormonal feedback in comparison to fetal life and childhood (Fig. 1). Whereas the follicles in the fetal, childhood, and postmenopausal phase develop until pre-antral follicle stage and become apoptotic thereafter, FSH is responsible for follicles developing beyond and that selected follicles reaching preovulatory status. The main action of FSH is protecting follicles from apoptosis. The follicles are now able to develop into and beyond late secondary or antral follicle stage into the mature tertiary follicle or Graafian follicle (Figs. 2 and 3). After the follicle has formed a fluid compartment (the antrum), it is referred to as an antral follicle. The maturing process of a follicle from a secondary follicle into a tertiary follicle takes 81 days. This last phase from tertiary follicle until Graafian follicle is gonadotrophin dependent. This last phase takes 14 days and it determines the menstrual cycle.

When the antrum develops, the oocyte lies eccentric in the follicle. The granulosa cells closely related to the oocyte are called cumulus cells. The granulosa cells in contact with the follicle fluid are the antral cells, and the granulosa cells at the outside in contact with the theca cells are the mural cells (Fig. 3).

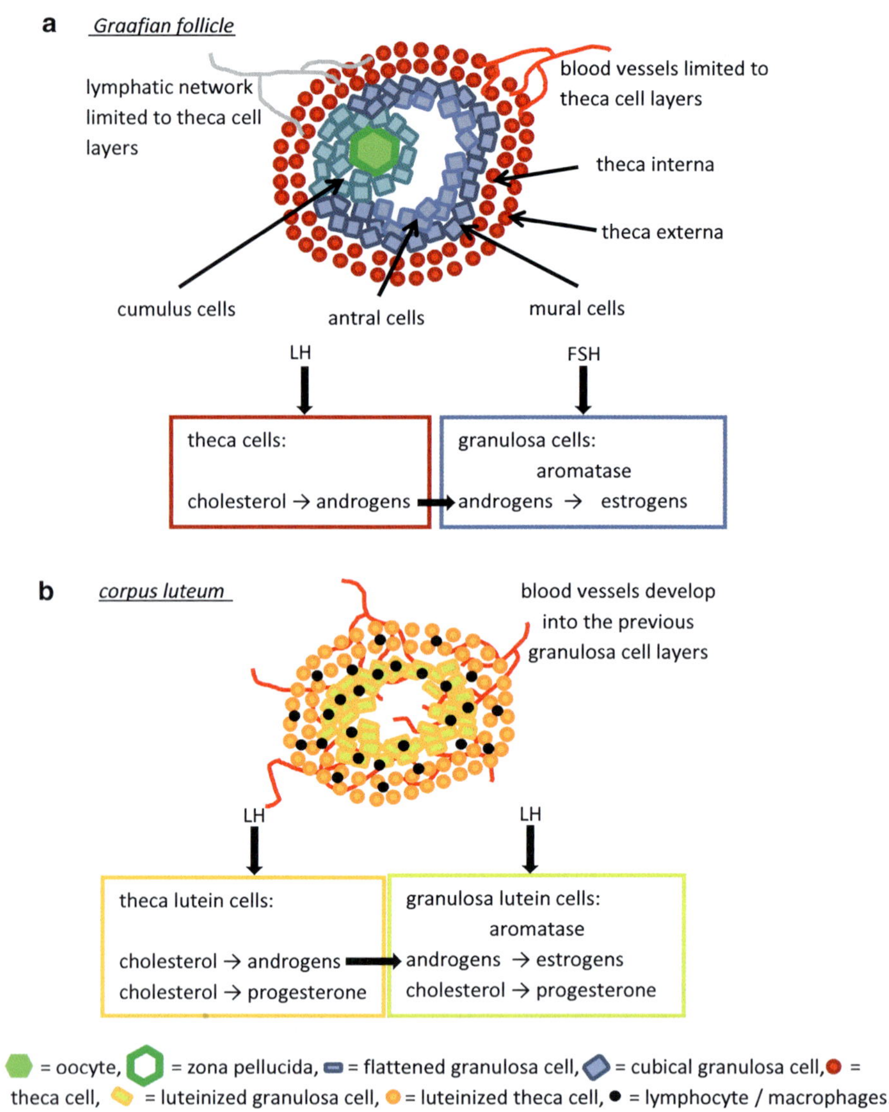

Fig. 3 Two cell two gonadotrophin system

Interaction Between Oocyte and Granulosa Cells

There is a close interaction between the oocyte and first layer of granulosa cells by gap junctions. This interaction is important for the growth of the follicle beyond pre-antral stage and for inhibiting the completion of the first meiotic division of the oocyte until ovulation. Furthermore, this interaction protects the oocyte from apoptosis and prevents the granulosa cells to change into lutein cells. Just like between

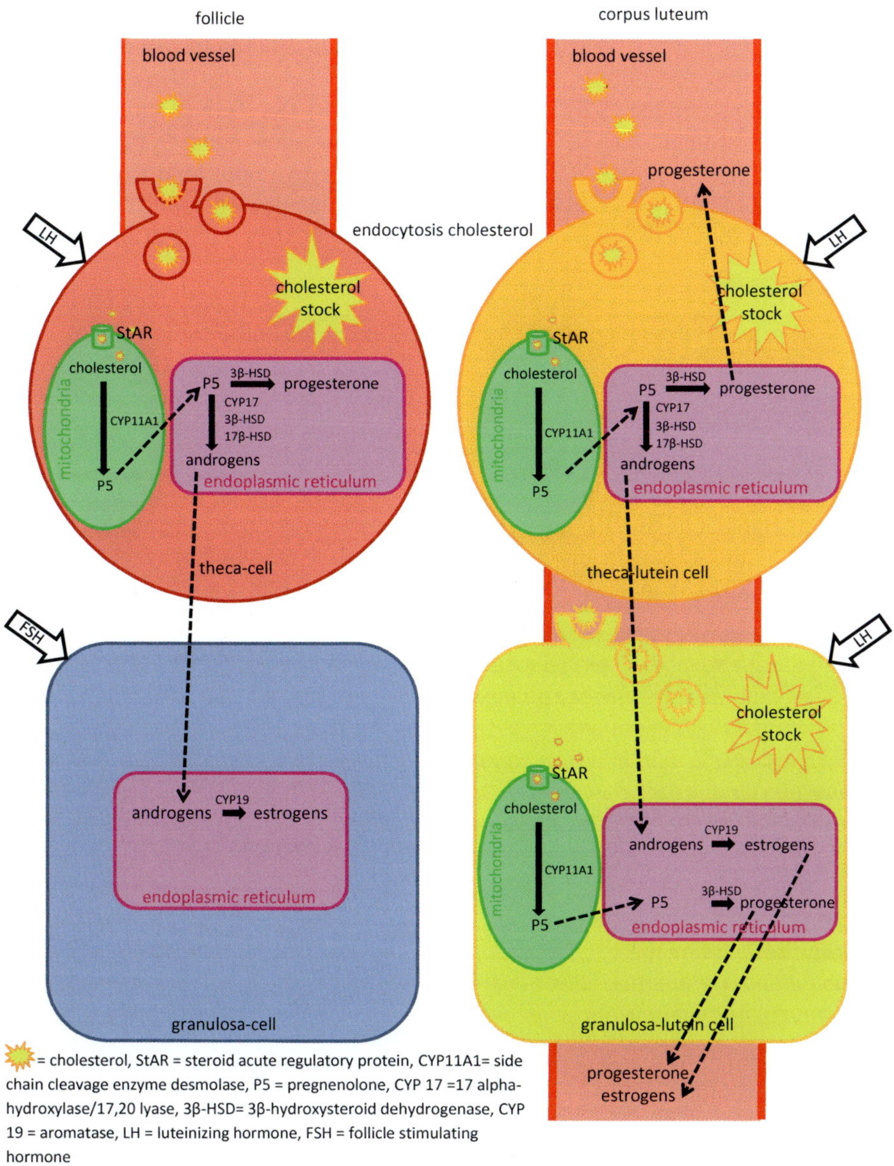

Fig. 4 Steroidogenesis

the oocyte and first row of granulosa cells, there are gap junctions present among granulosa cells. They play an important role in the viability and normal development of the oocyte.

The oocyte excretes a number of factors influencing its surrounding and regulating its survival among which R-spondin2 proteins being exclusively expressed in the oocyte of primary and larger follicles. R-spondin2 together with wingless (WNT) ligands stimulates WNT signaling pathway. R-spondin2 promotes primary follicle development into a secondary or pre-antral follicle (Cheng et al. 2013).

Other factors produced by the oocyte belong to the TGF-β superfamily of cysteine-knot proteins like activin, growth differentiation factor-9 (GDF9), and bone morphogenetic protein-15 (BMP15). The latter two both bind to the type II receptor serine kinase BMP receptor resulting in stimulation of downstream signaling enhancing follicle development (Juengel et al. 2004; Mazerbourg et al. 2004; Vitt et al. 2002).

GDF9 has an effect on both theca and granulosa cells. It promotes primordial follicle development into a primary follicle and small pre-antral follicle (Dong et al. 1996; Vitt et al. 2000). During later antral follicle development, GDF9 prevents apoptosis of the follicle (Orisaka et al. 2006). GDF9 prevents granulosa cells form luteinizing. Furthermore, it promotes theca cell proliferation and androgen production (Solovyeva et al. 2000; Spicer et al. 2008).

BMP15 promotes granulosa cell proliferation (Otsuka et al. 2000). In different species, mutations in BMP15 genes can increase ovulation rate, whereas others are associated with ovarian insufficiency (Davis et al. 1992; Galloway et al. 2000; Persani et al. 2014; Yan et al. 2001).

Hormone Production

Estradiol (Fig. 4)

One of the key functions of the ovary is the hormone production of androgens, estrogens, and progesterone (Fig. 4). The production of hormone is inseparably linked to follicle development. Granulosa cells and theca cells are the main producers of these hormones (Fig. 4).

The precursor of steroids is cholesterol. To obtain cholesterol, the cell can produce it de novo by 3-hydroxy-3methyl-glutaryl-CoA (HMG-CoA). However, this will not be the main source for steroidogenesis since HMG-CoA is in low concentrations present in theca cells (Gwynne and Strauss 1982). The main source of cholesterol will be endocytosis of low-density lipoprotein and maintain an esterified cholesterol store. It is possible that high-density lipoproteins are taken up by the cell as well as providing an extra source. Stimulated by gonadotrophins, cholesterol is taken up by the mitochondria. The steroid acute regulatory protein (StAR) plays an important role in this transportation from outside into the mitochondria (Fig. 4). The presence or absence of StAR is the rate-limited step in steroidogenesis (Stocco and Clark 1996; Strauss et al. 1999).

Inside the mitochondria, side-chain cleavage enzyme desmolase (CYP11A1) facilitates the change of cholesterol in pregnenolone (P5). In the smooth endoplasmic reticulum, 17α-hydroxylase/17,20 lyase (CYP17) and 3β-hydroxysteroid dehydrogenase (3β-HSD) convert P5 to DHEAS and androstenedione. Androstenedione can be turned into testosterone by 17β-HSD and into estrogens by aromatase (CYP19). Granulosa cells do not contain CYP17 and 3β-HSD and therefore are not able to produce androgens. They are supplied by androgens of their neighboring theca cells.

Androgens increase FSH receptor expression in granulosa cells (Shiina et al. 2006). Androgens are essential in follicular development (Hu et al. 2004; Shiina et al. 2006). Both FSH and androgens stimulate aromatase expression in mural granulosa cells and therefore estrogen production. During the maturation of the follicle, the importance of FSH declines and LH takes over. LH closes the gap junctions between granulosa cells and between the granulosa cumulus cells and oocyte.

Inhibins

Inhibins are heterodimeric peptides belonging to the TGF family. In the ovary, inhibin B is produced by the granulosa cells in the follicular phase, and inhibin A is produced in the luteal phase. Both under influence of FSH selectively suppress pituitary FSH secretion and act albeit as an important feedback factor (Hall et al. 1999).

AMH

AMH is produced by granulosa cells of pre-antral and small antral follicles and not by primordial follicles. When the diameter of the (pre)-antral follicle expands, the intrafollicular AMH concentration declines (Andersen et al. 2010). From the resting pool, a number of primordial follicles are selected and start to develop into primary or pre-antral follicles. At this stage, AMH plays a key role. It is thought that AMH reduces the number of follicles recruited from the resting pool by preventing primordial follicle to develop into primary follicles (Broekmans et al. 2008). By doing so, it prevents unnecessary follicle loss during the subsequent phase that leads to one single dominant follicle, and the others become atretic. The larger the originally recruited pool, the higher the number of follicles that will end up atretic. This process is independent from the stage of life and is not influenced by pregnancies, lactation, or oral contraceptive use.

While in early follicular development androgens and AMH play a more important role, FSH and estrogens take over in late follicular development (Dewailly et al. 2016). AMH is produced in primary follicles as soon as they are recruited in the growing pool. The AMH production is the highest in pre-antral follicles when the estrogens production is absent. The role of FSH in this stage seems less important, however, not insignificant (Arendsen de Wolff-Exalto 1982). It is postulated that FSH increases AMH concentrations based on studies that in FSH-deprived conditions, AMH is decreased compared to when FSH is normal (Chan and Liu 2014; Hagen et al. 2012). The opposite has been described as well (La et al. 2004; Weintraub et al. 2014). Furthermore, AMH reduces the sensitivity of pre-antral follicles for FSH (Durlinger et al. 2001). Pre-antral follicles will produce androgens when the theca cells are formed. These androgens will enhance FSH action by increasing FSH receptor expression. Both FSH and androgens increase estrogen production. Estrogens will inhibit AMH production making the follicle more FSH sensitive.

Cyclic Hormone Secretion

The first day of the cycle is defined as the first day of vaginal bleeding resulting from shedding of the endometrium that builds the previous cycle since no pregnancy was conceived. Estradiol, progesterone, and inhibin concentrations are low. The ovarian negative feedback is minimal resulting in a raised pituitary secretion of FSH (Fig. 5). FSH stimulates granulosa cell mitosis and aromatase activity and inhibin and LH receptor production. The aromatase activity is needed for the transformation of androgens into estrogens. The FSH stimulates inhibin B which in turn suppresses FSH. Furthermore, FSH increases gap junction formation in the dominant follicle increasing the contact between the oocyte and cumulus cells.

The concentration of FSH determines the amount of follicles that potentially develop into a Graafian follicle. When the recruited follicle will develop, the production of inhibin B will increase. This will lower FSH secretion by the pituitary resulting in mono-follicular growth of the most FSH-sensitive follicle. A follicle reaching dominance suppresses FSH sensitivity of other growing follicles by unknown mechanisms. The communication of the oocyte with its environment via paracrine signaling will probably play an important role. The oocyte communicating most effectively with its surrounding will have the highest chance of survival. It is hypothesized that inhibin B plays an

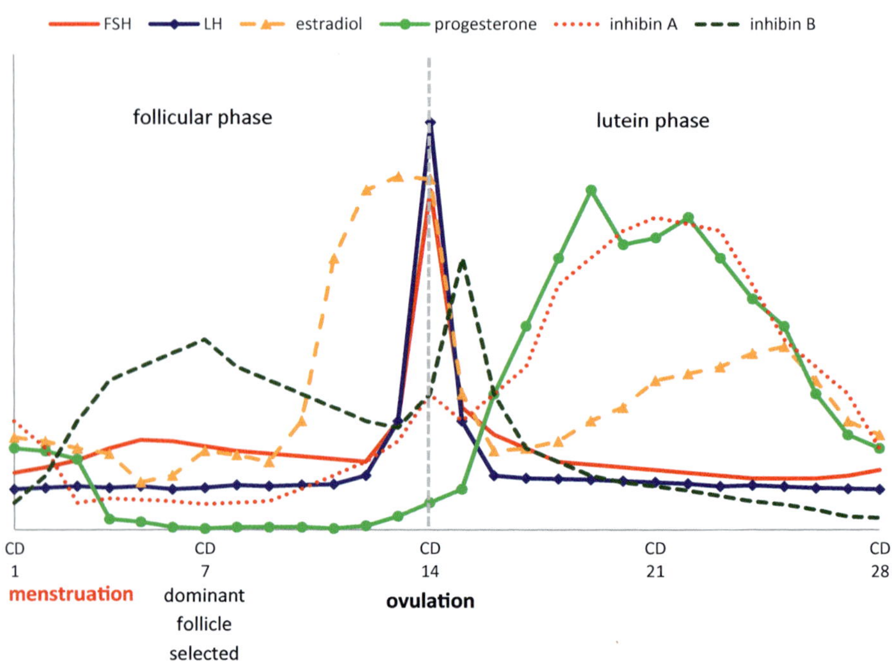

Fig. 5 Schematic graph of hormone levels throughout reproductive cycle. Plasma concentrations of follicle stimulating hormone (*FSH*), luteinizing hormone (*LH*), estradiol, progesterone, inhibin A and inhibin B throughout the menstrual cycle in ovulating women. After Groome et al. (1996 #109)

important role in this selection. The diameter of the follicle in this stage is 10–12 mm. While the estrogen concentrations start to increase a few days later, FSH concentrations start to decline simultaneously with inhibin B concentration increase (Fig. 5). It is suggested that inhibin B is a more prominent FSH inhibitor than estrogens. This signaling that has to be blood born in order to reach the other ovary. By maintaining and raising FSH levels as within ovarian hyperstimulation protocols in assisted reproductive technique will not enlarge the recruited pool but will protect follicles from apoptosis and enables more follicle than one to develop into a Graafian follicle.

Ovulation

Ovulation completes successful follicle development. This is the process of releasing the oocyte granulosa cumulus cells from the follicle and the granulosa cells (antral and mural), and theca cells left behind will luteinize and form the corpus luteum. Ovulation is put in motion by the LH surge. The interval between the start of the LH surge and ovulation is 36–42 h. Factors and processes leading to LH surge are not completely understood. While low estrogen and progesterone levels have an inhibitory effect on LH secretion, the increase in estrogens and subtle end follicular phase progesterone increase enormously enhance pituitary sensitivity of GnRH resulting in LH surge. Here, progesterone is an important cofactor next to the estrogen levels. Progesterone is produced in low quantities in follicular phase under the influence of LH in theca cells (Micevych and Sinchak 2011). So, the key feature of the timing of the mid-cycle LH surge is the progressive increase of pituitary sensitivity to GnRH triggered by positive feedback signals from the ovary that the follicle has reached ovulatory status. The LH surge is accompanied by an FSH surge. The function of this FSH surge is not clarified yet (Fig. 5).

Is there a hypothalamic neuropeptide surge at time of ovulation? Kisspeptin has been identified as important neuropeptide in the regulation of GnRH (Millar et al. 2010; Pineda et al. 2010). It increases the concentration of LH secretion via GnRH stimulation and in many species regulates a GnRH surge followed by the LH surge. However, this is uncertain in humans. It should be noted that women with hypogonadotropic anovulation treated with pulsatile GnRH do not need an increase in GnRH dosage or pulse frequency to enable ovulation.

The LH surge has several important effects. It closes the gap junction between the oocyte and the granulose cumulus cells. High concentrations of cyclic adenosine (cAMP) in the oocyte are important for inhibiting meiosis. The LH surge reduces cAMP levels resulting in resumption and completion of the first meiosis of the oocyte that started in fetal life. This timing is important in order to have a fertilizable oocyte at the moment of release.

Furthermore, the LH surge induces release of proteolytic factors that cause follicular rupture. The process of release of the oocyte cumulus cell complex takes 2–5 min. Inflammatory cells and proteolytic factors weaken the epithelial surface over the follicle. Increased blood flow and edema provide the intrafollicular pressure for the oocyte cumulus complex to leave the follicle.

Corpus Luteum

Besides luteinized granulosa and theca cells, the corpus luteum consists of endothelial, immune, and fibroblast cells (Retamales et al. 1994). It is a transient endocrine gland producing estrogens, inhibin A, and particularly progesterone.

Straight after the LH surge, progesterone strongly increases. This increase is on account of the theca cells in which the enzymatic system for progesterone production (StAR, CYP11A1, and 3βHSD) is already present at the time of the LH surge. The LH surge increases StAR expression in luteal granulosa cells together with the forming of the rest of the enzymatic system. Together with the vascularization of the complete corpus luteum, it enables the luteal granulosa cells to produce progesterone as well (Figs. 4 and 5). In the end, the luteal theca cells remain to be the most important producer of androgens which are aromatized producing estrogens in the luteal granulosa cells. So the two cell system for estrogen production remains after corpus luteum formation (Fig. 3). However, both the luteal theca cell and the luteal granulosa cell are stimulated by LH.

LH is crucial for the development of the corpus luteum and its maintenance. However, LH does not prevent corpus luteum demise. If no pregnancy is conceived in the cycle, the corpus luteum undergoes luteolysis in the absence of placental chorionic gonadotrophin (HCG) which encompasses the loss of structural and functional integration (Stocco et al. 2007). This deterioration is probably due to less responsiveness of the senescent corpus luteum on LH (Zeleznik 1998). In the older corpus luteum, a decrease in StAR expression is seen together with a decrease in progesterone production. This decrease in progesterone production is preceded by cell death of the corpus luteum. When progesterone decreases, the endometrium will not be maintained which will shed resulting in a menstruation, and the monthly cycle will begin again (Fig. 5).

If pregnancy occurs, HCG produced by the trophoblasts preserves the corpus luteum (Zeleznik 1998). Progesterone produced by the corpus luteum is important for endometrial conditioning allowing implantation and maintenance of the intrauterine pregnancy until the placenta will take over by approximately 12 weeks of gestation.

Toward and Beyond Menopause

Menopause is defined as the point in time of the last vaginal bleeding from the endometrium induced by influence of hormones produced by the ovaries. Women experience a physiological menopause on average at the age of 51 years (McKinlay et al. 1992). The age of menopause is largely genetically established (Stolk et al. 2009). Certain gene variations are associated with increased decline in ovarian reserve. After the age of 30 years, the fecundity decreases. Both the quantity and quality of the remaining oocytes are poorer in the aging ovary than in young ovaries resulting in lower chance of conception and implantation and higher chance of spontaneous abortions and chromosomal aberrant offspring.

The follicle pool continues to reduce, and in the aging ovary, this results in lower inhibin B production, as important inhibitor of FSH secretion (Sherman et al. 1976), and furthermore AMH concentrations decline (Bentzen et al. 2013; Welt and Schneyer 2001). Subsequently FSH concentrations increase. Both decreased AMH and increased FSH concentrations lead to a higher percentage of growing follicles relative to the resting pool (Gosden and Faddy 1994; Gougeon 1998; Gougeon et al. 1994). This phenomenon results in an acceleration of follicle depletion. Reduced AMH concentrations in combination with increased FSH concentrations lead to an increased aromatase activity resulting in increased estrogen concentrations (di Clemente et al. 1994). Despite ovarian aging a normal menstrual pattern will be maintained for a long period because of this increased follicle recruitment and increased estrogen production.

The first clinical sign of aging ovaries in women is shortening of the cycle. Higher FSH concentrations cause earlier follicle recruitment. This starts in the final stages of the previous cycle before menstruation resulting in a virtually shorter follicular phase of the following cycle and higher estradiol concentrations at cycle day 3 (Klein et al. 1996). Paradoxically, while the poor quantity and quality of the remaining oocytes lead to reduced fecundity, the high FSH levels can lead to multiple follicle growth resulting in a net higher percentage of multiple births in aging women (Beemsterboer et al. 2006).

Approximately, 1 year prior to menopause, 60–70% of the menstrual cycles become anovulatory or have a prolonged follicular phase. In this period, estrogen concentrations fluctuate strongly from undetectable up to many times normal. These irregular fluctuations are insufficient to trigger an LH surge, and persisting follicles occur (Keye and Jaffe 1975).

When the resting pool of oocytes consists of 1,000 follicles or less, the ovary is not able to maintain the cyclic hormonal production for regulation of the normal menstrual cycle, menopause occurs, and the postmenopausal life starts (Richardson 1993). FSH concentrations will increase and are stable 2–8 years after menopause (Fig. 1) (Randolph et al. 2011). Between 50 and 75 years of age, FSH gradually declines until it reaches 30% less than its highest value (Hall 2007). After menopause estrogens will decrease until they reach their lowest point 2 years after the final menstruation (Randolph et al. 2011). LH will increase after estrogens starts to decrease (Overlie et al. 1999). Inhibins A and B are undetectable after menopause (Verhoeven et al. 2009). In contrast androgen production is barely changed (Sluijmer et al. 1995, 1998). While estrogen production is dependent on follicular development, androgens are produced by the ovarian stroma as well. These androgens are aromatized into estrogens in the peripheral fat which is the only source for estrogen levels in postmenopausal women.

Summary

We discussed ovarian processes starting in the uterine life and subsequently across the following phases: from birth until puberty, the pubertal period itself, then from post puberty until menopause, and finally during menopause and the postmenopausal phase. The ovary has three important functions: first oocyte and follicle formation and storage, second oocyte and follicle development resulting in ovulation, and third reproductive hormone production. The hormone production is inseparable from follicular development. The various processes were described in each of the different phases of life.

Cross-References

▶ Growth Hormones and Aging
▶ The Endocrinology of Puberty

References

Adhikari D, Liu K. Molecular mechanisms underlying the activation of mammalian primordial follicles. Endocr Rev. 2009;30(5):438–64.

Adhikari D, Liu K. mTOR signaling in the control of activation of primordial follicles. Cell Cycle. 2010;9(9):1673–4.

Andersen CY, Schmidt KT, Kristensen SG, Rosendahl M, Byskov AG, Ernst E. Concentrations of AMH and inhibin-B in relation to follicular diameter in normal human small antral follicles. Hum Reprod. 2010;25(5):1282–7.

Anderson RA, McLaughlin M, Wallace WH, Albertini DF, Telfer EE. The immature human ovary shows loss of abnormal follicles and increasing follicle developmental competence through childhood and adolescence. Hum Reprod. 2014;29(1):97–106.

Apter D, Cacciatore B, Alfthan H, Stenman UH. Serum luteinizing hormone concentrations increase 100-fold in females from 7 years to adulthood, as measured by time-resolved immunofluorometric assay. J Clin Endocrinol Metab. 1989;68(1):53–7.

Arendsen de Wolff-Exalto E. Influence of gonadotrophins on early follicle cell development and early oocyte growth in the immature rat. J Reprod Fertil. 1982;66(2):537–42.

Baker TG, Scrimgeour JB. Development of the gonad in normal and anencephalic human fetuses. J Reprod Fertil. 1980;60(1):193–9.

Beemsterboer SN, Homburg R, Gorter NA, Schats R, Hompes PG, Lambalk CB. The paradox of declining fertility but increasing twinning rates with advancing maternal age. Hum Reprod. 2006;21(6):1531–2.

Bentzen JG, Forman JL, Johannsen TH, Pinborg A, Larsen EC, Andersen AN. Ovarian antral follicle subclasses and anti-mullerian hormone during normal reproductive aging. J Clin Endocrinol Metab. 2013;98(4):1602–11.

Broekmans FJ, Visser JA, Laven JS, Broer SL, Themmen AP, Fauser BC. Anti-Mullerian hormone and ovarian dysfunction. Trends Endocrinol Metab. 2008;19(9):340–7.

Castrillon DH, Miao L, Kollipara R, Horner JW, DePinho RA. Suppression of ovarian follicle activation in mice by the transcription factor Foxo3a. Science. 2003;301(5630):215–8.

Chan C, Liu K. Clinical pregnancy in a woman with idiopathic hypogonadotropic hypogonadism and low AMH: utility of ovarian reserve markers in IHH. J Assist Reprod Genet. 2014;31(10):1317–21.

Cheng Y, Kawamura K, Takae S, Deguchi M, Yang Q, Kuo C, et al. Oocyte-derived R-spondin2 promotes ovarian follicle development. FASEB J. 2013;27(6):2175–84.

Davis GH, McEwan JC, Fennessy PF, Dodds KG, McNatty KP, WS O. Infertility due to bilateral ovarian hypoplasia in sheep homozygous (FecXI FecXI) for the inverdale prolificacy gene located on the X chromosome. Biol Reprod. 1992;46(4):636–40.

Dewailly D, Robin G, Peigne M, Decanter C, Pigny P, Catteau-Jonard S. Interactions between androgens, FSH, anti-Mullerian hormone and estradiol during folliculogenesis in the human normal and polycystic ovary. Hum Reprod Update. 2016;22:709–24.

di Clemente N, Goxe B, Remy JJ, Cate R, Josso N, Vigier B, et al. Inhibitory effect of AMH upon aromatase activity and LH receptors of granulosa cells of rat and porcine immature ovaries. Endocrine. 1994;2(6):553–8.

Dickerman Z, Prager-Lewis R, Laron Z. Response of plasma LH and FSH to synthetic LH-RH in children at various pubertal stages. Am J Dis Child. 1976;130(6):634–8.

Dong J, Albertini DF, Nishimori K, Kumar TR, Lu N, Matzuk MM. Growth differentiation factor-9 is required during early ovarian folliculogenesis. Nature. 1996;383(6600):531–5.

Donnez J, Silber S, Andersen CY, Demeestere I, Piver P, Meirow D, et al. Children born after autotransplantation of cryopreserved ovarian tissue. a review of 13 live births. Ann Med. 2011;43(6):437–50.

Durlinger AL, Gruijters MJ, Kramer P, Karels B, Kumar TR, Matzuk MM, et al. Anti-Mullerian hormone attenuates the effects of FSH on follicle development in the mouse ovary. Endocrinology. 2001;142(11):4891–9.

Farquhar C, Brown J, Marjoribanks J. Laparoscopic drilling by diathermy or laser for ovulation induction in anovulatory polycystic ovary syndrome. Cochrane Database Syst Rev. 2012;6, CD001122.

Fraser IS, Baird DT. Endometrial cystic glandular hyperplasia in adolescent girls. J Obstet Gynaecol Br Commonw. 1972;79(11):1009–15.

Fraser IS, Michie EA, Wide L, Baird DT. Pituitary gonadotropins and ovarian function in adolescent dysfunctional uterine bleeding. J Clin Endocrinol Metab. 1973;37(3):407–14.

Gallardo TD, John GB, Shirley L, Contreras CM, Akbay EA, Haynie JM, et al. Genomewide discovery and classification of candidate ovarian fertility genes in the mouse. Genetics. 2007;177(1):179–94.

Galloway SM, McNatty KP, Cambridge LM, Laitinen MP, Juengel JL, Jokiranta TS, et al. Mutations in an oocyte-derived growth factor gene (BMP15) cause increased ovulation rate and infertility in a dosage-sensitive manner. Nat Genet. 2000;25(3):279–83.

Gosden RG, Faddy MJ. Ovarian aging, follicular depletion, and steroidogenesis. Exp Gerontol. 1994;29(3–4):265–74.

Gougeon A. Regulation of ovarian follicular development in primates: facts and hypotheses. Endocr Rev. 1996;17(2):121–55.

Gougeon A. Ovarian follicular growth in humans: ovarian ageing and population of growing follicles. Maturitas. 1998;30(2):137–42.

Gougeon A, Testart J. Germinal vesicle breakdown in oocytes of human atretic follicles during the menstrual cycle. J Reprod Fertil. 1986;78(2):389–401.

Gougeon A, Ecochard R, Thalabard JC. Age-related changes of the population of human ovarian follicles: increase in the disappearance rate of non-growing and early-growing follicles in aging women. Biol Reprod. 1994;50(3):653–63.

Groome NP, Illingworth PJ, O'Brien M, Pai R, Rodger FE, Mather JP, McNeilly AS. Measurement of dimeric inhibin B throughout the human menstrual cycle. J Clin Endocrinol and Metab. 1996; 81(4):1401–1402.

Gwynne JT, Strauss 3rd JF. The role of lipoproteins in steroidogenesis and cholesterol metabolism in steroidogenic glands. Endocr Rev. 1982;3(3):299–329.

Hagen CP, Aksglaede L, Sorensen K, Main KM, Boas M, Cleemann L, et al. Serum levels of anti-Mullerian hormone as a marker of ovarian function in 926 healthy females from birth to adulthood and in 172 Turner syndrome patients. J Clin Endocrinol Metab. 2010;95 (11):5003–10.

Hagen CP, Aksglaede L, Sorensen K, Mouritsen A, Andersson AM, Petersen JH, et al. Individual serum levels of anti-Mullerian hormone in healthy girls persist through childhood and adolescence: a longitudinal cohort study. Hum Reprod. 2012a;27(3):861–6.

Hagen CP, Sorensen K, Anderson RA, Juul A. Serum levels of anti mullerian hormone in early maturing girls before, during, and after suppression with GnRH agonist. Fertil Steril. 2012b;98 (5):1326–30.
Halder G, Johnson RL. Hippo signaling: growth control and beyond. Development. 2011;138 (1):9–22.
Hall JE. Neuroendocrine changes with reproductive aging in women. Semin Reprod Med. 2007;25 (5):344–51.
Hall JE, Welt CK, Cramer DW. Inhibin A and inhibin B reflect ovarian function in assisted reproduction but are less useful at predicting outcome. Hum Reprod. 1999;14(2):409–15.
Halpin DM, Charlton HM, Faddy MJ. Effects of gonadotrophin deficiency on follicular development in hypogonadal (hpg) mice. J Reprod Fertil. 1986;78(1):119–25.
Hergovich A, Hemmings BA. Hippo signalling in the G2/M cell cycle phase: lessons learned from the yeast MEN and SIN pathways. Semin Cell Dev Biol. 2012;23(7):794–802.
Hsueh AJ, Kawamura K, Cheng Y, Fauser BC. Intraovarian control of early folliculogenesis. Endocr Rev. 2015;36(1):1–24.
Hu YC, Wang PH, Yeh S, Wang RS, Xie C, Xu Q, et al. Subfertility and defective folliculogenesis in female mice lacking androgen receptor. Proc Natl Acad Sci U S A. 2004;101(31):11209–14.
Huang L, Wang ZB, Jiang ZZ, Hu MW, Lin F, Zhang QH, et al. Specific disruption of Tsc1 in ovarian granulosa cells promotes ovulation and causes progressive accumulation of corpora lutea. PLoS ONE. 2013;8(1), e54052.
Juengel JL, Bodensteiner KJ, Heath DA, Hudson NL, Moeller CL, Smith P, et al. Physiology of GDF9 and BMP15 signalling molecules. Anim Reprod Sci. 2004;82–83:447–60.
Kawamura K, Cheng Y, Suzuki N, Deguchi M, Sato Y, Takae S, et al. Hippo signaling disruption and Akt stimulation of ovarian follicles for infertility treatment. Proc Natl Acad Sci U S A. 2013;110(43):17474–9.
Keye WR, Jr., Jaffe RB. Strength-duration characteristics of estrogen effects on gonadotropin response to gonadotropin-releasing hormone in women. I. Effects of varying duration of estradiol.
Klein NA, Battaglia DE, Fujimoto VY, Davis GS, Bremner WJ, Soules MR. Reproductive aging: accelerated ovarian follicular development associated with a monotropic follicle-stimulating hormone rise in normal older women. J Clin Endocrinol Metab. 1996;81(3):1038–45.
Kuijper EA, Ket JC, Caanen MR, Lambalk CB. Reproductive hormone concentrations in pregnancy and neonates: a systematic review. Reprod Biomed Online. 2013;27(1):33–63.
Kuiri-Hanninen T, Kallio S, Seuri R, Tyrvainen E, Liakka A, Tapanainen J, et al. Postnatal developmental changes in the pituitary-ovarian axis in preterm and term infant girls. J Clin Endocrinol Metab. 2011;96(11):3432–9.
Kuiri-Hanninen T, Haanpaa M, Turpeinen U, Hamalainen E, Seuri R, Tyrvainen E, et al. Postnatal ovarian activation has effects in estrogen target tissues in infant girls. J Clin Endocrinol Metab. 2013;98(12):4709–16.
Kumar TR, Wang Y, Lu N, Matzuk MM. Follicle stimulating hormone is required for ovarian follicle maturation but not male fertility. Nat Genet. 1997;15(2):201–4.
La MA, Malmusi S, Giulini S, Tamaro LF, Orvieto R, Levratti P, et al. Anti-Mullerian hormone plasma levels in spontaneous menstrual cycle and during treatment with FSH to induce ovulation. Hum Reprod. 2004;19(12):2738–41.
Lashen H, Dunger DB, Ness A, Ong KK. Peripubertal changes in circulating antimullerian hormone levels in girls. Fertil Steril. 2013;99(7):2071–5.
Mazerbourg S, Klein C, Roh J, Kaivo-Oja N, Mottershead DG, Korchynskyi O, et al. Growth differentiation factor-9 signaling is mediated by the type I receptor, activin receptor-like kinase 5. Mol Endocrinol. 2004;18(3):653–65.
McGee EA, Perlas E, LaPolt PS, Tsafriri A, Hsueh AJ. Follicle-stimulating hormone enhances the development of preantral follicles in juvenile rats. Biol Reprod. 1997;57(5):990–8.
McKinlay SM, Brambilla DJ, Posner JG. The normal menopause transition. Maturitas. 1992;14 (2):103–15.

Micevych P, Sinchak K. The neurosteroid progesterone underlies estrogen positive feedback of the LH surge. Front Endocrinol (Lausanne). 2011;2:90.

Millar RP, Roseweir AK, Tello JA, Anderson RA, George JT, Morgan K, et al. Kisspeptin antagonists: unraveling the role of kisspeptin in reproductive physiology. Brain Res. 2010;1364:81–9.

Mouritsen A, Aksglaede L, Soerensen K, Hagen CP, Petersen JH, Main KM, et al. The pubertal transition in 179 healthy Danish children: associations between pubarche, adrenarche, gonadarche, and body composition. Eur J Endocrinol. 2013;168(2):129–36.

Naftolin F, et al. In: Ferin M et al., editors. Biorhytms and human reproduction. New York: Wiley; 1974. p. 219–38.

Orisaka M, Orisaka S, Jiang JY, Craig J, Wang Y, Kotsuji F, et al. Growth differentiation factor 9 is antiapoptotic during follicular development from preantral to early antral stage. Mol Endocrinol. 2006;20(10):2456–68.

Otsuka F, Yao Z, Lee T, Yamamoto S, Erickson GF, Shimasaki S. Bone morphogenetic protein-15. Identification of target cells and biological functions. J Biol Chem. 2000;275(50):39523–8.

Overlie I, Moen MH, Morkrid L, Skjaeraasen JS, Holte A. The endocrine transition around menopause – a five years prospective study with profiles of gonadotropines, estrogens, androgens and SHBG among healthy women. Acta Obstet Gynecol Scand. 1999;78(7):642–7.

Persani L, Rossetti R, Di Pasquale E, Cacciatore C, Fabre S. The fundamental role of bone morphogenetic protein 15 in ovarian function and its involvement in female fertility disorders. Hum Reprod Update. 2014;20(6):869–83.

Peters H, Byskov AG, Grinsted J. Follicular growth in fetal and prepubertal ovaries of humans and other primates. Clin Endocrinol Metab. 1978;7(3):469–85.

Pineda R, Garcia-Galiano D, Roseweir A, Romero M, Sanchez-Garrido MA, Ruiz-Pino F, et al. Critical roles of kisspeptins in female puberty and preovulatory gonadotropin surges as revealed by a novel antagonist. Endocrinology. 2010;151(2):722–30.

Randolph Jr JF, Zheng H, Sowers MR, Crandall C, Crawford S, Gold EB, et al. Change in follicle-stimulating hormone and estradiol across the menopausal transition: effect of age at the final menstrual period. J Clin Endocrinol Metab. 2011;96(3):746–54.

Reddy P, Liu L, Adhikari D, Jagarlamudi K, Rajareddy S, Shen Y, et al. Oocyte-specific deletion of Pten causes premature activation of the primordial follicle pool. Science. 2008;319(5863):611–3.

Richardson SJ. The biological basis of the menopause. Baillieres Clin Endocrinol Metab. 1993;7 (1):1–16.

Retamales I, Carrasco I, Troncoso JL, Las Heras J, Devoto L, Vega M. Morpho-functional study of human luteal cell subpopulations. Hum Reprod. 1994;9(4):591–6.

Sherman BM, West JH, Korenman SG. The menopausal transition: analysis of LH, FSH, estradiol, and progesterone concentrations during menstrual cycles of older women. J Clin Endocrinol Metab. 1976;42(4):629–36.

Shiina H, Matsumoto T, Sato T, Igarashi K, Miyamoto J, Takemasa S, et al. Premature ovarian failure in androgen receptor-deficient mice. Proc Natl Acad Sci U S A. 2006;103(1):224–9.

Sizonenko PC. Preadolescent and adolescent endocrinology: physiology and physiopathology. II. Hormonal changes during abnormal pubertal development. Am J Dis Child. 1978;132 (8):797–805.

Sluijmer AV, Heineman MJ, De Jong FH, Evers JL. Endocrine activity of the postmenopausal ovary: the effects of pituitary down-regulation and oophorectomy. J Clin Endocrinol Metab. 1995;80(7):2163–7.

Sluijmer AV, Heineman MJ, Koudstaal J, Theunissen PH, de Jong FH, Evers JL. Relationship between ovarian production of estrone, estradiol, testosterone, and androstenedione and the ovarian degree of stromal hyperplasia in postmenopausal women. Menopause. 1998;5 (4):207–10.

Solovyeva EV, Hayashi M, Margi K, Barkats C, Klein C, Amsterdam A, et al. Growth differentiation factor-9 stimulates rat theca-interstitial cell androgen biosynthesis. Biol Reprod. 2000;63 (4):1214–8.

Spicer LJ, Aad PY, Allen DT, Mazerbourg S, Payne AH, Hsueh AJ. Growth differentiation factor 9 (GDF9) stimulates proliferation and inhibits steroidogenesis by bovine theca cells: influence of follicle size on responses to GDF9. Biol Reprod. 2008;78(2):243–53.

Stocco DM, Clark BJ. Role of the steroidogenic acute regulatory protein (StAR) in steroidogenesis. Biochem Pharmacol. 1996;51(3):197–205.

Stocco C, Telleria C, Gibori G. The molecular control of corpus luteum formation, function, and regression. Endocr Rev. 2007;28(1):117–49.

Stolk L, Zhai G, van Meurs JB, Verbiest MM, Visser JA, Estrada K, et al. Loci at chromosomes 13, 19 and 20 influence age at natural menopause. Nat Genet. 2009;41(6):645–7.

Strauss 3rd JF, Kallen CB, Christenson LK, Watari H, Devoto L, Arakane F, et al. The steroidogenic acute regulatory protein (StAR): a window into the complexities of intracellular cholesterol trafficking. Recent Prog Horm Res. 1999;54:369–94. discussion 94–5.

Tarnawa ED, Baker MD, Aloisio GM, Carr BR, Castrillon DH. Gonadal expression of Foxo1, but not Foxo3, is conserved in diverse Mammalian species. Biol Reprod. 2013;88(4):103.

Verhoeven MO, van der Mooren MJ, Teerlink T, Verheijen RH, Scheffer PG, Kenemans P. The influence of physiological and surgical menopause on coronary heart disease risk markers. Menopause. 2009;16(1):37–49.

Vitt UA, McGee EA, Hayashi M, Hsueh AJ. In vivo treatment with GDF-9 stimulates primordial and primary follicle progression and theca cell marker CYP17 in ovaries of immature rats. Endocrinology. 2000;141(10):3814–20.

Vitt UA, Mazerbourg S, Klein C, Hsueh AJ. Bone morphogenetic protein receptor type II is a receptor for growth differentiation factor-9. Biol Reprod. 2002;67(2):473–80.

Weintraub A, Margalioth EJ, Chetrit AB, Gal M, Goldberg D, Alerhand S, et al. The dynamics of serum anti-Mullerian-hormone levels during controlled ovarian hyperstimulation with GnRH-antagonist short protocol in polycystic ovary syndrome and low responders. Eur J Obstet Gynecol Reprod Biol. 2014;176:163–7.

Welt CK, Schneyer AL. Differential regulation of inhibin B and inhibin a by follicle-stimulating hormone and local growth factors in human granulosa cells from small antral follicles. J Clin Endocrinol Metab. 2001;86(1):330–6.

Winter JS, Faiman C. The development of cyclic pituitary-gonadal function in adolescent females. J Clin Endocrinol Metab. 1973;37(5):714–8.

Yan C, Wang P, DeMayo J, DeMayo FJ, Elvin JA, Carino C, et al. Synergistic roles of bone morphogenetic protein 15 and growth differentiation factor 9 in ovarian function. Mol Endocrinol. 2001;15(6):854–66.

Young JM, McNeilly AS. Theca: the forgotten cell of the ovarian follicle. Reproduction. 2010;140 (4):489–504.

Zeleznik AJ. In vivo responses of the primate corpus luteum to luteinizing hormone and chorionic gonadotropin. Proc Natl Acad Sci U S A. 1998;95(18):11002–7.

Zhao B, Tumaneng K, Guan KL. The Hippo pathway in organ size control, tissue regeneration and stem cell self-renewal. Nat Cell Biol. 2011;13(8):877–83.

Part V

Nonclassical Endocrine Organs

The Endocrine Gut

19

Jens F. Rehfeld

Abstract

The gut is the largest endocrine organ in the body, both in terms of size and number of endocrine cells and hormones produced. More than 30 hormone genes are currently known to be expressed in the gastrointestinal tract. In order to overview the many hormonal peptides, it may be feasible to conceive the hormones under five headings: The *structural homology* groups a majority of the hormones into nine families, each of which is assumed to originate from one ancestral gene. The individual hormone gene often has *multiple phenotypes* due to alternative splicing, tandem organization, or cell-specific maturation of hormone precursors. By a combination of these mechanisms, more than 100 different hormonally active peptides are released from the gut. Gut hormone genes, however, are also *widely expressed in cells outside the gut*, some only in extraintestinal endocrine cells and neurons but others also in other cell types. The extraintestinal cells may synthesize different bioactive peptide fragments of the same prohormone due to *cell-specific biosynthetic pathways*. Moreover, endocrine cells, neurons, myocytes, cancer cells, and, for instance, spermatozoa *release the peptides differentially* (autocrine, endocrine, myocrine, neurocrine, paracrine, spermiocrine secretion, etc.), so the same peptide may act as a blood-borne hormone, a neurotransmitter, a local growth factor, or a fertility factor. The molecular targets of each bioactive peptide are specific receptors expressed in the cell membranes of the target cells. Also the target cells of gut hormones occur widespread outside the digestive tract.

J.F. Rehfeld (✉)
Department of Clinical Biochemistry, Rigshospitalet, University of Copenhagen, Copenhagen, Denmark
e-mail: jens.f.rehfeld@regionh.dk

A. Belfiore, D. LeRoith (eds.), *Principles of Endocrinology and Hormone Action*, Endocrinology, https://doi.org/10.1007/978-3-319-44675-2_19

Keywords
Biosynthesis • Cell biology • Digestion • Endocrine cells • Gastrointestinal tract • Growth factors • Hormones • Hormone genes • Hormone receptors • Neuropeptides • Peptides

Contents

Introduction

The blood-borne regulation by specific messenger molecules was discovered early in the previous century (Bayliss and Starling 1902). Based on the notion that acidification in the upper small intestine stimulates pancreatic secretion, Bayliss and Starling extracted from the duodenal mucosa a substance that released bicarbonate from the denervated pancreas when injected into blood. They named the substance secretin. Three years later, it was suggested that the antral mucosa contained a stimulator of gastric acid secretion, named "gastric secretin" or simply gastrin (Edkins 1906). Hence, the first two known blood-borne "chemical messengers," secretin and gastrin, were both of gastrointestinal origin. Subsequently, Starling proposed the word *hormone* from Greek *hormoa* ("I arouse to activity") as a general designation for blood-borne messengers (Starling 1905). In other words, endocrinology as such was actually born in the gut.

In the following decades, however, other types of hormones came into focus – steroids from the adrenals, ovaries, and testes; protein hormones from the pituitary gland; the thyronins from the thyroid gland; and insulin from the pancreatic islets. The often lifesaving effects of these discoveries made the interest for secretin and gastrin fade. Subsequently, only a small priesthood of physiologists studied endocrine control of digestion. Among them are Ivy and his assistant, who found a gallbladder-emptying hormone in the proximal small intestine, cholecystokinin (CCK) (Ivy and Oldberg 1928). Harper and Raper later described a stimulator of pancreatic enzyme secretion, pancreozymin (1943). But in the 1960s, it was shown that CCK and pancreozymin were one and the same hormone (Jorpes and Mutt 1966) for which the acronym CCK is now used.

Secretin, gastrin, and CCK constitute the classical troika of gut hormones, but in the latter half of the twentieth century, many more were discovered (Fig. 1). In order not to lose overview, this chapter summarizes the gut hormones, and their targets major biological activities in Tables 1, 2, and 3, but otherwise presents general principles governing structure and biogenesis of gastrointestinal hormones. Readers interested in details about individual hormones and their effects should consult multiauthor volumes comprising the full range of gut endocrinology (Schultz et al. 1989; Walsh and Dockray 1994; Taché et al. 2002).

It should be added that gut endocrinology is also worth considering in general from an evolutionary point of view. Thus, life in multicellular organisms began as a small tube with one opening, as illustrated by coelenterates (Fig. 2). They live in water that runs into their lumen, from which nutrients are absorbed into the epithelial cell lining. Coelenterates have no blood vessels, but a delicate regulatory system of primitive neurons spread out on the luminal wall. Apparently, these neurons release small peptides. Thus, multicellular life began as an isolated "gut" whose function was controlled by hormone-like peptides. Consequently, phylogenetically speaking, endocrine organs are all derivatives of the primordial gut.

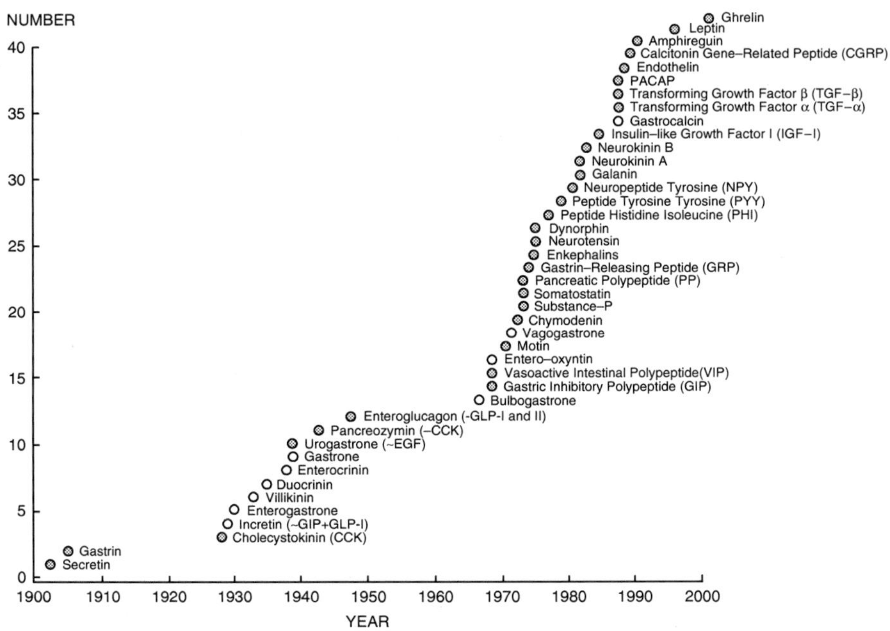

Fig. 1 Discovery and identification of regulatory peptides in the gastrointestinal tract 1900–2000. Discovery is indicated by year of first report. *Solid circles* indicated structural identification, and *open circles* indicated hormonal activities that still require structural identification. Some of the unidentified hormonal activities are explained by later identified hormones. For instance, the incretin activity is partly due to gastric inhibitory polypeptide (GIP) and glucagon-like peptide I (GLP-I). Commonly used acronyms are indicated in brackets after full name, except for PACAP, which is an acronym for pituitary adenylate cyclase-activating peptide

Table 1 Peptide hormone, neuropeptide, and growth factor families in the gastrointestinal tract and the pancreas

Families and members	Major regulatory activity
Secretin family	
Secretin	Stimulates pancreatic bicarbonate secretion
Glucagon	Increases glucose production and amino acid metabolism
Glucagon-like peptide 1 (GLP-1)	Stimulates insulin and inhibits glucagon secretion and gastric emptying
Glucagon-like peptide 2 (GLP-2)	Stimulates mucosal cell growth in intestinal crypts
Gastric inhibitory polypeptide (GIP)	Enhances glucose-stimulated insulin secretion and inhibits gastric secretion
Vasoactive intestinal polypeptide (VIP)	Inhibits gastrointestinal motility and stimulates fluid secretion
Peptide histidine isoleucine (PHI)	VIP-like actions
Growth hormone-releasing hormone	Stimulates growth hormone secretion
Pituitary adenylyl cyclase-activating peptide (PACAP)	Contributes to the regulation of gastric acid secretion and gastrointestinal motor function
Gastrin family	
Gastrin	Stimulates gastric acid secretion and gastric mucosal cell growth
Cholecystokinin (CCK)	Stimulates pancreatic enzyme secretion, cell growth, and gallbladder emptying, but inhibits gastric acid secretion
Caerulein, Cionin } Not expressed in mammals	Cholecystokinin-like activities
Tachykinin family	
Substance P	Stimulates motility
Neurokinin A	Stimulates motility
Neurokinin B	Stimulates motility
Ghrelin family	
Ghrelin	Stimulates appetite and growth hormone secretion
Obestatin	Suppresses food intake (?)
Motilin	Contracts gastrointestinal smooth muscles to stimulate motility
PP-fold family	
Pancreatic polypeptide (PP)	Involved in feeding behavior (?)
Peptide YY (PYY)	Reduces gastric emptying and pancreatic exocrine secretion and delays intestinal transit
Neuropeptide Y (NPY)	Modulates the contractility in smooth muscle cells
Somatostatin family	
Somatostatin	Inhibits gastric acid, gastrin secretion, and other gut functions through endocrine, paracrine, and neurocrine release
Cortistatin	Somatostatin-like activities
Insulin family	
Insulin	Establishes energy resources in fat, liver, and muscle cells

(*continued*)

Table 1 (continued)

Families and members	Major regulatory activity
Insulin-like growth factor I (IGF-I)	Stimulates growth and differentiation in interaction with other growth factors
Insulin-like growth factor II (IGF-II)	Stimulates growth and differentiation in interaction with other growth factors
Relaxin	Function in the gastrointestinal tract uncertain
EGF family	
Epidermal growth factor (EGF)	Stimulates growth of epithelial cells and inhibition of gastric acid secretion
Transforming growth factor α (TGFα)	EGF-like activities
Amphiregulin	Growth regulation of epithelial cells
Heparin-binding EGF-like growth factor	EGF-like activities
Opioid peptide family	
Enkephalins	Modulates transmitter activity from nerveplexes
β-endorphins	Modulates transmitter activity from nerveplexes
Dynorphins	Modulates transmitter activity from nerveplexes

General Features of Gut Hormones

The Structural Homology

The gut expresses a large number of hormones, neuropeptides, and growth factors. Not only have new hormones been found in gut extracts, but also peptides from the central nervous system and hormones first identified in other endocrine organs have been found in endocrine cells and/or neurons in the gut. Moreover, peptides originally believed to be classical hormones but later shown to be neurotransmitters have been isolated from gut extracts. The complexity is high, also because several genes for gut peptides encode different peptides released in a cell-specific manner.

In addition, there are still hormonal activities in the gut that are not yet structurally identified. Some of the activities can be explained by already identified peptides. Hence, the stimulation of insulin secretion from the gut, originally called "incretin," is today explained by two hormones – glucose-dependent insulinotropic peptide (GIP) and glucagon-like peptide-1 (GLP-1) – probably in combination with other gut hormones such as gastrin and CCK (Rehfeld 2011), whereas intestinal inhibition of gastric secretion, the gastrone effect, may be explained by combinations of CCK, somatostatin, and GIP. However, activities named villikinin, duocrinin, enterocrinin, and gastrocalcin still await structural identification. The complexity of hormones may jeopardize an overview of the endocrine gut. Fortunately, however, structural identifications have shown striking homologies between groups of peptides. Consequently, many of the biologically active gut peptides can now be classified into nine families (Table 1). The expression of several hormone genes both in the gut and

Table 2 Singular peptide hormones, neuropeptides, and growth hormones in the gastrointestinal tract

Hormones and growth factors	Major regulatory activity
Apelin	Stimulates gastric mucosal growth and cholecystokinin secretion
Bradykinin	Contributes to control alkaline secretion in the duodenal mucosa
Calcitonin gene-related peptide (CGRP)	Modulates blood flow, secretion, and motility
Cocaine and amphetamine-regulated transcript (CART)	Increases satiety
Galanin	Stimulates motility and luminal secretion
Gastrin-releasing peptide (GRP)	Stimulates antral gastrin secretion
Neurotensin	Increases the ileal brake
Orexin	Stimulates gut motility (?)
Transforming growth factor β (TGFβ)	Growth, differentiation, and inflammation
Thyrotropin-releasing hormone (TRH)	Releases TSH from epithelial cells in the gut

pancreas reflects the intestinal origin of the pancreas. The nature of the homology varies. It may be an overall similarity in the primary structure as, for example, the PP-fold family (Glover et al. 1984). Another type of homology is that of the gastrin family which, in addition to mammalian gastrin and CCK, also consists of the protochordean neuropeptide cionin (Johnsen and Rehfeld 1990) and frog skin peptide cerulein (Anastasi et al. 1968). The decisive homology of this family is concentrated to the structure of the active site, the C-terminal tetrapeptide sequence. Comparison between propeptide and gene structures also reveals some similarity, but the family is still defined primarily by the conserved active site sequence.

The frequent occurrence of homology among hormones, neuropeptides, and growth factors is not specific for peptides in the gut. It is a common feature among all kinds of hormonal peptides, enzymes, and other proteins in the organism (Doolittle et al. 1996). Each family is assumed to reflect the phylogenetic evolution by duplication and subsequent mutations of an ancestral gene. The phylogenetic story shows that gut hormones are indeed very old, maybe several hundred million years. So far, the data also support the idea that each hormone family has evolved from a single ancestor. An associated trait is that gut hormones have preserved their tissue-specific sites of expression during evolution (Rourke et al. 1997). Accordingly, evolution emphasizes the general significance of gut hormones as intercellular messenger molecules. At present, a few hormonal peptides in the gut have no relatives or family (Table 2). Time will show whether gut hormones still awaiting discovery will be related to these peptides.

The Multiple Phenotypes

Three decades ago, one gene was believed to encode one hormonal peptide in accordance with what we have learned about the master hormone, insulin. However,

Table 3 Receptors and receptor subtypes for some gastrointestinal hormones

Hormones	Receptors and subtypes
Atrial natriuretic peptide (ANP)	NP_A, NP_B, NP_C
Brain natriuretic peptide (BNP)	NP_A, NP_B, NP_C
C-type natriuretic peptide (CNP)	NP_A, NP_B, NP_C
Calcitonin	Calcitonin-R
Calcitonin gene-related peptide (CGRP)	$CGRP_1$, $CGRP_2$
Cholecystokinin (CCK)	CCK_A, CCK_B
Gastric inhibitory polypeptide (GIP)	GIP-R
Gastrin	Gastrin/CCK_B
Gastrin-releasing peptide (GRP)	GRP-R
Ghrelin	Ghrelin-R
Glucagon-like peptide-1 (GLP-1)	GLP-1-R
Motilin	Motilin-R
Neurotensin	NTR1, NTR2, NTR3
Parathyroid hormone-related protein (PTHrP)	PTH-R
Pituitary adenylate cyclase-activating peptide (PACAP)	PAC_1
Peptide tyrosine tyrosine (PYY)	Y_1, Y_2, Y_3, Y_4, Y_5
Secretin	Secretin-R
Somatostatin	sst_1, sst_{2A}, sst_{2B}, sst_3, sst_4, sst_5
Substance P	NK_1, NK_2, NK_3
Vasoactive intestinal polypeptide (VIP)	$VPAC_1$, $VPAC_2$

more intricate dimensions were added when it became obvious that a hormone gene often expresses different bioactive peptides. Today, we know three ways in which a gut hormone gene can vary its expression into peptides.

1. Alternative splicing of transcripts.
   Alternative splicing was discovered when it was shown that the calcitonin gene generates mRNAs encoding either calcitonin peptides or calcitonin gene-related peptides (CGRPs) (Amara et al. 1982). CGRPs are now known also to be abundantly expressed in intestinal neurons. Moreover, a tachykinin gene transcript (Nawa et al. 1984) and the transcript encoded by the secretin gene (Kopin et al. 1991) are also spliced alternatively in the gut.
2. Multiple products of prohormones with one active sequence.
   The somatostatin and gastrin families represent peptide systems in which the gene encodes only one prohormone that contains only one active site, but where the prohormone is processed in a way to release peptides of different lengths with the same active C-terminus. Although the different products of the same precursor are bound to the same receptor, their varying clearances from circulation affect their hormonal significance. Hence, it matters whether proCCK is processed mainly to CCK-58 or to CCK-8 (Fig. 3), or whether prosomatostatin is processed to somatostatin-28 or somatostatin-14. So far, the biosynthesis of gastrin in antral G cells has been examined particularly thoroughly. It is, therefore, a useful

Fig. 2 Scheme of the structure of coelenterates with endoderm (*En*), ectoderm (*Ek*), footplate (*Fp*), gaster (stomach *Ga*), mouth (*M*), and tentacles (*Te*)

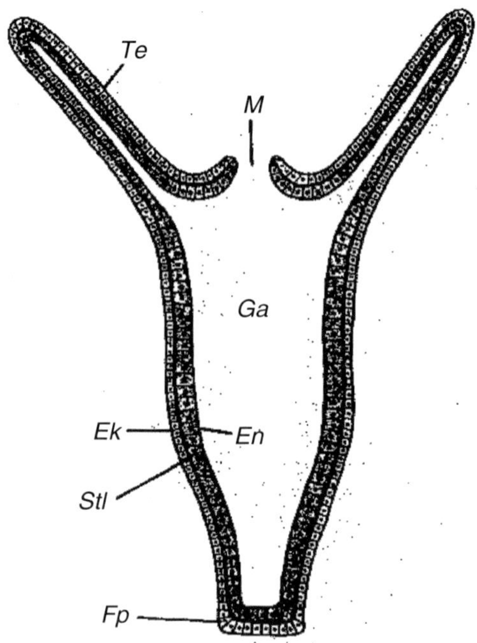

illustration of the second way in which one hormone gene can encode different bioactive peptides (Rehfeld 1998).

3. Differential processing of prohormones containing two or more active sequences. A third way in which one gene can express different bioactive peptides occurs when the gene encodes a propeptide containing different but often homologous peptide hormones or neuropeptides. Gut hormones and neuropeptides comprise many examples of such genes of which the opioid peptide genes, some of the tachykinin genes, the VIP gene, and the glucagon gene amply illustrate the phenomenon. Some of the genes not only encode a peptide precursor containing different bioactive peptides, which is then subjected to tissue-specific processing, but the primary transcripts of these gene(s) may also undergo tissue-specific alternative splicing.

Proglucagon is an example of a polyprotein precursor that contains three similar peptide sequences in mammals (Fig. 3, Bell et al. 1983). In pancreatic α-cells, proglucagon is processed to release the well-known pancreatic glucagon, whereas the C-terminal part of proglucagon remains silent. The L cells of the gut also express proglucagon but process it in a different way to release GLP-I and GLP-II (Holst et al. 1987; Mojsov et al. 1987). Although glucagon and, for instance, GLP-I are highly homologous and both glucoregulatory, they have separate activities and receptors. Proglucagon also tells another story, namely, that bioactive peptide

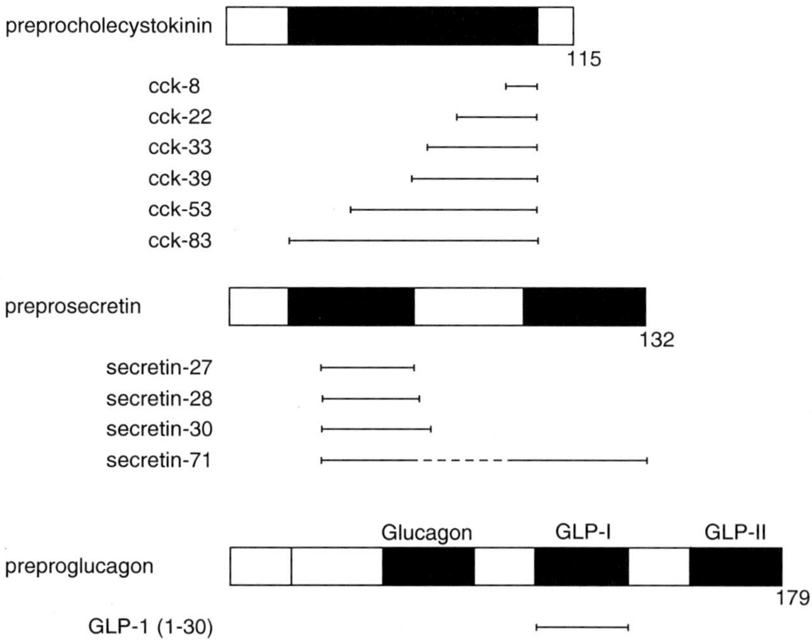

Fig. 3 Multiple phenotypes of three gut hormone genes. The cholecystokinin (CCK) gene encodes a prepropeptide which is processed to six CCK peptides varying in length from 83 to 8 amino acid residues through differentiated endoproteolytic cleavage. The six peptides have the same C-terminal bioactive octapeptide sequence. The secretin gene encodes a prepropeptide that through endoproteolytic cleavages and variable C-terminal trimming is processed to three bioactive secretin peptides of almost similar size (secretin-27, secretin-28, and secretin-30). In addition, bioactive secretion-71 is produced by splicing out RNA, encoding the midsequence of preprosecretin (i.e., broken line of secretin-71). The glucagon gene encodes a prepropeptide that through cell-specific endoproteolytic cleavages is processed to either genuine pancreatic glucagon (in pancreatic α-cells) or to glucagon-like peptides I and II (GLP-I, GLP-II) (Rehfeld 1998)

structures cannot be predicted from cDNA and protein precursor sequences. Identification requires exact examination of amino acid sequence and derivatizations of the released peptides and studies of their activities.

Widespread Gene Expression

The expression cascade for gut hormones involves many processing steps. Each step may control whether the initial gene transcription results in a bioactive peptide. Transcription can occur without the translation of the transcript, and the lack of parallelism between mRNA, propeptide, and the mature bioactive peptide has also been encountered.

All gut hormones are expressed in tissues outside the gastrointestinal tract, some mainly in neurons and endocrine cells. However, several gut hormones are also expressed in other cell types and tissues. The literature on extraintestinal expression of gut hormones has become overwhelming. Therefore, the phenomenon will be described for a single hormonal system only.

The gastrin gene is expressed in several other cells than the gastric G cells. Quantitatively, these other cells release only little gastrin to the blood in the normal adult organisms because the extra-antral secretion may serve local purposes. Besides that, biosynthetic processing is often so different that bioactive gastrins may not even be synthesized. So far, extra-gastric expression of the gastrin gene has been encountered in the distal small intestinal and colorectal mucosa, endocrine cells in the neonatal pancreas, pituitary corticotrophs and melanotrophs, hypothalamo-pituitary and vagal neurons, and spermatozoes (for review, see Rehfeld 1998).

The meaning of extraintestinal synthesis of gut hormones is often unknown, but local growth stimulation is a possibility. It is also possible that the low concentration is without significant function in the adult, but is a relic of a more comprehensive fetal synthesis. A third possibility is that low cellular concentration reflects constitutive secretion where the peptides are not stored in secretory granules.

Cell-Specific Prohormone Processing

Gut prohormone processing is so elaborate that the result of gene expression is unpredictable. Hence, the cellular equipment with processing enzymes and their cofactors determine the structure of the particular hormone. This cell-specific processing of prohormones applies to all gut hormones. But again, gastrin is also one of the most extensively studied hormones in this respect.

Almost every tissue in which progastrin is expressed has its own processing pattern. Four different patterns are shown in Fig. 4. For members of the gastrin family, the processing varies with respect to endoproteolytic processing and amino

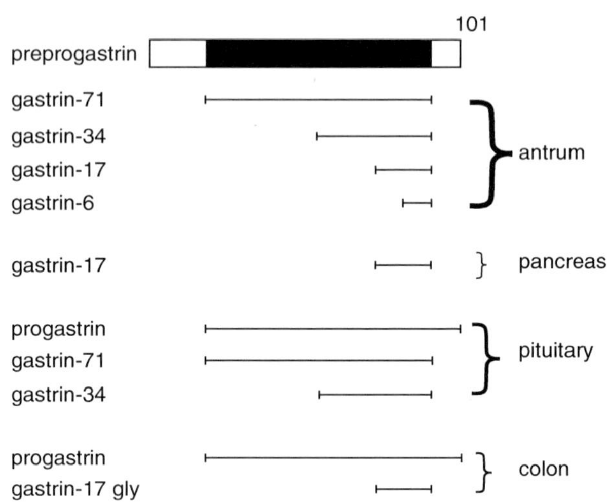

Fig. 4 Schematic illustration of cell-specific processing of preprogastrin in antral G cells, G cells in fetal and neonatal pancreas, in pituitary corticotrophic cells, and in unidentified cells in the colorectal mucosa (Rehfeld 1998)

acid derivatizations such as tyrosyl sulfations and phenylalanyl amidations. In this context it is worth realizing that the different types of processing may influence each other. Thus, tyrosyl sulfation, the earliest posttranslational modification for the gastrin family of prohormones, increases endoproteolytic cleavage efficiency (Bundgaard et al. 1995).

Cell-Specific Peptide Release

To understand the specific effects of gut hormones, it is necessary to realize that the different types of cells that express the genes also release the peptides in different ways. Secretion of gut hormones was supposed to be endocrine only, until 40 years ago. But today, three alternative routes of secretion to neighboring cells and one to the secretory cell itself have been discovered (Fig. 5). Firstly, the peptides synthesized in neurons are released from synaptosomal vesicles in the

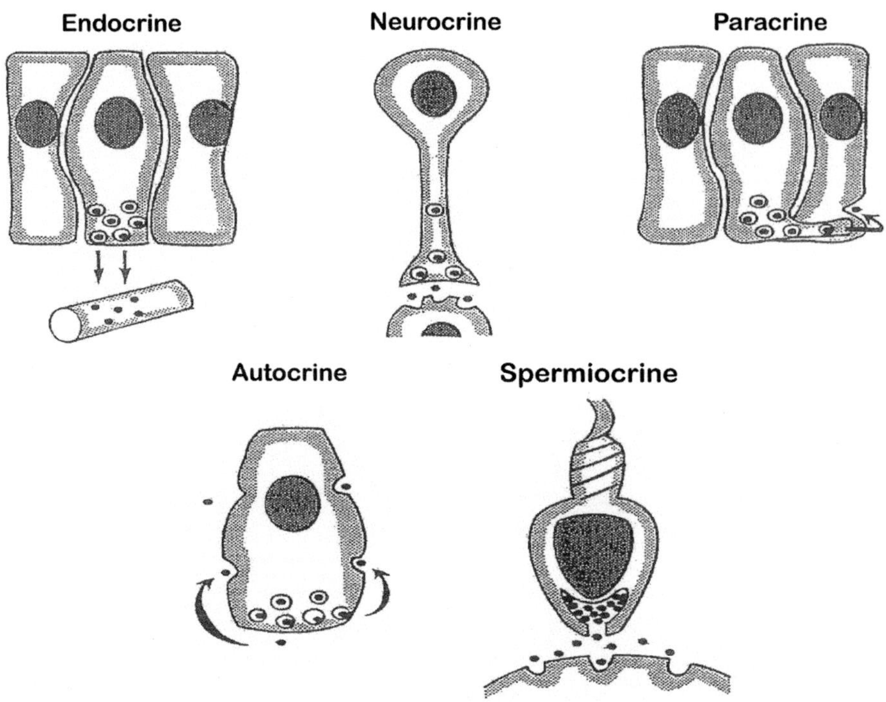

Fig. 5 Different types of cell-specific release of regulatory gut peptides: (1) endocrine release to capillaries from classic endocrine cells in the gastrointestinal mucosa, (2) neurotransmitter release from central or peripheral neurons to the synaptic cleft, (3) paracrine release to neighboring cells through short cellular processes, (4) autocrine release to receptors on membrane of the same cell that synthesizes and releases the peptides, and (5) spermiocrine release from acrosomal granule of spermatozoa to receptors on egg cell membranes (Rehfeld 1998)

nerve terminals to the receptors of adjacent target cells as neurotransmitters. It is also possible that some peptidergic neurons expressing gut hormonal peptides, such as hypothalamo-pituitary neurons, release the peptides directly to blood vessels as neurocrine secretion. Secondly, it has been shown that there are specific paracrine cells that release, for instance, somatostatin in the gastrointestinal mucosa (Larsson et al. 1979). These cells carry peptidergic granules through cytoplasmic extensions to specific target cells in the neighborhood.

Cells stimulate their own growth through autocrine secretion. Trophic peptides bind to specific receptors in the membranes of cells in which they are also synthesized (Fig. 5). Autocrine secretion is supposed to play a decisive role in tumor and cancer development (Sporn and Roberts 1985).

Cellular release of gastrointestinal peptides also occurs in a fifth way (Fig. 5): spermatozoes in mammals express gastrin, CCK, and pituitary adenylate cyclase-activating peptide (PACAP) genes (Li et al. 2000; Persson et al. 1989). The peptides are concentrated in the acrosome. In accordance with the acrosomal reaction, the peptides are released from the spermatozoon by contact with the jelly coat of the egg and subsequently bound to receptors in the egg membrane. Defects of the reproductive functions have now been found in PACAP-deficient mice (Shintani et al. 2002). The release of bioactive peptides from acrosomal granules could be termed *spermiocrine* release (Fig. 5).

General Features of Gut Hormone Targets

Target Cells

The molecular targets of gut hormones are specific G protein-coupled receptors expressed on a variety of cell membranes in the body. Many of the target cells are located in the gut: neurons (including the coordinating myenteric and submucosal nerveplexes); other endocrine gut cells; smooth muscles; secretory cells that release enzymes, amines, acid, and bicarbonate; etc. The hormonal control of intestinal cells ensures that digestion, growth, and motility of the gut occur in a coordinated manner in order to optimize the utilization of food and the subsequent energy delivery to the body. However, cells of many extraintestinal organs in the body also express receptors for gut hormones, which teleologically may explain why hormonal peptides from the gut are released to the general circulation. The extraintestinal organs include endocrine glands (the pituitary, thyroid C cells, parathyroid glands, islets of Langerhans, etc.), the liver, the gallbladder, the pancreas, the cardiovascular system, and the lungs. At low level most other tissues in the body also express gut hormone receptors, the significance of which is still unknown. Finally, many gastrointestinal and extraintestinal cancers express both gut hormones and their receptors whereby these cancers are equipped with their own autocrine and/or paracrine growth machine (Reubi 2003). The functions of each gut hormone are outlined in Tables 1 and 2.

Receptors

The receptors for gut hormones are as mentioned of the G protein-coupled type. The protein chain is often heavily derivatized by, for instance, phosphorylations and glycosylations sites. Receptors structurally identified so far are listed in Table 3 in relation to their hormonal ligand. The relationship is often complex because a specific ligand may bind several different receptors.

Detection of G protein-coupled receptors in normal tissues is difficult since the number of receptors on normal target cells is small, compared, for instance, to the amount of hormones synthesized in comparable sites. Therefore, the detection methods for receptors are limited. Several different in vitro techniques have been used to detect G protein-coupled receptors: measurement of receptor mRNA by PCR techniques is widely used with the limitations, however, that it is not the receptor protein that is detected and that the morphological correlate is missing (except for in vitro hybridization techniques). The lack of morphology and the high sensitivity of mRNA measurement by PCR imply that small amounts of normal cells expressing the receptors may erroneously suggest that they are the main target. Since most tissue samples are highly heterogeneous from a cellular point of view, it is better to use a morphological method for receptor analysis. It is also preferable to detect the receptor protein itself and, if possible, the receptor-binding sites in these proteins, since the binding sites represent the functional molecular basis for peptide hormones. A "gold standard" example is in vitro quantitative somatostatin receptor autoradiography on frozen tissue sections that combines morphology, binding site detection, and receptor quantification. Because of limited cellular resolution, receptor autoradiography is optimal for the detection of receptors in larger cell groups. An attractive alternative is immunohistochemical analysis of the receptors on formalin-fixed tissues with the limitations that quantification is not possible and that an epitope that may be different from the binding site is identified. The existence of subtypes for G protein-coupled receptors has made the evaluation of receptors more complex.

Perspective

The endocrine gut was developed and also recognized before the so-called classic endocrine organs. It was the discovery of secretin by Bayliss and Starling that founded the concept of endocrinology and hormones. Nevertheless, gut endocrinology has for decades been considered only an appendix to general endocrinology. Today, however, we know that the gut releases more than 100 hormone-like peptides expressed in a cell-specific manner all over the body. The peptides participate in intercellular regulation from the local control of growth and cell differentiation to acute systemic effects on metabolism all over the body. Thus, a revolution has changed the fundamental concepts over the last decades and opened wide perspectives for therapy with gut hormone analogues in human diseases.

Gut hormones must be viewed as evolutionarily conserved intercellular messengers of general significance. There are no obvious boundaries between their role in food intake and digestion and their function in other bodily regulations. Most regulatory peptides (cytokines, growth factors, hormones, myokines, and neuropeptides) are probably expressed in the gut, at least at some stage in the phylogenetic or ontogenetic development. Hence, gut endocrinology may continue to grow. On the other hand, such extension almost deprives the concept of *gut* endocrinology of its meaning. And that is exactly what it is about: gut hormones should be viewed not only as local hormones of specific interest to digestive physiologists and clinical gastroenterologists. They are chemical messengers integrated in the coordination and regulation of many or most bodily functions. Thus, it is not surprising that today gut hormones are studied not only in physiology and cell biology but also by microbiologists, psychiatrists, zoologists, cardiologists, diabetologists, and others.

Summary

This chapter emphasizes that the gastrointestinal tract is the largest and oldest endocrine organ in the body. It enlists individual gut hormones, their defining activities and their receptors, but it also describes general biological features of the hormones such as the structural homology, multiple phenotypes, extraintestinal expression, cell-specific prohormone processing and differentiated secretion. The concluding message is that gut hormonal peptides should be viewed as general intercellular messengers rather than just local regulators confined to the gut.

Acknowledgment The skillful and patient secretarial assistance of Connie Bundgaard is gratefully acknowledged.

Cross-References

- ▶ G Protein-Coupled Receptors
- ▶ Synthesis, Secretion, and Transport of Peptide Hormones
- ▶ Targeting of Steroid Hormone Receptor Function in Breast and Prostate Cancer
- ▶ The Endocrine Pancreas
- ▶ The Endocrine System

References

Amara SG, Jonas V, Rosenfeld MG, Onges ES, Evans RM. Alternative RNA processing in calcitonin gene expression generates mRNAs encoding different polypeptide products. Nature. 1982;298:240–4.

Anastasi A, Erspamer V, Endean R. Isolation and amino acid sequence of caerulein, the active decapeptide of the skin of hyla caerulea. Arch Biochem Biophys. 1968;125:57–68.

Bayliss WM, Starling EH. The mechanism of pancreatic secretion. J Physiol. 1902;28:325–53.

Bell GI, Santerre RF, Müllenbach GT. Hamster preproglucagon contains the sequence of glucagon and two related peptides. Nature. 1983;302:716–8.

Bundgaard JR, Vuust J, Rehfeld JF. Tyrosine O-sulfation promotes proteolytic processing of progastrin. EMBO J. 1995;14:3073–9.

Doolittle RF, Feng DF, Tsang S, Cho G, Little E. Determining divergence times of the major kingdoms of living organisms with a protein clock. Science. 1996;271:470–7.

Edkins JS. The chemical mechanism of gastric secretion. J Physiol. 1906;34:133–44.

Glover ID, Barlow DJ, Pitts JE, Wood SP, Tickle IJ, Blundell TL, et al. Conformational studies on the pancreatic polypeptide hormone family. Eur J Biochem. 1984;142:379–85.

Harper AA, Raper HS. Pancreozymin, a stimulation of the secretion of pancreatic enzymes in extracts of the small intestine. J Physiol. 1943;102:115–25.

Holst JJ, Ørskov C, Nielsen OV, Schwartz TW. Truncated glucagon-like peptide-I, an insulin-releasing hormone from the distal gut. FEBS Lett. 1987;211:169–74.

Ivy AC, Oldberg E. A hormone mechanism for gallbladder contraction and evacuation. Am J Physiol. 1928;86:599–613.

Johnsen AH, Rehfeld JF. Cionin: a di-sulfotyrosyl hybrid of cholecystokinin and gastrin from the protochordate, Ciona intestinalis. J Biol Chem. 1990;265:3054–8.

Jorpes JE, Mutt V. Cholecystokinin and pancreozymin, one single hormone? Acta Physiol Scand. 1966;66:196–202.

Kopin AS, Wheeler MB, Nishtani J, McBride EW, Chang TM, Chey WY, et al. The secretin gene: evolutionary history, alternative splicing and developmental regulation. Proc Natl Acad Sci U S A. 1991;88:5335–9.

Larsson LI, Goltermann N, de Magistris L, Rehfeld JF, Schwartz TW. Somatostatin cell processes as pathways for paracrine secretion. Science. 1979;205:1393–5.

Li M, Mbikay M, Nakayama K, Miyata A, Arimura A. Prohormone convertase PC4 processes the precursor of PACAP in the testis. Ann N Y Acad Sci. 2000;921:333–9.

Mojsov S, Weir GC, Habener JF. Insulintropin: glucagon-like peptide I (7-37) co-encoded in the glucagon gene is a potent stimulator of insulin release in the perfused rat pancreas. J Clin Invest. 1987;79:616–9.

Nawa H, Kotani H, Nakanishi S. Tissue-specific generation of two preprotachykinin mRNAs from one gene by alternative RNA splicing. Nature. 1984;312:729–34.

Persson H, Rehfeld JF, Ericsson A, Schalling M, Pelto-Huikko M, Hökfelt T. Transient expression of the cholecystokinin gene in male germ cells and accumulation of the peptide in the acrosomal granule: possible role of cholecystokinin in fertilization. Proc Natl Acad Sci U S A. 1989;86:6166–70.

Rehfeld JF. The new biology of gastrointestinal hormones. Physiol Rev. 1998;78:1087–108.

Rehfeld JF. Incretin physiology beyond glucagon-like peptide 1 and glucose-dependent insulinotropic polypeptide: cholecystokinin and gastrin peptides. Acta Physiol (Oxf). 2011;201:405–11.

Reubi JC. Peptide receptors as molecular targets for cancer diagnosis and therapy. Endocr Rev. 2003;24:389–427.

Rourke IJ, Rehfeld JF, Møller M, Johnsen AH. Characterization of the cholecystokinin and gastrin genes from the bullfrog, Rana catesbeiana: evolutionary conservation of primary and secondary sites of gene expression. Endocrinology. 1997;138:1719–27.

Schultz SG, Mackhlouf GM, Rauner BB, editors. Handbook of physiology. The gastrointestinal system. Neural and endocrine biology. Bethesda: American Physiology Society; 1989.

Shintani N, Mori W, Hashimoto H, Imai M, Tanaka K, Tomomoto S, et al. Defects in reproductive functions in PACAP-deficient female mice. Regul Pept. 2002;109:45–8.

Sporn MB, Roberts AB. Autocrine growth factors and cancer. Nature. 1985;313:745–7.

Starling EH. The Croonian lecture on the chemical correlation of the function of the body. Lancet. 1905;II:399–41.

Taché Y, Goto Y, Ohning G, editors. Gut-brain peptides in the new millennium. Los Angeles: Cure Foundation; 2002.

Walsh JH, Dockray GJ, editors. Gut peptides. New York: Raven; 1994.

The Endocrine Heart

20

Adolfo J. de Bold, John C. Burnett Jr., and Jens Peter Goetze

Abstract

Mammalian hearts express and secrete natriuretic peptides. Atrial natriuretic peptide (ANP) was the first to be identified in atria of rodents, and today the cardiac peptides consist of also the structurally related B-type natriuretic peptide – or BNP. Both peptide hormones have important hemodynamic properties including regulation of blood pressure and intravascular fluid hemostasis. As biomarkers, biosynthetic precursor fragments have gained a robust function in the assessment of human heart failure, where the markers are used primarily as exclusion markers. As drugs, both ANP and BNP, and derivatives of these peptides, seem promising as therapy in heart failure patients and in hypertension. Moreover, the cardiac peptide hormones may also possess organ-protective effects, where kidney function and cardiac remodeling seem in particular relevant.

Keywords

ANP • BNP • Heart • Heart failure • Natriuretic peptide • Regulatory peptide

---

A.J. de Bold (✉)
Department of Pathology and Laboratory Medicine, University of Ottawa, Faculty of Medicine, and the University of Ottawa, Heart Institute, Ottawa, ON, Canada
e-mail: adebold@bell.net

J.C. Burnett Jr.
Department of Cardiovascular Diseases, Cardiorenal Research Laboratory, Rochester, MN, USA
e-mail: burnett.john@mayo.edu

J.P. Goetze
Department of Clinical Biochemistry, Rigshospitalet, and University of Aarhus, Copenhagen, Denmark

Department of Clinical Medicine, Aarhus University, Aarhus, Denmark
e-mail: JPG@dadlnet.dk

A. Belfiore, D. LeRoith (eds.), *Principles of Endocrinology and Hormone Action*, Endocrinology, https://doi.org/10.1007/978-3-319-44675-2_20

Contents

Looking Back on Atrial Natriuretic Factor

Electron microscopic observations on cardiomyocytes of the atria of the mammalian heart during the early 1960s revealed cellular features additional to those earlier associated by light microscopy with classical striated cardiac muscle cell properties including excitation, conduction, and contraction. These additional features evident at the structural level included an abundant amount of rough endoplasmic reticulum, a highly developed Golgi complex, and storage granules, named specific atrial granules (Kisch 1963; Jamieson and Palade 1964) (Fig. 1). Morphologists associated these differentiations with a secretory function based on similarities with ultrastructural features found in cell types known to produce polypeptide hormones. However, the actual functional meaning of these cytological features in atrial cardiomyocytes remained a mystery for many years. That the heart produces polypeptide hormones that are secreted from atrial cardiomyocytes displaying bona fide morphological differentiations associated with polypeptide hormone-producing cells became established beginning with several findings based on new investigative techniques and the discovery of the natriuretic activity associated with atrial muscle extracts and the characterization of the natriuretic peptide (NP) family of hormones (de Bold 1978, 1979; de Bold et al. 1978, 1981; de Bold and Bencosme 1973, 1975a, b).

The four premises that led to the discovery of the natriuretic activity of atrial (rat) myocardium extracts obtained by injecting such extracts into bioassay rats were as follows: (1) Histochemical and radioautographic investigations suggested that the specific atrial granules contained a basic polypeptide with a random coil conformation, sulfur amino acids, and tryptophan (de Bold et al. 1978; de Bold and Bencosme 1975a, b). (2) An unbiased morphometric technique (de Bold 1978) showed that the number of specific atrial granules changed with manipulations of the water and electrolyte balance in rats (de Bold 1979). (3) The hypothesis that, because the specific number of granules changed with water and electrolyte balance, a hypothetical hormone contained in the granules might be related to kidney function given the pivotal role of this organ in the homeostatic control of such balance. (4) Extracts of the ventricles, which display no granules in the bulk of cardiomyocytes, would provide for a control injection into the bioassay rats.

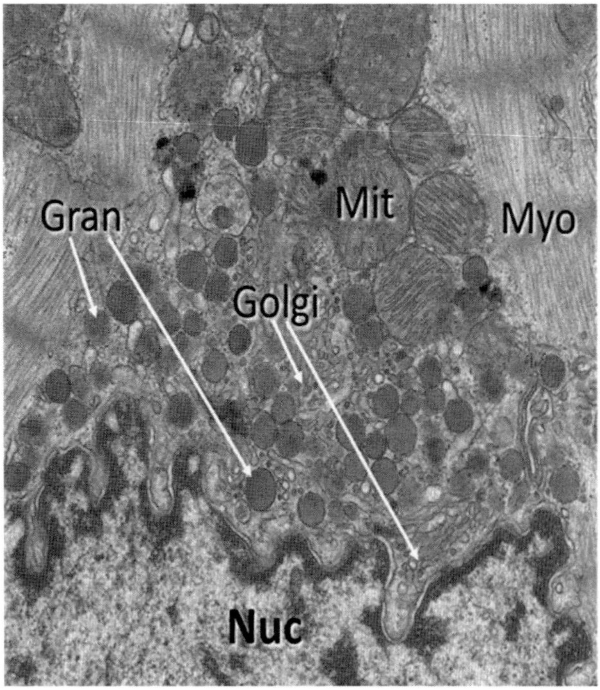

Fig. 1 Transmission electron microscopy of a portion of a mouse atrial cardiomyocyte showing a portion of the nucleus (*Nuc*) as well as mitochondria (*Mit*), myofibrils (*Myo*), Golgi complex (*Golgi*), and specific atrial granules (*Gran*). Original magnification: 5,000×

The renal response to an injection of atrial extract into bioassay rats was nothing short of spectacular in terms of diuresis and natriuresis, while little or no response was seen after injection of ventricular extracts (de Bold et al. 1981). It was quite obvious that an atrial natriuretic factor (ANF) was found. The potential importance of ANF resulted in a flurry of research on the physiological, pharmacological, biochemical, and other aspects of the discovery, resulting in an enormous amount of literature (Table 1). Also, the efforts to impose names on the new substance were numerous, but at present perhaps the most commonly used name is ANP even though the nomenclature agreed upon the designated name ANF as the official one (Dzau et al. 1987a, b).

In 1983, ANP – a 28-amino acid peptide that is the circulating form of this hormone – was isolated, purified, and sequenced from rat atrial tissue (de Bold and Flynn 1983; Flynn et al. 1983; Kennedy et al. 1984). The following year, ANP was isolated from human atria (Kangawa and Matsuo 1984). Tissue fractionation studies and immunocytochemistry demonstrated that ANP was associated with the specific atrial granules, thus confirming the view that these organelles contained a polypeptide hormone (de Bold 1982; de Bold and de Bold 1985). Following the discovery of ANP, structurally related peptides, including brain natriuretic peptide (BNP) (Sudoh et al. 1988) and C-type natriuretic peptide (CNP) (Kojima et al. 1990), were identified, thus establishing a natriuretic peptide (NP) family. NPs form a family of hormones based on the shared presence of a 17-amino acid ring structure

Table 1 The principal biological actions of ANP and BNP

Kidney	Glomerular filtration ↑
	Collecting duct sodium reabsorption ↓
	Diuresis and natriuresis ↑
Nervous system	Sympathetic nerve activity ↓
	Salt and water appetite ↓
Vasopressin ↓	
Heart	Cardiomyocyte hypertrophy ↓
	Cardiac fibrosis ↓
Vascular	Vascular smooth muscle proliferation ↓
	Vascular smooth muscle tone ↓
	Vascular regeneration ↑
RAAS[a]	RAAS ↓
Adipose tissue	Lipolysis ↑
Immune system	Pro-inflammatory cytokines↓

[a]*RAAS* renin angiotensin aldosterone system

formed by an intramolecular disulfide linkage. CNP is mainly expressed in the central nervous system and the endothelium. Even though these peptides are referred to as NPs, CNP lacks natriuretic activity due to the lack of a C-terminal sequence that is required for such activity to be present. CNP is also considered to be an autocrine or paracrine acting hormone. On the other hand, ANP and BNP are true cardiac (atrial in mammals) hormones. However, some degree of NP expression is found in virtually all cell types. Curiously, in the specific atrial granules, ANP is stored as the 28-amino acid-circulating hormone, while BNP is stored as its prohormone (proBNP). The circulating form of ANP is highly homologous among different mammalian species. Circulating BNPs from different species have a relatively lower degree of evolutionary homology. CNP displays the highest degree of homology among mammalian species (Table 2) and is considered to be the ancestor gene.

By northern blot analysis, immunocytochemistry, in situ hybridization, radioimmunoassay, and oligonucleotide array, ANP and BNP are far more abundant in the atria than the ventricles. Within the atria, ANP is by order of magnitude more abundant than BNP. The expression of NP in the ventricles is significant in the mammalian fetal heart and in the hypertrophic ventricles. However, the level of expression in the latter is still below that of the atria. BNP is sometimes characterized as a ventricular hormone, while ANP is viewed as an atrial hormone. This is an erroneous concept. The ANP concentration in normal subjects in atrium and ventricle is 9,600 and 37 pmol/g, respectively, whereas the BNP concentration in the atria and ventricles is 250 and 18 pmol/g, respectively (Mukoyama et al. 1991). Even taking into account the differences in mass between atria and ventricles, it is not possible to conclude that BNP is a ventricular hormone. Transcript abundance for atrial and ventricular ANP and BNP closely mirrors peptide abundance (Bianciotti and de Bold 2001; Yokota et al. 1995).

Table 2 Primary structure of various mammalian natriuretic peptides

Name	Sequence of mature hormones	Ref.
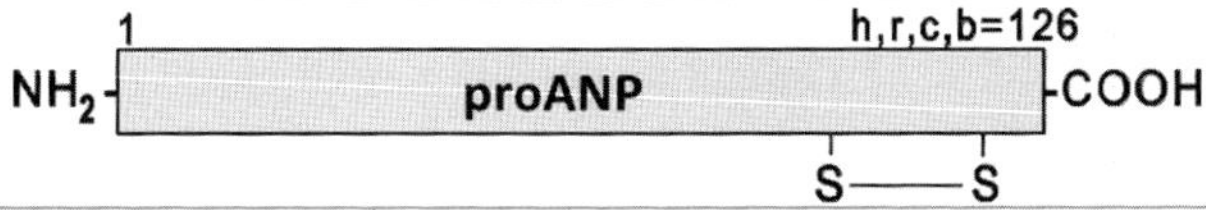		
$rANF_{99\text{-}126}$, rat (rodent)	Ser-Leu-Arg-Arg-Ser-Ser-**Cys**-Phe-Gly-Gly-Arg-Ile-Asp-Arg-Ile-Gly-Ala-Gln-Ser-Gly-Leu-Gly-**Cys**-Asn-Ser-Phe-Arg-Tyr	Burnett et al. (1986)
$hANF_{99\text{-}126}$ human, canine, bovine	Ser-Leu-Arg-Arg-Ser-Ser-**Cys**-Phe-Gly-Gly-Arg-Met-Asp-Arg-Ile-Gly-Ala-Gln-Ser-Gly-Leu-Gly-**Cys**-Asn-Ser-Phe- Arg-Tyr	Canaff et al. (1996)
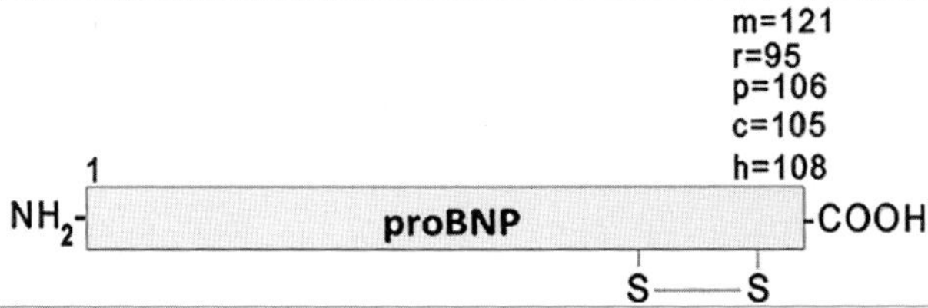		
BNP 45, rat = $rBNP_{51\text{–}95}$	Ser-Gln-Asp-Ser-Ala-Phe-Arg-Ile-Gln-Glu-Arg-Leu-Arg-Asn-Ser-Lys-Met-Ala-His-Ser-Ser-Ser-**Cys**-Phe-Gly-Gln-Lys-Ile-Asp-Arg-Ile-Gly-Ala-Val-Ser-Arg-Leu-Gly-**Cys**-Asp-Gly-Leu-Arg-Leu-Phe	Dschietzig et al. (2001)
BNP 32, human = $hBNP_{77\text{–}108}$	Ser-Pro-Lys-Met-Val-Gln-Gly-Ser-Gly-**Cys**-Phe-Gly-Arg-Lys-Met-Asp-Arg-Ile-Ser-Ser-Ser-Ser-Gly-Leu-Gly-**Cys**-Lys-Val-Leu-Arg-Arg-His	Dzau et al. (1987a, b)
BNP 32 canine = $cBNP_{74\text{–}105}$	Ser-Pro-Lys-Met-Met-His-Lys-Ser-Gly-**Cys**-Phe-Gly-Arg-Arg-Leu-Asp-Arg-Ile-Gly-Ser-Leu-Ser-Gly-Leu-Gly-**Cys**-Asn-Val-Leu-Arg-Lys-Tyr	Dzau et al. (1987b)
BNP 45, mouse = $mBNP_{77\text{–}121}$	Ser-Gln-Gly-Ser-Thr-Leu-Arg-Val-Gln-Gln-Arg-Pro-Gln-Asn-Ser-Lys-Val-Thr-His-Ile-Ser-Ser-**Cys**-Phe-Gly-His-Lys-Ile-Asp-Arg-Ile-Gly-Ser-Val-Ser-Arg-Leu-Gly-**Cys**-Asn-Ala-Leu-Lys-Leu-Leu	Edwards et al. (1988)
Porcine $BNP_{75\text{–}106}$	Ser-Pro-Lys-Thr-Met-Arg-Asp-Ser-Gly-**Cys**-Phe-Gly-Arg-Arg-Leu-Asp-Arg-Ile-Gly-Ser-Leu-Ser-Gly-Leu-Gly-**Cys**-Asn-Val-Leu-Arg-Arg-Tyr	Cataliotti et al. (2008)
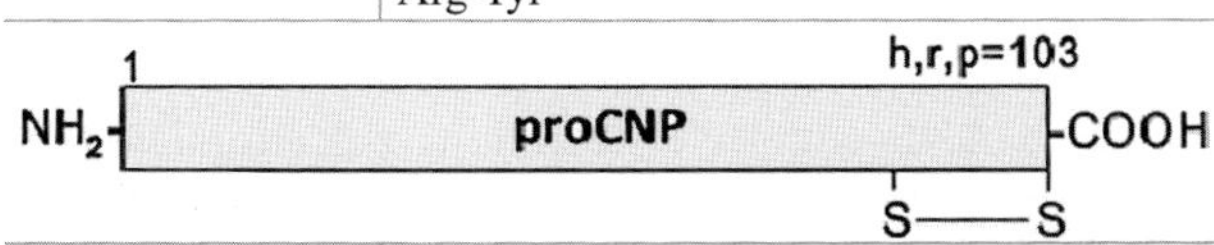		
CNP 22, h, r, p = $CNP_{82\text{–}103}$	Gly-Leu-Ser-Lys-Gly-**Cys**-Phe-Gly-Leu-Lys-Leu-Asp-Arg-Ile-Gly-Ser-Met-Ser-Gly-Leu-Gly-**Cys**	Cataliotti et al. (2011) and Flynn et al. (1983)

c canine, *h* human, *m* mouse, *p* porcine, *r* rat

Humans with left ventricular (LV) hypertrophy show that the abnormal circulating levels of ANP and BNP are significantly derived from atrial sources (Murakami et al. 2002). Lastly, replacement of the failing ventricle in orthotropic heart transplantation in humans does not result in normalization of either ANP or BNP even after other endocrine and cardiovascular parameters return to normal (Masters et al. 1993). These findings underscore that while there may be a good correlation between parameters such as ventricular hypertrophy, systolic failure, or ischemic events and ANP or BNP secretion, this secretion may not be considered of solely ventricular origin. In addition, physiopathologically ascribing increases of circulating ANP or BNP to increases in cardiac pressure or stretch are likely to be an oversimplification, as pressure without stretch does not result in increases in cardiac NP secretion as shown by investigations on cardiac tamponade (Klopfenstein et al. 1990; Vierhapper et al. 1989; Stokhof et al. 1994). Also, pathologies such as heart failure are well known to be associated with profound changes in the neuroendocrine environment that confound a hemodynamic-only interpretation of changes in NP concentrations in circulation during disease. Indeed, it can be demonstrated that there is a load-dependent and a load-independent component to the increase in NP gene expression in the hypertrophic heart (Ogawa et al. 1996) and that the correlation of NP blood levels with intracardiac pressures break down in advanced heart failure (Ogawa et al. 2005).

The ample spectrum of physiological effects of NP correlates well with the presence of their receptors in virtually all tissues (Kuhn 2003, 2004). The biologically active NP receptors are membrane-bound guanylyl cyclases-denominated "NPR-A" and "NPR-B." An NPR-C receptor appears to function as a clearance receptor (Ogawa et al. 1996; Ogawa and de Bold 2014). Oddly, the membrane-bound guanylyl cyclase was an orphan receptor until ANP was discovered (Chinkers et al. 1989). The NPR-A receptor binds both ANP and BNP, while the NPR-B receptor binds CNP. Activation of these receptors by their ligands induces production of intracellular cyclic GMP (cGMP), which, in turn, regulates the activity of various cGMP-sensitive effectors including ion channels, phosphodiesterases, and protein kinases. An increase in circulating cGMP, which is the result of cellular spillover of NP-receptor interaction in target cells, is thus a hallmark of such an interaction.

It is still an unsolved curiosity that ANP and BNP that share biological properties as well as storage site also share the same receptor type. It is, however, possible that a differentiation between these two NPs is made at the level of secretory stimuli as follows. Both ANP and BNP secretions are stimulated by regulatory peptides that signal through Gq-coupled receptors (e.g., endothelin, angiotensin II) and by muscle stretch, which is transduced by mechanisms involving Gi/o signaling (Ogawa et al. 1999; Bensimon et al. 2004). Unlike ANP, however, BNP secretion is also stimulated by some cytokines. This secretion is p38 MAPK inhibition sensitive (Ogawa and de Bold 2012; Ma et al. 2004; Meirovich et al. 2008). Striking examples of the differential secretory response of BNP vs ANP to cytokine stimulation may be seen in inflammatory states such as during human cardiac allograft rejection, lipopolysaccharide treatment, and in autoimmune myocarditis (Ogawa et al. 2005, 2008; Ogawa and de Bold 2012; Ma et al. 2004). These differences should possibly be of interest to those working on therapeutic applications of NP as well as those using NP blood levels as biomarkers of cardiovascular health (Ramos and de Bold 2006).

Circulating ANP and BNP in Heart Failure: The Birth of Heart Failure Biomarkers

Following de Bold's discovery of the heart as an endocrine organ and the production of atrial natriuretic peptide (ANP) with its natriuretic properties, our group at Mayo Clinic sought to first define circulating ANP in human heart failure (HF) (de Bold et al. 1981). Initially, studies in a hamster model of dilated cardiomyopathy suggested that ANP was deficient in HF with reduced atrial granules in the failing heart, which was mistakenly interpreted as reduced ANP production (Chimoskey et al. 1984). Specifically, our group developed a highly sensitive radioimmunoassay to measure circulating ANP concentrations and performed key studies in normal humans and in humans with mild, moderate, and severe HF including determining atrial pressures using cardiac catheterization (Burnett et al. 1986). In this seminal work, the progressive increase in circulating ANP associated with increasing atrial pressures and atrial stretch was reported (Fig. 2). These studies established the activation of the ANP hormonal system in human HF, followed by multiple studies by independent groups that B-type natriuretic peptide (BNP) is also increased in human HF plasma, including increased production in the ventricular myocardium in contrast to ANP (Muriokaya et al. 1992; (Edwards et al. 1988; Wei et al. 1993). Unlike ANP and BNP, circulating CNP is not increased in human HF (Wei et al. 1993).

The elevation of ANP and BNP in HF raised the question of the role of natriuretic peptide (NP) activation in a disease syndrome characterized by sodium and water retention and congestion. Physiological studies were thus performed in large animal models of HF that were designed to induce reductions in cardiac output but also to inhibit or impair the release of ANP (Lee et al. 1989; Stevens et al. 1995). When

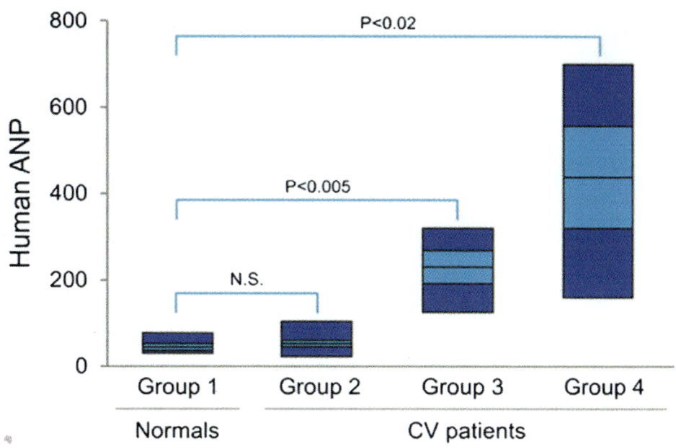

Fig. 2 Circulating ANP in normal humans and in humans with increasing severity of heart failure

cardiac output was reduced in a canine model of HF, and atrial stretch and ANP release were prevented, impaired renal function with sodium retention with activation of aldosterone was noted. When ANP was infused into the model of low ANP to produce circulating levels of ANP observed in HF, sodium retention and increases in aldosterone were reversed. In a second study in experimental HF, surgically removed atrial appendages of the heart, in order to limit the release of ANP, were examined (Stevens et al. 1995). When chronic HF was induced, the onset of sodium retention was more rapid with greater activation of both renin release by the kidney and aldosterone release by the adrenal glands in the ANP-deficient model. Furthermore, infusion of an NP receptor antagonist blocking the ANP receptor (NPR-A) in the atrial appendage also resulted in sodium retention and RAAS activation. Taken together, early activation of ANP in the evolution of HF has a compensatory role to maintain renal function and sodium homeostasis and retard RAAS despite reductions in cardiac output. During the transition to overt and severe experimental HF, the kidney, with more chronic reductions in renal perfusion pressure, right ventricular failure, and high venous pressure and gradual activation of the RAAS, is characterized by a relative renal resistance to ANP through impaired second messenger production (i.e., cGMP) in the kidney (Margulies et al. 1991; Supaporn et al. 1996). Thus, in end-stage HF, there is a relative renal escape from the renoprotective actions of ANP.

Altered Processing and Molecular Forms of Natriuretic Peptides in Heart Failure

The elevations of circulating ANP and BNP, including their precursor structures proANP and proBNP in HF, have contributed to their development as biomarkers in the diagnosis and prognosis of HF. Yet, contributing to an impaired compensatory role in maintaining overall cardiorenal function in HF has been the release of altered molecular forms of the NPs in advanced human HF with reduced biological activity contributing to a concept of the "natriuretic peptide endocrine paradox" (Goetze et al. 2003).

One of the first insights into altered processing as well as degradation of the NPs in HF was the key study of Hawkridge (Hawkridge et al. 2005). Here, mass spectrometry was used to characterize the presence or absence of mature BNP in plasma of patients with advanced HF with a high circulating BNP concentration by the use of conventional assays, the latter of which are insensitive to altered molecular forms of BNP. We reported the absence of mature BNP in human HF. This led to the conclusion that commonly used diagnostic assays to measure BNP must cross-react with precursor molecular forms such as proBNP. Indeed, studies have clearly established that proBNP is the predominant molecular form of the NPs that circulate in HF (Liang et al. 2007). Further, repeated studies have established that proBNP has markedly reduced NP receptor-activating properties when compared to mature BNP, underscoring that in HF altered molecular forms of BNP with reduced biological activity may be a mechanism for impaired renal function and RAAS activation

(Heublein et al. 2007; Huntley et al. 2015). Studies are ongoing to better define proANP in human HF. Most importantly, proANP in contrast to proBNP is a robust activator of the NPR-A which may have both diagnostic and therapeutic implications in HF (Ichiki et al. 2015). Nonetheless, the altered processing and degradation of molecular forms of the NPs in HF support the rational for the therapeutic use of either native NPs or the development of novel new generation designer NPs.

Therapeutic Use of ANP and BNP in Heart Failure

Recombinant ANP and BNP are, respectively, carperitide and nesiritide that have been approved for the treatment of acute HF. Based on initial studies from large clinical trials such as the VMAC Trial (Intravenous nesiritide, J Am Med Assoc 2002), BNP (nesiritide) was approved in the USA and widely used as an acute intravenous agent for acute HF. Approval of recombinant BNP (nesiritide) was based upon an improvement of dyspnea and a reduction in cardiac filling pressure compared to the vasodilator nitroglycerine that also acts through the second messenger cyclic GMP. Further clinical trials – especially the ASCEND trials which consisted of 7,000 subjects worldwide with acute HF who were randomized to either nesiritide or conventional therapy – reported there were no safety issues with nesiritide but that nesiritide therapy was neither superior to conventional therapy with a major adverse effect of hypotension (O'Connor et al. 2011).

A strategic advancement, however, in the further development of BNP as an NPR-A activator in HF was the realization that chronic BNP delivered locally to the heart or systemically through subcutaneous administration resulted in structural and functional improvements in the setting of experimental or human HF. In experimental hypertensive heart disease, which is present in the spontaneously hypertensive rat, novel gene delivery of proBNP which was processed then to mature BNP using an AAV9 cardiotropic gene delivery vector overexpressed BNP production in the rodent heart for 9 months following one injection systemically (Cataliotti et al. 2011). Chronic overexpression of BNP in the heart improved myocardial structure and function and also improved survival in this genetic model of hypertension. A seminal advance was in human HF in which Chen et al. treated patients with stable chronic HF with subcutaneous injection of BNP twice daily for 8 weeks (Chen et al. 2012). Endpoints were safety, clinical status, renal function, and myocardial function and structure. In this placebo controlled, randomized clinical study, chronic subcutaneous BNP improved LV mass by MRI and improved cardiac volumes in both systole and diastole. Symptoms were improved, renal function was preserved, and there was suppression of the renin angiotensin system. Most recently, studies have reported that 3 months of subcutaneous BNP to patients with preclinical systolic and diastolic dysfunction improved renal function and cardiorenal response to intravascular volume overload (McKie et al. 2016). Thus, chronic stimulation of NPR-A with native NPs have a therapeutic potential in the treatment of preclinical and symptomatic HF changing the paradigm of peptide therapeutics for human HF.

A key feature and requirement for successful NP therapeutics is the delivery of the peptide especially to facilitate chronic delivery. While still in early stages, in key studies by Cataliotti, the development of orally administered BNP by novel pegylation technology has been reported in experimental models (Cataliotti et al. 2007). A novel formation of pegylated BNP was readily absorbed and activated NPR-A with increases in plasma and urinary cyclic GMP and reductions in blood pressure. Further studies demonstrated that oral delivery of BNP could also have therapeutic potential in cardiovascular disease states such as experimental hypertension (Cataliotti et al. 2008). Natriuretic effects complimented enhancing actions on cyclic GMP and blood pressure.

Designer Natriuretic Peptides for Heart Failure

Advances in peptide engineering have provided strategies and technologies to modify native peptides to enhance receptor activation and/or to produce enhancements in pharmacokinetics or unique biological actions not present in native peptides. Cenderitide (CDNP) represents the most clinically advanced designer NP currently under clinical development for HF (Lisy et al. 2008; (Lee et al. 2009). Designed at the Mayo Clinic, Cenderitide was engineered to coactivate the NPR-A receptor but also the NPR-B receptor, the latter that is the target of the endothelial derived peptide C-type natriuretic peptide (CNP) (Dickey et al. 2009). A major goal was to produce a peptide that was less hypotensive than BNP or ANP that are more potent activators of NPR-A compared to Cenderitide as it is also well known that CNP is less hypotensive than ANP or BNP. Limiting hypotension in the treatment of HF would have more favorable renal actions, as marked reductions in renal perfusion pressure may impair renal function. Further, the design of Cenderitide also recognized that CNP lacks renal natriuretic actions (Clavell et al. 1993). Furthermore, as NPR-A activation also has aldosterone suppressing actions while NPR-B activation has endothelium enhancing and anti-fibrotic properties, Cenderitide represents a transformational advance in NP engineering.

The structure of Cenderitide (Fig. 3) fuses the mature 22-amino acid CNP with the 15-amino acid C-terminus of DNP which is derived from the mature peptide DNP isolated from the green mamba snake and a potent NPR-A activator (Schweitz et al. 1992). Extensive modeling and production of CDNP mutants demonstrated the superiority of CDNP to other novel CDNP like peptides establishing the structural requirement of the full mature CNP with the 15-amino acid sequence of DNP as a prerequisite for co-receptor activation (Lee et al. 2016). Further, this recent study demonstrated that Cenderitide activates cyclic GMP in isolated glomeruli and possesses potent GFR enhancing and natriuretic effects in addition to suppression of aldosterone, unlike CNP via NPR-B. These properties were clearly demonstrated in the first-in-human study of Cenderitide in normal human volunteers (Lee et al. 2009).

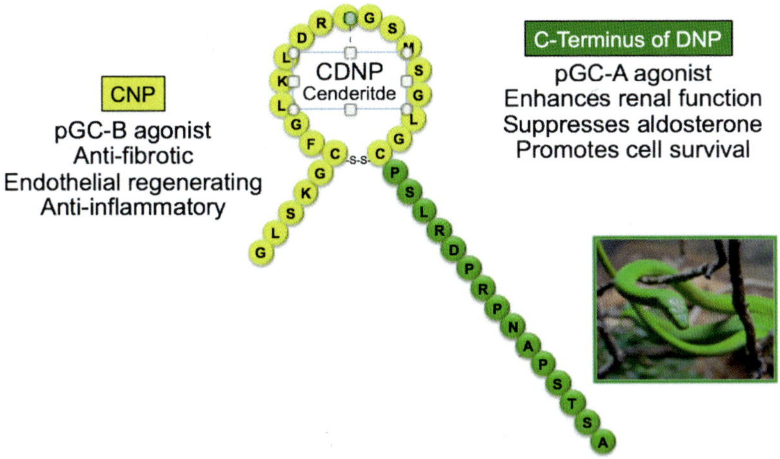

Fig. 3 Structure of Cenderitide (*CDNP*). Fusion of mature 22-amino acid CNP with the C-terminus of DNP resulting in a novel designer peptide which coactivates NPR-A and NPR-B

In experimental studies in human failing myocardium, the rational for CDNP in HF is strengthened by the upregulation of the NPR-B receptor and reduced production of CNP as recently reported by Ichiki et al. (2015). Further, Cenderitide compared to either BNP or CNP was also superior in inhibiting collagen production in human cardiac fibroblasts. In the model of mild left ventricular diastolic dysfunction with early mild cardiac fibrosis, chronic Cenderitide suppressed the development of both cardiac fibrosis and diastolic dysfunction (Martin et al. 2012). Several clinical studies are underway related to Cenderitide in HF. These include the targeting of patients with post-acute HF and impaired renal function to preserve renal function and delay the progression of HF. Studies are also underway to administer Cenderitide to patients with acute myocardial infarction to preserve LV systolic function and prevent the development of post-acute HF. Finally, it is now recognized that left ventricular assist mechanical devices (LVADs) while improving cardiac hemodynamics may induce further cardiac fibrosis and remodeling. Therefore, studies are also underway to assess the therapeutic potential of Cenderitide as a co-therapy with LVAD therapy to reduce the development of cardiac fibrosis and remodeling as well as to facilitate possible myocardial recovery.

Like oral delivery of BNP, novel delivery systems are being developed for Cenderitide. In current clinical trials, the OmniPod insulin delivery system is being employed to chronically administer subcutaneous Cenderitide in patients with HF. In experimental models of cardiovascular disease, novel nanoparticle gel polymer strategies are being tested (Lim et al. 2013). Further, novel film delivery system in which Cenderitide is released from a patch-like device around the heart is also being tested (XW et al. 2013). With the advent of highly innovative delivery systems, chronic delivery of Cenderitide or designer NPs will continue to emerge.

MANP for the Prevention of Heart Failure

Hypertension remains the leading cause of HF, and strategies to reduce HF are a high health care priority. The newest generation designer NP currently entering clinical trials is MANP which is a best-in-class NPR-A activator. The goal in the development of MANP was to engineer a designer NP to prevent HF by targeting high-risk populations who are at increased risk of future HF (McKie et al. 2012). MANP recently completed a first-in-human study in resistant-like hypertensive subjects. This initial trial recognizes resistant hypertension as the leading risk for the development of future HF, far exceeding other comorbidities (Calhoun et al. 2008).

Based upon genomic insights, MANP was engineered as a 40-amino acid peptide with the structure of the mature 28-amino acid ANP fused to a novel 12-amino acid carboxyl terminal extension (McKie et al. 2009). This novel C-terminal extension renders MANP highly resistant to degradation by neprilysin and thus represents an alternative to a nonspecific neprilysin enzyme inhibitor strategy (Dickey et al. 2009). MANP has the attractive biological properties of both resistance to neprilysin degradation with specific and direct ligand activation of NPR-A. MANP also has more sustained natriuretic, aldosterone suppressing, and blood pressure-lowering actions than native ANP (McKie et al. 2009). MANP markedly increases circulating and urinary cyclic GMP and is highly effective in reducing blood pressure in experimental hypertension (McKie et al. 2010). Both experimental and first-in-human studies suggest that MANP is a potent aldosterone inhibitor reducing the secretion of aldosterone. Experimental studies with native ANP and its interaction with the mineralocorticoid receptor (MR) would also suggest that MANP might also have direct actions to inhibit the MR (Nakagawa et al. 2014). Further, in a model of acute HF in the setting of hypertension, MANP is more effective than nitroglycerine in augmenting sodium excretion and preserving GFR, unloading the heart and suppressing aldosterone (McKie et al. 2014, 2016).

As important to peptide therapeutics as peptide design is the need to develop novel peptide delivery platforms (Fosgerau and Hoffmann 2015). Studies are underway to develop novel strategies to chronically deliver MANP in a formulation which results in sustained delivery. Like antidiabetic drugs such as GLP1 analogs, fatty acids can be linked to MANP, resulting in sustained delivery and prolonged activation of cyclic GMP. Ongoing studies also suggest that advanced peptide engineering can also result in gain of function of MANP to the NPR-A (Buglioni et al. 2016). Thus, in these exciting days of biotechnology, engineering peptides such as MANP provide potentially greater clinical efficacy in the treatment of human disease and yet retain highly specific receptor-mediated actions that contribute to safety as well as efficacy.

From Prohormone to Natriuretic Peptide

Human atrial (ANP) and B-type natriuretic peptide (BNP) are encoded by two genes colocated on chromosome 1 (Yang-Feng et al. 1985; Arden et al. 1995). The overall gene structure resembles other peptide hormone genes in size and composition with three exons separated by two introns. For both ANP and BNP, the major part of the coding sequence is located in exon 2. Genetic polymorphism has been reported in both genes as well as in the corresponding receptor genes (Lanfear 2010). Although the impact of genetic variation in the natriuretic peptide systems remains to be fully explored, it seems that it affects plasma concentrations in a heritable manner, which has been demonstrated in the general population (Wang et al. 2003). A common polymorphism in the BNP promoter region has also been associated to the prevalence of type 2 diabetes (Meirhaeghe et al. 2007). Conversely, diabetes mellitus induces increased risk for the development of cardiovascular disease with concomitant changes in cardiac natriuretic peptide expression (Christoffersen et al. 2007). A frameshift mutation in the ANP gene has been noted in heritable atrial fibrillation, where the frameshift introduces a C-terminally extended ANP peptide (Hodgson-Zingman et al. 2008).

Human proBNP comprises 108-amino acid residues. Mammalian precursor sequences have been deduced from cDNA sequences that encode the entire preprostructure (Sudoh et al. 1989; Steinhelper 1993; (Asano et al. 1999; Liu et al. 2002). Amino acid homology between species is confined to the amino- and carboxy-terminal regions, whereas the remaining prostructure varies considerably between animals (which as earlier noted is in contrast to a well-conserved primary structure of proANP). In addition to proBNP, human preproBNP contains an N-terminal hydrophobic signal peptide of 26-amino acid residues. As with most regulatory peptides, this sequence is removed during translation before the synthesis of the C-terminal part of the precursor is completed. PreproBNP does, therefore, not circulate as a separate entity but is only a theoretical structure. On the other hand, proBNP is an existing polypeptide, which has been indicated by chromatographic profiling and sequence-specific immunoassays (Hunt et al. 1995; Schulz et al. 2001; (Goetze et al. 2002; Giuliani et al. 2006; Seferian et al. 2007; Liang et al. 2007). The precursor molecule still remains to be purified together with the processing intermediates thereof – apart from the C-terminal cleavage product, i.e., BNP 32, and the N-terminal region of the precursor (Hino et al. 1990; Minamino et al. 1988; Flynn et al. 1989; Aburaya et al. 1989; Kambayashi et al. 1990).

The posttranslational phase of proBNP expression has become a subject of renewed interest. Recent advances through mass spectrometry combined with the development of sequence-specific antibodies have revealed a surprisingly complex cardiac biosynthesis of natriuretic peptides. The human proBNP structure, for instance, appears simple at first glance. It is divided into two principal regions by a cleavage site in position 73–76 (Arg-Ala-Pro-Arg) (Fig. 4). One region thus comprises the N-terminal fragment proBNP 1–76, and the second region is the bioactive part, e.g., the C-terminal BNP 32 (proBNP 77–108). The C-terminal region contains a ring structure formed by a disulfide bond between the cystyl residues in position 86 and 102, respectively. This modification in both ANP and BNP syntheses takes place in the endoplasmic reticulum and may be considered the first step in posttranslational processing, apart from the cleavage of the signal peptide, which happens during translation. The protein disulfide isomerase family and thiol-disulfide oxidoreductases are candidate enzymes involved in this disulfide bond

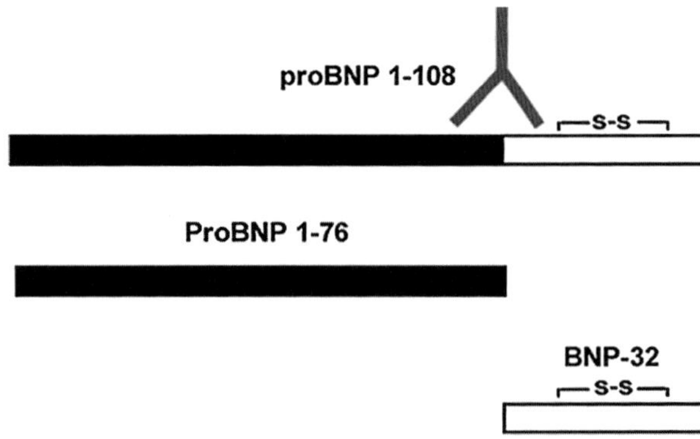

Fig. 4 Immunoassay for the detection of unprocessed human proBNP. The assay utilizes antibody recognition of an epitope spanning the Arg-Ala-Pro-Arg site (proBNP 74–76) thought to be cleaved by Corin Giuliani et al. (2006)

formation, where cardiac expression of the isomerase transcript has been reported to be upregulated in cardiac disease (Severino et al. 2007). Cellular experiments also suggest a direct cardioprotective effect of this regulation, which may relate to natriuretic peptide synthesis. Regulation of protein disulfide isomerase has been classified as "endoplasmic reticulum stress," which is a hallmark of several pathological disorders including ischemic heart disease (Azfer et al. 2006).

Larger forms of BNP (big big BNP) than the purified BNP 32 were first noted in gel filtration studies of tissue and plasma from patients with cardiac disease (Hunt et al. 1995; Schulz et al. 2001; Goetze et al. 2002; Shimizu et al. 2002, 2003). Some data also suggested forms larger than the predicted precursor. A singular report suggested that proANP and proBNP can oligomerize through a leucine zipper-like motif in the mid-region (Seidler et al. 1999). Whether the odd elution patterns were mere artifacts or represented peptide binding to other molecules was nevertheless put aside when it was demonstrated that proBNP is an O-linked glycoprotein (Schellenberger et al. 2006). In the precursor structure, the mid-region (proBNP 36–71) contains seven seryl and threonyl residues, where O-linked glycosylation occurs either fully or partially (Fig. 5). This major modification of a polypeptide does apparently not affect the overall structure of the precursor (Crimmins and Kao 2008). No specific immunoassay has yet been developed against the glycosylated forms, and the ratio between glycosylated and non-glycosylated proBNP products can only be deduced from assays that specifically measure the non-glycosylated forms or cross-react with both forms. It should also be noted that the ANP precursor may be subject for glycosylation, albeit no report has so far documented such events.

The next step in posttranslational processing is endoproteolysis. Human proBNP was first suggested to be cleaved by the ubiquitous endoprotease furin (Sawada et al. 1995, Sawada et al. 1997b). The Arg-Ala-Pro-Arg motif in position 73–76 in human proBNP has been shown to be a target for furin-mediated cleavage. In fact, endoproteolytical processing can be blocked in vitro by inhibition of furin, and furin has been shown to be essential for maturation of the structurally related CNP (Wu et al. 2003). A novel protease named corin has been identified in human heart cDNA (Yan et al. 1999; Hooper et al. 2000). Corin is a serine protease that can cleave both proANP and proBNP in vitro, presumably at a similar cleavage site (Yan et al. 2000;

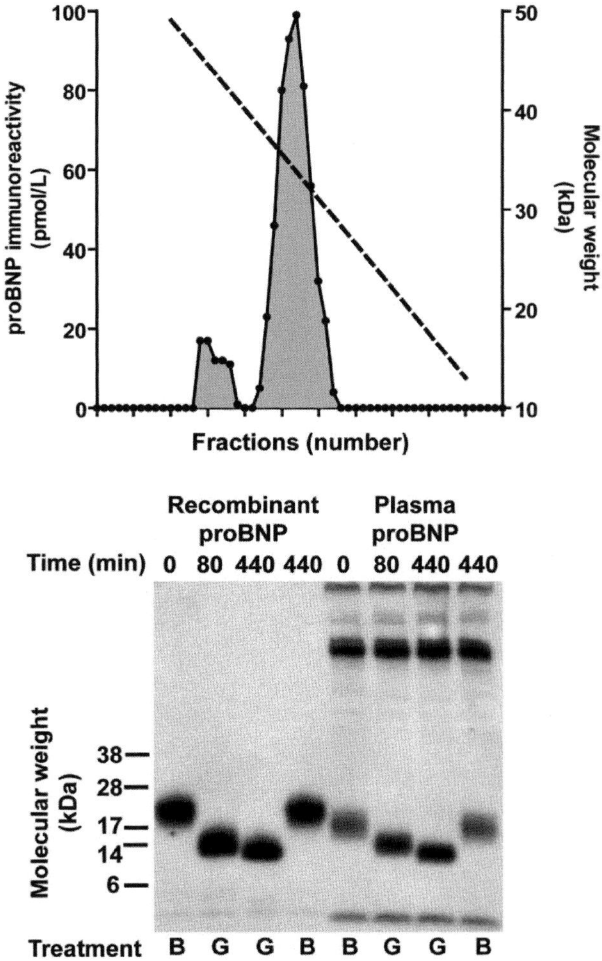

Fig. 5 The *upper panel* shows a chromatographic profile of proBNP immunoreactivity in human atrial tissue. Cardiac tissue extract was subjected to size-exclusion HPLC. Molecular size calibrators were eluted in a separate run. The proBNP immunoreactivity eluted in positions approximately three times higher than the theoretical molecular weight of intact proBNP. The lower panel displays western blotting of recombinant (*left*) and patient (*right* (*proBNP*) in buffer (*B*) or after deglycosylation (*G*). The incubation time is also listed (Modified from Schellenberger et al. 2006)

Wu et al. 2002). Corin contains a transmembrane domain anchored in the cell membrane and is thought to cleave the precursors upon secretion. The enzymatic activity does apparently not require the transmembrane domain, as a mutant soluble form is also capable of processing proANP (Knappe et al. 2003). A role of corin in the biosynthesis of cardiac natriuretic peptides in vivo has been further substantiated by genetic coupling of corin mutations to clinical phenotypes that can be explained by reduced ANP and BNP bioactivity in circulation, i.e., hypertension (Dries et al. 2005; Wang et al. 2008). Corin thus seems to be a relevant candidate for cardiac biosynthesis of natriuretic peptides generating N-terminal processing fragments and C-terminal bioactive peptides (Wu 2007). Of note, no study has yet demonstrated exactly where corin cleaves the proBNP structure. Moreover, atrial posttranslational processing of proANP and proBNP is likely to differ from ventricular processing, as isolated atrial granules have been reported to contain both unprocessed proANP and mature BNP 32 (Yokota et al. 1995). Corin activity alone can therefore not fully explain the endoproteolytical maturation of cardiac natriuretic propeptides.

Other processing enzymes deeply involved in prohormone maturation are the proprotein/prohormone convertases (PCs). In addition to furin, the subtilisin-like endoproteases PC1/3 and PC2 are expressed in the mammalian heart (Bloomquist et al. 1991; Beaubien et al. 1995), and PC1/3 expression has been demonstrated both in normal and pathological human cardiac tissue (Dschietzig et al. 2001). Atrial myocytes transfected with an adenoviral vector expressing PC1/3 process proANP to both mature ANP and a truncated form (Marx and Mains 1997). Although the precise cleavage site was not established and the processing capacity was somewhat inefficient, this report underscores that other proteases than furin and corin may be involved in the posttranslational endoproteolysis of proANP and proBNP. PC1/3 is active in secretory granules and could therefore be an important regulator of atrial proBNP processing. Cardiac PC1/3 expression has been reported to be upregulated at the transcriptional level in heart disease (Jin et al. 2004). Unfortunately, there are no data yet on other proBNP-derived fragments stemming from endoproteolytical processing. The precursor sequence contains several basic amino acid residues that potentially could represent cleavage sites for the PCs, and the molecular characterization may not be complete when it comes to processing intermediates from the natriuretic peptide precursors.

N-Terminal trimming of proBNP-derived peptides seems to be a biological feature, as both the N-terminus of the biosynthetic precursor and the C-terminal bioactive BNP product contain motifs for aminopeptidase cleavage. Both the N-terminus of proBNP and BNP 32 (proBNP 77–108) contain a prolyl residue in position 2 (His-Pro and Ser-Pro, respectively). While prolyl residues are important for peptide structure and folding, they can also be involved in exoproteolytic trimming if located near the N-terminus (Vanhoof et al. 1995). N-terminal trimming has been demonstrated for BNP in vitro (Brandt et al. 2006). Synthetic BNP 32 (proBNP 77–108) incubated with dipeptidyl peptidase (DPP)-IV removes the N-terminal Ser-Pro residues. DPP-IV is, however, an enzyme located mainly on endothelial cells and in the circulation with a preference for cleaving N-termini with either prolyl or alanyl residues in the second position (Ahrén 2007). Thus, this DPP-IV cleavage is not a part of the biosynthesis but rather related to the elimination phase from the circulation. An N-terminally trimmed form of proBNP lacking the His-Pro residues in position 1–2 has also been reported in heart failure patients (Lam et al. 2007). This report demonstrated that a truncated proBNP 3–108 form circulates in increased concentrations in heart failure patients. In extension, an initial report on glycosylated proBNP in a recombinant expression system (CHO cells) also identified a truncated proBNP 3–108 form in cellular extracts (Schellenberger et al. 2006). While this finding may be explained by experimental handling of extracts and medium, it could also imply that N-terminal exoproteolysis is a biosynthetic event. In mammalian cells, intracellular aminopeptidase activity has been reported in compartments different from the lysosomes suggesting N-terminal trimming as a possible part of the biosynthetic peptide maturation (Underwood et al. 1999;

Chiravuri et al. 2000). Whether trimming of natriuretic peptides and their precursors serves an actual regulatory function in cardiac physiology remains a question for future molecular research.

As stated earlier in this chapter, BNP gene expression is a feature of both atrial and ventricular myocytes. In the normal heart, the main site of BNP expression is in the atrial myocardium (Luchner et al. 1998; (Christoffersen et al. 2002). Ventricular BNP gene expression increases markedly in disease that affects the ventricles, i.e., congestive heart failure (Mukoyama et al. 1991). Atrial and ventricular myocytes, however, differ considerably with respect to their endocrine phenotypes, and it is reasonable to expect major differences in both peptide storage and secretion (Doyama et al. 1998; Goetze et al. 2006). Atrial granules contain both intact precursors and biosynthetic end products, i.e., bioactive ANP-28 and proBNP. In contrast, normal ventricular myocytes do not seem to express such granules, and ventricular myocytes do not contain proBNP-derived peptides (Christoffersen et al. 2002). A few reports have observed granules and proBNP-derived peptides in ventricular myocytes sampled from pathological hearts (Hasegawa et al. 1993; Nicolau et al. 1997; Takemura et al. 1998). Thus, ventricular myocytes not only regulate the BNP gene at the transcriptional and posttranslational level but also seem to differentiate with respect to the biosynthetic apparatus per se. One report even suggests the presence of different classes of granules, where one class contains only ANP-related products and the other class contains both ANP and BNP peptides (Hasegawa et al. 1991). The proANP structure has also been implicated in granule formation through calcium-mediated aggregation in the trans-Golgi network, where substitution of the acidic residues in the N-terminal region changes both the size and the shape of intracellular vesicles and their ability to dock with the plasma membrane (Canaff et al. 1996; Baertschi et al. 2001). In extension to these findings, it should be noted that atrial myocytes from ANP gene-deficient mice do not contain secretory granules on electron microscopy (John et al. 1995). Cardiac BNP expression in ANP-deficient mice is also affected with decreased BNP mRNA contents in the atria and increased expression in the ventricles (Tse et al. 2001). BNP peptide contents in these tissues paralleled the mRNA findings with no peptide in atrial regions and borderline detectable contents in ventricular samples. The formation of granules in atrial and ventricular myocytes consequently differs and may be dependent on the two cardiac natriuretic peptide systems. Finally, other cells within the heart also express the BNP gene. For instance, cardiac fibroblasts have been shown to produce and secrete cardiac natriuretic peptides (Tsuruda et al. 2002), and the coronary vasculature expresses all three natriuretic peptide genes, at least in coronary atherosclerosis (Casco et al. 2002). The biosynthesis of natriuretic peptides in these cells still remains to be elucidated.

ProBNP-derived peptides are secreted by cardiac myocytes and circulate in plasma. Their heterogeneity has primarily been characterized by chromatography and sequence-specific immunoassays. Much of our present conception of the cellular synthesis is still derived from the plasma phase, which represents the sum of both secretion and metabolism. The picomolar concentrations in plasma limit the possibilities for full biochemical identification and underscore a careful understanding of epitope recognition by the immunoassays. With this in mind, it is established that bioactive BNP is secreted from the heart and circulates without binding to plasma proteins (Hawkridge et al. 2008). Synthetic BNP 32 (proBNP 77–108) is trimmed when incubated in whole blood generating a BNP form lacking the two N-terminal amino acid residues (Shimizu et al. 2002; Hawkridge et al. 2005). As mentioned earlier, this form can also be generated by enzymatic trimming by DPP-IV (Brandt et al. 2006) and possibly other aminopeptidases. Further processing of plasma BNP seems to involve degradation with a loss of bioactivity though the disruption of the ring structure is mediated by neutral endopeptidase (NEP 24.11) – or by receptor-mediated uptake. The metabolic fate of BNP 32 has been reported to be 13–20 min (Richards et al. 1993; Smith et al. 2000). Immunoreactive BNP is also excreted in urine, but the precise contribution of renal excretion to renal metabolism is probably of minor relevance. A small degree of hepatic clearance has also been shown, which is not significantly altered in patients with liver failure (Henriksen et al. 2003).

In addition to bioactive BNP, other proBNP-derived fragments circulate in plasma (Goetze 2004, 2012). These fragments are commonly referred to as "N-terminal proBNP," but the molecular heterogeneity also includes the intact precursor, in particular in heart failure patients (Fig. 4) (Hunt et al. 1995, 1997a, b; Goetze et al. 2005). Cardiac secretion of proBNP and its N-terminal fragments has been demonstrated by blood sampling from the coronary sinus. The molar ratio of secreted proBNP 1–76 to intact proBNP is likely to depend on cardiac status, i.e., more unprocessed precursor compared to biosynthetic cleavage products in severe heart failure. On the metabolic phase, there are still discrepancies in the suggested half-life of N-terminal precursor fragments, which at least partially reflects the epitope recognition in the assays. Theoretically, the half-life of proBNP 1–76 in circulation should be around 25 min (Kroll et al. 2007) and should thus not differ greatly from the established metabolism of BNP 32 (proBNP 77–108). One report, however, suggested a considerably longer half-life (~90 min after cardiac pacing), which would explain the higher plasma concentrations of N-terminal proBNP fragments compared to bioactive BNP (Pemberton et al. 2000).

Summary

Cardiac natriuretic peptides and their molecular precursor structures have gained a robust role in clinical assessment of chronic heart failure. At first, the ANP gene attracted most interest, where BNP (and proBNP) measurement dominated the early 2000s. As of today, renewed interest in the ANP gene and the ANP physiology has been raised, where new peptide-based drugs may soon play an important therapeutic role in maintaining normal blood pressure and preservation of organ function at a local level.

References

Aburaya M, Hino J, Minamino N, Kangawa K, Matsuo H. Isolation and identification of rat brain natriuretic peptides in cardiac atrium. Biochem Biophys Res Commun. 1989;163:226–32.

Ahrén B. DPP-4 inhibitors. Best Pract Res Clin Endocrinol Metab. 2007;21:517–33.

Arden KC, Viars CS, Weiss S, Argentin S, Nemer M. Localization of the human B-type natriuretic peptide precursor (NPPB) gene to chromosome 1p36. Genomics. 1995;26:385–9.

Asano K, Murakami M, Endo D, Kimura T, Fujinaga T. Complementary DNA cloning, tissue distribution, and synthesis of canine brain natriuretic peptide. Am J Vet Res. 1999;60:860–4.

Azfer A, Niu J, Rogers LM, Adamski FM, Kolattukudy PE. Activation of endoplasmic reticulum stress response during the development of ischemic heart disease. Am J Physiol Heart Circ Physiol. 2006;291:H1411–20.

Baertschi AJ, Monnier D, Schmidt U, Levitan ES, Fakan S, Roatti A. Acid prohormone sequence determines size, shape, and docking of secretory vesicles in atrial myocytes. Circ Res. 2001;89: e23–9.

Beaubien G, Schafer MK, Weihe E, Dong W, Chretien M, Seidah NG, Day R. The distinct gene expression of the pro-hormone convertases in the rat heart suggests potential substrates. Cell Tissue Res. 1995;279:539–49.

Bensimon M, Chang A, Kuroski-de Bold ML, Ponce A, Carreras D, de Bold AJ. Participation of G proteins in natriuretic peptide hormone secretion from heart atria. Endocrinology. 2004;145:5313–21.

Bianciotti LG, de Bold AJ. Modulation of cardiac natriuretic peptide gene expression following endothelin type A receptor blockade in renovascular hypertension. Cardiovasc Res. 2001;49:808–16.

Bloomquist BT, Eipper BA, Mains RE. Prohormone-converting enzymes: regulation and evaluation of function using antisense RNA. Mol Endocrinol. 1991;5:2014–24.

Brandt I, Lambeir AM, Ketelslegers JM, Vanderheyden M, Scharpé S, De Meester I. Dipeptidyl-peptidase IV converts intact B-type natriuretic peptide into its des-SerPro form. Clin Chem. 2006;52:82–7.

Buglioni A, Sangaralingham SJ, Huntley BK, Harders GE, McCormick DJ, Winaver J, Chen HH, Burnett JC. ZD100 in a genetic model of essential hypertension and characterization of the role of the C-terminus of this novel designer peptide. J Am Soc of Hypertens. 2016;10:e10–3.

Burnett Jr JC, Kao PC, Hu DC, Heser DW, Heublein D, Granger JP, Opgenorth TJ, Reeder GS. Atrial natriuretic peptide elevation in congestive heart failure in the human. Science. 1986;231:1145–7.

Calhoun DA, Jones D, Textor S, et al. Resistant hypertension: diagnosis, evaluation, and treatment: a scientific statement from the American Heart Association Professional Education Committee of the Council for High Blood Pressure Research. Circulation. 2008;117:e510–26.

Canaff L, Brechler V, Reudelhuber TL, Thibault G. Secretory granule targeting of atrial natriuretic peptide correlates with its calcium-mediated aggregation. Proc Natl Acad Sci U S A. 1996;93:9483–7.

Casco VH, Veinot JP, Kuroski de Bold ML, Masters RG, Stevenson MM, de Bold AJ. Natriuretic peptide system gene expression in human coronary arteries. J Histochem Cytochem. 2002;50:799–809.

Cataliotti A, Chen HH, James KD, Burnett Jr JC. Oral brain natriuretic peptide: a novel strategy for chronic protein therapy for cardiovascular disease. Trends Cardiovasc Med. 2007;17:10–4.

Cataliotti A, Chen HH, Schirger JA, Martin FL, Boerrigter G, Costello-Boerrigter LC, James KD, Polowy K, Miller MA, Malkar NB, Bailey KR, Burnett Jr JC. Chronic actions of a novel oral B-type natriuretic peptide conjugate in normal dogs and acute actions in angiotensin II-mediated hypertension. Circulation. 2008;118:1729–36.

Cataliotti A, Tonne JM, Bellavia D, Martin FL, Oehler EA, Harders GE, Campbell JM, Peng KW, Russell SJ, Malatino LS, Burnett Jr JC, Ikeda Y. Long-term cardiac pro-B-type natriuretic

peptide gene delivery prevents the development of hypertensive heart disease in spontaneously hypertensive rats. Circulation. 2011;123:1297–305.
Chen HH, Glockner JF, Schirger JA, Cataliotti A, Redfield MM, Burnett Jr JC. Novel protein therapeutics for systolic heart failure: chronic subcutaneous B-type natriuretic peptide. J Am Coll Cardiol. 2012;60:2305–12.
Chimoskey JE, Spielman WS, Brandt MA, Heidenan SR. Cardio-atria of the Bio 14.6 hamsters are deficient in natriuretic factor. Science (Wash DC). 1984;223:820–2.
Chinkers M, Garbers DL, Chang MS, Lowe DG, Chin HM, Goeddel DV, Schulz S. A membrane form of guanylate cyclase is an atrial natriuretic peptide receptor. Nature. 1989;338:78–83.
Chiravuri M, Agarraberes F, Mathieu SL, Lee H, Huber BT. Vesicular localization and characterization of a novel post-proline-cleaving aminodipeptidase, quiescent cell proline dipeptidase. J Immunol. 2000;165:5695–702.
Christoffersen C, Goetze JP, Bartels ED, Larsen MO, Ribel U, Rehfeld JF, Nielsen LB. Chamber-dependent expression of brain natriuretic peptide and its mRNA in normal and diabetic pig heart. Hypertension. 2002;40:54–60.
Christoffersen C, Hunter I, Jensen AL, Goetze JP. Diabetes and the endocrine heart. Eur Heart J. 2007;28:2427–9.
Clavell AL, Stingo AJ, Wei CM, Heublien DM, Burnett Jr JC. C-type natriuretic peptide: a selective cardiovascular peptide. Am J Physiol. 1993;264:R290–5.
Crimmins DL, Kao JL. A glycosylated form of the human cardiac hormone pro B-type natriuretic peptide is an intrinsically unstructured monomeric protein. Arch Biochem Biophys. 2008;475:36–41.
de Bold AJ. Morphometric assessment of granulation in rat atrial cardiocytes: effect of age. J Mol Cell Cardiol. 1978;10:717–24.
de Bold AJ. Heart atria granularity effects of changes in water-electrolyte balance. Proc Soc Exp Biol Med. 1979;161:508–11.
de Bold AJ. Tissue fractionation studies on the relationship between an atrial natriuretic factor and specific atrial granules. Can J Physiol Pharmacol. 1982;60:324–30.
de Bold AJ, Bencosme SA. Studies on the relationship between the catecholamine distribution in the atrium and the specific granules present in atrial muscle cells: 1. Isolation of a purified specific granule subfraction. Cardiovasc Res. 1973;7:351–63.
de Bold AJ, Bencosme SA. Selective light microscopic demonstration of the specific granulation of the rat atrial myocardium by lead-hematoxylin-tartrazine. Stain Technol. 1975a;50: 203–5.
de Bold AJ, Bencosme SA. Autoradiographic analysis of label distribution in mammalian atrial and ventricular cardiocytes after exposure to tritiated leucine. In: Roy P-E, Harris P, editors. Recent advances in studies on cardiac structure and metabolism. The cardiac sarcoplasm. Baltimore: University Park Press; 1975b. p. 129–38.
de Bold ML, de Bold AJ. Immunocytochemical demonstration of cardionatrins in human atrial myocardium. In: Russo J, editor. Immunocytochemistry in tumor diagnosis. Boston: Martinus Nijhoss Publishing; 1985. p. 203–7.
de Bold AJ, Flynn TG. Cardionatrin I – a novel heart peptide with potent diuretic and natriuretic properties. Life Sci. 1983;33:297–302.
de Bold AJ, Raymond JJ, Bencosme SA. Atrial specific granules of the rat heart: light microscopic staining and histochemical reactions. J Histochem Cytochem. 1978;26:1094–102.
de Bold AJ, Borenstein HB, Veress AT, Sonnenberg H. A rapid and potent natriuretic response to intravenous injection of atrial myocardial extract in rats. Life Sci. 1981;28:89–94.
Dickey DM, Yoder AR, Potter LR. A familial mutation renders atrial natriuretic peptide resistant to proteolytic degradation. J Biol Chem. 2009;284:19196–202.
Doyama K, Fukumoto M, Takemura G, Tanaka M, Oda T, Hasegawa K, Inada T, Ohtani S, Fujiwara T, Itoh H, Nakao K, Sasayama S, Fujiwara H. Expression and distribution of brain natriuretic peptide in human right atria. J Am Coll Cardiol. 1998;32:1832–8.

Dries DL, Victor RG, Rame JE, Cooper RS, Wu X, Zhu X, Leonard D, Ho SI, Wu Q, Post W, Drazner MH. Corin gene minor allele defined by 2 missense mutations is common in blacks and associated with high blood pressure and hypertension. Circulation. 2005;112: 2403–10.

Dschietzig T, Richter C, Bartsch C, Laule M, Armbruster FP, Baumann G, Stangl K. The pregnancy hormone relaxin is a player in human heart failure. FASEB J. 2001;15:2187–95.

Dzau VJ, Baxter JD, Cantin M, de Bold AJ, Ganten D, Gross K, Husain A, Inagami T, Menard J, Poole S, et al. Nomenclature for atrial peptides. N Engl J Med. 1987a;316:1278–9.

Dzau VJ, Baxter JA, Cantin M, de Bold AJ, Ganten D, Gross K, Husain A, Inagami T, Menard J, Poole S, Robertson JI, Tang J, Yamamoto K. Report of the Joint Nomenclature and Standardization Committee of the International Society of Hypertension, American Heart Association and the World Health Organization. J Hypertens. 1987b;5:507–11.

Edwards BS, Ackermann DM, Lee ME, Reeder GS, Wold LE, Burnett Jr JC. Identification of atrial natriuretic factor within ventricular tissue in hamsters and humans with congestive heart failure. J Clin Invest. 1988;81:82–6.

Flynn TG, de Bold ML, de Bold AJ. The amino acid sequence of an atrial peptide with potent diuretic and natriuretic properties. Biochem Biophys Res Commun. 1983;117:859–65.

Flynn TG, Brar A, Tremblay L, Sarda I, Lyons C, Jennings DB. Isolation and characterization of iso-rANP, a new natriuretic peptide from rat atria. Biochem Biophys Res Commun. 1989;161:830–7.

Fosgerau K, Hoffmann T. Peptide therapeutics: current and future directions. Drug Discov. 2015;200:122–8.

Giuliani I, Rieunier F, Larue C, Delagneau JF, Granier C, Pau B, Ferrière M, Saussine M, Cristol JP, Dupuy AM, Merigeon E, Merle D, Villard S. Assay for measurement of intact B-type natriuretic peptide prohormone in blood. Clin Chem. 2006;52:1054–61.

Goetze JP. Biochemistry of pro-B-type natriuretic peptide-derived peptides: the endocrine heart revisited. Clin Chem. 2004;50:1503–10.

Goetze JP. B-type natriuretic peptide: from post-translational processing to clinical measurement. Clin Chem. 2012;58:83–91.

Goetze JP, Kastrup J, Pedersen F, Rehfeld JF. Quantification of pro-B-type natriuretic peptide and its products in human plasma by use of an analysis independent of precursor processing. Clin Chem. 2002;48:1035–42.

Goetze JP, Kastrup J, Rehfeld JF. The paradox of increased natriuretic hormones in congestive heart failure patients: does the endocrine heart also fail in heart failure? Eur Heart J. 2003;24:1471–2.

Goetze JP, Rehfeld JF, Videbaek R, Friis-Hansen L, Kastrup J. B-type natriuretic peptide and its precursor in cardiac venous blood from failing hearts. Eur J Heart Fail. 2005;7:69–74.

Goetze JP, Friis-Hansen L, Rehfeld JF, Nilsson B, Svendsen JH. Atrial secretion of B-type natriuretic peptide. Eur Heart J. 2006;27:1648–50.

Hasegawa K, Fujiwara H, Itoh H, Nakao K, Fujiwara T, Imura H, Kawai C. Light and electron microscopic localization of brain natriuretic peptide in relation to atrial natriuretic peptide in porcine atrium. Immunohistocytochemical study using specific monoclonal antibodies. Circulation. 1991;84:1203–9.

Hasegawa K, Fujiwara H, Doyama K, Mukoyama M, Nakao K, Fujiwara T, Imura H, Kawai C. Ventricular expression of atrial and brain natriuretic peptides in dilated cardiomyopathy. An immunohistocytochemical study of the endomyocardial biopsy specimens using specific monoclonal antibodies. Am J Pathol. 1993;142:107–16.

Hawkridge AM, Heublein DM, Bergen 3rd HR, Cataliotti A, Burnett Jr JC, Muddiman DC. Quantitative mass spectral evidence for the absence of circulating brain natriuretic peptide (BNP-32) in severe human heart failure. Proc Natl Acad Sci U S A. 2005;102:17442–7.

Hawkridge AM, Muddiman DC, Hebulein DM, Cataliotti A, Burnett Jr JC. Effect of plasma protein depletion on BNP-32 recovery. Clin Chem. 2008;54:933–4.

Henriksen JH, Goetze JP, Fuglsang S, Christensen E, Bendtsen F, Møller S. Increased circulating pro-brain natriuretic peptide (proBNP) and brain natriuretic peptide (BNP) in patients with cirrhosis: relation to cardiovascular dysfunction and severity of disease. Gut. 2003;52:1511–7.

Heublein DM, Huntley BK, Boerrigter G, Cataliotti A, Sandberg SM, Redfield MM, Burnett Jr JC. Immunoreactivity and guanosine 3′,5′-cyclic monophosphate activating actions of various molecular forms of human B-type natriuretic peptide. Hypertension. 2007;49:1114–9.

Hino J, Tateyama H, Minamino N, Kangawa K, Matsuo H. Isolation and identification of human brain natriuretic peptides in cardiac atrium. Biochem Biophys Res Commun. 1990;167:693–700.

Hodgson-Zingman DM, Karst ML, Zingman LV, Heublein DM, Darbar D, Herron KJ, Ballew JD, de Andrade M, Burnett Jr JC, Olson TM. Atrial natriuretic peptide frameshift mutation in familial atrial fibrillation. N Engl J Med. 2008;359:158–65.

Hooper JD, Scarman AL, Clarke BE, Normyle JF, Antalis TM. Localization of the mosaic transmembrane serine protease corin to heart myocytes. Eur J Biochem. 2000;267:6931–7.

Hunt PJ, Yandle TG, Nicholls MG, Richards AM, Espiner EA. The amino-terminal portion of pro-brain natriuretic peptide (Pro-BNP) circulates in human plasma. Biochem Biophys Res Commun. 1995;214:1175–83.

Hunt PJ, Espiner EA, Nicholls MG, Richards AM, Yandle TG. The role of the circulation in processing pro-brain natriuretic peptide (proBNP) to amino-terminal BNP and BNP-32. Peptides. 1997a;18:1475–81.

Hunt PJ, Richards AM, Nicholls MG, Yandle TG, Doughty RN, Espiner EA. Immunoreactive amino-terminal pro-brain natriuretic peptide (NT-PROBNP): a new marker of cardiac impairment. Clin Endocrinol. 1997b;47:287–96.

Huntley BK, Sandberg SM, Heublein DM, Sangaralingham SJ, Burnett Jr JC, Ichiki T. Pro-B-type natriuretic peptide-1-108 processing and degradation in human heart failure. Circ Heart Fail. 2015;8:89–97.

Ichiki T, Huntley BK, Sangaralingham SJ, Burnett Jr JC. Pro-atrial natriuretic peptide: a novel guanylyl cyclase receptor activator that goes beyond atrial and b-type natriuretic peptide. J Am Coll Cardiol Heart Fail. 2015;3:715–23.

Intravenous nesiritide vs nitroglycerin for treatment of decompensated congestive heart failure: a randomized controlled trial. JAMA. 2002;287:1531–40.

Jamieson JD, Palade GE. Specific granules in atrial muscle cells. J Cell Biol. 1964;23:151–72.

Jin H, Fedorowicz G, Yang R, Ogasawara A, Peale F, Pham T, Paoni NF. Thyrotropin-releasing hormone is induced in the left ventricle of rats with heart failure and can provide inotropic support to the failing heart. Circulation. 2004;109:2240–5.

John SW, Krege JH, Oliver PM, Hagaman JR, Hodgin JB, Pang SC, Flynn TG, Smithies O. Genetic decreases in atrial natriuretic peptide and salt-sensitive hypertension. Science. 1995;267:679–81.

Kambayashi Y, Nakao K, Mukoyama M, Saito Y, Ogawa Y, Shiono S, Inouye K, Yoshida N, Imura H. Isolation and sequence determination of human brain natriuretic peptide in human atrium. FEBS Lett. 1990;259:341–5.

Kangawa K, Matsuo H. Purification and complete amino acid sequence of alpha-human atrial natriuretic polypeptide (alpha-hANP). Biochem Biophys Res Commun. 1984;118:131–9.

Kennedy BP, Marsden JJ, Flynn TG, de Bold AJ, Davies PL. Isolation and nucleotide sequence of a cloned cardionatrin cDNA. Biochem Biophys Res Commun. 1984;122:1076–82.

Kisch B. A significant electron microscopic difference between the atria and the ventricles of the mammalian heart. Exp Med Surg. 1963;21:193–221.

Klopfenstein HS, Mathias DW, Bernath GA, Cogswell TL. Increasing atrial pressure during cardiac tamponade does not elevate plasma levels of the peptide ANP in conscious dogs. J Physiol. 1990;421:309–19.

Knappe S, Wu F, Masikat MR, Morser J, Wu Q. Functional analysis of the transmembrane domain and activation cleavage of human corin: design and characterization of a soluble corin. J Biol Chem. 2003;278:52363–70.

Kojima M, Minamino N, Kangawa K, Matsuo H. Cloning and sequence analysis of a cDNA encoding a precursor for rat C-type natriuretic peptide (CNP). Febs Lett. 1990;276:209–13.

Kroll MH, Twomey PJ, Srisawasdi P. Using the single-compartment ratio model to calculate half-life, NT-proBNP as an example. Clin Chim Acta. 2007;380:197–202.

Kuhn M. Structure, regulation, and function of mammalian membrane guanylyl cyclase receptors, with a focus on guanylyl cyclase-A. Circ Res. 2003;93:700–9.

Kuhn M. Molecular physiology of natriuretic peptide signaling. Basic Res Cardiol. 2004;99:76–82.

Lam CS, Burnett Jr JC, Costello-Boerrigter L, Rodeheffer RJ, Redfield MM. Alternate circulating pro-B-type natriuretic peptide and B-type natriuretic peptide forms in the general population. J Am Coll Cardiol. 2007;49:1193–202.

Lanfear DE. Genetic variation in the natriuretic peptide system and heart failure. Heart Fail Rev. 2010;15:219–28.

Lee MU, Miller W, Edwards B, Burnett Jr JC. Role of endogenous atrial natriuretic factor in acute heart failure. J Clin Invest. 1989;84:1962–6.

Lee CY, Chen HH, Lisy O, Swan S, Cannon C, Lieu HD, Burnett Jr JC. Pharmacodynamics of a novel designer natriuretic peptide, CD-NP, in a first-in-human clinical trial in healthy subjects. J Clin Pharmacol. 2009;49:668–73.

Lee CYW, Huntley BK, McCormick DJ, Ichiki T, Sangaralingham SJ, Burnett Jr JC. Cenderitide: structural requirements for the creation of a novel dual particulate guanylyl cyclase receptor agonist with renal enhancing in vivo and ex vivo actions. Eur Heart J CVP. 2016;2:98–105.

Liang F, O'Rear J, Schellenberger U, Tai L, Lasecki M, Schreiner GF, Apple FS, Maisel AS, Pollitt NS, Protter AA. Evidence for functional heterogeneity of circulating B-type natriuretic peptide. J Am Coll Cardiol. 2007;49:1071–8.

Lim SG, Venkatraman SS, Burnett Jr JC, Chen HH. In-vivo evaluation of an in situ polymer precipitation delivery system for a novel natriuretic peptide. PLoS One. 2013;8:e52484.

Lisy O, Huntley BK, McCormick DJ, Kurlansky PA, Burnett Jr JC. Design, synthesis, and actions of a novel chimeric natriuretic peptide: CD-NP. J Am Coll Cardiol. 2008;52:60–8.

Liu ZL, Wiedmeyer CE, Sisson DD, Solter PF. Cloning and characterization of feline brain natriuretic peptide. Gene. 2002;292:183–90.

Luchner A, Stevens TL, Borgeson DD, Redfield M, Wei CM, Porter JG, Burnett Jr JC. Differential atrial and ventricular expression of myocardial BNP during evolution of heart failure. Am J Physiol. 1998;274:H1684–9.

Ma KK, Ogawa T, de Bold AJ. Selective upregulation of cardiac brain natriuretic peptide at the transcriptional and translational levels by pro-inflammatory cytokines and by conditioned medium derived from mixed lymphocyte reactions via p38 MAP kinase. J Mol Cell Cardiol. 2004;36:505–13.

Ma KK, Banas K, de Bold AJ. Determinants of inducible brain natriuretic peptide promoter activity. Regul Pept. 2005;128:169–76.

Margulies KB, Heublein DM, Perrella MA, Burnett Jr JC. ANF-mediated renal cGMP generation in congestive heart failure. Am J Physiol. 1991;260:F562–8.

Martin FL, Sangaralingham SJ, Huntley BK, McKie PM, Ichiki T, Chen HH, Korinek J, Harders GE, Burnett Jr JC. CD-NP: a novel engineered dual guanylyl cyclase activator with anti-fibrotic actions in the heart. PLoS One. 2012;7:e52422.

Marx R, Mains RE. Adenovirally encoded prohormone convertase-1 functions in atrial myocyte large dense core vesicles. Endocrinology. 1997;138:5108–18.

Masters RG, Davies RA, Keon WJ, Walley VM, Koshal A, de Bold AJ. Neuroendocrine response to cardiac transplantation. Can J Cardiol. 1993;9:609–17.

McKie PM, Cataliotti A, Huntley BK, Martin FL, Olson TM, Burnett Jr JC. A human natriuretic peptide gene mutation reveals a novel peptide with enhanced blood pressure lowering, renal enhancing, and aldosterone suppressing actions. J Am Coll Cardiol. 2009;254:1024–32.

McKie PM, Cataliotti A, Boerrigter G, Chen HH, Sangaralingham SJ, Ichiki T, Martin FL, Burnett Jr JC. A novel atrial natriuretic peptide based therapeutic in experimental angiotensin II mediated acute. Hypertension. 2010;56:1152–9.

McKie PM, Ichiki T, Burnett Jr JC. M-atrial natriuretic peptide: a novel antihypertensive protein therapy. Curr Hypertens Rep. 2012;14:62–9.
McKie PM, Cataliotti A, Ichiki T, Sangaralingham SJ, Chen HH, Burnett Jr JC. M-atrial natriuretic peptide and nitroglycerin in a canine model of experimental acute hypertensive heart failure: differential actions of 2 cGMP activating therapeutics. J Am Heart Assoc. 2014;3:e000206.
McKie PM, Schirger JA, Benike SL, Harstad LK, Slusser JP, Hodge DO, Redfield MM, Burnett Jr JC, Chen HH. Chronic subcutaneous brain natriuretic peptide therapy in asymptomatic systolic heart failure. Eur J Heart Fail. 2016;18:433–41.
Meirhaeghe A, Sandhu MS, McCarthy MI, de Groote P, Cottel D, Arveiler D, Ferrières J, Groves CJ, Hattersley AT, Hitman GA, Walker M, Wareham NJ, Amouyel P. Association between the T-381C polymorphism of the brain natriuretic peptide gene and risk of type 2 diabetes in human populations. Hum Mol Genet. 2007;16:1343–50.
Meirovich YF, Veinot JP, de Bold ML, Haddad H, Davies RA, Masters RG, Hendry PJ, de Bold AJ. Relationship between natriuretic peptides and inflammation: proteomic evidence obtained during acute cellular cardiac allograft rejection in humans. J Heart Lung Transplant. 2008;27:31–7.
Minamino N, Aburaya M, Ueda S, Kangawa K, Matsuo H. The presence of brain natriuretic peptide of 12,000 daltons in porcine heart. Biochem Biophys Res Commun. 1988;155:740–6.
Mukoyama M, Nakao K, Hosoda K, Suga S, Saito Y, Ogawa Y, Shirakami G, Jougasaki M, Obata K, Yasue H. Brain natriuretic peptide as a novel cardiac hormone in humans. Evidence for an exquisite dual natriuretic peptide system, atrial natriuretic peptide and brain natriuretic peptide. J Clin Invest. 1991;87:1402–12.
Murakami Y, Shimada T, Inoue S, Shimizu H, Ohta Y, Katoh H, Nakamura K, Ishibashi Y. New insights into the mechanism of the elevation of plasma brain natriuretic polypeptide levels in patients with left ventricular hypertrophy. Can J Cardiol. 2002;18:1294–300.
Nakagawa H, Oberwinkler H, Nikolaev V, Gaßner B, Umbenhauer S, Wagner H, Saito Y M.D., Baba H, Stefan Frantz S, Kuhn M. Atrial natriuretic peptide locally counteracts the deleterious effects of cardiomyocyte mineralocorticoid receptor activation. Circ Heart Fail. 2014;7:814–21.
Nicolau N, Butur G, Laky D. Electronmicroscopic observations regarding the presence of natriuretic granules in the ventricle of patients with cardiopathies. Rom J Morphol Embryol. 1997;43:119–37.
O'Connor CM, Starling RC, Hernandez AF, Armstrong PW, Dickstein K, Hasselblad V, et al. Effect of nesiritide in patients with acute decompensated heart failure. N Engl J Med. 2011;365:32–43.
Ogawa T, de Bold AJ. Uncoordinated regulation of atrial natriuretic factor and brain natriuretic peptide in lipopolysaccharide-treated rats. Biomarkers. 2012;17:140–9.
Ogawa T, de Bold AJ. The heart as an endocrine organ. Endocr Connect. 2014;3:R31–44.
Ogawa T, Linz W, Stevenson M, Bruneau BG, Kuroski de Bold ML, Chen JH, Eid H, Schölkens BA, de Bold AJ. Evidence for load-dependent and load-independent determinants of cardiac natriuretic peptide production. Circulation. 1996;93:2059–67.
Ogawa T, Vatta M, Bruneau BG, de Bold AJ. Characterization of natriuretic peptide production by adult heart atria. Am J Physiol Heart Circ Physiol. 1999;276:H1977–86.
Ogawa T, Veinot JP, Davies RA, Haddad H, Smith SJ, Masters RG, Hendry PJ, Starling R, de Bold MK, Ponce A, Ma KK, Williams K, de Bold AJ. Neuroendocrine profiling of humans receiving cardiac allografts. J Heart Lung Transplant. 2005;24:1046–54.
Ogawa T, Veinot JP, Kuroski de Bold ML, Georgalis T, Bold AJ de. Angiotensin II receptor antagonism reverts the selective cardiac BNP upregulation and secretion observed in myocarditis. Am J Physiol Heart Circ Physiol. 2008;294:H2596–603.
Pemberton CJ, Johnson ML, Yandle TG, Espiner EA. Deconvolution analysis of cardiac natriuretic peptides during acute volume overload. Hypertension. 2000;36:355–9.
Ramos H, de Bold AJ. Gene expression, processing and secretion of natriuretic peptides: physiologic and diagnostic implications. Heart Fail Clin. 2006;2:255–68.
Richards AM, Crozier IG, Holmes SJ, Espiner EA, Yandle TG, Frampton C. Brain natriuretic peptide: natriuretic and endocrine effects in essential hypertension. J Hypertens. 1993;11:163–70.

Sawada Y, Inoue M, Kanda T, Sakamaki T, Tanaka S, Minamino N, Nagai R, Takeuchi T. Co-elevation of brain natriuretic peptide and proprotein-processing endoprotease furin after myocardial infarction in rats. FEBS Lett. 1997a;400:177–82.

Sawada Y, Suda M, Yokoyama H, Kanda T, Sakamaki T, Tanaka S, Nagai R, Abe S, Takeuchi T. Stretch-induced hypertrophic growth of cardiocytes and processing of brain-type natriuretic peptide are controlled by proprotein-processing endoprotease furin. J Biol Chem. 1997b;272:20545–54.

Schellenberger U, O'Rear J, Guzzetta A, Jue RA, Protter AA, Pollitt NS. The precursor to B-type natriuretic peptide is an O-linked glycoprotein. Arch Biochem Biophys. 2006;451:160–6.

Schulz H, Langvik TA, Lund SE, Smith J, Ahmadi N, Hall C. Radioimmunoassay for N-terminal probrain natriuretic peptide in human plasma. Scand J Clin Lab Invest. 2001;61:33–42.

Schweitz H, Vigne P, Moinier D, Frelin C, Lazdunski M. A new member of the natriuretic peptide family is present in the venom of the green mamba (Dendroaspis angusticeps). J Biol Chem. 1992;267:13928–32.

Seferian KR, Tamm NN, Semenov AG, Mukharyamova KS, Tolstaya AA, Koshkina EV, Kara AN, Krasnoselsky MI, Apple FS, Esakova TV, Filatov VL, Katrukha AG. The brain natriuretic peptide (BNP) precursor is the major immunoreactive form of BNP in patients with heart failure. Clin Chem. 2007;53:866–73.

Seidler T, Pemberton C, Yandle T, Espiner E, Nicholls G, Richards M. The amino terminal regions of proBNP and proANP oligomerise through leucine zipper-like coiled-coil motifs. Biochem Biophys Res Commun. 1999;255:495–501.

Severino A, Campioni M, Straino S, Salloum FN, Schmidt N, Herbrand U, Frede S, Toietta G, Di Rocco G, Bussani R, Silvestri F, Piro M, Liuzzo G, Biasucci LM, Mellone P, Feroce F, Capogrossi M, Baldi F, Fandrey J, Ehrmann M, Crea F, Abbate A, Baldi A. Identification of protein disulfide isomerase as a cardiomyocyte survival factor in ischemic cardiomyopathy. J Am Coll Cardiol. 2007;50:1029–37.

Shimizu H, Masuta K, Aono K, Asada H, Sasakura K, Tamaki M, Sugita K, Yamada K. Molecular forms of human brain natriuretic peptide in plasma. Clin Chim Acta. 2002;316:129–35.

Shimizu H, Masuta K, Asada H, Sugita K, Sairenji T. Characterization of molecular forms of probrain natriuretic peptide in human plasma. Clin Chim Acta. 2003;334:233–9.

Smith MW, Espiner EA, Yandle TG, Charles CJ, Richards AM. Delayed metabolism of human brain natriuretic peptide reflects resistance to neutral endopeptidase. J Endocrinol. 2000;167:239–46.

Steinhelper ME. Structure, expression, and genomic mapping of the mouse natriuretic peptide type-B gene. Circ Res. 1993;72:984–92.

Stevens T, Burnett Jr JC, Kinoshita M, Matsuda Y, Redfield MM. A functional role for endogenous atrial natriuretic peptide in a canine model of early left ventricular dysfunction. J Clin Invest. 1995;95:1101–8.

Stokhof AA, Overduin LM, Mol JA, Rijnberk A. Effect of pericardiocentesis on circulating concentrations of atrial natriuretic hormone and arginine vasopressin in dogs with spontaneous pericardial effusion. Eur J Endocrinol. 1994;130:357–60.

Sudoh T, Kangawa K, Minamino N, Matsuo H. A new natriuretic peptide in porcine brain. Nature. 1988;332:78–81.

Sudoh T, Maekawa K, Kojima M, Minamino N, Kangawa K, Matsuo H. Cloning and sequence analysis of cDNA encoding a precursor for human brain natriuretic peptide. Biochem Biophys Res Commun. 1989;159:1427–34.

Supaporn T, Sandberg S, Borgeson D, Heublein D, Luchner A, Wei CM, Dousa TP, Burnett Jr JC. Blunted cGMP response to agonists and enhanced glomerular cyclic 3′,5′-nucleotide phosphodiesterase activities in experimental congestive heart failure. Kidney Int. 1996;50:1718–25.

Takemura G, Takatsu Y, Doyama K, Itoh H, Saito Y, Koshiji M, Ando F, Fujiwara T, Nakao K, Fujiwara H. Expression of atrial and brain natriuretic peptides and their genes in hearts of patients with cardiac amyloidosis. J Am Coll Cardiol. 1998;31:754–65.

Tse MY, Watson JD, Sarda IR, Flynn TG, Pang SC. Expression of B-type natriuretic peptide in atrial natriuretic peptide gene disrupted mice. Mol Cell Biochem. 2001;219:99–105.

Tsuruda T, Boerrigter G, Huntley BK, Noser JA, Cataliotti A, Costello-Boerrigter LC, Chen HH, Burnett Jr JC. Brain natriuretic Peptide is produced in cardiac fibroblasts and induces matrix metalloproteinases. Circ Res. 2002;91:1127–34.

Underwood R, Chiravuri M, Lee H, Schmitz T, Kabcenell AK, Yardley K, Huber BT. Sequence, purification, and cloning of an intracellular serine protease, quiescent cell proline dipeptidase. J Biol Chem. 1999;274:34053–8.

Vanhoof G, Goossens F, De Meester I, Hendriks D, Scharpé S. Proline motifs in peptides and their biological processing. FASEB J. 1995;9:736–44.

Vierhapper H, Rokitansky A, Nowotny P, Losert U, Waldhäusl W. Effect of cardiac tamponade on plasma concentrations of atrial natriuretic peptide (ANP) in calves. Exp Clin Endocrinol. 1989;94:324–8.

Wang TJ, Larson MG, Levy D, Benjamin EJ, Corey D, Leip EP, Vasan RS. Heritability and genetic linkage of plasma natriuretic peptide levels. Circulation. 2003;108:13–6.

Wang W, Liao X, Fukuda K, Knappe S, Wu F, Dries DL, Qin J, Wu Q. Corin variant associated with hypertension and cardiac hypertrophy exhibits impaired zymogen activation and natriuretic peptide processing activity. Circ Res. 2008;103:502–8.

Wei C-M, Heublein DM, Perrella MA, Lerman A, Rodeheffer RJ, McGregor CGA, Edwards WD, Schaff HV, Burnett Jr JC. Natriuretic peptide system in human heart failure. Circulation. 1993;88:1004–9.

Wu Q. The serine protease corin in cardiovascular biology and disease. Front Biosci. 2007;12:4179–90.

Wu F, Yan W, Pan J, Morser J, Wu Q. Processing of pro-atrial natriuretic peptide by corin in cardiac myocytes. J Biol Chem. 2002;277:16900–5.

Wu C, Wu F, Pan J, Morser J, Wu Q. Furin-mediated processing of Pro-C-type natriuretic peptide. J Biol Chem. 2003;278:25847–52.

XW N, Huang Y, Chen HH, Burnett Jr JC, Boey FY, Venkatraman SS. Cenderitide-eluting film for potential cardiac patch applications. PLoS One. 2013;8:e68346.

Yan W, Sheng N, Seto M, Morser J, Wu Q. Corin, a mosaic transmembrane serine protease encoded by a novel cDNA from human heart. J Biol Chem. 1999;274:14926–35.

Yan W, Wu F, Morser J, Wu Q. Corin, a transmembrane cardiac serine protease, acts as a pro-atrial natriuretic peptide-converting enzyme. Proc Natl Acad Sci U S A. 2000;97:8525–9.

Yang-Feng TL, Floyd-Smith G, Nemer M, Drouin J, Francke U. The pronatriodilatin gene is located on the distal short arm of human chromosome 1 and on mouse chromosome 4. Am J Hum Genet. 1985;37:1117–28.

Yokota N, Bruneau BG, Fernandez BE, de Bold ML, Piazza LA, Eid H, de Bold AJ. Dissociation of cardiac hypertrophy, myosin heavy chain isoform expression, and natriuretic peptide production in DOCA-salt rats. Am J Hypertens. 1995;8:301–10.

21 Endocrine Functions of Bone

Mathieu Ferron

Abstract

Significant discoveries made within the past 15 years have revealed that bone, as an organ, is not only a target of several endocrine signals but by itself acts as an unpredicted but nevertheless important endocrine tissue. Indeed, bone cells are secreting at least two hormones, FGF23 and osteocalcin, which are implicated in the regulation of phosphate homeostasis and of energy metabolism, respectively. FGF23 is secreted specifically by the cells of the osteoblast-osteocyte lineage and inhibits phosphate reabsorption in the kidney proximal tubule mainly by reducing the expression of sodium-phosphate co-transporters. FGF23 also suppresses 1,25-dihydroxyvitamin D_3 synthesis in the proximal tubule and thereby impacts calcium and phosphate absorption as well. Osteocalcin is expressed and secreted by differentiated osteoblasts in bone and acts as a blood glucose-lowering hormone by stimulating insulin secretion by β-cells and by favoring insulin sensitivity in muscle, liver, and white adipose tissue. As we shall see in this chapter, the discovery that bone, like many other organs, possesses endocrine functions has opened new and exciting areas of research.

Keywords

Bone • Osteoblast • Osteoclast • Osteocyte • FGF23 • Osteocalcin • Fibroblast growth factor 23 • BGLAP • Insulin • Phosphate • Glucose • Insulin sensitivity • Energy metabolism

M. Ferron (✉)
Institut de recherches cliniques de Montréal (IRCM), Montréal, QC, Canada
e-mail: mathieu.ferron@ircm.qc.ca

A. Belfiore, D. LeRoith (eds.), *Principles of Endocrinology and Hormone Action*, Endocrinology, https://doi.org/10.1007/978-3-319-44675-2_21

Contents

FGF23, an Osteocyte-Derived Hormone Regulating Phosphate Homeostasis

Fibroblast growth factor 23 (FGF23), as indicated by his name, is a member of the fibroblast growth factors family. This is a relatively large class of secreted proteins, which include 18 members (FGF1–FGF10 and FGF16–FGF23). FGF11–FGF14 have been originally classified as FGFs based on sequence homology; however, they are not considered as genuine FGFs because they lack the residues implicated in the binding to the FGF receptors and, more importantly, they are intracellular proteins (Ornitz and Itoh 2015).

The secreted FGFs have pleiotropic functions during human development and in regulating metabolism postnatally (Ornitz and Marie 2015), but all FGFs signal to their target cells through the binding and activation of either one of the four FGF receptor tyrosine kinases (FGFR1-4; see ▶ Chap. 6, "Receptor Tyrosine Kinases and the Insulin Signaling System"). Of the 18 FGFs, 15 have been grouped into 5 subfamilies of paracrine-acting FGFs: the so-called FGF1, FGF7, FGF4, FGF8, and FGF9 subfamilies. The remaining three other FGFs, i.e., FGF19, FGF21, and FGF23, are members of the endocrine-acting FGF subfamily, which is also called the FGF19 subfamily (Itoh et al. 2015).

A unique feature of the endocrine FGFs is that they lack the strong affinity for heparan sulfates characterizing the paracrine FGFs. As a result, endocrine FGFs can diffuse freely in the extracellular matrix that is rich in heparan sulfates and reach blood circulation. The differences in the heparan sulfate-binding domain of the endocrine FGFs also reduce considerably the binding affinity for the FGFRs. As a result of this particularity and as explained with more details later in this chapter (see section "FGF23 Receptor and Co-receptor"), members of the FGF19 subfamily require specific co-receptors, named α and βklotho, in order to bind and activate FGFRs. Hence, we can consider endocrine FGFs as true humoral factors, i.e., hormones, as they circulate and act on distant organs through the activation of specific receptor complexes.

FGF19, called FGF15 in mice, is produced by the ileum in response to bile acid absorption and regulates new bile acid synthesis through an FGFR4/βklotho receptor complex in the liver. FGF21 secretion from the liver rises in fasting conditions and modulates glucose uptake in adipocytes via signaling through an FGFR1/βklotho receptor complex. Finally, FGF23, which we will review in details in the first half of this chapter, is secreted by osteocytes in the bone in response to high concentrations of calcitriol (1,25-dihydroxyvitamin D_3) and probably by increased serum phosphate and acts on the kidney to reduce reabsorption and thereby increases excretion of phosphate. The FGF23 receptor complex is composed of FGFR1c and of αklotho.

Identification of FGF23

In humans, phosphate represents about 1% of the entire body weight, 85% of which is stored in bones, while 14% is in cells and merely 1% is available in the serum. The serum phosphate levels have to be tightly regulated and maintained in a normal range in order to allow normal bone mineralization without causing ectopic phosphate deposition in arteries or other non-osseous tissues. Three factors determine the serum phosphate concentration: the absorption of phosphate from the diet in the intestine, its storage in the bone as hydroxyapatite mineral, and its urinary excretion. It is the proximal tubule of the nephron that is responsible for reabsorbing the phosphate in the urine and hence is the principal regulator of phosphate homeostasis in the organism. In steady-state conditions, approximately 85% of the phosphate filtered by the glomerulus is reabsorbed through sodium-phosphate co-transporters (NaPi2a and NiPi2c) localized in the proximal tubule basolateral membrane.

Prader and his colleagues were the first to predict the existence of one or several circulating factors actively promoting phosphate wasting in 1959 (Prader et al. 1959). Following the observation that a young girl with rickets, a disease characterized by defective bone mineralization, was cured after a giant cell granuloma in the rib was removed; they postulated that the tumor was producing a substance acting like an antagonist of vitamin D and/or as a phosphoric agent. This substance was termed "phosphatonin," and evidence for its existence was further provided in animals when it was shown that the hypophosphatemia observed in the *Hyp* mutant mice could be "transmitted" to wild-type mice through parabiosis but not through kidney transplantation (Meyer 1989). FGF23 was finally identified as a phosphatonin when mutations in this gene were found to be responsible for autosomal dominant hypophosphatemic rickets (ADHR) in humans (ADHRConsortium 2000). As we shall see in more detail in this chapter, FGF23 was later found to be implicated in other human pathologies of phosphate metabolism besides ADHR.

Actions of FGF23 as a Phosphatonin

FGF23's physiological action is to control phosphate metabolism. Although FGF1Rc, the receptor of FGF23, is expressed in several cell types, the main target tissues of FGF23 are the kidney and the parathyroid gland (Ben-Dov et al. 2007; Quarles 2008). This specificity of action is explained by the restricted expression pattern of αklotho, the obligatory co-receptor of FGF23.

The most important physiological target of FGF23 is the kidney and more precisely the cells of the proximal tubule of the nephron. On these cells, binding of FGF23 to αklotho/FGFR1 complexes inhibits the transcription of *Slc34a1* and *Slc34a3* the genes encoding NaPi2a and NaPi2c sodium-phosphate co-transporters. Consequently, excess of active FGF23 results in decreased phosphate reuptake in the kidney proximal tubule causing phosphate wasting and hypophosphatemia (Fig. 1).

Another critical action of FGF23 on the kidney is the suppression of the production of vitamin D. The active form of vitamin D, 1,25-dihydroxyvitamin D_3 (1,25 $(OH)_2D$), is produced in the kidney from an inactive precursor, 25-hydroxyvitamin D_3. This conversion is accomplished by the 1α-hydroxylase enzyme (CYP27B1). On the other hand, the vitamin D 24-hydroxylase encoded by the *Cyp24a1* gene is expressed in the proximal tubule and inactivates 1,25$(OH)_2D$. FGF23 suppresses the expression of *Cyp27b1* and at the same time increases *Cyp24a1* expression, leading to a net decrease in 1,25$(OH)_2D$ production and concentration. One important action of 1,25$(OH)_2D$ is to increase phosphate and calcium absorption in the small intestine. Hence, the suppression of 1,25$(OH)_2D$ production by FGF23 also results in a reduction of intestinal phosphate absorption (Fig. 1).

In accordance with these molecular outputs of FGF23 action on the kidney, *Fgf23* deficiency in mice results in increased serum levels of phosphate and 1,25$(OH)_2D$, extra-osseous calcifications, growth retardation, anomalies in bone mineralization, and a reduced life span (Shimada et al. 2004). In contrast, transgenic mice overexpressing FGF23 in the osteoblast lineage are characterized by osteomalacia and disturbed phosphate homeostasis (Larsson et al. 2004). At the moment, it is still not clear whether the effect of FGF23 on life span is dependent on its action on phosphate metabolism or whether FGF23 influences longevity through another yet to be identified pathway, but there is evidence that the reduced longevity of the FGF23 deficient mice is mediated by vitamin D (Razzaque et al. 2006).

The exact role of FGF23 signaling in the parathyroid gland remains somehow uncertain since some studies found that it increases parathyroid hormone (PTH) secretion, while others found the opposite effect (Ben-Dov et al. 2007; Brownstein et al. 2008).

FGF23 Receptor and Co-receptor

FGF23 is 32 kDa protein characterized in its N-terminal region by an FGF-homology domain and in C-terminus by a novel 71-amino acid motif. According to in vitro experiments, FGF23 can bind and activate FGFR1, FGFR3,

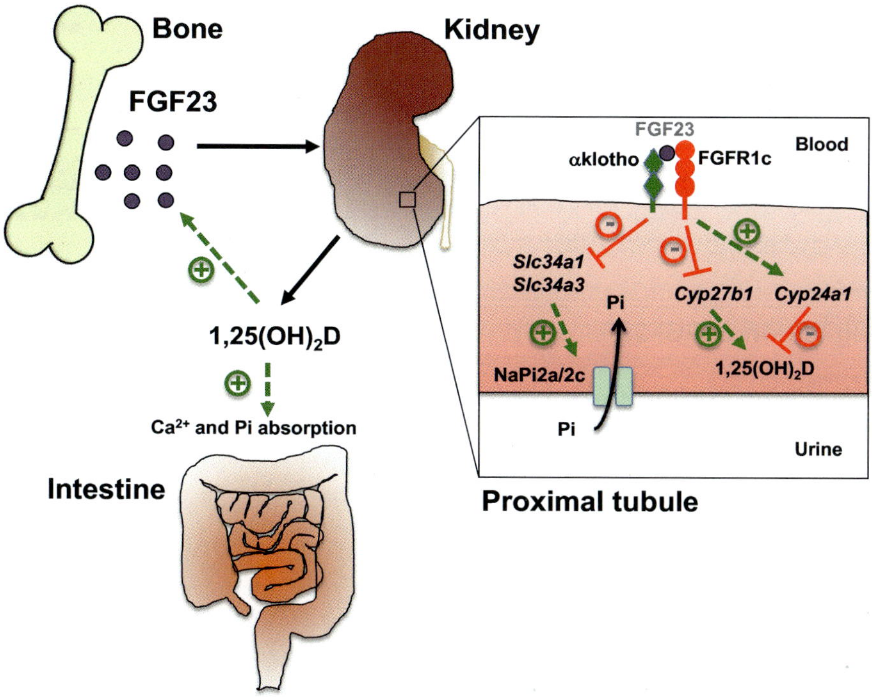

Fig. 1 FGF23 action on the kidney. FGF23 produced by osteocytes in bones acts principally on the kidney to modulate phosphate metabolism. In the proximal tubule of the nephron, FGF23 binds and activates its receptor complex composed of αklotho and FGFR1c. This activation leads to the repression of the expression of *Slc34a1* and *Slc34a3*, which encode two sodium-phosphate co-transporters (NaPi2a and NiPi2c) responsible for the reuptake of phosphate. Hence, the net effect of FGF23 action on the kidney is increased phosphate excretion in the urine. In addition, FGF23 reduces the production of 1,25-dihydroxyvitamin D ($1{,}25(OH)_2D$) in the same organ. This occurs through the repression of the expression of CYP27B1, which is responsible for the production of $1{,}25(OH)_2D$ and the increase expression of CYP24A1, which convert $1{,}25(OH)_2D$ to its inactive form. $1{,}25(OH)_2D$ promotes Ca^{2+} and phosphate absorption in the intestine. Finally, closing this bone-kidney endocrine loop, $1{,}25(OH)_2D$ is promoting FGF23 production

and FGFR4 at physiological concentrations only in the presence of the αklotho protein. αklotho which is encoded by the *KL* gene is a type I membrane β-glycosidase-like protein, which acts as an essential cofactor for the binding and activation of FGFRs by FGF23 (Urakawa et al. 2006). Although in vitro experiments suggest that FGF23 can bind FGFR1, FGFR3, and FGFR4, FGFR1c appears to be the bona fide FGFR responsible for FGF23 signaling in vitro. Supporting this includes the observation that FGF23 can still induce its phosphaturic effects in mice lacking FGFR3 or FGFR4 (Liu et al. 2008).

Mechanistically, the N-terminal FGF domain of FGF23 binds to canonical FGFRs, while its C-terminus interacts with αklotho, which also bind the FGFR, creating this unique and specific FGF23 receptor complex. As mentioned previously, this mechanism of activation of FGFR by FGF23 is different from the classical FGFs that require extracellular acidic glycosaminoglycans for receptor activation. Importantly, the ablation of *Kl* gene in mice results in FGF23 insensitivity in all organs and particularly in the kidney. Consequently, the *Kl−/−* mice display hyperphosphatemia, elevated 1,25(OH)$_2$D levels, early mortality, and soft tissue calcification (Kuro-o et al. 1997). These phenotypes are highly reminiscent of the ones observed in the *Fgf23−/−* mice and therefore add genetic credence to the conclusion that αklotho is absolutely required for FGF23-dependent signaling in vivo.

Regulation of FGF23

Although low levels of expression of *Fgf23* have been reported in other tissues like bone marrow, brain, and thymus, the main source of circulating FGF23 is widely accepted as being osteocytes. FGF23 production and secretion by osteocytes are controlled both at the transcriptional and posttranslational levels (Fig. 2).

At the transcriptional level, 1,25(OH)$_2$D stimulates directly the expression of *Fgf23* in osteocytes through a vitamin D response element (VDRE) present in the *Fgf23* promoter (Liu et al. 2006a). Because FGF23 suppresses 1,25(OH)$_2$D production in the kidney, the induction of FGF23 directly by 1,25(OH)$_2$D effectively closes this bone-kidney endocrine feedback loop (Figs. 1 and 2). A possible regulation by phosphate and/or calcium of FGF23 production by osteocytes was speculated based on the premise that, since FGF23 is a phosphaturic hormone, phosphate levels should regulate its levels. However, the clinical and experimental evidence supporting a direct regulation of this hormone by phosphate and calcium are conflicting. Notably, neither extracellular phosphate nor calcium is able to stimulate FGF23 production by osteocytes or osteoblasts in culture, suggesting that if a regulation of FGF23 by these ions exists, it is most likely indirect.

FGF23 protein is also regulated posttranslationally through three important mechanisms (Fig. 2). The first and most characterized one is an inactivating proteolysis by a subtilisin-like proprotein convertase at a conserved Arg-His-Thr-Arg/Ser-Ala-Glu dibasic motif located between amino acids 176 and 179 in human FGF23. Cleavage of FGF23 at this specific site by a furin-like proprotein convertase generates inactive N- and C-terminal fragments of this hormone. Autosomal dominant hypophosphatemic rickets (ADHR) is caused by missense mutations, which substitute R176 or R179 for unrelated amino acid resulting in non-cleavable or stabilized FGF23. Therefore, cleavage of FGF23 by one or more proprotein convertases in osteocytes represents an important mechanism regulating the bioactivity of this hormone. In vitro assays using osteosarcoma cell lines suggest that furin may be the proprotein convertase responsible for FGF23 cleavage, but it remains undetermined whether this is also the case in vivo in osteocytes (Tagliabracci et al. 2014).

O-Glycosylation is another posttranslational modification regulating FGF23 biological activity (Fig. 2). Familial tumoral calcinosis, a syndrome characterized by hyperphosphatemia and severe ectopic calcification, can be caused by loss-of-

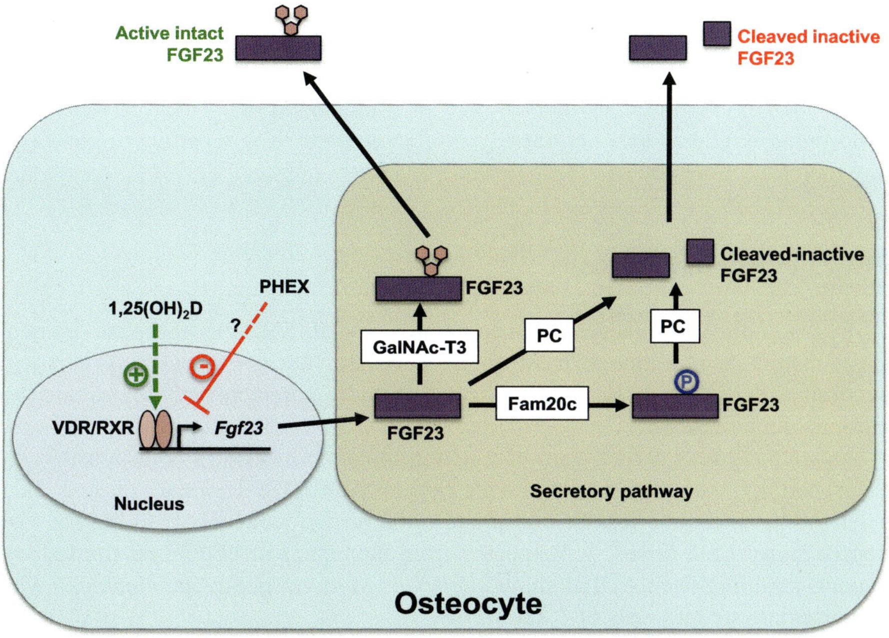

Fig. 2 Regulation of FGF23 production and activity in osteocytes. *Fgf23* gene transcription is promoted by 1,25-dihydroxyvitamin D (1,25$(OH)_2$D) through the activation of the vitamin D nuclear receptor (VDR) that functions in heterodimer with RXR. PHEX inhibit *Fgf23* transcription through an unknown mechanism. The FGF23 protein is regulated through a series of posttranslational mechanisms in the secretory pathway. *O*-Glycosylation by GalNAc-T3 prevents FGF23 cleavage and inactivation by a proprotein convertase (PC). In contrast, phosphorylation by Fam20c prevents FGF23 *O*-glycosylation and therefore favors its inactivation through proprotein convertase cleavage

function mutation in polypeptide N-acetylgalactosaminyltransferase 3 (GalNAc-T3 or *GALNT3*), a glycosyltransferase that *O*-glycosylates FGF23 at Thr178 within the proprotein convertase cleavage site. In the absence of GalNAc-T3, *O*-glycosylation of FGF23 is prevented, and this results in a hormone more easily cleaved by proprotein convertases (Kato et al. 2006). Hence, when FGF23 fails to be produced in its *O*-glycosylated form, it is mainly secreted as inactive cleaved fragments.

Finally, phosphorylation of FGF23 by a specific kinase located within the secretory pathway also appears to play an important role in the regulation of this hormone (Fig. 2). Family with sequence similarity 20, member C (Fam20C) is a kinase that phosphorylates secreted proteins on Ser-X-Glu motifs. Raine syndrome is a severe and often lethal osteosclerotic bone dysplasia caused by loss-of-function mutations in human *FAM20C* gene. Interestingly, a subset of patients with Raine syndrome survives through adulthood and develops hypophosphatemia due to elevated levels of active intact FGF23. Similarly, mice lacking *Fam20c* are characterized by increased circulating active FGF23, renal phosphate wasting, and hypophosphatemic rickets. It appears that Fam20c phosphorylates FGF23 directly on Ser120, which is located next to the proprotein convertase cleavage site. Phosphorylation of FGF23 prevents its *O*-glycosylation by GalNAc-T3, hence making it more susceptible to proteolysis by proprotein convertases (Tagliabracci et al. 2014). Therefore, in the absence of Fam20c, as it is the case in Raine syndrome, FGF23 is more efficiently *O*-glycosylated, less sensitive to cleavage, and therefore more active.

FGF23 in Human Diseases

FGF23 is implicated in several human pathologies, all linked to phosphate homeostasis disturbance. Although most of these diseases are rare genetically inherited syndrome, FGF23 may also be implicated in more common pathologies such as chronic kidney disease.

As we have seen earlier, gain-of-function mutation in FGF23 is responsible for autosomal dominant hypophosphatemic rickets (ADHR), a hereditary disease characterized by excessive loss of phosphate in the urine, which leads to rickets, i.e., poorly mineralized bones. As expected from the action of FGF23 on the kidney, patients suffering from ADHR show low levels of serum phosphate combined with inappropriate serum levels of 1,25$(OH)_2$D.

Hyperphosphatemic familial tumoral calcinosis (HFTC), or familial tumoral calcinosis, is another uncommon recessive disorder, which is characterized by hyperphosphatemia and the progressive deposition of calcium phosphate crystals in periarticular and soft tissues. Hence, even though they are called tumoral calcinosis, these lesions are not true neoplasms, as they do not include dividing cells. Genetic studies have established that HFTC is caused by loss-of-function mutation in *FGF23*, *KL*, or *GALNT3*, with most cases being associated with mutation in the later (Ichikawa et al. 2007a, b). As will be expected from a FGF23 or a αklotho deficiency, patients suffering HFTC have elevated serum phosphorus and 1,25 $(OH)_2$D levels. As we have seen earlier, loss-of-function mutations in *GALNT3* results in HFTC because FGF23 is inactivated by proteolysis by proprotein convertases when it is not *O*-glycosylated by GalNAc-T3.

Tumor-induced osteomalacia or oncogenic hypophosphatemic osteomalacia is another rare disease resulting in excessive renal phosphate wasting, hypophosphatemia, and osteomalacia. This disorder is characterized by low serum phosphate and phosphaturia, i.e., high urine phosphate. Although the exact pathophysiology of tumor-induced osteomalacia is not fully understood, it appears that at least in some instances this paraneoplastic syndrome is secondary to the presence of a tumor of mesenchymal origin producing FGF23 (White et al. 2001).

X-linked hypophosphatemia (XLH), the most frequent genetic form of rickets or osteomalacia, is caused by loss-of-function mutations in *PHEX* gene, which encodes phosphate-regulating gene with homologies to endopeptidases on the X chromosome. Patients or mice with mutations in the *PHEX* gene are both characterized by hypophosphatemia, abnormal vitamin D metabolism, and rickets or osteomalacia. Interestingly, serum FGF23 is markedly increased in patients suffering from XLH and in the *Hyp* mice, which lack *Phex*. Moreover, deletion of *Fgf23* in the *Hyp* mice is sufficient to correct their phenotypes, suggesting that FGF23 is indeed implicated in the pathology of XLH (Liu et al. 2006b). PHEX being an endopeptidase highly expressed in osteoblasts and osteocytes, it was initially speculated that it might be responsible of cleaving and inactivating FGF23. However, this could not be demonstrated and it remains unclear how PHEX regulates FGF23 production. Based on these observations, FGF23-blocking antibodies have been developed with the objective of treating XLH and have shown some efficacy in normalizing serum phosphate levels in a clinical trial (Carpenter et al. 2014).

Secondary or adaptive increases in FGF23 have been proposed to be involved in the pathophysiology of other human disorders. For instance, serum FGF23 rises in the early stages of chronic kidney diseases. In this setting, the increase in FGF23 results in diminished 1,25(OH)$_2$D production and ultimately may contribute to the development of secondary hyperparathyroidism (see ► Chap. 14, "The Parathyroids" by Kovacs, C). Increased serum FGF23 levels have been associated with increased mortality in patients suffering from end-stage renal disease (Gutierrez et al. 2005, 2008).

Osteocalcin, an Osteoblast-Derived Hormone Regulating Energy Metabolism

The discovery of an endocrine regulation of phosphate homeostasis by bone was retrospectively and at a certain level expected given the importance of phosphate for bone structure. As explained with more details below, osteoblasts produce another hormone, osteocalcin, which promotes insulin secretion by the pancreas, insulin sensitivity in peripheral organs, and overall energy expenditure. The subsequent uncovering of a bone endocrine action on glucose and energy metabolism was at a first sight more surprising.

Clinical and Experimental Observations Support the Existence of an Endocrine Link Between Bone and Energy Metabolism

When put in perspective with some clinical observations and the biology of bone itself, the existence of a regulation of energy metabolism by a bone-derived hormone could in fact be predicted.

One can assume that bone remodeling, the process by which bone tissue is renewed through subsequent cycles of bone resorption by osteoclasts and bone formation by osteoblasts, is costly in terms of energy for the rest of the body. This implies that the process of bone remodeling is extremely dependent on the energetic status of the organism. This hypothesis is supported by clinical observations: patients suffering from anorexia nervosa and insulin-dependent diabetes mellitus are often characterized by osteoporosis and/or by an increased risk of fracture, while in contrast an increased bone mass is observed in people with a higher body mass index (BMI) (Kemink et al. 2000; Legroux-Gerot et al. 2005; Misra and Klibanski 2011; Ravn et al. 1999; Tremollieres et al. 1993). Also supporting a link between energy metabolism and bone turnover is the finding that impairing glucose uptake in osteoblasts through the deletion of the gene encoding the glucose transporter GLUT1 results in delayed bone formation during development and severe osteoporosis in adult mice (Wei et al. 2015). Similarly, reduced glycolysis or fatty acid oxidation in osteoblasts through the inactivation of the WNT signaling pathway also results in markedly reduced bone acquisition and low bone mass in mice (Esen et al. 2013; Frey et al. 2015).

Together, these observations suggested the existence of hormones or systemic factors regulating bone and energy metabolism in a coordinated manner. Such factors have been identified and included two fat-derived adipokines, leptin and adiponectin, which are both implicated in the regulation of bone remodeling and of energy metabolism (Ducy et al. 2000; Kajimura et al. 2013). Insulin is also known to influence bone formation in addition to its important role on glucose metabolism (Ferron et al. 2010; Fulzele et al. 2010; Riddle et al. 2014) (see also ▶ Chap. 16, "The Endocrine Pancreas"). Finally, gut-derived hormones and factor such as glucagon-like peptides 1 and 2 (GLP-1 and GLP-2) and serotonin are also known to influence both bone and energy metabolism (Henriksen et al. 2009; Ma et al. 2013; Sumara et al. 2012; Yadav et al. 2009).

The existence of an endocrine regulation of bone mass by circulating factors originally characterized for their role in energy metabolism, combined with the notion of endocrine feedback loops, suggested an intriguing hypothesis: bone itself may produce hormone(s) affecting some aspect of glucose homeostasis. Pursuing this hypothesis a group of researchers were able to demonstrate that osteocalcin, a protein produced exclusively by osteoblasts, was a bona fide bone-derived hormone implicated in the control of energy metabolism.

Osteocalcin Is a Bone-Derived Hormone Modulating Glucose Homeostasis

Osteocalcin is a secreted protein expressed exclusively by fully differentiated osteoblasts. Although initially identified as a bone extracellular matrix protein, both loss- and gain-of-function in vivo experiments have failed to demonstrate a critical function for osteocalcin in extracellular matrix mineralization (Ducy et al. 1996; Murshed et al. 2004). While it is detected at high concentration in the bone extracellular matrix (ECM), osteocalcin also possesses several characteristics of a hormone: it is a short protein (46 and 49 amino acids in mouse and human, respectively), it is produced as a prepro-protein, and, more importantly, its mature form is present in the blood in fair amounts (between 10 and 40 ng/ml in humans).

The phenotypic characterization of mice lacking osteocalcin (*Ocn−/−* mice) revealed that the absence of this gene results in a marked reduction in glucose tolerance, which can be ascribed to a decrease both in insulin sensitivity and in insulin secretion. These mutant mice also accumulate more fat and have reduced whole-body energy expenditure. Hence, the deletion of a gene expressed only in osteoblasts and encoding for a protein present in the circulation resulted in glucose metabolism abnormalities, suggesting that osteocalcin may possess endocrine functions. Conversely, animals later characterized as a gain-of-function model of this hormone, the *Esp−/−* mice, or mice treated with recombinant osteocalcin displayed improved glucose tolerance, insulin sensitivity and secretion, reduced fat mass and protection against diet-induced obesity and insulin resistance (Lee et al. 2007).

Before it is secreted by osteoblasts, the osteocalcin precursor is γ-carboxylated on three specific glutamic acid residues (Glu 17, Glu 21, and Glu 24 in human osteocalcin) converting them into γ-carboxyglutamic acid (Gla). This process is dependent on vitamin K, since the enzyme responsible for γ-carboxylation, the γ-glutamyl carboxylase, requires reduced vitamin K as a cofactor (Fig. 3a). This posttranslational modification increases the affinity of osteocalcin for hydroxyapatite, the mineral component of bone, and consequently the γ-carboxylated form of osteocalcin is extremely abundant in the bone extracellular matrix. For this reason, osteocalcin is also named "bone Gla protein" (BGP or BGLAP). In the blood, uncarboxylated, undercarboxylated, as well as fully carboxylated forms of osteocalcin are present. Several studies in vivo and in vitro have shown that undercarboxylated osteocalcin and the uncarboxylated osteocalcin represent truly active forms of this hormone with regard to glucose metabolism (see Ferron and Lacombe 2014 for a review). In support of this conclusion, mice in which *Ggcx*, the gene encoding the γ-glutamyl carboxylase, was inactivated specifically in osteoblasts displayed increased levels of uncarboxylated osteocalcin in the serum and improved glucose tolerance (Ferron et al. 2015). As we will see later (section "Regulation of Osteocalcin Activity by Bone Resorption and Other Factors"), in physiological conditions, bone resorption by osteoclasts appears to be responsible for the generation and release of undercarboxylated active osteocalcin from the bone matrix.

Effects of Osteocalcin on Insulin Secretion

As mentioned previously, in vivo studies suggested that osteocalcin favors insulin secretion. In fact, osteocalcin has multiple independent biological effects on pancreatic β-cells, which result altogether in a net increase in insulin secretion in response to glucose. Indeed, osteocalcin promotes β-cell proliferation and thereby increases the β-cell pool, but it also promotes insulin synthesis and secretion directly, as well as indirectly through GLP-1 (Fig. 4).

Osteocalcin stimulates β-cell proliferation by stimulating the expression of critical genes implicated in β-cell division, including cyclin D1, cyclin D2, and Cdk4 (Ferron et al. 2008). Osteocalcin's effect on β-cell proliferation can be observed in adult mice treated with daily injections of the recombinant undercarboxylated form of this protein for 4 months, which are characterized by a 50% increase in β-cell mass and an improved insulin secretion in response to glucose (Ferron et al. 2012). Osteocalcin also appears to play an important role in the perinatal expansion of the

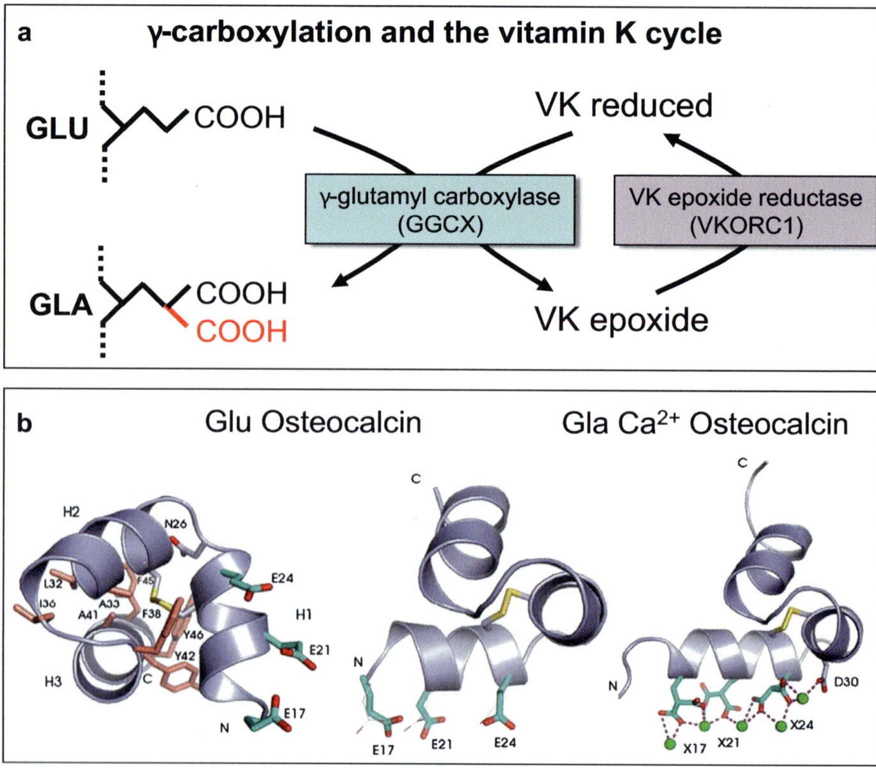

Fig. 3 Osteocalcin γ-carboxylation and structure. (**a**) γ-Carboxylation is the addition of a carboxyl group to the glutamic acid (*GLU*) residue of a protein to generate a γ-carboxyglutamic acid (*GLA*) residue. This reaction relies on GGCX and requires vitamin K. The oxidized vitamin K epoxide generated by this reaction can be reduced by VKORC1 to allow another γ-carboxylation cycle to take place. (**b**) Comparative 3D structure of bovine 3 Glu-OCN (*left two panels*) and porcine 3 Gla Ca^{2+}-OCN (*right*). On the *left* end image, we can see the relative orientation of the main helices (H1–H3) as well as the disulfide bridge (C23–C29, *yellow bond*) and the hydrophobic side-chain interactions within the hydrophobic core (*pink*). In the structural comparison between bovine 3 Glu-OCN (*left*) and porcine 3 Gla $Ca2^{+}$-OCN (right), the Glu and Gla side chains are *colored cyan*. The calcium ions complexed by the Gla osteocalcin are shown as *green* spheres (Courtesy of Dr. Terry L. Dowd, Brooklyn College of the City University of New York)

β-cell pool. Interestingly, serum levels of active undercarboxylated osteocalcin rise sharply between embryonic day 17.5 and postnatal day 10 in mice, a period during which the β-cell pool undergoes a massive expansion. In addition, the absence of osteocalcin or of its receptor GPRC6A (see section "Regulation of Osteocalcin Activity by Bone Resorption and Other Factors") impaired the proliferation index of pancreatic β-cells in mouse embryos and neonates and resulted in a reduced β-cell mass and glucose intolerance in adults (Wei et al. 2014).

Osteocalcin also promotes insulin secretion and production from β-cells. This occurs through two distinct signaling pathways. First, osteocalcin stimulates directly,

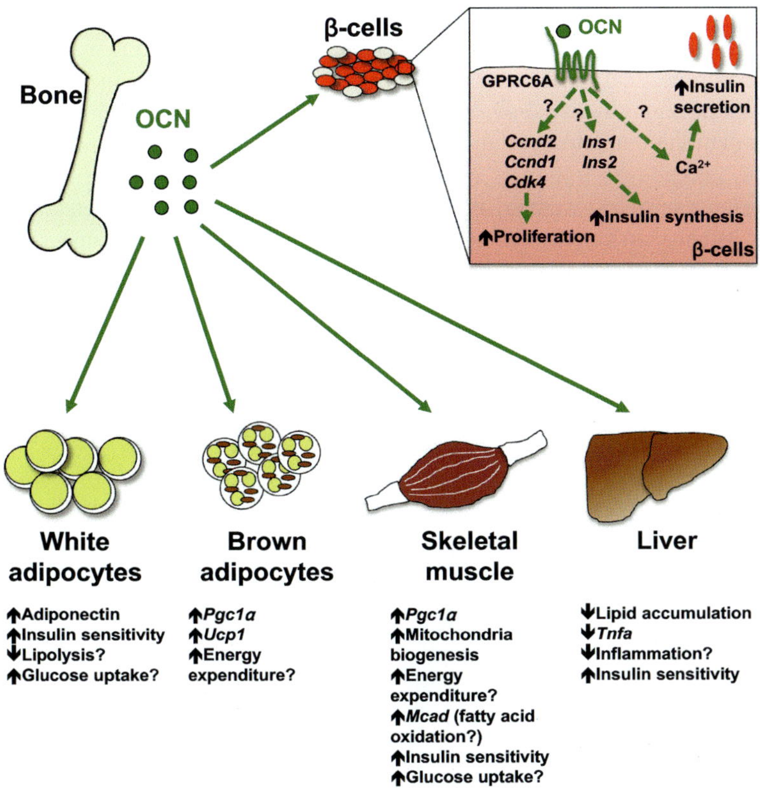

Fig. 4 Endocrine functions of osteocalcin. Once released in the blood stream, undercarboxylated osteocalcin affects glucose metabolism mainly in two ways. First, osteocalcin directly affects β-cell function by binding to the receptor GPRC6A and increasing their capacity to proliferate as well as to synthetize and secrete insulin. Second, osteocalcin improves insulin sensitivity and energy expenditure through multiple mechanisms. Osteocalcin stimulates energy expenditure by increasing mitochondrial biogenesis in the muscle and by regulating the expression of genes implicated in energy consumption in brown adipose tissue and skeletal muscle. Osteocalcin also affects insulin sensitivity possibly by increasing adiponectin expression in white fat and decreasing lipid accumulation and inflammation in steatotic liver. A direct impact of osteocalcin as an insulin-sensitizing hormone is speculative and remains to be established

within minutes, insulin secretion by β-cells. Second, osteocalcin promotes within a few hours the expression at the mRNA levels of the two genes encoding insulin in mice, *Ins1* and *Ins2* (Ferron et al. 2008; Wei et al. 2014). Both of these effects are dependent on the presence of a functional GPRC6A at the surface of β-cells, since osteocalcin is unable to induce insulin secretion or insulin gene expression in pancreatic islets lacking *Gprc6a* (Pi et al. 2011; Wei et al. 2014). Mechanistically, the acute effect of osteocalcin on insulin secretion appears to be mediated through the generation of cAMP in the cells following activation of GPRC6A. This increased cAMP levels in turn may promote an increase in the cytosolic content of Ca^{2+} which is known to promote the release of insulin granules from β-cells (Hinoi et al. 2008).

Finally, there is evidence that osteocalcin promotes insulin secretion indirectly through glucagon-like peptide-1 (GLP-1). GLP-1 is a member of the incretin family, a group of intestinal hormones which promotes insulin secretion by β-cells in conditions of high glucose only (see also ▶ Chap. 16, “The Endocrine Pancreas”). The stimulation of an intestinal endocrine cell line with osteocalcin promotes GLP-1 secretion, and administration of recombinant osteocalcin by repeated injections in mice caused a surge in serum GLP-1 levels (Mizokami et al. 2013). Interestingly, this effect of osteocalcin can also be observed when this hormone is administered orally, suggesting that osteocalcin is bioavailable through the oral route. Of note, the osteocalcin receptor GPRC6A was detected in intestinal endocrine cells expressing GLP-1 (Mizokami et al. 2014).

Effects of Osteocalcin on Fat Metabolism, Energy Expenditure and Insulin Sensitivity

In addition to its effect on β-cells, osteocalcin also affect fat accumulation, energy expenditure and insulin sensitivity (Fig. 4). Absence of osteocalcin in mice results in increased fat mass, adipocyte numbers and serum triglyceride levels. On the contrary, a gain-of-function of osteocalcin, *Esp−/−* mice (see section “Regulation of Osteocalcin Activity by Bone Resorption and Other Factors”) causes a reduction of fat mass, adipocyte numbers and serum triglycerides (Lee et al. 2007). Likewise, infusion or injections of osteocalcin in WT mice is associated with a decrease in their fat mass, their serum triglyceride levels and the expression of genes implicated in lipolysis (*Tgl* and *Perilipin*) in fat (Ferron et al. 2008). It is currently unknown by which mechanism osteocalcin influences fat mass. Nonetheless, there is evidence that osteocalcin can directly induce expression of adiponectin in cultured adipocyte, suggesting the presence of a functional osteocalcin receptor on these cells. Adiponectin is an adipokine potentially implicated in the regulation of systemic insulin sensitivity (Yamauchi et al. 2001), hence it was suggested that osteocalcin might be improving insulin sensitivity through the induction of adiponectin in adipocytes.

In parallel to these effects on fat metabolism, osteocalcin can also directly increase glucose transport in adipocytes and can suppress the secretion of pro-inflammatory cytokines and induce the secretion of anti-inflammatory cytokines as well as adiponectin (Hill et al. 2014). Although the absence of a functional *GPRC6A* in mice and humans also results in an increased fat mass (Oury et al. 2013a; Pi et al. 2008), it still needs to be determined if GPRC6A is the osteocalcin receptor in adipocytes.

Another possibility is that the effect of osteocalcin on fat metabolism is indirect and secondary to alternative physiological functions of this hormone. Indeed, two gain-of-function models of osteocalcin ($Esp^{-/-}$ mice and *Ggcx*-osteoblast specific knockout mice) are characterized by increased energy expenditure, whereas the *Ocn−/−* mice displayed the opposite phenotype. Moreover, wild-type mice fed a high fat diet and injected daily with osteocalcin have increased energy expenditure, but normal food intake. At the mechanistic level, it appears that osteocalcin promotes energy expenditure in part by stimulating mitochondria biogenesis in muscle. Indeed, the number of mitochondria is increased in muscles isolated from *Esp*$^{-/-}$ mice or from WT mice fed a high fat diet and injected with osteocalcin (Ferron et al. 2011). Furthermore, osteocalcin induces the expression of *Pgc1α*, *Nrf1* and *Mcad*, three genes implicated in mitochondrial biogenesis in the muscle. Osteocalcin infusion in mice also increases, in brown adipose tissue, the expression of *Pgc1α* and *Ucp1*, two genes involved in thermogenesis. Osteocalcin might also be affecting insulin-dependent glucose uptake in skeletal muscle (Tsuka et al. 2015). Altogether, these observations suggested that the protective effect of osteocalcin on obesity and insulin resistance might be, at least in part, due to its capacity to increase energy expenditure in brown adipose tissue and skeletal muscle.

High-fat diet induces insulin resistance, but also liver steatosis, a condition characterized by an abnormal accumulation of lipids in this organ. This condition is also known as nonalcoholic fatty liver disease (NAFLD) in human and can progress to hepatocellular carcinoma in some cases. Interestingly, osteocalcin injection in mice protected their liver from steatosis. More precisely, limited amount of lipids were detected in livers from osteocalcin-treated mice, and the expression of the gene encoding tumor necrosis factor alpha (*Tnfa*) was rescued back to normal levels by osteocalcin treatment suggesting that the inflammatory state habitually associated with liver steatosis was not present in these mice (Ferron et al. 2012). The exact mechanism through which lipid accumulation in the liver is prevented by osteocalcin is still unknown. Nonetheless, we can speculate that it is dependent on the receptor GPRC6A since *Gprc6a−/−* mice also exhibit features of hepatic steatosis. Moreover, osteocalcin affects the expression of genes implicated in glucose metabolism in the liver (*Foxa2*, *Pepck*) consistent with a role for osteocalcin as an insulin-sensitizing hormone. Of note, cross-sectional studies in humans found an inverse relationship between serum osteocalcin levels and the presence of NAFLD (Luo et al. 2015; Sinn et al. 2015).

Overall, these studies using mouse models support the concept that osteocalcin regulates fat mass, insulin secretion, and energy expenditure through multiple mechanisms (Fig. 4). The main targets of osteocalcin appear to be pancreatic β-cells through the activation of GPRC6A and adipose tissues, skeletal muscles, and the liver through unidentified receptor(s).

Other Endocrine Functions of Osteocalcin

Like many other hormones, it appears that osteocalcin affects a number of physiological functions. Indeed, further phenotypic characterization of the *Ocn−/−* mice has uncovered two additional roles for osteocalcin in male reproductive function and in brain development.

The importance of gonad-derived sex steroid in bone homeostasis is well established (see ► Chaps. 17, "The Physiology of the Testis" and ► 18, "Ovarian Physiology").

It is therefore not so surprising that a bone-derived hormone can in turn modulate reproductive function. Indeed, it appears that osteocalcin promotes testosterone production by Leydig cells from the testis. This occurs through the transcriptional induction of several genes involved in testosterone synthesis including the steroidogenic acute regulatory protein (*StAR*), cholesterol side-chain cleavage enzyme (*Cyp11a*), cytochrome P-450 17 alpha (*Cyp17*), 3-β-hydroxysteroid dehydrogenase (*3β-HSD*), aromatase enzyme (*Cyp19*), and 17-β-hydroxysteroid dehydrogenase (*HSD-17*). Consequently, *Ocn−/−* male mice have reduced testosterone levels, decreased spermatozoid counts, and are subfertile (Oury et al. 2011).

Osteocalcin has also some effects on brain function and development. In adults, this hormone crosses the blood-brain barrier; binds to neurons of the brainstem, midbrain, and hippocampus; increases the synthesis of monoamine neurotransmitters; blocks GABA synthesis; prevents anxiety and depression; and at the same time promotes learning and memory. Interestingly, osteocalcin also seems to play an important role during brain development. Maternally derived osteocalcin crosses the placenta during pregnancy and inhibits neuronal apoptosis before embryos begin to synthesize this hormone themselves (Oury et al. 2013b).

The discovery of these new functions for osteocalcin in the brain and testis suggests that this hormone potentially may have other still unknown and unexpected functions.

Gprc6a Is an Osteocalcin Receptor in β-Cells and in Leydig Cells

Originally described as a cation and amino acid-sensing receptor, the G protein-coupled receptor GPRC6A is expressed in many tissues including the liver, skeletal muscle, brain, testis, bone, and pancreatic β-cells. Remarkably, mice lacking GPRC6A (*Gprc6a*$^{-/-}$ mice) are characterized by an increased mass of white adipose tissue compared to WT animals, are glucose intolerant, are insulin resistant, and exhibit histological features of liver steatosis and declining testosterone levels (Pi et al. 2008). Because *Gprc6a*$^{-/-}$ mice phenocopied *Ocn*$^{-/-}$ mice with regard to their metabolic abnormalities, it suggested that GPRC6A might mediate osteocalcin function, at least in pancreatic islets. Supporting this contention, the inactivation of *Gprc6a* specifically in pancreatic tissue caused glucose intolerance in mice due to an impaired capacity of β-cells to secrete insulin in response to glucose. It was also established that osteocalcin effect on pancreatic islets depends solely on GPRC6A since the capacity of this hormone to promote insulin secretion was abolished in *Gprc6a*$^{-/-}$ islets (Pi et al. 2016; Wei et al. 2014). *Gprc6a*$^{-/-}$ pancreases have decreased β-cell area and β-cell mass similarly to *Ocn*$^{-/-}$ pancreases. Other experiments have established that GPRC6A is the receptor mediating the function of osteocalcin in Leydig cells, where osteocalcin promotes testosterone production and male fertility (Oury et al. 2011). Intriguingly, additional genetic manipulations in mice have shown that GPRC6A is not responsible for mediating osteocalcin action on the brain, suggesting that a different osteocalcin receptor(s) is present in this organ (Oury et al. 2013b).

Regulation of Osteocalcin Activity by Bone Resorption and Other Factors

As mentioned earlier (see section "Osteocalcin is a Bone-Derived Hormone Modulating Glucose Homeostasis"), γ-carboxylation of osteocalcin appears to be an important mechanism through which the biological activity of this hormone is regulated (Fig. 3a). The structures of fully carboxylated osteocalcin (GLA) and of undercarboxylated osteocalcin (GLU) were both determined using X-ray crystallography (Hoang et al. 2003; Malashkevich et al. 2013). It appears that there are resemblances but also dissimilarities between the structural regulations of these two forms. GLU and GLA osteocalcin structures are related, consisting of three α-helices surrounding a hydrophobic core with a disulfide bond between two of the helices (Fig. 3b). Nonetheless, in contrast to GLA osteocalcin, the undercarboxylated form of this protein does not bind Ca^{2+} and does not require high Ca^{2+} concentration to fold into a helical structure, while GLA osteocalcin requires 5 mM Ca^{2+} to be fully folded (Dowd et al. 2001; Hauschka and Carr 1982). These observations suggest that at Ca^{2+} concentration of approximately 1 mM as usually found in cell culture media or in vivo in blood and interstitial fluid, only GLU osteocalcin will exhibit a helical conformation and presumably be able to activate its receptor(s). These data provide a structural elucidation for the lack of biological activity of GLA osteocalcin in energy metabolism.

One critical regulator of osteocalcin carboxylation levels is the osteotesticular protein tyrosine phosphatase (OST-PTP also called ESP or PTPRV), a receptor-type tyrosine phosphatase expressed mainly in osteoblasts and in the Sertoli cells of the testis. Remarkably, the deletion of *Esp*, the gene encoding for OST-PTP in mice, does not cause any obvious bone defect but rather resulted in abnormal glucose metabolism (Lee et al. 2007). Indeed, $Esp^{-/-}$ mice are characterized by improved glucose tolerance, increased insulin sensitivity, and augmented insulin secretion in response to glucose. Moreover, these mutant animals are protected from obesity and glucose intolerance normally induced by a high-fat and high-sucrose diet. Notably, these phenotypes were detected both in a global knockout and in an osteoblast-specific knockout of OST-PTP, demonstrating that this protein affects energy metabolism essentially through its expression in osteoblast (Lee et al. 2007). These phenotypes parallel the ones of mice lacking osteocalcin, and molecular analyses revealed that osteocalcin carboxylation levels are decreased in $Esp^{-/-}$ mice compared to wild-type mice, implying that the inactivation of OST-PTP resulted in a gain-of-function mouse model of osteocalcin. This conclusion was further supported by a genetic experiment where deletion of one allele of *Ocn* in $Esp^{-/-}$ mice was shown to be sufficient to correct their metabolic abnormalities (Lee et al. 2007).

Although these initial studies suggested that OST-PTP negatively regulates osteocalcin through carboxylation, the mechanism by which a tyrosine phosphatase could regulate the carboxylation of this secreted molecule was still unknown. An answer to this question was provided by the identification of the insulin receptor (InsR) as an OST-PTP substrate in osteoblasts (Ferron et al. 2010). These observations suggested that insulin signaling in osteoblasts might be implicated in the regulation of osteocalcin activation and of glucose metabolism. Confirming this hypothesis, it was observed that animals lacking *InsR* in osteoblasts only (*InsR*^{osb}$-/-$ mice) presented impaired glucose tolerance, insulin sensitivity, and insulin secretion. In addition, these mice have reduced energy expenditure and are fatter. Decreased serum levels of undercarboxylated active osteocalcin were observed in *InsR*^{osb}$-/-$ mice (Ferron et al. 2010; Fulzele et al. 2010), suggesting that insulin signaling in osteoblasts regulates energy homeostasis by modulating osteocalcin carboxylation.

Inactivating *InsR* in osteoblasts also results in decreased bone formation and most importantly in reduced bone resorption in vivo. This decreased osteoclastic activity is caused by increased osteoblastic expression of *Osteoprotegerin* (*Opg*), an inhibitor of bone resorption. It was found that the transcription factor FoxO1 controls *Opg* expression in osteoblasts and that insulin signaling repressed *Opg* expression by inducing FoxO1 phosphorylation which results in its nuclear export (see Fig. 5). Additional work led to the conclusion that the metabolic phenotype of the *InsR*^{osb}$-/-$ mice is secondary to their defective bone resorption.

How osteoclasts activity may be linked to the regulation of osteocalcin and of glucose metabolism? This question led to the identification of a previously unknown mechanism by which osteocalcin could be decarboxylated in vivo. In fact, the low pH generated by osteoclasts in the resorption lacuna during the process of bone resorption is a sufficient means to decarboxylate and activate osteocalcin molecules embedded in the bone ECM. Therefore, it is by increasing bone resorption that insulin signaling in osteoblasts increases osteocalcin bioavailability (see Fig. 5). Overall, the study of *InsR*^{osb}$-/-$ mice identified osteoblasts as a new and physiologically important target of insulin and raised the prospect that osteoclastic bone resorption may be a critical determinant of glucose homeostasis.

The role of bone resorption on energy metabolism and on osteocalcin carboxylation was further addressed in vivo using osteoclast gain- and loss-of-function model. *Opg*$^{-/-}$ mice are characterized by an increased number of active osteoclasts and display improved glucose tolerance. Conversely, ablation of osteoclasts in mice through the expression of the diphtheria toxin fragment A (DTA) in cathepsin K-positive cells, i.e., in osteoclasts, resulted in reduced glucose tolerance. Importantly, undercarboxylated osteocalcin levels are augmented in *Opg*$-/-$ mice and decreased in osteoclast-depleted animals, suggesting that osteoclasts are regulating glucose metabolism at least in part by promoting the decarboxylation of osteocalcin (Lacombe et al. 2013).

The studies reviewed so far suggest that osteocalcin and insulin increase each other's activity or secretion in a feed-forward loop. Therefore, negative regulators of osteocalcin must exist to maintain glucose homeostasis. Studies in mice have revealed that leptin and glucocorticoids are two important negative hormonal regulators of osteocalcin activity. Leptin acts in the brain to increase the sympathetic nervous system activity which results ultimately in the induction of the expression of *Esp*, the gene encoding OST-PTP, in osteoblasts. Hence, in the absence of leptin, in *ob/ob* mice, OST-PTP expression is reduced and more

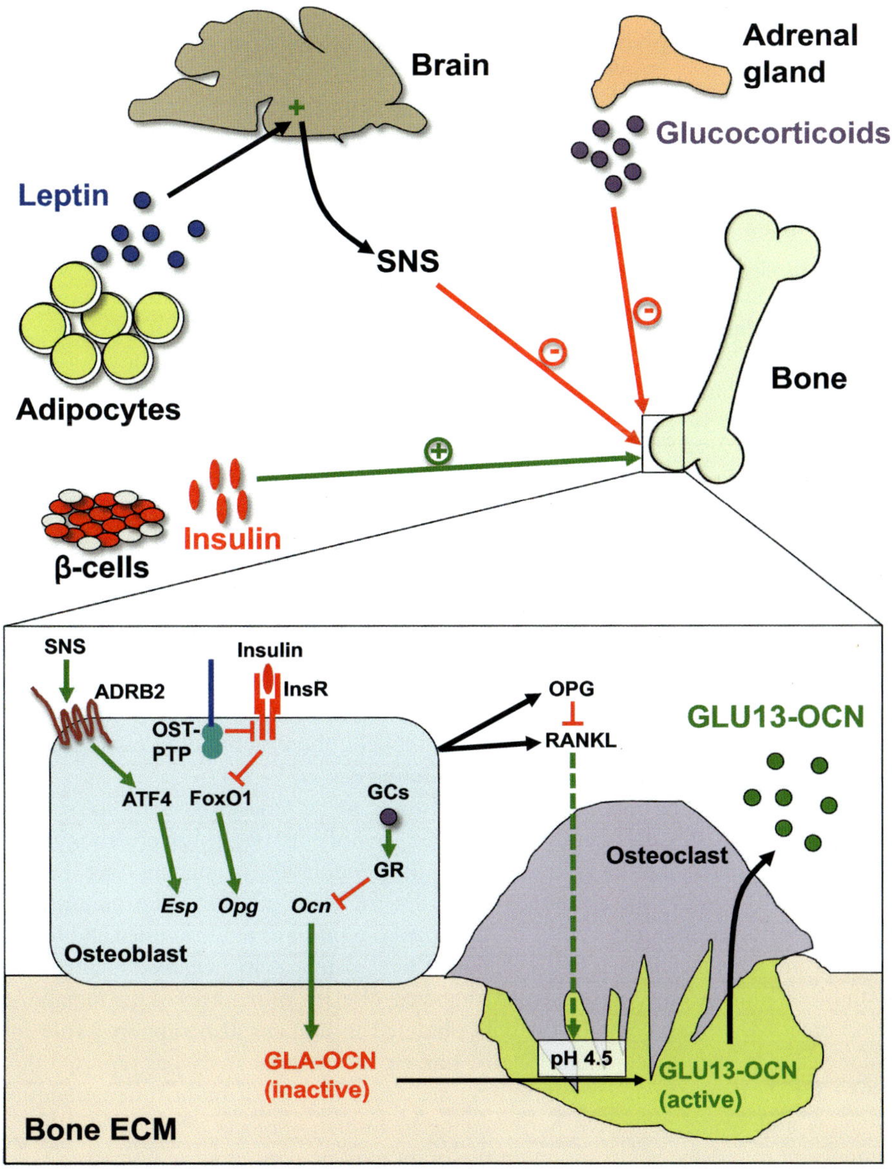

Fig. 5 Regulation of osteocalcin activity. Once γ-carboxylated and secreted by osteoblasts, osteocalcin is stored in the bone extracellular matrix in an inactive form. To fulfill its beneficial effects on glucose metabolism, osteocalcin has to be activated, i.e., decarboxylated. This is accomplished through osteoclastic bone resorption which generates the acid pH necessary for osteocalcin decarboxylation. Insulin signaling in osteoblasts affects osteocalcin activity by increasing bone resorption through osteoprotegerin (*Opg*) downregulation. Since osteocalcin stimulates insulin secretion, a feed-forward loop exists between osteocalcin and insulin activity, and negative regulators of osteocalcin are in place to counteract this amplification. Leptin secretion by adipocytes

undercarboxylated active osteocalcin is produced. It is believed that this mechanism may partly explain the hyperinsulinemia observed in the leptin-deficient animals (Hinoi et al. 2008).

The use of glucocorticoids as anti-inflammatory agents has been associated with the development of insulin resistance, type 2 diabetes, and dyslipidemia. It is also well known that glucocorticoids have undesirable effects on bone where they suppress osteoblast activity, which results in decreased osteocalcin secretion. Interestingly, the detrimental effect of glucocorticoids on glucose metabolism can in part be explained by its negative action on osteocalcin production (Brennan-Speranza et al. 2012). In contrast to WT mice, mice overexpressing the glucocorticoid-inactivating enzyme 11β-hydroxysteroid dehydrogenase type 2 (11bHSD2) specifically in osteoblasts do not develop insulin resistance and obesity following corticosterone treatment. Moreover, glucocorticoid treatment reduces serum undercarboxylated osteocalcin in wild-type mice, but not in transgenic mice with disrupted glucocorticoid signaling in osteoblasts. Finally, ectopic expression of osteocalcin from hepatocytes greatly improved the metabolic abnormalities induced by glucocorticoids in mice, suggesting that suppression of osteocalcin production is an important mediator of the adverse effect of glucocorticoids on insulin sensitivity.

Osteocalcin and Glucose Metabolism in Humans

Although most of the work characterizing osteocalcin function in energy metabolism was performed using genetically modified models, there is building evidence that osteocalcin may have a similar function in humans.

Regardless of a few contradictory publications, so far most cross-sectional studies provide support to the notion that bone, mainly through undercarboxylated osteocalcin, contributes to glucose metabolism regulation in humans (see Ferron and Lacombe (2014) for an extensive review of these studies). The majority of studies conducted in human subjects confirmed the findings made in mice and found that serum levels of undercarboxylated or total osteocalcin negatively correlated with blood glucose, insulin resistance, diabetes, obesity, or markers of the metabolic syndrome. Moreover, some of the data obtained in humans also support a role for osteocalcin in insulin secretion. Finally, one cross-sectional study has reported that lower serum osteocalcin concentrations are associated with brain microstructural changes and worse cognitive performance in human subjects (Puig et al. 2015), suggesting that osteocalcin action on the brain may be conserved in human.

Of particular interest are a series of meta-analyses combining all studies investigating the link between osteocalcin and glucose metabolism in humans. A first meta-

Fig. 5 (continued) stimulates the sympathetic nervous system in the brain, which then signals to osteoblasts to increase Esp expression through ATF4. OST-PTP, the gene product of Esp, negatively regulates insulin receptor signaling and decreases osteocalcin activity. Glucocorticoids decrease osteocalcin activity by suppressing osteoblast function and osteocalcin production

analysis demonstrated that both undercarboxylated and total osteocalcin serum levels are negatively correlated with fasting plasma glucose and hemoglobin A1c (HbA1c), a marker of uncontrolled hyperglycemia (Liu et al. 2015b). Two other meta-analyses observed that levels of total serum osteocalcin negatively correlate with the risk of adverse metabolic outcomes such as type 2 diabetes and metabolic syndrome (Kunutsor et al. 2015; Liu et al. 2015a).

At the genetic level, a heterozygous and dominant mutation in *GPRC6A*, the gene encoding the human homologue of the osteocalcin receptor, has been found in two individuals characterized by peripheral testicular insufficiency coupled to glucose intolerance, insulin resistance, and increased BMI (Oury et al. 2013a). The striking resemblances between the clinical presentation of these patients and the phenotypes of the $Ocn^{-/-}$ and the $Gprc6a^{-/-}$ mice suggest a conservation of the OCN/GPRC6A signaling pathway between mice and humans (Lee et al. 2007; Oury et al. 2013a; Pi et al. 2008). An association between variants in *BGLAP*, the gene encoding for osteocalcin in human, and BMI in healthy individual was documented, suggesting that variations in osteocalcin genomic region may affect body composition in humans (Korostishevsky et al. 2012). A nonsynonymous single nucleotide polymorphism (SNP) in *BGLAP* exon 4 (R94Q) was found to be associated with insulin sensitivity and glucose disposal in African Americans (Das et al. 2010), although the same *BGLAP* variant was found not to be a major risk factor for type 2 diabetes in Caucasians.

Finally, it should be noted that additional studies suggest that the mechanism by which osteocalcin is decarboxylated and activated by osteoclasts may also be preserved in humans. For example, it was shown that patients treated with bisphosphonates have a decreased undercarboxylated osteocalcin level in the serum (Aonuma et al. 2009; Iwamoto et al. 2004; Mokuda et al. 2012; Schafer et al. 2011) and that serum undercarboxylated osteocalcin levels and/or markers of insulin secretion or sensitivity are positively associated with markers of bone resorption in humans (Basu et al. 2011; Thrailkill et al. 2012; Winhofer et al. 2012). Moreover, patients suffering from a dominant form of osteopetrosis caused by a defect in osteoclasts activity were characterized by reduced serum levels of undercarboxylated osteocalcin and hypoinsulinemia (Ferron et al. 2010). One study found that changes in osteocalcin serum levels following the initiation of bisphosphonates treatment were correlated with changes in body weight and fat mass (Schafer et al. 2011). However, others failed in detecting any changes in glucose or insulin following treatment with the same class of drugs (Hong et al. 2013) or to observe a correlation between antiresorptive therapies and the risk of developing diabetes (Schwartz et al. 2013). Therefore, additional work is needed to clearly ascertain whether bone resorption also influences glucose metabolism in human.

Summary

Traditionally, bone has been viewed as a relatively static tissue, serving as a mere scaffold for the other organs and as a phosphate and calcium store. In the past decade however, mainly through the study of rare human diseases or the use of mouse genetics, a more complex picture of bone physiology has emerged. It is now clear that bone integrity and normal function depend upon, but also affect, other organs. In particular, a series of key discoveries made in the early 2000s revealed that bone possesses important endocrine functions. Osteoblasts and osteocytes, two bone cells otherwise implicated in the formation and maintenance of the bone extracellular matrix, secrete two hormones, FGF23 and osteocalcin, which have significant impact on the control of phosphate and glucose homeostasis, respectively. Importantly, like it is the case for other endocrine tissues, this endocrine function of bone is itself subjected to tight and complex regulations by other hormones. This chapter will review the basic biology of FGF23 and osteocalcin functions; the signal regulating their expression, secretion, and biological activity; and their respective implication in human pathologies.

Conclusion

Like many other organs, bone has emerged in recent years, as an unsuspected endocrine tissue. Bone cells secrete at least two hormones, osteocalcin and FGF23, which accomplish several physiological functions. A better and more complete understanding of all the roles and the regulation of these two bone-derived hormones must be achieved before FGF23- or osteocalcin-based therapies for phosphate or glucose metabolism disorders can be developed for humans. Nevertheless, wherever the future research on bone endocrine function will take us, it is clear that our view of bone has already been irremediably affected and transformed.

Cross-References

▸ G Protein-Coupled Receptors
▸ Synthesis, Secretion, and Transport of Peptide Hormones
▸ The Endocrine Pancreas
▸ The Endocrine Regulation of Energy and Body Weight
▸ The Physiology of the Testis

References

ADHRConsortium. Autosomal dominant hypophosphataemic rickets is associated with mutations in FGF23. Nat Genet. 2000;26(3):345–8.

Aonuma H, Miyakoshi N, Hongo M, Kasukawa Y, Shimada Y. Low serum levels of undercarboxylated osteocalcin in postmenopausal osteoporotic women receiving an inhibitor of bone resorption. Tohoku J Exp Med. 2009;218(3):201–5.

Basu R, Peterson J, Rizza R, Khosla S. Effects of physiological variations in circulating insulin levels on bone turnover in humans. J Clin Endocrinol Metab. 2011;96(5):1450–5.

Ben-Dov IZ, Galitzer H, Lavi-Moshayoff V, Goetz R, Kuro-o M, Mohammadi M, et al. The parathyroid is a target organ for FGF23 in rats. J Clin Invest. 2007;117(12):4003–8.

Brennan-Speranza TC, Henneicke H, Gasparini SJ, Blankenstein KI, Heinevetter U, Cogger VC, et al. Osteoblasts mediate the adverse effects of glucocorticoids on fuel metabolism. J Clin Invest. 2012;122(11):4172–89.

Brownstein CA, Adler F, Nelson-Williams C, Iijima J, Li P, Imura A, et al. A translocation causing increased alpha-klotho level results in hypophosphatemic rickets and hyperparathyroidism. Proc Natl Acad Sci U S A. 2008;105(9):3455–60.

Carpenter TO, Imel EA, Ruppe MD, Weber TJ, Klausner MA, Wooddell MM, et al. Randomized trial of the anti-FGF23 antibody KRN23 in X-linked hypophosphatemia. J Clin Invest. 2014;124(4):1587–97.

Das SK, Sharma NK, Elbein SC. Analysis of osteocalcin as a candidate gene for type 2 diabetes (T2D) and intermediate traits in Caucasians and African Americans. Dis Markers. 2010;28 (5):281–6.

Dowd TL, Rosen JF, Mints L, Gundberg CM. The effect of Pb(2+) on the structure and hydroxyapatite binding properties of osteocalcin. Biochim Biophys Acta. 2001;1535(2):153–63.

Ducy P, Desbois C, Boyce B, Pinero G, Story B, Dunstan C, et al. Increased bone formation in osteocalcin-deficient mice. Nature. 1996;382(6590):448–52.

Ducy P, Amling M, Takeda S, Priemel M, Schilling AF, Beil FT, et al. Leptin inhibits bone formation through a hypothalamic relay: a central control of bone mass. Cell. 2000;100 (2):197–207.

Esen E, Chen J, Karner CM, Okunade AL, Patterson BW, Long F. WNT-LRP5 signaling induces Warburg effect through mTORC2 activation during osteoblast differentiation. Cell Metab. 2013;17(5):745–55.

Ferron M, Hinoi E, Karsenty G, Ducy P. Osteocalcin differentially regulates beta cell and adipocyte gene expression and affects the development of metabolic diseases in wild-type mice. Proc Natl Acad Sci U S A. 2008;105(13):5266–70.

Ferron M, Wei J, Yoshizawa T, Del Fattore A, DePinho RA, Teti A, et al. Insulin signaling in osteoblasts integrates bone remodeling and energy metabolism. Cell. 2010;142(2):296–308.

Ferron M, Boudiffa M, Arsenault M, Rached M, Pata M, Giroux S, et al. Inositol polyphosphate 4-phosphatase B as a regulator of bone mass in mice and humans. Cell Metab. 2011;14 (4):466–77.

Ferron M, McKee MD, Levine RL, Ducy P, Karsenty G. Intermittent injections of osteocalcin improve glucose metabolism and prevent type 2 diabetes in mice. Bone. 2012;50(2):568–75.

Ferron M, Lacombe J. Regulation of energy metabolism by the skeleton: Osteocalcin and beyond. Archives of biochemistry and biophysics. 2014 Nov 1;561C:137–46. PubMed PMID: 24893146.

Ferron M, Lacombe J, Germain A, Oury F, Karsenty G. GGCX and VKORC1 inhibit osteocalcin endocrine functions. J Cell Biol. 2015;208(6):761–76.

Frey JL, Li Z, Ellis JM, Zhang Q, Farber CR, Aja S, et al. Wnt-Lrp5 signaling regulates fatty acid metabolism in the osteoblast. Mol Cell Biol. 2015;35(11):1979–91.

Fulzele K, Riddle RC, DiGirolamo DJ, Cao X, Wan C, Chen D, et al. Insulin receptor signaling in osteoblasts regulates postnatal bone acquisition and body composition. Cell. 2010;142 (2):309–19.

Gutierrez O, Isakova T, Rhee E, Shah A, Holmes J, Collerone G, et al. Fibroblast growth factor-23 mitigates hyperphosphatemia but accentuates calcitriol deficiency in chronic kidney disease. J Am Soc Nephrol. 2005;16(7):2205–15.

Gutierrez OM, Mannstadt M, Isakova T, Rauh-Hain JA, Tamez H, Shah A, et al. Fibroblast growth factor 23 and mortality among patients undergoing hemodialysis. N Engl J Med. 2008;359 (6):584–92.

Hauschka PV, Carr SA. Calcium-dependent alpha-helical structure in osteocalcin. Biochemistry. 1982;21(10):2538–47.

Henriksen DB, Alexandersen P, Hartmann B, Adrian CL, Byrjalsen I, Bone HG, et al. Four-month treatment with GLP-2 significantly increases hip BMD: a randomized, placebo-controlled, dose-ranging study in postmenopausal women with low BMD. Bone. 2009;45(5):833–42.

Hill HS, Grams J, Walton RG, Liu J, Moellering DR, Garvey WT. Carboxylated and uncarboxylated forms of osteocalcin directly modulate the glucose transport system and inflammation in adipocytes. Horm Metab Res = Horm Stoffwechselforschung = Horm Metab. 2014;46(5):341–7.

Hinoi E, Gao N, Jung DY, Yadav V, Yoshizawa T, Myers Jr MG, et al. The sympathetic tone mediates leptin's inhibition of insulin secretion by modulating osteocalcin bioactivity. J Cell Biol. 2008;183(7):1235–42.

Hoang QQ, Sicheri F, Howard AJ, Yang DS. Bone recognition mechanism of porcine osteocalcin from crystal structure. Nature. 2003;425(6961):977–80.

Hong SH, Koo JW, Hwang JK, Hwang YC, Jeong IK, Ahn KJ, et al. Changes in serum osteocalcin are not associated with changes in glucose or insulin for osteoporotic patients treated with bisphosphonate. J Bone Metab. 2013;20(1):37–41.

Ichikawa S, Guigonis V, Imel EA, Courouble M, Heissat S, Henley JD, et al. Novel GALNT3 mutations causing hyperostosis-hyperphosphatemia syndrome result in low intact fibroblast growth factor 23 concentrations. J Clin Endocrinol Metab. 2007a;92(5):1943–7.

Ichikawa S, Imel EA, Kreiter ML, Yu X, Mackenzie DS, Sorenson AH, et al. A homozygous missense mutation in human KLOTHO causes severe tumoral calcinosis. J Clin Invest. 2007b;117(9):2684–91.

Itoh N, Ohta H, Konishi M. Endocrine FGFs: evolution, physiology, pathophysiology, and pharmacotherapy. Front Endocrinol (Lausanne). 2015;6:154.

Iwamoto J, Takeda T, Sato Y. Effect of treatment with alendronate in osteogenesis imperfecta type I: a case report. Keio J Med. 2004;53(4):251–5.

Kajimura D, Lee HW, Riley KJ, Arteaga-Solis E, Ferron M, Zhou B, et al. Adiponectin regulates bone mass via opposite central and peripheral mechanisms through FoxO1. Cell Metab. 2013;17 (6):901–15.

Kato K, Jeanneau C, Tarp MA, Benet-Pages A, Lorenz-Depiereux B, Bennett EP, et al. Polypeptide GalNAc-transferase T3 and familial tumoral calcinosis. Secretion of fibroblast growth factor 23 requires *O*-glycosylation. J Biol Chem. 2006;281(27):18370–7.

Kemink SA, Hermus AR, Swinkels LM, Lutterman JA, Smals AG. Osteopenia in insulin-dependent diabetes mellitus; prevalence and aspects of pathophysiology. J Endocrinol Invest. 2000;23(5):295–303.

Korostishevsky M, Malkin I, Trofimov S, Pei Y, Deng HW, Livshits G. Significant association between body composition phenotypes and the osteocalcin genomic region in normative human population. Bone. 2012;51(4):688–94.

Kunutsor SK, Apekey TA, Laukkanen JA. Association of serum total osteocalcin with type 2 diabetes and intermediate metabolic phenotypes: systematic review and meta-analysis of observational evidence. Eur J Epidemiol. 2015;30(8):599–614.

Kuro-o M, Matsumura Y, Aizawa H, Kawaguchi H, Suga T, Utsugi T, et al. Mutation of the mouse klotho gene leads to a syndrome resembling ageing. Nature. 1997;390(6655):45–51.

Lacombe J, Karsenty G, Ferron M. In vivo analysis of the contribution of bone resorption to the control of glucose metabolism in mice. Mol Metab. 2013;2(4):498–504.

Larsson T, Marsell R, Schipani E, Ohlsson C, Ljunggren O, Tenenhouse HS, et al. Transgenic mice expressing fibroblast growth factor 23 under the control of the alpha1(I) collagen promoter exhibit growth retardation, osteomalacia, and disturbed phosphate homeostasis. Endocrinology. 2004;145(7):3087–94.

Lee NK, Sowa H, Hinoi E, Ferron M, Ahn JD, Confavreux C, et al. Endocrine regulation of energy metabolism by the skeleton. Cell. 2007;130(3):456–69.

Legroux-Gerot I, Vignau J, Collier F, Cortet B. Bone loss associated with anorexia nervosa. Joint Bone Spine. 2005;72(6):489–95.

Liu S, Tang W, Zhou J, Stubbs JR, Luo Q, Pi M, et al. Fibroblast growth factor 23 is a counter-regulatory phosphaturic hormone for vitamin D. J Am Soc Nephrol. 2006a;17 (5):1305–15.
Liu S, Zhou J, Tang W, Jiang X, Rowe DW, Quarles LD. Pathogenic role of Fgf23 in Hyp mice. Am J Physiol Endocrinol Metab. 2006b;291(1):E38–49.
Liu S, Vierthaler L, Tang W, Zhou J, Quarles LD. FGFR3 and FGFR4 do not mediate renal effects of FGF23. J Am Soc Nephrol. 2008;19(12):2342–50.
Liu C, Wo J, Zhao Q, Wang Y, Wang B, Zhao W. Association between serum total osteocalcin level and type 2 diabetes mellitus: a systematic review and meta-analysis. Horm Metab Res. 2015a;47 (11):813–9.
Liu DM, Guo XZ, Tong HJ, Tao B, Sun LH, Zhao HY, et al. Association between osteocalcin and glucose metabolism: a meta-analysis. Osteoporos Int. 2015b;26(12):2823–33.
Luo YQ, Ma XJ, Hao YP, Pan XP, Xu YT, Xiong Q, et al. Inverse relationship between serum osteocalcin levels and nonalcoholic fatty liver disease in postmenopausal Chinese women with normal blood glucose levels. Acta Pharmacol Sin. 2015;36(12):1497–502.
Ma X, Meng J, Jia M, Bi L, Zhou Y, Wang Y, et al. Exendin-4, a glucagon-like peptide-1 receptor agonist, prevents osteopenia by promoting bone formation and suppressing bone resorption in aged ovariectomized rats. J Bone Miner Res. 2013;28(7):1641–52.
Malashkevich VN, Almo SC, Dowd TL. X-ray crystal structure of bovine 3 Glu-osteocalcin. Biochemistry. 2013;52(47):8387–92.
Meyer Jr RA. Humoral abnormalities in X-linked hypophosphatemic mice. Nephron. 1989;53 (4):293–6.
Misra M, Klibanski A. The neuroendocrine basis of anorexia nervosa and its impact on bone metabolism. Neuroendocrinology. 2011;93(2):65–73.
Mizokami A, Yasutake Y, Gao J, Matsuda M, Takahashi I, Takeuchi H, et al. Osteocalcin induces release of glucagon-like peptide-1 and thereby stimulates insulin secretion in mice. PLoS One. 2013;8(2):e57375.
Mizokami A, Yasutake Y, Higashi S, Kawakubo-Yasukochi T, Chishaki S, Takahashi I, et al. Oral administration of osteocalcin improves glucose utilization by stimulating glucagon-like peptide-1 secretion. Bone. 2014;69:68–79.
Mokuda S, Okuda Y, Onishi M, Sawada N, Matoba K, Yamada A, et al. Post-menopausal women with rheumatoid arthritis who are treated with raloxifene or alendronate or glucocorticoids have lower serum undercarboxylated osteocalcin levels. J Endocrinol Invest. 2012;35(7):661–4.
Murshed M, Schinke T, McKee MD, Karsenty G. Extracellular matrix mineralization is regulated locally; different roles of two gla-containing proteins. J Cell Biol. 2004;165(5):625–30.
Ornitz DM, Itoh N. The fibroblast growth factor signaling pathway. Wiley Interdiscip Rev Dev Biol. 2015;4(3):215–66.
Ornitz DM, Marie PJ. Fibroblast growth factor signaling in skeletal development and disease. Genes Dev. 2015;29(14):1463–86.
Oury F, Sumara G, Sumara O, Ferron M, Chang H, Smith CE, et al. Endocrine regulation of male fertility by the skeleton. Cell. 2011;144(5):796–809.
Oury F, Ferron M, Huizhen W, Confavreux C, Xu L, Lacombe J, et al. Osteocalcin regulates murine and human fertility through a pancreas-bone-testis axis. J Clin Invest. 2013a;123(6):2421–33.
Oury F, Khrimian L, Denny CA, Gardin A, Chamouni A, Goeden N, et al. Maternal and offspring pools of osteocalcin influence brain development and functions. Cell. 2013b;155(1):228–41.
Pi M, Chen L, Huang MZ, Zhu W, Ringhofer B, Luo J, et al. GPRC6A null mice exhibit osteopenia, feminization and metabolic syndrome. PLoS One. 2008;3(12):e3858.
Pi M, Wu Y, Quarles LD. GPRC6A mediates responses to osteocalcin in beta-cells in vitro and pancreas in vivo. J Bone Miner Res. 2011;26(7):1680–3.
Pi M, Kapoor K, Ye R, Kenneth Nishimoto S, Smith JC, Baudry J, et al. Evidence for osteocalcin binding and activation of GPRC6A in beta-cells. Endocrinology. 2016;157:1866–80. en20152010.

Prader A, Illig R, Uehlinger E, Stalder G. Rickets following bone tumor. Helv Paediatr Acta. 1959;14:554–65.

Puig J, Blasco G, Daunis-i-Estadella J, Moreno M, Molina X, Alberich-Bayarri A, et al. Lower serum osteocalcin concentrations are associated with brain microstructural changes and worse cognitive performance. Clin Endocrinol (Oxf). 2016 May;84(5):756–63. PubMed PMID: 26406918.

Quarles LD. Endocrine functions of bone in mineral metabolism regulation. J Clin Invest. 2008;118 (12):3820–8.

Ravn P, Cizza G, Bjarnason NH, Thompson D, Daley M, Wasnich RD, et al. Low body mass index is an important risk factor for low bone mass and increased bone loss in early postmenopausal women. Early Postmenopausal Intervention Cohort (EPIC) study group. J Bone Miner Res. 1999;14(9):1622–7.

Razzaque MS, Sitara D, Taguchi T, St-Arnaud R, Lanske B. Premature aging-like phenotype in fibroblast growth factor 23 null mice is a vitamin D-mediated process. FASEB J. 2006;20 (6):720–2.

Riddle RC, Frey JL, Tomlinson RE, Ferron M, Li Y, DiGirolamo DJ, et al. Tsc2 is a molecular checkpoint controlling osteoblast development and glucose homeostasis. Mol Cell Biol. 2014;34(10):1850–62.

Schafer AL, Sellmeyer DE, Schwartz AV, Rosen CJ, Vittinghoff E, Palermo L, et al. Change in undercarboxylated osteocalcin is associated with changes in body weight, fat mass, and adiponectin: parathyroid hormone (1–84) or alendronate therapy in postmenopausal women with osteoporosis (the PaTH study). J Clin Endocrinol Metab. 2011;96(12):E1982–9.

Schwartz AV, Schafer AL, Grey A, Vittinghoff E, Palermo L, Lui LY, et al. Effects of antiresorptive therapies on glucose metabolism: results from the FIT, HORIZON-PFT, and FREEDOM trials. J Bone Miner Res. 2013;28(6):1348–54.

Shimada T, Kakitani M, Yamazaki Y, Hasegawa H, Takeuchi Y, Fujita T, et al. Targeted ablation of Fgf23 demonstrates an essential physiological role of FGF23 in phosphate and vitamin D metabolism. J Clin Invest. 2004;113(4):561–8.

Sinn DH, Gwak GY, Rhee SY, Cho J, Son HJ, Paik YH, et al. Association between serum osteocalcin levels and non-alcoholic fatty liver disease in women. Digestion. 2015;91(2):150–7.

Sumara G, Sumara O, Kim JK, Karsenty G. Gut-derived serotonin is a multifunctional determinant to fasting adaptation. Cell Metab. 2012;16(5):588–600.

Tagliabracci VS, Engel JL, Wiley SE, Xiao J, Gonzalez DJ, Nidumanda Appaiah H, et al. Dynamic regulation of FGF23 by Fam20C phosphorylation, GalNAc-T3 glycosylation, and furin proteolysis. Proc Natl Acad Sci U S A. 2014;111(15):5520–5.

Thrailkill KM, Jo CH, Cockrell GE, Moreau CS, Lumpkin Jr CK, Fowlkes JL. Determinants of undercarboxylated and carboxylated osteocalcin concentrations in type 1 diabetes. Osteoporos Int. 2012;23(6):1799–806.

Tremollieres FA, Pouilles JM, Ribot C. Vertebral postmenopausal bone loss is reduced in overweight women: a longitudinal study in 155 early postmenopausal women. J Clin Endocrinol Metab. 1993;77(3):683–6.

Tsuka S, Aonuma F, Higashi S, Ohsumi T, Nagano K, Mizokami A, et al. Promotion of insulin-induced glucose uptake in C2C12 myotubes by osteocalcin. Biochem Biophys Res Commun. 2015;459(3):437–42.

Urakawa I, Yamazaki Y, Shimada T, Iijima K, Hasegawa H, Okawa K, et al. Klotho converts canonical FGF receptor into a specific receptor for FGF23. Nature. 2006;444(7120):770–4.

Wei J, Hanna T, Suda N, Karsenty G, Ducy P. Osteocalcin promotes beta-cell proliferation during development and adulthood through Gprc6a. Diabetes. 2014;63(3):1021–31.

Wei J, Shimazu J, Makinistoglu MP, Maurizi A, Kajimura D, Zong H, et al. Glucose uptake and Runx2 synergize to orchestrate osteoblast differentiation and bone formation. Cell. 2015;161 (7):1576–91.

White KE, Jonsson KB, Carn G, Hampson G, Spector TD, Mannstadt M, et al. The autosomal dominant hypophosphatemic rickets (ADHR) gene is a secreted polypeptide overexpressed by tumors that cause phosphate wasting. J Clin Endocrinol Metab. 2001;86(2):497–500.

Winhofer Y, Kiefer FW, Handisurya A, Tura A, Klein K, Schneider B, et al. CTX (crosslaps) rather than osteopontin is associated with disturbed glucose metabolism in gestational diabetes. PLoS One. 2012;7(7):e40947.

Yadav VK, Oury F, Suda N, Liu ZW, Gao XB, Confavreux C, et al. A serotonin-dependent mechanism explains the leptin regulation of bone mass, appetite, and energy expenditure. Cell. 2009;138(5):976–89.

Yamauchi T, Kamon J, Waki H, Terauchi Y, Kubota N, Hara K, et al. The fat-derived hormone adiponectin reverses insulin resistance associated with both lipoatrophy and obesity. Nat Med. 2001;7(8):941–6.

Part VI

The Regulatory Role of Endocrine System

The Endocrine Regulation of Energy and Body Weight

22

Valentina Lo Preiato, Valentina Vicennati, Alessandra Gambineri, and Uberto Pagotto

Abstract

The regulation of body weight is governed by a delicate balance between complex mechanisms controlling food intake and energy expenditure. In this scenario, hormones of peripheral origins and of neuronal production, nutrients, and other factors including information generated by the sensory experience of eating are integrated by the brain to define the energy requirement of the body to consequently modify the experience of hunger and satiety, respectively. However, this sophisticated balance regulating feeding and energy expenditure may become partially compromised or even totally altered, leading to consequent pathological changes in body weight. Adaptations to body weight changes include modifications at the level of circulating appetite-related hormones that, in turn, may profoundly interact with the homeostatic and hedonistic neural centers. The homeostatic control system makes it possible to maintain energy reserves through signals of hunger stimulation that are usually downregulated when the body receives an adequate caloric intake. However, this homeostatic system is asymmetrical, showing greater effectiveness in defending against energy deficit in the light of a reduced efficiency in the defense against the energy excess. Furthermore, the homeostatic system is strongly influenced by hedonic signals, based on reward mechanisms, frequently causing food intake even in the absence of biological needs. This review will summarize the role of the main central and peripheral hormones involved in controlling energy balance.

V. Lo Preiato • V. Vicennati
Bologna, Italy

A. Gambineri • U. Pagotto (✉)
Division of Endocrinology, Department of Medical and Surgical Sciences, Centre for Applied Biomedical Research (C.R.B.A.), S. Orsola-Malpighi Hospital, Alma Mater Studiorum University of Bologna, Bologna, Italy
e-mail: uberto.pagotto@unibo.it

A. Belfiore, D. LeRoith (eds.), *Principles of Endocrinology and Hormone Action*, Endocrinology, https://doi.org/10.1007/978-3-319-44675-2_22

Keywords
Hormone • Hypothalamus • Food intake • Mesolimbic system • Brainstem • Gut • Adipose tissue • Endocrine pancreas

Contents

The Homeostatic Control of Food Intake

The homeostatic control of food intake is mainly exercised by the hypothalamus and the brainstem. These cerebral areas integrate acute satiation signals, mainly arising in the gut and secreted phasically during meals, with more tonically active signals to appropriately adjust nutrient intake and energy expenditure coming from peripheral organs such as adipose tissue and endocrine pancreas. Indeed, several hormones are secreted by the gastrointestinal tract, most of them signal satiety such as cholecystokinin (CCK), glucagon-like peptide-1 (GLP-1), glucagon-like peptide-2 (GLP-2), oxyntomodulin (OXM), and peptide YY (PYY). Only ghrelin, produced in the stomach, is able to stimulate hunger. Other peripheral hormones such as insulin and leptin may exert tonically anorectic effects by directly interacting with the hypothalamus and the brainstem. These two cerebral areas are strongly linked to other brain regions and in particular to those involved in the mechanisms of hedonic food intake control.

The Hypothalamus

The hypothalamus is located at the base of the brain, around the third ventricle, and is divided into various nuclei, each of these being involved in the regulation of a number of fundamental biological processes, including energy balance control. The hypothalamic nuclei have many synaptic connections among themselves, but they also receive neural afferents and hormonal signals from the periphery in order to generate an integrative message to be released to the higher brain centers to definitively control food intake and energy expenditure. The hypothalamic nuclei involved in the homeostatic control of food intake include the arcuate nucleus (ARC), the paraventricular nucleus (PVH), the ventromedial nucleus (VMN), the dorsomedial nucleus (DMN), and the lateral hypothalamic area (LHA).

Arcuate Nucleus

The ARC is located at the foot of the hypothalamus, near to the median eminence. In this area, the blood-brain barrier (BBB) is not present; thus, due to the anatomical location, the ARC is considered to be a hypothalamic area primarily sensing peripheral hormonal and metabolic nutrient signals. In the ARC, various populations of first-order neurons have been described such as neuropeptide Y (NPY) and agouti-related peptide (AgRP) co-expressing neurons stimulating food intake, therefore exhibiting anabolic properties, and proopiomelanocortin (POMC) and cocaine- and amphetamine-regulated transcript (CART) co-expressing neurons suppressing hunger and consequently exhibiting catabolic actions (Morton et al. 2014).

AgRP/NPY neurons release not only AgRP and NPY (Hahn et al. 1998; Tong et al. 2008) but also γ-aminobutyric acid (GABA), and through the action of this neurotransmitter, they inhibit adjacent anorectic POMC neurons (Cowley et al. 2001). In rats, intracerebroventricular (IVC) infusion of AgRP or NPY determines food intake increase and delay of the onset of satiety (Stanley et al. 1985). NPY effects are mediated by six specific subtypes of receptors (Fetissov et al. 2004; Lin et al. 2005); among these, Y1 and Y5 interact synergistically to convey the orexigenic effect of NPY (Mashiko et al. 2009). AgRP released from the terminals of AgRP/NPY neurons to the synaptic space of neurons of the second order counteracts the anorexigenic effect of MSH, being a potent and selective antagonist of type 3 melanocortin receptor (MC3R) and type 4 melanocortin receptor (MC4R) (Ollmann et al. 1997). The AgRP/NPY neurons receive influences from the periphery, being stimulated by ghrelin, while inhibited by amylin, insulin, leptin, and serotonin (5-HT) (Harrold et al. 2012). Importantly, fasting increases AgRP neuron GABAergic inputs on POMC neurons (Vong et al. 2011) resulting in POMC activity neuron reduction and promotion of food intake (Cowley et al. 2001). In addition, the AgRP neurons can interact with the reward corticolimbic system, increasing the motivation for eating behavior (Krashes et al. 2011).

POMC/CART neurons belong to the melanocortin system, comprising of agonist peptides and specific receptors. Cleavage of the precursor protein POMC produces α-melanocyte-stimulating hormone (α-MSH) that is released from presynaptic terminals of POMC neurons and binds to MC3R and MC4R, G protein-coupled receptors highly expressed in the hypothalamus on the second-order neurons mainly located at the level of PVH (Mountjoy 2015; Krashes et al. 2016). In this way, α-MSH activates catabolic pathways reducing food intake and enhancing energy expenditure (Krashes et al. 2016). MC4R is thought to have a major role in suppressing food intake compared to MC3R. MC4R knockout mice have hyperphagia and obesity (Huszar et al. 1997). In humans, MC4R mutations account for 6% of early-onset obesity, clearly warranting the pivotal role of the central melanocortin system in the control of energy metabolism (Krashes et al. 2016). In contrast, MC3R null mice develop obesity in the absence of elevated food intake, indicating a role in fat homeostasis (Chen et al. 2000). Interestingly, being located on ARC melanocortin neurons, MC3R also appears to play the role of an autoreceptor (Lee et al. 2008). POMC neurons also project to the VMN, where α-MSH stimulates the expression of anorexigenic brain-derived neurotrophic factor (BDNF) (Xu et al. 2003), and to the nucleus of tractus solitarius (NTS), promoting satiety (Zheng et al. 2005, 2010). The expression level of POMC and the release of α-MSH from POMC neurons are regulated by nutrient signals and adiposity. Glucose stimulates the α-MSH release (Parton et al. 2007), whereas leptin stimulates the expression of both POMC and CART (Fan et al. 1997; Kristensen et al. 1998). Moreover, a subpopulation of POMC neurons (distinct from POMC neurons expressing leptin receptors) expresses the 5-HT subtype 2c receptor (5-HT_{2C}) that binds the endogenous neurotransmitter 5-HT. 5-HT, released from the raphe nuclei, stimulates MSH release (Heisler et al. 2002); indeed, 5-HT_{2C}R-deficient mice are hyperphagic and obese (Tecott et al. 1995; Nonogaki et al. 1998; Sohn et al. 2011). Moreover, POMC/CART neurons extend their terminals to the dopaminergic neurons in the nucleus accumbens (NAc), suggesting that they mediate messages between the homeostatic and the hedonic system controlling food intake (Krashes et al. 2016).

As described above, POMC/CART neurons also produce CART, a peptide representing the third most abundant transcript identified within the hypothalamus. Its abundant mRNA distribution within the hypothalamus and NAc evokes a role for CART in the control of food intake (Lau and Herzog 2014). The physiological role of CART in energy homeostasis has not yet been fully defined, although an involvement of this peptide has been proposed in a variety of mechanisms impacting on food intake. In rats, central administration of CART to rodents determines suppression of food intake (Yang and Shieh 2005), whereas blocking CART action by central infusion of anti-CART antibodies has been shown to increase food intake (Lau and Herzog 2014). Administration of CART inhibits NPY-induced feeding, while administration of leptin increases CART mRNA in the ARC (Kristensen et al. 1998). Additionally, there is evidence for interactions between CART and endocannabinoids and dopamine, key players in the hedonic regulatory circuitry (Osei-Hyiaman et al. 2005; Lage et al. 2015; Jaworsky et al. 2003). On the other hand, CART appears to have a role in energy expenditure as the injection of CART in the PVH or ARC determines a dramatic increase in the uncoupling protein-1 transcription in rats' brown adipose tissue (Wang et al. 2000; Kong et al. 2003).

The ARC has extensive reciprocal connections with other hypothalamic appetite-regulating regions including the PVH, VMH, DMH, and LHA, also receiving afferent information via the NTS.

Paraventricular Nucleus

The main function of the PVH is the integration of signals from many neuronal pathways involved in the regulation of energy intake. For many years, it has been known that lesions of the PVH result in hyperphagia, reduced energy expenditure, and obesity (Shor-Posner et al. 1986); this means that the neuropeptides secreted at PVH level exhibit a catabolic effect, as a whole. These neuropeptides include thyrotropin-releasing hormone (TRH), corticotropin-releasing hormone (CRH), and oxytocin (Rui 2013). The main catabolic action of TRH is due to its stimulation of the TSH-thyroid hormones axis, producing an increase in the basal metabolic rate. The action of CRH neurons in hunger regulation is still under discussion. The CRH-ACTH-glucocorticoid system is involved in stressful situation management. Generally, acute and intense stress leads to a reduction of hunger, while chronic stress tends to increase the intake of food in rodents, monkeys, and humans (Ulrich-Lai et al. 2007; Willner et al. 1996; Bartolomucci et al. 2009; Michopoulos et al. 2012; Bellisle et al. 1990; Rutters et al. 2009; Wardle et al. 2000; Vicennati et al. 2011). On the other hand, glucocorticoids promote the activation of AgRP neurons and inhibition of POMC neurons (Gyengesi et al. 2010), therefore promoting an anabolic action. Importantly, glucocorticoids seem to be involved in food choices. In particular, in stressful situations, numerous studies in animals and humans have shown that highly palatable foods are favored (Francis et al. 2013; George et al. 2010). Oxytocin, produced in the PVH but also in the supraoptic nucleus, has an anorectic function as demonstrated by the inhibition of food intake after its central administration in rodents (Onaka et al. 2012) and by the hyperphagia caused by blocking oxytocin release (Zhang et al. 2011). Oxytocin increases the NTS sensitivity to satiety signals (Matarazzo et al. 2012; Blevins et al. 2004), also reducing the AgRP neurons' action. Satiety signals arising from the gastrointestinal system may result in an increase of oxytocin release (Onaka et al. 2012; Matarazzo et al. 2012).

Ventromedial Nucleus

The VMN plays a fundamental role in the integration of hunger and satiety signals, such as receiving neuronal projections from the ARC and, in turn, projecting the glutamatergic axons to the ARC, the LHA, and the brainstem. VMN neurons produce the anorectic factor BDNF, which acts at the level of the PVH, increasing the production of CRH and MC4R expression (Toriya et al. 2010; Cordeira and Rios 2011; Noble et al. 2011; Jeanneteau et al. 2012). Importantly, VMN neurons act as sensors of glucose and leptin and in rats and VMN destruction causes obesity, hyperphagia, and hyperglycemia (Shimizu et al. 1987). For these reasons, VMN is regarded as a crucial area to stabilize satiety and to maintain glucose homeostasis in the physiological ranges.

Dorsomedial Nucleus

The DMN contains abundant orexigenic NPY neurons which project to the PVH and LHA; NPY therefore seems to be the neuropeptide playing a pivotal role in the DMN. Increased NPY expression in the DMN has been detected under diet-induced obesity (Guan et al. 1998; Bi et al. 2003; Lee et al. 2013), NPY administration into the DMH increases food intake (Bi et al. 2012), and overexpression of NPY in the same nucleus also increases food intake and body weight in rats (Yang et al. 2009). Neurons in the DMN express CCK1 receptors, and injection of CCK into the DMN decreases food intake (Bi et al. 2004), suggesting that DMN neurons may integrate satiety signals arriving from peripheral sites. Destruction of the DMN results in hyperphagia and obesity (Bernardis et al. 1987).

Lateral Hypothalamic Area

In contrast to the PVN, VMN, and DMN, destruction of the LHA leads to weight loss and hypophagia. LHA neurons produce two neuropeptides: orexin (hypocretin) and melanin-concentrating hormone (MCH). Orexin is present in two isoforms: A and B that act in several brain areas. In fact, orexin receptors (OX_1R and OX_2R) are widely expressed in the brain (Sakurai et al. 1998). Stimulation of these receptors causes increased food intake (Parise et al. 2011). Moreover, orexin-producing neurons are also involved in the control of blood pressure and body temperature and more importantly in the regulation of sleep-awake cycles (Plazzi et al. 2011). An impairment of the hypocretin neurotransmission causes narcolepsy, a chronic sleep disorder characterized by cataplexy and excessive daytime sleepiness (Plazzi et al. 2011). In addition to its stimulation on food intake, orexin-A increases oxygen consumption and energy expenditure, thus preventing weight gain. This is why narcoleptic patients, who usually completely lose brain orexin signaling, do show increased body weight. Glucose is a very important peripheral nutrient signal that appears to regulate orexin neuronal activity; indeed, orexin neurons are stimulated by low levels of glycemia (Burdakov et al. 2013). The orexin neurons also activate the MCH neurons in the LHA (Tsujino and Sakurai 2009).

Numerous studies have demonstrated the endogenous orexigenic action of MCH. Indeed, MCH overexpression is associated with obesity (Ludwig et al. 2001). Conversely, transgenic mice that are deficient in MCH receptors or MCH are lean (Marsh et al. 2002). NPY/AgRP and α-MSH immunoreactive terminals from ARC neurons are in close contact with orexin and MCH expression of LHA neurons; at the same time, large populations of orexigenic neurons from the LHA project to the mesolimbic area to connect homeostatic with hedonic circuits.

Brainstem

Peripheral signals such as those represented by the hormones produced by the gastrointestinal tract may influence food intake at three sites: the hypothalamus, the vagus nerve, and the brainstem. Within the brainstem, the dorsal vagal complex (DVC) plays a crucial role in relaying these peripheral signals to the hypothalamus. The DVC includes the NTS, the dorsal motor nucleus of the vagus nerve (DVN), and the area postrema (AP). The NTS receives extensive neuronal projections from the PVN of the hypothalamus and vice versa; furthermore, afferent sensory information from the mouth (carried by the cranial nerves), including taste, also converges on this region, thus generating a key site for integration of various afferent signals and for relaying such signals to further CNS integratory sites. Like the ARC, the NTS is located in an ideal position to integrate peripheral signals due to its close proximity to the AP, which has an incomplete BBB. Indeed, numerous peripheral hormones act on the NTS, such as CCK (Moriarty et al. 1997), ghrelin (Lawrence et al. 2002), GLP-1 (Nakagawa et al. 2004), and leptin (Burdyga et al. 2002). It has been observed that the effects of various peripheral hormones on food intake are attenuated by lesions of the AP (van der Kooy 1984) or vagotomy (Schwartz et al. 1978; Date et al. 2002; Abbott et al. 2005a; Koda et al. 2005), indicating the importance of this brainstem area in controlling energy balance and in particular in determining the size of the meal. The sectioning of all vagal fibers causes an increase in the amount of food consumed and the duration of the outage.

Hedonic Control of Food Intake

Hedonic control of food intake refers to the involvement of cognitive and emotional factors in the eating regulation. In such case, the rewarding properties of food override the homeostatic requirements; thus, fuel depletion does not represent the motivation to eat, whereas palatability and pleasure constitute the most powerful motivators of eating. The neuronal circuitries involved in the hedonic control of food intake are complex. They mainly involve the insula and orbitofrontal cortex (brain areas controlling emotional experience of pleasure, also defined as "liking") and subcortical limbic structures like the amygdala, ventro-tegmental area (VTA), and NAc (brain structures involved in the motivational processes toward food, a process named as "wanting") (Nicola 2016). Dopaminergic neuron projections to the NAc, usually excited by glutamate and inhibited by GABAergic fibers, respectively, have been strongly implicated in food reward with the potential to exert their crucial role in translating motivation into action. The importance of this neuronal system is demonstrated by numerous observations in rodents and humans. Mice lacking dopamine caused by the selective inactivation of tyrosine hydroxylase develop fatal hypophagia, and this effect will disappear if dopamine is centrally injected (Szczypka et al. 2001). In addition, a study using PET has suggested that obese individuals have decreased DA dopamine 2 (D2) receptor availability in the striatum (Wang et al. 2001). Moreover, individuals carrying a genetic polymorphism thought to attenuate dopamine signaling in this region (TaqIA A1 allele) may overeat to compensate for a hypofunctioning dorsal striatum, as demonstrated by functional magnetic resonance imaging (fMRI) (Stice et al. 2008). Along the same lines, it has been shown that the lower D2 receptors correlate with a higher body mass index (BMI) in obese subjects (Haltia et al. 2007). These findings are consistent with the hypothesis that diminished D2 receptor activity promotes feeding and the risk of obesity (Volkow et al. 2011).

Opioids and endocannabinoids, together with dopamine, appear to make a significant contribution to the control of reward-related food intake. Opioids are involved in food choices; indeed, the administration of μ-opioid receptor agonists in the NAc stimulates the intake of highly palatable foods, characterized by either sweetness or high fat content (Zhang et al. 1998). Conversely, the administration of opioid antagonists in patients with binge eating behavior evokes a substantial reduction of sweet food consumption (Drewnowski et al. 1992; Yeomans and Gray 1996). Opioid antagonist administration seems to more the pleasantness of food affect than modifying the sense of hunger or the sensory evaluation of food (Yeomans and Gray 1996). This is why it is known that opioids affect the "liking" more than the "wanting"; indeed, the impact of opioids on the intake of palatable food is orientated more toward the maintenance and termination of feeding rather than on the initiation of feeding.

Studies carried out in the last 20 years clearly showed that also cannabinoids of both endogenous and exogenous origin may play an important role in the hedonic aspect of eating. These findings originally derive from epidemiological evidence reporting the strong impulse promoted by the use of marijuana toward highly palatable food (Cota et al. 2003; Silvestri and Di Marzo 2013). Marijuana is a recreational drug known to contain Δ9-tetrahydrocannabinol (Δ9-THC), an exogenous cannabinoid. After the identification of the two major endogenous cannabinoids – 2-arachidonylglycerol (2-AG) and anandamide (AEA) – a series of experiments showed that the activation of cannabinoid type 1 receptor (CB1) by Δ9-THC or synthetic CB1 agonists stimulates feeding (Jamshidi and Taylor 2001; Kirkham et al. 2002). On the other hand, CB1 antagonists have been shown to reduce food intake and body weight in rodents and humans (Cota et al. 2006). At the level of the mesolimbic system, endocannabinoids strongly interact with both dopaminergic and opioidergic pathways, resulting in strong stimulation toward highly palatable food (Verty et al. 2004; Cota et al. 2006; Melis et al. 2007). AEA injection into the NAc has been shown to increase liking reactions to sucrose (Mahler et al. 2007), whereas the release of dopamine in the NAc in response to palatable food is inhibited by the CB1 antagonist rimonabant (Melis et al. 2007). In response to fasting, an increased amount of endocannabinoids is produced in the NAc, returning to normal after refeeding (Kirkham et al. 2002). A similar increase is described in the hypothalamus (Kirkham et al. 2002), under the influence of two main feeding-regulated hormones, i.e., leptin (Di Marzo et al. 2002) and ghrelin (Kola et al. 2008). This is one of the pieces of evidence supporting a role for the endocannabinoid system not only in the hedonic processes regulating food intake but also in the homeostatic mechanisms controlling energy balance (Wenger et al. 1997; Jamshidi and Taylor 2001; Verty et al. 2009). However, cerebral functions related to mesolimbic or even superior centers such as liking and wanting may also be modulated by peripheral hormones. Leptin acts on the dopaminergic neurons in the VTA to suppress feeding (Hommel et al. 2006), presumably by decreasing hedonic and incentive values of food and food ingestion (Hommel et al. 2006; Fulton et al. 2006). Insulin also directly suppresses dopamine neuron activity in the VTA, which contributes to insulin's anorexigenic effects (Labouebe et al. 2013). In contrast, ghrelin activates the corticolimbic reward system in humans and increases hedonic and incentive valences of food-related cues (Malik et al. 2008).

The Role of the Peripheral Hormones in the Control of Food Intake

Tonic and episodic peripheral factors from the gastrointestinal tract, adipose tissue, and pancreas are integrated in the brain to influence food intake. Tonic factors are usually hormones presumed to influence metabolic needs over the long term, whereas episodic factors are short-term signals of various origin influencing hunger and satiety (Halford and Blundell 2000). Hunger is defined as the stimulus to seek and eat food, initiating a feeding episode. Conversely, satiation can be explained as the feeling of fullness that contributes to the decision to stop eating. This ultimately leads to a state of satiety that may be described as the prolongation of the interval until hunger or the drive to eat reappears (Harrold et al. 2012). Food smell and/or sight, as well as food taste and/or textures, may represent important hunger signals that anticipate consumption of food (McCrickerd and Forde 2016). The sensory information continues with the oral phase, in which contact of the food with the oral mucosa is notified and transmitted to the brainstem via the cranial nerves. The perception of food taste and smell is modified by a series of hormonal signals such as leptin, insulin, GLP-1, endocannabinoids (Soria-Gomez et al. 2014), and many others (Berthoud 2011). Leptin is able to reduce the perception of sweet taste by acting on tongue taste cells (Shigemura et al. 2004) and to modulate the smell of food by changing the mucus production in the olfactory mucosa cells (Badonnel et al. 2009). GLP-1 stimulates the intake of sweet foods, at the same time reducing salty food intake (Martin et al. 2009). Subsequently, the passage of food in the stomach results in gastric distension and production of a series of peptidergic hormones by enteroendocrine cells. The gastrointestinal tract releases more than 20 different regulatory peptide hormones that influence food intake by decreasing hypothalamic orexigenic signaling and increasing anorectic signaling directly or via vagal afferent nerve activation (Lean and Malkova 2016). Another effect of these peptides is to mediate inhibitory feedback mechanisms on intestinal transit, contributing to prolonged gastric distension, and increased satiety between meals. On the other hand, nutrients like lipids and glucose and some neurotransmitter precursors are, once absorbed, also able to directly interact in key regulatory sites of the brain.

Signals from the Gastrointestinal Tract in the Control of Food Intake

Ghrelin

Ghrelin is an octanoylated peptide showing a unique orexigenic property among the hormones produced by the gastrointestinal tract (Tschöp et al. 2000). This has been proved by the experiments in which central or peripheral infusion of ghrelin stimulated food intake in rodents and humans (Wren et al. 2000, 2001). However, some recent data do not favor a role of peripheral ghrelin in the regulation of food intake (Lippl et al. 2012). Indeed, ghrelin circulating levels peak in response to fasting and anticipation of the coming meal; thus, the role attributed to this hormone is to initiate and promote eating (Cummings et al. 2001). Consequently, serum ghrelin levels are shown to be decreased by refeeding. In humans, circulating ghrelin levels are negatively correlated with BMI (Lean and Malkova 2016), and more importantly, compared with lean subjects, obese subjects demonstrated less suppression of ghrelin following the meal (English et al. 2002). This flattened ghrelin profile around mealtimes may be a factor in the altered eating behavior pattern reported in obese subjects. Ghrelin is principally secreted by gastric oxyntic gland cells but also by the intestine, pancreas, colon, and brain (Müller et al. 2015). Being expressed within the ARC and PVH of the hypothalamus, ghrelin may also act as a neurotransmitter (Cowley et al. 2003). Ghrelin's action is vagally mediated; in fact, its receptor GHS-R has been found to be expressed in the vagus nerve (Page et al. 2007), although a direct ghrelin action on the CNS via stimulation of NPY/AgRP neurons within the ARC has been hypothesized (Wang et al. 2002). Indeed, the total ablation of both NPY and AgRP hypothalamic neurons completely abolishes ghrelin's orexigenic action (Chen et al. 2004). Furthermore, a recent large body of evidence suggests that, via activation of its receptor in the VTA, ghrelin may impact on mesolimbic dopamine circuitry to enhance the motivation for highly palatable food (Dickson et al. 2011).

CCK

CCK is a 27-amino-acid peptide able to trigger short-term satiation processes in the upper gastrointestinal tract. Indeed, CCK is secreted postprandially by the I cell of the duodenal and jejunal mucosa in response to fat- and protein-containing meals, rising in the plasma within 15 min after meal ingestion and not beginning to fall until 3–5 h after food intake (Murphy and Bloom 2006). CCK acts by binding to its receptors, CCK-1 and CCK-2, differently distributed at the peripheral levels and in the CNS (Moran et al. 1986). Physiological functions of CCK include stimulating the release of enzymes from the pancreas and gallbladder, promoting intestinal motility, delaying gastric emptying, stimulating gallbladder contraction, and reducing gastric acid secretion (Moran and Kinzig 2004). Moreover, a large body of evidence showed that CCK infusion reduces meal quantity in rodents, monkeys, and humans (Gibbs et al. 1973; Hirosue et al. 1993; Figlewicz et al. 1992; Kissileff et al. 1981). This anorectic effect seems to be mainly mediated by CCK-1 receptors, in particular by receptors endowed in the vagus nerve (Beglinger et al. 2001). The importance of the vagus nerve is highlighted by some studies that show that bilateral vagotomy reduces the anorectic actions of CCK. However, vagotomy does not cause the complete absence of CCK's anorectic effects. This suggests that CCK may also act independently of the vagus nerve (Zhang and Ritter 2012). Indeed, the CCK-1 receptors are also found in the hypothalamus (Blevins et al. 2000), and CCK administration to fasted rats has been demonstrated to induce expression changes in neuropeptides and their receptors involved in food intake (Dockray and Burdyga 2011).

GLP-1

GLP-1 is a gut hormone resulting from the cleavage of the pre-proglucagon precursor peptide. Differential tissue-specific posttranslational processing of proglucagon in the pancreas and in the gut and brain via proteolytic cleavage by prohormone convertases 1 and 2 occurs. In the pancreas, processing yields the glucagon sequence, whereas the region containing the GLP-1 and GLP-2 peptides is secreted as a single inactive fusion called major proglucagon fragment (MPGF) or GLP-1 and GLP-2. Posttranslational processing in the gut and brain results in the secretion of GLP-1 and GLP2, while the glucagon sequence remains in a larger peptide, glicentin or glicentin-related pancreatic peptide, and OXM (Pocai 2012). GLP-1 and OXM are expressed in L-cells and glucagon in pancreatic α-cells (Cho et al. 2014). Throughout the intestine, GLP-1 is stored in L-cell granules and invariably co-secreted with another peptide called PYY in response to nutrient ingestion. Among macronutrients, sugars and lipids are the more potent stimulators of GLP-1 secretion. GLP-1 has two biologically active forms: GLP-1_{7-37} and GLP-1_{7-36} both showing a short plasma half-life (1–2 min), partly because

GLP-1 undergoes rapid enzymatic degradation by dipeptil-peptidase IV (DPP-IV), partly due to the renal clearance (Cho et al. 2014; Campbell and Drucker 2013). Circulating GLP-1 levels rise postprandially and fall in fasted state; however, it has recently been demonstrated that GLP-1 blood levels rise in anticipation of a meal (Vahl et al. 2010). GLP-1_{7-36} is widely distributed within the CNS. Immunoreactive neurons for GLP-1_{7-36} are located in the NTS, PVN, DMN, DVC, and pituitary (Larsen et al. 1997). GLP-1 exerts its effect through activation of the GLP-1 receptor (GLP-1R), a G protein-coupled receptor. GLP-1R is widely distributed in the gastrointestinal tract, in the pancreas, in the nodose ganglion, and, importantly, in the brain, in particular in hypothalamus glial cells, in POMC neurons, and in the striatum, brainstem, substantia nigra, subventricular zone, and amygdala (Holst 2007). GLP-1, along with glucose-dependent insulinotropic polypeptide (GIP), is responsible for the "incretin" effect, a mechanism by which insulin secretion is enhanced in response to oral but not to intravenous glucose administration (Campbell and Drucker 2013). Together with this action that is lost or firmly reduced in association with type 2 diabetes mellitus, GLP-1 has other physiological functions such as inhibition of glucagon secretion and reduction of gastric emptying rate (Deane et al. 2010). Indeed, GLP-1 contributes to the "ileal brake" by delaying gastric emptying to decelerate nutrient absorption (Campbell and Drucker 2013). The "ileal brake" is a negative feedback mechanism that inhibits the motility of the upper gastrointestinal tract when unabsorbed dietary components are present in the colon in order to allow efficient digestion and nutrient uptake (Spreckley and Murphy 2015). The inhibition of gastric emptying induced by GLP-1 partially explains the anorectic effect of this hormone, an effect that is probably mediated by local GLP-1 action on vagal nerve afferents in the GI tract or by GLP-1 central action on vagal efferents (Plamboeck et al. 2013). Nevertheless, there is strong evidence that circulating GLP-1 has appetite-suppressing effects through direct activation of energy homeostatic centers in the brain (De Silva et al. 2011; Sisley et al. 2014). Moreover, consistent with the neuroanatomical location in areas that mediate hedonic control of food intake, functional studies support a role for GLP-1R signaling in regulating food reward (Heppner and Perez-Tilve 2015). Recent fMRI studies in obese and obese diabetic patients have demonstrated that intravenous infusion of GLP-1 agonist decreases the activation of brain regions involved in mediating food reward (van Bloemendaal et al. 2014). Due to the action on insulin secretion and for the anorectic effect attributed to GLP-1, pharmacotherapies based on GLP-1 analogues represent milestones in the treatment of type 2 diabetes mellitus and obesity (Pi-Sunyer et al. 2015; Marso et al. 2016).

GLP-2

GLP-2 is a 33-amino-acid peptide co-secreted with GLP-1 by L-cells in response to a meal. As GLP-1, it is also rapidly degraded by DPP-IV. GLP-2 reduces gastric motility and acid secretion, induces crypt cell proliferation and contributes to improve nutrient absorption (Spreckley and Murphy 2015). However, its role in energy balance regulation seems to be less important than the role of GLP-1.

OXM

OXM is a longer isoform of glucagon produced by L-gut cells. Like GLP-1, OXM is also rapidly degraded by DPP-IV. OXM is a dual agonist of the GLP-1 and glucagon receptors but with a 10- to 100-fold lower affinity than the native ligands. OXM has been shown to delay gastric emptying and to reduce gastric acid secretion. Moreover, this peptide has been demonstrated to decrease food intake and in the longer term to decrease weight gain in rodents (Dakin et al. 2001) and humans (Wynne et al. 2005) by suppressing food intake but also by increasing energy expenditure. Indeed, the effects attributed to OXM potentially combine its effect on GLP-1R to reduce food intake and on the glucagon receptor to increase energy expenditure. On the other hand, the activation of the glucagon receptor is classically associated with an elevation in glucose levels, while the hypoglycemic properties of GLP-1R agonism counteract this effect. OXM thus represents a therapeutic target for obesity treatment (Heppner and Perez-Tilve 2015).

PYY

Like NPY and pancreatic polypeptide (PP), PYY belongs to the "PP-fold" family of proteins. PYY is released by L-distal intestine cells in response to ingested nutrients. There are two forms of PYY: PPY_{1-36} and PYY_{3-36}, this latter being the product of PYY_{1-36} degradation by DPP-IV. PYY_{3-36} is released at the very end of the meal or immediately after, thereafter determining a decrease in gastric emptying and consequently a reduction in food intake (Manning and Batterham 2014). PYY has also been reported to regulate energy expenditure, reduce acid secretion, and inhibit gallbladder contraction and pancreatic exocrine secretions (Suzuki et al. 2012). In normal-weight and obese human subjects, high-protein intake induced the greatest release of PYY_{3-36} (Batterham et al. 2006), whereas studies of circulating levels of PYY in obese and lean people reported inconsistent results (Batterham et al. 2003; Pfluger et al. 2007). PPY_{1-36} acts on all NPY Y receptors, while PYY_{3-36} acts primarily on NPY Y_2 receptors of the vagus nerve and hypothalamus. Peripheral administration of PYY_{3-36} has been shown in a number of studies to reduce food intake and weight gain in rodents (Batterham et al. 2002; Chelikani et al. 2005; Vrang et al. 2006) and humans (Batterham et al. 2003). However, the anorectic effect of PYY_{3-36} in rodents has been critically discussed by others (Tschop et al. 2004). The peripheral anorectic effect of PYY_{3-36} seems to be due to a direct action of presynaptic inhibitory NPY Y_2 receptors located on the ARC, and these receptors may act in an auto-inhibitory fashion for NPY. However, it has also been suggested that PYY_{3-36} acts to reduce food intake via the vagal afferent nerves (Broberger et al. 1997; Abbott et al. 2005b). Similarly to other hormones produced in the gastrointestinal tract, PYY_{3-36} has been demonstrated to be able to modulate neural activity not only in brain areas associated with homeostatic appetite control but also within higher cortical areas associated with reward and hedonic control (Batterham et al. 2007).

Signals from Pancreas and Adipose Tissue in the Control of Food Intake

Whereas gastrointestinal signals usually provide information about acutely ingested nutrients, the adiposity signals leptin, mainly produced by white adipose tissue, and insulin, synthesized in the ß cells of the pancreas, provide accurate information about the stored fuel. Thus, both hormones are implicated in the long-term regulation of energy balance, their circulating levels being in positive correlation with adipose tissue mass within the body. These hematic hormonal increases lead to reduced food intake and increased energy expenditure, in the attempt to restore body fat to normal (Belgardt and Brüning 2010).

Insulin

Insulin is synthesized in the ß cells of the pancreas and rapidly secreted after a meal. Together with its well-known hypoglycemic action, insulin also acts as an anorexigenic hormone at the level of the brain. Insulin enters the CNS through a saturable receptor-mediated transport process (Baura et al. 1993) and at the level of the brain interacts with insulin receptors expressed in the hypothalamic nuclei such as the ARC, PVH, and DMN to act as an anorectic agent (Corp et al. 1986). Intrahypothalamic insulin infusion in rodents results in a reduction of food intake (Menéndez and Atrens 1991). Although the mechanism of insulin-mediated anorexia has not been fully elucidated, NPY seems to be involved, because a fasting-induced increase in NPY mRNA expression in the PVN and ARC in rodents has been shown to be blocked by ICV administration of insulin. This suggests that fasting increases NPY biosynthesis through an ARC-PVN pathway in the hypothalamus via a mechanism which is dependent on low insulin levels. Moreover, insulin also has the ability to modify the activation of mesolimbic centers involved in the hedonic control of food intake; indeed, insulin also directly suppresses dopamine neuron activity in the VTA, which contributes to insulin's anorexigenic effects (Labouebe et al. 2013).

Leptin

Leptin, identified by Friedman and coworkers (Zhang et al. 1994), is probably the most important tonically acting adiposity signal; it is produced mainly by white adipose tissue. Its secretion increases as body lipid content rises, acting as an afferent signal to the receptors in the hypothalamus to counteract any increase in fat mass in order to maintain a constant body weight. Leptin's actions are mediated by three receptors: the long form (OB-Rb), the secreted form (OB-Rc), and the short intracellular domain receptor (OB-Ra). Among those, the Ob-Rb receptor, highly expressed in the hypothalamus (Fei et al. 1997), acts as the main receptor involved in appetite control. Rodents and humans with mutations in the leptin or leptin-receptor gene suffer extreme early-onset obesity and have endocrine defects (Farooqi and O'Rahilly 2008). In both animals and humans, long-term leptin replacement therapy for leptin deficiency has shown striking results, clearly demonstrating that leptin has a key function in the regulation of energy balance in humans (Campfield et al. 1995; Farooqi and O'Rahilly 2008). In humans, leptin circulating concentrations correlate with total fat mass, demonstrating the ability of leptin to respond to weight gain. Indeed, most obese humans have elevated plasma leptin levels, implying they may have leptin resistance rather than leptin deficiency. Thus, in the presence of obesity, leptin shows little influence on energy intake. Indeed, this resistance leptin state insensitivity has been proposed to be a result of defective leptin entry into the CNS (Caro et al. 1996). Leptin crosses the BBB via a saturable transport system to enter the mediobasal hypothalamus and ARC. Leptin resistance might derive from saturation of leptin transporters at the BBB (Wauman and Tavernier 2011); on the other hand, high levels of circulating or intrahypothalamic proinflammatory cytokines may impair leptin transport in obese subjects (De Git and Adan 2015). Leptin acts via activation of Janus kinase 2-STAT3 and inhibition of AMP-activated protein kinase activity on the ARC NPY/AgRP and POMC/CART neurons expressing leptin receptors (Munzberg 2010). Leptin induces an increase of POMC/CART and a decrease of NPY/AgRP neuronal activity resulting in reduced food intake and increased energy expenditure (Schwartz et al. 2000; Sahu 2003). Leptin is also able to amplify the gut satiating effect of CCK, acting synergistically to decrease food intake via activation of leptin receptors located in the brainstem and in the vagal afferents (Peters et al. 2006). Interestingly, leptin also affects the thresholds of sweet taste perception in the tongue (Nakamura et al. 2008). Leptin influence on eating behaviors may also be partially mediated through the regulation of the mesolimbic and/or nigrostriatal dopaminergic pathways (Farooqi et al. 2007) and by activating the hippocampus, an area of the brain that controls learning and memory function (Kanoski et al. 2011). These reward and cognitive processes may importantly contribute to leptin's inhibition of food intake.

Conclusions

Since the discovery of leptin, an explosive increase has been observed in the number of studies into the regulation of food intake and body weight in reply to the dramatic epidemiological alarm triggered by the exponential increase of obesity, worldwide. It is now clear that the eating pattern is orchestrated by a complex brain-peripheral interaction, by which gastrointestinal, pancreatic, and adipose tissue-derived hormones directly influence distinct areas of the CNS. Recent studies have shown that the traditional homeostatic approach to food intake regulation must be regarded alongside the hedonic aspect of appetite control. Indeed, profound interactions exist between these two regulatory pathways, so that the recent epidemic of obesity has been partially attributed to an alteration of the hedonic system. The great provision and promotion of energy-dense food may blunt satiety signals and override homeostatic control to mediate a persistent drive to eat, contributing to further expanding the global pandemic of obesity. Ongoing research will further increase our understanding of the effects of gut, pancreatic, and adipose tissue hormones on body weight homeostasis, potentially enabling us to exploit pharmacological therapeutics which might lead to sustained weight loss for patients affected by obesity.

References

Abbott CR, Monteiro M, Small CJ, et al. The inhibitory effects of peripheral administration of peptide YY 3-36 and glucagon-like peptide-1 on food intake are attenuated by ablation of the vagal-brainstem-hypothalamic pathway. Brain Res. 2005a;1044:127–31.

Abbott CR, Small CJ, Kennedy AR, et al. Blockade of the neuropeptide Y Y2 receptor with the specific antagonist BIIE0246 attenuates the effect of endogenous and exogenous peptide YY (3–36) on food intake. Brain Res. 2005b;1043:139–44.

Badonnel K, Durieux D, Monnerie R, et al. Leptin-sensitive OBP-expressing mucous cells in rat olfactory epithelium: a novel target for olfaction-nutrition crosstalk? Cell Tissue Res. 2009;338:53–66.

Bartolomucci A, Cabassi A, Govoni P. Metabolic consequences and vulnerability to diet-induced obesity in male mice under chronic social stress. PLoS One. 2009;4:e4331.

Batterham RL, Cowley MA, Small CJ, et al. Gut hormone PYY(3–36) physiologically inhibits food intake. Nature. 2002;418:650–4.

Batterham RL, Cohen MA, Ellis SM, et al. Inhibition of food intake in obese subjects by peptide YY3–36. N Engl J Med. 2003;349:941–8.

Batterham RL, Heffron H, Kapoor S, et al. Critical role for peptide YY in protein-mediated satiation and body-weight regulation. Cell Metab. 2006;4:223–33.

Batterham RL, Ffytche DH, Rosenthal JM, et al. PYY modulation of cortical and hypothalamic brain areas predicts feeding behaviour in humans. Nature. 2007;450:106–9.

Baura GD, Foster DM, Porte Jr D, et al. Saturable transport of insulin from plasma into the central nervous system of dogs in vivo. A mechanism for regulated insulin delivery to the brain. J Clin Invest. 1993;92:1824–30.

Beglinger C, Degen L, Matzinger D, D'Amato M, Drewe J. Loxiglumide, a CCK-A receptor antagonist, stimulates calorie intake and hunger feelings in humans. Am J Physiol Regul Integr Comp Physiol. 2001;280:R1149–54.

Belgardt BF, Brüning JC. CNS leptin and insulin action in the control of energy homeostasis. Ann N Y Acad Sci. 2010;1212:97–113.

Bellisle F, Louis-Sylvestre J, Linet N, et al. Anxiety and food intake in men. Psychosom Med. 1990;52:452–7.

Bernardis LL, McEwen G, Kodis M, Feldman MJ. Pair-feeding of sham-operated controls to rats with dorsomedial hypothalamic lesions: new evidence for an 'organismic' set point. Behav Brain Res. 1987;26:99–108.

Berthoud HR. Metabolic and hedonic drives in the neural control of appetite: who's the boss? Curr Opin Neurobiol. 2011;21:888–96.

Bi S, Robinson BM, Moran TH. Acute food deprivation and chronic food restriction differentially affect hypothalamic NPY mRNA expression. Am J Physiol Regul Integr Comp Physiol. 2003;285:R1030–6.

Bi S, Scott KA, Kopin AS, Moran TH. Differential roles for cholecystokinin a receptors in energy balance in rats and mice. Endocrinology. 2004;145:3873–80.

Bi S, Kim YJ, Zheng F. Dorsomedial hypothalamic NPY and energy balance control. Neuropeptides. 2012;46:309–14.

Blevins JE, Stanley BG, Reidelberger RD. Brain regions where cholecystokinin suppresses feeding in rats. Brain Res. 2000;860:1–10.

Blevins JE, Schwartz MW, Baskin DG. Evidence that paraventricular nucleus oxytocin neurons link hypothalamic leptin action to caudal brain stem nuclei controlling meal size. Am J Physiol Regul Integr Comp Physiol. 2004;287:R87–96.
Broberger C, Landry M, Wong H, Walsh JN, Hokfelt T. Subtypes Y1 and Y2 of the neuropeptide Y receptor are respectively expressed in proopiomelanocortin- and neuropeptide-Y-containing neurons of the rat hypothalamic arcuate nucleus. Neuroendocrinology. 1997;66:393–408.
Burdakov D, Karnani MM, Gonzalez A. Lateral hypothalamus as a sensor-regulator in respiratory and metabolic control. Physiol Behav. 2013;121:117–24.
Burdyga G, Spiller D, Morris R, et al. Expression of the leptin receptor in rat and human nodose ganglion neurons. Neuroscience. 2002;109:339–47.
Campbell JE, Drucker DJ. Pharmacology, physiology, and mechanisms of incretin hormone action. Cell Metab. 2013;17:819–37.
Campfield LA, Smith FJ, Guisez Y, Devos R, Burn P. Recombinant mouse OB protein: evidence for a peripheral signal linking adiposity and central neural networks. Science. 1995;269:546–9.
Caro JF, Kolaczynski JW, Nyce MR, et al. Decreased cerebrospinal-fluid/serum leptin ratio in obesity: a possible mechanism for leptin resistance. Lancet. 1996;348:159–61.
Chelikani PK, Haver AC, Reidelberger RD. Intravenous infusion of peptide YY(3–36) potently inhibits food intake in rats. Endocrinology. 2005;146:879–88.
Chen AS, Marsh DJ, Trumbauer ME, et al. Inactivation of the mouse melanocortin-3 receptor results in increased fat mass and reduced lean body mass. Nat Genet. 2000;26:97–102.
Chen HY, Trumbauer ME, Chen AS, et al. Orexigenic action of peripheral ghrelin is mediated by neuropeptide Y and agouti-related protein. Endocrinology. 2004;145:2607–12.
Cho YM, Fujita Y, Kieffer TJ. Glucagon-like peptide-1: glucose homeostasis and beyond. Annu Rev Physiol. 2014;76:535–59.
Cordeira J, Rios M. Weighing in the role of BDNF in the central control of eating behavior. Mol Neurobiol. 2011;44:441–8.
Corp ES, Woods SC, Porte Jr D, Dorsa DM, Figlewicz DP, Baskin DG. Localization of 125I-insulin binding sites in the rat hypothalamus by quantitative autoradiography. Neurosci Lett. 1986;70:17–22.
Cota D, Marsicano G, Lutz B, et al. Endogenous cannabinoid system as a modulator of food intake. Int J Obes Relat Metab Disord. 2003;27:289–301.
Cota D, Tschoep MH, Horvath T, Levine AS. Cannabinoids, opioids and eating behavior: the molecular face of hedonism? Brain Res Rev. 2006;51:85–107.
Cowley MA, Smart JL, Rubinstein M, et al. Leptin activates anorexigenic POMC neurons through a neural network in the arcuate nucleus. Nature. 2001;411:480–4.
Cowley MA, Smith RG, Diano S, et al. The distribution and mechanism of action of ghrelin in the CNS demonstrates a novel hypothalamic circuit regulating energy homeostasis. Neuron. 2003;37:649–61.
Cummings DE, Purnell JQ, Frayo RS, Schmidova K, Wisse BE, Weigle DS. A preprandial rise in plasma ghrelin levels suggests a role in meal initiation in humans. Diabetes. 2001;50:1714–9.
Dakin CL, Gunn I, Small CJ, et al. Oxyntomodulin inhibits food intake in the rat. Endocrinology. 2001;142:4244–50.
Date Y, Murakami N, Toshinai K, et al. The role of the gastric afferent vagal nerve in ghrelin-induced feeding and growth hormone secretion in rats. Gastroenterology. 2002;123:1120–8.
de Git KC, Adan RA. Leptin resistance in diet-induced obesity: the role of hypothalamic inflammation. Obes Rev. 2015;16:207–24.
De Silva A, Salem V, Long CJ, et al. The gut hormones PYY 3–36 and GLP-1 7–36 amide reduce food intake and modulate brain activity in appetite centers in humans. Cell Metab. 2011;14:700–6.
Deane AM, Nguyen NQ, Stevens JE, et al. Endogenous glucagon-like peptide-1 slows gastric emptying in healthy subjects, attenuating postprandial glycemia. J Clin Endocrinol Metab. 2010;95:215–21.

Di Marzo V, Goparaju SK, Wang L, et al. Leptin-regulated endocannabinoids are involved in maintaining food intake. Nature. 2001;410:822–5.

Dickson SL, Egecioglu E, Landgren S, Skibicka KP, Engel JA, Jerlhag J. The role of the central ghrelin system in reward from food and chemical drugs. Mol Cell Endocrinol. 2011;340:80–7.

Dockray GJ, Burdyga G. Plasticity in vagal afferent neurones during feeding and fasting: mechanisms and significance. Acta Physiol (Oxf). 2011;201(3):313–21.

Drewnowski A, Krahn DD, Demitrack MA, Nairn K, Gosnell BA. Taste responses and preferences for sweet high-fat foods: evidence for opioid involvement. Physiol Behav. 1992;51:371–9.

English PJ, Ghatei MA, Malik IA, Bloom SR, Wilding JP. Food fails to suppress ghrelin levels in obese humans. J Clin Endocrinol Metab. 2002;87:2984.

Fan W, Boston BA, Kesterson RA, Hruby VJ, Cone RD. Role of melanocortinergic neurons in feeding and the agouti obesity syndrome. Nature. 1997;385:165–8.

Farooqi IS, O'Rahilly S. Mutations in ligands and receptors of the leptin-melanocortin pathway that lead to obesity. Nat Clin Pract Endocrinol Metab. 2008;4:569–77.

Farooqi IS, Bullmore E, Keogh J, Gillard J, O'Rahilly S, Fletcher PC. Leptin regulates striatal regions and human eating behavior. Science. 2007;317:1355.

Fei H, Okano HJ, Li C, et al. Anatomic localization of alternatively spliced leptin receptors (Ob-R) in mouse brain and other tissues. Proc Natl Acad Sci U S A. 1997;94:7001–5.

Fetissov SO, Kopp J, Hökfelt T. Distribution of NPY receptors in the hypothalamus. Neuropeptides. 2004;38(4):175–88.

Figlewicz DP, Nadzan AM, Sipols AJ, et al. Intraventricular CCK-8 reduces single meal size in the baboon by interaction with type-A CCK receptors. Am J Physiol. 1992;263:R863–7.

Francis L, Granger D, Susman EJ. Adrenocortical regulation, eating in the absence of hunger and BMI in young children. Appetite. 2013;64:32–8.

Fulton S, Pissios P, Manchon RP, et al. Leptin regulation of the mesoaccumbens dopamine pathway. Neuron. 2006;51:811–22.

George S, Khan S, Briggs H, Abelson JL. CRH-stimulated cortisol release and food intake in healthy, non-obese adults. Psychoneuroendocrinology. 2010;35:607–12.

Gibbs J, Young RC, Smith GP. Cholecystokinin decreases food intake in rats. J Comp Physiol Psychol. 1973;84:488–95.

Guan XM, Yu H, Trumbauer M, Frazier E, Van der Ploeg LH, Chen H. Induction of neuropeptide Y expression in dorsomedial hypothalamus of diet-induced obese mice. Neuroreport. 1998;9:3415–9.

Gyengesi E, Liu Z-W, D'Agostino G, et al. Corticosterone regulates synaptic input organization of POMC and NPY/AgRP neurons in adult mice. Endocrinology. 2010;151:5395–402.

Hahn TM, Breininger JF, Baskin DG, Schwartz MW. Coexpression of AgRP and NPY in fasting-activated hypothalamic neurons. Nat Neurosci. 1998;1:271–2.

Halford JC, Blundell JE. Separate systems for serotonin and leptin in appetite control. Ann Med. 2000;32:222–32.

Haltia LT, Rinne JO, Merisaari H, et al. Effects of intravenous glucose on dopaminergic function in the human brain in vivo. Synapse. 2007;61:748–56.

Harrold JA, Dovey TM, Blundell JE, Halford JC. CNS regulation of appetite. Neuropharmacology. 2012;63:3–17.

Heisler LK, Cowley MA, Tecott LH, et al. Activation of central melanocortin pathways by fenfluramine. Science. 2002;297:609–11.

Heppner KM, Perez-Tilve D. GLP-1 based therapeutics: simultaneously combating T2DM and obesity. Front Neurosci. 2015;9:92. doi:10.3389/fnins.2015.0009.

Hirosue Y, Inui A, Teranishi A, et al. Cholecystokinin octapeptide analogues suppress food intake via central CCK-A receptors in mice. Am J Physiol. 1993;265:R481–6.

Holst JJ. The physiology of glucagon-like peptide 1. Physiol Rev. 2007;87:1409–39.

Hommel JD, Trinko R, Sears RM, et al. Leptin receptor signaling in midbrain dopamine neurons regulates feeding. Neuron. 2006;51:801–10.

Huszar D, Lynch CA, Fairchild-Huntress V, et al. Targeted disruption of the melanocortin-4 receptor results in obesity in mice. Cell. 1997;88:131–41.

Jamshidi N, Taylor DA. Anandamide administration into the ventromedial hypothalamus stimulates appetite in rats. Br J Pharmacol. 2001;134:1151–4.

Jaworski JN, Vicentic A, Hunter RG, Kimmel HL, Kuhar MJ. CART peptides are modulators of mesolimbic dopamine and psychostimulants. Life Sci. 2003;73:741–7.

Jeanneteau FD, Lambert WM, Ismaili N, et al. BDNF and glucocorticoids regulate corticotrophin-releasing hormone (CRH) homeostasis in the hypothalamus. Proc Natl Acad Sci U S A. 2012;109:1305–10.

Kanoski SE, Hayes MR, Greenwald HS, et al. Hippocampal leptin signaling reduces food intake and modulates food-related memory processing. Neuropsychopharmacology. 2011;36:1859–70.

Kirkham TC, Williams CM, Fezza F, Di Marzo V. Endocannabinoid levels in rat limbic forebrain and hypothalamus in relation to fasting, feeding and satiation: stimulation of eating by 2-arachidonoyl glycerol. Br J Pharmacol. 2002;136:550–7.

Kissileff HR, Pi-Sunyer FX, Thornton J, Smith GP. C-terminal octapeptide of cholecystokinin decreases food intake in man. Am J Clin Nutr. 1981;34:154–60.

Koda S, Date Y, Murakami N, et al. The role of the vagal nerve in peripheral PYY3–36-induced feeding reduction in rats. Endocrinology. 2005;146:2369–75.

Kola B, Farkas I, Christ-Crain M, et al. The orexigenic effect of ghrelin is mediated through central activation of the endogenous cannabinoid system. PLoS One. 2008;3:e1797.

Kong WM, Stanley S, Gardiner J, et al. A role for arcuate cocaine and amphetamine regulated transcript in hyperphagia, thermogenesis, and cold adaptation. FASEB J. 2003;17:1688–90.

Krashes MJ, Koda S, Ye C, et al. Rapid, reversible activation of AgRP neurons drives feeding behavior in mice. J Clin Invest. 2011;121:1424–8.

Krashes MJ, Lowell BB, Garfield AS. Melanocortin-4-receptor regulated energy homeostasis. Nat Neurosci. 2016;19:206–19.

Kristensen P, Judge ME, Thim L, et al. Hypothalamic CART is a new anorectic peptide regulated by leptin. Nature. 1998;393:72–6.

Labouebe G, Liu S, Dias C, et al. Insulin induces long-term depression of ventral tegmental area dopamine neurons via endocannabinoids. Nat Neurosci. 2013;16:300–8.

Lage R, Parisi C, Seoane-Collazo P et al (2015) Lack of hypophagia in CB1 null mice is associated to decreased hypothalamic POMC and CART expression. Int J Neuropsychopharmacol 18. pii: pyv011. doi: 10.1093/ijnp/pyv011.

Larsen PJ, Tang-Christensen M, Holst JJ, Orskov C. Distribution of glucagon-like peptide-1 and other preproglucagon-derived peptides in the rat hypothalamus and brainstem. Neuroscience. 1997;77:257–70.

Lau J, Herzog H. CART in the regulation of appetite and energy homeostasis. Front Neurosci. 2014;8:313. doi:10.3389/fnins.2014.00313. eCollection 2014.

Lawrence CB, Snape AC, Baudoin FM, Luckman SM. Acute central ghrelin and GH secretagogues induce feeding and activate brain appetite centers. Endocrinology. 2002;143:155–62.

Lean MEJ, Malkova D. Altered gut and adipose tissue hormones in overweight and obese individuals: cause or consequence? Int J Obes (Lond). 2016;40:622–32.

Lee M, Kim A, Conwell IM, et al. Effects of selective modulation of the central melanocortin-3-receptor on food intake and hypothalamic POMC expression. Peptides. 2008;29:440–7.

Lee SJ, Kirigiti M, Lindsley SR, et al. Efferent projections of neuropeptide Y-expressing neurons of the dorsomedial hypothalamus in chronic hyperphagic models. J Comp Neurol. 2013;521:1891–914.

Lin S, Boey D, Couzens M, Lee N, Sainsbury A, Herzog H. Compensatory changes in [125I]-PYY binding in Y receptor knockout mice suggest the potential existence of further Y receptor(s). Neuropeptides. 2005;39:21–8.

Lippl F, Erdmann J, Steiger A, et al. Low-dose ghrelin infusion – evidence against a hormonal role in food intake. Regul Pept. 2012;174:26–31.

Ludwig DS, Tritos NA, Mastaitis JW, et al. Melanin-concentrating hormone overexpression in transgenic mice leads to obesity and insulin resistance. J Clin Invest. 2001;107:379–86.

Mahler SV, Smith KS, Berridge KC. Endocannabinoid hedonic hotspot for sensory pleasure: anandamide in nucleus accumbens shell enhances 'liking' of a sweet reward. Neuropsychopharmacology. 2007;32:2267–78.
Malik S, McGlone F, Bedrossian D, Dagher A. Ghrelin modulates brain activity in areas that control appetitive behavior. Cell Metab. 2008;7:400–9.
Manning S, Batterham RL. The role of gut hormone peptide YY in energy and glucose homeostasis: twelve years on. Annu Rev Physiol. 2014;76:585–60.
Marsh DJ, Weingarth DT, Novi DE, et al. Melanin-concentrating hormone 1 receptor-deficient mice are lean, hyperactive, and hyperphagic and have altered metabolism. Proc Natl Acad Sci U S A. 2002;99:3240–5.
Marso SP, Daniels GH, Brown-Frandsen K, et al. Liraglutide and cardiovascular outcomes in type 2 diabetes. N Engl J Med. 2016;375:311–22.
Martin B, Dotson CD, Shin YK, et al. Modulation of taste sensitivity by GLP-1 signaling in taste buds. Ann N Y Acad Sci. 2009;1170:98–101.
Mashiko S, Moriya R, Ishihara A, et al. Synergistic interaction between neuropeptide Y1 and Y5 receptor pathways in regulation of energy homeostasis. Eur J Pharmacol. 2009;615:113–7.
Matarazzo V, Schaller F, Nedelec E, et al. Inactivation of Socs3 in the hypothalamus enhances the hindbrain response to endogenous satiety signals via oxytocin signaling. J Neurosci. 2012;32:17097–107.
McCrickerd K, Forde CG. Sensory influences on food intake control: moving beyond palatability. Obes Rev. 2016;17:18–29.
Melis T, Succu S, Sanna F, Boi A, Argiolas A, Melis MR. The cannabinoid antagonist SR 141716A (Rimonabant) reduces the increase of extra-cellular dopamine release in the rat nucleus accumbens induced by a novel high palatable food. Neurosci Lett. 2007;419:231–5.
Menéndez JA, Atrens DM. Insulin and the paraventricular hypothalamus: modulation of energy balance. Brain Res. 1991;555:193–201.
Michopoulos V, Toufexis D, Wilson ME. Social stress interacts with diet history to promote emotional feeding in females. Psychoneuroendocrinology. 2012;37:1479–90.
Moran TH, Kinzig KP. Gastrointestinal satiety signals II. Cholecystokinin. Am J Physiol Gastrointest Liver Physiol. 2004;286:G183–8.
Moran TH, Robinson PH, Goldrich MS, McHugh PR. Two brain cholecystokinin receptors: implications for behavioral actions. Brain Res. 1986;362:175–9.
Moriarty P, Dimaline R, Thompson DG, Dockray GJ. Characterization of cholecystokinin (A) and cholecystokinin (B) receptors expressed by vagal afferent neurons. Neuroscience. 1997;79:905–13.
Morton GJ, Meek TH, Schwartz MW. Neurobiology of food intake in health and disease. Nat Rev Neurosci. 2014;15:367–78.
Mountjoy KG. Pro-opiomelanocortin (POMC) neurones, POMC-derived peptides, melanocortin receptors and obesity: how understanding of this system has changed over the last decade. J Neuroendocrinol. 2015;27:406–18.
Müller TD, Nogueiras R, Andermann ML, et al. Ghrelin. Mol Metab. 2015;4:437–60.
Munzberg H. Leptin-signaling pathways and leptin resistance. Forum Nutr. 2010;63:123–32.
Murphy KG, Bloom SR. Gut hormones and the regulation of energy homeostasis. Nature. 2006;444:854–9.
Nakagawa A, Satake H, Nakabayashi H, et al. Receptor gene expression of glucagon-like peptide-1, but not glucose-dependent insulinotropic polypeptide, in rat nodose ganglion cells. Auton Neurosci. 2004;110:36–43.
Nakamura Y, Sanematsu K, Ohta R, et al. Diurnal variation of human sweet taste recognition thresholds is correlated with plasma leptin levels. Diabetes. 2008;57:2661–5.
Nicola SM. Reassessing wanting and liking in the study of mesolimbic influence on food intake. Am J Physiol Regul Integr Comp Physiol. 2016. doi:10.1152/ajpregu.00234.2016 [Epub ahead of print].
Noble EE, Billington CJ, Kotz CM, Wang C. The lighter side of BDNF. Am J Physiol Regul Integr Comp Physiol. 2011;300:R1053–69.

Nonogaki K, Strack AM, Dallman MF, Tecott LH. Leptin-independent hyperphagia and type 2 diabetes in mice with a mutated serotonin 5-HT2C receptor gene. Nat Med. 1998;4:1152–6.
Ollmann MM, Wilson BD, Yang YK, et al. Antagonism of central melanocortin receptors in vitro and in vivo by agouti-related protein. Science. 1997;278:135–8.
Onaka T, Takayanagi Y, Yoshida M. Roles of oxytocin neurones in the control of stress, energy metabolism, and social behaviour. J Neuroendocrinol. 2012;24:587–98.
Osei-Hyiaman D, Depetrillo M, Harvey-White J, et al. Cocaine- and amphetamine-related transcript is involved in the orexigenic effect of endogenous anandamide. Neuroendocrinology. 2005;81:273–82.
Page AJ, Slattery JA, Milte C, et al. Ghrelin selectively reduces mechanosensitivity of upper gastrointestinal vagal afferents. Am J Physiol Gastrointest Liver Physiol. 2007;292:G1376–84.
Parise EM, Lilly N, Kay K, et al. Evidence for the role of hindbrain orexin-1 receptors in the control of meal size. Am J Physiol Regul Integr Comp Physiol. 2011;301:R1692–9.
Parton LE, Ye CP, Coppari R, et al. Glucose sensing by POMC neurons regulates glucose homeostasis and is impaired in obesity. Nature. 2007;449:228–32.
Peters JH, Simasko SM, Ritter RC. Modulation of vagal afferent excitation and reduction of food intake by leptin and cholecystokinin. Physiol Behav. 2006;89:477–85.
Pfluger PT, Kampe J, Castaneda T, et al. Effect of human body weight changes on circulating levels of peptide YY and peptide YY3-36. J Clin Endocrinol Metab. 2007;92:583–8.
Pi-Sunyer X, Astrup A, Fujioka K, et al. A randomized, controlled trial of 3.0 mg of Liraglutide in weight management. N Engl J Med. 2015;373:11–22.
Plamboeck A, Veedfald S, Deacon CF, et al. The effect of exogenous GLP-1 on food intake is lost in male truncally vagotomized subjects with pyloroplasty. Am J Physiol Gastrointest Liver Physiol. 2013;304:G1117–27.
Plazzi G, Moghadam KK, Maggi LS, et al. Autonomic disturbances in narcolepsy. Sleep Med Rev. 2011;15:187–96.
Pocai A. Unraveling oxyntomodulin, GLP1's enigmatic brother. J Endocrinol. 2012;215:335–46.
Rui L. Brain regulation of energy balance and body weight. Rev Endocr Metab Disord. 2013;14:387–407.
Rutters F, Nieuwenhuizen AG, Lemmens SGT, Born JM, Westerterp-Plantenga MS. Acute stress-related changes in eating in the absence of hunger. Obesity (Silver Spring). 2009;17:72–7.
Sahu A. Leptin signaling in the hypothalamus: emphasis on energy homeostasis and leptin resistance. Front Neuroendocrinol. 2003;24:225–53.
Sakurai T, Amemiya A, Ishii M, et al. Orexins and orexin receptors: a family of hypothalamic neuropeptides and G protein-coupled receptors that regulate feeding behavior. Cell. 1998;92:573–85.
Schwartz TW, Holst JJ, Fahrenkrug J, et al. Vagal, cholinergic regulation of pancreatic polypeptide secretion. J Clin Invest. 1978;61:781–9.
Schwartz MW, Woods SC, Porte Jr D, Seeley RJ, Baskin DG. Central nervous system control of food intake. Nature. 2000;404:661–71.
Shigemura N, Ohta R, Kusakabe Y, et al. Leptin modulates behavioral responses to sweet substances by influencing peripheral tastestructures. Endocrinology. 2004;145:839–47.
Shimizu N, Oomura Y, Plata-Salamán CR, Morimoto M. Hyperphagia and obesity in rats with bilateral ibotenic acid-induced lesions of the ventromedial hypothalamic nucleus. Brain Res. 1987;416:153–6.
Shor-Posner G, Azar AP, Jhanwar-Uniyal M, Filart R, Leibowitz SF. Destruction of noradrenergic innervation to the paraventricular nucleus: deficits in food intake, macronutrient selection, and compensatory eating after food deprivation. Pharmacol Biochem Behav. 1986;25:381–92.
Silvestri C, Di Marzo V. The endocannabinoid system in energy homeostasis and the etiopathology of metabolic disorders. Cell Metab. 2013;17(4):475–90.
Sisley S, Gutierrez-Aguilar R, Scott M, D'Alessio DA, Sandoval DA, Seeley RJ. Neuronal GLP1R mediates liraglutide's anorectic but not glucose-lowering effect. J Clin Invest. 2014;124:2456–63.

Sohn JW, Xu Y, Jones JE, Wickman K, Williams KW, Elmquist JK. Serotonin 2C receptor activates a distinct population of arcuate proopiomelanocortin neurons via TRPC channels. Neuron. 2011;71:488–97.

Soria-Gomez E, Bellocchio L, Marsicano G. New insights on food intake control by olfactory processes: the emerging role of the endocannabinoid system. Mol Cell Endocrinol. 2014;397:59–66.

Spreckley E, Murphy KG. The L-cell in nutritional sensing and the regulation of appetite. Front Nutr. 2015;2:23. doi:10.3389/fnut.2015.00023.

Stanley BG, Chin AS, Leibowitz SF. Feeding and drinking elicited by central injection of neuropeptide Y: evidence for a hypothalamic site(s) of action. Brain Res Bull. 1985;14:521–4.

Stice E, Spoor S, Bohon C, Small DM. Relation between obesity and blunted striatal response to food is moderated by TaqIA A1 allele. Science. 2008;322:449–52.

Suzuki K, Jayasena CN, Bloom SR. Obesity and appetite control. Exp Diabetes Res. 2012;2012:824305.

Szczypka MS, Kwok K, Brot MD, et al. Dopamine production in the caudate putamen restores feeding in dopamine-deficient mice. Neuron. 2001;30:819–28.

Tecott LH, Sun LM, Akana SF, et al. Eating disorder and epilepsy in mice lacking 5-HT2c serotonin receptors. Nature. 1995;374:542–6.

Tong Q, Ye C, Jones JE, Elmquist JK, Lowell BB. Synaptic release of GABA by AgRP neurons is required for normal regulation of energy balance. Nat Neurosci. 2008;11:998–1000.

Toriya M, Maekawa F, Maejima Y, et al. Long-term infusion of brain-derived neurotrophic factor reduces food intake and body weight via a corticotrophin releasing hormone pathway in the paraventricular nucleus of the hypothalamus. J Neuroendocrinol. 2010;22:987–95.

Tschöp M, Smiley DL, Heiman ML. Ghrelin induces adiposity in rodents. Nature. 2000;407:908–13.

Tschöp M, Castañeda TR, Joost HG, et al. Physiology: does gut hormone PYY3–36 decrease food intake in rodents? Nature. 2004;430:165.

Tsujino N, Sakurai T. Orexin/hypocretin: a neuropeptide at the interface of sleep, energy homeostasis, and reward system. Pharmacol Rev. 2009;61:162–76.

Ulrich-Lai YM, Ostrander MM, Thomas IM, et al. Daily limited access to sweetened drink attenuates hypothalamic-pituitary-adrenocortical axis stress responses. Endocrinology. 2007;148:1823–34.

Vahl TP, Drazen DL, Seeley RJ, D'Alessio DA, Woods SC. Meal-anticipatory glucagon-like peptide-1 secretion in rats. Endocrinology. 2010;151:569–75.

van Bloemendaal L, IJzerman RG, Ten Kulve JS, et al. GLP-1 receptor activation modulates appetite- and reward-related brain areas in humans. Diabetes. 2014;63:4186–96.

van der Kooy D. Area postrema: site where cholecystokinin acts to decrease food intake. Brain Res. 1984;295:345–7.

Verty AN, McGregor IS, Mallet PN. The dopamine receptor antagonist SCH 23390 attenuates feeding induced by Delta9-tetrahydrocannabinol. Brain Res. 2004;1020:188–95.

Verty AN, Boon WM, Mallet PE, McGregor IS, Oldfield BJ. Involvement of hypothalamic peptides in the anorectic action of the CB receptor antagonist rimonabant (SR 141716). Eur J Neurosci. 2009;29:2207–16.

Vicennati V, Pasqui F, Cavazza C, et al. Cortisol, energy intake, and food frequency in overweight/obese women. Nutrition. 2011;27:677–80.

Volkow ND, Wang GJ, Baler RD. Reward, dopamine and the control of food intake: implications for obesity. Trends Cogn Sci. 2011;15:37–46.

Vong L, Ye C, Yang Z, Choi B, Chua Jr S, Lowell BB. Leptin action on GABAergic neurons prevents obesity and reduces inhibitory tone to POMC neurons. Neuron. 2011;71:142–54.

Vrang N, Madsen AN, Tang-Christensen M, Hansen G, Larsen PJ. PYY(3–36) reduces food intake and body weight and improves insulin sensitivity in rodent models of diet-induced obesity. Am J Physiol Regul Integr Comp Physiol. 2006;291:R367–75.

Wang CF, Billington CJ, Levine AS, Kotz CM. Effect of CART in the hypothalamic paraventricular nucleus on feeding and uncoupling protein gene expression. Neuroreport. 2000;11:3251–5.
Wang GJ, Volkow ND, Logan J, et al. Brain dopamine and obesity. Lancet. 2001;357:354–7.
Wang L, Saint-Pierre DH, Tach Y. Peripheral ghrelin selectively increases Fos expression in neuropeptide Y – synthesizing neurons in mouse hypothalamic arcuate nucleus. Neurosci Lett. 2002;325:47–51.
Wardle J, Steptoe A, Oliver G, Lipsey Z. Stress, dietary restraint and food intake. J Psychosom Res. 2000;48:195–202.
Wauman J, Tavernier J. Leptin receptor signaling: pathways to leptin resistance. Front Biosci (Landmark Ed). 2011;16:2771–93.
Wenger T, Jamali K, Juaneda C, Leonardelli J, Tramu G. Arachidonyl ethanolamide (anandamide) activates the parvocellular part of hypothalamic paraventricular nucleus. Biochem Biophys Res Commun. 1997;237:724–8.
Willner P, Moreau JL, Nielsen CK, Papp M, Sluzewska A. Decreased hedonic responsiveness following chronic mild stress is not secondary to loss of body weight. Physiol Behav. 1996;60:129–34.
Wren AM, Small CJ, Abbott CR, et al. Ghrelin causes hyperphagia and obesity in rats. Diabetes. 2000;50:2540–7.
Wren AM, Seal LJ, Cohen MA, et al. Ghrelin enhances appetite and increases food intake in humans. J Clin Endocrinol Metab. 2001;86:5992.
Wynne K, Park AJ, Small CJ, et al. Subcutaneous oxyntomodulin reduces body weight in overweight and obese subjects: a double-blind, randomized, controlled trial. Diabetes. 2005;54:2390–5.
Xu B, Goulding EH, Zang K, et al. Brain-derived neurotrophic factor regulates energy balance downstream of melanocortin-4 receptor. Nat Neurosci. 2003;6:736–42.
Yang SC, Shieh KR. Differential effects of melanin concentrating hormone on the central dopaminergic neurons induced by the cocaine- and amphetamine-regulated transcript peptide. J Neurochem. 2005;92:637–46.
Yang L, Scott KA, Hyun J, et al. Role of dorsomedial hypothalamic neuropeptide Y in modulating food intake and energy balance. J Neurosci. 2009;29:179–90.
Yeomans MR, Gray RW. Selective effects of naltrexone on food pleasantness and intake. Physiol Behav. 1996;60:439–46.
Zhang J, Ritter RC. Circulating GLP-1 and CCK-8 reduce food intake by capsaicin-insensitive, nonvagal mechanisms. Am J Physiol Regul Integr Comp Physiol. 2012;302:R264–73.
Zhang Y, Proenca R, Maffei M, Barone M, Leopold L, Friedman JM. Positional cloning of the mouse obese gene and its human homologue. Nature. 1994;372:425–32.
Zhang M, Gosnell BA, Kelley AE. Intake of high fat food is selectively enhanced by Mu opioid receptor stimulation within the nucleus accumbens. J Pharmacol Exper Therap. 1998;285:908–14.
Zhang G, Bai H, Zhang H, et al. Neuropeptide exocytosis involving synaptotagmin-4 and oxytocin in hypothalamic programming of body weight and energy balance. Neuron. 2011;69:523–35.
Zheng H, Patterson LM, Phifer CB, Berthoud HR. Brain stem melanocortinergic modulation of meal size and identification of hypothalamic POMC projections. Am J Physiol Regul Integr Comp Physiol. 2005;289:R247–58.
Zheng H, Patterson LM, Rhodes CJ, et al. A potential role for hypothalamo-medullary POMC projections in leptin-induced suppression of food intake. Am J Physiol Regul Integr Comp Physiol. 2010;298:R720–8.

The Endocrine Regulation of Blood Pressure 23

Massimo Mannelli, Gian Paolo Rossi, Paul-Emmanuel Vanderriele, and Gabriele Parenti

Abstract

Blood pressure is a vital parameter controlled by very complex mechanisms mainly involving neuronal and endocrine effectors. The sympathetic-adrenal system (SAS) and the renin-angiotensin-aldosterone system (RAAS), besides paracrine mechanisms in the vessel wall, are the main players of these complex networks that permit the maintenance of blood pressure, sufficient for the perfusion of organs and tissues. These systems regulate the cardiac pump, the circulating volume, and the peripheral resistances. They are the targets of almost all the drugs prescribed to hypertensive patients.

In addition to these major neurohormonal systems, many other factors can modulate blood pressure participating in the control of the blood volume or the peripheral resistances. These factors include, among the others, natriuretic peptides, dopamine, nitric oxide, endothelin-1, vasopressin, and cortisol.

Keywords

Blood pressure • Sympathetic-adrenal system • Renin • Angiotensins • Aldosterone • Vasopressin • Nitric oxide • Endothelin-1 • Dopamine • Natriuretic peptides • Cortisol

M. Mannelli (✉)
Department of Experimental and Clinical Biomedical Sciences "Mario Serio", University of Florence, Florence, Italy
e-mail: massimo.mannelli@unifi.it

G.P. Rossi • P.-E. Vanderriele
Clinica dell'Ipertensione Arteriosa – Department of Medicine, Internal Medicine 4 DIME, University of Padova, Padova, Italy
e-mail: gianpaolo.rossi@unipd.it; paulemmanuelv@yahoo.fr

G. Parenti
Endocrinology Unit, Department of Medicine and Geriatrics, Azienda Ospedaliera-Universitaria di Careggi, Careggi Hospital, Florence, Italy
e-mail: gabrieleparenti@libero.it

A. Belfiore, D. LeRoith (eds.), *Principles of Endocrinology and Hormone Action*, Endocrinology, https://doi.org/10.1007/978-3-319-44675-2_23

Contents

Introduction

Cells, tissue, and organs need blood supply to survive and function. Blood circulates in a closed system constituted by arteries and veins, because of pressure gradients generated by the contractile activity of the heart. The blood pressure (BP) warrants the perfusion of the tissues and is the results of cardiac output, blood volume, and peripheral resistances. It is continuously monitored and controlled by a complex network of integrated systems regulating these three main factors. Among these, the sympathetic-adrenal system (SAS) and the renin-angiotensin-aldosterone system (RAAS) play a major role in BP control although many other factors participate in this extremely complex regulation acting at the central (aortic) as well as the peripheral (tissue) levels. As a consequence, almost all the most widely used antihypertensive drugs are aimed at lowering the blood volume and the activity of the SAS and the RAAS.

In this paper we will review the physiology of these two systems and we will briefly mention the many other "minor" factors influencing BP.

The Sympathetic-Adrenal System (SAS)

The SAS is part of the autonomic nervous system that also includes the parasympathetic nervous system. It is involved in the homeostasis of many vital functions such as the cardiovascular (Goldstein 1995).

The anatomical and chemical characteristics of the SAS allow very rapid responses to the internal and external stimuli, and therefore the SAS is the quickest system devoted to the maintenance of cardiovascular homeostasis.

The SAS is functionally integrated with other homeostatic systems such as the endocrine system, whose responses, which are slow-onset but more persistent, may, in turn, modulate the SAS function (Goldstein et al. 1998).

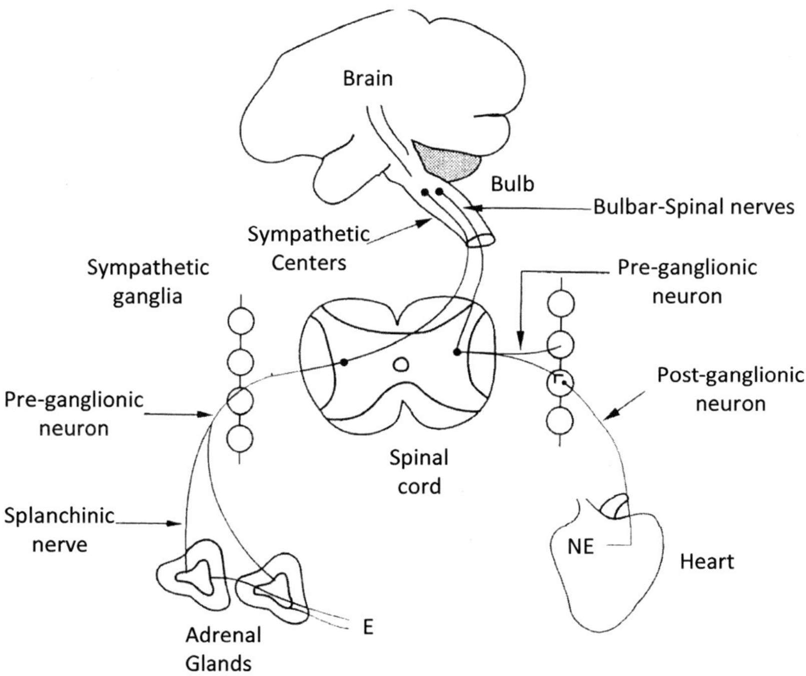

Fig. 1 Schematic representation of the anatomical organization of the sympathetic-adrenal system

The SAS has two effector branches constituted by a neuronal and an endocrine one: the first is represented by the sympathetic nerves releasing the neurotransmitter norepinephrine (NE) in the synaptic cleft; the second is represented by the chromaffin cells of the adrenal medulla secreting the hormone epinephrine (E) in the blood stream (Fig. 1).

The effector branch unit of the sympathetic system is composed by two neurons: a preganglionic neuron whose cell body is in the mediolateral area of the spinal cord and a postganglionic neuron, innervated by the previous one in the sympathetic ganglion. The cell bodies of the preganglionic neurons are located in the spinal cord at the level of the first thoracic vertebra down to the second lumbar one. The sympathetic ganglia are localized at the same levels on both sides of the column. The postganglionic neurons innervate peripheral vessels, tissues, and organs diffusely. The neurotransmitter released by the preganglionic nerve is acetylcholine, while the postganglionic nerve releases NE.

The activity of the sympathetic nerves is strictly controlled by neurons of the sympathetic centers located in the medulla oblongata. The activity of these sympathetic centers is, in turn, regulated by nervous pathways coming from the periphery of the body, as well as from higher centers of the brain. As a whole, the activity of the SAS is the final result of the integration of all the stimuli impinging on the medullary sympathetic centers (Goldstein 1995).

Among the most important factors modulating the activity of these centers are the afferent inputs from sites of the peripheral circulation, such as the arterial high-pressure and cardiac baroreceptors that are stretch receptors located in the walls of the arteries (especially important is the carotid sinus at the bifurcation of the common carotid artery) and cardiac/venous low-pressure receptors located in the walls of the cardiac atria.

The arterial high-pressure baroreceptors monitor the stretching of the arterial walls and elicit reflex responses that control arterial BP. The low-pressure baroreceptors monitor the stretch of the cardiac and pulmonary arterial walls and elicit reflex responses that maintain central blood volume (Goldstein 1995).

The SAS is differently activated by stressors: standing up elicits the response of the neuronal branch of the SAS characterized by NE release from the sympathetic nerve terminals, whereas hypoglycemia preferentially causes E release from the adrenal medulla. Both the branches are highly activated in case of a profound hypotension.

Sympathetic nerve stimulation causes a rapid constriction of arterioles, increasing regional resistance to blood flow and shifting the blood to other regions with lower resistance.

The arteriole vasoconstriction is mediated by the adrenergic α-receptors. At the cardiac level, the sympathetic discharge-induced NE release activates the β-receptors, thus increasing heart rate and contractility. Therefore, a diffuse sympathetic stimulation causes a BP increase due to increased cardiac output and peripheral resistances.

At the kidney level, sympathetic activation leads to a decrease in sodium excretion and, through β-receptor activation, to an increase in renin release by the juxtaglomerular cells (see below).

The hormonal branch of the SAS includes preganglionic neurons, which innervate the chromaffin cells of the adrenal medulla that may be considered a modified sympathetic ganglion. Chromaffin cells do not possess neuritis but secrete catecholamines, mainly E, in the circulation. An increase in E plasma levels causes a rapid increase in the heart rate and contractility, an increase in renin release, and a redistribution of blood volume toward the heart, brain, and skeletal muscles and away from the kidneys, skin, and gut.

A pathological catecholamine release in the blood circulation, as well as an abrupt neuronal sympathetic discharge, causes a rise in BP, sometimes to very high levels. Such conditions are exemplified by the catecholamine release by pheochromocytoma/paraganglioma (Lenders et al. 2005) and also by the sympathetic activation in panic disorders. Increased sympatho-neuronal outflow associated to hypertension is present also in various neurologic syndromes such as autonomic epilepsy, baroreceptor deafferentation, Guillain-Barre syndrome, generalized seizures, and bladder stimulation in tetraplegic patients (Goldstein 1995).

Conversely, a pathological decrease in sympathetic outflow induces a decrease in BP that, when profound, causes a vasodepressor syncope with fainting. Neurogenic orthostatic hypotension is present in diseases such as pure autonomic failure, multiple system atrophy, and dopamine-β-hydroxylase deficiency.

The Renin-Angiotensin-Aldosterone System

Over a century after the identification of a "renin-like" activity in the canine kidney by Tigerstedt and Bergman (Tigerstedt and Bergman 1898), and more than 50 years after the purification of the vasoactive peptide angiotensin II (Ang II), carried out independently by Page and Braun-Menendez (Braun-Menendez and Page 1958), the characterization of the renin-angiotensin-aldosterone system (RAAS) continues relentless, thus broadening our understanding of the function of this key hormonal system, which has paramount clinical and therapeutic implications. The RAAS is currently regarded as both an endocrine and a paracrine system (Rocha and Stier 2001). The circulating RAAS entails a coordinated hormonal cascade, which begins with the biosynthesis of prohormone (prorenin) that undergoes proteolytic cleavage of the prosegment N-terminus peptide to give the bioactive renin. The latter is a secretory glycoprotein mainly made by the juxtaglomerular cells (JG) that line the afferent arteriole of the renal glomerulus. Renin is stored in granules of the JG cells and released first into the renal circulation and then, systemically, through a highly regulated exocytic process. Besides and in parallel to this, the kidney constitutively releases prorenin, which can be activated at the level of the pro(renin) receptor (Rocha and Stier 2001). Compelling evidence now indicates that the RAAS also acts as a paracrine system, which is directly involved in regulating the function of many organs, such as the adrenal gland, the reproductive system, the visceral adipose tissue, the vascular tissue, the eyes, the heart, and the brain.

Control of renin secretion is a key determinant of the RAAS activity, because renin regulates the initial and rate-limiting step of the RAAS by cleaving the N-terminal portion of the renin substrate (angiotensinogen) to form the biologically inert decapeptide angiotensin I (Ang I). Although mainly produced in the liver, angiotensinogen is also synthesized locally in tissues, such as the vessel wall and adipocytes. These sites might attain importance in disease conditions, as shown by the observation that adipocyte angiotensinogen deficiency, while not affecting plasma angiotensinogen levels under normal conditions, greatly reduced circulating Ang II under high-fat diets.

Ang I, the inactive decapeptide formed by renin, is hydrolyzed by the angiotensin-converting enzyme type 1 (ACE 1), which removes the C-terminal His-Leu dipeptide to form the octapeptide Ang II (Ang 1–8), which, alongside aldosterone, is the major mediator of the RAAS. Ang II was initially held to act via two different receptors, angiotensin II type 1 receptor (AT1R) and type 2 receptor (AT2R), which belong to the G-protein-coupled receptor (GPCR) family and share 34% of sequence homology. Upon stimulation these receptors induce effects that are altogether different and, most of the times, opposite: AT1R mediates the most known effects of Ang II, including vasoconstriction, cell growth, oxidative stress generation, inflammation, and vascular and cardiac hypertrophy. Moreover, in the adrenal cortex zona glomerulosa, AT1R activation increases inositol triphosphate formation, thus leading to release of Ca^{2+} from the endoplasmic reticulum, transcription of the aldosterone synthase (*CYP11B2*) gene, and aldosterone biosynthesis.

The AT2R is expressed in fetus, where it plays a major role in organ development, but also in adults, mainly in the adrenals, kidneys, uterus, ovary, heart, and specialized nuclei in the brain. Notwithstanding this, its role in adult animals and humans remained uncertain for decades, owing to the fact that specific agonists for AT2R were not available. Therefore, concomitant stimulation of the AT1R could not be avoided when using the AT2R natural ligand Ang II, which binds to AT1R and AT2R with almost equal affinity. Hence, given the higher abundance of the AT1R receptors in many organs, Ang II usually induces predominant AT1R effects. Moreover, the synthetic peptide CGP42112A, which was used to identify the AT2R, was thereafter found to have AT2R agonistic and antagonistic effects depending on its concentration. With the use of the first non-peptide AT2R agonist, compound 21 (C21), more information on the role of AT2R has been recently obtained. Thus, activation of the AT2R was found to result in vasodilatation, inhibition of cell proliferation, induction of apoptosis, extracellular matrix remodeling, and axonal regeneration. Moreover, this receptor was found to be upregulated in various pathological conditions, suggesting that it can serve a counter-regulatory role when overactivation of the AT1R occurs. Thus, the RAAS has a dual action in cardiovascular disease, playing both a detrimental and a protective role (Foulquier et al. 2012; Padia and Carey 2013). Accordingly, AT2R agonists are being tested for preventing hypertension-induced vascular and other end-organ damage.

Along the same line, accumulating evidence exists that other metabolites of Ang I and II may have significant biological activity, particularly in tissues. Ang III (Ang-(2–8)) and Ang IV (Ang-(3–8)) are formed by the sequential removal of amino acids from the N-terminus of Ang II by the action of aminopeptidases. Moreover, Ang-(1–7) is formed from Ang II by the action of carboxypeptidases including the angiotensin-converting enzyme type 2 (ACE 2) as shown in Fig. 2.

Unlike ACE 1, this enzyme does not convert Ang I to Ang II; moreover, its activity is not blunted by ACE inhibitors. Ang-(1–7), which is detectable in the kidney of various species at levels comparable to those of Ang II, has a low affinity for AT1R and AT2R but a very high affinity for an additional Ang receptor defined as Mas receptor (MasR), whose role remains poorly known.

Nowadays, it is well established that in pathological conditions some of these new players such as ACE2, the peptides made by this enzyme – Ang-(1–7) and Ang-(1–9) – and MasR can counteract Ang II. For instance, the acute infusion of Ang-(1–7) increases glomerular filtration rate (GFR) and renal blood flow. Moreover, Ang-(1–7) induces vasodilation, acutely stimulates the formation of NO, and reduces oxidative stress by blunting components of the NAD(P)H oxidase complex in the afferent vessels that was associated with lower cortical oxygenated radical (ROS) and 8-isoprostane excretion. This new regulatory system is named the protective RAAS (McKinney et al. 2014; Passos-Silva et al. 2013).

Pathological activation of the RAAS, such as in renal artery stenosis or the very rare occurrence of a reninoma (tumor of the juxtaglomerular cells), causes arterial hypertension. Moreover, the RAAS plays a detrimental role in cardiovascular

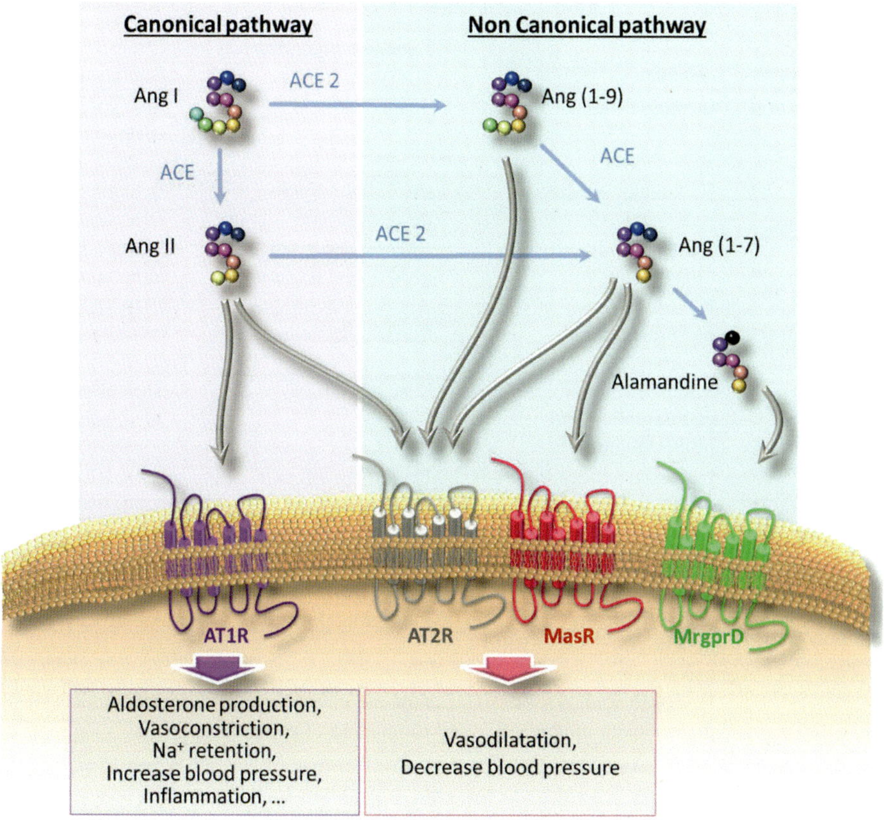

Fig. 2 Canonical and noncanonical pathways of the RAAS. The peptides are shown in *black* and the enzymes in *light blue*

damage in hypertension, including left ventricular hypertrophy (Dahlof et al. 2002), in renal damage (Keane et al. 2003), and also in heart failure as shown by randomized clinical trials with both ACE inhibitors (Swedberg et al. 1990) and mineralocorticoid receptor antagonists (the RALES investigators 1996).

Finally, as mentioned above, a fundamental component of the RAAS is aldosterone, which plays a key role for controlling sodium, potassium, and water balance, and ultimately blood pressure. Its major physiological targets are the epithelial cells, particularly those located in the distal nephron, colon, and salivary gland. At these sites aldosterone increases Na^+ reabsorption, in exchange for K^+ and H^+ excretion. Besides the actions on Na^+ balance, body fluid volumes, and blood pressure, aldosterone influences the function of the cardiovascular system by acting on the heart, vessels, and central nervous system. Accordingly, the key enzyme for aldosterone synthesis – aldosterone synthase – is regulated (besides Ang II) by several factors, including serum K^+, endothelin-1, dopamine, atrial natriuretic peptide

Table 1 Role of RAAS in cardiovascular diseases

RAAS component	Biochemical effects	Functional/pathological effects	Clinical manifestations
Angiotensin II	Increased intracellular Ca^{2+}	Vasoconstriction	Renovascular HBP, renin essential HBP
	Endothelin synthesis	Increased oxidative stress, vasoconstriction	Ischemia, infarction
	Decreased nitric oxide (NO) production	Inflammation, plaque growth and rupture	HBP, ischemia, infarction
	Release of pro-inflammatory mediators	Arterial hypertrophy, fibrosis, stiffening	HBP, ischemia, infarction
	Vascular smooth muscle cell migration and proliferation	Vascular fibrosis	Thrombosis, atherosclerosis
	Increased extracellular matrix formation	Plaque growth and rupture, cardiac remodeling	HBP, HF, and congestion
	Thromboxane A2 release	Clotting, platelet aggregation	Isolated systolic HBP
	Enhanced matrix metalloproteinase (MMP) production	Platelet aggregation	Atherosclerosis
	Increased synthesis of plasminogen inhibitor-1 (PAI-1)	Inflammation (via stimulation of production of monocyte chemoattractant protein (MCP)-1), increased activity of MMP-1 and MMP-3	Atherothrombosis
	Renovascular HBP, high renin essential HBP	Sodium retention	Atherosclerosis, HF
	Low-density lipoprotein (LDL) oxidation		Thrombosis,
	Stimulation of aldosterone production		Atherosclerosis
	Excess autonomous production		Atherosclerosis
			Thrombosis
			HBP, HF, congestion
Aldosterone	Excess autonomous production	Bilateral adrenal hyperplasia, aldosterone-producing adenoma	Primary aldosteronism
	Increased endothelial Na channel (ENAC)	Sodium and water retention	HBP, HF, congestion
	Hypokalemia and hypomagnesemia	Reentry mechanisms	Arrhythmias

(*continued*)

Table 1 (continued)

RAAS component	Biochemical effects	Functional/pathological effects	Clinical manifestations
	Increased oxidative stress and activation of inflammatory pathways	Inflammation, oxidative damage to DNA	Vascular and myocardial tissue damage Atherosclerosis
	Increased synthesis of collagen I and III and fibronectin	NO release	Atrial fibrillation, HF, and congestion HBP, HF
	Vascular smooth muscle cell migration and proliferation	Fibrosis, LVH	Vascular damage
		Vascular remodeling, hypertrophy, artery stiffness	Atherosclerosis

Foulquier et al. 2012; Gaddam et al. 2009; McKinney et al. 2014; Padia and Carey 2013; Passos-Silva et al. 2013; Rocha and Stier 2001; Willerson and Ridker 2004
HBP high blood pressure, *HF* heart failure, *LVH* left ventricular hypertrophy

(ANP), brain natriuretic peptide (BNP), urotensin II, and serotonin. When produced in excess and under conditions of high-to-normal Na^+ intake, aldosterone causes oxidative stress, inflammation, fibrosis, and oxidative damage to DNA. Hence, its production must be tightly controlled to maintain ion and fluid homeostasis and avoid hyperaldosteronism. Table 1 summarizes the fundamental role played by the RAAS in many cardiovascular diseases.

Excessive aldosterone biosynthesis autonomous from these regulators occurs in primary aldosteronism (PA), the most common form of secondary hypertension with an estimated prevalence of about 11.2% in referred patients and about 2% in primary care and as high as 20% in patients with resistant hypertension (Douma et al. 2008). The two major causes of PA are unilateral aldosterone-producing adenoma (APA) and bilateral adrenal hyperplasia (BAH), accounting together for 95% of cases (Boulkroun et al. 2015).

Conversely, hypoaldosteronism, mainly due to Addison disease, in spite of increased renin and angiotensin release, causes hypotension. Hyporeninemic hypoaldosteronism due to nonsteroidal anti-inflammatory drugs usually manifests itself with hyperkalemia rather than hypotension.

In summary, with the discoveries of new pathways, including the protective ones, and novel actions of the RAAS component, several potential new targets for therapeutic interventions have been identified and are currently under testing with the final goal to develop new drugs to combat hypertension and cardiovascular disease. In fact, drugs currently in clinical trials include C21, encapsulated Ang-(1–7), novel mineralocorticoid receptor antagonists, and aldosterone synthase inhibitors. They might eventually provide additional weapons besides the well-established RAAS inhibitors as beta-blockers, ACE inhibitors, AT1R antagonists, and renin inhibitors.

Other Factors Influencing Blood Pressure Control

Natriuretic Peptides

Natriuretic peptides (NP) belong to a family of hormones all sharing a common 17 amino acid ring and differing for NH2 and COOH residues outside the ring (Nakao et al. 1992). All family members are characterized by a similar molecular structure and similar biological effects mainly exerted at the cardiovascular level (Levin et al. 1998).

Atrial natriuretic peptide (ANP) is released by the cardiac atria when their wall tension increases. B-type natriuretic peptide (BNP) derives from a precursor (Pro-BNP) mainly synthesized and released by the cardiac ventricles in response to an increase in ventricular wall tension.

Once released, Pro-BNP is cleaved in two fragments: the C-terminal (BNP) is constituted by 32 amino acids and is biologically active, while the N-terminal, constituted by 76 amino acids, is not but is measured as a biomarker of activation of BNP synthesis.

C-type natriuretic peptide (CNP) derives from a 122 amino acid precursor and is characterized by 22 amino acids. It is secreted in the central nervous system, the kidney, and the endothelial tissue in response to shear stress.

The main physiological actions of NP occur in the kidney, where they exert a potent vasodilatory effect and regulate blood volume through sodium and water excretion, thus contributing to BP homeostasis.

They also cause, by paracrine and autocrine actions, relaxation of the vascular muscle walls, thus inducing vasodilation and decrease in BP. Finally, NP inhibit the secretion of other vasoactive hormones such as renin, aldosterone, vasopressin, and endothelin-1.

In summary, NP participate in cardiovascular homeostasis counteracting acute and chronic volume overload and exerting opposite actions to those elicited by the SAS and the RAAS.

Dopamine

Dopamine (DA) is a catecholamine acting at different levels in the body. In the central and peripheral nervous system, DA acts as a neurotransmitter, whereas in the kidney it acts as a paracrine hormone at the tubular level where the high activity of the enzyme DOPA decarboxylase transforms circulating L-DOPA into DA. Urinary DA reflects tubular synthesis. Activation of dopaminergic receptors at the periphery increases natriuresis and diuresis by several mechanisms: acting on DA1 receptors on vascular smooth muscle cells, DA causes increase in renal blood flow, augmenting glomerular filtration of sodium; acting on DA2 presynaptic receptors, DA inhibits NE release from the sympathetic nerve terminals, thus reducing the sympathetic-mediated vasoconstriction, and aldosterone release from the adrenal cortex, thus preventing its pressor actions (Rossitto et al. 2016). Finally, in the kidney, DA acts as a paracrine hormone at DA1 receptors on proximal convoluted tubular cells, inhibiting Na/K ATPase and reducing sodium reabsorption (Carey et al. 1990). Thus, on the whole, endogenous DA acts as a natriuretic and hypotensive hormone.

Nitric Oxide

Nitric oxide (NO) is a small molecule, composed by a nitrogen and oxygen atom, synthesized from its precursor L-arginine by the activity of NO synthase (NOS), an enzyme present in activated inflammatory cells (inducible NOS – iNOS) and in neuronal (nNOS) and endothelial (eNOS) cells where it is constitutively produced and secreted (Lowenstein et al. 1994).

NO has a very short half-life of about 30 s. Among the different NOS isoforms, the most important at the cardiovascular level is eNOS: by releasing NO it induces vasodilation, thus regulating local blood pressure, and inhibits platelet aggregation. Endothelial NO is the main factor mediating vasodilation in response to the shear stress caused by a local flow increase (Corretti et al. 2002). NO is also an important endothelial factor counteracting the vasoconstriction induced by angiotensin II and endothelin-1.

Endothelin-1

Endothelium has to be regarded as a paracrine organ regulating vascular tone as well as other functions such as platelet aggregation and vascular cell proliferation (Behrendt and Ganz 2002). It secretes not only vasodilating agent such as NO but also vasoconstrictor factors such as endothelin-1 (ET).

Endothelins are a group of peptides of 21 amino acids, which include three different isoforms (ET-1, ET-2, and ET-3) (Inoue et al. 1989). ET-1 is the most represented isoform at the vascular level, where it exerts a potent vasoconstriction, acting on type A receptors (ET_A) located in the vascular smooth muscle cells.

ET-1 exerts additional relevant cardiovascular effects acting at different organs. In the vascular bed, ET-1 also acts on ET_B receptors, located on the endothelial cells, where it causes vasodilation. In the heart, ET-1 exerts a chronotropic and inotropic effect in vitro, whereas in vivo it decreases cardiac output, due to baroreceptor-mediated decrease in heart rate and increased afterload. In the kidney, ET-1 causes constriction of both afferent and efferent arterioles and decrease in glomerular filtration rate and renal plasma flow, through ET_A receptors. At the tubular level, ET-1 decreases sodium and water reabsorption through ET_B receptors. Moreover, ET-1, by acting on ET_B receptors, mediates the epithelial mesenchymal transition induced by Ang II, a process whereby tubular epithelial cells transform into fibroblasts, which produce extracellular matrix proteins, ultimately leading to hypertensive nephroangiosclerosis (Seccia et al. 2016). Hence, ET-1 is held to play a key role in the progression of hypertensive renal disease to chronic kidney disease and ultimately end-stage kidney failure.

ET-1 affects also the RAAS, stimulating ACE activity and enhancing aldosterone release from the adrenal cortex. In fact, the adrenocortical zona glomerulosa cells can produce ET-1 and express both ET_A and ET_B receptors (Rossi et al. 1994); the latter mediate a potent secretagogue effect of ET-1 on aldosterone (Belloni et al. 1996).

As a whole, ET causes increase in BP through regional and systemic vasoconstriction (Clarke et al. 1989) contributing to the occurrence of diseases such as essential hypertension, pulmonary hypertension, chronic renal failure, and chronic heart failure.

Arginine Vasopressin

Arginine vasopressin (AVP), also known as antidiuretic hormone, is a nonapeptide primarily secreted by the supraoptic and paraventricular nuclei of the hypothalamus. The regulation of AVP synthesis and secretion involves two processes, osmotic and pressure-volume. The first is very sensitive in that hypothalamic osmoreceptors may perceive even small changes in plasma osmolality, thus regulating AVP secretion. The pressure and volume regulation is mediated by specific receptors located in the carotid sinus/aortic arch and atria/pulmonary venous system, respectively; these pathways regulate AVP release through a tonic inhibitory action that decreases with significant fall in blood volume and pressure (about >10–20%). The most important physiologic action of AVP is to influence the rate of water excretion at the level of renal collecting tubules by promoting concentration of the urine. Other functions of AVP include contraction of smooth muscle in blood vessels, stimulation of ACTH secretion, and regulation of glycogenolysis in the liver. The effects of AVP are mediated through interaction with specific receptors, named V1a, V1b, and V2: the latter mediates the antidiuretic effect, while the remaining functions are mediated by the other receptors. In physiological conditions, AVP does not seem to play a significant role in the maintenance of BP (Gavras et al. 1982); moreover, disorders with excess or deficit of AVP secretion/action are characterized primarily by abnormalities of osmolality induced by abnormal excretion or retention of water, without significant effects on blood pressure. Thus, the pressure and volume regulation of AVP secretion probably plays a minor role in physiological conditions, but attains a major role in acute and large disturbance of hemodynamic states. In fact, in severe hypovolemic shock, when AVP release is very high, the hormone does contribute to the compensatory increase in systemic vascular resistance. In addition to activation of V1a receptors, AVP may induce vasoconstriction by other mechanisms such as modulation of ATP-sensitive K^+-channels, modulation of NO, and potentiation of adrenergic and other vasoconstrictor agents (den Ouden and Meinders 2005). Based on these concepts, vasopressin is commonly used as an adjunct to catecholamines to support blood pressure in refractory hypovolemic shock.

Cortisol

Cortisol, the major human glucocorticoid, is produced by the adrenocortical zona fasciculate; it is essential for the maintenance of body internal environment, the so-called homeostasis. Cortisol affects virtually all body organs influencing, regulating, or modulating the changes that occur in the body in response to stress, including heart contraction and blood vessel tone. Cortisol participates in the maintenance of normal BP, as suggested by the observation that disorders of cortisol secretion, either in excess or deficit, are characterized by significant changes of BP levels, e.g., hypertension or hypotension, respectively. Cortisol may increase BP by several mechanisms: in vascular smooth muscle, it increases sensitivity to other pressor agents such as catecholamines and angiotensin II while interferes with NO-mediated endothelial dilatation (Grunfeld and Eloy 1987). In the kidney, cortisol shows high affinity for mineralocorticoid receptors and, depending on the activity of type 2 isoenzyme of 11-beta-hydroxysteroid-dehydrogenase, which converts cortisol to inactive cortisone, may exert a mineralocorticoid action with sodium retention, potassium loss, and volume expansion (Stewart 1999). At the heart level, cortisol increases cardiac output (Whitworth et al. 2005); moreover, it increases hepatic synthesis of the renin substrate angiotensinogen (Saruta et al. 1986).

Summary

BP is a vital physical parameter, which is essential to warrant blood supply to organs and tissues in any conditions, as different posture (supine or upright) or different behavior (rest or exercise). Therefore, not surprisingly, its regulation is extremely complex, depending on several strictly interconnected and finely regulated systems, which are able to control and adjust this parameter continuously on a beat-to-beat basis. BP, generated by heart action, depends on vascular peripheral resistances, generated by arterial contraction. However, it critically depends also on blood volume, mainly dependent on salt intake and kidney function. Blood volume, in turn, affects cardiac output. All these functions need a permanent control by sensors located in different sites of the cardiovascular tree (arteries, veins, heart). This continuous setting (and resetting) needs both rapid and long-lasting responses elicited by neuronal and hormonal mechanisms controlling heart activity, blood volume, and peripheral resistances. The two major systems responsible for BP control are the SAS and the RAAS. Their main role is to avoid a fall in BP and therefore their activation increases BP. When not regulated by the counteracting mechanisms, their activation is responsible for the occurrence of hypertension and, in the long run, cardiovascular damages.

Their activation is maximal in conditions of a profound hypotension, such as during large hemorrhage and dehydration: in these situations additional factors, such as vasopressin and cortisol release, may be recruited to maintain tissue perfusion.

Blood volume mostly depends on sodium and water reabsorption in the kidney. Both the SAS and the RAAS play a pivotal role at this level where other systems, such as natriuretic peptides and dopamine, counteract their sodium- and water-retaining action in an attempt to avoid excessive volume expansion.

Lastly, blood flow needs also a local, peripheral adjustment depending on tissue demands. This fine regulation is attained by means of local, mainly endothelial, vasodilating or vasoconstrictor factors, among which NO and endothelin-1 are the main players.

References

Behrendt D, Ganz P. Endothelial function. From vascular biology to clinical applications. Am J Cardiol. 2002;90:40L–8.

Belloni AS, Rossi GP, Andreis PG, Neri G, Albertin G, Pessina AC, Nussdorfer GG. Endothelin adrenocortical secretagogue effect is mediated by the B receptor in rats. Hypertension. 1996;27:1153–9.

Boulkroun S, Fernandes-Rosa FL, Zennaro MC. Molecular and cellular mechanisms of aldosterone producing adenoma development. Front Endocrinol (Lausanne). 2015;6:95.

Braun-Menendez E, Page IH. Suggested revision of nomenclature – angiotensin. Science. 1958;127:242.

Carey RM, Siragy HM, Felder RA. Physiological modulation of renal function by the renal dopaminergic system. J Auton Pharmacol. 1990;10 Suppl 1:s47–51.

Clarke JG, Benjamin N, Larkin SW, Webb DJ, Davies GJ, Maseri A. Endothelin is a potent long-lasting vasoconstrictor in men. Am J Physiol. 1989;257:H2033–5.

Corretti MC, Anderson TJ, Benjamin EJ, Celermajer D, Charbonneau F, Creager MA, Deanfield J, Drexler H, Gerhard-Herman M, Herrington D, Vallance P, Vita J, Vogel R. Guidelines for the ultrasound assessment of endothelial-dependent flow-mediated vasodilation of the brachial artery: a report of the international brachial artery reactivity task force. J Am Coll Cardiol. 2002;39:257–65.

Dahlof B, Devereux RB, Kjeldsen SE, Julius S, Beevers G, de Faire U, Fyhrquist F, Ibsen H, Kristiansson K, Lederballe-Pedersen O, Lindholm LH, Nieminen MS, Omvik P, Oparil S, Wedel H. Cardiovascular morbidity and mortality in the losartan intervention for endpoint reduction in hypertension study (LIFE): a randomised trial against atenolol. Lancet. 2002;359:995–1003.

den Ouden DT, Meinders AE. Vasopressin: physiology and clinical use in patients with vasodilatory shock: a review. Neth J Med. 2005;63:4–13.

Douma S, Petidis K, Doumas M, Papaefthimiou P, Triantafyllou A, Kartali N, Papadopoulos N, Vogiatzis K, Zamboulis C. Prevalence of primary hyperaldosteronism in resistant hypertension: a retrospective observational study. Lancet. 2008;371:1921–6.

Foulquier S, Steckelings UM, Unger T. Impact of the AT(2) receptor agonist C21 on blood pressure and beyond. Curr Hypertens Rep. 2012;14:403–9.

Gaddam KK, Pimenta E, Husain S, Calhoun DA. Aldosterone and cardiovascular disease. Curr Probl Cardiol. 2009;34:51–84.

Gavras H, Hatzinikolaou P, North WG, Bresnahan M, Gavras I. Interaction of the sympathetic nervous system with vasopressin and renin in the maintenance of blood pressure. Hypertension. 1982;4:400–5.

Goldstein DS. Stress, catecholamines and cardiovascular disease. New York: Oxford University Press; 1995.

Goldstein DS, Eisenhofer G, McCarty R, editors. Catecholamines. Bridging basic science with clinical medicine. San Diego: Academic Press; 1998.

Grunfeld JP, Eloy L. Glucocorticoids modulate vascular reactivity in the rat. Hypertension. 1987;10:608–18.

Inoue A, Yanagisawa M, Kimura S, Kasuya Y, Miyauchi T, Goto K, Masaki T. The human endothelin family: three structurally and pharmacologically distinct isopeptides predicted by three separate genes. Proc Natl Acad Sci U S A. 1989;86:2863–7.

RALES Investigators. Effectiveness of spironolactone added to an angiotensin-converting enzyme inhibitor and a loop diuretic for severe chronic congestive heart failure (the randomized aldactone evaluation study [RALES]). Am J Cardiol. 1996;78:902–7.

Keane WF, Brenner BM, de Zeeuw D, Grunfeld JP, McGill J, Mitch WE, Ribeiro AB, Shahinfar S, Simpson RL, Snapinn SM, Toto R, RENAAL Study Investigators. The risk of developing end-stage renal disease in patients with type 2 diabetes and nephropathy: the RENAAL study. Kidney Int. 2003;63:1499–507.

Lenders JW, Eisenhofer G, Mannelli M, Pacak K. Phaeochromocytoma. Lancet. 2005;366:665–75.

Levin ER, Gardner DG, Samson WK. Natriuretic peptides. N Engl J Med. 1998;339:321–8.

Lowenstein CJ, Dinerman JL, Snyder SH. Nitric oxide: a physiologic messenger. Ann Intern Med. 1994;120:227–37.

McKinney CA, Fattah C, Loughrey CM, Milligan G, Nicklin SA. Angiotensin-(1–7) and angiotensin-(1–9): function in cardiac and vascular remodelling. Clin Sci (Lond). 2014;126:815–27.

Nakao K, Ogawa Y, Suga S, Imura H. Molecular biology and biochemistry of the natriuretic peptide system. I: natriuretic peptides. J Hypertens. 1992;10:907–12.

Padia SH, Carey RM. AT2 receptors: beneficial counter-regulatory role in cardiovascular and renal function. Pflugers Arch. 2013;465:99–110.

Passos-Silva DG, Verano-Braga T, Santos RA. Angiotensin-(1–7): beyond the cardio-renal actions. Clin Sci (Lond). 2013;124:443–56.

Rocha R, Stier Jr CT. Pathophysiological effects of aldosterone in cardiovascular tissues. Trends Endocrinol Metab. 2001;12:308–14.

Rossi G, Albertin G, Belloni A, Zanin L, Biasolo MA, Prayer-Galetti T, Bader M, Nussdorfer GG, Palu G, Pessina AC. Gene expression, localization, and characterization of endothelin A and B receptors in the human adrenal cortex. J Clin Invest. 1994;94:1226–34.

Rossitto G, Miotto D, Battistel M, Barbiero G, Maiolino G, Bisogni V, Sanga V, Rossi GP. Metoclopramide unmasks potentially misleading contralateral suppression in patients undergoing adrenal vein sampling for primary aldosteronism. J Hypertens. (2016) [Epub ahead of print]

Saruta T, Suzuki H, Handa M, Igarashi Y, Kondo K, Senba S. Multiple factors contribute to the pathogenesis of hypertension in cushing's syndrome. J Clin Endocrinol Metab. 1986;62:275–9.

Seccia TM, Caroccia B, Gioco F, Piazza M, Buccella V, Guidolin D, Guerzoni E, Montini B, Petrelli L, Pagnin E, Ravarotto V, Belloni AS, Calò LA, Rossi GP. Endothelin-1 drives epithelial-mesenchymal transition in hypertensive nephroangiosclerosis. J Am Heart Assoc. 2016;5(7):e003888. doi:10.1161/JAHA.116.003888.

Stewart PM. Mineralocorticoid hypertension. Lancet. 1999;353:1341–7.

Swedberg K, Eneroth P, Kjekshus J, Wilhelmsen L. Hormones regulating cardiovascular function in patients with severe congestive heart failure and their relation to mortality. Circulation. 1990;82:1730–6. CONSENSUS Trial Study Group.

Tigerstedt R, Bergmann PG. Niere und kreislauf. Skand Arch Physiol. 1898;8:223–7.

Whitworth JA, Williamson PM, Mangos G, Kelly JJ. Cardiovascular consequences of cortisol excess. Vasc Health Risk Manag. 2005;1:291–9.

Willerson JT, Ridker PM. Inflammation as a cardiovascular risk factor. Circulation. 2004;109: II2–10.

The Endocrinology of Puberty

24

Sara A. DiVall and Carolina DiBlasi

Abstract

The hypothalamic-pituitary-gonadal axis is unique among the hypothalamic-pituitary hormonal systems in that it undergoes dramatic changes in biologic activity during fetal, childhood, and adult development. Unlike the other pituitary hormonal systems, the axis is quiescent for much of childhood, becoming active at the developmental stage that defines puberty. Puberty begins when the gonadotropin-releasing hormone (GnRH) neurons of the hypothalamus secrete GnRH in a pulsatile manner. Pulsatile GnRH causes pituitary gonadotrophs to synthesize and release luteinizing hormone (LH) and follicle-stimulating hormone (FSH). LH and FSH in turn induce steroidogenesis and gametogenesis in the gonads. Steroid production then causes the physical and physiological changes associated with puberty. A single pathway or factor that triggers this hormonal cascade at puberty has not been found, although several pathways have been identified that affect GnRH neuron function at puberty. This chapter will first discuss the physiology of the reproductive axis in intrauterine life and childhood, detailing the hormonal signals and receptor function of normal puberty. Next, genes implicated in pubertal timing will be discussed in context of the disease processes that result from the genetic derangement. Finally, secular trends in pubertal timing will be discussed.

Keywords

GnRH • Kisspeptin • Hypogonadotropic hypogonadism • Precocious puberty

S.A. DiVall (✉) • C. DiBlasi
Division of Pediatric Endocrinology, Seattle Children's Hospital/University of Washington, Seattle, WA, USA
e-mail: sara.divall@seattlechildrens.org; Carolina.DiBlasi@seattlechildrens.org

A. Belfiore, D. LeRoith (eds.), *Principles of Endocrinology and Hormone Action*, Endocrinology, https://doi.org/10.1007/978-3-319-44675-2_25

Contents

Reproductive Axis Development

The reproductive axis undergoes dramatic changes during fetal life, infancy, and childhood. Because the hypothalamic-pituitary-gonadal axis (Fig. 1) is active in the fetus and newborn then enters a quiescent state during childhood, a discussion of the factors involved in puberty is best started with a review of the development of the neuroendocrine axis and the activity of the axis in various stages of infancy and childhood.

Fetal Life

The hypothalamic peptide kisspeptin plays a role in triggering GnRH pulsatile release at puberty (detailed below). Timing of kisspeptin neuron development in humans is unknown, but the sequence of events can be inferred from rodent studies. In adults, there are two populations of kisspeptin neurons in the hypothalamus, one in the arcuate nucleus (ARC) and a different population in the preoptic area (POA). Kisspeptin neurons of the arcuate nucleus seem to arise from proopiomelanocortin (POMC) precursor cells (Sanz et al. 2015). The expression of the kisspeptin and its receptor, GPR54 genes, starts in the midgestation period after GnRH expression is

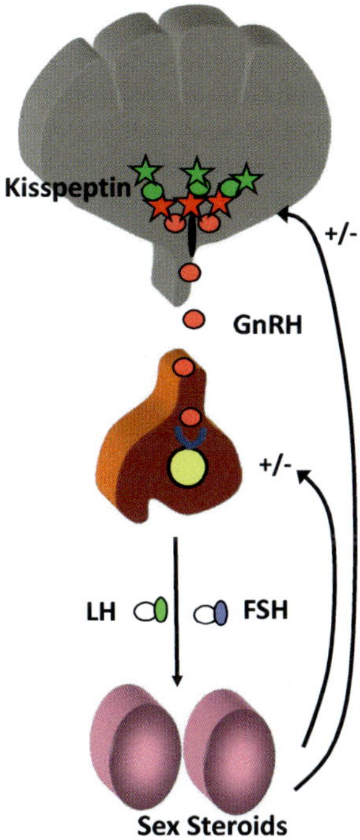

Fig. 1 Schematic of the hypothalamic-pituitary-gonadal (HPG) axis. Kisspeptin neurons (*green stars*) secrete kisspeptin (*green circles*) that induces gonadotropin-releasing hormone (GnRH) neurons (*red starts*) to secrete GnRH hormone (*red circles*). GnRH in turn induces the pituitary gonadotrophs to synthesize and secrete luteinizing hormone (LH) and follicle-stimulating hormone (FSH). LH and FSH then induce Leydig cells of the testes to produce testosterone or theca and granulosa cells to produce estradiol. The sex steroids result in secondary sex characteristics of puberty

detected. There seems to be a sexual dimorphism in kisspeptin expression, with females having greater amounts of kisspeptin expression (Knoll et al. 2013). Kisspeptin neuron axons extend to the GnRH neuron with presumed established synaptic connections in utero.

GnRH neurons are unique among neurons in that they arise outside of the neuroectoderm in the olfactory pit. This occurs at week 6 postconception in humans. The GnRH neuron begins to synthesize and secrete GnRH shortly thereafter. The neurons then migrate via the forebrain, arriving at the hypothalamus by week 9 (Schwanzel-Fukuda et al. 1996). The location, number of GnRH neurons, and projection to the median eminence are similar to adult animals. Migration is supported by the gene products of the signaling proteins *Kal1* (anosmin), *PROK1* (prokineticin 1), *FGF8* (fibroblast growth factor 8), as well as genes that encode receptors such as *FGFR1*, *PROKR2*, and *CHD7* (Bhagavath and Layman 2007). Disorders caused by alterations in these genes will be discussed later in the chapter. GnRH neuron migration is independent from kisspeptin neuron development and is not dependent upon kisspeptin signaling.

The anterior pituitary gland arises from Rathke's pouch, an invagination of neuroectoderm, beginning at week 3 postconception. Supported by early-expressing transcription factors such as bone morphogenetic protein 4 (BMP4), FGF8, FGF10, Wnt 4, and Wnt 5, cells of Rathke's pouch differentiate into pituitary cell lineage precursors. Further differentiation into specific hormone-releasing cells occurs by week 12 postconception with the support of transcription factors such as Prop1, LHx3/4, and Sox2/3. Thus, by week 12, gonadotrophs are synthesizing both the common alpha and unique beta subunits of LH and FSH (Dattani and Gevers 2016). In addition to the pituitary transcription factors required for differentiation into the other pituitary secreting cells, gonadotroph development also requires the genes steroidogenic factor 1 (*SF1*) and *DAX1*.

Gonadal development occurs completely separately from neuroendocrine development. Before gestational week 6, the genital duct systems for male and female duct systems coexist with an indifferent (bipotential) gonad. The presence or absence of the Y chromosome, and thus the gene *SRY*, is the determining factor directing development of the bipotential gonad into either testes or ovaries, respectively. *SRY* is expressed by week 6 of gestation. *SRY* directs the expression of many genes that direct the differentiation of the bipotential gonad into the Leydig (testosterone producing) cells of the testes as well as the Sertoli cells (Achermann and Hughes 2016). *SRY* also induces expression of the gene *SF1*. *SF1* in turn acts to induce expression of anti-Mullerian hormone (AMH), which induces regression of the female (Mullerian) duct structures. Mullerian structures include the fallopian tubes, uterus, and upper third of the vagina. In the presence of two normal X chromosomes, ovarian differentiation commences although less is known about ovarian development. Formation of the bipotential gonad into testes or ovaries is complete by week 8 gestation, while differentiation of the genital duct systems into the male or female internal reproductive organs is complete by week 9 gestation (Achermann and Hughes 2016).

External development of male or female structures is determined by the presence or absence of testosterone (and thus the *SRY* gene). Further conversion of testosterone to dihydrotestosterone (DHT) is necessary for normal development of the penis and prostate gland. In the absence of DHT, the lower two-thirds of the vagina and the labia minora and majora develop.

Placental human chorionic gonadotropin (HCG) directs testosterone secretion by the ever-expanding Leydig cell population after week 14 gestation. Testosterone, in effect, directs formation of the external genitalia. LH and FSH are reaching peak levels at midgestation, about 20–24 weeks. The testes and ovaries are responsive to LH and FSH by week 20, and some primary follicles are seen in ovaries. However, placental estrogen predominates, so estrogen secretion by the fetal ovary is thought to be minimal. LH-directed testosterone synthesis is required for normal testicular descent from the abdomen into the scrotal sac in late gestation as well as further lengthening of the penis in late gestation. By the last half of the third trimester, placental estrogen production provides negative feedback to the axis to cause LH and FSH levels to decrease (Kaplan et al. 1976).

Kisspeptin expression slowly diminishes in late gestation, but GnRH expression remains at the same level throughout gestation. Neuron secretion of these peptides during gestation, however, is unknown given the difficulty in quantifying peptide secretion from fetal neurons. It is believed that despite gene expression and translation, release of the neuropeptides does not occur.

Neonatal Life

At birth, LH and FSH levels are low, but begin to increase again upon withdrawal of placental estrogens. LH and FSH levels rise in the first few months of life, with FSH levels higher in female infants than in male infants. Negative steroid regulation of the axis is intact during this time, because agonadal human and primate infants exhibit LH and FSH levels similar to that of agonadal adults (and higher than intact persons) (Conte et al. 1975). In girls, LH and FSH levels fall to nearly undetectable levels by the age of 2 years, while in boys the LH and FSH fall sooner, by 12–18 months of life. This effect is independent of steroid feedback because agonadal toddlers also experience the decrease in gonadotropin levels (Ross et al. 1983). This fall in gonadotropin levels is thought to be due to suppressive influences of the central nervous system that develop during the first years of life.

The prolonged postnatal LH surge occurs only in primate species, and whether hypothalamic events mediate these physiological events is not known. In rodents, LH and testosterone levels are elevated in the first 4 h of life and then decrease and remain low until the pubertal period. It is debated whether this event is mediated by hypothalamic events or not. Postnatal GnRH and kisspeptin gene expression in primates and rodents is sustained in early infancy and prepubertally (Knoll et al. 2013). In the immediate postnatal period, murine GnRH neurons release GnRH at high frequency but low amplitude (as measured by calcium-dependent voltage changes across the membrane); this effect was noted in neurons of late gestational and neonatal pups up to 1 week of age, sharply diminishing in two-week-old pups. Amplitude of GnRH release increased in peripubertal animals, but frequency did not change appreciably using this technique (Glanowska et al. 2014). This high-frequency GnRH release is not dependent upon kisspeptin signaling, and the pituitary does not release LH in response to the high-frequency GnRH release.

Early Childhood

The precise inhibitory mechanisms that diminish GnRH and LH release after the perinatal period are not known. In addition, the activity of the HPG axis is not well characterized between early infancy and the peripubertal period. However, the axis seems to have detectable activity, at least in humans. Multiple groups have shown that prepubertal children as young as 5 years of age have infrequent, low-level LH and FSH peaks during sleep. Using ultrasensitive immunofluorometric assays to measure LH and FSH, peaks have been detected in boys and girls 3 years prior to the first physical signs of puberty (Apter et al. 1993; Mitamura et al. 2000; Wu et al. 1996). FSH peaks are higher than LH peaks, and the gonadotropin peaks do not result in detectable steroid hormone levels.

Peripuberty

Girls. About 1 year prior to breast budding, prepubertal girls begin to experience more frequent and higher peaks of LH exclusively during sleep. Brief nocturnal increases in estradiol, barely above detectable, are noted. In a population sample, this was manifested as an increase in estradiol concentration by ultrasensitive means detectable in the morning. At the time that breast budding becomes detectable, LH peak amplitude increases about tenfold, while FSH pulse amplitude doubles. These changes produce a smaller FSH/LH ratio (Oerter et al. 1990). The augmentation of LH pulse amplitude occurs because of increased pituitary responsiveness to GnRH. There is a priming effect of GnRH on LH release by the gonadotroph and an increase in the number of GnRH receptors on the gonadotroph. Pulse frequency increases to a lesser extent and pulses become diurnal. Increases in estradiol also become more prolonged. This is manifested in a population sample as average higher morning estradiol levels.

Boys. Prepubertally, boys also have greater amount of detectable serum FSH than LH (Wu et al. 1996). Boys exhibit a similar pattern of nighttime LH pulsation, with an increase in LH amplitude about a year prior to achieving physical evidence of pubertal onset. Very early pubertal boys also have further augmentation of nocturnal LH pulse amplitude. LH pulses then become diurnal as puberty progresses. Similar to girls, the LH pulses that become diurnal result in higher baseline testosterone levels, which is manifested in a population sample as average higher morning testosterone levels (Oerter et al. 1990).

Puberty

Girls. Subsequent changes in hormonal patterns are most readily discussed with reference to standards developed by Tanner for staging female puberty on the basis of physical changes of the breast and appearance of pubic hair (Tanner 1952). The pubertal progression from Tanner stage 2 (breast budding) to 3 (increasing amount of breast tissue and differing contour of the areola) is marked by further increases in LH pulse amplitude, 20–40-fold increase from levels detected prepubertally (Oerter et al. 1990). LH pulse frequency increases to a far lesser extent (e.g., twofold). The highest pulse amplitudes occur during sleep, but detectable LH pulses become present during the day, with basal LH levels detectable at all times of day. Estradiol levels become detectable at all hours as well. Girls without gonadal function do not experience the day-night variation in LH pulse frequency, suggesting that ovarian hormones be involved in inhibition of daytime gonadotropin pulses of early puberty. Upon progression to breast Tanner stage 4, the pattern of gonadotropin release is not appreciably different, but estradiol levels continue to rise. This suggests that ovarian responsiveness to gonadotropins has increased, possibly via gonadotropin-induced increase in enzymes necessary for steroidogenesis. Ovary release of the molecule inhibin also rises during this time, possibly mediating some degree of negative feedback on the axis (Sehested et al. 2000). In mid-late pubertal girls, FSH levels rise at night, whereas LH levels are detectable night and day. The degree of FSH rise is only threefold from prepubertal levels, in contrast to the 10–20-fold increase in LH levels. This is thought to be due to the inhibin negative feedback. Coincident with the rise in nighttime FSH level is a lowering of activin A levels from daytime highs. At this time, the LH and FSH secretion pattern resembles that of adult women, in which pulses have higher amplitude during day than during the night. Menarche occurs at mid-end of stage 4, after a year-long rise in daily estradiol output (Legro et al. 2000). After menarche, high estradiol levels can exert negative feedback on the axis to suppress it, leading to cyclic estradiol levels and uterine bleeding. At the time of menarche, positive feedback of estradiol on the axis (to induce the LH surge) is not established, so ovulation usually does not occur. Uterine bleeding occurs with varying cyclicity until the mechanism of estradiol-induced LH surge is mature, leading to regular ovulatory cycles. This process can take a year or more after menarche to become fully established.

Boys. As in girls, the change in hormonal patterns of puberty is discussed in the context of pubertal staging standards of Tanner (1952). Traditionally, testicular volumes of 3 or 4 ml have both been described as predictive of the onset of gonadotropin activation at puberty, with 4 ml being more predictive than 3 ml. However, 10–20% of boys will exhibit these size testicles and not experience progressive puberty (Rosenfield et al. 2012). For most boys, however, the evolution of LH and FSH secretion during puberty is the same as girls. Early puberty is marked by increases in nocturnal LH pulse amplitude and lesser increases in pulse frequency, becoming diurnal by Tanner stage 4 (Wu et al. 1996). It is noted that the diurnal pattern of LH pulsation is experienced earlier in puberty in girls than in boys. Testosterone secretion is nocturnal in early puberty, becoming detectable during the day upon stage 4 and 5 of puberty (Wu et al. 1996). Testicular size increases gradually as puberty progresses; as testicular size is associated with sleep LH, it is theorized that the LH-induced testosterone production leads to seminiferous tubule development contributing to testicular size. Intratesticular testosterone is important for spermatogenesis. A critical testosterone level that is associated with genesis of viable sperm is not known, but it is generally accepted that sperm of an adult male concentration and motility is not synthesized until late in puberty, Tanner stage 5. Testosterone also induces changes to the larynx, resulting in the deeper voice of men. This starts to occur in Tanner stages 3 and 4, when testosterone becomes detectable during the day as well.

Modulation by Obesity

The modulation of the gonadotropin release pattern by obesity has been studied more in girls than in boys, given the observed trend of earlier onset of breast development in obese girls. The limited studies show that early-mid pubertal obese girls do not experience the vast difference in LH secretion between day and night that normal-weight girls experience. In general, their wake LH secretion is lower than that in normal-weight girls, while their nighttime LH secretion does not increase appreciably or to a lesser extent (Rosenfield and Bordini 2010). After menarche, obese girls do not experience the full evolution of LH pulsatility to the adult female pattern; their nighttime LH does not decrease to an extent that the LH of normal girls does. This effect seems to be associated with hyperandrogenism both pre- and post-menarche, as obese girls without hyperandrogenism have an LH pulse pattern similar to normal-weight girls (Collins et al. 2014).

There has been only one study investigating the LH pulse pattern in obese boys. In the low number of boys studied, no differences in LH pulsation were noted between lean and obese boys (Rosenfield et al. 2012). Obese boys seem to experience similar increases in morning testosterone with pubertal progression until Tanner stage 5, when their total testosterone levels are lower than lean boys. Later in puberty, testicular volume also does not seem to increase to the same extent in obese as in lean boys. The mechanisms underlying this difference are not known at this time.

Adrenarche

Coincident with sex steroid production by the gonads during puberty, the adrenal glands begin to secrete androgens that cause pubic and axillary hair development. This androgen output by the adrenal gland is called adrenarche and is associated with the development of the zona reticularis. Pubic hair generally develops at breast Tanner stage 3 in girls, with 20% of normal girls experiencing pubic hair development earlier in puberty or prepubertally. Pubic hair development generally occurs in late in genital stage Tanner 2 in boys with a far lower percentage experiencing a disordered timing of adrenarche. The factors causing development of the zona reticularis and subsequent adrenal gland steroid production are unknown. Although androgen production by the adrenal gland and sex steroid production by the gonad coincide, they appear to be separate processes that are regulated independently. If timing of adrenarche varies from the norm, it can be indicative of pathologic adrenal secretion.

Hypothalamic Events of Puberty

In the late 1970s, Wildt and Knobil established that pulsatile GnRH is essential for initiating puberty by inducing pulsatile LH and subsequent estradiol secretion and physical changes in a prepubertal monkey upon pulsatile GnRH administration (Wildt et al. 1980). Research since that time is centered on trying to tease out the sequence and orchestration of hypothalamic events that results in the “reawakening” of the GnRH neuron at puberty. It is postulated that the machinery within the GnRH neuron is ready to reinitiate GnRH release, as application of various stimuli can induce GnRH pulsatile secretion in a juvenile primate. Thus, it is viewed that events and cells afferent to the GnRH neuron network integrate signals to initiate pubertal onset and that possibly a biological “brake” on GnRH release is in effect prior to pubertal onset that is independent of gonadal steroids (Terasawa et al. 2013). This postulated "brake" may be due to tonic inhibitory factor(s) or lack of stimulatory input(s) or a combination of both. It is controversial whether rodent species experience a similar phenomenon, as it is unclear whether the decrease in gonadotropin during the juvenile period is dependent or independent of gonadal steroids. Nevertheless, studies in rodents have yielded a wealth of data and will be discussed in tandem with primate studies. Inhibitory, stimulatory, and nutrition-dependent signals have been identified. Equally important, though less studied, is the hypo-responsiveness of the pituitary gonadotroph to GnRH. Decades of research have demonstrated that absence (or presence) of one factor within the experimental model of puberty may not consistently modulate puberty; thus, redundant systems are in place to regulate pubertal timing. This section discusses the signals postulated to play a role in the reawakening of the GnRH neuron to result in puberty and the emerging understanding of the hypothalamic network involved in controlling GnRH neuron function.

Kisspeptin

The crucial role of kisspeptin and its receptor, GPR54, in the release of GnRH at puberty was established by two independent research groups. Humans (and mice) with mutations in the GPR54 gene leading to loss-of-receptor function have hypogonadotropic hypogonadism. Gonadotrope release in these patients was induced by exogenous GnRH, implying that the GPR54 acts upstream of GnRH to signal its release (deRoux et al. 2003; Seminara et al. 2003). Before this seminal discovery, the kisspeptin gene (*KISS1*) was cloned in 1996 at Pennsylvania State College of Medicine in Hershey, Pennsylvania, also home to the famous chocolate product, Hershey's Kisses, from which the gene derives its name. As the resultant peptide was found to initially suppress proliferation of cancerous cell lines, it was named metastin. The Gq protein-coupled receptor, GPR54, was subsequently found to bind metastin to mediate its effects.

In the ensuing decade, much work was done to investigate that cellular signaling and pathways involved in GPR54-mediated GnRH neuron function. The culmination of this work is presented here as the function and biology of the kisspeptin neuron which releases kisspeptin into the hypothalamic neuronal network, as well as the events and signals that modulate kisspeptin expression and secretion.

The Kisspeptin Neuron

In rodents, primates, and other mammals, the administration of exogenous kisspeptin quickly induces GnRH and gonadotropin release in prepubertal and adult animals; thus, it is a major stimulating factor for GnRH release (Seminara 2006). As GnRH antagonists block the stimulatory effect on gonadotropins, it is believed that kisspeptin acts exclusively through GnRH to induce gonadotropin release.

Mammalian kisspeptin neurons are found in the arcuate nucleus (ARC) of the medial basal hypothalamus (or species-specific equivalent) (Terasawa et al. 2013). In all mammals studied, females exhibit greater kisspeptin neuron cell number and axonal fiber density. Kisspeptin neurons contact GnRH neuron cell bodies and dendrites via axonal projections that approximate the GnRH neurons. Female rodents also have a second population of kisspeptin neurons in the anteroventral periventricular nucleus (AVPV) of the preoptic area of the hypothalamus; it is controversial whether primates exhibit a similar population of neurons (Terasawa et al. 2013). In general, expression of *KISS1* in the ARC starts to increase prior to puberty in rodents, with female mice exhibiting a more dramatic increase in *KISS1* expression than male rodents. Whether the increase in *KISS1* expression is steroid dependent varies between studies. In the AVPV of rodents, kisspeptin neuron number in females increases until the age of puberty and is dependent upon estradiol. In primates, KISS1 expression in the ARC increases with puberty in both sexes (Terasawa et al. 2013). GPR54 expression also seems to undergo an increase at the time of puberty. Gain of function mutations in GPR54 in humans has been reported to cause precocious activation of pubertal development (Macedo et al. 2014).

Studies in primates have characterized the pattern of kisspeptin release in relation to GnRH around the time of puberty, as kisspeptin peptide (like GnRH peptide) can be detected in the median eminence. These *in vivo* studies indicate that kisspeptin release is pulsatile, and is not detectable in juvenile monkeys until pubertal age. Kisspeptin increases in amplitude and frequency upon puberty in tandem with GnRH release. The increase in kisspeptin pulsation is also observed in agonadal animals, but it is to a greater extent, indicating that the puberty-related increase in kisspeptin pulsation is independent of gonadal steroids (Terasawa et al. 2013). The greater extent of the pulsation indicates that sex steroid negative feedback can temper kisspeptin release. Whether kisspeptin pulsatile release precedes GnRH release upon pubertal onset is unknown. Studies in primates also indicate that the same dose of administered kisspeptin induces a greater GnRH surge in pubertal vs. prepubertal animals. Thus, it is postulated that the sensitivity of GPR54 to hypothalamic kisspeptin also increases upon puberty. This sensitivity of GPR54 to kisspeptin also seems to be enhanced by sex steroids (Terasawa et al. 2013).

A subpopulation of kisspeptin neurons in the arcuate nucleus also contains the proteins neurokinin B (NKB) and dynorphin (DYN). These neurons are dubbed KNDy neurons and have extensive projections to other KNDy neurons and regular kisspeptin neurons. NKB is important for human reproduction, as individuals with mutations in its gene, *TAC3* or the NKB receptor (*TACR3*), have hypogonadotropic hypogonadism and absent puberty (Lippincott et al. 2013). Dynorphin is present in few human kisspeptin cells, so it is unclear whether it plays a similar role to what is proposed in other mammals. A theoretical model developed based upon studies in female rodents and sheep posits that the KNDy neurons generate the pulsatile release of kisspeptin from the larger cell population by the reciprocal interaction of NKB, which stimulates peptide release, and DYN, which inhibits peptide release (Grachev et al. 2014). The release of both stimulatory and inhibitory neuropeptides by the KNDy neuron causes surrounding kisspeptin neurons and KNDy neurons to release kisspeptin in an intermittent (e.g., pulsatile) manner, which then results in GnRH pulsatile release from downstream GnRH neurons. As this pulse generator model was developed based on studies in adult female rodents and sheep, it remains to be seen whether it applies to primates, males, and peripubertal mammals. Studies using agonists of NKB suggest that the physiological response of the hypothalamic-pituitary system (as determined by serum LH changes) to acute activation of the NKB receptor may depend upon the steroid milieu, sex, animal species, and pubertal status of the animal. Indeed, unlike humans, mice with aberrations of their *TAC3* gene have normal pubertal timing (Lippincott et al. 2013).

The KNDy neurons contain the estrogen receptor-α, androgen receptor, and the progesterone receptor. This is in contrast to GnRH neurons, which have not been definitely shown to contain the major estrogen receptor, ER-α. Thus, it has been postulated that the kisspeptin neuron is the locus of negative feedback regulation of estrogen on the HPG axis in adult females (Garcia-Galiano et al. 2012). Support for this notion comes from studies that show that kisspeptin gene expression increases in the absence of estradiol, decreasing with reintroduction of estradiol. Additionally, animals lacking kisspeptin or GPR54 do not experience the post-gonadectomy rise in gonadotropins. In female rodents the second population of kisspeptin neurons in the AVPV also expresses the sex steroid receptors; this kisspeptin neuron population does not synthesize NKB or DYN. There is evidence that this population of kisspeptin neurons participates in the preovulatory GnRH/LH surge present in adult females (Garcia-Galiano et al. 2012). Kisspeptin expression increases in response to estradiol in this population of neurons, and kisspeptin antagonists can block the LH surge.

Sex steroid effect on kisspeptin physiology during puberty in the APVP is characterized most in rodents; studies have suggested that estradiol is necessary for kisspeptin expression in this region during puberty. When rodents are gonadectomized in the juvenile period, there is a blunted increase in kisspeptin during the pubertal and adult times compared to intact rodents; kisspeptin expression is restored to intact levels if low-dose estradiol is given post gonadectomy (Clarkson 2013). The lack of robust increase in kisspeptin during the pubertal age is also seen in mice with hypogonadotropic hypogonadism due to perturbations in GPR54 or GnRH and thus has lifelong low sex steroid levels (Clarkson 2013). Interestingly, female mice that lack ER-α specifically in their kisspeptin neurons have precocious puberty, implying that estradiol signaling is necessary to serve as a pubertal "brake" (Dubois et al. 2016). Clearly, sex steroid regulation of kisspeptin during the pubertal transition is complex and may involve both stimulatory and inhibitory mechanisms at different developmental time points.

Glutamate

Glutamate is a major excitatory neurotransmitter in the hypothalamus. Glutamate stimulates GnRH release via N-methyl-D-aspartic acid (NMDA) receptors, α-amino-3-hydroxy-5-methyl-4-isoxazolepropionate (AMPA), or kainite receptors.

Glutamate stimulates GnRH release, as inferred by LH release, in prepubertal monkeys and rodents. Stimulation of NMDA receptors induces precocious puberty in rats and monkeys (Claypool et al. 2000), and NMDA receptor blockers delay, but do not prevent puberty in rodents. It is unknown which neuron or site within the hypothalamus induces the response to glutamate, but it may be the GnRH neuron itself. GnRH neurons contain NMDA and kainite receptors, which cluster on dendritic spines opposite to presynaptic active zones (Iremonger et al. 2010). The neuron(s) responsible for upstream release of glutamate is also not known. Glutamate receptor expression within the GnRH neuron increases upon puberty. However, glutamate activity on GnRH neurons is not a primary driver of puberty, as mice with a GnRH neuron-specific deletion of NMDA and AMPA receptors have normal puberty and fertility. Thus, the details of how glutamate influences reproductive function have yet to be elucidated.

Growth Factors

Astroglia adjacent to GnRH neurons synthesize and release growth factors such as transforming growth factor alpha and –beta (TGF-α and TGF–β), fibroblast growth factor (FGF), epidermal growth factor (EGF), and insulin-like growth factor 1 (IGF-1). The hypothalamic expression of TGF and its receptor, erbB1, increases at the time of puberty (Ojeda et al. 2006). Transgenic mice overexpressing TGF in the hypothalamus experience precocious puberty. Additionally, defective erbB1 signaling has been implicated in the pathogenesis of hypothalamic hamartomas.

IGF-1 has been found to play a role in puberty in rodents. Intravascular infusion of IGF-1 induces puberty in rates, while intraventricular infusion of IGF-1 antibody delays puberty. IGF-1 increases GnRH expression in vitro, and mice that lack the IGF-1 receptor on GnRH neurons have delayed pubertal onset associated with delayed maturation of GnRH neuron dendritic pruning and development of spines to receive afferent input in the pubertal period (Divall et al. 2010).

Gamma-Aminobutyric Acid (GABA)

GABA is made by specialized neurons of the hypothalamus and is a major inhibitory neurotransmitter of the hypothalamus. GABA receptors are ligand-gated ion channels, most notably for chloride ions. The change in electrochemical gradient induced by the chloride flux leads to depolarization or hyperpolarization of the neuron, depending upon the direction of the flux of chloride neurons (into or out of the cell, respectively). In most instances, GABA receptor stimulation leads to hyperpolarization of membrane potential and thus decreases in intrinsic pulsatile release of neuropeptides. Interestingly, neuronal response to GABA switches from depolarization to hyperpolarization during early postnatal development.

In primates, a reduction in GABA inhibition is thought to play a role in pubertal onset. GABA secretion to the median eminence decreases at the onset of puberty in primates. Additionally, release of GABA inhibition by infusing $GABA_A$ receptor antagonists to prepubertal animals results in pulsatile GnRH secretion to a greater extent in prepubertal than pubertal animals, indicating that GABAergic tone is higher in prepubertal animals. Treatment of prepubertal primates with $GABA_A$ receptor antagonists results in precocious puberty (Keen et al. 1999). Associated with an increase in GnRH secretion upon $GABA_A$ receptor antagonist infusion is an increase in kisspeptin secretion. Mouse studies have indicated that both GnRH and kisspeptin neurons contain $GABA_A$ receptors. Thus, it is quite possible that the release of GABA inhibition of GnRH secretion is mediated via kisspeptin (Terasawa et al. 2013). This supposition seems to be supported by the observation that mice that lack $GABA_A$ receptor signaling in their GnRH neurons have no change in pubertal timing (Herbison and Moenter 2011).

GABA signaling in GnRH neurons has been extensively studied in vitro. Whether GABA has an inhibitory or stimulatory effect on GnRH neuron activity is dependent upon experimental conditions, hormonal milieu, and even the cellular location of the stimulus (soma vs. dendrite) (Herbison and Moenter 2011). The in vitro effects of GABA on kisspeptin function are far less studied, but also seem to be affected by steroid milieu and experimental conditions.

Nutritional Signals

That nutrition status affects pubertal onset is undisputed as many observations support this supposition. In humans, children with chronic malnutrition and disease states associated with malabsorption experience delayed puberty. The dramatic decrease in age of menarche over the industrial age is thought to be due to improved nutrition. In 1970, Frisch hypothesized that a threshold weight and fat mass must be achieved before menarche can occur (Frisch and Revelle 1970). The site of integration of metabolic signals to the reproductive axis is at the hypothalamus, as studies in nonprimates indicate that food deprivation dampens GnRH pulse frequency. Many candidate metabolic signals have been studied for a possible role in pubertal timing; some are discussed below.

Leptin. Leptin is a signal of nutritional status to the hypothalamus; thus, it has been most extensively studied. Cumulative work indicates that leptin plays a permissive, rather than primary active role in pubertal onset. Humans with defects in leptin production or signaling have delayed, not absent puberty. Yet in women with anorexia (a low leptin state) and amenorrhea, menses return upon leptin administration (Welt et al. 2004). Intraventricular leptin does not advance puberty in primates. In mice, the effect of leptin on function of the reproductive axis is more pronounced. Administration of leptin can induce puberty in mice in some studies but not others (Sanchez-Garrido and Tena-Sempere 2013). Mice with congenital absence of leptin have obesity and hypogonadotropic hypogonadism; leptin treatment improves reproductive axis function before significant weight loss occurs. The site of leptin action is likely the hypothalamus, as leptin-deficient mice can achieve ovulation upon administration of gonadotropins. Many different mouse models have been developed with cell-specific absence of leptin signaling to elucidate the site of action of leptin on reproductive axis function (Sanchez-Garrido and Tena-Sempere 2013). The GnRH neuron does not contain leptin receptors. Although the kisspeptin neuron contains leptin receptors, mice with absence of the leptin receptor in their kisspeptin neurons do not have altered pubertal timing or fertility. Altered leptin signaling in other hypothalamic neurons, such as GABAergic neurons or POMC neurons, may play a role. However, whether these neurons act through the kisspeptin or GnRH neuron remains to be seen (Sanchez-Garrido and Tena-Sempere 2013).

Insulin. Intraventricular release of insulin induces GnRH release in food-deprived sheep and insulin-deficient rats. Mice with absence of the insulin receptor in neurons have hypogonadism that improves with GnRH administration, indicating a hypothalamic source for their reproductive dysfunction (Bruning et al. 2000). However, mice that lack the insulin receptor in their GnRH neurons have normal pubertal timing (Divall et al. 2010). Mice that lack the insulin receptor in the kisspeptin neurons have delayed puberty but with normal fertility, implying that insulin plays a role in kisspeptin neuron function (Qiu et al. 2013).

Other metabolic factors that have been studied include ghrelin, glucose, and free fatty acids. Additionally, cellular energy sensors such as the proteins mammalian target of rapamycin (mTOR), AMP-activated protein kinase (AMPK), and phosphatidylinositol 3-kinase (PI3K) have also been implicated and are areas of active investigation (Roa and Tena-Sempere 2014). However, the involved neurons and mechanisms regarding how these sensors are involved in the nutritional regulation of puberty are not known.

Disorders of Puberty: Insights into Physiology

The study of human individuals with variations in pubertal timing or inability to start or complete puberty has provided tremendous insight into the physiology of normal puberty. A number of these disorders, discussed in the context of the perturbation of pubertal timing, are discussed below.

Genetic Disorders of Absent Puberty

Delayed puberty is commonly defined as the lack of sexual maturation at an age greater than two SDs above the mean for a given population. In conventional clinical practice, this leads to evaluation of boys who have not achieved testicular volume of 4 ml (as an indicator of LH stimulation) or greater by 14 years of age and girls without breast development (as an indicator of estradiol production) by 13 years of age.

The most common cause of delayed puberty is the entity known as constitutional delay of growth and puberty (CDGP), in which children have delayed puberty and delayed longitudinal growth patterns. CDGP seems to be highly heritable, with 50–80% of patients having a positive family history of delayed puberty. In the absence of underlying conditions, delayed puberty is typically self-limited, and individuals progress through puberty before 18 years of age.

Greater than 30 genes have been implicated in the pathogenesis of idiopathic hypogonadotropic hypogonadism, and these genes regulate the development, migration, and secretory function of GnRH neurons (Table 1).

Congenital hypogonadotropic hypogonadism (CHH) is a rare reproductive disorder that is primarily caused by GnRH deficiency but with significant genetic heterogeneity (Kim 2015). In approximately 50% of cases, patients with CHH also present with reduced or absent sense of smell (hyposmia or anosmia, respectively), a condition termed Kallmann syndrome (KS). Although a rare disorder, CHH/KS is the most common form of gonadotropin deficiency. The reported frequency varies across studies, ranging from 1/8,000 males and 1/40,000 females. Patients with CHH are commonly diagnosed in late adolescence or early adulthood. Delayed puberty is defined as absence of breast development (Tanner stage 1) by 13 years in females and absence of testicular enlargement (testicular volume <4 ml) by 14 years in males. When either a micropenis (stretch penile length <2.5 cm) in 5–10% of cases or cryptorchidism (30% of cases) is present in infant males in conjunction with lack of HPG activation during the minipuberty of infancy, an early diagnosis of CHH can be made and later confirmed with further hormonal assessment. Significant progress in genetic research regarding CHH has led to the identification of more than 30 different putative loci for CHH, 17 of those are associated with KS. There is a variable phenotype among individuals carrying the same mutation. CHH/KS may present as either sporadic or familial form, following autosomal dominant, autosomal recessive, or X-linked modes of inheritance (Kim 2015).

In the last decade, a number of genetic defects at various sites have been identified as causing normosmic idiopathic hypogonadotropic hypogonadism (IHH), including *GnRHR* (de Roux et al. 1999), *KISS1R*/G protein-coupled receptor 54 (*GPR54*) (deRoux et al. 2003), nasal embryonic LHRH factor (*NELF*) (Miura et al. 2004), fibroblast growth factor receptor 1 (*FGFR1*) (Pitteloud et al. 2006), fibroblast growth factor 8 (*FGF8*) (Falardeau et al. 2008), and GnRH-1 (*GNRH1*) (Bouligand et al. 2009). Other forms of hypogonadotropic hypogonadism with known genetic mutations are associated with adrenal hypoplasia congenital (*DAX1*) and with severe infantile obesity (leptin and its receptor).

KISS1 and *KISS1R* (*GPR54*) *mutation*. The *GPR54* gene is located on chromosome 19 (19p13.3), initially described as an orphan receptor, and binds a 54-amino-acid peptide derived by proteolysis from the KISS1 protein. The receptor is found in the brain, pituitary, and placenta. GPR54 is formed of five exons. In 2003, two groups revealed the link between hypogonadotropic hypogonadism and mutations in GPR54. These studies showed that humans or mice in which GPR54 was mutated did not enter puberty.

The frequency of mutations in KISS1R (GPR54) as a cause of IHH is relatively low. To date, several mutations within the gene have been described. A hot spot of biological significance does not seem to exist in KISS1R, and mutations span the length of the gene, and almost every affected family has its own mutation. The clinical phenotype appears to mirror the severity of their hormonal deficiency.

Table 1 Genes associated with pubertal disorders

Gene	Gene product	Phenotypes upon gene disruption
KISS1	Kisspeptin	HH
		Gonadotropin-dependent precocious puberty
GPR54	Kisspeptin receptor	HH
		Gonadotropin-dependent precocious puberty
GnRH	GnRH	HH
GnRHR	GnRH receptor	HH
NELF/ NSMF	Nasal embryonic LHRH factor	±Anosmia, HH
TAC3	Tachykinin 3 (neurokinin B)	±Anosmia, HH
TACR3	Tachykinin 3 receptor	±Anosmia, HH
PROK2	Prokineticin 2	±Anosmia, HH
PROKR2	Prokineticin receptor 2	±Anosmia, HH, septo-optic dysplasia
FGFR1	Fibroblast growth factor receptor 1	±Anosmia, HH, limb defects, cleft lip/palate
FGF8	Fibroblast growth factor 8	±Anosmia, HH, craniofacial and limb defects
KAL1	Anosmin-1	Anosmia, HH
FEZF1	FEX family zinc finger 1	Anosmia, HH
IL17RD	Interleukin 17 receptor D	Anosmia, HH
SEMA3A	Semaphorin 3A	Anosmia, HH
SOX10	SRY-related HMG box 10	Anosmia, HH
DMXL2	Rabconnectin-3α	HH, polyendocrine-polyneuropathy syndrome
LEP	Leptin	Hyperphagia, obesity, extremely delayed puberty
LEPR	Leptin receptor	Hyperphagia, obesity, extremely delayed puberty
NR0B1 (DAX1)	Dax1	HH, X-linked congenital adrenal hypoplasia
OTUD4	OTU domain-containing protein 4	HH, Gordon Holmes syndrome
PCSK1	Proprotein convertase 1	HH, obesity, diarrhea, hypopituitarism
PNPLA6	Patatin-like phospholipase domain-containing protein 6	HH, ataxia, blindness
RNF216	Ring finger protein 216	HH, ataxia, dementia
AXL	AXL receptor tyrosine kinase	HH
CHD7	Chromodomain-helicase-DNA-binding protein 7	HH, CHARGE syndrome
FGF17	Fibroblast growth factor 17	HH
HS6ST1	Heparan sulfate 6-sulfotransferase-1	HH
SEMA7A	Semaphorin 7A	HH

(*continued*)

Table 1 (continued)

Gene	Gene product	Phenotypes upon gene disruption
WDR11	WD repeat protein 11	HH
MKRN3	Makorin ring finger protein 3	Gonadotropin-dependent precocious puberty
LHR	LH receptor	Familial male-limited precocious puberty
GNAS	Gs-α subunit	McCune-Albright syndrome

HH Hypogonadotropic hypogonadism

Underdeveloped external genitalia (cryptorchidism and micropenis) most likely reflect insufficient secretion of gonadotropins and testosterone during the prenatal period, although some male patients displayed intact external genitalia. This suggests that some mutations have a more deleterious effect on the gonadotropin axis activity, already expressed in the antenatal period (Nimri et al. 2011). According to Seminara et al., the testes of patients bearing a *GPR54* gene mutation may retain functional response to gonadotropins (Seminara et al. 2003).

In 2008, Teles et al. reported a girl with a *KISS1R* (*GRP54*)-activating mutation, causing prolongation of the intracellular signaling in response to kisspeptin, associated with central precocious puberty phenotype (Teles et al. 2008). In 2010, Silveira et al. identified a *KISS1* mutation associated with male central precocious puberty. The mutation resulted in higher kisspeptin resistance to degradation in vitro, suggesting greater kisspeptin bioavailability and a potential role in the precocious puberty (Silveira et al. 2010).

KAL1 (*ANOS1*) *mutation*. Anosmin-1, a secreted extracellular matrix protein encoded by *KAL1* (*ANOS1*) gene, was the first mutated gene to be identified on KS. Later it was shown that anosmin-1 binds to FGFR1 as a co-ligand. The classic form of Kallmann syndrome is characterized by anosmia/hyposmia, hypogonadotropic hypogonadism, and X-linked inheritance. *KAL1* is located on Xp22.3 locus of the X chromosome. The gene escapes X-inactivation. *KAL1* encodes a 680-amino-acid glycoprotein called anosmin-1, a neural adhesion molecule that guides the migration of GnRH neurosecretory neurons from the olfactory placode to the medial basal hypothalamus. The immunoreactive distribution of anosmin-1 in the human fetus demonstrates its widespread distribution including the olfactory placode, mesonephros, metanephros, inner ear, precartilaginous skeleton, and cerebellum. Inconsistently associated defects are cleft lip and/or palate, seizures, short metacarpal bone, pes cavus, neurosensory hearing loss, cerebellar ataxia, nystagmus, oculomotor abnormalities, renal aplasia, or dysplasia, and limited to the X-linked form is bimanual synkinesia (mirror movements of the upper extremities).

A variety of deletions and mutations causing Kallmann syndrome have been described and are shown in Table 1 (Kim 2015).

GnRHR. The action of GnRH is mediated through a G protein-coupled receptor with seven transmembrane segments, present in the cell membrane of gonadotropes. The human GnRHR gene encodes a 328-amino-acid protein. The gene was assigned to the long arm of chromosome 4. Activation of this receptor results in increased activity of phospholipase C leading to hydrolysis of phosphatidylinositol 4,5-bisphosphate (PIP2) and formation of inositol 1,4,5-trisphosphate (IP3) and diacylglycerol (DAG). These second messengers are required for intracellular calcium mobilization and protein kinase C activation. The mobilization of internal IP3-sensitive calcium stores is followed by external calcium influx via voltage sensitive calcium channels. The GnRHR also stimulates phospholipase A2 and D. Pulsatile and continuous administration of GnRH stimulates the transcription of the α-subunit gene. LH β-subunit gene transcription is only stimulated by pulsatile administration of GnRH.

De Roux et al. described mutations on the receptor gene (*GnRHR*) causing partial hypogonadotropic hypogonadism without anosmia (de Roux et al. 1999). These studies of natural mutations of *GnRHR* in patients with hypogonadotropic hypogonadism have highlighted three critical regions of the GnRHR: the first extracellular loop, the fifth transmembrane domain, and the third intracellular loop. The phenotype is a continuum between partial and complete hypogonadism. However, there is a highly variable degree of hypogonadism with the same mutation suggesting that other genetic or environmental factors may modulate the phenotypic expression of loss-of-function mutation of the *GnRHR*.

Other Genetic Disorders

Prader-Willi syndrome. Prader-Willi syndrome (PWS) is a multisystemic complex genetic disorder caused by lack of expression of genes on the paternally inherited chromosome 15q11-q13 region. PWS is recognized as a genomic imprinting disorder. Affected infants have significant hypotonia, feeding difficulties, and failure to thrive, followed later in early childhood by hyperphagia with gradual development of obesity, short stature and/or decreased growth velocity, intellectual disabilities, and behavioral problems: skin picking and temper tantrums. Hypothalamic dysfunction has been implicated in many manifestations of PWS including hyperphagia, temperature instability, sleep-disordered breathing, and hypogonadotropic hypogonadism. Depending on the age, clinical expression of hypogonadism is extremely variable and tends to be more prominent in males than females. Clinical signs of hypogonadism in boys are cryptorchidism in 93%, scrotal hypoplasia, micropenis, small testes volume, delayed or incomplete pubertal development, and infertility. Clitoral and labia minora hypoplasia occurs in females. Most patients with PWS are able to start puberty, but then have pubertal arrest (Radicioni et al. 2012). Interestingly, recent studies demonstrated normal minipuberty of infancy hormonal profile and a hormonal profile of testicular failure after the onset of puberty (elevated FSH and low inhibin B). The pattern of gonadal dysfunction in PWS females seems to be similar to those in males. Girls with PWS have normal or near normal secondary sexual characteristics including breast development and menses, indicating a lesser degree of hypothalamic-gonadal dysfunction.

Primary Gonadal Disorders

Gonadal dysgenesis (XO, XY). Gonadal dysgenesis (45, XO) due to deficiencies on the X chromosome is the most common cause of primary ovarian insufficiency. It is due to a large deletion of X chromosome material, which is associated with a variable phenotype called Turner syndrome. Fetuses with 45,XO karyotype undergo a rapid reduction in the number of follicles, causing gonadal streaks via an accelerated rate of apoptosis. Specific loci on the X chromosome are associated with primary ovarian insufficiency. Xp11.2, Xq harbors two independent loci, in addition to the fragile X premutation.

Klinefelter's syndrome is the most common chromosomal abnormality associated with primary testicular insufficiency and male infertility. The most prevalent karyotype is 47,XXY karyotype (97%). Parental origin of the extra X chromosome is equal. The 47,XXY karyotype results from nondisjunction during the first meiotic division in one of the parents. Nondisjunction of maternal chromosomes is the cause of 47,XXY karyotype in two-thirds of affected men. Advanced maternal age is a risk factor for nondisjunction. The mechanism by which the extra X chromosome renders infertility in males is not known. X-inactivation in primary spermatocytes is necessary for spermatogenesis to proceed through meiosis. It is possible that expression of some X chromosome genes is detrimental to spermatogenesis.

The clinical features are small firm testes, small penis, gynecomastia, and tall stature due to testosterone deficiency and an extra copy of the short stature homeobox-containing gene (SHOX). Academic and emotional difficulties are common. The extra X chromosome affects both Leydig and Sertoli cell function. Azoospermia is the rule in men with Klinefelter's syndrome who have the 47, XXY karyotype. Men with mosaicism might have germ cells in the testes. Testicular architecture is relatively normal in fetal and prepubertal testes. The gonads experience loss of germ cells over time, culminating in fibrosis and hyalinization of the seminiferous tubules causing infertility.

FMR premutation and ovary function. Fragile X syndrome accounts for about one-half of cases of X-linked mental retardation and is the second most common cause of mental impairment after trisomy 21, affecting 1/4,000 males and 1/8,000 females. Fragile X syndrome results from an expansion of the CGG repeat in the 5′ untranslated region of the *FMR1* gene. When the triplet repeat number exceeds 200, the gene is methylated (silenced). A repeat length of 55–200 is termed premutation, as it can expand to >200 repeats in progeny through the mother. The definition of premutation and intermediate alleles is based on the likelihood that the repeat will expand to a full mutation to cause fragile X syndrome in progeny, not to describe ovarian function. *FMR1* premutation repeat length of 55–200 can expand to full within one generation, whereas the intermediate repeats (45–54) will need two or more generations to expand to full mutation. There are different degrees of severity of decreased ovarian reserve (Karimov et al. 2011). Women who carry the premutation may develop fragile X-associated primary ovarian insufficiency (FXPOI). POI in all degrees of severity has been identified in women carrying the premutation.

Approximately 20% of women who carry the premutation experienced overt POI, in contrast with 1% of women in the general population. In addition, premutation carriers experience earlier menopause (by ~5 years). It was considered possible that FMR1 protein plays a role in oogenesis, because *FMR1* is highly expressed when oogenesis occurs.

Genetic Disorders of Precocious Puberty

Precocious puberty is defined as the development of secondary sexual characteristics before the age of 8 years in girls and 9 years in boys. There are several causes of precocious puberty. It is important to distinguish between central (gonadotropin-dependent) precocious puberty, resulting from premature activation of the hypothalamic-pituitary-gonadal axis, and gonadotropin-independent precocious puberty. The timing of pubertal development is driven in part by genetic factors, but only few rare molecular defects associated with precocious puberty have been identified.

MKRN3. Makorin ring finger 3 (*MKRN3*) was first cloned in 1999 during a study of the Prader-Willi/Angelman syndrome critical region. The role of *MKRN3* in pubertal initiation was first described in 2013 after the identification of deleterious *MKRN3* mutations in five families with central precocious puberty (Abreu et al. 2013). All affected persons inherited the mutations from their fathers. More recently, it was found that mutation in *MKRN3* causes sporadic cases of central precocious puberty (Macedo et al. 2014). *MKRN3* encodes the makorin ring finger protein 3. *MKRN3* is an intronless gene, located on chromosome 15q11.2 in the Prader-Willi syndrome critical region. This gene is maternally imprinted (silenced), and only the paternal allele is expressed. MKRN3 is associated with protein ubiquitination, in which a ubiquitin moiety is attached to a protein. Ubiquitination can have diverse effects on the protein substrate, varying from proteasome-dependent proteolysis to modulation of protein function and/or localization. Its precise function has not yet been determined. The structural features of this gene and its pattern of expression in the developing hypothalamus suggest that MKRN3 might function much like polycomb group proteins as silencers of downstream genes that activate puberty, such as *KISS1* (Ojeda and Lomniczi 2014). The similar incidence of central precocious puberty in association with MKRN3 mutations in the two sexes in the affected families is consistent with autosomal dominant inheritance with complete penetrance but with exclusive paternal transmission, consistent with nonallelic expression of MKRN3 (a maternally imprinted gene) (Macedo et al. 2014; Abreu et al. 2013). All patients with central precocious puberty carrying loss-of-function mutations in MKRN3 exhibited typical clinical and hormonal features of premature activation of the reproductive axis, including breast and testes development, pubic hair, accelerated linear growth, and advanced bone age. In patients with central precocious puberty due to *MKRN3* defects, the median age of pubertal onset was 6.0 years in girls (ranging from 3.0 to 7.5) and 8.25 years in boys (ranging from 5.9 to 9.0).

McCune-Albright syndrome. This disorder is caused by a somatic mutation at codon R201 in exon 8 of the *GNAS1* gene (20q13.2). The gene encodes for the Gs-α subunit protein that couples transmembrane receptors to adenylate cyclase. The mutation causes the prolongation of Gs-α activity with reduced hydrolysis of the protein due to dysfunction in the intrinsic GTPase domain in which the substitution resides, causing hyperfunction and proliferation of target tissues. The R201 substitutions are postzygotic somatic mutations, which occur at various times during embryogenesis and lead to cellular mosaicism with different proportion of mutated cells in each tissue. The mutation is nearly always a substitution of the residue arginine at position 201 by histidine or cysteine. Very infrequently, arginine is replaced by serine, glycine, or leucine. No differences in phenotype have been detected between the different substitutions (Weinstein 2006).

The McCune-Albright syndrome (MAS) is a sporadic disorder classically defined by the triad of café au lait skin pigmentation, fibrous bone dysplasia, and peripheral precocious puberty. Gonadotropin-independent precocious puberty is the most frequent endocrinopathy associated with MAS and usually presents between 2 and 6 years. Its estimated prevalence is between 1/100,000 and 1/1,000,000. LH receptor signaling involves Gs-α activity to stimulate steroidogenesis in theca and granulosa cells of the ovary. The GNAS mutation causes stimulation of the steroidogenesis pathways in the absence of LH, leading to unregulated estradiol production and gonadotropin-independent precocious puberty. The disease is very rare in males, but when males are affected, they can present with bilateral (rarely unilateral) macroorchidism, without other signs of precocious puberty. Testicular microlithiasis is present in 62%. The macroorchidism is due to Gs-α mutations in the Sertoli cells causing its hypertrophy. If the mutation occurs in Leydig cells (<15% of cases), it causes peripheral precocious puberty because of unregulated testosterone production. Various mechanisms have been described to account for the phenotypic features of the macroorchidism: Gs-α imprinting, a different early embryonic origin of precursors contributing to Sertoli and Leydig cell lineages, and over-expression of anti-Mullerian hormone (AMH) and its inhibitory effect on Leydig cell function and maturation.

McCune-Albright Syndrome can also include other endocrinopathies in endocrine tissues that rely on G proteins in signaling transduction. Other endocrinopathies include pituitary adenomas capable of producing LH, FSH, ACTH, GH, and/or prolactin. Hyperthyroidism is also reported, as is Cushing syndrome due to autonomous multinodular hyperplasia in the thyroid and adrenal gland, respectively. The *GNAS1* R201 mutation detection rate in patients with MAS can be influenced by different factors, such as the progressive nature of the disease, cellular mosaicism, and the unavailability of the affected tissues. The detection rate in peripheral blood is low when only one or two features of the classic triad are present. Testing on leukocytes DNA is possible, but it is unreliable. There is no known genotype/phenotype correlation.

Familial male-limited precocious puberty. The luteinizing hormone receptor (LHR) presents primarily in the ovary and testes. The receptor can bind either pituitary LH or the nearly identical placental hormone human chorionic gonadotropin (hCG). In postpubertal males, LHR stimulation activates (via Gs-α signaling cascade) testosterone synthesis by the Leydig cells of the testes. In postpubertal females, LHR signaling plays several roles. During the follicular phase, LHR signaling stimulates theca cells to synthetize androgens, later aromatized to estradiol by the granulosa cells under stimulation of follicle-stimulating hormone (FSH). The midcycle surge of LH induces follicular maturation and ovulation. During the luteal phase, LHR signaling induces the formation of the corpus luteum and stimulates progesterone synthesis.

LHR is composed of 11 exons, and the gene has been mapped to 2p21. The high-affinity binding of the hormone is mediated by the extracellular N-terminal domain of the receptor (Latronico and Segaloff 1999). The primary pathway of the LHR is the Gs/adenylyl cyclase/cAMP pathway. Naturally occurring mutations in G protein-coupled receptor genes can cause human disease by producing either gain- or loss-of-receptor function (Latronico and Segaloff 1999). Familial male-limited precocious puberty (FMPP), also known as testotoxycosis, is a gonadotropin-independent disorder that is inherited in an autosomal dominant, male-limited pattern. LH receptor is a member of the family G protein-coupled receptor. Several constitutively activating mutations of the LH receptor gene, resulting in high basal cyclic AMP levels, have been identified. Precocious puberty is observed only in males carrying activating mutations of the LHR gene and not in females. It has been suggested that females require the activation of both LHR and FSHR for the induction of puberty. The disease usually presents by age 1–4 years, with physical signs of puberty, rapid virilization, growth acceleration, skeletal advancement, and elevated testosterone levels despite prepubertal levels of LH.

Secular Trends in Pubertal Timing

Even though the tempo and series of events in puberty are remarkably conserved in different populations, the onset of puberty occurs across a wide range of ages in normal children. The age of pubertal transition has changed through the centuries. The age of menarche, a sentinel event of late female puberty, dramatically fell between the eighteenth and twentieth centuries, thought to be due to the improved nutrition associated with industrialization. Puberty in boys is not marked by such a sentinel event, so the trend over the centuries is more difficult to track. However, historical data on the age and composition of the Leipzig Boys Choir (soprano (no voice cracking), alto (some voice cracking), and tenor (full deep voice achieved)) suggested that in the 1700s, the average age of altos was 16, whereas in 1950s England it was 13.5 years (Daw 1970). In the twentieth and twenty-first centuries, data on age of menarche is available for more diverse populations and countries (Fig. 2); the secular trend of an earlier age of menarche is continuing, although measured in months, not years.

Reliable data on age of pubertal onset is more difficult to gather for both sexes, as the physical changes of early puberty are subtle. Longitudinal studies of English children by Marshall and Tanner in the 1960s established the median age of pubertal

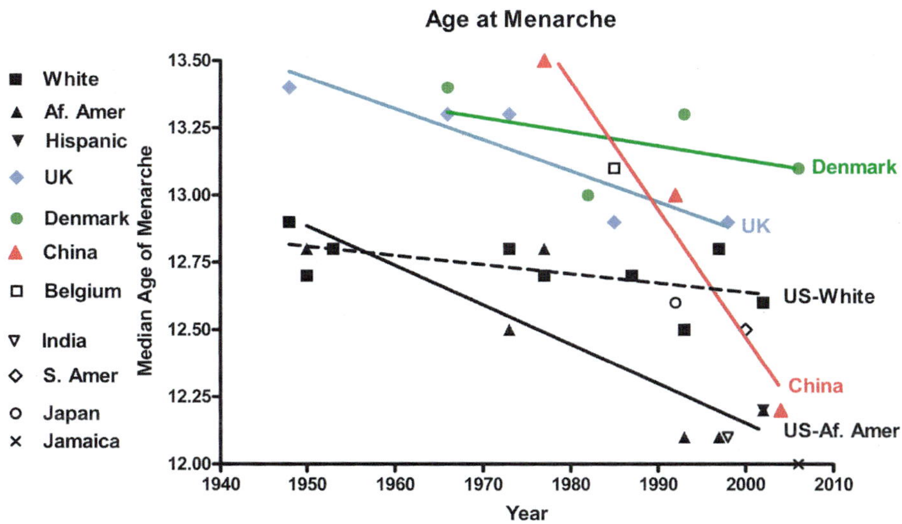

Fig. 2 Trend in median age of menarche in multiple countries from 1940 to 2010. If multiyear data is available for a particular country, it is depicted by a line connecting the years of available data (Data compiled from Sun et al. (2002), Wu et al. (2002), and (Parent et al. 2003))

onset (breast budding) in girls as around 10.75 years with a 3–97% range of 8.5–13 years (Marshall and Tanner 1969). Earlier studies (1940s) in North America suggested the median onset of breast development (as later defined by Tanner) as 10.5–10.75 years of age. Both studies were in Caucasian girls and used visual inspection. Studies in boys by Tanner in the 1960s established the median age of testicular volume enlargement to the pubertal threshold in males as age 11.5 years with a 3–97% range of 9.5–13.5 years. These studies were performed by visual inspection on <200 subjects (Marshall and Tanner 1970). Studies in North America for Caucasian boys suggested the median onset was 11.5 years as well. The definition of delayed and precocious puberty, based upon these studies, is pubertal onset outside of the 2.5 standard deviation from the mean. Thus, the age of precocious puberty in girls was defined as breast development before age 8 and testicular enlargement before age 9 in boys with delayed puberty in girls as no breast development by age 13 in girls and no testicular enlargement by age 14 in boys.

The age of pubertal onset in girls in the developing world was thought to be relatively stable over the last 50 years, but a controversial study published in 1997 put that belief into question. Herman-Giddens et al. published a cross-sectional study of 17,000 girls in the Pediatric Research in Office Settings (PROS) network (Herman-Giddens et al. 1997). Upon visual inspection of girls seen for regular office visits, 6.5% of white girls and 27.5% of black girls had breast or pubic hair development before the age of 8 years. Therefore, application of the traditional definitions of precocious puberty would result in a high number of potentially normal girls undergoing extensive and expensive testing for precocious puberty. Initial reaction to this study was mixed, as some experts supported the findings of this study and suggested revised guidelines (Kaplowitz et al. 1999), while others expressed uncertainty of the findings and conclusions because of concerns of ascertainment bias and the lack of palpation to verify the visual inspection (Finlay et al. 2000; Rosenfield et al. 2000).

In the ensuing nearly two decades since this study, this secular trend in girls has been studied more extensively in the USA and elsewhere (Fig. 3). In the USA, data from the National Health and Nutrition Examination Survey (NHANES), a recurrent cross-sectional study of participants designed to represent the diverse ethnic makeup of the US population in general, was analyzed. Data from these studies also showed an earlier trend toward pubertal onset in girls compared to NHANES studies from previous decades, but not as pronounced as the PROS study (Sun et al. 2002; Wu et al. 2002). Nonwhite girls and girls with higher BMI were noted to have a higher prevalence of breast development before age 8 in these studies (Kaplowitz et al. 2001; Rosenfield et al. 2009). Since the early 2000s, longitudinal studies have been initiated that have incorporated palpation in an attempt to more accurately assign girls with true thelarche versus lipomastia. A multicenter study in the US (Breast Cancer and the Environment Research Centers, BCERC) enrolled 1,200 girls aged 6–8 and assessed their growth and pubertal development over time. In this multi-ethnic study, it was found that the median age of breast development was 9.7 years in white girls, 9.3 years in Asian girls, and 8.8 years in black girls. For all ethnicities, girls with a higher BMI had an earlier onset of breast development by palpation (Biro et al. 2013). This study is ongoing; thus, the question of whether the tempo of puberty is also different is unknown. In Denmark, evaluation of breast development

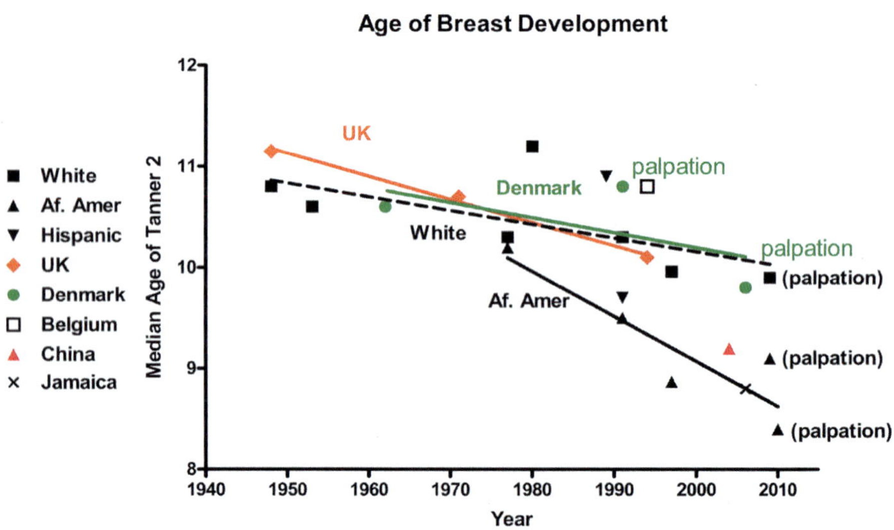

Fig. 3 Trend in median age of breast development (Tanner stage 2) in multiple countries from 1940 to 2010. If multiyear data is available for a particular country, it is depicted by a line connecting the years of available data (Data compiled from Sun et al. (2002); Wu et al. (2002); Aksglaede et al. (2009), Biro et al. (2013), and (Parent et al. 2003))

(using palpation) of 995 school-age girls from study dates 2006–2008 was compared to 1,100 girls from study dates 1991–1993 (Copenhagen Puberty Study). Using the same examiners in each decade, it was found that the mean age of breast development was 10.8 years in the 1991–1993 cohort and 9.8 years in 2006–2008 cohort (Aksglaede et al. 2009). The authors of the study posited that the decrease in age of breast development over the ~15 years was not due to overweight/obesity, as the prevalence of overweight/obesity was not different between the cohorts. In the Netherlands, the median age of breast development was 10.7 years in 1997 and 11.0 years in 1965 (Mul et al. 2001). Other studies documenting age of onset of breast development in girls use maternal or self-report of Tanner staging, which has variable concordance with clinical visual inspection and/or palpation.

There is far less data about the secular trend in pubertal onset in boys (Fig. 4). Sexual maturity in males is difficult to assign by visual inspection, as the demarcation between different stages is subtle. Additionally, the threshold in testicular size that is the hallmark of pubertal activation of testes in males is also difficult to detect by visual inspection and varies between studies as ≥3 ml or ≥4 ml. Using visual inspection, the Bogalusa study in the USA of 1,800 boys indicated that the median age of pubertal onset as determined by gonadal stage was age 11.8 for Caucasian boys and 11.2 for black boys in the years 1973–1974 (Foster et al. 1977). NHANESIII data, also by visual inspection, indicated that in the years 1988–1994, the median age of pubertal onset was 10.1 year in Caucasian boys, 9.3 years in black boys, and 10.3 years in Mexican-American boys (Herman-Giddens et al. 2001;

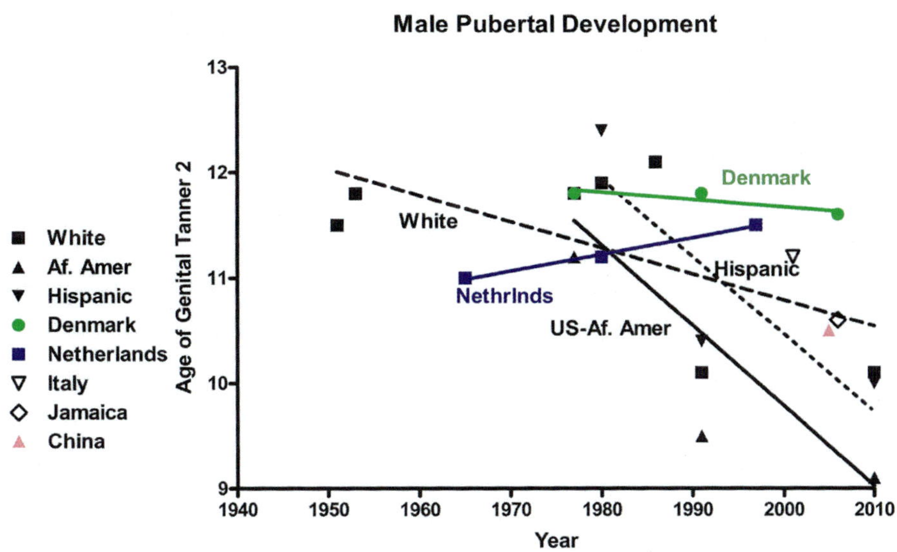

Fig. 4 Trend in median age of Tanner stage 2 genitalia development in boys in multiple countries from 1940 to 2010. If multiyear data is available for a particular country, it is depicted by a line connecting the years of available data (Data compiled from Herman-Giddens et al. (2012) and (Parent et al. 2003))

Karpati et al. 2002; Sun et al. 2002). In attempts to supply more accurate data on pubertal onset in boys using physical examination, the PROS network in the USA was again employed. This study of 4,131 boys between years 2005 and 2010 indicated that the median age of ≥3 ml testes was 9.9 in Caucasian males, 9.7 in African-American boys, and 9.63 in Hispanic boys, while median age of ≥4 ml was 11.5 years in Caucasian boys, 11.75 in African-American boys, and 11.29 years in Hispanic boys (Herman-Giddens et al. 2012). The genital maturity rating to stage 2 via visual inspection (most comparable to earlier studies) was 10.1 years in Caucasian boys, 9.14 in Caucasian boys, and 10.0 in Hispanic boys. This is the only study that presented data on achieved age of testicular volume of 3 ml vs. 4 ml.

In countries outside the USA, studies by Prader indicated that the threshold of ≥3 ml testes was indicative of central puberty (Largo and Prader 1983); this study of 142 Swiss boys in the late 1970s indicated that the median age of this size of the testes was 11.8 years. In Sweden, the median age of ≥3 ml testes in 55 boys was 12.3 years, which was correlated with increase in testosterone (Ankarberg-Lindgren and Norjavaara 2004). Using a testicular volume of ≥4 ml, the average age of mean age of attainment of pubertal onset in the Netherlands was 12.0 years in 1965 and 11.5 years in 1997 (Mul et al. 2001). The Copenhagen Puberty Study indicated that the mean age of attainment of testicular volume ≥3 ml was 11.9 in 1991–1993 and 11.66 in 2006–2008 (Sorensen et al. 2010).

Therefore, in both girls and boys, there is an earlier age of pubertal onset over the last 50 years or so, possibly more dramatically in the latter two decades of the twentieth century and into turn of the twenty-first century. It remains to be seen whether the tempo of puberty has also changed, as observations suggest that girls with early normal puberty may have a slower tempo of puberty (Marti-Henneberg and Vizmanos 1997). Indeed, the less dramatic change in age of menarche vs. age of breast development suggests that the duration of puberty may be longer. The longitudinal studies by Biro et al. will help to answer this question.

Hypotheses Regarding Changing Secular Trends of Puberty

As both boys and girls are entering puberty earlier, what would be the causal factors? Obesity is an obvious candidate, as the rate of obesity in children in the USA has increased dramatically since the 1970s (Broyles et al. 2010; Freedman et al. 2012). This secular trend toward increased childhood obesity is observed in 42 countries using data from the World Health Organization Burden of Disease Program (Wang and Lobstein 2006). Data from both the PROS study and BCERC study indicate that girls with a higher BMI have earlier breast development (Biro et al. 2013; Kaplowitz et al. 2001). However, it is controversial whether girls with a higher BMI have earlier menarche, as some studies note a trend (Rosenfield et al. 2009), while others do not (Anderson and Must 2005; Bau et al. 2009). Interpretation is complicated by the fact that girls at later stages of puberty have higher BMI. Interestingly, it appears that boys with overweight have earlier puberty, but those with obesity may have pubertal timing coincident with or later than their normal-weight peers (Lee et al. 2016).

The developmental origins of adult disease posit that fetal and/or early life environmental experiences influence metabolic phenotype in adulthood (Dyer and Rosenfeld 2011). This hypothesis is formed from the observational cohort studies showing that adults born small for gestational age (SGA) have higher rates of obesity, type 2 diabetes mellitus, and hyperlipidemia (reviewed in Dyer and Rosenfeld 2011). Extending this hypothesis to childhood and puberty, multiple studies have indicated that lower birth weight is associated with earlier menarche and pubertal development in girls (reviewed in Roth and DiVall 2016). It was also noted that children with rapid weight gain in early childhood also experience earlier pubertal development and/or menarche. There is also evidence of the same phenomenon in boys, but the data is less extensive.

Another hypothesis for the relatively rapid change in pubertal timing since the second half of the twentieth century is the increasing exposure to endocrine disrupting chemicals (EDCs). As detailed earlier in this chapter, the hypothalamic-pituitary-gonadal axis may be particularly sensitive to epigenetic regulation that ultimately affects pubertal timing. Much of the evidence gathered is from epidemiologic studies or rodent studies. Epidemiologic studies give data on population exposure and disease association, whereas rodent studies give insight into mechanisms of disease underlying the associations and the particular developmental window that conveys susceptibility to the exposure. Implicated EDCs include persistent organic pollutants that have long half-lives and persist for decades in soils and organic tissue. Chemicals in this class include pesticides, industrial by-products, and flame retardants. Short-lived EDCs include those chemicals used in plastics such as bisphenols or phthalates. EDCs can have estrogenic, androgenic, corticosteroidogenic, or leptogenic properties. Studies in rodents indicate exposure to a particular EDC during fetal or the immediate postnatal life can have an opposite effect on pubertal timing as when the exposure is closer to pubertal onset (reviewed in Parent et al. 2015). In addition to the developmental stage of the EDC exposure, the particular dose and route of administration of the EDC result in different effects on pubertal timing. Given the constant and extensive exposure to EDCs during human fetal and postnatal life, it is extremely difficult to tease out which of the different EDCs that children are potentially exposed lead to variations in pubertal timing.

Summary

The molecular mechanisms regulating initiation and timing of puberty are still largely unknown. "What triggers puberty" is a compelling research question that has driven myriads of scientists for decades. The answer to this question will be ascertained only with stepwise advances in biochemistry, molecular biology, genetics, physiology, population genetics, and clinical investigation. Clinical observation and characterization of patients with disorders of pubertal development have yielded information that has provided new directions in the field of puberty and reproduction research. This underscores the importance of the bedside-to-bench approach of translational investigation in advancing our knowledge of this very critical process – a process that is necessary for the propagation of our species.

Cross-References

▶ Steroid Hormones: Synthesis, Secretion, and Transport
▶ G Protein-Coupled Receptors
▶ The Physiology of the Testis
▶ Ovarian Physiology

References

Abreu AP, Dauber A, Macedo DB, Noel SD, Brito VN, Gill JC, Cukier P, Thompson IR, Navarro VM, Gagliardi PC, Rodrigues T, Kochi C, Longui CA, Beckers D, de Zegher F, Montenegro LR, Mendonca BB, Carroll RS, Hirschhorn JN, Latronico AC, Kaiser UB. Central precocious puberty caused by mutations in the imprinted gene MKRN3. N Engl J Med. 2013;368:2467–75.

Achermann JC, Hughes IA. Pediatric disorders of sex development. In: Melmed S, Polonsky KS, Larsen PR, Kronenberg HM, editors. Williams textbook of endocrinology. Elsevier, Philadelphia, PA, 13th edn. 2016

Aksglaede L, Sorensen K, Petersen JH, Skakkebaek NE, Juul A. Recent decline in age at breast development: the Copenhagen Puberty Study. Pediatrics. 2009;123:e932–9.

Anderson SE, Must A. Interpreting the continued decline in the average age at menarche: results from two nationally representative surveys of U.S. girls studied 10 years apart. J Pediatr. 2005;147:753–60.

Ankarberg-Lindgren C, Norjavaara E. Changes of diurnal rhythm and levels of total and free testosterone secretion from pre to late puberty in boys: testis size of 3 ml is a transition stage to puberty. Eur J Endocrinol. 2004;151:747–57.

Apter D, Butzow T, Laughlin G, Yen S. Gonadotropin-releasing hormone pulse generator activity during pubertal transition in girls: pulsatile and diurnal patterns of circulating gonadotropins. J Clin Endocrinol Metab. 1993;76:940–9.

Bau AM, Ernert A, Schenk L, Wiegand S, Martus P, Gruters A, Krude H. Is there a further acceleration in the age at onset of menarche? A cross-sectional study in 1840 school children focusing on age and bodyweight at the onset of menarche. Eur J Endocrinol. 2009;160:107–13.

Bhagavath B, Layman LC. The genetics of hypogonadotropic hypogonadism. Semin Reprod Med. 2007;25:272–86.

Biro FM, Greenspan LC, Galvez MP, Pinney SM, Teitelbaum S, Windham GC, Deardorff J, Herrick RL, Succop PA, Hiatt RA, Kushi LH, Wolff MS. Onset of breast development in a longitudinal cohort. Pediatrics. 2013;132:1019–27.

Bouligand J, Ghervan C, Tello JA, Brailly-Tabard S, Salenave S, Chanson P, Lombes M, Millar RP, Guiochon-Mantel A, Young J. Isolated familial hypogonadotropic hypogonadism and a GNRH1 mutation. N Engl J Med. 2009;360:2742–8.

Broyles S, Katzmarzyk PT, Srinivasan SR, Chen W, Bouchard C, Freedman DS, Berenson GS. The pediatric obesity epidemic continues unabated in Bogalusa, Louisiana. Pediatrics. 2010;125:900–5.

Bruning JC, Gautam D, Burks DJ, Gillette J, Schubert M, Orban PC, Klein R, Krone W, Muller-Wieland D, Kahn CR. Role of brain insulin receptor in control of body weight and reproduction. Science. 2000;289:2122–5.

Clarkson J. Effects of estradiol on kisspeptin neurons during puberty. Front Neuroendocrinol. 2013;34:120–31.

Claypool L, Kasuya E, Saitoh Y, Marzban F, Terasawa E. N-methyl D,L-aspartate induces the release of luteinizing hormone-releasing hormone in the prepubertal and pubertal female rhesus monkey as measured by in vivo push-pull perfusion in the stalk-median eminence. Endocrinology. 2000;141:219–28.

Collins JS, Beller JP, Burt Solorzano C, Patrie JT, Chang RJ, Marshall JC, McCartney CR. Blunted day-night changes in luteinizing hormone pulse frequency in girls with obesity: the potential role of hyperandrogenemia. J Clin Endocrinol Metab. 2014;99:2887–96.

Conte F, Grumbach M, Kaplan S. A diphasic pattern of gonadotropin secretion in patients with the syndrome of gonadal dysgenesis. J Clin Endocrinol Metab. 1975;40:670–4.

Dattani MT, Gevers EF. Endocrinology of fetal development. In: Melmed S, Polonsky KS, Larsen PR, Kronenberg HM, editors. Williams textbook of endocrinology. Elsevier, Philadelphia, PA, 13th edn. 2016. p. 849–92.

Daw SF. Age of boys' puberty in Leipzig, 1727–49, as indicated by voice breaking in J.S. Bach's choir members. Hum Biol. 1970;42:87–9.

de Roux N, Young J, Misrahi M, Schaison G, Milgrom E. Loss of function mutations of the GnRH receptor: a new cause of hypogonadotropic hypogonadism. J Pediatr Endocrinol Metab. 1999;12 Suppl 1:267–75.

deRoux N, Genin E, Carel J, Matsuda F, Chaussain J, Milgrom E. Hypogonadotropic hypogonadism due to loss of function of the KiSS1-derived peptide receptor GPR54. Proc Natl Acad Sci. 2003;100:10972–6.

Divall SA, Williams TR, Carver SE, Koch L, Bruning JC, Kahn CR, Wondisford F, Radovick S, Wolfe A. Divergent roles of growth factors in the GnRH regulation of puberty in mice. J Clin Invest. 2010;120:2900–9.

Dubois SL, Wolfe A, Radovick S, Boehm U, Levine JE. Estradiol restrains prepubertal gonadotropin secretion in female mice via activation of ERalpha in kisspeptin neurons. Endocrinology. 2016;157:1546–54.

Dyer JS, Rosenfeld CR. Metabolic imprinting by prenatal, perinatal, and postnatal overnutrition: a review. Semin Reprod Med. 2011;29:266–76.

Falardeau J, Chung WC, Beenken A, Raivio T, Plummer L, Sidis Y, Jacobson-Dickman EE, Eliseenkova AV, Ma J, Dwyer A, Quinton R, Na S, Hall JE, Huot C, Alois N, Pearce SH, Cole LW, Hughes V, Mohammadi M, Tsai P, Pitteloud N. Decreased FGF8 signaling causes deficiency of gonadotropin-releasing hormone in humans and mice. J Clin Invest. 2008;118:2822–31.

Finlay F, Jones R, Kaplowitz P, Oberfield S. Precocious puberty. Pediatrics. 2000;106:162b–3.

Foster TA, Voors AW, Webber LS, Frerichs RR, Berenson GS. Anthropometric and maturation measurements of children, ages 5 to 14 years, in a biracial community – the Bogalusa Heart Study. Am J Clin Nutr. 1977;30:582–91.

Freedman DS, Goodman A, Contreras OA, DasMahapatra P, Srinivasan SR, Berenson GS. Secular trends in BMI and blood pressure among children and adolescents: the Bogalusa Heart Study. Pediatrics. 2012;130:e159–66.

Frisch RE, Revelle R. Height and weight at menarche and a hypothesis of critical body weights and adolescent events. Science. 1970;169:397–9.

Garcia-Galiano D, Pinilla L, Tena-Sempere M. Sex steroids and the control of the kiss1 system: developmental roles and major regulatory actions. J Neuroendocrinol. 2012;24:22–33.

Glanowska KM, Burger LL, Moenter SM. Development of gonadotropin-releasing hormone secretion and pituitary response. J Neurosci. 2014;34:15060–9.

Grachev P, Millar RP, O'Byrne KT. The role of neurokinin B signalling in reproductive neuroendocrinology. Neuroendocrinology. 2014;99:7–17.

Herbison AE, Moenter SM. Depolarising and hyperpolarising actions of GABA(A) receptor activation on gonadotrophin-releasing hormone neurones: towards an emerging consensus. J Neuroendocrinol. 2011;23:557–69. doi:10.1111/j.1365-2826.2011.02145.x.

Herman-Giddens M, Slora E, Wasserman R, Bourdony C, Bhapkar M, Koch G, Hasemeier C. Secondary sexual characteristics and menses in young girls seen in office practice: a study from the pediatric research in office settings network. Pediatrics. 1997;99:505–12.

Herman-Giddens ME, Wang L, Koch G. Secondary sexual characteristics in boys: estimates from the national health and nutrition examination survey III, 1988–1994. Arch Pediatr Adolesc Med. 2001;155:1022–8.

Herman-Giddens ME, Steffes J, Harris D, Slora E, Hussey M, Dowshen SA, Wasserman R, Serwint JR, Smitherman L, Reiter EO. Secondary sexual characteristics in boys: data from the Pediatric Research in Office Settings Network. Pediatrics. 2012;130:e1058–68.

Iremonger KJ, Constantin S, Liu X, Herbison AE. Glutamate regulation of GnRH neuron excitability. Brain Res. 2010;1364:35–43.

Kaplan SL, Grumbach MM, Aubert ML. The ontogenesis of pituitary hormones and hypothalamic factors in the human fetus: maturation of central nervous system regulation of anterior pituitary function. Recent Prog Horm Res. 1976;32:161–243.

Kaplowitz P, Oberfield S, The Drug and Therapeutics and Executive Committees of the Laws on Wilkins Pediatric Endocrine Society. Reexamination of the age limit for defining when puberty is precocious in girls in the United States: implications for evaluation and treatment. Pediatrics. 1999;104:936–41.

Kaplowitz PB, Slora EJ, Wasserman RC, Pedlow SE, Herman-Giddens ME. Earlier onset of puberty in girls: relation to increased body mass index and race. Pediatrics. 2001;108:347–53.

Karimov CB, Moragianni VA, Cronister A, Srouji S, Petrozza J, Racowsky C, Ginsburg E, Thornton KL, Welt CK. Increased frequency of occult fragile X-associated primary ovarian insufficiency in infertile women with evidence of impaired ovarian function. Hum Reprod. 2011;26:2077–83.

Karpati AM, Rubin CH, Kieszak SM, Marcus M, Troiano RP. Stature and pubertal stage assessment in American boys: the 1988–1994 Third National Health and Nutrition Examination Survey1. J Adolesc Health. 2002;30:205–12.

Keen K, Burich A, Mitsushima D, Kasuya E, Terasawa E. Effects of pulsatile infusion of the GABAA receptor blocker bicuculline on the onset of puberty in female rhesus monkeys. Endocrinology. 1999;140:5257–66.

Kim SH. Congenital hypogonadotropic hypogonadism and kallmann syndrome: past, present, and future. Endocrinol Metab (Seoul). 2015;30:456–66.

Knoll JG, Clay CM, Bouma GJ, Henion TR, Schwarting GA, Millar RP, Tobet SA. Developmental profile and sexually dimorphic expression of kiss1 and kiss1r in the fetal mouse brain. Front Endocrinol (Lausanne). 2013;4:140.

Largo RH, Prader A. Pubertal development in Swiss boys. Helv Paediatr Acta. 1983;38:211–28.

Latronico AC, Segaloff DL. Naturally occurring mutations of the luteinizing-hormone receptor: lessons learned about reproductive physiology and G protein-coupled receptors. Am J Hum Genet. 1999;65:949–58.

Lee JM, Wasserman R, Kaciroti N, Gebremariam A, Steffes J, Dowshen S, Harris D, Serwint J, Abney D, Smitherman L, Reiter E, Herman-Giddens ME. Timing of puberty in overweight versus obese boys. Pediatrics. 2016;137:1–10.

Legro R, Lin H, Demers L, Lloyd T. Rapid maturation of the reproductive axis during perimenarche independent of body composition. J Clin Endocrinol Metab. 2000;85:1021–5.

Lippincott MF, True C, Seminara SB. Use of genetic models of idiopathic hypogonadotrophic hypogonadism in mice and men to understand the mechanisms of disease. Exp Physiol. 2013;98:1522–7.

Macedo DB, Abreu AP, Reis AC, Montenegro LR, Dauber A, Beneduzzi D, Cukier P, Silveira LF, Teles MG, Carroll RS, Junior GG, Filho GG, Gucev Z, Arnhold IJ, de Castro M, Moreira AC, Martinelli Jr CE, Hirschhorn JN, Mendonca BB, Brito VN, Antonini SR, Kaiser UB, Latronico AC. Central precocious puberty that appears to be sporadic caused by paternally inherited mutations in the imprinted gene makorin ring finger 3. J Clin Endocrinol Metab. 2014;99: E1097–103.

Marshall WA, Tanner JM. Variations in pattern of pubertal changes in girls. Arch Dis Child. 1969;44:291–303.

Marshall WA, Tanner JM. Variations in the pattern of pubertal changes in boys. Arch Dis Child. 1970;45:13–23.

Marti-Henneberg C, Vizmanos B. The duration of puberty in girls is related to the timing of its onset. J Pediatr. 1997;131:618–21.

Mitamura R, Yano K, Suzuki N, Ito Y, Makita Y, Okuno A. Diurnal rhythms of luteinizing hormone, follicle-stimulating hormone, testosterone, and estradiol secretion before the onset of female puberty in short children. J Clin Endocrinol Metab. 2000;85:1074–80.

Miura K, Acierno Jr JS, Seminara SB. Characterization of the human nasal embryonic LHRH factor gene, NELF, and a mutation screening among 65 patients with idiopathic hypogonadotropic hypogonadism (IHH). J Hum Genet. 2004;49:265–8.

Mul D, Fredriks AM, van Buuren S, Oostdijk W, Verloove-Vanhorick SP, Wit JM. Pubertal development in The Netherlands 1965–1997. Pediatr Res. 2001;50:479–86.

Nimri R, Lebenthal Y, Lazar L, Chevrier L, Phillip M, Bar M, Hernandez-Mora E, de Roux N, Gat-Yablonski G. A novel loss-of-function mutation in GPR54/KISS1R leads to hypogonadotropic hypogonadism in a highly consanguineous family. J Clin Endocrinol Metab. 2011;96:E536–45.

Oerter K, Uriarte M, Rose S, Barnes K, Cutler Jr G. Gonadotropin secretory dynamics during puberty in normal girls and boys. J Clin Endocrinol Metab. 1990;71:1251–8.

Ojeda SR, Lomniczi A. Puberty in 2013: unravelling the mystery of puberty. Nat Rev Endocrinol. 2014;10:67–9.

Ojeda S, Lomniczi A, Mastronardi C, Heger S, Roth C, Parent A, Matagne V, Mungenast A. Minireview: the neuroendocrine regulation of puberty: is the time ripe for a systems biology approach? Endocrinology. 2006;147:1166–74.

Parent AS, et al. The timing of normal puberty and the age limits of sexual precocity: variations around the world, secular trends, and changes after migration. Endocr Rev. 2003;24:669–93.

Parent A, Franssen D, Fudvoye J, Gérard A, Bourguignon J. Developmental variations in environmental influences including endocrine disruptors on pubertal timing and neuroendocrine control: revision of human observations and mechanistic insight from rodents. Front Neuroendocrinol. 2015;38:12–36.

Pitteloud N, Acierno Jr JS, Meysing A, Eliseenkova AV, Ma J, Ibrahimi OA, Metzger DL, Hayes FJ, Dwyer AA, Hughes VA, Yialamas M, Hall JE, Grant E, Mohammadi M, Crowley Jr WF. Mutations in fibroblast growth factor receptor 1 cause both Kallmann syndrome and normosmic idiopathic hypogonadotropic hypogonadism. Proc Natl Acad Sci. 2006;103:6281–6.

Qiu X, Dowling AR, Marino JS, Faulkner LD, Bryant B, Bruning JC, Elias CF, Hill JW. Delayed puberty but normal fertility in mice with selective deletion of insulin receptors from kiss1 cells. Endocrinology. 2013;154:1337–48.

Radicioni AF, Di Giorgio G, Grugni G, Cuttini M, Losacco V, Anzuini A, Spera S, Marzano C, Lenzi A, Cappa M, Crino A. Multiple forms of hypogonadism of central, peripheral or combined origin in males with Prader-Willi syndrome. Clin Endocrinol (Oxf). 2012;76:72–7.

Roa J, Tena-Sempere M. Connecting metabolism and reproduction: roles of central energy sensors and key molecular mediators. Mol Cell Endocrinol. 2014;397:4–14.

Rosenfield RL, Bordini B. Evidence that obesity and androgens have independent and opposing effects on gonadotropin production from puberty to maturity. Brain Res. 2010;1364:186–97.

Rosenfield R, Bachrach L, Chernausek S, Gertner J, Gottschalk M, Hardin D, Pescovitz O, Saenger P, Herman-Giddens M, Slora E, Wasserman R. Current age of onset of puberty. Pediatrics. 2000;106:622–3.

Rosenfield RL, Lipton RB, Drum ML. Thelarche, Pubarche, and Menarche attainment in children with normal and elevated body mass index. Pediatrics. 2009;123:84–8.

Rosenfield RL, Bordini B, Yu C. Comparison of detection of normal puberty in boys by a hormonal sleep test and a gonadotropin-releasing hormone agonist test. J Clin Endocrinol Metab. 2012;97:4596–604.

Ross J, Loriaux D, Cutler Jr G. Developmental changes in neuroendocrine regulation of gonadotropin secretion in gonadal dysgenesis. J Clin Endocrinol Metab. 1983;57:288–93.
Roth CL, DiVall S. Consequences of early life programing by genetic and environmental influences: a synthesis regarding pubertal timing. Endocr Dev. 2016;29:134–52.
Sanchez-Garrido MA, Tena-Sempere M. Metabolic control of puberty: roles of leptin and kisspeptins. Horm Behav. 2013;64:187–94.
Sanz E, Quintana A, Deem JD, Steiner RA, Palmiter RD, McKnight GS. Fertility-regulating kiss1 neurons arise from hypothalamic pomc-expressing progenitors. J Neurosci. 2015;35:5549–56.
Schwanzel-Fukuda M, Crossin KL, Pfaff DW, Bouloux PM, Hardelin JP, Petit C. Migration of luteinizing hormone-releasing hormone (LHRH) neurons in early human embryos. J Comp Neurol. 1996;366:547–57.
Sehested A, Juul A, Andersson A, Petersen J, Jensen T, Muller J, Skakkebaek N. Serum inhibin A and inhibin B in healthy prepubertal, pubertal, and adolescent girls and adult women: relation to age, stage of puberty, menstrual cycle, follicle-stimulating hormone, luteinizing hormone, and estradiol levels. J Clin Endocrinol Metab. 2000;85:1634–40.
Seminara SB. Mechanisms of disease: the first kiss-a crucial role for kisspeptin-1 and its receptor, G-protein-coupled receptor 54, in puberty and reproduction. Nat Clin Pract Endocrinol Metab. 2006;2:328–34.
Seminara S, Messager S, Chatzidaki E, Thresher R, Acierno Jr J, Shagoury J, Bo-Abbas Y, Kuohung W, Schwinof K, Hendrick A, Zahn D, Dixon J, Kaiser U, Slaugenhaupt S, Gusella J, O'Rahilly S, Carlton ML, Crowley Jr W, Aparicio SJR, Colledge W. The GPR54 gene as a regulator of puberty. N Engl J Med. 2003;349:1614–27.
Silveira LG, Noel SD, Silveira-Neto AP, Abreu AP, Brito VN, Santos MG, Bianco SD, Kuohung W, Xu S, Gryngarten M, Escobar ME, Arnhold IJ, Mendonca BB, Kaiser UB, Latronico AC. Mutations of the KISS1 gene in disorders of puberty. J Clin Endocrinol Metab. 2010;95:2276–80.
Sorensen K, Aksglaede L, Petersen JH, Juul A. Recent changes in pubertal timing in healthy Danish boys: associations with body mass index. J Clin Endocrinol Metab. 2010;95:263–70.
Sun S, Schubert C, Chumlea W, Roche A, Kulin H, Lee P, Himes J, Ryan A. National estimates of the timing of sexual maturation and racial differences among US children. Pediatrics. 2002;110:911–9.
Tanner JM. The assessment of growth and development in children. Arch Dis Child. 1952;27:10–33.
Teles MG, Bianco SDC, Brito VN, Trarbach EB, Kuohung W, Xu S, Seminara SB, Mendonca BB, Kaiser UB, Latronico AC. A GPR54-activating mutation in a patient with central precocious puberty. N Engl J Med. 2008;358:709–15.
Terasawa E, Guerriero KA, Plant TM. Kisspeptin and puberty in mammals. Adv Exp Med Biol. 2013;784:253–73.
Wang Y, Lobstein T. Worldwide trends in childhood overweight and obesity. Int J Pediatr Obes. 2006;1:11–25.
Weinstein LS. G(s)alpha mutations in fibrous dysplasia and McCune-Albright syndrome. J Bone Miner Res. 2006;21 Suppl 2:P120–4.
Welt CK, Chan JL, Bullen J, Murphy R, Smith P, DePaoli AM, Karalis A, Mantzoros CS. Recombinant human leptin in women with hypothalamic amenorrhea. N Engl J Med. 2004;351:987–97.
Wildt L, Marshall G, Knobil E. Experimental induction of puberty in the infantile female rhesus monkey. Science. 1980;207:1373–5.
Wu F, Butler G, Kelnar C, Huhtaniemi I, Veldhuis J. Ontogeny of pulsatile gonadotropin releasing hormone secretion from midchildhood, through puberty, to adulthood in the human male: a study using deconvolution analysis and an ultrasensitive immunofluorometric assay. J Clin Endocrinol Metab. 1996;81:1798–805.
Wu T, Mendola P, Buck G. Ethnic differences in the presence of secondary sex characteristics and menarche among US girls: the Third National Health and Nutrition Examination Survey, 1988–1994. Pediatrics. 2002;110:752–7.

The Endocrine Control of Human Pregnancy 25

Kelly Kuo, David Hackney, and Sam Mesiano

Abstract

The endocrinology of human pregnancy is dominated by multiple placental hormones that induce physiologic changes in the mother in favor of pregnancy. Hormones synthesized by the placenta include chorionic gonadotropin which prevents regression of the ovarian corpus luteum during the first several weeks of pregnancy and progesterone which promotes uterine quiescence. Placental somatotrophins such as placental lactogen and placental growth hormone generate maternal metabolic changes in the mother that are favorable to the fetus, though in some cases can contribute to gestational diabetes. In addition to metabolic changes, pregnancy can impact a wide range of other maternal endocrine systems including thyroid function and the renin-angiotensin-aldosterone system. The placenta is also an extremely vascular organ and thus also secretes several angiogenic factors, many of which may play a role in the development of pre-eclampsia. Understanding the broad and complex hormonal changes that occur in pregnancy is important understanding the pathophysiology of pregnancy and for clinicians who providers care to reproductive age women.

K. Kuo
Department of Obstetrics and Gynecology, Oregon Health and Science University, Portland, OR, USA

D. Hackney
Department of Obstetrics and Gynecology, Case Western Reserve University, Cleveland, OH, USA

Department of Obstetrics and Gynecology, University Hospitals of Cleveland, Cleveland, OH, USA

S. Mesiano (✉)
Department of Reproductive Biology, Case Western Reserve University, Cleveland, OH, USA
e-mail: sam.mesiano@case.edu

A. Belfiore, D. LeRoith (eds.), *Principles of Endocrinology and Hormone Action*, Endocrinology, https://doi.org/10.1007/978-3-319-44675-2_26

Keywords
Endocrinology • Parturition • Placental hormones • Pregnancy

Contents

Introduction

Perhaps no other medical event exists which generates as many profound physiologic changes in as wide a range of organ systems as occurs in pregnancy, with alterations to the endocrine system being among the most important. Not only does pregnancy impact all of the existing maternal endocrine glands but the placenta itself is a complicated endocrine organ, the optimal function of which bears responsibility for nothing less than the continued propagation of the species. Even if a clinician does not deliver babies or practice obstetrics, an understanding of maternal physiology is crucial for any physician called upon to care for pregnant women with endocrinopathies. This chapter covers the endocrine function of the placenta, physiologic endocrine changes of the mother, and the endocrinology of pregnancy maintenance and parturition. The endocrinology of ovulation, conception, and implantation as well as the endocrine development of the fetus and neonate is not covered. Other excellent reviews and texts are available for these areas.

Fetal Contributions to the Endocrinology of Pregnancy

The Placenta

Known hormones synthesized within and secreted by the human placenta are listed in Table 1. Given the breadth and depth of this list, an argument can be made for the placenta being the most complicated of all human endocrine organs. Hormone production begins shortly after conception and even before implantation, as evidenced by the identification in maternal serum of chorionic gonadotropin (CG) only a few days after ovulation in a fertile cycle. During the early stages of blastocyst formation, the cells which will form the placenta, the trophoblasts, distinguish themselves from the cells which will form the embryo and are referred to at this stage as cytotrophoblasts. During implantation and villi formation, the cytotrophoblasts which are in direct contact with the maternal blood supply begin to fuse their collective cell membranes and become a large, singular multinucleated structure known as the syncytiotrophoblast. The syncytiotrophoblast is the primary source of subsequent placental hormone synthesis, the products of which are secreted directly into the maternal circulation. It is not a two-way street, however, and the syncytiotrophoblast blocks the majority of maternal hormones (as well as pharmaceuticals and many other agents)

Table 1 Hormones synthesized by the human placenta

Neuropeptides	Pituitary-like hormones	Steroid hormones	Monoamines and adrenal-like peptides
CRH	ACTH	Progesterone	Epinephrine
TRH	TSH	Estradiol	Norepinepherine
GnRH	GH	Estrone	Dopamine
Melatonin	PL	Estriol	Serotonin
Cholecystokinin	CG	Estetrol	Adrenomedullin
Met-enkephalin	LH	2-Methoxyestradiol	
Dynorphin	FSH	Allopregnanolone	
Neurotensin	B-Endorphin	Pregnenolone	
VIP	Prolactin	5α-Dihydroprogesterone	
Galanin	Oxytocin		
Somatostatin	Leptin		
CGRP	Activin		
Neuropeptide Y	Follistatin		
Substance P	Inhibin		
Endothelin			
ANP			
Renin			
Angiotensin			
Urocortin			

From Reis and Petraglia (2001)
VIP vasoactive intestinal peptide, *CGRP* calcitonin gene-related peptide, *ANP* atrial natriuretic peptide

from crossing into the fetal circulation. Thus the fetus can enjoy its own endocrine homeostasis according to its developmental program. In addition to the syncytiotrophoblast, the maternal endometrium that is in contact with the placenta and fetal membranes, known as the decidua, also becomes an important source of hormone synthesis. Decidual hormones include several agents that are secreted across the fetal membranes or into the uterine muscle (the myometrium) and help control of onset of labor. These include relaxin, prostaglandins (PGs), and cytokines.

Chorionic Gonadotropin

No other placental hormone is as quintessential as CG (commonly referred to as human (h)CG) if for no other reason than the fact that it is clinically used to diagnose pregnancy and is the earliest clinically recognized hormone secreted by the new conceptus. Like all gonadotropins it is a glycoprotein heterodimer with an α and β subunit. CG is structurally similar to LH and predominantly functions through the LH receptor. Its primary importance is immediately after conception and during the first several weeks of pregnancy when it prevents regression of the ovarian corpus luteum and as such promotes continued generation of progesterone. Progesterone is necessary for the establishment and continuation of pregnancy, and in the first several weeks, it prevents sloughing of the endometrial lining and allows implantation to advance. Thus, the initial stages of pregnancy are dependent on the corpus luteum as the primary source of progesterone. At around the sixth to tenth week of pregnancy, however, the syncytiotrophoblast of the placenta becomes a major source of progesterone obviating the need for the ovarian corpus luteum for the remainder of pregnancy. After its rapid rise through the first half of pregnancy, CG concentrations subsequently plateau. Maternal LH and FSH levels are low (essentially undetectable) during pregnancy due to negative feedback effect of placental steroids (see below) on the maternal hypothalamic-pituitary axis.

Measurement of CG in pregnancy has multiple useful clinical applications, the most basic of which is the diagnosis of pregnancy. Additionally, serial quantitative CG measurements in early pregnancy can assist in establishing the viability of an uncertain gestation as well as a possible ectopic pregnancy. The trophoblasts of genetically abnormal conceptions, such as those with trisomies 13, 18, and 21, secrete either abnormally high or low levels of CG, and thus it is included in the first and second trimester maternal serum genetic screening. Additionally, choriocarcinomas and molar gestations generate very high concentrations of CG, and in turn declining and subsequently undetectable serum concentrations of CG can be used to monitor treatment and recurrence.

Placental Steroids

Progesterone: The human placenta synthesizes and secretes estrogens and progesterone from precursors supplied by the mother and fetus (Fig. 1). The most important of the placenta steroids is progesterone. Though CG may be the most quintessential

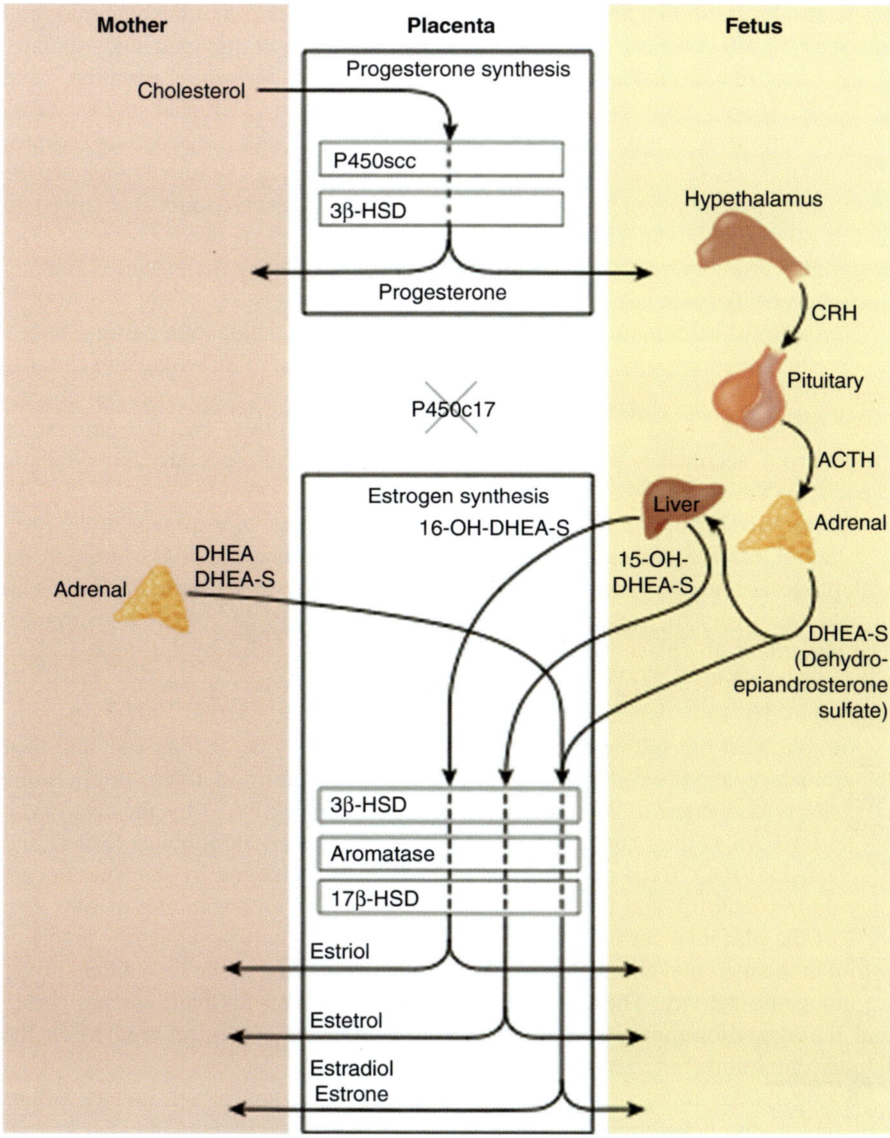

Fig. 1 Biosynthesis of progesterone and estrogens by the human placenta. Progesterone is produced mainly from maternal cholesterol. P450c17 is not expressed in the human placenta, and therefore, progesterone cannot be converted to C19 androgens. Instead, estrogens are biosynthesized from C19-androgen precursors (mainly DHEAS) provided by the maternal and fetal adrenals (From Mesiano (2001); Artwork from Boron and Boulpaep, *Medical Physiology*, 3rd edition)

placental hormone, progesterone is necessary for the maintenance of pregnancy at all stages and promotes numerous physiologic changes required for the success of pregnancy. A major function of progesterone during pregnancy is to promote myometrial relaxation and quiescence and immunosuppression of the maternal-fetal interface by affecting decidual cell function. Its importance for pregnancy maintenance is not just embedded in its name (a condensation of "pro," "gestation," and "steroid hormone") but more importantly is demonstrated by clinical studies showing that inhibition of progesterone activity by treatment with progesterone receptor (PR) antagonists (e.g., mifepristone) terminates pregnancy by augmenting uterine contractility and inducing the full parturition cascade (Christin-Maitre et al. 2000). In fact, in all viviparous species examined so far, studies of progesterone receptor (PR) antagonists show that progesterone is essential for pregnancy maintenance and any disruption of its synthesis or action induces parturition.

During most of human pregnancy, the placenta is the major source of progesterone producing approximately 250–300 mg/day at the peak of its production (Strauss et al. 1996). The human placenta synthesizes progesterone from maternal cholesterol. Synthesis of progesterone appears to be constitutive, and the amount of progesterone secreted is a function of placental mass and especially the synthetic capacity of the syncytiotrophoblast.

Estrogens: The human placenta produces large amounts of estrogens in the form of estradiol, estrone, and estriol, especially during the second and third trimesters. As with progesterone, the syncytiotrophoblast cannot synthesize estrogens de novo and instead has a very high capacity for aromatization of C19 androgens to estrogens. The precursors for placental estrogen synthesis are provided by the fetal adrenal cortex that produces large amounts of dehydroepiandrosterone sulfate (DHEAS) after the 10–15th week of gestation (Mesiano and Jaffe 1997). In syncytiotrophoblast the sulfate moiety, via the sulfatase enzyme, is removed, and then the aromatase enzyme converts DHEA to estradiol and estrone. Interestingly, some DHEAS is converted to 16-hydroxy-DHEAS (16OH-DHEAS) by the fetal liver. 16OH-DHEAS is then converted to estriol by the syncytiotrophoblast (Siiteri and MacDonald 1966). Expression of the 16-hydroxylase enzyme by the liver occurs only during fetal life and is lost soon after delivery. Estriol constitutes greater than 90% of the placental estrogens in the maternal circulation. Consequently, levels of estriol in the maternal circulation are therefore an indication of the fetal adrenal/liver steroidogenic activity. The functional interaction between the fetal adrenal cortex and the syncytiotrophoblast for the synthesis of estrogens is referred to as the fetoplacental unit (Siiteri and MacDonald 1963).

Estrogens are important stimulants of uterine growth and blood flow as well as maternal breast development in preparation for lactation. Insight into the role of placental estrogens in the regulation of human pregnancy can be gained from congenital conditions that disrupt the fetoplacental unit. In congenital adrenal hyperplasia, DHEAS production by the fetal adrenal cortex is increased and consequently so too is placental estrogen production (Miller and Levine 1987; Morel and Miller 1991; New 1998). These pregnancies are normal with normal parturition at term suggesting that higher estrogens are not detrimental to pregnancy outcome (Price et al. 1971). Pregnancy and parturition timing are also not affected by abnormalities that decrease placental estrogen production such as anencephaly or placental aromatase deficiency (Milic and Adamsons 1969; Honnebier and Swaab

1973; Shozu et al. 1991; Harada et al. 1992; Mullis et al. 1997). It should be noted, however, that conditions of placental estrogen deficiency do not exclude a role for estrogens in the physiology of human pregnancy since the levels of maternal estrogens, although low compared with normal pregnancies, are similar to levels reached in the mid-cycle and luteal phases. Estrogen is produced by other sources (e.g., ovarian follicles and adipose tissue) in the maternal compartment. Thus, despite conditions that affect placental estrogen synthesis, there are no natural conditions in which pregnancy and normal parturition occur in the complete absence of estrogens.

Glucocorticoid metabolism: In addition to steroid hormone synthesis, the syncytiotrophoblast also plays an important role in catalyzing existing maternal steroid hormones in order to prevent them from entering the fetal circulation. Specifically the placenta expresses 11β-hydroxysteroid dehydrogenase type 2 (11β-HSD2) which inactivates cortisol, the normal concentration of which is several times higher in the maternal than fetal circulation (Sun et al. 1999). This barrier to maternal glucocorticoid is likely essential for the normal development of the fetal hypothalamic-pituitary-adrenal axis.

The barrier, however, has clinical implication since administration of glucocorticoid to the fetus is desired in cases of threatened preterm birth to stimulate maturation of the fetal lungs and in rare cases to provide direct fetal endocrine therapy. To circumvent the placental barrier, synthetic glucocorticoids such as betamethasone and dexamethasone, which are not metabolized by 11ß-HSD2, are used clinically.

Somatotrophins

In addition to steroid synthesis and CG, the placenta also produces an array of somatotrophins which are structurally and genetically similar to growth hormone. The primary placental somatotrophins are placental lactogen (PL) and placental growth hormone (PGH). The word "lactogen" in PL is a historical remnant from the original assays used for its detection. Ironically it is unclear if PL has any actual impact on lactation, which is predominantly controlled by prolactin, oxytocin, and sex steroids, and the administration of PL to nonpregnant adults does not generate lactation. Instead both somatotrophins activate the growth hormone (GH) receptor and stimulate maternal metabolic changes, which in turn promote fetal growth. Their maternal peripheral concentrations increase progressively through pregnancy in concert with increasing total placental mass. In much the same manner that placental CG makes maternal pituitary LH and FSH virtually undetectable during pregnancy, the increasing concentrations of placental somatotrophins eventually make maternal pituitary GH undetectable.

Placental somatotrophins are responsible for many of the maternal metabolic changes of pregnancy including impaired glucose tolerance, decreased insulin sensitivity, and increased circulating free fatty acids (Samaan et al. 1968). In an otherwise healthy mother, these changes are all advantageous as they ensure an appropriate supply of energy to the rapidly growing fetus. In women with borderline insulin resistance at conception, however, these changes can generate overt though transient diabetes (i.e., gestational diabetes). Additionally, for patients with pre-existing diabetes, the further increase in insulin resistance and mobilization of free fatty acids during pregnancy can both worsen the blood sugar control overall and generate a predisposition to ketogenesis. Diabetic ketogenic acidosis (DKA), a major life-threatening complication of diabetes, occurs mainly in patients with type I disease, but may also occur in patients with type II disease; of note, the underlying predisposition to ketogenesis in pregnancy allows DKA to develop at serum blood glucose levels which are only slightly elevated (Cullen et al. 1996). DKA can have potentially devastating impacts on the mother and fetus, and thus providers of clinical care for pregnant patients should be cautious regarding its potential occurrence.

Angiogenic Factors

The placenta is an extremely vascular organ, and thus the 40 weeks from conception to delivery during which it dramatically increases in size is obviously an intense period of angiogenesis. Likewise the placenta produces several angiogenic factors, including platelet-derived endothelial cell growth factor and vascular endothelial growth factor (VEGF), among others. The placenta, however, also produces several anti-angiogenic factors, which may guard against placental overgrowth or even invasion. Significant advancements have occurred in the last 20 years in our understanding of placental angiogenic factors and their roles, particularly with regard to preeclampsia (Levine et al. 2004).

Preeclampsia is an elusive and mysterious disease which is limited to pregnant humans and currently lacks an optimal clinical treatment, though the condition resolves after delivery of the placenta. The clinical criteria include hypertension and proteinuria with more severe manifestations including headache, pulmonary edema, seizures (eclampsia), and platelet and hepatic impairment. The root cause of all of these manifestations, however, is endothelial dysfunction which is now known to primarily stem from excessive placental anti-angiogenic factors (Zhou et al. 2002; Tsatsaris et al. 2003). Specifically, the human placenta secretes the soluble variant of the fms-like tyrosine kinase-1 (sflt-1) receptor into the maternal circulation. The full-length flt-1 is a membrane protein which is a receptor for VEGF and whose signaling on endothelial cells broadly serves to promote angiogenesis and optimal endothelial cell function. In contrast sflt-1 is a truncated version which lacks the intramembrane portion of the protein and is thus soluble. In the maternal circulation, it binds VEGF and as such functions as a competitive VEGF inhibitor and anti-angiogenic factor. Maternal serum concentrations of sflt-1 are increased both during preeclamspia and are even increased earlier in pregnancy in patients who are known to have subsequently developed preeclampsia at a later date (McKeeman et al. 2004). In vitro human trophoblast will increase sflt-1 production in response to hypoxia (Nagamatsu et al. 2004), and it is hypothesized that in vivo conditions which generate impaired trophoblast oxygenation increase sflt-1 secretion and thus in turn clinical preeclampsia. Potential causes of trophoblast hypoxia include the known risk factors for preeclampsia itself such as vascular disease secondary to diabetes, hypertension, or thrombosis. The discovery of sflt-1 and its role in preeclampsia has tremendous clinical potential with regard to both early screening tests and treatments.

Other Hormones

Though CG, sex steroids, somatotrophins, and angiogenic factors account for the majority of the clinical manifestations attributable to the placenta, the total number of placental hormones is extensive as evidenced in Table 1. A full description of all hormonal products generated by the placenta is beyond the capacity of this chapter, and in many cases their actual physiologic roles, if any, have not yet been elucidated. In a broader sense, it is unclear why the placenta generates such a vast array of hormonal products. It is possible that some of them represent evolutionary holdovers which no longer have a specific function. Many of them, however, have redundant functions. For example, in addition to the two primary somatotrophins, many other placental hormones, such as leptin and neuropeptide Y, alter maternal metabolism in manners favorable to the fetus. Given the profound evolutionary importance of securing appropriate fetal nutrition, the benefits of such redundancy would be logical. In many cases, however, the functions of different hormonal products are explicitly antagonistic toward one another. In addition to the described angiogenic and anti-angiogenic factors, another clear example would be the inhibins and activins which are both secreted and have exact opposite functions. In these cases, the placenta can potentially exert exact control over a physiologic process by increasing or decreasing antagonistic hormones. Likewise many of these agonist/antagonist pairs regulate vascular and endothelial functions, which must be carefully balanced to ensure appropriate placental perfusion while also protecting maternal health. Given the system complexity and current lack of understanding of many hormonal pathways, the placenta will likely remain a very fertile area of research for years to come.

Physiologic Changes of the Maternal Endocrine System in Pregnancy

Glucose Metabolism

Normal pregnancy is characterized by significant alterations in glucose metabolism. Basal hepatic glucose production increases by approximately 30% by late pregnancy, while insulin-mediated glucose uptake decreases by 50–60% (Catalano et al. 1991). These changes are driven in part by placental hormone production and cytokine release, with the overall effect of increasing insulin resistance and nutrient shunting to the fetus, particularly in the third trimester. In healthy nondiabetic women, this progressive increase in insulin resistance is matched by an increase in insulin secretion. In response to a glucose load, insulin secretion increases by 200–250% above basal levels in order to suppress hepatic gluconeogenesis and to maintain euglycemia (Catalano et al. 1999). However, in women with underlying insulin resistance or a genetic predisposition toward developing diabetes, the longitudinal changes in insulin secretion and sensitivity that occur over the course of pregnancy may result in overt or subclinical diabetes.

The mechanism of insulin resistance in normal pregnancy is multifactorial. Hormonal control has historically been attributed to PL, which increases up to 30-fold during gestation and acts as an insulin secretagogue in cultured islet cells (Brelje et al. 1993; Lombardo et al. 2011), in addition to estrogen, progesterone, and cortisol. In euglycemic-hyperinsulinemic clamp studies, however, changes in maternal placental hormone levels do not correlate directly with changes in insulin responsiveness (Kirwan et al. 2002). Increasing evidence now exists for a physiologic blunting of insulin signaling pathways that occurs due to local cytokine production, altered fatty acid metabolism, and increased lipolysis, which together produce a state of low-grade, chronic inflammation (Hotamisligil et al. 1994; Liu et al. 1998; Kirwan et al. 2002; Yu et al. 2002; Barbour et al. 2007). Tumor necrosis factor alpha (TNF-α), an inflammatory cytokine, likely plays a key role in this process through both transcriptional regulation and cell signaling pathways (Moller 2000; Kirwan et al. 2002).

At the cellular level, the ability of insulin to stimulate glucose uptake is dependent on multiple steps: tyrosine phosphorylation of the insulin receptor (IR); activation of downstream signaling via insulin receptor substrate-1 (IRS-1), protein kinase B, and phosphoinositide 3-kinase (PI3K); and translocation of glucose transporter type 4 (GLUT4) from the cytoplasm to the plasma membrane (Czech and Corvera 1999; Pessin and Saltiel 2000). Inhibition of this signaling process may occur at multiple levels, thereby decreasing the cellular response to insulin. Placental secretion of tumor necrosis factor alpha (TNF-α) has been shown to inhibit IRS-1 signaling through phosphorylation of IR and IRS-1 and also through induction of free fatty acids, which also inhibits signaling through PI3K (Hotamisligil et al. 1994; Liu et al. 1998; Moller 2000; Yu et al. 2002). At the transcriptional level, TNF-α downregulates genes required for normal insulin action and inhibits expression of adiponectin, a key insulin-sensitizing hormone, in maternal adipocytes (Moller 2000; Bruun et al. 2003).

The longitudinal changes in insulin sensitivity and resistance that occur during pregnancy are also a reflection of the prepregnant metabolic state (Fig. 2). Lean women usually have greater pre-gravid insulin sensitivity as compared with obese women and are more likely to be able to maintain normoglycemia during pregnancy despite a similar 50–60% increase in insulin resistance (Catalano et al. 1991, 1999). In the setting of obesity, however, increased production of cytokines and fatty acids from adipose tissue contributes to increased systemic inflammation and further dampening of insulin signaling pathways. Obesity is further associated with decreased mRNA and protein expression of GLUT4 in both skeletal muscle and adipose tissue (Colomiere et al. 2010). Obese women have a three- to tenfold

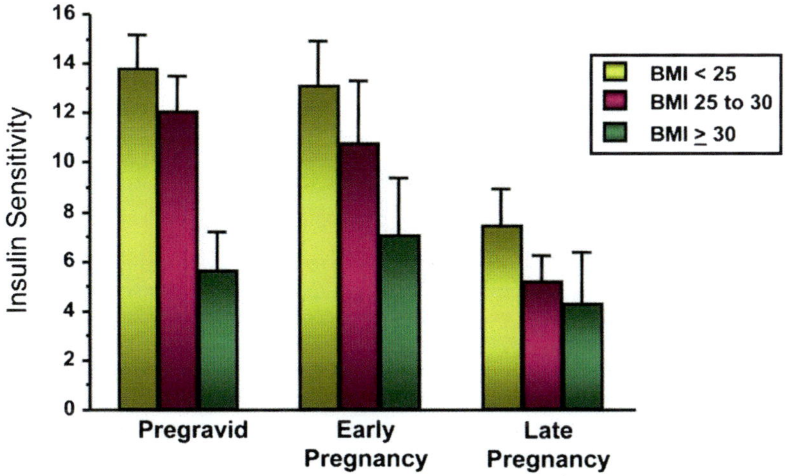

Fig. 2 The longitudinal changes in insulin sensitivity in average (BMI<25), overweight (BMI 25–30), and obese (BMI>30) women over time (*BMI* body mass index) (Adapted from Catalano and Ehrenberg (2006))

increased risk of developing gestational diabetes mellitus (GDM) as compared to women of normal weight (Sebire et al. 2001), with significant implications for maternal and fetal health. A continuous positive association exists between increasing plasma glucose concentrations and the risk of fetal macrosomia and cesarean section (Group et al. 2008; Hartling et al. 2012). Poorly controlled maternal hyperglycemia is associated with an increased risk of congenital anomalies, preterm delivery, and intrauterine demise (Cundy et al. 2000; Biggio et al. 2010). The insulin resistance of pregnancy reverses rapidly after delivery. However, women who develop GDM carry an increased lifetime risk of type II diabetes and cardiovascular disease, while their offspring have higher rates of childhood obesity and metabolic syndrome (Lee et al. 2007; Moore 2010).

Thyroid Function

Significant alterations in maternal thyroid function occur in pregnancy due to increased metabolic demand and hormonal stimulation of the hypothalamic-pituitary-thyroid axis. Triiodothyronine (T3) and thyroxine (T4) syntheses increase by 30–100% above nonpregnant levels (Fantz et al. 1999), largely due to the thyrotropic effects of CG and to increasing levels of thyroxine-binding globulin (TBG), the main carrier of T4 in the bloodstream.

In early pregnancy, rising CG levels directly stimulate thyroid hormone production via binding of the CG β-subunit to maternal thyroid stimulating hormone (TSH) receptors (Yoshimura and Hershman 1995). Total T3 and T4 levels peak at 10–15 weeks gestation, in parallel with the normal CG peak that occurs near the end of the first trimester; TSH levels nadir concurrently due to feedback loop inhibition (Haddow et al. 2008; Grun et al. 1997). In approximately 3–5% of pregnancies, a transient and self-limited hyperthyroidism occurs at this time in association with hyperemesis gravidarum, a syndrome of excessive nausea, vomiting, electrolyte disturbance, and weight loss in pregnancy (Tan et al. 2002). Levels of TBG rise due to estrogen-induced sialylation and decreased hepatic clearance, doubling by 16–20 weeks (Ain et al. 1987; Yoshimura and Hershman 1995; Glinoer 1999). Decreased levels of unbound T3 and T4 in turn trigger additional feedback stimulation and TSH secretion to maintain normal circulating levels of free thyroid hormone. The maternal thyroid gland enlarges in size by 10–15%, while iodine uptake increases in order to compensate for ongoing urinary excretion and the continual transfer of T4 and iodine to the fetoplacental unit (Rasmussen et al. 1989; Liberman et al. 1998; Glinoer 1999, 2001; Pearce 2008).

The sustained, higher output demand of pregnancy constitutes a stress test for the maternal thyroid. As a result, women with low thyroid reserve or relative iodine deficiency may develop hypothyroidism during the course of pregnancy; similarly, pregnancy may unmask or exacerbate underlying autoimmune dysfunction (Galofre et al. 2010). The use of pregnancy- and trimester-specific reference ranges is recommended for the diagnosis of hypo- or hyperthyroidism, given the normal physiologic and longitudinal changes that occur (Soldin et al. 2004; Stagnaro-Green et al. 2011). If trimester-specific reference ranges for TSH are unavailable in the laboratory, the following reference ranges are recommended by the American Thyroid Association: 0.1–2.5 mIU/L in the first trimester, 0.2–3.0 mIU/L in the second trimester, and 0.3–3.0 mIU/L in the third trimester (Stagnaro-Green et al. 2011).

The regulation of placental deiodination and transfer of maternal T4 is essential for normal fetal growth and is particularly important for the early stages of fetal brain development. T4 is converted to T3 and reaches adult levels in the fetal cerebral cortex by mid-gestation. Differential expression of iodothyronine deiodinases is likely needed for spatial and temporal regulation of T3 bioavailability, according to the varying needs of different brain structures over the course of pregnancy (de Escobar et al. 2004). A population-based study in the Netherlands reported that both maternal hypothyroidism and hyperthyroidism during pregnancy were associated with lower IQ in childhood and decreased cortical volume on MRI, independent of neonatal TSH levels or thyroid peroxidase antibodies (Korevaar et al. 2015). In animal models, neuronal migration into cortical layers, early synaptogenesis, cell differentiation, and myelination can be disrupted even by transient periods of moderate hypothyroxinemia; conversely, premature differentiation and impaired function are associated with hyperthyroxinemia (Noguchi and Sugisaki 1984; Adamo et al. 1990; Auso et al. 2004; de Escobar et al. 2004; Bernal 2007). However, screening for subclinical thyroid deficiencies in early pregnancy does not lead to improved neurologic outcomes in clinical trials (Lazarus et al. 2012) and is thus not recommended by professional organizations (American College of Obstetricians and Gynecologists. Practice bulletin no. 148: 2015).

Renin-Angiotensin-Aldosterone System

The renin-angiotensin-aldosterone system (RAAS) plays an essential role in the regulation of systemic blood pressure, electrolytes, and fluid balance. In response to low circulating blood volume and sodium levels, renin is rapidly synthesized and released from renal juxtaglomerular cells (Johnston 1976; Thurau et al. 1982). Renin cleaves angiotensinogen to produce angiotensin I (ANG I), which is then cleaved by angiotensin-converting enzyme (ACE) to the biologically active angiotensin II (ANG II). ANG II signals primarily through its type 1 receptor (AT_1R) subtype, which is expressed abundantly on vascular smooth muscle cells and adrenal glomerulosa cells. ANG II binding induces vasoconstriction as well as aldosterone secretion, with the net effect of increasing sodium resorption, intravascular volume, and blood pressure. ANG II signaling through its type 2 receptor (AT_2R) has the opposing effect of vasodilation (de Gasparo et al. 2000; Carey and Siragy 2003). While AT_2R is minimally expressed in systemic vasculature, it is the predominant ANG II receptor found in the myometrium and uterine arteries (Cox et al. 1996; Matsumoto et al. 1996), suggesting a biologic role in the hemodynamic regulation of pregnancy. Local tissue-specific RAAS has also been identified in cardiac, ovarian, placental, and decidual tissue, with local production of angiotensins which likely modulate circulatory RAAS function (Poisner 1998; Kumar et al. 2007; Irani and Xia 2008).

Numerous hemodynamic changes occur during pregnancy, including an approximate 40% increase in total blood volume, 30% decrease in systemic vascular resistance (SVR), and a 10- to 12-fold increase in uteroplacental blood flow (Ueland 1976; Krishna and Bhalerao 2011; Mahendru et al. 2014). Significant RAAS activation is therefore required, with estrogen-mediated increases in hepatic production of angiotensinogen beginning early in the first trimester (Lumbers and Pringle 2014). Endogenous progesterone functions as a potent mineralocorticoid receptor antagonist, and the increased urinary excretion of sodium triggers a compensatory increase in renin secretion, ATII production, and plasma aldosterone (Oelkers 1996). Ovarian, placental, and decidual secretion of prorenin also directly contributes to increased RAAS activity (Itskovitz et al. 1987; Downing et al. 1996; Pringle et al. 2015). Despite significant sodium retention with a net gain of approximately 1,000 mg prior to delivery, the increased pituitary secretion of antidiuretic hormone (vasopressin) that occurs during pregnancy contributes to even greater water retention and the characteristic hyponatremic hypervolemia of pregnancy (Cheung and Lafayette 2013).

In the setting of major RAAS upregulation, the mechanisms through which maternal blood pressures are maintained in a state of relative hypotension during normal pregnancy are incompletely understood. As compared to systemic blood vessels, uteroplacental vessels demonstrate less sensitivity to ANG II-induced vasoconstriction (Cox et al. 1996), potentially due to predominant expression of AT_2R on uterine artery smooth muscle; however, uteroplacental vessels are much more sensitive than systemic vasculature to norepinephrine-induced vasoconstriction. Increasing evidence has accumulated over the past two decades for a new branch of the RAAS regulatory pathway, which may function to counter the ACE/ANG II/AT1R receptor axis. Both ANG I and ANG II can be cleaved by ACE2, an enzyme homologous to ACE, to produce ANG 1–7, a heptapeptide with vasodilatory, natriuretic, and antiproliferative effects. In animal models, ACE2 gene expression is activated by both acute and chronic inflammation, and studies suggest that it may be required for normal development of both the kidney and the microvascular capillary bed of the heart (Zhang et al. 2001; Burrell et al. 2005; Zisman 2005). ACE2 knockout mice demonstrate greater sensitivity to both ANG II and phenylephrine-induced arterioconstriction, placental hypoxia, and reduced umbilical blood flow velocity (Yamaleyeva et al. 2015). The effects of ANG 1–7 are conflicting, but may depend on the context. In pregnant rats, for example, ANG 1–7 induces diuresis associated with downregulation of aquaporin-1, while opposite effects of water retention and aquaporin-1 upregulation are seen in virgin rats (Joyner et al. 2008).

Aberrant RAAS signaling is implicated in the development of preeclampsia. ANG 1–7 levels are decreased in preeclamptic women as compared with normotensive pregnant women (Brosnihan et al. 2000). An AT_1R autoantibody with agonist activity has been identified in both human and animal models of preeclampsia, which may contribute to impaired angiogenesis, adrenal dysfunction, and the complement-mediated inflammatory cascade (Zhou et al. 2008; Wang et al. 2012; Siddiqui et al. 2013).

Calcium Metabolism

Calcium homeostasis is an important aspect of maternal and fetal physiology during pregnancy. Ongoing placental transfer of calcium is required for fetal skeletal mineralization, with net deposition of approximately 25–30 g over the course of pregnancy, 80% of which occurs in the third trimester. Increased fetal requirements are met through increased maternal intestinal absorption of calcium, with minimal contribution from the maternal skeleton (Kovacs 2001).

The changes in mineral absorption and calciotropic hormones that occur during pregnancy are well characterized (Kovacs and Kronenberg 1997; Kovacs 2001). A clinically insignificant drop in total serum calcium occurs in the first trimester due to physiologic hemodilution and decreased serum albumin levels; however, levels of ionized calcium, phosphate, and magnesium remain constant. Parathyroid hormone (PTH) may decrease to low-normal values in the first trimester, increasing back to mid-normal ranges by term in normal women with calcium-replete diets; in women with extremely calcium-deficient diets, however, secondary hyperparathyroidism may occur. A twofold increase in 1,25-dihydroxyvitamin D (calcitriol) occurs starting in early pregnancy; this increase appears to be independent of PTH and driven instead by PTH-related protein (PTHrP), estradiol, prolactin, and placental lactogen-mediated 1α-hydroxylase activity in the maternal kidneys (Fleischman et al. 1980; Turner et al. 1988). While increased glomerular filtration leads to increased urinary calcium excretion, a doubling of intestinal calcium absorption by 12 weeks of gestation compensates for renal losses (Kovacs 2001).

Limited data exist on the effect of pregnancy-related hormones on bone metabolism and calcium homeostasis. Nuclear progesterone receptors (PRs) are present in both osteoclasts and osteoblasts, with increased osteogenesis and total bone mass seen in PR knockout mice (Yao et al. 2010). Prolactin may have a similar inhibitory effect on bone mineralization by decreasing osteoblast differentiation (Seriwatanachai et al. 2009). Conversely, osteoclasts are inhibited by both estradiol and oxytocin (Colucci et al. 2002; Oursler 2003; Tamma et al. 2009). Urinary markers of bone turnover are increased as early as 10 weeks of gestation, although maternal-fetal transfer of calcium in the first trimester is minimal; of note, these markers of bone turnover are not significantly elevated even in the third trimester when fetal calcium requirements are at a peak. Sequential imaging studies of maternal bone density have been mixed in regard to whether or not significant bone loss actually occurs during pregnancy (Kovacs 2001; Pearson et al. 2004; Salari and Abdollahi 2014). Hence, while maternal bone metabolism may provide some contribution to fetal calcium demands, upregulation of intestinal calcium absorption appears to be much more significant.

Cortisol Secretion

Significant activation of the hypothalamic-pituitary-adrenal (HPA) axis occurs during pregnancy, accompanied by profound suppression of the stress response. In response to normal stressors, corticotrophin-releasing hormone (CRH) is released from the paraventricular nucleus of the hypothalamus. CRH in turn stimulates release of adrenocorticotrophin hormone (ACTH) from the anterior pituitary, and ACTH stimulates secretion of cortisol from the adrenal cortex. The physiologic hypercortisolemia of pregnancy is driven in part by high levels of estrogen (Coe et al. 1986), which lead to an increase in corticosteroid-binding globulin (CBG) and an increase in free cortisol levels. Maternal cortisol also stimulates placental synthesis of CRH, which drives additional adrenal secretion of cortisol in a positive feedback cycle (Mastorakos and Ilias 2003). Circulating cortisol levels are increased by approximately 200% by the third trimester. At the same time, however, hypothalamic production of CRH is significantly depressed secondary to feedback inhibition by high serum cortisol levels. Allopregnanolone, a neuroactive progesterone metabolite, may also indirectly inhibit norepinephrine release in the paraventricular nucleus to further suppress maternal CRH production (Brunton et al. 2009). The ability of the maternal HPA axis to respond to physiologic stress in pregnancy is thus significantly decreased.

Although maternal cortisol increases by two- to fourfold over the course of pregnancy (Mastorakos and Ilias 2003; Sandman et al. 2006), only a small fraction crosses the placenta to reach the fetus. Approximately 80–90% of maternal cortisol is inactivated by placental 11β-hydroxysteroid dehydrogenase type 2 (11β-HSD2), which serves as a partial barrier against excessive fetal cortisol exposure. Levels of placental 11β-HSD2 decrease rapidly toward the end of the third trimester, when increased cortisol is required for fetal lung maturation and surfactant production

(Edwards et al. 1996; Sun et al. 1997; Ma et al. 2003; Togher et al. 2014). Although the fetal adrenal gland is also a functional source of cortisol, the extent to which fetal cortisol regulates in utero development is uncertain; of note, fetuses with markedly decreased endogenous cortisol production due to congenital adrenal hyperplasia are generally born at term without apparent signs of lung immaturity (Byers et al. 2012).

Growing evidence suggests an important role for dysregulation of the maternal HPA axis in fetal "programming" of disease. Maternal HPA activity and 11β-HSD2 expression are affected by both acute and chronic stress, malnutrition, injury, and illness and may result in increased placental transfer of cortisol. Higher glucocorticoid exposure in utero is associated with preterm birth and lower birth weight and may also be correlated with lower cognitive skills in offspring, changes in brain volume, and higher incidence of neuropsychiatric disorders (Lesage et al. 2001; LeWinn et al. 2009).

The Endocrine Control of Parturition

The Process of Parturition

For most of pregnancy, the uterus serves to house, contain, and protect the developing conceptus (fetus, placenta, membranes, and amniotic fluid). The uterine cervix remains closed and rigid, and the myometrium (major component of the uterine wall) is in a state of relaxed quiescence and grows and distends to accommodate the growing conceptus. At some time, however, pregnancy must end and the fetus must be born. This process, referred to as parturition, involves dramatic biophysical changes in the uterus and gestational tissues such that the fetus and associated tissues are actively ejected. Three distinct processes occur:

(1) The extracellular matrix of the uterine cervix remodels so that the cervix no longer restricts the uterine outlet but instead softens and stretches in response to increased intrauterine pressure and eventually dilates enough to allow passage of the fetus and placenta (i.e., the gateway opens).
(2) The uterine myometrium transitions from a relaxed and quiescent state to the highly excitable and contractile state to produce the rhythmic contraction of labor (i.e., the engine for birth is activated) forcing the contents of the uterus against the cervix to further promote dilation.
(3) The amnion membrane, especially the zone overlying the cervix, weakens such that it ruptures in response to increased intra-amniotic pressure.

These processes are controlled by a balance between hormones that modulate uterine function and growth, known as uterotropins (e.g., estrogens, progesterone), and hormones that directly affect myometrial contractility, known as uterotonins (e.g., oxytocin, $PGF_{2\alpha}$, PGI_2). For most of pregnancy, progesterone and relaxatory uterotonins promote myometrial quiescence, uterine growth, and distensibility, and cervical closure prevail. At parturition, the balance shifts to favor estrogens and prolabor uterotropins that promote myometrial contractions and cervical softening. Some of the key hormones controlling the functional state of the gravid uterus especially in the context of parturition are discussed below.

Progesterone

Arpad Csapo, in the 1950s, proposed the "progesterone block" hypothesis, which posits that progesterone maintains pregnancy by promoting myometrial relaxation, cervical closure, and decidual quiescence and that progesterone withdrawal initiates parturition. Indeed, in most animals, parturition is preceded and triggered by a systemic decrease in maternal circulating progesterone levels (Young et al. 2010). In women, however, maternal progesterone levels do not decrease prior to the onset of labor at term or preterm, but instead the placenta continues to produce large amount of progesterone throughout pregnancy and until it is delivered at parturition (Tulchinsky et al. 1972; Okada et al. 1974). In this regard, human parturition is distinct from other species in that it is not triggered by a systemic progesterone withdrawal. Instead, human parturition is thought to be triggered by a functional progesterone withdrawal, whereby progesterone target cells (myometrial, cervical, and decidual cells) desensitize to the pro-pregnancy action of progesterone. In all species studied to date, including human, interventions that block PR signaling increase myometrial contractility and promote cervical softening and dilation to induce parturition at all stages of pregnancy (Chwalisz and Garfield 1994). Thus, it is clear that the progesterone block to parturition operates, at least in part, through progesterone-/PR-mediated mechanisms and that parturition in women can be induced by a functional withdrawal (or modulation) of PR-mediated progesterone actions in myometrial, cervical, and decidual cells. Several mechanisms for PR-mediated functional progesterone withdrawal have been proposed including PR isoform switching (Mesiano et al. 2002; Merlino et al. 2007; Tan et al. 2012), decrease in PR transcriptional coactivators (Condon et al. 2003), and inhibition of PR signaling by other transcription factors (Kalkhoven et al. 1996; Lindstrom and Bennett 2005). Progesterone withdrawal also may be mediated by the conversion of progesterone to a less active form with diminished progestin activity in target cells (Mahendroo et al. 1999; Andersson et al. 2008; Williams et al. 2012).

Progesterone Therapy to Prevent Preterm Birth

The discovery that progesterone maintains pregnancy naturally led to the idea that preterm birth could be prevented by treating women with progesterone (Csapo 1956). Early studies showed that high doses of progesterone administered to women in active labor decreased contraction frequency and responsiveness to oxytocin (Hendricks et al. 1961; Pinto et al. 1965). Although those data supported the core idea that progesterone therapy suppresses labor, subsequent clinical trials of chronic progestin therapy to prevent preterm birth produced mixed outcomes

(Johnson et al. 1975; Hartikainen-Sorri et al. 1980; Hauth et al. 1983; Yemini et al. 1985) and were underpowered to produce statistically meaningful data. The issue was readdressed in the early 2000s using larger randomized trials. Those trials showed prophylactic treatment with progesterone administered vaginally (DeFranco et al. 2007), or 17α-hydroxyprogesterone caproate (17HPC) given as a long-acting intramuscular injection (Meis et al. 2003) decreased the incidence of preterm birth and improved neonatal outcome. However, the effect was detected only in women with an increased risk for preterm birth (based on a prior preterm birth); no benefit was found in the general population. Subsequent studies showed that the preterm birth rate was not affected by progesterone administered vaginally (O'Brien et al. 2007) and that 17HPC failed to alter the preterm birth rate in twin pregnancies (Rouse et al. 2007). A recent large clinical trial also failed to show any beneficial effects of vaginal progesterone prophylaxis for the prevention of preterm birth (Norman et al. 2016). The only positive data to emerge from recent clinical trials is that vaginal progesterone therapy decreased the incidence of preterm birth in women with a short cervix, which is also an indication of heightened preterm birth risk (DeFranco et al. 2007; Fonseca et al. 2007; Hassan et al. 2011; Romero et al. 2012; Conde-Agudelo et al. 2013; Conde-Agudelo and Romero 2016). Thus, prophylactic progesterone supplementation therapy to prevent preterm, although widely used, may be effective only in small subset of women at increased risk for preterm birth. The mechanism for this effect remains a conundrum since the PRs in uterine target cells are saturated by high levels of placental progesterone throughout pregnancy (Tulchinsky and Okada 1975). Other mechanisms of progesterone action, possibly via PRs distinct from the classical nuclear PRs, may operate. Further research is needed to resolve this issue. Nonetheless, progesterone/PR signaling remains a logical therapeutic target to clinical control parturition and prevent preterm birth.

Estrogens

Estrogens are potent uterotropic agents that promote growth and blood flow in the myometrium, decidua, and cervix (Pepe and Albrecht 1995; Mesiano and Jaffe 1997; Albrecht et al. 2000). These effects are clearly necessary for the maintenance of pregnancy, and it is noteworthy that no naturally occurring conditions are known in which human pregnancy exists in the complete absence of estrogens. The placenta is the main source of estrogens for most of pregnancy, but pregnancy is not compromised if placental estrogen synthesis fails (Shozu et al. 1991; Harada et al. 1992; Harada 1993). This may be because low, but physiologically relevant, levels of estrogens are produced by the maternal tissues (e.g., adipocytes). Thus, it is generally considered that for most of pregnancy, estrogens, like progesterone, exert pro-pregnancy actions.

At parturition, estrogens appear to oppose the actions of progesterone to promote the expression of genes in myometrial, decidual, and cervical cells whose products increase contractility and promote cervical ripening and membrane rupture. This implies that estrogenic action on the uterus increases as part of the parturition process. This is clearly apparent in most species where estrogen levels are low during most of pregnancy and increase in conjunction with systemic progesterone withdrawal prior to parturition (Pasqualini and Kincl 1985). In women, however, estrogen levels are high during the second and third trimesters and increase exponentially during the final weeks of gestation (Tulchinsky et al. 1972), yet the uterine tissue appears to be refractory to its prolabor effects. To explain this inconsistency, it is proposed that prolabor actions of estrogens on the uterine tissues are controlled by modulation of target cell responsiveness in much the same manner as progesterone actions are regulated to facilitate functional progesterone withdrawal (Mesiano et al. 2002). In this case, however, the modulation causes functional activation of prolabor actions. According to this scenario, the absolute levels of estrogens in the maternal system are less important than target cell responsiveness provided that sufficient hormone is present when responsiveness to the prolabor estrogenic actions is activated. This may explain why pregnancy and parturition are normal in cases where estrogen levels are low due to decreased placental estrogen production but sufficient to affect responsive cells (Shozu et al. 1991; Harada et al. 1992; Harada 1993).

Cortisol

In contrast to its critical role in inducing parturition in sheep (Liggins 1974), cortisol does not appear to be involved in the human parturition process. It is, however, crucial for the maturation of fetal organ systems prior to birth, and as such administration of synthetic glucocorticoid is used to promote fetal lung development in cases of threatened preterm birth. Although clinical administration of synthetic glucocorticoids does not advance the parturition process, it does not rule out the possibility that cortisol from maternal or fetal origin is involved in triggering parturition onset. However, human parturition occurs normally at term in pregnancies where the fetus cannot produce cortisol suggesting that unlike the sheep, human parturition is not dependent on cortisol from the fetal compartment (Price et al. 1971; Honnebier and Swaab 1973).

Oxytocin

Oxytocin (OT), a small nine amino acid peptide, is a potent uterotonin that increases the frequency and force of myometrial contractions. OT is synthesized by magnocellular neurosecretory cells in the supraoptic and paraventricular nuclei of the hypothalamus whose axons terminate in the posterior pituitary. It is also produced by the decidua, amnion, and chorion, although at low levels compared with the amount released by the posterior pituitary during active labor and in response to cervical distention. The production of OT by the maternal hypothalamic-pituitary axis likely represents a mechanism for maternal control of parturition in response to factors such as circadian cycles and environmental stressors. OT is also secreted as part of the milk letdown reflex during lactation and therefore is critical for nurturing of the neonate.

OT secretion from the maternal posterior pituitary is triggered by cervical and vaginal distention during labor. This is part of a positive feedback loop whereby distention of the cervix due to the contractions of labor induces the release of OT that stimulates myometrial contraction to further distend the cervix. This direct uterotonic effect of OT occurs predominantly during the expulsive phase of labor, and the positive feedback interaction plays key role in successful parturition.

OT is administered to augment labor. However, because of its potent uterotonic effects, risk for uterine abruption and hemorrhagic detachment of the placenta from the uterine wall increases if excessive amounts of OT are administered (Golan et al. 1980). OT is far less effective as an uterotonin when administered before the onset of active labor. This is because the uterus is relatively insensitive to OT at this time due to low levels of OT receptor (OXTR) expression. In the myometrium expression of OXTR is increased at term and in response to estrogens and progesterone withdrawal (Fuchs et al. 1982; Soloff et al. 1983). Distention also increases OXTR expression in myometrial cells (Terzidou et al. 2005). Thus, the parturition process includes increased OXTR expression in the myometrium in response to progesterone withdrawal, increased estrogenic stimulation, and stretch to augment uterine responsiveness to OT. In experimental animals inhibition of OXTR signaling represses labor and delays parturition, and clinical trials of OXTR antagonist demonstrate limited effectiveness in repressing preterm labor without any benefit to neonatal health (Romero et al. 2000).

Despite the unequivocal effects of OT as a stimulatory uterotonin during labor, studies of women with posterior pituitary dysfunction and in animal models lacking OT show that it is not essential for successful parturition but absolutely required for lactation (Schellenberg 1995; Renfree et al. 1996). The current consensus, therefore, is that OT is essential for lactation, but redundant mechanism operates to allow successful parturition in its absence.

Tissue-Level Inflammation

Human parturition is associated with significant sterile tissue-level inflammation in each of the uterine compartments (Kelly 1996; Romero et al. 2007). Increased edema, neutrophil infiltration, activation of resident macrophages, and expression of pro-inflammatory cytokines, chemokines, and PGs occur in the myometrium, cervix, and decidua during the prepartum period (Young et al. 2002; Osman et al. 2003, 2006). Tissue-level inflammation is considered causal to labor onset. Preterm birth is commonly associated with intrauterine infection (Gomez et al. 1995), clinically silent upper genital tract infection, and bacterial vaginosis (Romero et al. 2007), and normal term birth is preceded by increased inflammation, especially in the myometrium, decidua, and cervix (Thomson et al. 1999; Osman et al. 2003). Multiple studies in animal models show that administration of pro-inflammatory cytokines or factors that induce a pro-inflammatory response initiates preterm labor (Romero et al. 1991; Hirsch et al. 1995; Sadowsky et al. 2006). The process appears to involve a tissue-level positive feedback inflammatory loop that amplifies the inflammatory state. The pro-inflammatory nuclear factor-κB (NF-κB) transcription factor complex appears to be a key mediator of this loop. Studies in myometrial cells suggest that progesterone prevents the pro-inflammatory feedback loop by inhibiting NF-κB activity (Tan et al. 2012). This implies that progesterone promotes uterine relaxation in part by preventing inflammation. The concept that progesterone promotes pregnancy by suppressing pro-inflammatory responses in the gestational tissues was proposed by Siiteri and colleagues in the 1970s (Siiteri et al. 1977). Recent studies have shown that progesterone via the PRs inhibits responsiveness of myometrial cells to pro-inflammatory stimuli and that this anti-inflammatory effect is abolished by a switch in the PR isoform ratio (Hardy et al. 2006; Tan et al. 2012). However, studies also have shown that pro-inflammatory stimuli such as $PGF_{2\alpha}$ and interleukin 1ß (IL-1ß) affect the expression and activity of the PR-A isoform such that its capacity to repress the transcriptional activity of PR-B is increased to cause functional progesterone withdrawal (Madsen et al. 2004). Thus, it is possible that for most of pregnancy, progesterone acting via the type-B PR isoform (PR-B) promotes uterine quiescence in part by repressing responsiveness to prolabor/pro-inflammatory stimuli (e.g., uterine distention). However, as pregnancy advances, the net inflammatory load from multiple prolabor/pro-inflammatory stimuli (e.g., uterine distention, fetal stress, placental senescence) gradually increases until it reaches a threshold, whereby local inflammatory cytokines activate the trans-repressive activity of PR-A to inhibit PR-B activity. This may produce a local pro-inflammatory positive feedback state leading to tissue-level inflammation and the production of multiple inflammatory cytokines, including uterotonic PGs (especially PGE_2 and $PGF_{2\alpha}$) and IL-1ß that promote cervical softening, myometrial contractions, and membrane weakening (Fig. 3).

Prostaglandins

PGs are potent uterotonins (stimulatory and relaxatory) and act locally within uterine/gestational tissues to play critical roles in the control of parturition. The principal PGs involved in parturition are PGE_2 and $PGF_{2\alpha}$. Levels of PGE_2 and $PGF_{2\alpha}$ in the amniotic fluid increase prior to the onset of labor, and treatment with agents that inhibit PG function (PG synthesis inhibitors or PG receptor antagonists) suppresses labor and inhibits parturition (Gibb 1998). Thus, the production and action of PGs in the gestational tissues is a pivotal step in the parturition cascade. Administration of $PGF_{2\alpha}$ induces parturition at all stages of human pregnancy (Thiery 1979). This suggests that PGs (especially $PGF_{2\alpha}$) are capable of inducing the full parturition cascade. In the context of tissue-level inflammation, this becomes an important issue because it raises the possibility that locally produced $PGF_{2\alpha}$ can reach a critical level where it induces a positive feedback cycle that amplifies inflammation within the uterine tissues to overcome the progesterone block and transform the uterus to the laboring state.

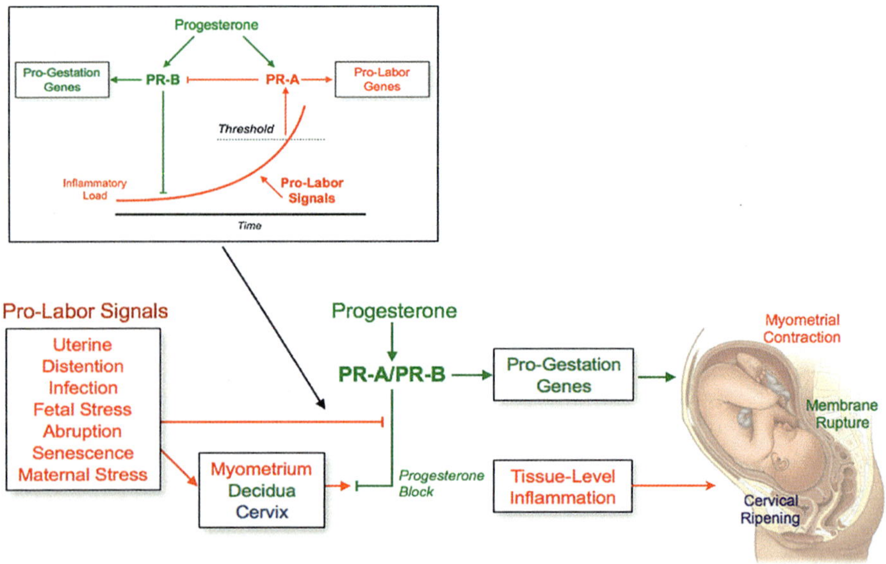

Fig. 3 Proposed model for the interaction of inflammation with progesterone signaling in the control of human parturition. Prolabor signals comprise multiple pro-inflammatory stimuli on the myometrium, decidua, and cervix, the net effect of which is to exert an inflammatory load on the pregnancy uterus. For most of pregnancy, progesterone prevents the inflammatory load from reaching a level that induces the tissue-level inflammation leading to the onset of labor. However, an inflammatory load threshold exists above which the transcriptional activity of PR-A is modulated such that it causes a tissue-level functional progesterone withdrawal. This leads to amplification of local inflammation leading to increase local PG levels that transform the uterine tissue to the laboring state

Placental Corticotrophin-Releasing Hormone

In general, most hormones produced by the placenta affect maternal physiology in favor of maintaining pregnancy and providing resources to the developing fetus. One placental hormone, corticotrophin-releasing hormone (CRH), however, may play a key role in the control of parturition and mediating fetal stress signals to the parturition trigger mechanism.

Placental CRH, which is identical to hypothalamic CRH, is produced by the syncytiotrophoblast, fetal membranes, and decidua (Frim et al. 1988). Placental CRH is secreted into the maternal compartment and can be detected in the maternal circulation from as early as the 10–15th week of gestation. Its levels then increase markedly until term (McLean et al. 1995). The rate of maternal CRH increase with advancing gestation is predictive of gestation length, with a rapid rise indicative of eventual preterm birth, and a slow rise indicative of post-term birth (McLean et al. 1995). Although the exact function of placental CRH in the control of human pregnancy and parturition is not known, its role as a potential biomarker for preterm birth risk is well established.

Given the role of hypothalamic CRH as a key mediator of the stress response, it is possible that placental CRH mediates a fetal/placental stress response to trigger the parturition process. This may occur when its levels in the maternal compartment reach preset threshold. Thus, the faster the rise in CRH, the earlier in gestation the parturition trigger threshold is reached, and vice versa. CRH receptors have been identified on myometrial cells, decidual cells, and amnion cells, and in vitro studies show that it affects myometrial contractility and PG production by decidua and amnion (Quartero and Fry 1989). The exact mechanism by which it contributes to the parturition process however remains unclear.

Interestingly, unlike hypothalamic CRH production which is inhibited by glucocorticoid, a distinguishing feature of placental CRH is that its production by the syncytiotrophoblast is increased by glucocorticoid (Robinson et al. 1988; Korebrits et al. 1998). This may be part of a positive feedback endocrine loop whereby placental CRH stimulates the maternal and/or fetal pituitary-adrenal axis to secrete cortisol which in turn stimulates more CRH secretion from the placenta. In the fetus, this would cause an increase in cortisol and DHEAS production by the fetal adrenal cortex which are both induced by adrenocorticotropin (ACTH). CRH also increases the basal- and ACTH-induced production of DHEAS by human fetal adrenal cortical cells directly suggesting that it affects the function of the feto-placental steroidogenic unit (Smith et al. 1998; Chakravorty et al. 1999; Ibanez et al. 1999).

Cross-References

▶ Endocrine Functions of Bone
▶ The Thyroid
▶ The Endocrine Pancreas
▶ The Hypothalamus–Pituitary Axis

References

Adamo AM, Aloise PA, Soto EF, Pasquini JM. Neonatal hyperthyroidism in the rat produces an increase in the activity of microperoxisomal marker enzymes coincident with biochemical signs of accelerated myelination. J Neurosci Res. 1990;25(3):353–9.

Ain KB, Mori Y, Refetoff S. Reduced clearance rate of thyroxine-binding globulin (TBG) with increased sialylation: a mechanism for estrogen-induced elevation of serum TBG concentration. J Clin Endocrinol Metab. 1987;65(4):689–96.

Albrecht ED, Aberdeen GW, Pepe GJ. The role of estrogen in the maintenance of primate pregnancy. Am J Obstet Gynecol. 2000;182(2):432–8.

American College of Obstetricians and Gynecologists. Practice bulletin no. 148: thyroid disease in pregnancy. Obstet Gynecol. 2015;125(4):996–1005.

Andersson S, Minjarez D, Yost NP, Word RA. Estrogen and progesterone metabolism in the cervix during pregnancy and parturition. J Clin Endocrinol Metab. 2008;93(6):2366–74.

Auso E, Lavado-Autric R, Cuevas E, Del Rey FE, Morreale De Escobar G, Berbel P. A moderate and transient deficiency of maternal thyroid function at the beginning of fetal neocorticogenesis alters neuronal migration. Endocrinology. 2004;145(9):4037–47.

Barbour LA, McCurdy CE, Hernandez TL, Kirwan JP, Catalano PM, Friedman JE. Cellular mechanisms for insulin resistance in normal pregnancy and gestational diabetes. Diabetes Care. 2007;30 Suppl 2:S112–9.

Bernal J. Thyroid hormone receptors in brain development and function. Nat Clin Pract Endocrinol Metab. 2007;3(3):249–59.

Biggio Jr JR, Chapman V, Neely C, Cliver SP, Rouse DJ. Fetal anomalies in obese women: the contribution of diabetes. Obstet Gynecol. 2010;115(2 Pt 1):290–6.

Brelje TC, Scharp DW, Lacy PE, Ogren L, Talamantes F, Robertson M, Friesen HG, Sorenson RL. Effect of homologous placental lactogens, prolactins, and growth hormones on islet B-cell division and insulin secretion in rat, mouse, and human islets: implication for placental lactogen regulation of islet function during pregnancy. Endocrinology. 1993;132(2):879–87.

Brosnihan KB, Karoly M, Merrill D. Plasma angiotensin-(1-7) is decreased in preeclampsia. Hypertension. 2000;36 Suppl 1:696.

Brunton PJ, McKay AJ, Ochedalski T, Piastowska A, Rebas E, Lachowicz A, Russell JA. Central opioid inhibition of neuroendocrine stress responses in pregnancy in the rat is induced by the neurosteroid allopregnanolone. J Neurosci. 2009;29(20):6449–60.

Bruun JM, Lihn AS, Verdich C, Pedersen SB, Toubro S, Astrup A, Richelsen B. Regulation of adiponectin by adipose tissue-derived cytokines: in vivo and in vitro investigations in humans. Am J Physiol Endocrinol Metab. 2003;285(3):E527–33.

Burrell LM, Risvanis J, Kubota E, Dean RG, MacDonald PS, Lu S, Tikellis C, Grant SL, Lew RA, Smith AI, Cooper ME, Johnston CI. Myocardial infarction increases ACE2 expression in rat and humans. Eur Heart J. 2005;26(4):369–75.

Byers HM, Dagle JM, Klein JM, Ryckman KK, McDonald EL, Murray JC, Borowski KS. Variations in CRHR1 are associated with persistent pulmonary hypertension of the newborn. Pediatr Res. 2012;71(2):162–7.

Carey RM, Siragy HM. Newly recognized components of the renin-angiotensin system: potential roles in cardiovascular and renal regulation. Endocr Rev. 2003;24(3):261–71.

Catalano PM, Ehrenberg HM. The short- and long-term implications of maternal obesity on the mother and her offspring. BJOG. 2006;113(10):1126–33. Review. PubMed PMID: 16827826.

Catalano PM, Tyzbir ED, Roman NM, Amini SB, Sims EA. Longitudinal changes in insulin release and insulin resistance in nonobese pregnant women. Am J Obstet Gynecol. 1991;165(6 Pt 1):1667–72.

Catalano PM, Huston L, Amini SB, Kalhan SC. Longitudinal changes in glucose metabolism during pregnancy in obese women with normal glucose tolerance and gestational diabetes mellitus. Am J Obstet Gynecol. 1999;180(4):903–16.

Chakravorty A, Mesiano S, Jaffe RB. Corticotropin-releasing hormone stimulates P450 17alpha-hydroxylase/17,20-lyase in human fetal adrenal cells via protein kinase C. J Clin Endocrinol Metab. 1999;84(10):3732–8.

Christin-Maitre S, Bouchard P, Spitz IM. Medical termination of pregnancy. N Engl J Med. 2000;342(13):946–56.

Chwalisz K, Garfield RE. Antiprogestins in the induction of labor. Ann N Y Acad Sci. 1994;734:387–413.

Coe CL, Murai JT, Wiener SG, Levine S, Siiteri PK. Rapid cortisol and corticosteroid-binding globulin responses during pregnancy and after estrogen administration in the squirrel monkey. Endocrinology. 1986;118(1):435–40.

Colomiere M, Permezel M, Lappas M. Diabetes and obesity during pregnancy alter insulin signalling and glucose transporter expression in maternal skeletal muscle and subcutaneous adipose tissue. J Mol Endocrinol. 2010;44(4):213–23.

Colucci S, Colaianni G, Mori G, Grano M, Zallone A. Human osteoclasts express oxytocin receptor. Biochem Biophys Res Commun. 2002;297(3):442–5.

Conde-Agudelo A, Romero R. Vaginal progesterone to prevent preterm birth in pregnant women with a sonographic short cervix: clinical and public health implications. Am J Obstet Gynecol. 2016;214(2):235–42.

Conde-Agudelo A, Romero R, Nicolaides K, Chaiworapongsa T, O'Brien JM, Cetingoz E, da Fonseca E, Creasy G, Soma-Pillay P, Fusey S, Cam C, Alfirevic Z, Hassan SS. Vaginal progesterone vs. cervical cerclage for the prevention of preterm birth in women with a sonographic short cervix, previous preterm birth, and singleton gestation: a systematic review and indirect comparison metaanalysis. Am J Obstet Gynecol. 2013;208(1):42 e41–18.

Condon JC, Jeyasuria P, Faust JM, Wilson JW, Mendelson CR. A decline in the levels of progesterone receptor coactivators in the pregnant uterus at term may antagonize progesterone receptor function and contribute to the initiation of parturition. Proc Natl Acad Sci U S A. 2003;100(16):9518–23.

Cox BE, Word RA, Rosenfeld CR. Angiotensin II receptor characteristics and subtype expression in uterine arteries and myometrium during pregnancy. J Clin Endocrinol Metab. 1996;81 (1):49–58.

Csapo A. Progesterone block. Am J Anat. 1956;98(2):273–91.

Cullen MT, Reece EA, Homko CJ, Sivan E. The changing presentations of diabetic ketoacidosis during pregnancy. Am J Perinatol. 1996;13(7):449–51.

Cundy T, Gamble G, Townend K, Henley PG, MacPherson P, Roberts AB. Perinatal mortality in type 2 diabetes mellitus. Diabet Med. 2000;17(1):33–9.

Czech MP, Corvera S. Signaling mechanisms that regulate glucose transport. J Biol Chem. 1999;274(4):1865–8.

de Escobar GM, Obregon MJ, del Rey FE. Maternal thyroid hormones early in pregnancy and fetal brain development. Best Pract Res Clin Endocrinol Metab. 2004;18(2):225–48.

de Gasparo M, Catt KJ, Inagami T, Wright JW, Unger T. International union of pharmacology. XXIII. The angiotensin II receptors. Pharmacol Rev. 2000;52(3):415–72.

DeFranco EA, O'Brien JM, Adair CD, Lewis DF, Hall DR, Fusey S, Soma-Pillay P, Porter K, How H, Schakis R, Eller D, Trivedi Y, Vanburen G, Khandelwal M, Trofatter K, Vidyadhari D, Vijayaraghavan J, Weeks J, Dattel B, Newton E, Chazotte C, Valenzuela G, Calda P, Bsharat M, Creasy GW. Vaginal progesterone is associated with a decrease in risk for early preterm birth and improved neonatal outcome in women with a short cervix: a secondary analysis from a randomized, double-blind, placebo-controlled trial. Ultrasound Obstet Gynecol. 2007;30 (5):697–705.

Downing GJ, Maulik D, Poisner AM. Human chorionic gonadotropin stimulates placental prorenin secretion: evidence for autocrine/paracrine regulation. J Clin Endocrinol Metab. 1996;81 (3):1027–30.

Edwards CR, Benediktsson R, Lindsay RS, Seckl JR. 11 beta-hydroxysteroid dehydrogenases: key enzymes in determining tissue-specific glucocorticoid effects. Steroids. 1996;61(4):263–9.

Fantz CR, Dagogo-Jack S, Ladenson JH, Gronowski AM. Thyroid function during pregnancy. Clin Chem. 1999;45(12):2250–8.

Fleischman AR, Rosen JF, Cole J, Smith CM, Deluca HF. Maternal and fetal serum 1,25-dihydroxyvitamin D levels at term. J Pediatr. 1980;97(4):640–2.

Fonseca EB, Celik E, Parra M, Singh M, Nicolaides KH. Progesterone and the risk of preterm birth among women with a short cervix. N Engl J Med. 2007;357(5):462–9.

Frim DM, Emanuel RL, Robinson BG, Smas CM, Adler GK, Majzoub JA. Characterization and gestational regulation of corticotropin-releasing hormone messenger RNA in human placenta. J Clin Invest. 1988;82:287–92.

Fuchs AR, Fuchs F, Husslein P, Soloff MS, Fernstrom MJ. Oxytocin receptors and human parturition: a dual role for oxytocin in the initiation of labor. Science. 1982;215(4538):1396–8.

Galofre JC, Haber RS, Mitchell AA, Pessah R, Davies TF. Increased postpartum thyroxine replacement in Hashimoto's thyroiditis. Thyroid. 2010;20(8):901–8.

Gibb W. The role of prostaglandins in human parturition. Ann Med. 1998;30(3):235–41.

Glinoer D. What happens to the normal thyroid during pregnancy? Thyroid. 1999;9(7):631–5.

Glinoer D. Pregnancy and iodine. Thyroid. 2001;11(5):471–81.

Golan A, Sandbank O, Rubin A. Rupture of the pregnant uterus. Obstet Gynecol. 1980;56 (5):549–54.

Gomez R, Ghezzi F, Romero R, Munoz H, Tolosa JE, Rojas I. Premature labor and intra-amniotic infection. Clinical aspects and role of the cytokines in diagnosis and pathophysiology. Clin Perinatol. 1995;22(2):281–342.

Grun JP, Meuris S, De Nayer P, Glinoer D. The thyrotrophic role of human chorionic gonadotrophin (hCG) in the early stages of twin (versus single) pregnancies. Clin Endocrinol (Oxf). 1997;46 (6):719–25.

Haddow JE, McClain MR, Lambert-Messerlian G, Palomaki GE, Canick JA, Cleary-Goldman J, Malone FD, Porter TF, Nyberg DA, Bernstein P, D'Alton ME. Variability in thyroid-stimulating hormone suppression by human chorionic [corrected] gonadotropin during early pregnancy. J Clin Endocrinol Metab. 2008;93(9):3341–7.

HAPO Study Cooperative Research Group, Metzger BE, Lowe LP, Dyer AR, Trimble ER, Chaovarindr U, Coustan DR, Hadden DR, McCance DR, Hod M, McIntyre HD, Oats JJ, Persson B, Rogers MS, Sacks DA. Hyperglycemia and adverse pregnancy outcomes. N Engl J Med. 2008;358(19):1991–2002.

Harada N. Genetic analysis of human placental aromatase deficiency. J Steroid Biochem Mol Biol. 1993;44(4–6):331–40.

Harada N, Ogawa H, Shozu M, Yamada K. Genetic studies to characterize the origin of the mutation in placental aromatase deficiency. Am J Hum Genet. 1992;51(3):666–72.

Hardy DB, Janowski BA, Corey DR, Mendelson CR. Progesterone receptor plays a major anti-inflammatory role in human myometrial cells by antagonism of nuclear factor-kappaB activation of cyclooxygenase 2 expression. Mol Endocrinol. 2006;20(11):2724–33.

Hartikainen-Sorri AL, Kauppila A, Tuimala R. Inefficacy of 17 alpha-hydroxyprogesterone caproate in the prevention of prematurity in twin pregnancy. Obstet Gynecol. 1980;56(6):692–5.

Hartling L, Dryden DM, Guthrie A, Muise M, Vandermeer B, Aktary WM, Pasichnyk D, Seida JC, Donovan L. Screening and diagnosing gestational diabetes mellitus. Evid Rep Technol Assess (Full Rep). 2012;210:1–327.

Hassan SS, Romero R, Vidyadhari D, Fusey S, Baxter JK, Khandelwal M, Vijayaraghavan J, Trivedi Y, Soma-Pillay P, Sambarey P, Dayal A, Potapov V, O'Brien J, Astakhov V, Yuzko O, Kinzler W, Dattel B, Sehdev H, Mazheika L, Manchulenko D, Gervasi MT, Sullivan L, Conde-Agudelo A, Phillips JA, Creasy GW. Vaginal progesterone reduces the rate of preterm birth in women with a sonographic short cervix: a multicenter, randomized, double-blind, placebo-controlled trial. Ultrasound Obstet Gynecol. 2011;38(1):18–31.

Hauth JC, Gilstrap 3rd LC, Brekken AL, Hauth JM. The effect of 17 alpha-hydroxyprogesterone caproate on pregnancy outcome in an active-duty military population. Am J Obstet Gynecol. 1983;146(2):187–90.

Hendricks CH, Brenner WE, Gabel RA, Kerenyi T. The effect of progesterone administered intra-amniotically in late human pregnancy. Brook Lodge symposium: progesterone. Augusta: The Upjohn Company; 1961.

Hirsch E, Saotome I, Hirsh D. A model of intrauterine infection and preterm delivery in mice. Am J Obstet Gynecol. 1995;172(5):1598–603.

Honnebier WJ, Swaab DF. The influence of anencephaly upon intrauterine growth of fetus and placenta and upon gestation length. J Obstet Gynaecol Br Commonw. 1973;80:577–88.

Hotamisligil GS, Murray DL, Choy LN, Spiegelman BM. Tumor necrosis factor alpha inhibits signaling from the insulin receptor. Proc Natl Acad Sci U S A. 1994;91(11):4854–8.

Ibanez L, Potau N, Marcos MV, de Zegher F. Corticotropin-releasing hormone as adrenal androgen secretagogue. Pediatr Res. 1999;46(3):351–3.

Irani RA, Xia Y. The functional role of the renin-angiotensin system in pregnancy and preeclampsia. Placenta. 2008;29(9):763–71.

Itskovitz J, Sealey JE, Glorioso N, Rosenwaks Z. Plasma prorenin response to human chorionic gonadotropin in ovarian-hyperstimulated women: correlation with the number of ovarian follicles and steroid hormone concentrations. Proc Natl Acad Sci. 1987;84(20):7285–9.

Johnson JW, Austin KL, Jones GS, Davis GH, King TM. Efficacy of 17alpha-hydroxyprogesterone caproate in the prevention of premature labor. N Engl J Med. 1975;293(14):675–80.

Johnston CI. Effect of antihypertensive drugs on the renin-angiotensin system. Drugs. 1976;12 (4):274–91.

Joyner J, Neves LAA, Stovall K, Ferrario CM, Brosnihan KB. Angiotensin-(1-7) serves as an aquaretic by increasing water intake and diuresis in association with downregulation of aquaporin-1 during pregnancy in rats. Am J Physiol Regul Integr Comp Physiol. 2008;294 (3):R1073–80.

Kalkhoven E, Wissink S, van der Saag PT, van der Burg B. Negative interaction between the RelA (p65) subunit of NF-kappaB and the progesterone receptor. J Biol Chem. 1996;271 (11):6217–24.

Kelly RW. Inflammatory mediators and parturition. Rev Reprod. 1996;1(2):89–96.

Kirwan JP, Hauguel-De Mouzon S, Lepercq J, Challier JC, Huston-Presley L, Friedman JE, Kalhan SC, Catalano PM. TNF-alpha is a predictor of insulin resistance in human pregnancy. Diabetes. 2002;51(7):2207–13.

Korebrits C, Yu DH, Ramirez MM, Marinoni E, Bocking AD, Challis JR. Antenatal glucocorticoid administration increases corticotrophin-releasing hormone in maternal plasma. Br J Obstet Gynaecol. 1998;105(5):556–61.

Korevaar TI, Muetzel R, Medici M, Chaker L, Jaddoe VW, de Rijke YB, Steegers EA, Visser TJ, White T, Tiemeier H, Peeters RP. Association of maternal thyroid function during early pregnancy with offspring IQ and brain morphology in childhood: a population-based prospective cohort study. Lancet Diabetes Endocrinol. 2015;4(1):35–43.

Kovacs CS. Calcium and bone metabolism in pregnancy and lactation*. J Clin Endocrinol Metabol. 2001;86(6):2344–8.

Kovacs CS, Kronenberg HM. Maternal-fetal calcium and bone metabolism during pregnancy, puerperium, and lactation. Endocr Rev. 1997;18(6):832–72.

Krishna U, Bhalerao S. Placental insufficiency and fetal growth restriction. J Obstet Gynaecol India. 2011;61(5):505–11.

Kumar R, Singh VP, Baker KM. The intracellular renin-angiotensin system: a new paradigm. Trends Endocrinol Metab. 2007;18(5):208–14.

Lazarus JH, Bestwick JP, Channon S, Paradice R, Maina A, Rees R, Chiusano E, John R, Guaraldo V, George LM, Perona M, Dall'Amico D, Parkes AB, Joomun M, Wald NJ. Antenatal thyroid screening and childhood cognitive function. N Engl J Med. 2012;366 (6):493–501.

Lee AJ, Hiscock RJ, Wein P, Walker SP, Permezel M. Gestational diabetes mellitus: clinical predictors and long-term risk of developing type 2 diabetes: a retrospective cohort study using survival analysis. Diabetes Care. 2007;30(4):878–83.

Lesage J, Blondeau B, Grino M, Breant B, Dupouy JP. Maternal undernutrition during late gestation induces fetal overexposure to glucocorticoids and intrauterine growth retardation, and disturbs the hypothalamo-pituitary adrenal axis in the newborn rat. Endocrinology. 2001;142 (5):1692–702.

Levine RJ, Maynard SE, Qian C, Lim KH, England LJ, Yu KF, Schisterman EF, Thadhani R, Sachs BP, Epstein FH, Sibai BM, Sukhatme VP, Karumanchi SA. Circulating angiogenic factors and the risk of preeclampsia. N Engl J Med. 2004;350(7):672–83.

LeWinn KZ, Stroud LR, Molnar BE, Ware JH, Koenen KC, Buka SL. Elevated maternal cortisol levels during pregnancy are associated with reduced childhood IQ. Int J Epidemiol. 2009;38 (6):1700–10.

Liberman CS, Pino SC, Fang SL, Braverman LE, Emerson CH. Circulating iodide concentrations during and after pregnancy. J Clin Endocrinol Metab. 1998;83(10):3545–9.

Liggins GC. Parturition in the sheep and the human. Basic Life Sci. 1974;4(PT. B):423–43.

Lindstrom TM, Bennett PR. The role of nuclear factor kappa B in human labour. Reproduction. 2005;130(5):569–81.

Liu LS, Spelleken M, Rohrig K, Hauner H, Eckel J. Tumor necrosis factor-alpha acutely inhibits insulin signaling in human adipocytes: implication of the p80 tumor necrosis factor receptor. Diabetes. 1998;47(4):515–22.

Lombardo MF, De Angelis F, Bova L, Bartolini B, Bertuzzi F, Nano R, Capuani B, Lauro R, Federici M, Lauro D, Donadel G. Human placental lactogen (hPL-A) activates signaling pathways linked to cell survival and improves insulin secretion in human pancreatic islets. Islets. 2011;3(5):250–8.

Lumbers ER, Pringle KG. Roles of the circulating renin-angiotensin-aldosterone system in human pregnancy. Am J Physiol Regul Integr Comp Physiol. 2014;306(2):R91–101.

Ma XH, Wu WX, Nathanielsz PW. Gestation-related and betamethasone-induced changes in 11beta-hydroxysteroid dehydrogenase types 1 and 2 in the baboon placenta. Am J Obstet Gynecol. 2003;188(1):13–21.

Madsen G, Zakar T, Ku CY, Sanborn BM, Smith R, Mesiano S. Prostaglandins differentially modulate progesterone receptor-A and -B expression in human myometrial cells: evidence for prostaglandin-induced functional progesterone withdrawal. J Clin Endocrinol Metab. 2004;89 (2):1010–3.

Mahendroo MS, Porter A, Russell DW, Word RA. The parturition defect in steroid 5alpha-reductase type 1 knockout mice is due to impaired cervical ripening. Mol Endocrinol. 1999;13(6):981–92.

Mahendru AA, Everett TR, Wilkinson IB, Lees CC, McEniery CM. A longitudinal study of maternal cardiovascular function from preconception to the postpartum period. J Hypertens. 2014;32(4):849–56.

Mastorakos G, Ilias I. Maternal and fetal hypothalamic-pituitary-adrenal axes during pregnancy and postpartum. Ann N Y Acad Sci. 2003;997:136–49.

Matsumoto T, Sagawa N, Mukoyama M, Tanaka I, Itoh H, Goto M, Itoh H, Horiuchi M, Dzau VJ, Mori T, Nakao K. Type 2 angiotensin II receptor is expressed in human myometrium and uterine leiomyoma and is down-regulated during pregnancy. J Clin Endocrinol Metab. 1996;81 (12):4366–72.

McKeeman GC, Ardill JE, Caldwell CM, Hunter AJ, McClure N. Soluble vascular endothelial growth factor receptor-1 (sFlt-1) is increased throughout gestation in patients who have pre-eclampsia develop. Am J Obstet Gynecol. 2004;191(4):1240–6.

McLean M, Bisits A, Davies J, Woods R, Lowry P, Smith R. A placental clock controlling the length of human pregnancy. Nat Med. 1995;1:460–3.

Meis PJ, Klebanoff M, Thom E, Dombrowski MP, Sibai B, Moawad AH, Spong CY, Hauth JC, Miodovnik M, Varner MW, Leveno KJ, Cariti SN, Iams JD, Wapner RJ, Conway D, O'Sullivan MJ, Carpenter M, Mercer B, Ramin SM, Thorp JM, Peaceman AM, Gabbe S, National Institute of Child Health and Human Development Maternal-Fetal Medicine Units Network. Prevention of recurrent preterm delivery by 17 alpha-hydroxyprogesterone caproate. N Engl J Med. 2003;348(24):2379–85.

Merlino AA, Welsh TN, Tan H, Yi LJ, Cannon V, Mercer BM, Mesiano S. Nuclear progesterone receptors in the human pregnancy myometrium: evidence that parturition involves functional progesterone withdrawal mediated by increased expression of progesterone receptor-A. J Clin Endocrinol Metab. 2007;92(5):1927–33.

Mesiano S. Roles of estrogen and progesterone in human parturition. Front Horm Res. 2001;27:86.

Mesiano S, Jaffe RB. Developmental and functional biology of the primate fetal adrenal cortex. Endocr Rev. 1997;18(3):378–403.

Mesiano S, Chan EC, Fitter JT, Kwek K, Yeo G, Smith R. Progesterone withdrawal and estrogen activation in human parturition are coordinated by progesterone receptor A expression in the myometrium. J Clin Endocrinol Metab. 2002;87(6):2924–30.

Milic AB, Adamsons K. The relationship between anencephaly and prolonged pregnancy. J Obstet Gynaecol Br Commonw. 1969;76(2):102–11.

Miller W, Levine L. Molecular and clinical advances in congenital adrenal hyperplasia. J Pediatr. 1987;111:1–71.

Moller DE. Potential role of TNF-alpha in the pathogenesis of insulin resistance and type 2 diabetes. Trends Endocrinol Metab. 2000;11(6):212–7.

Moore TR. Fetal exposure to gestational diabetes contributes to subsequent adult metabolic syndrome. Am J Obstet Gynecol. 2010;202(6):643–9.

Morel Y, Miller W. Clinical and molecular genetics of congenital adrenal hyperplasia due to 21-hydroxylase deficiency. Adv Hum Genet. 1991;20:1–68.
Mullis PE, Yoshimura N, Kuhlmann B, Lippuner K, Jaeger P, Harada H. Aromatase deficiency in a female who is compound heterozygote for two new point mutations in the P450arom gene: impact of estrogens on hypergonadotropic hypogonadism, multicystic ovaries, and bone densitometry in childhood. J Clin Endocrinol Metab. 1997;82(6):1739–45.
Nagamatsu T, Fujii T, Kusumi M, Zou L, Yamashita T, Osuga Y, Momoeda M, Kozuma S, Taketani Y. Cytotrophoblasts up-regulate soluble fms-like tyrosine kinase-1 expression under reduced oxygen: an implication for the placental vascular development and the pathophysiology of preeclampsia. Endocrinology. 2004;145(11):4838–45.
New MI. Diagnosis and management of congenital adrenal hyperplasia. Annu Rev Med. 1998;49:311–28.
Noguchi T, Sugisaki T. Hypomyelination in the cerebrum of the congenitally hypothyroid mouse (hyt). J Neurochem. 1984;42(3):891–3.
Norman JE, Marlow N, Messow CM, Shennan A, Bennett PR, Thornton S, Robson SC, McConnachie A, Petrou S, Sebire NJ, Lavender T, Whyte S, Norrie J, OPPTIMUM Study Group. Vaginal progesterone prophylaxis for preterm birth (the OPPTIMUM study): a multicentre, randomised, double-blind trial. Lancet. 2016;387(10033):2106–16.
O'Brien JM, Adair CD, Lewis DF, Hall DR, Defranco EA, Fusey S, Soma-Pillay P, Porter K, How H, Schackis R, Eller D, Trivedi Y, Vanburen G, Khandelwal M, Trofatter K, Vidyadhari D, Vijayaraghavan J, Weeks J, Dattel B, Newton E, Chazotte C, Valenzuela G, Calda P, Bsharat M, Creasy GW. Progesterone vaginal gel for the reduction of recurrent preterm birth: primary results from a randomized, double-blind, placebo-controlled trial. Ultrasound Obstet Gynecol. 2007;30(5):687–96.
Oelkers WK. Effects of estrogens and progestogens on the renin-aldosterone system and blood pressure. Steroids. 1996;61(4):166–71.
Okada DM, Tulchinsky D, Ross JW, Hobel CJ. Plasma estrone, estradiol, estriol, progesterone, and cortisol in normal labor. Am J Obstet Gynecol. 1974;119(4):502–7.
Osman I, Young A, Ledingham MA, Thomson AJ, Jordan F, Greer IA, Norman JE. Leukocyte density and pro-inflammatory cytokine expression in human fetal membranes, decidua, cervix and myometrium before and during labour at term. Mol Hum Reprod. 2003;9(1):41–5.
Osman I, Young A, Jordan F, Greer IA, Norman JE. Leukocyte density and proinflammatory mediator expression in regional human fetal membranes and decidua before and during labor at term. J Soc Gynecol Investig. 2006;13(2):97–103.
Oursler MJ. Direct and indirect effects of estrogen on osteoclasts. J Musculoskelet Neuronal Interact. 2003;3(4):363–6; discussion 381.
Pasqualini JR, Kincl F. Hormones and the fetus. Oxford: Pergamin Press; 1985.
Pearce EN. Iodine in pregnancy: is salt iodization enough? J Clin Endocrinol Metab. 2008;93 (7):2466–8.
Pearson D, Kaur M, San P, Lawson N, Baker P, Hosking D. Recovery of pregnancy mediated bone loss during lactation. Bone. 2004;34(3):570–8.
Pepe GJ, Albrecht ED. Actions of placental and fetal adrenal steroid hormones in primate pregnancy. Endocr Rev. 1995;16(5):608–48.
Pessin JE, Saltiel AR. Signaling pathways in insulin action: molecular targets of insulin resistance. J Clin Invest. 2000;106(2):165–9.
Pinto RM, Montuori E, Lerner U, Baleiron H, Glauberman M, Nemirovsky H. Effect of progesterone on the oxytocic action of estradiol-17-beta. Am J Obstet Gynecol. 1965;91:1084–9.
Poisner AM. The human placental renin-angiotensin system. Front Neuroendocrinol. 1998;19 (3):232–52.
Price HV, Cone BR, Keogh M. Length of gestation in congenital adrenal hyperplasia. J Obstet Gynecol Br Commonw. 1971;78:430–4.
Pringle KG, Wang Y, Lumbers ER. The synthesis, secretion and uptake of prorenin in human amnion. Physiol Rep. 2015;3(4).

Quartero HW, Fry CH. Placental corticotrophin releasing factor may modulate human parturition. Placenta. 1989;10(5):439–43.
Rasmussen NG, Hornnes PJ, Hegedus L. Ultrasonographically determined thyroid size in pregnancy and post partum: the goitrogenic effect of pregnancy. Am J Obstet Gynecol. 1989;160 (5 Pt 1):1216–20.
Reis FM, Petraglia F. The placenta as a neuroendocrine organ. Front Horm Res. 2001;27:216.
Renfree MB, Parry LJ, Shaw G. Infusion with an oxytocin receptor antagonist delays parturition in a marsupial. J Reprod Fertil. 1996;108(1):131–7.
Robinson BG, Emanuel RL, Frim DM, Majzoub JA. Glucocorticoid stimulates expression of corticotropin-releasing hormone gene in human placenta. Proc Natl Acad Sci U S A. 1988;85 (14):5244–8.
Romero R, Mazor M, Tartakovsky B. Systemic administration of interleukin-1 induces preterm parturition in mice. Am J Obstet Gynecol. 1991;165(4 Pt 1):969–71.
Romero R, Sibai BM, Sanchez-Ramos L, Valenzuela GJ, Veille JC, Tabor B, Perry KG, Varner M, Goodwin TM, Lane R, Smith J, Shangold G, Creasy GW. An oxytocin receptor antagonist (atosiban) in the treatment of preterm labor: a randomized, double-blind, placebo-controlled trial with tocolytic rescue. Am J Obstet Gynecol. 2000;182(5):1173–83.
Romero R, Espinoza J, Goncalves LF, Kusanovic JP, Friel L, Hassan S. The role of inflammation and infection in preterm birth. Semin Reprod Med. 2007;25(1):21–39.
Romero R, Nicolaides K, Conde-Agudelo A, Tabor A, O'Brien JM, Cetingoz E, Da Fonseca E, Creasy GW, Klein K, Rode L, Soma-Pillay P, Fusey S, Cam C, Alfirevic Z, Hassan SS. Vaginal progesterone in women with an asymptomatic sonographic short cervix in the midtrimester decreases preterm delivery and neonatal morbidity: a systematic review and metaanalysis of individual patient data. Am J Obstet Gynecol. 2012;206(2):124 e121–119.
Rouse DJ, Caritis SN, Peaceman AM, Sciscione A, Thom EA, Spong CY, Varner M, Malone F, Iams JD, Mercer BM, Thorp J, Sorokin Y, Carpenter M, Lo J, Ramin S, Harper M, Anderson G. A trial of 17 alpha-hydroxyprogesterone caproate to prevent prematurity in twins. N Engl J Med. 2007;357(5):454–61.
Sadowsky DW, Adams KM, Gravett MG, Witkin SS, Novy MJ. Preterm labor is induced by intraamniotic infusions of interleukin-1beta and tumor necrosis factor-alpha but not by interleukin-6 or interleukin-8 in a nonhuman primate model. Am J Obstet Gynecol. 2006;195 (6):1578–89.
Salari P, Abdollahi M. The influence of pregnancy and lactation on maternal bone health: a systematic review. J Fam Reprod Health. 2014;8(4):135–48.
Samaan N, Yen SC, Gonzalez D, Pearson OH. Metabolic effects of placental lactogen (HPL) in man. J Clin Endocrinol Metab. 1968;28(4):485–91.
Sandman CA, Glynn L, Schetter CD, Wadhwa P, Garite T, Chicz-DeMet A, Hobel C. Elevated maternal cortisol early in pregnancy predicts third trimester levels of placental corticotropin releasing hormone (CRH): priming the placental clock. Peptides. 2006;27(6):1457–63.
Schellenberg JC. The effect of oxytocin receptor blockade on parturition in guinea pigs. J Clin Invest. 1995;95(1):13–9.
Sebire NJ, Jolly M, Harris J, Wadsworth J, Joffe M, Beard R, Regan L, Robinson S. Maternal obesity and pregnancy outcome: a study of 287,213 pregnancies in London. Int J Obes Relat Metab Disord: J Int Assoc Study Obes. 2001;25(8):1175–82.
Seriwatanachai D, Krishnamra N, van Leeuwen JP. Evidence for direct effects of prolactin on human osteoblasts: inhibition of cell growth and mineralization. J Cell Biochem. 2009;107 (4):677–85.
Shozu M, Akasofu K, Harada T, Kubota Y. A new cause of female pseudohermaphroditism: placental aromatase deficiency. J Clin Endocrinol Metab. 1991;72(3):560–6.
Siddiqui AH, Irani RA, Zhang W, Wang W, Blackwell SC, Kellems RE, Xia Y. Angiotensin receptor agonistic autoantibody-mediated soluble fms-like tyrosine kinase-1 induction contributes to impaired adrenal vasculature and decreased aldosterone production in preeclampsia. Hypertension. 2013;61(2):472–9.

Siiteri P, MacDonald P. The utilization of circulating dehydroepiandrosterone sulfate for estrogen synthesis during human pregnancy. Steroids. 1963;2:713–30.

Siiteri PK, MacDonald PC. Placental estrogen biosynthesis during human pregnancy. J Clin Endocrinol Metab. 1966;26(7):751–61.

Siiteri PK, Febres F, Clemens LE, Chang RJ, Gondos B, Stites D. Progesterone and maintenance of pregnancy: is progesterone nature's immunosuppressant? Ann N Y Acad Sci. 1977;286:384–97.

Smith R, Mesiano S, Chan EC, Brown S, Jaffe RB. Corticotropin-releasing hormone directly and preferentially stimulates dehydroepiandrosterone sulfate secretion by human fetal adrenal cortical cells. J Clin Endocrinol Metab. 1998;83(8):2916–20.

Soldin OP, Tractenberg RE, Hollowell JG, Jonklaas J, Janicic N, Soldin SJ. Trimester-specific changes in maternal thyroid hormone, thyrotropin, and thyroglobulin concentrations during gestation: trends and associations across trimesters in iodine sufficiency. Thyroid. 2004;14 (12):1084–90.

Soloff MS, Fernstrom MA, Periyasamy S, Soloff S, Baldwin S, Wieder M. Regulation of oxytocin receptor concentration in rat uterine explants by estrogen and progesterone. Can J Biochem Cell Biol. 1983;61(7):625–30.

Stagnaro-Green A, Abalovich M, Alexander E, Azizi F, Mestman J, Negro R, Nixon A, Pearce EN, Soldin OP, Sullivan S. Guidelines of the American Thyroid Association for the diagnosis and management of thyroid disease during pregnancy and postpartum. Thyroid. 2011;21 (10):1081–125.

Strauss JF, Martinez F, Kiriakidou M. Placental steroid hormone synthesis: unique features and unanswered questions. Biol Reprod. 1996;54(2):303–11.

Sun K, Yang K, Challis JR. Differential expression of 11 beta-hydroxysteroid dehydrogenase types 1 and 2 in human placenta and fetal membranes. J Clin Endocrinol Metab. 1997;82 (1):300–5.

Sun K, Adamson SL, Yang K, Challis JR. Interconversion of cortisol and cortisone by 11beta-hydroxysteroid dehydrogenases type 1 and 2 in the perfused human placenta. Placenta. 1999;20 (1):13–9.

Tamma R, Colaianni G, Zhu LL, DiBenedetto A, Greco G, Montemurro G, Patano N, Strippoli M, Vergari R, Mancini L, Colucci S, Grano M, Faccio R, Liu X, Li J, Usmani S, Bachar M, Bab I, Nishimori K, Young LJ, Buettner C, Iqbal J, Sun L, Zaidi M, Zallone A. Oxytocin is an anabolic bone hormone. Proc Natl Acad Sci U S A. 2009;106(17):7149–54.

Tan JY, Loh KC, Yeo GS, Chee YC. Transient hyperthyroidism of hyperemesis gravidarum. BJOG. 2002;109(6):683–8.

Tan H, Yi L, Rote NS, Hurd WW, Mesiano S. Progesterone receptor-A and -B have opposite effects on proinflammatory gene expression in human myometrial cells: implications for progesterone actions in human pregnancy and parturition. J Clin Endocrinol Metab. 2012;97(5):E719–30.

Terzidou V, Sooranna SR, Kim LU, Thornton S, Bennett PR, Johnson MR. Mechanical stretch up-regulates the human oxytocin receptor in primary human uterine myocytes. J Clin Endocrinol Metab. 2005;90(1):237–46.

Thiery J. Induction of labor with prostaglandins. In: Keirse M, Anderson A, Benebroek-Gravenhorst J, editors. Human parturition. The Hague: Martinus Nijhoff; 1979. p. 155–64.

Thomson AJ, Telfer JF, Young A, Campbell S, Stewart CJ, Cameron IT, Greer IA, Norman JE. Leukocytes infiltrate the myometrium during human parturition: further evidence that labour is an inflammatory process. Hum Reprod. 1999;14(1):229–36.

Thurau K, Gruner A, Mason J, Dahlheim H. Tubular signal for the renin activity in the juxtaglomerular apparatus. Kidney Int Suppl. 1982;12:S55–62.

Togher KL, Togher KL, O'Keeffe MM, O'Keeffe MM, Khashan AS, Khashan AS, Gutierrez H, Gutierrez H, Kenny LC, Kenny LC, O'Keeffe GW, O'Keeffe GW. Epigenetic regulation of the placental HSD11B2 barrier and its role as a critical regulator of fetal development. Epigenetics. 2014;9(6):816–22.

Tsatsaris V, Goffin F, Munaut C, Brichant JF, Pignon MR, Noel A, Schaaps JP, Cabrol D, Frankenne F, Foidart JM. Overexpression of the soluble vascular endothelial growth factor receptor in preeclamptic patients: pathophysiological consequences. J Clin Endocrinol Metab. 2003;88(11):5555–63.

Tulchinsky D, Okada D. Hormones in human pregnancy: IV. Plasma progesterone. Am J Obstet Gynecol. 1975;121:293–9.

Tulchinsky D, Hobel CJ, Yeager E, Marshall JR. Plasma estrone, estradiol, estriol, progesterone, and 17-hydroxyprogesterone in human pregnancy. I. Normal pregnancy. Am J Obstet Gynecol. 1972;112(8):1095–100.

Turner M, Barre PE, Benjamin A, Goltzman D, Gascon-Barre M. Does the maternal kidney contribute to the increased circulating 1,25-dihydroxyvitamin D concentrations during pregnancy? Miner Electrolyte Metab. 1988;14(4):246–52.

Ueland K. Maternal cardiovascular dynamics. VII. Intrapartum blood volume changes. Am J Obstet Gynecol. 1976;126(6):671–7.

Wang W, Irani RA, Zhang Y, Ramin SM, Blackwell SC, Tao L, Kellems RE, Xia Y. Autoantibody-mediated complement C3a receptor activation contributes to the pathogenesis of preeclampsia. Hypertension. 2012;60(3):712–21.

Williams KC, Renthal NE, Condon JC, Gerard RD, Mendelson CR. MicroRNA-200a serves a key role in the decline of progesterone receptor function leading to term and preterm labor. Proc Natl Acad Sci U S A. 2012;109(19):7529–34.

Yamaleyeva LM, Pulgar VM, Lindsey SH, Yamane L, Varagic J, McGee C, daSilva M, Lopes Bonfa P, Gurley SB, Brosnihan KB. Uterine artery dysfunction in pregnant ACE2 knockout mice is associated with placental hypoxia and reduced umbilical blood flow velocity. Am J Physiol Endocrinol Metab. 2015;309(1):E84–94.

Yao W, Dai W, Shahnazari M, Pham A, Chen Z, Chen H, Guan M, Lane NE. Inhibition of the progesterone nuclear receptor during the bone linear growth phase increases peak bone mass in female mice. PLoS One. 2010;5(7):e11410.

Yemini M, Borenstein R, Dreazen E, Apelman Z, Mogilner BM, Kessler I, Lancet M. Prevention of premature labor by 17 alpha-hydroxyprogesterone caproate. Am J Obstet Gynecol. 1985;151 (5):574–7.

Yoshimura M, Hershman JM. Thyrotropic action of human chorionic gonadotropin. Thyroid. 1995;5(5):425–34.

Young A, Thomson AJ, Ledingham M, Jordan F, Greer IA, Norman JE. Immunolocalization of proinflammatory cytokines in myometrium, cervix, and fetal membranes during human parturition at term. Biol Reprod. 2002;66(2):445–9.

Young IR, Renfree MB, Mesiano S, Shaw G, Jenkin G, Smith R. The comparative physiology of parturition in mammals: hormones and parturition in mammals. In: Norris D, Lopez K, editors. Hormones and reproduction in vertebrates. London: Academic; 2010. p. 5.

Yu C, Chen Y, Cline GW, Zhang D, Zong H, Wang Y, Bergeron R, Kim JK, Cushman SW, Cooney GJ, Atcheson B, White MF, Kraegen EW, Shulman GI. Mechanism by which fatty acids inhibit insulin activation of insulin receptor substrate-1 (IRS-1)-associated phosphatidylinositol 3-kinase activity in muscle. J Biol Chem. 2002;277(52):50230–6.

Zhang H, Wada J, Hida K, Tsuchiyama Y, Hiragushi K, Shikata K, Wang H, Lin S, Kanwar YS, Makino H. Collectrin, a collecting duct-specific transmembrane glycoprotein, is a novel homolog of ACE2 and is developmentally regulated in embryonic kidneys. J Biol Chem. 2001;276 (20):17132–9.

Zhou Y, McMaster M, Woo K, Janatpour M, Perry J, Karpanen T, Alitalo K, Damsky C, Fisher SJ. Vascular endothelial growth factor ligands and receptors that regulate human cytotrophoblast survival are dysregulated in severe preeclampsia and hemolysis, elevated liver enzymes, and low platelets syndrome. Am J Pathol. 2002;160(4):1405–23.

Zhou CC, Zhang Y, Irani RA, Zhang H, Mi T, Popek EJ, Hicks MJ, Ramin SM, Kellems RE, Xia Y. Angiotensin receptor agonistic autoantibodies induce pre-eclampsia in pregnant mice. Nat Med. 2008;14(8):855–62.

Zisman LS. ACE and ACE2: a tale of two enzymes. Eur Heart J. 2005;26(4):322–4.

Growth Hormones and Aging

26

Changhan D. Lee and Valter D. Longo

Abstract

The endocrine system coordinates and regulates various physiological functions and has a profound influence on the aging process. Studies from multiple model organisms indicate that hormones that regulate growth and metabolism can also play central roles in aging and the incidence of age-related diseases. The growth hormone (GH) and insulin-like growth factor 1 (IGF-1) signaling pathways represent perhaps the most potent and best characterized pro-aging axis. In mammals, GH and IGF-1 activity also contributes to age-related diseases, including cancer and diabetes. Growth factors can affect disease progress, in part, by regulating cellular resistance to stress and by the inhibiting stem cell-dependent regeneration. Here, we discuss the GH-IGF-1 axis, its connections with the recently identified mitochondrial-derived endocrine factor, and their effect on aging and age-related diseases.

Keywords

Growth hormone • Insulin-like growth factor 1 (IGF-1) • Caloric restriction • Mitochondrial-derived peptides • Humanin • MOTS-c

C.D. Lee (✉)
Davis School of Gerontology, University of Southern California, Los Angeles, CA, USA
e-mail: changhan.lee@usc.edu

V.D. Longo (✉)
Davis School of Gerontology, University of Southern California, Los Angeles, CA, USA

IFOM, FIRC Institute of Molecular Oncology, Milano, Italy
e-mail: vlongo@usc.edu

A. Belfiore, D. LeRoith (eds.), *Principles of Endocrinology and Hormone Action*,
Endocrinology, https://doi.org/10.1007/978-3-319-44675-2_27

Contents

Introduction

Aging is accompanied by a progressive dysfunction of the endocrine system that ultimately affects hormone levels. Based on studies from model organisms, hormones, particularly those involved in growth, can regulate the rate of aging and incidence of age-related diseases. The growth hormone (GH) and insulin-like growth factor 1 (IGF-1) (GH/IGF-1) axis includes a set of genes, which have well characterized pro-aging functions in various model organisms. In mice and possibly humans, high GH/IGF-1 axis activity also contributes to diseases, including cancer and diabetes. One possible connection between growth factors and diseases is their effect on both the sensitization to stress of a variety of cell types and their role in the inhibition of stem cell-dependent regeneration. Here, we discuss the GH/IGF-1 axis, its effect on aging and age-related diseases, and its connections with the recently identified mitochondrial-derived endocrine factors in the regulation of aging.

The Somatotropic Axis

The GH/IGF-1 Axis Overview

Growth hormone (GH), also called somatotropin, is synthesized and secreted by somatotropic cells in the anterior pituitary gland in a pulsatile manner. Release of GH in humans, which is strongly associated with sleep, exercise, and metabolism, begins to decline after age 20 (Bartke et al. 2013). Its secretion is largely regulated by the hypothalamic growth hormone-releasing hormone (GHRH) and somatostatin (SST). A key role of GH is to induce IGF-1 expression in the liver via specific receptors, which are also expressed in other cell types including adipocytes and muscle (156, 208). Hepatic production accounts for >80% of circulating IGF-1, which is known to be a major mediator of many GH actions. The sharp age-related fall in GH secretion and serum concentration is accompanied by the decline in circulating IGF-1 levels (Bartke et al. 2013; Ho et al. 1987; Iranmanesh et al. 1991; Zadik et al. 1985; Juul et al. 1994), which is affected by protein intake (Levine et al. 2014) (Fig. 1).

GH exerts mitogenic and metabolic effects both directly and through the stimulation of IGF-1 and the inhibition of insulin actions. The GH/IGF-1 axis is a major regulator of fetal and postnatal growth (Baker et al. 1993; Cohen et al. 2010; Randhawa and Cohen 2005). Also, when nutrients are abundant, the GH-induced stimulation of IGF-1 and insulin is important for anabolic storage and growth of lean body mass (LBM), adipose tissue, and glycogen reserves (Kaplan and Cohen 2007). However, under nutrient-restricted conditions, such as fasting, GH acts as a lipolytic factor that largely targets adipose tissue, leading to an increased release of free fatty acids (FFAs) into the circulation (Vijayakumar et al. 2010; Gormsen et al. 2007; Moller et al. 2003).

GH/IGF-1 Axis and Aging

The GH/IGF-1 axis is strongly implicated in the regulation of aging and age-related diseases. Mice with congenital GH deficiency experience a dwarf phenotype and significantly extended lifespan and healthspan. Ames, Snell, and little mice carry mutations (*prop-1*, *pit-1*, *Ghrhr*, respectively) that cause GH deficiency, leading to dwarfism and extended lifespan (>50%, >40%, and >20%, respectively) (Brown-Borg et al. 1996; Flurkey et al. 2001). GH receptor/binding protein (GHR/BP) knockout mice (GHRKO), which were initially developed to model the human Laron syndrome, exhibit a 90% reduction in circulating IGF-1 levels and dwarfism

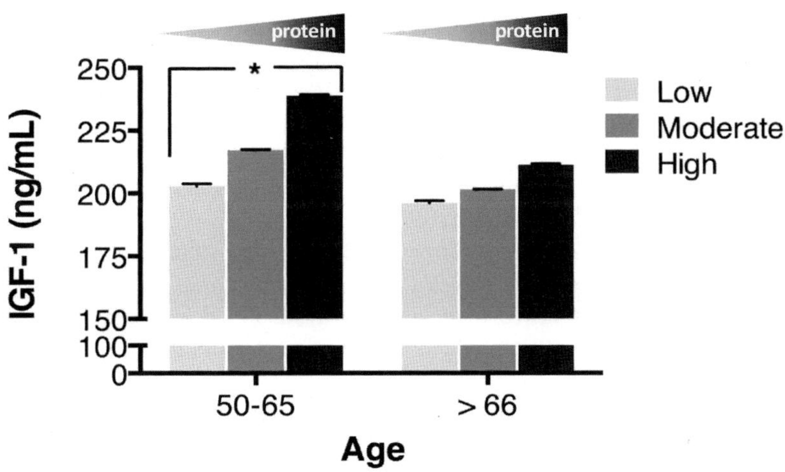

Fig. 1 Circulating IGF-1 levels of subjects with different protein consumptions among 50–65 and >66 years of age. IGF-1 levels were measured in 2,253 participants of NHANES III, a nationally representative, cross-sectional study. Subjects were categorized by percent of calorie intake from protein into a (i) high-protein group (20% or more of calories from proteins), a (ii) moderate-protein group (10–19% of calories from proteins), or a (iii) low-protein group (less than 10% of calories from proteins). Data points represent the mean ± SEM. $*p < 0.01$ (Figure adapted from Levine et al. 2014)

and an approximately 50% increase in lifespan (Zhou et al. 1997; Coschigano et al. 2000). On the contrary, GH-overexpressing transgenic mice can exhibit a 50% decrease in mean lifespan (Bartke 2003) and experience kidney dysfunction, increased age-dependent liver alterations, and neoplasms (Wolf et al. 1993). IGF-1 is potentially a major mediator of the effects of GH on aging, and inhibiting its signaling can result in lifespan extension. Notably, a common characteristic of the GH-deficient and GHRKO mice is the significant decrease of circulating IGF-1 levels. The heterozygous deletion of IGF-1 receptor (IGF-1R) extends lifespan in female, but not male, mice (Holzenberger et al. 2003). In contrast, transgenic mice expressing an antagonistic analog of GH, which has a very modest reduction in serum IGF-1 and eventually reach normal body size, are not long-lived (Coschigano et al. 2003). However, mice with liver-specific *IGF-1* gene deletion (LID) or inactivation at 1-month postnatal (LI-IGF-1 −/−), which lead to ~75% reduction in circulating IGF-1 and a compensatory increase in GH levels, are slightly smaller and only live longer (16%) if they are female (Sjogren et al. 1999; Yakar et al. 1999; Svensson et al. 2011). Because both GH- and GHR-deficient mice live over 40% longer and considering that they affect both IGF-1 and insulin, as well as many other pathways, it is likely that IGF-1 signaling is only an effector of the pro-aging role of GH. In humans, GHR deficiency also causes severe IGF-1 deficiency and has been shown to protect against cancer (Guevara-Aguirre et al. 2011; Steuerman et al. 2011) and diabetes (Guevara-Aguirre et al. 2011, 2015), but data on lifespan is yet to be collected.

At the cellular level, IGF-1 acts through its specific receptor (IGF-1R) and, with less affinity, to the structurally related insulin receptors (IRs) in various tissues (Slaaby 2015). Insulin receptor substrates 1 and 2 (IRS-1 and IRS-2) transduce signals from the IGF-1R and the IR that activate several signaling cascades. The global deletion of *Irs1* (*Irs1*$^{-/-}$) caused a 17% increase in lifespan in female mice (Selman et al. 2008a, 2011), and the global deletion of *Irs2* (*Irs2*$^{-/-}$) significantly shortened lifespan, largely due to diabetes (Selman et al. 2008a). In contrast, mice carrying a heterozygous mutant *Irs2* (*Irs2*$^{+/-}$) have been reported to experience an increase in mean lifespan of 17% by one group (Taguchi et al. 2007), but not by another group due to unresolved differences (Selman et al. 2008b). The insulin/IGF-1 signaling (IIS) pathway also involves a highly conserved nutrient-sensing network, which includes PI3K/AKT, the target of rapamycin (TOR) kinase and its downstream S6 kinase (S6K), all implicated as pro-aging factors (Fontana et al. 2010). Recently, IGF-1 signaling has also been connected to another pro-aging enzyme implicated in aging in both yeast and mice: the protein kinase A (PKA) (Fabrizio et al. 2001; Cheng et al. 2014).

In yeast, which does not express an IGF-1-like gene, deleting the orthologs of genes functioning in mammalian GH/IGF-1 signaling causes a major extension of longevity (Fabrizio et al. 2001). Mutations in *RAS* (*RAS2*) and/or *TOR-S6K* (*TOR-SCH9*) increase lifespan by more than 200% while elevating stress resistance against oxidants, genotoxins, and heat shock (Longo and Finch 2003). Similarly, in *C. elegans*, mutations in the human homologs of insulin/IGF-1 receptor (*daf-2*) and PI3K (*age-1*) extend lifespan to 200% and show increased resistance to thermal and oxidative stress (Kleemann and Murphy 2009). In *D. melanogaster*, mutations in the insulin receptor substrate (*Chico*) lead to a 150% lifespan extension (Giannakou and Partridge 2007). In humans, a functional mutation in the IGF-1R, which confers partial IGF-1 resistance, was more prevalent in centenarians, as compared to controls without familial longevity (Suh et al. 2008). Further, in exceptionally long-lived individuals (nonagenarians), low levels of circulating IGF-1 were correlated with their prolonged survival in cancer-free females, but not males, and in both sexes with a history of cancer (Milman et al. 2014). Another study showed that the offspring of centenarians had relatively lower circulating IGF-1 bioactivity compared to offspring-matched controls, which was inversely related to insulin sensitivity (Vitale et al. 2012).

Dietary Restriction (DR) GH/IGF-1 Signaling and Aging

Caloric restriction (CR), which if it includes a restriction of protein intake reduces also both insulin and IGF-1 levels, is the most effective and reproducible intervention known to decelerate the rate of aging and increase healthspan in model organisms ranging from yeast to worms, flies, rodents, and nonhuman primates (Fontana et al. 2010). In 1934, Crowell and McCay reported that white rats fed with a calorie-restricted diet with sufficient nutrients from the time of weaning resulted in lifespans nearly doubling (McCay et al. 1989). A 30+ year longitudinal adult-onset CR study in rhesus monkeys performed at the Wisconsin National Primate Research Center (WNPRC) shows that CR (30%) delays disease onset and mortality, with a 50% decrease in cancer incidence (Colman et al. 2009, 2014). However, a comparable 20 + year study performed at the National Institute on Aging (NIA) does not show extended lifespan in CR monkeys, although this dietary intervention reduces the incidence of diabetes and cancer and thus improves healthspan (Mattison et al. 2012). The disparities between the WNPRC and NIA studies were largely attributed to differences in diet composition and the genetic origin of the monkeys. However, there are multiple trade-offs resulting from a severe and chronic CR, which include impaired wound healing (Hunt et al. 2012) and immune responses (Kristan 2008). Also, because proteins and amino acids are the major regulators of GH/IGF-1 axis activity, it is not clear whether CR without protein restriction can actually be effective in lifespan and healthspan. In both mice and humans, a high-protein intake combined with CR reversed its beneficial effects (Brandhorst et al. 2013; Fontana et al. 2008).

The long-lived GH/IGF-1 mutant mice and wild-type mice on CR share several phenotypes, including reduced levels of circulating IGF-1 and enhanced insulin sensitivity (Lee and Longo 2011; Masternak et al. 2009; Bonkowski et al. 2009; Dominici et al. 2002). They are also both protected against several age-related pathologies and conditions, such as cancer and insulin resistance (Omodei and Fontana 2011; Ikeno et al. 2013). The anticancer effect of CR on spontaneous and induced tumors can be mediated, at least in part, by the reduction in IGF-1 levels and an increase in corticosteroid levels (Longo and Fontana 2010). GHRKO mice do not benefit from further lifespan extension and improved insulin sensitivity by CR, suggesting overlapping mechanisms (Bonkowski et al. 2009; Arum et al. 2009), whereas the GH-deficient Ames mice showed further increase in lifespan by CR (Bartke et al. 2001). These studies suggest that the GH/IGF-1 axis and CR affect aging in overlapping, but not identical, mechanisms, and additional components, such as diet and metabolic signals, should be carefully considered.

Although CR can extend lifespan and/or healthspan, it is undoubtedly a very challenging dietary regimen with potential malnutrition. Thus, a CR-mimicking diet that delivers the beneficial effects without severe abstinence from food would be an exciting field of investigation. A recent report showed that a fasting-mimicking diet (FMD), designed based on its ability to reduce IGF-1, increases IGFBP-1, reduces glucose, and increases ketone bodies comparably to water-only fasting, while maximizing nourishment, and minimizing adverse effects, showed significant increase in median lifespan (25.5 vs. 28.3 months) in mice (Brandhorst et al. 2015). A pilot randomized clinical trial in which subjects consumed an FMD for five consecutive days every month for 3 months and returned to normal diet in between FMDs showed a significant reduction of circulating IGF-1 (~24%) and had beneficial effects on fasting glucose, the inflammatory marker CRP, and abdominal fat (Brandhorst et al. 2015). Notably, the FMD reduced body weight without loss of lean mass relative to total weight (Brandhorst et al. 2015).

Interventions Targeting the GH/IGF-1 Axis

Interventions to inhibit the GH/IGF-1 axis to increase lifespan and healthspan are promising but should be approached with caution. As mentioned above, this axis is integrated with other endocrine systems, such as insulin, and, thus, targeted interventions may lead to diabetic symptoms. For instance, somatostatin analogs, which lower GH production and reduce circulating IGF-1 levels, also suppress insulin secretion. A more promising approach may be to target the GHR using compounds similar to pegvisomant, a dominant negative GH mimetic that is FDA approved for the treatment of acromegaly. Pegvisomant reduces serum IGF-1 levels by up to 90% (20 mg/day for 12 weeks) (Trainer et al. 2000) and also acts as an insulin sensitizer that counters the diabetogenic action of GH and thus improves glucose metabolism (Thankamony et al. 2014; Higham et al. 2009).

GH/IGF-1 Axis and Mitochondrial-Derived Endocrine Factors

Mitochondrial dysfunction is strongly implicated in aging, but the mechanistic details are poorly understood. Mitochondria are increasingly being appreciated as signaling organelles, especially in light of recent studies that clearly indicate the importance of a balanced mitochondrial-to-nuclear communication in coordinating homeostasis. Mitochondria have retained a semiautonomous genetic system, complete with its own independent genome known to encode for 13 proteins that are all part of the electron transport chain. The recently discovered two peptides (MDPs), as described below, expand the mitochondrial genetic repertoire and provide a novel category of hormones that may influence aging and age-related diseases. Notably, MDPs may represent a novel mitochondrial component of the GH/IGF-1 signaling pathway that regulates longevity.

Humanin

Humanin was the first short open reading frame (sORFs) to be identified in the mtDNA, suggesting the existence of a larger mitochondrial genetic repertoire (Lee et al. 2013; Hashimoto et al. 2001a; Guo et al. 2003). Humanin is a conserved polypeptide (Guo et al. 2003) encoded as a 75 bp polycistronic sORF within the 16S rRNA, discovered in 2001 from an unbiased functional screen using a cDNA library created from the surviving brain fraction of an Alzheimer's disease (AD) patient (Hashimoto et al. 2001a, b). Its expression is age dependent (Bachar et al. 2010; Muzumdar et al. 2009) and found in various tissues and also in circulation in rodents and humans (Hashimoto et al. 2001a). Humanin is secreted from cells and found in circulation (Hashimoto et al. 2001a; Muzumdar et al. 2010) and is proposed to act through two different types of receptors (Ying et al. 2004; Hashimoto et al. 2009). Humanin binds to IGF-binding protein 3 (IGFBP-3), which regulates IGF-1 bioactivity, with high affinity and specificity (Ikonen et al. 2003). Notably, circulating humanin levels are (i) negatively correlated with circulating IGF-1 levels and (ii) positively correlated with longevity (Lee et al. 2014). The long-lived Ames mice and Laron syndrome patients, mentioned above, had elevated circulating humanin levels, whereas short-lived GH-transgenic mice had reduced levels (Lee et al. 2014). Furthermore, GH or IGF-1 treatment reduced circulating humanin levels in both mice and human subjects (Lee et al. 2014). This suggests a potential coordinated mitochondrial element to the GH/IGF-1 regulation of aging. At the cellular level, humanin acts as an antiapoptotic factor that binds to and inhibits the activity of the proapoptotic protein BAX (Guo et al. 2003). Its cytoprotective effects were first tested and confirmed in vitro against mutant forms of amyloid precursor protein (APP) and presenilins 1 and 2 (PS1/2), which cause familial AD, in neurons (Hashimoto et al. 2001a). A wide range of in vitro and in vivo studies, which cause variable levels of oxidative stress, now indicate that humanin protects against various types of stress or disease states, including AD, cancer, and type 1 diabetes (Lee et al. 2013; Yen et al. 2013).

MOTS-c

MOTS-c (mitochondrial ORF of the 12S rRNA-c) is a recently identified MDP. As its name implies, it is encoded as a polycistronic 51 bp gene within the 12S rRNA of the mtDNA, yielding a 16-amino acid peptide (Lee et al. 2015; Zarse and Ristow 2015). It is detected in various tissues and in circulation in an age-dependent manner

(Lee et al. 2015). Its primary target organ appears to be the skeletal muscle, and its cellular actions inhibit the folate cycle and its tethered de novo purine biosynthesis, causing a significant accumulation of AICAR and consequent AMPK activation; MOTS-c shares strikingly similar effects with the pro-longevity diabetes drug metformin (Martin-Montalvo et al. 2013; Hall 2015), which has also shown to target the folate/purine cycle (Cabreiro et al. 2013; Corominas-Faja et al. 2012). The intracellular effect of MOTS-c on glucose metabolism is mediated by AMPK and SIRT1 (Lee et al. 2015), two major proteins that work in concert with the GH/IGF-1 pathway to regulate aging (Lopez-Otin et al. 2013). This suggests that MOTS-c, similar to Humanin, may be a mitochondrial signal that is integrated with the GH/IGF-1 axis. In mice, MOTS-c regulates glucose homeostasis and significantly improves insulin sensitivity in aged and high-fat diet-fed mice, largely by targeting skeletal muscle (Lee et al. 2015). Notably, the mitochondrial m.1382A>C polymorphism, which is found specifically in the D4b2 haplogroup that is associated with exceptional longevity in the Japanese population (Alexe et al. 2007), causes a Lys14Gln variation that may have functional alterations (Fuku et al. 2015). Further studies are required to test if MOTS-c, and its analogs, can positively extend healthspan and/or lifespan in model organisms.

Conclusion

The GH/IGF-1 axis and its conserved downstream IIS pathways have been central to aging research and have provided much mechanistic insight into the regulation of lifespan and healthspan. Recent discoveries of additional age-dependent humoral factors, such as mitokines and MDPs, further expand the mechanistic breadth of the aging process. As mentioned above, the GH/IGF-1 axis seems to have overlapping, but not identical, mechanisms with CR on longevity, suggesting additional metabolism-related factors to be involved. Connecting these novel endocrine factors with DR and the GH/IGF-1 axis may unveil a more integrated multicomponent regulatory system of aging and also provide insight into the coordination of differential aging rates of various tissue types. Further, these endocrine factors can be used as biomarkers for the development of interventions that extend healthy lifespan.

References

Alexe G, et al. Enrichment of longevity phenotype in mtDNA haplogroups D4b2b, D4a, and D5 in the Japanese population. Hum Genet. 2007;121(3–4):347–56.

Arum O, Bonkowski MS, Rocha JS, Bartke A. The growth hormone receptor gene-disrupted mouse fails to respond to an intermittent fasting diet. Aging Cell. 2009;8(6):756–60.

Bachar AR, et al. Humanin is expressed in human vascular walls and has a cytoprotective effect against oxidized LDL-induced oxidative stress. Cardiovasc Res. 2010;88(2):360–6.

Baker J, Liu JP, Robertson EJ, Efstratiadis A. Role of insulin-like growth factors in embryonic and postnatal growth. Cell. 1993;75(1):73–82.

Bartke A. Can growth hormone (GH) accelerate aging? Evidence from GH-transgenic mice. Neuroendocrinology. 2003;78(4):210–6.

Bartke A, et al. Extending the lifespan of long-lived mice. Nature. 2001;414(6862):412.

Bartke A, Sun LY, Longo V. Somatotropic signaling: trade-offs between growth, reproductive development, and longevity. Physiol Rev. 2013;93(2):571–98.

Bonkowski MS, et al. Disruption of growth hormone receptor prevents calorie restriction from improving insulin action and longevity. PLoS One. 2009;4(2):e4567.

Brandhorst S, Wei M, Hwang S, Morgan TE, Longo VD. Short-term calorie and protein restriction provide partial protection from chemotoxicity but do not delay glioma progression. Exp Gerontol. 2013;48(10):1120–8.

Brandhorst S, et al. A periodic diet that mimics fasting promotes multi-system regeneration, enhanced cognitive performance, and healthspan. Cell Metab. 2015;22(1):86–99.

Brown-Borg HM, Borg KE, Meliska CJ, Bartke A. Dwarf mice and the ageing process. Nature. 1996;384(6604):33.

Cabreiro F, et al. Metformin retards aging in C. elegans by altering microbial folate and methionine metabolism. Cell. 2013;153(1):228–39.

Cheng CW, et al. Prolonged fasting reduces IGF-1/PKA to promote hematopoietic-stem-cell-based regeneration and reverse immunosuppression. Cell Stem Cell. 2014;14(6):810–23.

Cohen P, et al. Variable degree of growth hormone (GH) and insulin-like growth factor (IGF) sensitivity in children with idiopathic short stature compared with GH-deficient patients: evidence from an IGF-based dosing study of short children. J Clin Endocrinol Metab. 2010;95(5):2089–98.

Colman RJ, et al. Caloric restriction delays disease onset and mortality in rhesus monkeys. Science. 2009;325(5937):201–4.

Colman RJ, et al. Caloric restriction reduces age-related and all-cause mortality in rhesus monkeys. Nat Commun. 2014;5:3557.

Corominas-Faja B, et al. Metabolomic fingerprint reveals that metformin impairs one-carbon metabolism in a manner similar to the antifolate class of chemotherapy drugs. Aging. 2012;4 (7):480–98.

Coschigano KT, Clemmons D, Bellush LL, Kopchick JJ. Assessment of growth parameters and life span of GHR/BP gene-disrupted mice. Endocrinology. 2000;141(7):2608–13.

Coschigano KT, et al. Deletion, but not antagonism, of the mouse growth hormone receptor results in severely decreased body weights, insulin, and insulin-like growth factor I levels and increased life span. Endocrinology. 2003;144(9):3799–810.

Dominici FP, Hauck S, Argentino DP, Bartke A, Turyn D. Increased insulin sensitivity and upregulation of insulin receptor, insulin receptor substrate (IRS)-1 and IRS-2 in liver of Ames dwarf mice. J Endocrinol. 2002;173(1):81–94.

Fabrizio P, Pozza F, Pletcher SD, Gendron CM, Longo VD. Regulation of longevity and stress resistance by Sch9 in yeast. Science. 2001;292(5515):288–90.

Flurkey K, Papaconstantinou J, Miller RA, Harrison DE. Lifespan extension and delayed immune and collagen aging in mutant mice with defects in growth hormone production. Proc Natl Acad Sci U S A. 2001;98(12):6736–41.

Fontana L, Weiss EP, Villareal DT, Klein S, Holloszy JO. Long-term effects of calorie or protein restriction on serum IGF-1 and IGFBP-3 concentration in humans. Aging Cell. 2008;7(5):681–7.

Fontana L, Partridge L, Longo VD. Extending healthy life span – from yeast to humans. Science. 2010;328(5976):321–6.

Fuku N, et al. The mitochondrial-derived peptide MOTS-c: a player in exceptional longevity? Aging Cell. 2015;14:921.

Giannakou ME, Partridge L. Role of insulin-like signalling in Drosophila lifespan. Trends Biochem Sci. 2007;32(4):180–8.

Gormsen LC, et al. Dose-response effects of free fatty acids on glucose and lipid metabolism during somatostatin blockade of growth hormone and insulin in humans. J Clin Endocrinol Metab. 2007;92(5):1834–42.

Guevara-Aguirre J, et al. Growth hormone receptor deficiency is associated with a major reduction in pro-aging signaling, cancer, and diabetes in humans. Sci Transl Med. 2011;3(70):70ra13.
Guevara-Aguirre J, et al. GH receptor deficiency in Ecuadorian adults is associated with obesity and enhanced insulin sensitivity. J Clin Endocrinol Metab. 2015;100(7):2589–96.
Guo B, et al. Humanin peptide suppresses apoptosis by interfering with Bax activation. Nature. 2003;423(6938):456–61.
Hall SS. A trial for the ages. Science. 2015;349(6254):1274–8.
Hashimoto Y, et al. A rescue factor abolishing neuronal cell death by a wide spectrum of familial Alzheimer's disease genes and Abeta. Proc Natl Acad Sci U S A. 2001a;98(11):6336–41.
Hashimoto Y, et al. Mechanisms of neuroprotection by a novel rescue factor humanin from Swedish mutant amyloid precursor protein. Biochem Biophys Res Commun. 2001b;283(2):460–8.
Hashimoto Y, Kurita M, Aiso S, Nishimoto I, Matsuoka M. Humanin inhibits neuronal cell death by interacting with a cytokine receptor complex or complexes involving CNTF receptor alpha/WSX-1/gp130. Mol Biol Cell. 2009;20(12):2864–73.
Higham CE, Rowles S, Russell-Jones D, Umpleby AM, Trainer PJ. Pegvisomant improves insulin sensitivity and reduces overnight free fatty acid concentrations in patients with acromegaly. J Clin Endocrinol Metab. 2009;94(7):2459–63.
Ho KY, et al. Effects of sex and age on the 24-hour profile of growth hormone secretion in man: importance of endogenous estradiol concentrations. J Clin Endocrinol Metab. 1987;64(1):51–8.
Holzenberger M, et al. IGF-1 receptor regulates lifespan and resistance to oxidative stress in mice. Nature. 2003;421(6919):182–7.
Hunt ND, et al. Effect of calorie restriction and refeeding on skin wound healing in the rat. Age (Dordr). 2012;34(6):1453–8.
Ikeno Y, et al. Do Ames dwarf and calorie-restricted mice share common effects on age-related pathology? Pathobiol Aging Age Relat Dis. 2013;3:20833.
Ikonen M, et al. Interaction between the Alzheimer's survival peptide humanin and insulin-like growth factor-binding protein 3 regulates cell survival and apoptosis. Proc Natl Acad Sci U S A. 2003;100(22):13042–7.
Iranmanesh A, Lizarralde G, Veldhuis JD. Age and relative adiposity are specific negative determinants of the frequency and amplitude of growth hormone (GH) secretory bursts and the half-life of endogenous GH in healthy men. J Clin Endocrinol Metab. 1991;73(5):1081–8.
Juul A, et al. Serum insulin-like growth factor-I in 1030 healthy children, adolescents, and adults: relation to age, sex, stage of puberty, testicular size, and body mass index. J Clin Endocrinol Metab. 1994;78(3):744–52.
Kaplan SA, Cohen P. The somatomedin hypothesis 2007: 50 years later. J Clin Endocrinol Metab. 2007;92(12):4529–35.
Kleemann GA, Murphy CT. The endocrine regulation of aging in *Caenorhabditis elegans*. Mol Cell Endocrinol. 2009;299(1):51–7.
Kristan DM. Calorie restriction and susceptibility to intact pathogens. Age (Dordr). 2008;30(2–3):147–56.
Lee C, Longo VD. Fasting vs dietary restriction in cellular protection and cancer treatment: from model organisms to patients. Oncogene. 2011;30(30):3305–16.
Lee C, Yen K, Cohen P. Humanin: a harbinger of mitochondrial-derived peptides? Trends Endocrinol Metab: TEM. 2013;24:222.
Lee C, et al. IGF-I regulates the age-dependent signaling peptide humanin. Aging Cell. 2014;13(5):958–61.
Lee C, et al. The mitochondrial-derived peptide MOTS-c promotes metabolic homeostasis and reduces obesity and insulin resistance. Cell Metab. 2015;21(3):443–54.
Levine ME, et al. Low protein intake is associated with a major reduction in IGF-1, cancer, and overall mortality in the 65 and younger but not older population. Cell Metab. 2014;19(3):407–17.
Longo VD, Finch CE. Evolutionary medicine: from dwarf model systems to healthy centenarians? Science. 2003;299(5611):1342–6.

Longo VD, Fontana L. Calorie restriction and cancer prevention: metabolic and molecular mechanisms. Trends Pharmacol Sci. 2010;31(2):89–98.

Lopez-Otin C, Blasco MA, Partridge L, Serrano M, Kroemer G. The hallmarks of aging. Cell. 2013;153(6):1194–217.

Martin-Montalvo A, et al. Metformin improves healthspan and lifespan in mice. Nat Commun. 2013;4:2192.

Masternak MM, Panici JA, Bonkowski MS, Hughes LF, Bartke A. Insulin sensitivity as a key mediator of growth hormone actions on longevity. J Gerontol A Biol Sci Med Sci. 2009;64(5):516–21.

Mattison JA, et al. Impact of caloric restriction on health and survival in rhesus monkeys from the NIA study. Nature. 2012;489(7415):318–21.

McCay CM, Crowell MF, Maynard LA. The effect of retarded growth upon the length of life span and upon the ultimate body size. 1935. Nutrition. 1989;5(3):155–71; discussion 172.

Milman S, et al. Low insulin-like growth factor-1 level predicts survival in humans with exceptional longevity. Aging Cell. 2014;13(4):769–71.

Moller N, Gjedsted J, Gormsen L, Fuglsang J, Djurhuus C. Effects of growth hormone on lipid metabolism in humans. Growth Horm IGF Res. 2003;13(Suppl A):S18–21.

Muzumdar RH, et al. Humanin: a novel central regulator of peripheral insulin action. PLoS One. 2009;4(7):e6334.

Muzumdar RH, et al. Acute humanin therapy attenuates myocardial ischemia and reperfusion injury in mice. Arterioscler Thromb Vasc Biol. 2010;30(10):1940–8.

Omodei D, Fontana L. Calorie restriction and prevention of age-associated chronic disease. FEBS Lett. 2011;585(11):1537–42.

Randhawa R, Cohen P. The role of the insulin-like growth factor system in prenatal growth. Mol Genet Metab. 2005;86(1–2):84–90.

Selman C, et al. Evidence for lifespan extension and delayed age-related biomarkers in insulin receptor substrate 1 null mice. FASEB J: Off Publ Fed Am Soc Exp Biol. 2008a;22(3):807–18.

Selman C, Lingard S, Gems D, Partridge L, Withers DJ. Comment on "Brain IRS2 signaling coordinates life span and nutrient homeostasis". Science. 2008b;320(5879):1012; author reply 1012.

Selman C, Partridge L, Withers DJ. Replication of extended lifespan phenotype in mice with deletion of insulin receptor substrate 1. PLoS One. 2011;6(1):e16144.

Sjogren K, et al. Liver-derived insulin-like growth factor I (IGF-I) is the principal source of IGF-I in blood but is not required for postnatal body growth in mice. Proc Natl Acad Sci U S A. 1999;96(12):7088–92.

Slaaby R. Specific insulin/IGF1 hybrid receptor activation assay reveals IGF1 as a more potent ligand than insulin. Sci Rep. 2015;5:7911.

Steuerman R, Shevah O, Laron Z. Congenital IGF1 deficiency tends to confer protection against post-natal development of malignancies. Eur J Endocrinol/Eur Fed Endocr Soc. 2011;164(4):485–9.

Suh Y, et al. Functionally significant insulin-like growth factor I receptor mutations in centenarians. Proc Natl Acad Sci U S A. 2008;105(9):3438–42.

Svensson J, et al. Liver-derived IGF-I regulates mean life span in mice. PLoS One. 2011;6(7): e22640.

Taguchi A, Wartschow LM, White MF. Brain IRS2 signaling coordinates life span and nutrient homeostasis. Science. 2007;317(5836):369–72.

Thankamony A, et al. Short-term administration of pegvisomant improves hepatic insulin sensitivity and reduces soleus muscle intramyocellular lipid content in young adults with type 1 diabetes. J Clin Endocrinol Metab. 2014;99(2):639–47.

Trainer PJ, et al. Treatment of acromegaly with the growth hormone-receptor antagonist pegvisomant. N Engl J Med. 2000;342(16):1171–7.

Vijayakumar A, Novosyadlyy R, Wu Y, Yakar S, LeRoith D. Biological effects of growth hormone on carbohydrate and lipid metabolism. Growth Horm IGF Res. 2010;20(1):1–7.

Vitale G, et al. Low circulating IGF-I bioactivity is associated with human longevity: findings in centenarians' offspring. Aging. 2012;4(9):580–9.

Wolf E, et al. Effects of long-term elevated serum levels of growth hormone on life expectancy of mice: lessons from transgenic animal models. Mech Ageing Dev. 1993;68(1–3):71–87.

Yakar S, et al. Normal growth and development in the absence of hepatic insulin-like growth factor I. Proc Natl Acad Sci U S A. 1999;96(13):7324–9.

Yen K, Lee C, Mehta H, Cohen P. The emerging role of the mitochondrial-derived peptide humanin in stress resistance. J Mol Endocrinol. 2013;50(1):R11–9.

Ying G, et al. Humanin, a newly identified neuroprotective factor, uses the G protein-coupled formylpeptide receptor-like-1 as a functional receptor. J Immunol. 2004;172(11):7078–85.

Zadik Z, Chalew SA, McCarter Jr RJ, Meistas M, Kowarski AA. The influence of age on the 24-hour integrated concentration of growth hormone in normal individuals. J Clin Endocrinol Metab. 1985;60(3):513–6.

Zarse K, Ristow M. A mitochondrially encoded hormone ameliorates obesity and insulin resistance. Cell Metab. 2015;21(3):355–6.

Zhou Y, et al. A mammalian model for Laron syndrome produced by targeted disruption of the mouse growth hormone receptor/binding protein gene (the Laron mouse). Proc Natl Acad Sci U S A. 1997;94(24):13215–20.

Principles of Endocrine Diseases

27

Elizabeth Lowden and Peter Kopp

Abstract

Broadly defined, endocrine diseases can be defined as disorders of (1) hormone deficiency, (2) hormone excess, (3) hormone resistance, (4) defects in transport proteins, and (5) benign or malignant tumors of the hormone-producing glands. These diseases can, in part, be caused by mutations in single genes (monogenic disorders), others result from the interaction of genetic predisposition and lifestyle factors (complex or multifactorial disorders), some are solely due to environmental factors (nutritional iodine deficiency), and several disorders are the result of a dysregulated immune system (autoimmune disorders). A detailed understanding of the underlying pathophysiology is of significant importance because it can provide means for an accurate diagnosis, therapy and intervention, and the development of novel therapeutic modalities.

Keywords

Hormone • Hormone receptor • Feedback loop • Hormone resistance • Binding proteins • Genetics • Endocrine neoplasia

Contents

E. Lowden • P. Kopp (✉)
Division of Endocrinology, Metabolism and Molecular Medicine, Feinberg School of Medicine, Northwestern University, Chicago, IL, USA
e-mail: p-kopp@northwestern.edu

A. Belfiore, D. LeRoith (eds.), *Principles of Endocrinology and Hormone Action*, Endocrinology, https://doi.org/10.1007/978-3-319-44675-2_28

Introduction

The endocrine system consists of several endocrine glands that secrete hormones into the blood stream. Hormones are chemical mediators that have been traditionally defined as exerting their action on one or several distant organs, but some can also exert local effects (Kronenberg et al. 2016; Jameson 2011). Together with the nervous and the immune system, the endocrine system plays a key role in the communication between different tissues in a multicellular organism and thus in the integration of fundamental physiologic processes such as development, growth, differentiation, reproduction, metabolism, circadian and other biological rhythms, and behavior.

Chemically, hormones are very diverse, and they can consist of amino acid derivatives (glycoproteins, peptides, modified amino acids, and amines), steroids, and eicosanoids. Some hormones require transport proteins to reach their site of action. Hormones exert their effect by binding to membrane receptors or intracellular cytosolic and nuclear receptors. Some but not all hormones exerting intracellular actions require transporters or channels to cross the plasma membrane, and defects in these transporters can result in diminished hormone action. Hormone effects can be of stimulatory or blocking nature, and they can be mediated through non-genomic or genomic actions. Some hormones have a multitude of target tissues, and their effect may vary between tissues and also depend on the developmental window, sex, age, or biorhythm. Other hormones have a single known target tissue. Some biological processes are under the control of several hormones with complex interactions, while others are regulated by a single hormone.

Categories of Disease

Very broadly defined, endocrine diseases can be defined as disorders of (1) hormone deficiency, (2) hormone excess, (3) hormone resistance, (4) defects in transport proteins, and (5) benign or malignant tumors of the hormone-producing glands. There is, however, frequent overlap between these categories. Many endocrine disorders are caused by mutations in single genes involved in the development or function of endocrine glands or hormone synthesis (monogenic disorders), while others result from the interaction of genetic predisposition and lifestyle factors (complex or multifactorial disorders) (Jameson and Kopp 2015a). Iodine deficiency, which can lead to endemic goiter and cretinism (abnormal development and mental impairment due to hypothyroidism), is an example of an isolated nutritional deficiency resulting in abnormal growth and dysfunction of an endocrine gland, the thyroid. Several chromosomal disorders can include endocrine abnormalities, among other manifestations.

Dysregulation of the immune system plays an important etiological role in common disorders such as autoimmune thyroid disease and diabetes mellitus type 1. A detailed understanding of the underlying pathophysiology resulting in endocrine disease is of significant importance because it can provide means for an accurate diagnosis, therapy and intervention, and the development of novel therapeutic modalities.

Hormone Deficiency

Insufficient hormone synthesis and secretion is a common phenomenon underlying endocrine disorders (Table 1). Deficiencies in hormone production by endocrine glands such as the thyroid, adrenal glands, ovaries, and testes are designated as primary deficiencies, whereas deficient pituitary or hypothalamic hormone secretion are often described as secondary or tertiary or central defects.

The mechanisms leading to hormone deficiency can consist in developmental defects of the endocrine organ; inborn defects in hormone synthesis; autoimmune processes that result in the disruption or stimulation of the hormonogenic process and/or inflammatory destruction of the gland; destruction of the gland by infectious,

Table 1 Selected examples of hormone deficiency disorders

	Hormone deficiency	Phenotypic manifestation
Hypothalamus	Vasopressin	Diabetes insipidus
	Growth hormone-releasing hormone (GHRH)	Dwarfism
	Gonadotropin-releasing hormone (GnRH)	Hypogonadotropic hypogonadism
Pituitary[a]	Growth hormone (GH)	Dwarfism
	Luteinizing hormone (LH) Follicle-stimulating hormone (FSH)	Hypogonadotropic hypogonadism
	Thyroid-stimulating hormone (TSH)	Central hypothyroidism
	Prolactin	Absent milk production
	Adrenocorticotropic hormone (ACTH)	Secondary adrenal insufficiency
Thyroid	Thyroxine (T4) Triiodothyronine (T3)	Hypothyroidism
Adrenal cortex	Cortisol	Adrenal insufficiency
Pancreas	Insulin	Diabetes mellitus
Ovaries	Estradiol Progesterone	Hypogonadism, amenorrhea, infertility
Testes	Testosterone	Hypogonadism, infertility

[a]Combined pituitary hormone deficiencies can include several or all anterior pituitary hormones

infiltrative, hemorrhagic, or malignant processes; or drugs that inhibit hormone synthesis or lead to partial or permanent tissue damage. For example, hypothyroidism, the insufficient production of thyroid hormones, is a common disorder caused by a multitude of mechanisms (Table 2). Most commonly, it is caused by an autoimmune thyroiditis (Hashimoto's thyroiditis) that leads to the destruction of the gland, most frequently after puberty (Tomer 2014). Hypothyroidism can, however, be congenital due to defects in the development of the thyroid gland or thyroid hormone biosynthesis. Similarly, defects in the hypothalamic-pituitary axis can also lead to isolated central hypothyroidism or hypothyroidism associated with other hormone deficiencies (combined pituitary hormone deficiency, CPHD). Therapy of hyperthyroidism with radioiodine or surgical removal of the thyroid can result in iatrogenic hypothyroidism.

The consequences of hormone deficiencies are generally well characterized, and the specific role of endocrine glands has historically been identified through the removal or destruction of these organs in experimental animals or human patients. For example, the preeminent role of thyroid in regulating growth and metabolism has been recognized after surgical removal of goiters in human patients. The resulting

Table 2 Examples of various etiologies of hypothyroidism

	Category	Comments
Congenital hypothyroidism	Developmental defects of the thyroid	Athyreosis Hemiagenesis Ectopic thyroid
	Defects in thyroid hormone synthesis	Multiple defects in the biochemical steps involved in thyroid hormone synthesis
	Isolated or combined pituitary defects resulting in deficient TSH secretion	Central hypothyroidism
	Partial or complete resistance to the stimulatory effects of TSH	Thyroid hypoplasia. Compensated or overt hypothyroidism
Acquired hypothyroidism	Autoimmune thyroid disease (Hashimoto's thyroiditis)	Blocking antibodies and/or destruction of the gland through inflammatory autoimmune process
	Destruction of the thyroid gland by radioiodine therapy or surgery	Consequence of therapy for hyperthyroidism or thyroid cancer
	Thyroiditis	Infectious or infiltrative processes Often preceded by hormone excess during the destructive process
	Drugs leading to inflammation and typically transient destruction of the gland Characteristic examples of involved drugs include amiodarone, interferon, tyrosine kinase inhibitors, immune checkpoint inhibitors	Often preceded by hormone excess during the destructive process

phenotype, termed *cachexia strumipriva* (cachexia caused by removal of a struma, i.e., an enlarged thyroid), led to recognition that cretinism (congenital thyroid hormone deficiency resulting in severe mental retardation) and myxedema (the historical designation for hypothyroidism) all result from absent or malfunctioning thyroid tissue. These observations then led to the first successful therapeutic attempts with extracts from animal thyroid tissue in the late nineteenth century, years before thyroxine (tetraiodothyronine, T4), the most abundant thyroid hormone, could be isolated and synthesized.

Similarly, diabetes mellitus type 1 is caused by the autoimmune destruction of the insulin-secreting pancreatic beta cells. The recognition that the annihilation of the pancreatic tail harboring the insulin-producing islets in animal models results in diabetes mellitus was essential for the subsequent isolation of insulin in 1921. The amino acid structure was then solved in the 1950s. The isolation of the coding sequence of the human *insulin (INS)* gene was the foundation for the synthesis of insulin by recombinant technologies, and, nowadays, biosynthetic recombinant insulin or insulin analogues with altered kinetic profiles have largely replaced insulin products obtained from animal sources.

Hormone deficiency can be partial or complete thereby resulting in a broad phenotypic spectrum ranging from very mild to very severe manifestations. While overt hormone deficiency is usually readily recognized, the detection of partial hormone deficiencies can, in part, be challenging, and it may need so-called dynamic testing.

Diagnosis of Hormone Deficiency

Hormone deficiencies are typically associated with characteristic signs and symptoms that permit to suspect the absence or decreased hormone levels. Mild deficiencies, particularly if developing insidiously over time, can be more difficult to recognize. In many instances, the direct measurement of hormones allows establishing the diagnosis (Sluss and Hayes 2016). Very often, this is combined with the determination of the associated pituitary hormones. For example, for the diagnosis of hypothyroidism, it is routine practice to measure thyroid stimulating hormone (TSH) and free or total thyroxine (T4). Because of the decrease in the negative feedback exerted by thyroid hormone on the pituitary thyrotrope cells, TSH is elevated while T4 levels are low. Some hormone measurements are only meaningful or more informative under conditions of dynamic testing (growth hormone (GH), cortisol). For example, partial adrenal insufficiency may only be apparent under conditions of stress, when the endogenous secretion of cortisol needs to increase in order to cover physiological needs. Dynamic testing for cortisol deficiency/adrenal insufficiency can be performed through injection of insulin and subsequent hypoglycemia in the *insulin-tolerance test*; under these conditions, cortisol levels should double and exceed a certain level.

In other instances, the diagnosis of hormone deficiency is established by measuring a key metabolite. This is best illustrated by diabetes mellitus, which results in elevated glucose levels. In the case of deficient vasopressin secretion, which leads to diabetes insipidus, the characterization of inappropriate volumes of dilute urine together with high fluid intake usually permits establishing the diagnosis.

Ancillary tests, for example, imaging studies of the hormone-secreting organ, can complement the biochemical characterization of hormone deficiencies in some instances (for details see ▶ Chaps. 6, "Receptor Tyrosine Kinases and the Insulin Signaling System," ▶ 7, "Cytokine Receptors," ▶ 8, "Steroid Hormone Receptors and Signal Transduction Processes," ▶ 9, "Thyroid Hormone Nuclear Receptors and Molecular Actions," ▶ 10, "Nongenomic Actions of Thyroid Hormones," ▶ 11, "The Hypothalamus–Pituitary Axis," ▶ 12, "The Posterior Pituitary," and ▶ 13, "The Thyroid").

Therapy of Hormone Deficiency

The therapy of hormone deficiencies is in general reasonably straightforward because many hormones or hormone derivatives are available for substitution therapy. For hormones with no or little circadian variation, replacement therapies can achieve serum levels that are similar to the physiological condition. For hormones that have variable circadian levels or that quickly respond to external stimuli, for example, cortisol, it is more difficult to approximate the physiological rhythmicity. In diabetes mellitus type 1, insulin substitution requires administration of so-called basal insulin, the insulin required during the fasting state, and prandial insulin, which is required to store glucose and lipids in the liver, muscle, and fat tissue.

Hormone Excess

Excessive hormone production can occur in essentially all hormone-producing glands (Table 3). The underlying etiologies are very diverse. They can include hypersecretion of hormones by benign or malignant tumors, activation of cellular growth, and hormone production by stimulating antibodies as exemplified by hyperthyroidism due to Graves' disease, constitutive activation of hormone-binding receptors or downstream signaling molecules by gain-of-function mutations, inappropriate release of hormone through the destruction by inflammatory processes, and ectopic hormone secretion in the context of paraneoplastic syndromes (see below).

Diagnosis of Hormone Excess

As with overt hormone deficiency, significant hormone excess is often readily recognized because it results in characteristic signs, symptoms, and abnormal physical findings. It can be more challenging to recognize mild forms or fluctuating hormone excess. The direct measurement of the suspected hormones is at the core of establishing the diagnosis (Sluss and Hayes 2016). For certain diagnoses (e.g., GH and cortisol excess), dynamic testing is often also required. For example, GH is physiologically released in pulses and single measurements are not clinically useful. Therefore, GH measurements to diagnose excessive hormone secretion are only informative under conditions of suppression. This can be performed by the administration of glucose, which should result in suppression of GH secretion. The measurement of metabolites is also used for the diagnosis of hormone excess. GH stimulates the secretion of insulin-like growth factor type 1 (IGF-1), which promotes the effects of GH on

Table 3 Selected examples of disorders caused by hormone excess

	Hormone	Phenotypic manifestation
Hypothalamus	Antidiuretic hormone/vasopressin	Syndrome of inappropriate antidiuretic hormone secretion (SIADH)
	GHRH	Acromegaly
Pituitary	Growth hormone (GH)	Acromegaly
	Luteinizing hormone (LH)	Interference with ovulation and conception
	Thyroid-stimulating hormone (TSH)	Central hyperthyroidism
	Prolactin	Galactorrhea, hypogonadism
	Adrenocorticotropic hormone (ACTH)	Cushing's disease
Thyroid	Thyroxine (T4) Triiodothyronine (T3)	Hyperthyroidism
Adrenal cortex	Cortisol	Cushing's syndrome
	Aldosterone	Hyperaldosteronism, hypertension
Adrenal medulla	Epinephrine Norepinephrine	Pheochromocytoma/ paraganglioma
Pancreas	Insulin	Insulinoma
	Glucagon	Diabetes mellitus
Ovaries	Estradiol Progesterone	Precocious puberty
	Androgens	Hirsutism, virilization
Testes	Testosterone	Precocious puberty
Paraneoplastic syndromes *(see* Table 9*)*	Ectopic secretion of hormones such as adrenocorticotropic hormone (ACTH), antidiuretic hormone (ADH)	ACTH: hypokalemia, metabolic alkalosis, Cushing's syndrome ADH: SIADH

peripheral tissues. In contrast to GH, IGF-1 levels are stable rather than pulsatile, and its measurement is useful for the diagnosis of GH excess or deficiency.

Therapy of Hormone Excess

The therapy of disorders caused by hormone excess is significantly more challenging and diverse than the therapy of hormone deficiency. Therapeutic modalities include surgical removal of the hormone-secreting gland, benign or malignant tumors within the affected gland, or treatment with drugs that block thyroid hormone synthesis or action. For a detailed discussion of therapeutic options, the reader should refer to the individual chapters covering these disorders.

Hormone Resistance

Although hormone resistance syndromes are rare, they have played an enormous role in the elucidation of the mechanisms involved in hormone action (Spiegel 1999).

The concept of hormone resistance was first described in 1942 by Fuller Albright (a preeminent endocrinologist who has characterized a large number of disease entities), who recognized end-organ insensitivity to the action of parathyroid hormone (PTH). In resistance to PTH, the serum PTH level is elevated, but it fails to exert its action at the level of the target cell, hence resulting in a phenotype mimicking hormone deficiency (Mantovani et al. 2016). Since the description of resistance to PTH, resistance to hormone action has been recognized for the majority of hormones (Table 4). The phenotypic spectrum is large and spans from complete resistance to mild resistance. For example, in the complete androgen insensitivity syndrome (CAIS, which has also been referred to as testicular feminization), XY male fetuses do not respond at all to the action of (dihydro) testosterone due to mutations in the nuclear androgen receptor (AR) (Mongan et al. 2015). This prevents the masculinization of the male genitalia in the developing fetus and the development of secondary sexual characteristics, and therefore the affected individuals have a female external appearance. However, the vagina consists only of a short blind pouch and the uterus and ovaries are absent. The testes are located intraabdominally or in the inguinal canal. In contrast, in the partial androgen insensitivity syndrome (PAIS, also referred to as Reifenstein syndrome), the virilization of the external genitalia is partial, resulting in a micropenis, often with hypospadias (a malformation of the penis with an incorrectly localized and malformed opening of the urethra). As another example, nephrogenic diabetes insipidus can be caused by an absent or impaired response of the kidney to the action of vasopressin (AVP). Nephrogenic diabetes insipidus can be hereditary due to mutations in the X-linked AVPR2 receptor or the aquaporin 2 water channels, or it can be acquired due to insults to the principal cells in the collecting ducts of the kidney.

Mechanistically, resistance syndromes are typically caused by mutations in membrane receptors, signaling molecules, or nuclear receptors. Loss-of-function mutations of both alleles are the norm for membrane receptors, and this can be associated with autosomal or X-linked recessive inheritance (Table 4). Mutations in nuclear receptors can result in dominant negative properties whereby the mutated allele impedes the action of the corresponding wild type allele. In this instance, the defect can be inherited in an autosomal dominant fashion. This is, for example, illustrated by mutations in the thyroid hormone receptors alpha (THRA) and beta (THRB). In other instances, the mechanisms of resistance are incompletely understood. This applies, for example, to diabetes mellitus type II which is characterized, at least in part, by an acquired insulin resistance that has a multifactorial origin involving genetic factors as well as lifestyle factors (Table 4).

Diagnosis and Therapy of Hormone Resistance

The diagnosis and therapy of resistance syndrome can be complex. The key to establishing the diagnosis is the recognition of a phenotype consistent with hormone deficiency at the levels of target organs in combination with elevated hormone

Table 4 Selected examples of resistance to hormone action

Site of resistance	Mechanism	Phenotypic manifestation
(A) Mutations in membrane receptors		
TRH receptor	Resistance to TRH Inactivating mutation in GPCR	Central hypothyroidism due to decreased secretion of TSH
GHRH receptor	Resistance to GHRH Inactivating mutation in GPCR	GH deficiency: short stature/dwarfism
GnRH receptor	Resistance to GnRH Inactivating mutation in GPCR	Hypogonadotropic hypogonadism
AVPR2 receptor	Resistance to vasopressin Inactivating mutation in GPCR	X-linked nephrogenic diabetes insipidus
TSH receptor	Resistance to TSH Inactivating mutation in GPCR	Thyroid hypoplasia Overt or compensated hypothyroidism
LH/CG receptor	Resistance to LH Inactivating mutation in GPCR	Females: primary or secondary amenorrhea and infertility Male: pseudohermaphroditism
FSH receptor	Resistance to FSH Inactivating mutation in GPCR	Females: delayed pubertal development, primary or secondary amenorrhea, premature ovarian failure Males: defect in spermatogenesis
ACTH receptor	Resistance to ACTH Inactivating mutation in GPCR	Adrenal insufficiency, high ACTH, hyperpigmentation
GH receptor	Resistance to GH Inactivating mutation in cytokine receptor	Short stature/dwarfism
Insulin receptor	Resistance to insulin Inactivating mutation in tyrosine kinase receptor	Insulin-resistant diabetes mellitus, acanthosis nigricans, leprechaunism, Rabson-Mendenhall syndrome
Anti-Müllerian hormone type II receptor	Resistance to Anti-Müllerian hormone Mutations in TGFbeta serine kinase receptor	Persistent Müllerian duct syndrome
(B) Mutations in signaling molecule		
Gsα	Resistance to PTH: Pseudohypoparathyroidism Resistance to TSH Resistance to FSH	Albright's hereditary osteodystrophy Hypocalcemia Hypothyroidism Hypogonadism

(continued)

Table 4 (continued)

Site of resistance	Mechanism	Phenotypic manifestation
C) Mutations in nuclear receptors		
Thyroid hormone receptor beta (THRB)	Resistance to thyroid hormone Dominant negative mutations in THRB	High T4 and T3, inappropriately high TSH, goiter, tachycardia
Thyroid hormone receptor alpha (THRA)	Resistance to thyroid hormone Dominant negative mutations in THRA	Low serum T4/T3 ratio; cognitive impairment, short lower limbs, skeletal dysplasia, delayed bone and dental development, constipation, anemia
Androgen receptor (AR)	Resistance to (dihydro) testosterone Completely or partially inactivating mutations in X-linked AR	Complete or partial androgen insensitivity syndrome
Estrogen receptor (ER)	Resistance to estrogen Inactivating mutations in ER	Osteoporosis Gigantism due to absent closure of epiphyses
Glucocorticoid receptor (GR)	Resistance to glucocorticoids Inactivating mutations in GR	Adrenal insufficiency
Mineralocorticoid receptor (MR)	Resistance to aldosterone Inactivating mutations in MR	Pseudohypoaldosteronism type 1 (PHA1): neonatal salt loss, hyponatremia, hyperkalemia, metabolic acidosis
Vitamin D receptor (VDR)	Resistance to vitamin D Inactivating mutations in VDR	Vitamin D-resistant rickets
D) Post-receptor defect		
Multifactorial	Resistance to insulin Genetic and environmental factors	Diabetes mellitus type 2

TRH TSH-releasing hormone, *GPCR* G-protein-coupled seven transmembrane receptor, *GHRH* GH-releasing hormone, *GnRH* gonadotropin-releasing hormone, *AVPR2* vasopressin 2 receptor, *TSH* thyroid-stimulating hormone, *LH/CG receptor* luteinizing hormone/chorionic gonadotropin receptor, *LH* luteinizing hormone, *FSH* follicle-stimulating hormone, *ACTH* adrenocorticotropic hormone, *GH* growth hormone, *TGFβ* transforming growth factor β, *PTH* parathyroid hormone, *Gsα* stimulatory G-protein subunit α

levels. Depending on the particular resistance syndrome, this may need ancillary biochemical studies, determination of the karyotype, imaging, and genetic testing.

In some instances, partial hormone resistance can be compensated by the administration of supra-physiological doses of the hormone. For example, in patients with X-linked nephrogenic diabetes insipidus, a subset of mutated AVPR2 receptors can be stimulated by pharmacologic doses of vasopressin, thereby decreasing the polyuria. In instances of complete resistance, therapeutic possibilities may be limited. For example, in the CAIS, the phenotype cannot be corrected, and affected individuals are raised as females. Affected individuals need appropriate psychological support if confronted with the diagnosis, and a careful discussion of the infertility and difficulties with sexual function associated with CAIS. The testes need to be removed because of the risk of developing germ cell tumors.

Alterations in Binding Proteins

Many hormones are bound to transport proteins in the serum. The bound hormone fraction results in a large hormone pool that can serve as a buffer system, while the very small free hormone pool exerts the biological actions.

Alterations in the concentration or the affinity of the bound hormone(s) can alter the total concentration of the respective hormone on biochemical testing, but in most instances, they have no other consequences. Binding protein abnormalities can be inherited or acquired. Recognition of these conditions is of clinical importance in order to prevent unnecessary treatments. Only rarely, the abnormal binding protein is associated with clinical abnormalities.

The best-studied binding proteins are the ones involved in thyroid hormone transport. They are characterized by abnormal total T4 or T3 concentrations with normal free hormone concentrations. Because of the normal free hormone concentrations, the individuals do not have any signs of hyper- or hypothyroidism. Thyroid hormones are bound to three major serum transport proteins: thyroxine-binding globulin (TBG), transthyretin (TTR), and human serum albumin (HSA) (Table 5). TBG has the strongest affinity for thyroid hormones. TBG deficiency (complete or partial) can be caused by inherited mutations in the X-linked *TBG* gene, and TBG excess can result from gene duplication or triplication. The diagnosis of inherited TBG defects requires genetic analysis. TBG concentrations can also be influenced by endogenous and exogenous hormones. For example, increased estrogen concentrations (pregnancy, therapy with oral contraceptives) lead to an increase in serum TBG because of a prolonged half-life of the protein. TTR mutations are divided into amyloidogenic and non-amyloidogenic variants. Autosomal dominant gain-of-function mutations that are associated with increased total T4 concentrations are non-amyloidogenic. The dominant amyloidogenic mutations do not alter thyroid hormone concentrations but cause familial amyloidotic polyneuropathy (FAP), which is characterized by neuropathy and cardiomyopathy due to amyloid deposition. Lastly, gain-of-function mutations in HSA can cause elevated total T4 levels (familial dysalbuminemic hyperthyroxinemia) or T3 levels (familial dysalbuminemic hypertriiodothyroninemia).

Sex hormone-binding globulin (SHBG) serves as the major transport protein for testosterone and estradiol. SHBG levels are regulated by numerous factors including, among others, diet and body weight, androgens and estrogens, thyroid hormone, insulin, liver function, and numerous drugs (Table 5). These variations impact the distribution between the protein-bound and the free fraction of the

Table 5 Selected examples of abnormal binding protein affinities or concentrations

Transport protein	Transported hormone	Phenotypic manifestation	Condition
Thyroxine-binding globulin	Thyroxine (T4)	Partial or complete deficiency: decreased total T4 concentration	X-linked: mutations in the *TBG* gene One family with autosomal dominant inheritance; defect not known
Thyroxine-binding globulin	Thyroxine (T4)	Excess: increased total T4 concentration	Duplication or triplication of the *TBG* gene
Thyroxine-binding globulin	Thyroxine (T4)	Excess: increased total T4 concentration	Endogenous estrogen increase: pregnancy Exogenous estrogen increase: oral contraceptives
Transthyretin	Thyroxine (T4)	Isolated total T4 elevation with normal free hormone levels, no other consequences	Autosomal dominant, non-amyloidogenic mutations in TTR
Transthyretin	Thyroxine (T4)	Familial amyloidotic polyneuropathy (FAP) with neuropathy and cardiomyopathy	Autosomal dominant, amyloidogenic mutations in TTR
Albumin	Thyroxine (T4)	Isolated total T4 elevation with normal free hormone levels, no other consequences	Autosomal dominant gain-of-function mutation: Familial dysalbuminemic hyperthyroxinemia
Albumin	Triiodothyronine	Isolated total T3 elevation with normal free hormone levels, no other consequences	Autosomal dominant gain-of-function mutation: Familial dysalbuminemic triiodothyroniemia
Sex-hormone binding globulin	Testosterone Estradiol	Decrease in total hormone concentrations	Obesity, nephrotic syndrome, hypothyroidism, glucocorticoids, androgen, progestins
Sex-hormone binding globulin	Testosterone Estradiol	Increase in total hormone concentrations	Aging, hepatic cirrhosis, hyperthyroidism, anticonvulsants, estrogens, HIV infection

TBG thyroxine-binding globulin, *TTR* transthyretin, *HIV* human immunodeficiency virus

respective hormones. Differences in plasma SHBG levels and activity are also influenced by polymorphisms in the coding region and the regulatory regions of the *SHBG* gene. Complete deficiency in SHBG due to biallelic missense mutations has been described; it does result in low total testosterone levels, but gonadal development and spermatogenesis are normal. Recent genetic studies suggest that specific polymorphisms in the *SHBG* gene influence the risk for diabetes mellitus type 2 and the metabolic syndrome.

Benign and Malignant Tumors of the Endocrine System

Neoplasms of the endocrine glands are quite common (Table 6). In the majority of cases, these are benign nodules or adenomas (monoclonal neoplasms) that are not secreting any hormones. However, benign and (more rarely) malignant tumors of all endocrine glands can synthesize and secrete excessive amounts of the respective hormones (Table 1).

Hormone deficiency associated with benign neoplasms of the endocrine system is less common but can, for example, be present in pituitary adenomas compressing the anterior pituitary cells.

The most common form of malignant tumors of the endocrine system is thyroid cancer, but malignant tumors can occur in all endocrine glands, albeit rarely. Thyroid cancer originates most commonly from thyroid follicular cells (papillary thyroid cancer (PTC) ~80–90%, follicular thyroid cancer (FTC) 5–10%), or calcitonin-producing parafollicular cells (medullary thyroid cancer (MTC) <5%) (Cabanillas et al. 2016). The highly aggressive anaplastic thyroid cancer is rare. Over the past three decades, the incidence of thyroid carcinomas in the United States has nearly tripled with 62,980 new cases diagnosed in 2014. This increase is mainly due to an increased diagnosis of small papillary thyroid carcinomas, which typically have a good prognosis in terms of long-term survival.

Malignant tumors of other endocrine glands are less common but can affect the ovaries, adrenal glands (cortex and medulla), pancreas, testes, and the pituitary.

Endocrine tumors can be part of tumor syndromes. This includes the Multiple Endocrine Neoplasia syndromes 1 and 2 (MEN1 and MEN2) and pheochromocytomas/paragangliomas (see below).

The pathogenesis of benign and malignant tumors involves *somatic* mutations (mutations limited to the affected tissue) in genes controlling cell growth, survival, and differentiation. The development of some endocrine tumors is associated with a predisposition conferred by hereditary *germline* mutations (Jameson and Kopp 2015a). The multiple endocrine neoplasia syndromes 1 and 2 (MEN1 and MEN2) are excellent examples to illustrate this.

Multiple Endocrine Neoplasia

MEN1 is an autosomal dominant tumor syndrome that includes parathyroid adenomas, pituitary adenomas, pancreatic tumors, and gastrinomas (Table 6). It is caused by biallelic mutations in the tumor suppressor gene *menin*. The germline mutation is inherited in an autosomal dominant fashion inactivating one the two *menin alleles*. If the second allele gets inactivated by a somatic mutation or by epigenetic silencing, this will lead to neoplastic growth (Knudson two-hit concept) (Jameson and Kopp 2015b). The need for the second hit provides an explanation for the fact that tumors only develop later in life and that the tumor burden can be different among affected individuals.

MEN2 is also an autosomal dominant tumor syndrome (Table 6). Multiple endocrine neoplasia type 2 is divided into three subtypes depending on its clinical manifestations: familial medullary thyroid carcinoma (FMTC), multiple endocrine

Table 6 Selected examples of benign and malignant tumors of the endocrine system

	Hormone	Phenotypic manifestation
Hypothalamus	Craniopharyngioma	Mass effect Anterior and posterior pituitary hormone deficiency
Pituitary	Non-secreting adenoma	Mass effect possible, hormone deficiencies
	Prolactinoma	Hypogonadotropic hypogonadism, galactorrhea
	GH-secreting adenoma	Acromegaly, gigantism
	ACTH-secreting adenoma	Cushing's disease
	TSH-secreting adenoma	Central hyperthyroidism
	FSH, LH, subunits	Mass effect, hypogonadism
Thyroid	Benign nodule with normal hormone secretion	None, mass effect
	Toxic adenoma: benign nodule with autonomous hormone secretion	Hyperthyroidism
	Papillary thyroid cancer	Thyroid mass. Locoregional and distant metastases possible
	Follicular thyroid cancer	Thyroid mass. Locoregional and distant metastases possible
	Medullary thyroid cancer	Thyroid mass. Locoregional and distant metastases possible
	Anaplastic thyroid cancer	Rapidly growing thyroid mass. Very aggressive malignancy, high lethality
Parathyroid	Parathyroid adenoma	Hyperparathyroidism, osteoporosis
	Parathyroid hyperplasia involving all glands	Hyperparathyroidism in the context of MEN1
	Parathyroid carcinoma	Hyperparathyroidism with significant hypercalcemia
Adrenal cortex	Non-secreting adenoma	Usually incidental finding
	Glucocorticoid-secreting adenoma	Cushing's syndrome
	Aldosterone-secreting adenoma	Hypertension, hypokalemia
	Adrenal cell carcinoma	Without or with excessive hormone secretion
Adrenal medulla	Pheochromocytoma	Hypertensive crises Malignant behavior in a subset of tumors
Pancreas	Insulinoma	Hypoglycemia
	Glucagonoma	Impaired glucose tolerance or diabetes mellitus, dermatitis, weight loss
	VIPoma	Watery diarrhea, hypokalemia, achlorhydria, flushing
	Somatostatinoma	Diabetes mellitus, gall stones, diarrhea, steatorrhea

(*continued*)

Table 6 (continued)

	Hormone	Phenotypic manifestation
Ovaries	Several forms of benign and malignant germ cell tumors	Mass effect
	Several forms of benign and malignant stromal cell tumors	Often hormone secreting. Precocious puberty dysfunctional bleeding, virilization possible.
Testes	Leydig cell adenoma	Precocious puberty
	Several forms of malignant tumors: seminoma and non-seminomas	Testicular mass. Locoregional and distant metastases possible

GH growth hormone, *ACTH* adrenocorticotropic hormone, *TSH* thyroid-stimulating hormone, *FSH* follicle-stimulating hormone, *LH* luteinizing hormone, *VIP* vasointestinal peptide

neoplasia type 2A (MTC, parathyroid hyperplasia, and pheochromocytomas), and multiple endocrine neoplasia type 2B (MTC, pheochromocytomas and ganglioneuromas). MEN2 is caused by gain-of-function mutations in a membrane tyrosine kinase receptor, the RET (rearranged in transformation) receptor. Given that the oncogenic event is driven by a gain-of-function mutation, only one allele needs to be affected, which contrasts with the situation in MEN1. The availability of mutational analysis of the *RET* gene in affected patients and their relatives is greatly facilitating carrier detection and clinical management. Importantly, specific *RET* mutations (genotype) are associated with the age of onset and aggressiveness of MTC and the development of other endocrine neoplasms (phenotype), a phenomenon referred to as genotype-phenotype correlation. The recognition of this phenomenon has allowed classifying all known mutations, and it permits making recommendations on the timing of prophylactic thyroidectomy and the screening for other manifestations of the syndrome. It is a classic example how molecular medicine can impact and improve patient care and an illustration of the potential of "precision medicine" (Collins and Varmus 2015).

Pheochromocytomas/Paragangliomas

Pheochromocytomas/paragangliomas can occur in a sporadic or inherited fashion (Table 6). It has become apparent that seemingly sporadic pheochromocytomas are relatively often associated with germline mutations in several genes (*RET*, VHL (von Hippel-Lindau), *succinate dehydrogenase type D and B (SDHD, SDHB)*, among others), and screening for these mutations is of increasing clinical importance because it permits early detection of these tumors through genetic testing in relatives (Castro-Vega et al. 2016).

As in other fields of medical oncology, a thorough understanding of the molecular events governing the development of endocrine malignancies is essential for the development of novel therapeutic modalities. For example, thyroid cancers derived from thyroid follicular cells frequently harbor mutations in the RAS-

BRAF-MAPK pathway. Therapy with tyrosine kinase inhibitors now provides a means to increase the progression-free survival of patients with advanced thyroid cancers. Similar strategies are under active investigation for other endocrine malignancies.

Diagnosis of Endocrine Tumors

Endocrine tumors are recognized because of the appearance of a mass, the incidental finding of a tumor on imaging studies for other purposes, or because of the diagnosis of hormone excess or hormone deficiencies. Pituitary adenomas that secrete hormones such as prolactin, GH, ACTH, or TSH are associated with characteristic clinical presentations. Non-secreting tumors of the pituitary can come to medical attention because of mass effects (headaches, compression of the optic chiasm with visual defects, leakage of cerebrospinal fluid) or because they compress the remainder of the pituitary resulting in anterior pituitary hormone deficiencies. Thyroid neoplasms are either found on palpation or through imaging studies of the neck region. Adrenal tumors manifest themselves through excessive secretion of hormones of the adrenal cortex (cortisol, aldosterone) or the adrenal medulla (adrenaline, noradrenaline), or they are detected incidentally on imaging studies of the abdomen. Hypersecretion of hormones of the pancreatic tail is relatively uncommon but can result in characteristic manifestations. Excessive sex steroid secretion by the gonads is also rare, and ovarian and testicular tumors are usually detected by demonstration of a mass.

Dedicated imaging studies (computerized tomography, magnetic resonance imaging, ultrasound, nuclear medicine studies) are essential to characterize size, features, and exact location of masses in endocrine tissues. Thyroid nodules that have suspicious features on ultrasound are evaluated with fine-needle aspiration. Cytological results of these aspirations often provide a definitive diagnosis. If the diagnosis remains indeterminate because of inconclusive findings, analysis of gene mutations or mRNA (messenger ribonucleic acid) expression profiles is now entering clinical practice and can provide further indication whether a lesion is benign or malignant.

Therapy of Endocrine Tumors

For a detailed discussion of the therapeutic modalities used for the treatment of endocrine tumors, the reader is referred to the individual chapters. Prolactinomas can be treated successfully in the majority of patients by administering dopamine agonists, which inhibit prolactin secretion and result in shrinkage of the tumor. Other pituitary tumors (non-secreting tumors, tumors secreting GH, ACTH, TSH) are most commonly surgically removed by transsphenoidal pituitary surgery. GH-secreting tumors can be treated with somatostatin analogues. Targeted radiation of pituitary tumors (cyber knife) can be used for tumors that have been incompletely excised or that recur.

Partial or total thyroidectomy is used for benign and malignant thyroid tumors. Thyroid carcinomas may be associated with metastases to locoregional lymph nodes, which requires appropriate dissection of the affected neck compartments. Thyroid carcinomas that originate from thyroid follicular cells (PTC, FTC) typically retain the ability to accumulate iodine. This permits to use radioiodine for the detection and therapy of residual or recurrent locoregional and metastatic disease, hence a very specific way of treating these carcinomas (Cabanillas et al. 2016). For advanced thyroid carcinomas (PTC, FTC, MTC, ATC), targeted therapy with kinase inhibitors can have a significant impact on progression-free survival. Parathyroid adenomas are treated surgically or, more rarely, with agonists targeting the calcium-sensing receptor (CASR). Adrenal tumors are removed through laparoscopic or open surgery. Adrenolytic drugs or drugs inhibiting glucocorticoid synthesis and action can be used in select cases of adrenal carcinomas secreting excessive amounts of cortisol or other steroids. Pancreatic islet tumors and gonadal tumors are typically treated with surgical excision.

Autoimmune Disorders and Autoimmune Polyglandular Syndromes

Autoimmune disorders play an important role as cause of endocrinopathies (Table 7). All endocrine glands can be targeted by the immune system through an autoimmune mechanism. This can result in dysfunction of individual glands or in polyglandular syndromes that also involve non-endocrine organs. Autoimmune disorders such as Hashimoto's thyroiditis, Graves' disease, and diabetes mellitus type are quite common, whereas lymphocytic hypophysitis, autoimmune hypoparathyroidism, adrenal insufficiency, and ovarian failure occur much more rarely. Hallmarks of these disorders include lymphocytic infiltration of the affected gland and the development of autoantibodies against several antigens (Tomer 2014). The etiology is multifactorial and includes genetic and environmental components. An association with certain human leukocyte antigen (HLA) variants is well established, and recent genome-wide association studies (GWAS) have identified other risk alleles.

The autoimmune polyglandular syndromes (APS) are diverse group of disorders that have, in part, endocrine components together with non-endocrine autoimmune manifestations (Table 7) (Michels and Gottlieb 2010). They include the monogenic APS I and complex genetic disorders such as APS II and APS III.

APS I manifests itself often already in infancy or early childhood. Hallmarks include hypoparathyroidism, adrenal insufficiency, and chronic candida infections. In addition, there are multiple other possible disease manifestations (Table 7). APSI is a rare autosomal recessive syndrome, but there are certain populations with an increased prevalence. It is caused by mutations in the autoimmune-suppressor gene (*AIRE,* for autoimmune regulator), which encodes a transcription factor that controls the expression of autoantigens by medullary thymic epithelial cells. Patients with APS I need replacement of deficient hormones and treatment of the candidiasis. These patients need close lifelong monitoring.

APS II (Schmidt's syndrome) is a more common disorder and consists of Addison's disease in combination with disorders such as hypothyroidism, diabetes mellitus type 1, pernicious anemia, celiac disease, and vitiligo. It is a complex

Table 7 Autoimmune disorders and autoimmune polyglandular syndromes

Disease entity	Phenotypic manifestation	Comments
Lymphocytic hypophysitis	Anterior pituitary hormone deficiency	
Hashimoto's thyroiditis	Hypothyroidism	Common More prevalent in females
Graves' disease	Hyperthyroidism	Relatively common More prevalent in females
Addison's disease	Adrenal insufficiency	
Diabetes mellitus type 1	Diabetes mellitus	
Oophoritis	Premature ovarian failure	
Autoimmune polyglandular syndrome type 1 (APS 1)	Adrenal insufficiency Hypoparathyroidism Mucocutaneous candidiasis Multiple other manifestations possible	Autosomal recessive Rare Childhood onset
Autoimmune polyglandular syndrome type 2 (APS 2)	Adrenal insufficiency Hashimoto's thyroiditis Multiple other manifestations possible	Polygenic/ multifactorial HLA-DR3 and HLA-DR4 associated Adult onset
Autoimmune polyglandular syndrome type 3 (APS 2)	Autoimmune thyroid disease Diabetes mellitus type 1 Multiple other manifestations possible	Polygenic/ multifactorial
IPEX: Immune dysregulation, polyendocrinopathy, enteropathy, X-linked syndrome	Early onset enteropathy, dermatitis, failure to thrive, and diabetes mellitus type 1, among others	X-linked Rare

genetic disorder that has been associated with particular human leukocyte antigen (HLA) alleles, and it is more common in females. Treatment includes hormone replacement as necessary. Glucocorticoids should be started before initiating therapy with levothyroxine in patients with Addison's disease and hypothyroidism. Patients with celiac disease need a gluten-free diet.

APS III is defined by the presence of autoimmune thyroid disease in combination with other autoimmune disorders except adrenal insufficiency, hypoparathyroidism, and chronic candidiasis.

Chromosomal Disorders

Several chromosomal disorders are associated with characteristic endocrine deficiencies (Table 8) (Jameson and Kopp 2015a). Among them, numerical abnormalities in sex chromosomes are relatively common and relevant from an endocrine

Table 8 Examples of chromosomal disorders associated with endocrine manifestations

	Chromosomal defect	Phenotypic manifestation
Klinefelter syndrome	47,XXY	Hypogonadism, tall stature
Turner syndrome	45,XO	Ovarian failure, short stature, autoimmune thyroid disease
Prader-Willi syndrome	del15 q11-13 (paternal copy) or maternal uniparental disomy	Hypogonadotropic hypogonadism, short stature, obesity, hyperphagia, mental retardation
Male-to-female sex reversal	X-chromosomal duplication involving *DAX1 (NROB1)*	Male-to-female sex reversal
Adrenal hypoplasia congenital	*DAX1 (NROB1)* deletion[a]	Congenital adrenal insufficiency, hypogonadotropic hypogonadism

[a]Can also be caused by point mutations in the *DAX1 (NROB1)* gene

perspective. Males with a 47,XXY karyotype have Klinefelter syndrome. In its typical presentation, the phenotype of these individuals is defined by small testicles, hypogonadism with sterility, increased and disproportionate height, and, in subset of patients, behavioral alterations. The 47,XXY can result from paternal or maternal non-disjunction during development of the gametes.

Females with a missing X chromosome and a X0 karyotype have Turner's syndrome, which is characterized by hypogonadism and sterility due to streak gonads, and stunted growth, among others. The 45,XO monosomy is present in 1–2% of all pregnancies but leads to spontaneous abortions in the majority of gestations. 45,X0 monosomy usually results from loss of the paternal sex chromosome.

The critical role of an appropriate dosage of the sex chromosomes is also illustrated by duplication or deletions of the X chromosomal region harboring the *DAX1 (NROB1)* gene. Duplication of this area causes dosage sensitive male-to-female sex reversal, while deletions (or point mutations within the gene) result in adrenal hypoplasia congenita (adrenal insufficiency due to abnormally developed adrenal glands) with hypogonadotropic hypogonadism in affected males.

Another classic example of a chromosomal disorder with endocrine manifestations is the Prader-Willi syndrome (PWS), which also illustrates the phenomenon of genomic imprinting (Jameson and Kopp 2015b). Genomic imprinting refers to the fact that certain genes or chromosomal regions are silenced in a parent-of-origin-specific way. This leads to the exclusive expression of the maternal allele if the paternal copy is imprinted, or expression of the paternal allele if the maternal equivalent is silenced. PWS is characterized by short stature, hypogonadotropic hypogonadism, obesity, hypotonia, and mental retardation. It can be caused by deletions involving the paternal copy of chromosome 15q leading to a contiguous gene syndrome (i.e., deletion of several adjacent genes). Because the homologous region on the maternal chromosome is imprinted and silenced, these genes are not expressed and cannot compensate for the loss of the paternal alleles. A distinct mechanism leading to PWS is uniparental disomy, the inheritance of two maternal copies of chromosome 15 instead of a maternal and a paternal copy.

Mosaicism

Mosaicism, the presence of two or more cell populations with different genotypes in a single individual, is caused by a mutation that occurs early in development of an embryo rather than in the germline (Jameson and Kopp 2015b). These mutations include both chromosomal disorders and point mutations. Organs and cells that descend from the initial mutated cell will carry the mutation, whereas the organs and cells that descend from the non-mutated cell will have normal genes. Thus, the affected individual is a *mosaic* of mutated and normal cells. The disorders caused by mosaicism can have a broad phenotypic spectrum depending on the stage in development at which the mutation occurred. In some individuals, very few tissues are involved; in others, the mutated cell type is abundant.

Chromosomal disorders such as Klinefelter syndrome (XXY cells in a background of normal male XY cells) or Turner syndrome (X0 cells in a background of normal female XX cells) can be present in mosaic form.

The McCune-Albright syndrome is a classic example of mosaicism (Jameson and Kopp 2015a). It is caused by a point mutation in the *GNAS1* gene during blastocyst development. The *GNAS1* gene encodes the stimulatory Gsα subunit, a signaling molecule that is essential for the transmission of signals by G-protein coupled transmembrane receptors. The manifestations of the syndrome include precocious puberty, fibrous dysplasia, café-au-lait spots, and a variety of endocrine disorders including hyperthyroidism, Cushing's syndrome, or acromegaly. The number of organ systems and hormonal signaling pathways that are affected depends on the initial number of cells that were mutated during blastocyst development.

Paraneoplastic Syndromes

Paraneoplastic syndromes are a rare manifestation associated with malignancies that arise from the secretion of humoral factors such as hormones, cytokines, or by immunologic alterations (Table 9). They most commonly occur in patients affected by cancers of the lung, breast, ovaries, and kidneys, as well as lymphomas. For example, small cell lung cancer (SCLC), which originates from neuroendocrine cells in the bronchus, can secrete hormones such as antidiuretic hormone (ADH) leading to the syndrome of inappropriate ADH secretion (SIADH), or they can secrete ACTH causing hypokalemia, metabolic alkalosis, and hypertension with or without Cushing's syndrome (ectopic ACTH syndrome) or parathyroid hormone-related peptide (PTHrP) which results in hypercalcemia (Kanaji et al. 2014). Paraneoplastic syndromes may be the first manifestation of a malignancy.

Table 9 Selected examples of endocrine paraneoplastic syndromes

Syndrome	Secreted hormone	Carcinomas secreting the hormone
Ectopic ACTH syndrome/Cushing's syndrome	ACTH	Small cell lung cancer Thymoma
SIADH	Antidiuretic hormone	Small cell lung cancer CNS malignancies
Hypercalcemia of malignancy	PTHrP	Squamous cell lung cancer Breast cancer Renal cell cancer
Hypoglycemia	Insulin	Insulinoma
Hypoglycemia	IGF-II	Mesenchymal tumors, sarcomas, hepatocellular carcinoma
Carcinoid syndrome (flushing and diarrhea, bronchoconstriction)	Serotonin, bradykinin	Bronchial carcinoid tumors Pancreatic carcinoma Gastric carcinoma

ACTH adrenocorticotropic hormone, *SIADH* syndrome of inappropriate antidiuretic hormone secretion, *CNS* central nervous system, *PRTHrP* parathyroid hormone-related peptide, *IGF-II* insulin-like growth factor type 2

Genes and Environment

Genetic components contribute to the pathogenesis of numerous endocrine and non-endocrine disorders. A large number of endocrine disorders can now be explained by single-gene mutations. Many common disorders such as diabetes mellitus type 2, obesity, hypertension, and heart disease, among others, have a complex or multifactorial pathogenesis involving genetic, nutritional, and lifestyle factors (Jameson and Kopp 2015a). During the last two decades, numerous genes and loci contributing to the pathogenesis of complex disorders have been identified through the analysis of candidate genes, GWAS, and more recently sequencing of the exome (all coding regions) or the whole genome. The identification of the genetic variations that predispose for or protect against the development of a complex disorder is of importance for the prediction of disease risk and for the development of novel therapeutic modalities.

However, it is important to emphasize that environmental factors can also have an important influence on the expression of a disease. Obesity is an ideal example to illustrate the interactions between gene and environment. At one end of the spectrum, very rare monogenic disorders can cause severe early onset obesity (Stears et al. 2012). For example, very severe early-onset obesity can be caused by mutations in the *leptin (LEP)* gene, and homozygous mutations in the (*leptin receptor (LEPR)* gene result in obesity, absent pubertal development, and impaired GH and TSH secretion. These observations indicate that leptin is an important physiological regulator of several endocrine functions in humans. At the other extreme of the spectrum, overweight and obesity can simply be induced by inappropriate energy homeostasis due to excessive caloric intake and insufficient expenditure. In between these two extremes, the combination of genetic predisposition and lifestyle factors (diet, interactions with the gastrointestinal microbiome, energy expenditure) can explain the development of excessive weight, and a number of genes associated with human obesity have been identified. A genetic predisposition is also supported by the high concordance of body weight among monozygotic twins.

Iodine deficiency serves as an impressive example how the deficiency of a micronutrient can result in endocrine disease. The synthesis of thyroid hormones is dependent on an adequate iodine intake. Iodide is rare in many parts of the world, and iodine deficiency results in the development of goiter and, in severe cases, cretinism (Pearce et al. 2013). Although iodine deficiency has been eradicated in many parts of the world through iodization of salt or other measures, it is still a major health problem affecting almost a third of the world population.

Summary

Endocrinology, the field of *internal secretion*, is concerned with the physiology and pathophysiology of glands and hormones. The term *hormone* is derived from the Greek verb *horman*, "that which sets in motion." Hormones are regulatory substances produced in an organism that are transported in tissue fluids such as blood to regulate other cells or organs. In addition to the classical endocrine glands (pituitary, thyroid, parathyroid, pancreatic islets, adrenal cortex and medulla, ovaries, testes), many other tissues secrete hormones, growth factors, or cytokines.

The endocrine system is primarily evaluated by the measurement of hormones or metabolites. Disorders such as diabetes mellitus and thyroid dysfunction are very prevalent in the general population, while other endocrine disorders are rare.

Hormone deficiency disorders can be treated with physiologic hormone replacement. Resistance to hormone action can mimic hormone deficiency. Hormone excess is amenable to therapy by blocking hormone synthesis or action, or through surgical removal of the hormone-secreting gland or adenomas within the affected organ. Many endocrine disorders are caused by a dysregulation of the immune system. This includes, among others, diabetes mellitus type 1 or autoimmune thyroid disease resulting in hypothyroidism (Hashimoto's disease) or hyperthyroidism (Graves' disease).

Thyroid nodules and papillary thyroid cancer are frequent; other benign and malignant tumors of the endocrine system are relatively uncommon. Tumors of the endocrine system often require surgical therapy, but certain tumors such as prolactinomas can be efficiently treated with medical treatments. In addition to surgery, malignant tumors of the endocrine glands may require additional therapeutic interventions, for example, with radioiodine in the case of thyroid tumors of follicular origin, radiation, chemotherapy, or targeted therapies with kinase inhibitors.

Malignancies of non-endocrine organs can occasionally also secrete hormones resulting in paraneoplastic syndromes.

The etiology of endocrine disorders is diverse and encompasses monogenic, polygenic, multifactorial, autoimmune, and environmental factors. The progress in identifying and characterizing the underlying pathogenesis is essential for improving diagnostic approaches, a rationale therapy, and the identification of novel therapeutic interventions.

References

Cabanillas ME, McFadden DG, Durante C. Thyroid cancer. Lancet. 2016;388(10061):2783–95.

Castro-Vega LJ, Lepoutre-Lussey C, Gimenez-Roqueplo AP, Favier J. Rethinking pheochromocytomas and paragangliomas from a genomic perspective. Oncogene. 2016;35(9):1080–9.

Collins FS, Varmus H. A new initiative on precision medicine. N Engl J Med. 2015;372(9):793–5.

Jameson J. Principles of endocrinology. In: Braunwald E, Fauci A, Kasper D, Hauser S, Longo D, Jameson J, editors. Harrison's principles of internal medicine. 2. New York: McGraw-Hill; 2011. p. 2866–75.

Jameson J, Kopp P. Applications of molecular biology and genetics in endocrinology. In: DeGroot L, Jameson J, editors. Endocrinology. 1. 7th ed. Philadelphia: WB Saunders; 2015a. p. 41–67.

Jameson J, Kopp P. Principles of human genetics. In: Braunwald E, Fauci A, Kasper D, Hauser S, Longo D, Jameson J, editors. Harrison's principles of internal medicine. 19th ed. New York: McGraw-Hill; 2015b. p. 425–45.

Kanaji N, Watanabe N, Kita N, Bandoh S, Tadokoro A, Ishii T, et al. Paraneoplastic syndromes associated with lung cancer. World J Clin Oncol. 2014;5(3):197–223.

Kronenberg H, Melmed S, Larsen P, Polonsky K. Principles of endocrinology. In: Melmed S, Polonsky K, Larsen P, Kronenberg H, editors. Williams textbook of endocrinology. 13th ed. Philadelphia: Elsevier; 2016. p. 2–11.

Mantovani G, Spada A, Elli FM. Pseudohypoparathyroidism and Gsalpha-cAMP-linked disorders: current view and open issues. Nat Rev Endocrinol. 2016;12(6):347–56.

Michels AW, Gottlieb PA. Autoimmune polyglandular syndromes. Nat Rev Endocrinol. 2010;6 (5):270–7.

Mongan NP, Tadokoro-Cuccaro R, Bunch T, Hughes IA. Androgen insensitivity syndrome. Best Pract Res Clin Endocrinol Metab. 2015;29(4):569–80.

Pearce EN, Andersson M, Zimmermann MB. Global iodine nutrition: where do we stand in 2013? Thyroid. 2013;23(5):523–8.

Sluss P, Hayes F. Laboratory techniques for recognition of endocrine disorders. In: Melmed S, Polonsky K, Larsen P, Kronenberg H, editors. Williams textbook of endocrinology. 13th ed. Philadelphia: Elsevier; 2016. p. 77–107.

Spiegel AM. Hormone resistance caused by mutations in G proteins and G protein-coupled receptors. J Pediatr Endocrinol Metab. 1999;12(Suppl 1):303–9.

Stears A, O'Rahilly S, Semple RK, Savage DB. Metabolic insights from extreme human insulin resistance phenotypes. Best Pract Res Clin Endocrinol Metab. 2012;26(2):145–57.

Tomer Y. Mechanisms of autoimmune thyroid diseases: from genetics to epigenetics. Annu Rev Pathol. 2014;9:147–56.

Genetic Disorders of Adrenocortical Function

28

Fady Hannah-Shmouni and Constantine A. Stratakis

Abstract

The first detailed description of the human adrenal glands was by Eustachius (1520–1574); their presence was confirmed by Piccolomini (1562–1605) and Casserius (1552–1616) (Vrezas et al. 2000). Their function, however, was largely unknown until the late nineteenth century. In the last 30 years, our growing understanding of adrenocortical development and function has led to the discovery of numerous genetic disorders that affect the adrenal glands. Developmental pathways have also been linked to the formation of adrenocortical tumors (ACTs), which represent a heterogeneous group of lesions of the adrenal cortex. ACTs have been found to be due to or associated with somatic or germline mutations in key molecular pathways, including the cyclic AMP (cAMP) and *Wnt* signaling pathways. In this chapter, we review the various genetic causes of adrenocortical disorders and focus on congenital causes of adrenal insufficiency associated with hypoplasia of the adrenal glands, genetic causes of autoimmunity that affect the adrenal glands, and genetic causes of benign and malignant ACT.

Keywords

Adrenal • Cortex • Congenital adrenocortical hypoplasia • Genes • Adrenocortical insufficiency • Molecular genetics • DAX1 • TPIT • SF1 • Glucocorticoid

---

Conflict of Interest Statement: The authors declare that the research was conducted in the absence of any potential conflict of interest.

Author and Contributors: All authors contributed equally to the conception or design of the work or the acquisition, analysis,or interpretation of data for the work, drafting the work or revising it critically for important intellectual content, final approval of the version to be published, and agreement to be accountable for all aspects of the work in ensuring that questions related to the accuracy or integrity of any part of the work are appropriately investigated and resolved.

F. Hannah-Shmouni • C.A. Stratakis (✉)
Section on Endocrinology and Genetics (SEGEN), National Institute of Child Health and Human Development (NICHD), National Institutes of Health (NIH), Bethesda, MD, USA
e-mail: fady.hannah-shmouni@nih.gov; stratakc@mail.nih.gov

A. Belfiore, D. LeRoith (eds.), *Principles of Endocrinology and Hormone Action*, Endocrinology, https://doi.org/10.1007/978-3-319-44675-2_29

resistance • Mineralocorticoid receptor • Sodium channel defects • Adrenocortical tumors • Adrenal hyperplasia • Cushing syndrome • Genetics • Carney complex • Cyclic AMP • PPNAD • Cancer • Mutations

Abbreviations

AC	Adenyl cyclase
ACTH	Adrenocorticotropic hormone
AIMAH	ACTH-independent macronodular adrenal hyperplasia
Alleles	Alternative forms of a gene
AMP/ATP	Adenosine monophosphate/adenosine triphosphate
BAH	Bilateral adrenocortical hyperplasia
BMAH	Bilateral macronodular adrenal hyperplasia
cAMP	Cyclic adenosine monophosphate
CNC	Carney complex
CS	Cushing syndrome
Genes	Units of inheritance at specific locations (loci) on a chromosome
GMP/GDP/GTP	Guanosine monophosphate/guanosine diphosphate/guanosine triphosphate
GPCRs	G protein-coupled receptors
Heterozygous	A genotype with two different alleles of a gene for a particular trait
Homozygous	A genotype with the same allele of a gene for a particular trait
MMAD	Massive macronodular adrenocortical disease
Mutations	Alteration of genetic material producing a new variation
PBAD	Primary bimorphic adrenocortical disease
PBMAH	Primary bilateral macronodular adrenocortical hyperplasia
PDEs	Phosphodiesterases
Phenotype	Detectable expression of a genotype
PKA	Protein kinase A
PPNAD	Primary pigmented nodular adrenocortical disease

Contents

Adrenal Gland Development

Following the formation of the adrenal cortex at the fourth week of human embryonic development, a blastema of undifferentiated cells of mesodermal origin forms from either the medial part of the urogenital ridge or mesoderm (Else and Hammer 2005). The adrenogonadal primordium cells undergo proliferation and invasion of the underlying mesenchyme that is dependent on the interplay between the transcriptional factors SF1 and DAX1 (see later) (Else and Hammer 2005; Hanley and Arlt 2006) that ultimately separates from the gonads by day 33 post conception. Further mesodermal cell proliferation, under the control of fetal adrenocorticotropic hormone (ACTH or corticotropin), forms the first evidence for zonation: a definitive zone (DZ) and a fetal zone (FZ) that arise from the celomic epithelium, while the transitional zone (TZ) originates from the mesonephron and arises from the region of Bowman's capsule (Else and Hammer 2005; Nguyen and Conley 2008). Between the 9th and 12th embryonic week, sinusoidal vascularization of the glands forms the framework for the zonation of the adult cortex (Else and Hammer 2005). Cortisol is produced from the rapidly growing FZ at about the sixth week of development, reaching a peak between the eighth and ninth week (Goto et al. 2006). Gradually, aldosterone and cortisol are made by DZ and TZ cells, whereas the FZ produces primarily dehydroepiandrosterone (DHEA) and dehydroepiandrosterone sulfate (DHEAS) that support estrogen production through the fetal-placental unit (Nguyen and Conley 2008).

By the ninth week, progenitor populations of the adult adrenal cortex encapsulate the adrenal glands, expressing *Nr5a1* and *Gli1* (Wood et al. 2013). Migrating neural crest cells forms the adrenal medulla and intermingles with cortical cells of the FZ, attaining a maximum adrenal size by the fourth month. Thereafter, the gradual receding of FZ, and expansion of DZ and TZ, gives rise to the adult zona glomerulosa (ZG) and zona fasciculata (ZF), respectively (Else and Hammer 2005; Nguyen and Conley 2008). After birth, FZ involutes and the corticomedullary junction separates between steroid hormone-producing and catecholamine-secreting cells (Else and Hammer 2005). A transition zone of primarily fibrous tissue separates the FZ from the remaining gland. By the end of the second year of life, the first evidence of an anatomically distinct zona reticularis (ZR) appears; however, steroidogenic activity of this zone is not present until the age of 5 years (Wood et al. 2013), concomitant with the onset of adrenarche. The adult adrenal cortex likely reaches maturity as early as 8 years of age to as late as after mid-puberty (Nguyen and Conley 2008; Suzuki et al. 2000; Merke and Stratakis 2006; Sucheston and Cannon 1968). The various developmental stages of the adrenal cortex are portrayed in Fig. 1 (Merke and Stratakis 2006).

Congenital Adrenal Insufficiency

Congenital adrenal insufficiency (CAI) represents a heterogeneous group of genetic disorders that affect adrenocortical development and function. The most frequent etiology of CAI is CAH, followed by non-autoimmune and autoimmune etiologies.

Congenital Adrenal Insufficiency due to Primary Adrenal Disorders

The proliferation and invasion of adrenogonadal primordium cells are dependent on the interplay between the transcriptional factors SF1 and DAX1 (Else and Hammer 2005; Hanley and Arlt 2006). Mice that are knockouts (KO) for *Sf1* have complete absence of the adrenal glands, whereas mice KO for *Dax1* have developmental adrenal gland defects without adrenal insufficiency (AI) (Else and Hammer 2005). Regardless of etiology, CAI due to primary adrenal disorders is characterized by hyponatremia, hyperkalemia, acidosis, and an elevated serum concentration of ACTH. In humans, X-linked *DAX1* (mutations in *NR0B1*) defects cause the most common human form of CAI (Muscatelli et al. 1994; Lin et al. 2006). DAX1 is an orphan nuclear receptor that is expressed in the adrenal glands, gonads, ventromedial hypothalamus (VMH), and the pituitary gonadotropes (Ferraz-de-Souza and Achermann 2008). Patients with CAI due to *DAX1* are usually 46,XY phenotypic boys and may have hypogonadotropic hypogonadism and a family history of male-only CAI. *DAX1* mutations are also described below under "adrenal hypoplasia congenita".

Humans with heterozygous *SF1* (coded by the *NR5A1* gene) mutations have AI and gonadal abnormalities (Zanaria et al. 1994). More recently, patients with isolated AI and heterozygous *NR5A1* mutations have been described. *SF1* gene mutations were also found in patients who also had isolated 46,XY gonadal dysgenesis (Zanaria et al. 1994) and have been rarely identified in patients with CAI without evidence of gonadal defects.

Some genes that have been implicated in hypoplastic adrenals with retention of adrenocortical function may present with mild functional defects in adrenarche and pubertal anomalies but without CAI. Such examples include defects in Wilms' tumor 1 (*WT1*), a transcriptional regulator that is mutated in Denys-Drash and Frasier syndromes (Melo et al. 2002), *WNT4*, and *WNT11*, which are members of the *frizzled*

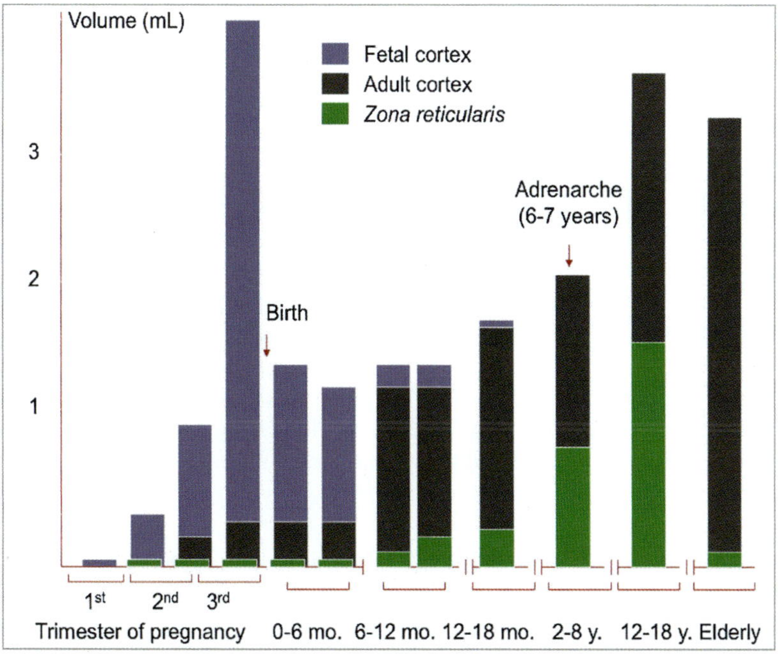

Fig. 1 **The development of the fetal and adult adrenal cortex**. Between the 9th and 12th embryonic week, sinusoidal vascularization of the adrenal glands forms the framework for the zonation of the adult cortex. Cortisol is produced from the rapidly growing fetal zone (*blue*) at about the sixth week reaching a peak between the eighth and ninth week of development. Gradually, aldosterone and cortisol are made by definitive zone and transitional zone, whereas the fetal zone produces primarily DHEA and DHEAS that support estrogen production through the fetal-placental unit. Migrating neural crest cells forms the adrenal medulla and intermingles with cortical cells of the fetal zone, attaining a maximum adrenal size by the fourth month. Thereafter, the gradual receding of fetal zone and expansion of the other zones give rise to the adult zona glomerulosa and zona fasciculata. After birth, fetal zone involutes, and the corticomedullary junction separates between steroid hormone-producing and catecholamine-secreting cells. A transition zone of primarily fibrous tissue separates the fetal zone from the remaining gland. By the end of the second year of life, the first evidence for an anatomically distinct zona reticularis appears; however, steroidogenic activity is not present until the age of 5 years, concomitant with the onset of adrenarche. The adult adrenal cortex likely reaches maturity as early as 8 years of age to as late as after mid-puberty (Modified from Merke and Stratakis (2006))

receptor family. A missense substitution of the *WNT4* gene causes an autosomal recessive syndrome designated as SerKAL (46,XX *se*x *r*eversal with dysgenesis of *k*idneys, *a*drenals, and *l*ungs) (Mandel et al. 2008).

Congenital Adrenal Insufficiency due to Metabolic Disorders

Several rare metabolic disorders may affect adrenocortical function in early life. X-linked adrenoleukodystrophy (X-ALD) is a neurodegenerative disorder that affects the nervous system white matter and the adrenal cortex due to impaired beta-oxidation of very long chain fatty acids (VLCFAs). This impairment is a result of mutations in a gene encoding a peroxisomal ATP-binding cassette (ABC) transporter (ALD protein) (Feigenbaum et al. 1996). X-ALD is the most common inherited peroxisomal disorder (and metabolic disorder causing CAI) that affects 1/15,000–20,000 males in the Caucasian population (Bezman et al. 2001). Three main phenotypes are seen in affected males: (i) a childhood cerebral form that manifests most commonly between ages 4 and 8 years due to progressive impairment of cognition, behavior, vision, hearing, and motor function leading to total disability within 2 years; (ii) adrenomyeloneuropathy (AMN) that manifests most commonly in the late twenties as progressive paraparesis, sphincter disturbances, sexual dysfunction, and, often, impaired adrenocortical function; and (iii) AI only that presents between age 2 years and adulthood although some degree of neurologic disability may manifest later. Approximately 20% of female carriers develop a milder AMN-like manifestation usually during their late adulthood.

Other metabolic causes of CAI include:

- Wolman disease (familial xanthomatosis) which is caused by defects in lysosomal acid cholesteryl ester hydrolase that may present with CAI and adrenal calcification (Kahana et al. 1968; Anderson et al. 1994).
- Smith-Lemli-Opitz syndrome (SLOS) which is a disorder of cholesterol biosynthesis that is associated with developmental delay, dysmorphic features, and male undervirilization and/or hypogonadism. SLOS may present with CAI, adrenal crisis, or more commonly compensated adrenocortical dysfunction (Chemaitilly et al. 2003; McKeever and Young 1990; Bianconi et al. 2011).
- Hereditary cystatin C amyloid angiopathy (HCCAA) which is a genetic amyloid disease that occurs frequently in Iceland and is caused by a mutation in cystatin C that causes amyloid deposition, predominantly in brain arteries and arterioles, but also in tissues outside the brain including the adrenal cortex, resulting in hemorrhage (Palsdottir et al. 2006).

Congenital Adrenal Insufficiency due to Autoimmunity

Adrenal gland failure in the context of autoimmune polyglandular syndrome (APS) usually presents after the first 2 years of life. APS is a rare polyendocrinopathy that exists in two major forms: APS-1, or otherwise known as autoimmune polyendocrinopathy-candidiasis-ectodermal dysplasia (APECED) syndrome, is an autosomal recessive disorder that is caused by mutations in the autoimmune regulator (*AIRE*) gene (Heino et al. 1999) and consists of chronic mucocutaneous candidiasis and/or acquired hypoparathyroidism, Addison's disease (autoimmune adrenalitis), chronic active hepatitis, malabsorption, juvenile onset pernicious anemia, alopecia, primary hypogonadism, and less commonly type 1 diabetes mellitus; autoimmune thyroid disease; ectodermal dystrophy, affecting the dental enamel and nails; vitiligo; or corneal disease (keratopathy). APS-2 is an autosomal dominant disorder with variable expressivity that manifests later in life with type 1 diabetes mellitus and/or autoimmune thyroid disease, among other endocrinopathies, and affects predominately females. A variability of age of onset exists in APS-1, from 6 months to 41 years with a peak around 13 years of age, with AI developing in 60–100% of patients with APECED and may be preceded by months to years of detectable adrenal cortex autoantibodies.

The genetic predisposition of both major types of APS differs. APS-2 involves HLA-B8, HLA-DR3, and HLA-DR4 (chromosome 6), cytotoxic T-lymphocyte antigen-4 (*CTLA-4*) gene (chromosome 2), and the protein tyrosine phosphatase non-receptor type 22 (*PTPN22*) genes (chromosome 1) (Kahaly 2012; Dittmar and Kahaly 2003). The gene for APECED is on chromosome 21q22.3 and encodes a 545 amino acid protein, AIRE (autoimmune regulator). AIRE is expressed in tissues that have important role in the maturation of immune system and development of immune tolerance, such as the thymus, lymph nodes, and fetal liver. APS-1 is more common in certain genetically isolate populations, with an incidence of 1:9,000 in Iranian Jews, 1:14,400 in Sardinians, and 1:25,000 in Finnish (Heino et al. 1999). A common Finnish mutation, p.R257X, was shown to be responsible for 82% of Finnish APS-1 cases, while the nonsense mutation, p.R139X, was the major mutation among Sardinians (Heino et al. 1999).

Congenital Adrenal Insufficiency due to Other Genetic Conditions

Mutations in a member of the T-box gene family lead to pituitary-dependent CAI without any other defects (isolated ACTH deficiency). All members of the T-box gene family encode an N-terminal DNA-binding domain (the T-box) and are important for the development of several, mostly mesodermal, tissues in the human and mouse embryo. TPIT (or TBX19), one of the members, is a transcription factor that is required for expression of the *POMC* gene in the differentiating pituitary corticotrophs. Mutations in *TPIT* are associated with autosomal recessive pituitary-dependent CAI (Lamolet et al. 2001), with a typical presentation in the neonate with very low, but not necessarily undetectable, ACTH and cortisol levels, hypoglycemia, seizures, and occasionally death. In one study, 65% of cases of neonatal CAI due to isolated ACTH deficiency were caused by *TPIT* mutations (Couture et al. 2012).

Hereditary resistance to ACTH action (R-ACTH) is an autosomal recessive disorder that is caused by defects of the ACTH receptor (ACTHR) (Tsigos et al. 1993). Disorders of R-ACTH have been described that are biochemically characterized by cortisol, but usually not mineralocorticoid, deficiency: familial glucocorticoid deficiency type 1 (FGD-1) due to inactivating *MC2R* gene mutations typically present in infancy with severe AI, hypoglycemia, and seizures or later in childhood with a milder form of AI and tall stature (patients end up being taller than their genetically determined final height potential) (Elias et al. 2000), and FGD-2 is caused by non-*MC2R* mutations in the gene encoding an accessory protein required for ACTH signaling (MC2 receptor accessory protein, MRAP) (Metherell et al. 2005) that lead to severe glucocorticoid deficiency and death if not recognized early. *MC2R* consists of one coding exon and is located on chromosome 18; FGD-1 due to *MC2R* mutations is seen in 25–40% of cases (Lin et al. 2007).

More recently, additional defects beyond *MC2R* and *MRAP* have been described to cause FGD. They are involved in replicative and oxidative stress, including the minichromosome maintenance-deficient 4 homologue (*MCM4*) (natural killer cell and glucocorticoid deficiency with DNA repair defect – NKGCD) and nicotinamide nucleotide transhydrogenase (*NNT*) genes (Meimaridou et al. 2013). Finally, genes involved in mitochondrial function such as thioredoxin reductase 2 (*TXNRD2*), glutathione peroxidase 1 (*GPX1*), and peroxiredoxin 3 (*PRDX3*) have also been found to cause FGD. In a recent study of a large cohort of patients with CAI, investigated by whole exome sequencing (WES), mutations in the genes listed here were found in only 17 of 43 patients, indicating that there are additional genetic defects to be discovered that cause this disease (Chan et al. 2015).

Allgrove or triple A syndrome (AAAS) is an autosomal recessive multisystem disorder that is characterized by R-ACTH AI, alacrima, achalasia, neurodegeneration, and autonomic dysfunction (Brooks et al. 2004). AI in AAAS may present with neonatal hypoglycemic seizures and adrenal crisis or can be late onset not requiring glucocorticoid replacement therapy until teenage years or later. As in other forms of CAI, rarely patients require mineralocorticoid replacement, as well. The most frequent genetic defect is a splicing mutation (IVS14+1G>A) of the *AAAS* gene (located on chromosome 12q13) (Brooks et al. 2005), which encodes for a 546 amino acid protein called ALADIN (for alacrima-achalasia-adrenal insufficiency neurologic disorder). Patients with missense mutations in one allele have delayed onset of AI as compared with truncation mutations in both alleles. The frequency of AI is significantly higher in patients with only truncation mutations (Ikeda et al. 2013).

Adrenal hypoplasia congenita (AHC) is a disorder that manifests with CAI in infancy. Two major histologic types exist: "cytomegalic" form, due to mutations in the *DAX1* gene that is inherited as X-linked recessive and typically presents in males with AI and hypogonadotropic hypogonadism (Achermann and Vilain 1993), and "miniature" form, which is a heterogenous genetic disorder that is autosomal recessive and often associated with other developmental defects including abnormalities of the pituitary gland and the central nervous system.

Several rare genetic causes of pituitary-dependent CAI exist in association with other developmental defects: mutations in *HESX1*, *LHX3*, *LHX4*, and *SOX3* genes; homozygote or compound heterozygote genetic defects of the ACTH precursor, pro-opiomelanocortin (*POMC*) gene, its processing enzyme (prohormone convertase 1 or *PC1*), and the product of the proprotein convertase subtilisin/kexin type 1 (*PCSK1*) gene (Hanley and Arlt 2006; Ferraz-de-Souza and Achermann 2008; Perry et al. 2005; Krude et al. 2003; Metherell et al. 2006; Jackson et al. 1997; Achermann et al. 1999); and defects that lead to other forms of hypopituitarism (ACTH deficiency in combination with other defects) (Karpac et al. 2007).

CAI may also be part of a number of developmental conditions caused by genes whose main action is not in the adrenal cortex. These include (i) IMAGe (intrauterine growth retardation, metaphyseal dysplasia, adrenal hypoplasia, genitourinary anomalies) due to mutations in *CDKN1C* (chromosome 11p15) (Arboleda et al. 2012); (ii) CHARGE syndrome (coloboma of the eye; heart anomaly; atresia, choanal; retardation of mental and somatic development; microphallus; ear abnormalities and/or deafness) due to mutations in the chromodomain helicase DNA-binding protein 7 (CHD7) gene (James et al. 2003; Jongmans et al. 2006); (iii) Meckel syndrome, a severe pleiotropic autosomal recessive developmental disorder caused by mutations in *MKS1* (chromosome 17q22) that leads to dysfunction of primary cilia during early embryogenesis (Hsia et al. 1971); or (iv) conditions associated with chromosomal defects, such as duplication in 5p (Chen et al. 1995), tetraploidy, triploidy, trisomy 19, trisomy 21, monosomy 7, and 11q syndrome.

Adrenocortical Tumors

The first report of cAMP pathway mutations causing ACTs was in patients with McCune-Albright syndrome (MAS) due to *GNAS* (encodes the alpha subunit (Gsα) of the stimulatory guanine nucleotide-binding protein) that resulted in adrenocortical hyperplasia and/or benign cortisol-producing adenomas (CPAs) (Weinstein et al. 1991; Stratakis and Boikos 2007). This was rapidly followed by other important discoveries in the genetics of ACT formation, including the regulatory subunit type 1-α (RIα) of protein kinase A (PKA, *PRKAR1A* gene) and phosphodiesterase 11A and phosphodiesterase 8B (*PDE11A* and *PDE8B* genes, respectively) in Carney complex (CNC) and isolated ACTs and/or adrenal hyperplasia, respectively (Stratakis and Boikos 2007). Recently, germline mutations in the tumor suppressor gene *ARMC5* (*armadillo repeat containing 5*) in primary bilateral macronodular adrenocortical hyperplasia (PBMAH) and somatic mutations in *KCNJ5* in aldosterone-producing adenomas (APA) further expanded our understanding of tumorigenesis in ACTs (Stratakis and Boikos 2007; Horvath and Stratakis 2008). In this section, we provide a comprehensive review of the genetics of mostly benign ACTs.

Classification of Adrenocortical Tumors

A comprehensive classification of ACT was proposed in 2007 (Tables 1, 2, and 3) (Stratakis and Boikos 2007). ACT is divided into adrenocortical adenomas (ACAs), adrenocortical hyperplasia, and adrenocortical cancer (ACC) (Stratakis and Boikos 2007). These lesions can be classified on their radiographic appearance as either unilateral or bilateral or on biochemistry as either functioning or nonfunctioning. ACAs are common incidental findings on imaging (5% of cases); however, adrenocortical hyperplasias are more frequently encountered on imaging (36% of cases) (Saeger et al. 1998) but are often misread as "normal adrenal glands".

Bilateral adrenocortical hyperplasias (BAH) are divided into micronodular (<1 cm in diameter) or macronodular (>1 cm in diameter) (Stratakis and Boikos 2007).

Table 1 Causes of congenital adrenal insufficiency

Congenital adrenal insufficiency	Gene (locus)	Mode of inheritance	Major features
Due to primary adrenal disorders			
DAX1	*NR0B1* (*DAX1*)	X-linked	*DAX1* mutations: 46,XY phenotypic boys, hypogonadotropic hypogonadism, and a family history of male-only CAI
SF1	*NR5A1* (*SF1*)	AR	*SF1* mutations: AI and gonadal abnormalities Occasionally heterozygous mutations act in AD fashion causing milder phenotypes, such as isolated CAI
Denys-Drash syndrome	*WT1*	AD	
Frasier syndrome	*WT1*	AD	
SerKA	*WNT4*	AD	
Due to metabolic disorders			
X-ALD	*ABCD1*	X-linked	X-ALD: progressive demyelination of the white matter with or without AI, with less than half of patients presenting with CAI, and some male carriers have no detectable disease until later in life or none at all
Wolman disease	*LIPA*	AR	Wolman disease (familial xanthomatosis): CAI and adrenal calcification
Smith-Lemli-Opitz syndrome	*DHCR7*	AR	Smith-Lemli-Opitz syndrome: developmental delay, dysmorphic features and male undervirilization and/or hypogonadism, CAI, adrenal crisis, or more commonly compensated adrenocortical dysfunction
Hereditary cystatin C amyloid angiopathy	*APP*	AR	Hereditary cystatin C amyloid angiopathy: most common mutation is in the *APP* and particularly seen in the Dutch, Italian, Arctic, Iowa, Flemish, and Piedmont populations. Mutations in the *CST3* cause the Icelandic type. Familial British and Danish dementia is caused by mutations in *ITM2B*. Causes adrenal hemorrhage and neurological manifestations
	CST3	Sporadic	
	ITM2B		

(*continued*)

Table 1 (continued)

Congenital adrenal insufficiency	Gene (locus)	Mode of inheritance	Major features
Due to autoimmune disease			
APS1	*AIRE*	AR	APS1: usually manifests in early childhood, consists of chronic mucocutaneous candidiasis and/or acquired hypoparathyroidism, Addison's disease, chronic active hepatitis, malabsorption, juvenile onset pernicious anemia, alopecia, primary hypogonadism, and infrequently type 1 diabetes mellitus; autoimmune thyroid disease; ectodermal dystrophy, affecting the dental enamel and nails; vitiligo; or corneal disease (keratopathy)
APS2	HLA-B8, HLA-DR3 and HLA-DR4, CTLA-4, PTPN22; chromosomes 6, 2, and 1	AD	APS2: type 1 diabetes mellitus and/or autoimmune thyroid disease has a later but variable age of onset and affects predominately females
Due to rare genetic syndromes			
T-box gene family	*TPIT*	AR	*TPIT* mutation: neonatal onset CAI, hypoglycemia, seizures, and occasionally death
Hereditary resistance to ACTH action		AR	
A – FGD type 1	*MC2R, MCM4, NNT*		FGD-1: infancy with severe AI (most require only glucocorticoid replacement), hypoglycemia, and seizures or later in childhood with a milder form of AI and are taller than their expected (by genetic target) height
B – FGD type 2	*MRAP*		FGD-2: severe glucocorticoid deficiency and death
Allgrove (triple A) syndrome	*AAAS*	AR	AAAS: AI, alacrima, achalasia, neurodegeneration, and autonomic dysfunction

(*continued*)

Table 1 (continued)

Congenital adrenal insufficiency	Gene (locus)	Mode of inheritance	Major features
Adrenal hypoplasia congenital:	*NR0B1* (*DAX1*)	X-linked recessive	Adrenal hypoplasia congenital: cytomegalic form: males with adrenal insufficiency and hypogonadotropic hypogonadism. Miniature" form: CAI, developmental defects including abnormalities of the pituitary gland and the central nervous system
A – Cytomegalic form			
B – Miniature form			
Intrauterine growth restriction, metaphyseal dysplasia, adrenal hypoplasia congenita, and genital anomalies (IMAGe)	*CDKN1C* (11p15)	AD with paternal imprinting	
Coloboma, heart defect, choanal atresia, retarded growth and development, genital abnormality, and ear abnormality (CHARGE syndrome)	*CHD7*	AD	
	Duplication in 5p	Sporadic	

AAAS: *AI* alacrima, achalasia, neurodegeneration, and autonomic dysfunction, *AI* adrenal insufficiency, *AD* autosomal dominant, *APS* autoimmune, polyglandular syndrome, *AR* autosomal recessive, *CAI* congenital adrenal insufficiency, *IMAGe intrauterine growth restriction, metaphyseal dysplasia, adrenal hypoplasia congenita, and genital anomalies, *CHARGE* coloboma, heart defect, choanal atresia, retarded growth and development, genital abnormality, and ear abnormality, *SerKA* female-to-male sex reversal and kidney, adrenal, and lung dysgenesis, FGD familial glucocorticoid deficiency.

Secondary bilateral adrenocortical hyperplasia is caused by excess ACTH and should be differentiated from primary causes, which are often due to genetic defects. The classification of BAH is summarized in Table 2. The micronodular subtypes are usually diagnosed in children and young adults and are either pigmented (c-PPNAD for primary pigmented nodular adrenocortical disease, familial as seen in CNC, or isolated, i-PPNAD) or not pigmented (iMAD for isolated micronodular adrenocortical disease) (Stratakis and Boikos 2007). The macronodular subtypes are usually diagnosed in adults and may be sporadic or familial. Syndromic forms are seen with mutations in *APC*, *MEN1*, *FH*, and other genes (see under "Familial Syndromes"). Other subtypes of macronodular hyperplasias include primary bimorphic adrenocortical disease (PBAD), as seen in MAS, and Beckwith-Wiedemann syndrome (BWS). Approximately 75–90% of ACTs leading to Cushing syndrome (CS) are due to a unilateral and benign CPA, with the remaining being caused by BAH (Lodish and Stratakis 2016). The different histopathologic characteristics of these lesions are summarized in Table 2.

PBMAH is a form of BAH that was first described in 1964 (Kirschner et al. 1964) and is estimated to affect 10% and 15% of CS in young adulthood and childhood, respectively (Stratakis and Boikos 2007), with likely higher figures in subclinical CS. PBMAH was previously called massive macronodular adrenocortical disease

Table 2 Classification and characteristics of adrenocortical tumors

Adrenocortical lesions	Genes (locus)	Histolopathology	Characteristics
ACA	*CTNNB1* (3p22.1)	ACA are small (<5 cm), well-circumscribed, bright yellow due to their enriched cytoplasmic lipid	Can be associated with MEN1, FAP, MAS, HLRCS, CNC, Carney triad, and others
	PRKAR1A (17q22-24)	Nonneoplastic adrenal cortical nodules may be difficult to differentiate from ACA; they may be multifocal and bilateral	
APA	*CTNNB1* (3p22.1)	APA is predominantly composed of cells similar to fasciculate; hyperplasia of the glomerulosa layer may be seen. Others may appear like fasciculata, glomerulosa, and reticularis admixed	Majority of APA harbor a *KCNJ5* mutation
	KCNJ5 (11q24.3)		
	ARMC5 (16p11.2)		Germline mutations in *ARMC5* gene may be seen in APA of patients from African-American decent
	ATP1A1 (1p13.1)		
	ATP2B3 (Xq28)		*ATP2B3* has been implicated in APA of females with a more severe phenotype
	CACNA1D (3p14.3)		*CACNA1D* mutants in APA are more common in males
	CACNA1H (16p13.3)		Germline mutations (p. M1549V) in *CACNA1H* were identified in early-onset PA and may represent a new subtype of familial hyperaldosteronism
CPA	*PRKACA* (19p13.1)	CPA is composed of cells similar to fasciculate, with adjacent cortical atrophy. Heterogeneity with lipid-depleted cells admixed may be present	Somatic-activating mutations of *PRKACA* (c.617A>G/p.L206R) with an estimated incidence of approximately 42% in CPA
	GNAS (20q13)		Somatic mutations in *GNAS* were identified in 5–17% of CPA
	PRKAR1A (17q22-24)		The somatic allelic losses of *PRKAR1A* were found in 23% of CPA that were smaller tumors and exhibited a paradoxical increase in urinary cortisol levels after dexamethasone suppression, due to increased glucocorticoid receptor expression in ACT
	CTNNB1 (3p22.1)		*CTNNB1* (S45P, S45F) in approximately 23.1% of CPA

(*continued*)

Table 2 (continued)

Adrenocortical lesions	Genes (locus)	Histolopathology	Characteristics
PBMAH	*ARMC5* (16p11.2)	Distinct adenomas (usually two or three), >1 cm, with internodular atrophy, or hyperplasia without atrophy	Middle age
	MEN1 (11q13)		Associated with MEN1, FAP, MAS, HLRCS, CNC, isolated (AD)
	FH (1q42.3-43)		Majority of lesions with ectopic GPCRs (vasopressin, serotonin, catecholamines, luteinizing hormone)
	APC (5q22.2)		PBMAH carry the ability of intra-adrenal production of ACTH with an autocrine/paracrine effect on cortisol production
	PRKAR1A (17q22-24)		
	PDE11A (2q31.2)		
	GNAS (20q13)		
PBAD	*GNAS* (20q13)	Distinct adenomas (>1 cm), with occasional microadenomas and internodular atrophy	Infants and very young children
			MAS
i-PPNAD	*PRKAR1A* (17q22-24)	Microadenomatous (<1 cm) hyperplasia with pigmentation	Children and young adults
	PDE11A (2q31.2)		Lentiginosis in few cases
	PDE8B (5q13)		
	PRKACB (1p31.1)		
c-PPNAD	*PRKAR1A* (17q22-24, CNC1 locus)	Microadenomatous (<1 cm) hyperplasia with (mostly) internodular atrophy and pigmentation	c.709-7del6 mutation and c.1A>G/p.M1V substitution in *PRKAR1A*
	PRKACB (1p31.1)		Children, young, and middle-aged adults
	2p16 (unkown gene; CNC2 locus)		Disease at a younger age and a higher frequency of myxomas, schwannomas, and thyroid and gonadal tumors than patients without *PRKAR1A* mutations
			In-frame deletion of exon 3 and the c.708 +1G>T mutation appears to confer a more severe CNC phenotype, while the splice

(*continued*)

Table 2 (continued)

Adrenocortical lesions	Genes (locus)	Histolopathology	Characteristics
			variant c.709(-7-2)del6 and the initiation alternating substitution c.1A>G/p.M1Vp have been associated with incomplete penetrance of CNC, as seen in i-PPNAD
			CNC1: The hotspot c.491-492delTG mutation is most closely associated with lentigines, cardiac myxoma, and thyroid tumors when opposed to all other *PRKAR1A* mutations
			Expressed RIα mutant protein present with more severe and aggressive CNC phenotype
			CNC2: Sporadic disease later in life with a lower frequency of myxomas, schwannomas, thyroid, and LCCSCT
iMAD	*PDE11A* (2q31.2)	Microadenomatous (<1 cm) hyperplasia with internodular hyperplasia and limited or absent pigmentation	Mostly children and young adults
	PDE8B (5q13)		May be associated with a paradoxical rise of glucocorticoid excretion during the Liddle's test
	PRKAR1A (2q31.2)		
	PRKACA (19p13.1)		
	2p12-p16		
	5q		

ACA adrenocortical adenoma, *APC* adenomatous polyposis coli gene, *c-PPNAD* CNC-associated PPNAD, *CPA* cortisol-producing adenoma, *CNC* Carney complex, *FAP* familial adenomatous polyposis, *GNAS* gene coding for the stimulatory subunit α of the G-protein (Gsα), *GPCR* G-protein-coupled receptor, *HLRCS* hereditary leiomyomatosis and renal cancer syndrome, *i-MAD* isolated micronodular adrenocortical disease, *i-PPNAD* isolated PPNAD, *MAS* McCune-Albright syndrome, *MEN1* multiple endocrine neoplasia type 1, *PBAD* primary bimorphic adrenocortical disease, *PBMAH* primary bilateral macronodular adrenocortical hyperplasia, *PDE8B* phosphodiesterase 8B gene, *PDE11A* phosphodiesterase 11A gene, *PPNAD* primary pigmented nodular adrenocortical disease, *PRKAR1A* protein kinase cAMP-dependent, regulatory, type I, α gene

(MMAD), bilateral macronodular adrenal hyperplasia (BMAH), and ACTH-independent macronodular adrenocortical hyperplasia (AIMAH); however, given the recent discovery of a local intra-adrenal secretion of adrenocorticotropic hormone (ACTH) (Louiset et al. 2013; Lefebvre et al. 2003), the term PBMAH was proposed. Secondary bilateral adrenocortical hyperplasia is caused by excess ACTH and should be differentiated from primary causes, as with PBMAH.

Table 3 Familial syndromes associated with adrenocortical tumors

Familial syndromes	Gene (locus)	Mode of inheritance	Major features
Carney complex	*PRKAR1A* (17q22-24, CNC1 locus)	AD	PPNAD
			Cardiac myxomas
			Pigmented skin lesions (lentiginosis and blue nevi)
			Somatotroph pituitary adenomas
			LCCSCT
			Benign thyroid nodules, differentiated thyroid cancer
			Melanocytic schwannomas
	PRKACB (1p31.1) and 2p16 (unkown gene; CNC2 locus)		ACT and rarely ACC
Multiple endocrine neoplasia type 1	*MEN1* (11q13)	AD	Primary hyperparathyroidism
			Pituitary adenomas
			Neuroendocrine tumors
Congenital adrenal hyperplasia	*CYP21A2* (6p21.3)	AR	Salt wasting (most severe)
	CYP11B1 (8q24)		Simple virilizing
	CYP17A1 (10q24.32)		Nonclassic (late onset)
			Cryptic
Familial adenomatous polyposis	*APC* (5q22.2)	AD	Large precancerous colorectal polyps in the second and third decades of life
			ACT, ACC
			Papillary thyroid carcinomas
			Lipomas
			Pancreatic carcinomas
Hereditary leiomyomatosis and renal cell cancer	*FH* (1q42.3-43)	AD	Hereditary leiomyomatosis
			Renal cancer
			ACT
Carney-Stratakis syndrome	*SDHB* (1p36)	AD	GIST
	SDHC (1q21)		Paragangliomas
	SDHD (11q23)		ACT
Carney triad	Unkown genetic defect	Sporadic	Pulmonary chondromas
			Pigmented skin lesions
			GIST
			Sarcomas
			PGL
			Esophageal leiomyoma
			ACT

(*continued*)

Table 3 (continued)

Familial syndromes	Gene (locus)	Mode of inheritance	Major features
Familial hyperaldosteronism	Type I (GRA): chimeric fusion of *CYP11B2* and *CYP11B1* (8q24.3)	AD	Type 1: severe early-onset hypertension with significant phenotypic and biochemical heterogeneity exists, and some individuals may never develop hypertension. Should be considered in patients with early-onset hypertension (<20 years) in the setting of a suppressed plasma renin activity, a family history of PA or early cerebral hemorrhage (<40 years) from intracranial aneurysms or hemorrhagic strokes
	Type II: mapped to 7p22		Type 2: affects adults and is characterized by hyperaldosteronism due to adrenocortical hyperplasia, an aldosterone-producing adenoma, or both, that is not glucocorticoid remediable
	Type III: heterozygous mutation in *KCNJ5* (11q2)		Type 3: presents earlier, in childhood, with severe hypertension and metabolic derangements
Li-Fraumeni syndrome	*TP53*	AD	The most frequent cancers are breast (25–30%), sarcoma (25–30%), and brain (9–16%). ACC is a less frequent manifestation accounting for 10–14% of cancers
			In southern Brazil, a specific germline *TP53* mutation (p. R33H) was identified in over 80% of children, and 13.5% of adults, with ACT, where the incidence of ACT is 15 times higher than the rest of the world
Beckwith-Wiedemann syndrome	epigenetic/genetic alterations on chromosome 11p15		The overall risk of tumor development in children is 7.5% (4–21%), with ACC being rare

(*continued*)

Table 3 (continued)

Familial syndromes	Gene (locus)	Mode of inheritance	Major features
	Mutations in the cyclin–dependent kinase inhibitor 1C (*CDKN1C*) gene		The most frequent clinical features are anterior abdominal wall defects (80%), macroglossia (97%), and overgrowth
	Microdeletions at imprinting center 1 (IC1) and microduplication at imprinting center 2 (IC2) in cases with germline defects		
	Uniparental disomy of 11p15		
	Gain of methylation at IC1		
	Loss of methylation at IC2		
Neurofibromatosis type 1	*NF1*	AD	About 50% of individuals have no family history of the disease
			The clinical hallmark is a predisposition to a variety of benign and malignant tumors: the most common malignant tumors are sarcomas (leiomyosarcoma and neurofibrosarcoma), breast, lung, and gastrointestinal tract tumors
			A few cases of ACC have been reported in patients with NF1; recently, a novel germline frameshift mutation (c.5452_5453delAT) in exon 37 of the *NF1* gene was associated with ACC development

ACC adrenocortical carcinoma, *ACT* adrenocortical tumor, *AD* autosomal dominant, *AR* autosomal recessive, *APC* adenomatous polyposis coli gene, *c-PPNAD* CNC-associated PPNAD, *CNC* Carney complex, *FAP* familial adenomatous polyposis, *GIST* gastrointestinal stromal tumors, *GNAS* gene coding for the stimulatory subunit α of the G-protein (Gsα), *GPCR* G-protein-coupled receptor, *GRA* glucocorticoid remediable aldosteronism, *HLRCS* hereditary leiomyomatosis and renal cancer syndrome, *i-MAD* isolated micronodular adrenocortical disease, *i-PPNAD* isolated PPNAD, *LCCSCT* benign large cell calcifying Sertoli cell tumor, *MAS* McCune-Albright syndrome, *MEN1* multiple endocrine neoplasia type 1, *PBAD* primary bimorphic adrenocortical disease, *PBMAH* primary bilateral macronodular adrenocortical hyperplasia, *PDE8B* phosphodiesterase 8B gene, *PDE11A* phosphodiesterase 11A gene, *PGL* paraganglioma, *PPNAD* primary pigmented nodular adrenocortical disease, *PRKAR1A* protein kinase, cAMP-dependent, regulatory, type I, α gene

ACCs are rare with an incidence of 0.5–2 million per year leading to 0.2% of all cancer deaths in the United States. ACCs are significantly more frequent in females (median age of diagnosis is at approximately 46 years across) and associated with a 16–44% 5-year survival rate (Fassnacht and Allolio 2009). An early peak of the disease between the ages of 5 and 7 years represents a clinically and molecularly different form of ACC (1.3% of the total number of cancers in children) (Fassnacht and Allolio 2009; Icard et al. 2001). ACCs may be non-secretory or cause hormone excess, including CS, hyperaldosteronism, or hyper-androgenism (Arlt et al. 2011).

Molecular Pathways in Adrenocortical Tumor Development

Two major molecular pathways contribute to ACT formation and share the downstream activation of certain oncogenic signals (Almeida et al. 2012). In the cAMP signaling pathway, activation of adenyl cyclase (AC) through the Gsα subunit (encoded by *GNAS*) generates cAMP that activates protein kinase A (PKA) (Fig. 1). PKA is a holoenzyme that consists of a tetramer of two homo- or heterodimer regulatory subunits (R1α, R1β, R2α, and R2β) and catalytic subunits (Cα, Cβ, Cγ, and PRKX) that are encoded by seperate genes (Taylor et al. 2012); their dissociation in the presence of cAMP enables phosphorylation of PKA targets, including gene expression to mediate cell growth, differentiation, and hormone production (e.g., cortisol). Alterations in any of these complex steps in the cAMP-dependent signaling pathway may predispose to the formation of ACT (Fig. 2) through constitutive activation by increasing the availability of the PKA catalytic subunits (Figs. 2 and 3). However, PKA signaling may either inhibit or stimulate cell proliferation depending on its specific role in the cell cycle (Robinson-White et al. 2006; Lania et al. 2004); this variability may explain, in part, why some biochemically active ACTs are small and difficult to detect clinically. The *Wnt* signaling pathway consists of a β-catenin-dependent and a β-catenin-independent pathway. A ligand binds to a series of Frizzled family receptors, such as LRP6 that activates phosphoproteins and inhibit the phosphorylation of β-catenin (Fig. 1). This in turn leads to the transcription of important genes, such as *WISP2*, *CTNNB1*, and *GSK3B*, as seen in PBMAH and PPNAD (Bourdeau et al. 2004).

Familial Syndromes Associated with Adrenocortical Tumors

Several familial syndromes have been described in association with benign and malignant ACTs. In the context of ACCs, a complex pattern of genetic defects from many chromosomal aberrations to somatic mutations in a number of genes has been described (Lerario et al. 2014). Moreover, high levels of estrogens have been suggested to increase the incidence of ACC based on the observation of ACC development during pregnancy, higher frequency of ACC in females, and in vitro studies showing growth-promoting effects of estrogen on the ACC (Sirianni et al. 2012). In this section, we present the various familial syndromes that are associated with benign ACTs and/or ACCs.

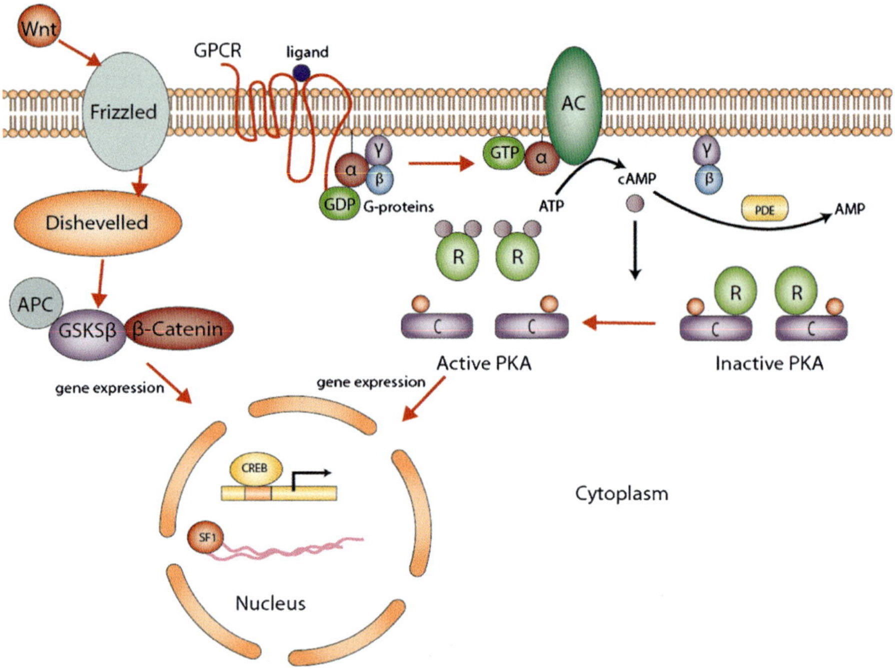

Fig. 2 The cyclic AMP and *Wnt* signaling pathways in adrenocortical tumors. In the cAMP signaling pathway, activation of adenyl cyclase (AC) through the Gsα subunit (encoded by *GNAS*) generates cAMP that activates protein kinase A (PKA). PKA is a holoenzyme that consists of a tetramer of two homo- or heterodimer regulatory subunits (R1α, R1β, R2α, and R2β) and catalytic subunits (Cα, Cβ, Cγ, and PRKX) that are encoded by seperate genes; their dissociation in the presence of cAMP enables phosphorylation of PKA targets, including gene expression to mediate cell growth, differentiation, and hormone production (e.g., cortisol). Alterations in any of these complex steps in the cAMP-dependent signaling pathway may predispose to the formation of ACT through constitutive activation by increasing the availability of the PKA catalytic subunits. However, PKA signaling may either inhibit or stimulate cell proliferation depending on its specific role in the cell cycle; this variability may explain, in part, why some biochemically active ACTs are small and difficult to detect clinically. The *Wnt* signaling pathway consists of a β-catenin-dependent and a β-catenin-independent pathway. A ligand binds to a series of Frizzled family receptors, such as LRP6 that activates phosphoproteins and inhibit the phosphorylation of β-catenin. This in turn leads to the transcription of important genes, such as *WISP2*, *CTNNB1*, and *GSK3B*, as seen in PBMAH and PPNAD. *Abbreviations*: *AC* adenylyl cyclase; *C* catalytic subunit of protein kinase A; *cAMP* cyclic AMP; *CREB* cyclic AMP response element binding protein, a transcription factor; *GPCR* G-protein-coupled receptor; *Gsα* stimulatory subunit α of the G-protein; *GSK3β* glycogen synthase kinase 3β; *PKA* cAMP-dependent protein kinase; *R* regulatory subunit; *SF1* steroidogenic factor 1; *WNT* wingless-type MMTV integration site family (Courtesy of Stratakis Laboratory, NICHD, NIH)

Carney Complex (CNC)

Carney complex (CNC) is an autosomal dominant (AD) syndrome that predisposes to multiple neoplasias. CNC is caused mostly by germline inactivating mutations in *PRKAR1A* (17q22-24, CNC1 locus), an apparent tumor suppressor

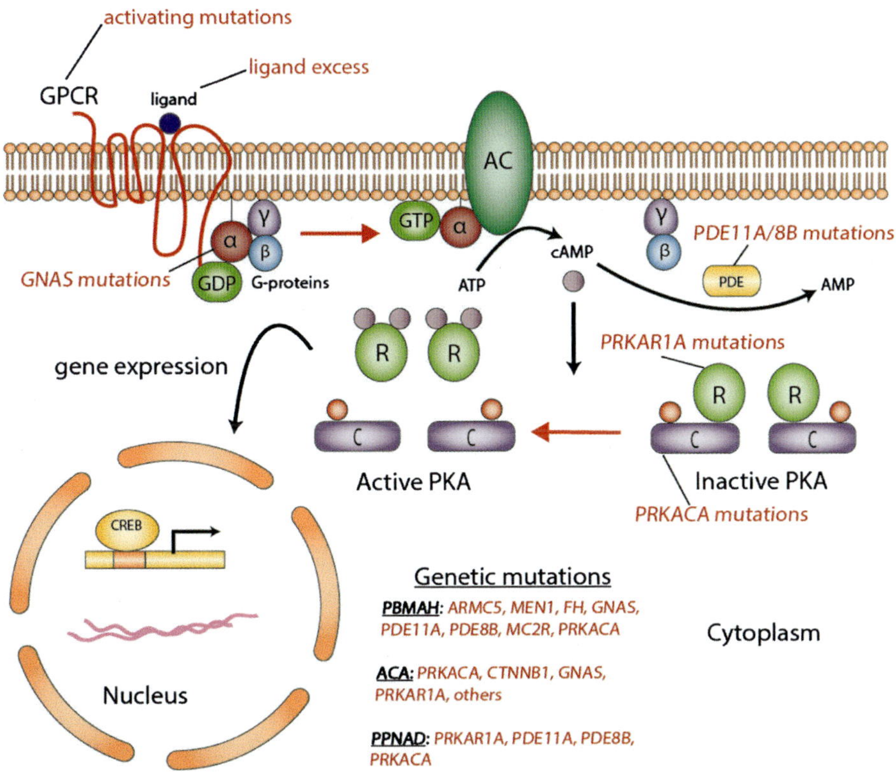

Fig. 3 Aberrations in the cyclic AMP-dependent signaling pathways in adrenocortical tumors. The first report of mutations causing ACTs was found in patients with McCune-Albright syndrome (MAS) due to *GNAS* that resulted in adrenocortical hyperplasia and/or benign cortisol-producing adenomas (CPA). This was rapidly followed by other important discoveries in the genetics of ACT formation, including the regulatory subunit type 1-α (RIα) of protein kinase A (PKA, *PRKAR1A* gene) and phosphodiesterase 11A and phosphodiesterase 8B (*PDE11A* and *PDE8B* genes, respectively) in Carney complex (CNC) and isolated ACTs and/or adrenal hyperplasia, respectively. Recently, germline mutations in the tumor suppressor gene *ARMC5* (*armadillo repeat containing 5*) were discovered in the majority of primary bilateral macronodular adrenocortical hyperplasia (PBMAH) cases. *Abbreviations*: *AC* adenyl cyclase; *C* catalytic subunit of protein kinase A; *cAMP* cyclic AMP; *CREB* cyclic AMP response element-binding protein, a transcription factor; *GPCR* G protein-coupled receptor; *Gsα* stimulatory subunit α of the G protein; *PDE11A* phosphodiesterase 11A; *PKA* cAMP-dependent protein kinase A; *R* regulatory subunit (Courtesy of Stratakis Laboratory, NICHD, NIH)

gene which encodes for the R1α subunit of PKA that carries an overall penetrance of over 95% by the age of 50 (Stratakis et al. 2001), and less commonly due to a yet-unidentified gene on chromosome 2p16 (CNC2) or *PRKACB* amplification on chromosome 1p31.1 (Kirschner et al. 2000; Horvath et al. 2010; Forlino et al. 2014). The clinical manifestations of CNC are broad, and the diagnosis is established if two or more of the following exists: CS from

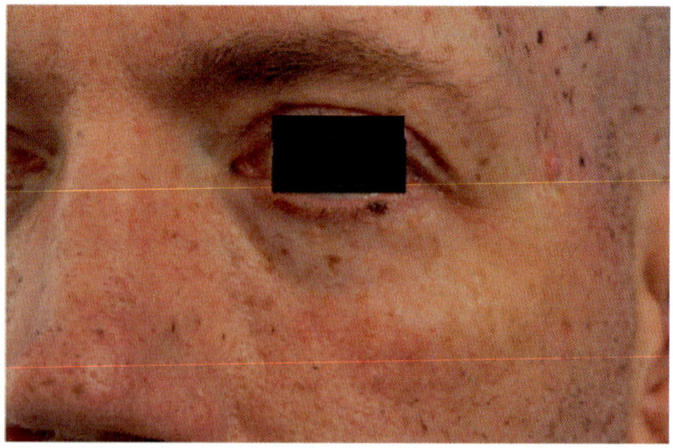

Image 1 Spotty skin pigmentations in a male patient with Carney complex (Courtesy of Stratakis Laboratory, NICHD, NIH)

PPNAD (the most frequent finding), cardiac myxomas, pigmented skin lesions (lentiginosis and blue nevi, Image 1), somatotroph pituitary adenomas, benign large cell calcifying Sertoli cell tumor (LCCSCT) of the testis, benign thyroid nodules, differentiated thyroid cancer, and melanocytic schwannomas. In-frame deletion of exon 3 and the c.708 +1G>T mutation appears to confer a more severe CNC phenotype, while the splice variant c.709(-7-2)del6 and the initiation-alternating substitution c.1A>G/p.M1Vp lead to an incomplete penetrance of CNC (Groussin et al. 2006). The hot spot c.491-492delTG mutation is most closely associated with lentigines, cardiac myxoma, and thyroid tumors when opposed to all other *PRKAR1A* mutations. CNC2 occurs later in life with a lower frequency of myxomas, schwannomas, thyroid tumors, and LCCSCT. Some patients may present with mild disease with i-PPNAD, with or without accompanied lentiginosis, and this “subtype” of CNC is usually diagnosed before 8 years of age and may be due to pathogenic mutations in *PRKAR1A*, particularly c.709 (-7-2) del6 or c.1A>G/p.M1V, in approximately 50% of cases.

Multiple Endocrine Neoplasia Type 1 (MEN1)

Multiple endocrine neoplasia type 1 (MEN1) is also an AD syndrome due to a heterozygous inactivating germline mutation of the tumor suppressor gene *MEN1* (11q13) (Chandrasekharappa et al. 1997) that is found in approximately 90% of affected individuals. The clinical features of MEN1 include primary hyperparathyroidism due to parathyroid hyperplasia, pituitary adenomas, neuroendocrine tumors, and facial angiofibromas, among others (Thakker et al. 2012). Nonfunctional ACTs are seen in approximately 20% of patients with MEN1 (Gatta-Cherifi et al. 2012), while functional ACTs are rare (primarily primary aldosteronism) (Gatta-Cherifi et al. 2012; Simonds et al. 2012).

Congenital Adrenal Hyperplasia (CAH)

Congenital adrenal hyperplasia (CAH) refers to a group of autosomal recessive disorders due to single gene defects in the various steps of cortisol biosynthesis. CAH represents a continuous phenotypic spectrum with over 95% of all cases caused by 21-hydroxylase deficiency that is classified into classic salt wasting, classic simple virilizing, and nonclassic (Speiser et al. 2010). Patients with CAH are predisposed to benign ACT, including adrenocortical adenomas, myelolipomas, and bilateral hyperplasia, due to a compensatory increase in ACTH secretion from pituitary corticotrophs that promotes proliferation of ACT.

Familial Adenomatous Polyposis (FAP)

Familial adenomatous polyposis (FAP) is an AD disorder due to genetic defects in the tumor suppressor gene *APC* (5q22.2) that predisposes to large precancerous colorectal polyps in the second and third decades of life. Bi-allelic inactivation of *APC* (copresence of germline and somatic mutations) leads to tumorigenesis through activation of the *Wnt*/β-catenin pathway. Extra-colonic manifestations are common and include ACT and adrenocortical hyperplasias, PBMAH (Hsiao et al. 2009), ACC, papillary thyroid carcinomas, lipomas, and pancreatic carcinomas (Gaujoux et al. 2010; Berthon et al. 2012).

Hereditary Leiomyomatosis and Renal Cell Cancer (HLRCC)

Hereditary leiomyomatosis and renal cell cancer (HLRCC) is an AD disorder caused by inactivating mutations of the tumor suppressor gene fumarate hydratase (*FH*, 1q42.3-43) that predispose to hereditary leiomyomatosis, renal cancer, and ACT (approximately 8%). Bi-allelic inactivation of *FH* leads to increased tumorigenesis through the activation of the hypoxia-induced factor 1 (HIF1) pathway that results in alterations in glycolytic activity, neovascularization, and downregulation of apoptotic mechanisms in tumor tissue. PBMAH or isolated adrenal nodularity has been reported in HLRCC (Matyakhina et al. 2005), where loss of heterozygosity for *FH* was confirmed in tumor tissue (Matyakhina et al. 2005).

Carney-Stratakis Syndrome (CCS)

Carney-Stratakis syndrome (CSS) is an AD disorder that predisposes to the formation of gastrointestinal tumors (GIST), paragangliomas (PGL), and ACT (Carney and Stratakis 2002). Germline mutations in *SDHB* (1p36), *SDHC* (1q21), and *SDHD* (11q23) that were known to be involved in inherited PGL and pheochromocytoma but were not previously involved in familial GIST or in ACTs have been linked to CSS. ACTs including PBMAH and nonfunctional tumors are rare in CSS.

Carney Triad (CT)

Carney triad (CT) is a sporadic condition that predisposes to hamartomatous lesions in various organs (pulmonary chondromas and pigmented and other skin lesions), GIST, sarcomas, PGL, esophageal leiomyoma, and ACA. CT is the only known adrenal disease that has among its clinical manifestations adrenocortical and medullary involvement, such as coexisting PBMAH or ACA, often non-functional, and pheochromocytomas or PGL (Carney et al. 1977). The genetics of CT is complex; a subset of patients may carry germline variants in the *SDHA*, *SDHB*, or *SDHC*, including loss of regions on the short arm (1p) and the long arm (1q) of chromosome 1 (Boikos et al. 2016), or recurrent aberrant dense DNA methylation at the gene locus of *SDHC* that leads to a reduced mRNA expression of SDHC and concurrent loss of the SDHC subunit on the protein level (Haller et al. 2014). Various ACT including subclinical Cushing syndrome due to ACT were proposed as the fourth component of the Carney triad (Carney et al. 2013).

Familial Hyperaldosteronism (FH)

Familial hyperaldosteronism (FH) is a group of AD disorders consists of three types. Type I (also known as glucocorticoid-remediable aldosteronism, GRA) is characterized by a chimeric fusion of *CYP11B2* and *CYP11B1* (8q24.3), rendering the aldosterone synthase hybrid gene to be under the regulation of ACTH rather than the renin-angiotensin system (Lifton et al. 1992), and should be considered in patients with early-onset hypertension (<20 years) in the setting of a suppressed plasma renin activity, a family history of PA, or early cerebral hemorrhage (<40 years) from intracranial aneurysms or hemorrhagic strokes. Type II (mapped to chromosome 7p22) typically affects adults and is characterized by hyperaldosteronism due to adrenocortical hyperplasia, an aldosterone-producing adenoma (APA), or both that is not glucocorticoid remediable (Torpy et al. 1998; Lafferty et al. 2000). Type III presents earlier, in childhood, with severe hypertension and metabolic derangements and is due to a heterozygous mutation in *KCNJ5* (11q2) (Geller et al. 2008).

Li-Fraumeni Syndrome (LFS)

Li-Fraumeni syndrome (LFS) is an autosomal dominant syndrome due to germline mutations in the tumor suppressor gene *TP53* that predisposes to cancers by age 30. The most frequent cancers are breast (25–30%), sarcoma (25–30%), and brain (9–16%) (Sorrell et al. 2013; Palmero et al. 2010). Early-onset cancers are caused by mutations in the DNA-binding portion of the gene, while slower rates of tumor development are seen with mutations outside the core DNA-binding domain (Varley et al. 1999). ACC is a less frequent manifestation accounting for 10–14% of cancers (Palmero et al. 2010) but are usually larger and associated with advanced stage, shorter disease-free survival, greater resistance to chemotherapy and radiation therapy, and overall higher rates of relapse, when compared to cases without *TP53* mutations (Fernandez-Cuesta et al. 2012). Germline mutations of *TP53* are found in 70%, 50–80%, and 3–6% of cases with LFS (Bachinski et al. 2005), adult ACT (Herrmann et al. 2012), and child ACT (Varley et al. 1999), respectively. In southern Brazil, a specific germline *TP53* mutation (p.R33H) of the p53 protein was identified in over 80% of children, and 13.5% of adults, with ACT, where the incidence of ACT is 15 times higher than the rest of the world (Giacomazzi et al. 2013; Petitjean et al. 2007; Ribeiro et al. 2001).

Beckwith-Wiedemann Syndrome (BWS)

Beckwith-Wiedemann syndrome (BWS) is a pediatric overgrowth disorder with an estimated incidence of 1 in 13,700 neonates due to epigenetic/genetic alterations on chromosome 11p15 (Weksberg et al. 2010). BWS usually occurs sporadically (85%), although familial transmission can also occur in 15% of the cases (Weksberg et al. 2010). Other genetic defects include mutations in the cyclin-dependent kinase inhibitor 1C (*CDKN1C*) gene or microdeletions at imprinting center 1 (IC1) and rarely microduplication at imprinting center 2 (IC2) in cases with germline defects (Hatada et al. 1997), uniparental disomy of 11p15 or gain of methylation at IC1 (associated with highest risk for Wilms' tumor and hepatoblastoma), and loss of methylation at IC2 (associated with a lower risk for tumor development). The overall risk of tumor development in children is 7.5% (4–21%), with ACC being rare (Rump et al. 2005). The most frequent clinical features of BWS are anterior abdominal wall defects (80%), macroglossia (97%), and overgrowth (Weksberg et al. 2010). Increased insulin growth factor 2 (IGF2) signaling is the main molecular cause of the phenotype associated with BWS, and IGF2 overexpression has also been linked with the development and progression of sporadic ACCs (Boulle et al. 2001). The most frequent ACT in BWS is hyperplasia (Carney et al. 2012), but rarely some patients develop ACC.

Neurofibromatosis Type 1 (NF1)

Neurofibromatosis type 1 (NF1) is an autosomal dominant disease with an incidence of 1 in 3,000 cases that results from a loss-of-function mutation or deletion in the *NF1* gene. About 50% of individuals with NF1 have no family history of the disease. The clinical hallmark of NF1 is a predisposition to a variety of benign and malignant tumors. The most common malignant tumors are sarcomas (leiomyosarcoma and neurofibrosarcoma) and breast, lung, and gastrointestinal tract tumors. A few cases of ACC have been reported in patients with NF1 (Menon et al. 2014; Fraumeni and Miller 1967; Fienman and Yakovac 1970); recently, a novel germline frameshift mutation (c.5452_5453delAT) in exon 37 of the *NF1* gene was associated with ACC development (Menon et al. 2014).

Genetic Aberrations in Common Benign Adrenocortical Tumors

Adrenocortical Adenomas (ACAs)

Adrenocortical adenomas (ACAs) represent the commonest form of ACT and are often detected incidentally on imaging. Approximately 10% of ACAs are functioning (primarily aldosterone-producing adenomas (APAs) or CPA) and comprise of a small (<5 cm), well-circumscribed, solitary lesions (but may be multiple) that are histologically bright yellow due to their enriched cytoplasmic lipid. These lesions should be differentiated from nonneoplastic ACA due to old age, hypertension, or diabetes mellitus that are either dominant, multifocal, or bilateral nodularity.

The *Wnt*/β-catenin and cAMP signaling pathways are activated in nonfunctional ACA and in most cases due to mutations in *CTNNB1* (3p22.1); somatic allelic losses of *PRKAR1A*, leading to inactivation with resultant decreased PKA (Bertherat et al. 2003); or other aberrations. Aberrant GPCRs detected by in vivo stimulation tests appear to be common in these lesions (Reznik et al. 2004). In the case of APA, somatic mutations in the *KCNJ5* gene (11q24.3) have been implicated in the majority (30–65%) (Choi et al. 2011). Recently, germline mutations in *ARMC5* (16p11.2) have also been implicated in PA and particularly in patients from African-American decent (Zilbermint et al. 2015). A second somatic genetic event, either 16p loss of heterozygosity or a second somatic mutation in the coding region of the gene, is required in addition to the germline mutation in *AMRC5* to mediate tumorigenesis leading to polyclonal nodularity (Faucz et al. 2014; Correa et al. 2015). Other genes that have been implicated in APA formation include *ATP1A1* (1p13.1) (Beuschlein et al. 2013; Williams et al. 2014), *ATP2B3* gene (Xq28) (Beuschlein et al. 2013; Williams et al. 2014), and *CACNA1D* (3p14.3) (Scholl et al. 2013). *PRKACA* mutations are very rare findings in APA (Rhayem et al. 2016).

Unlike APAs, the majority of CPAs are caused by aberrations in the cAMP-dependent signaling pathway, including somatic activating mutations of *PRKACA* with an estimated incidence of approximately 42% (86 of 206 tumors studied to date) (Beuschlein et al. 2014; Cao et al. 2014; Goh et al. 2014), somatic mutations in *GNAS* (5–17%) (Fragoso et al. 2003), and somatic allelic losses of *PRKAR1A* (23%). Defects in *Wnt* signaling have been reported in CPA, with *CTNNB1* in approximately 23% of cases (Thiel et al. 2015). The coexistence of two different ACTs causing the concurrent diagnosis of PA and Cushing syndrome due to different genetic alterations (coexisting mutations in *PRKACA* and *KCNJ5* in different nodules) is possible (Nanba et al. 2016). There are many unknown genetic defects that lead to CPA or APA formation and are under current investigation.

Primary Bilateral Macronodular Adrenocortical Hyperplasia (PBMAH)

Primary bilateral macronodular adrenocortical hyperplasia (PBMAH) represents a heterogeneous benign disorder that is often associated with subclinical CS in adults over a number of years and accounts for less than 2% of all endogenous CS (Lacroix 2009). Non-mutated aberrant receptors (e.g., gastrointestinal peptide, vasopressin, serotonin, catecholamines, luteinizing hormone, or autocrine/paracrine ACTHs) may stimulate cortisol, aldosterone, and estrogen either singly or in combination (Bourdeau et al. 2001; Lacroix et al. 2010). Mutations in the tumor suppressor *ARMC5* gene were identified in over 50% of apparent sporadic and familial PBMAH cases, where both alleles carried one germline and one somatic mutation each (Assie et al. 2013; Faucz et al. 2014; Alencar et al. 2014). Other genetic aberrations in PBMAH have been described, including *GNAS* (without features of MAS) (Hsiao et al. 2009; Fragoso et al. 2003), *PDE11A* gene variants (Libé et al. 2011; Hsiao et al. 2009), germline duplications of *PRKACA* resulting in copy number gains (Beuschlein et al. 2014), and germline mutations in *FH*, *MEN1*, and *APC* (Hsiao et al. 2009; Fragoso et al. 2003). The clinical spectrum and genetic aberrations in PBMAH are heterogeneous, and further studies are required to better elucidate the molecular mechanisms involved in its tumorigenesis.

Alterations of Phosphodiesterases (PDEs)

Phosphodiesterases (PDEs) are key enzymes in the cAMP signaling pathway that function through the hydrolyzation of cAMP (PDE isoforms 4, 7, and 8) and cGMP (PDE isoforms 5, 6, and 9) into their respective AMP and GMP (Francis et al. 2011; Azevedo et al. 2014). *PDE8B* and *PDE11A* have been implicated in ACT formation; an inactivating mutation in *PDE8B* (5q14.1) was reported in a 2-year-old girl with iMAD that she had inherited from her father (Horvath et al. 2008), and inactivating mutations in the highly polymorphic *PDE11A* (2q31.2) were reported in patients with PPNAD or iMAD (Libé et al. 2011). Genetic variations in *PDE8B* and *PDE11A* may be low penetrance alleles (with a relative frequency in the general population), which may predispose for the development of ACT.

McCune-Albright Syndrome (MAS)

McCune-Albright syndrome (MAS) is caused by postzygotic gain-of-function point mutations in *GNAS* that lead to polyostotic fibrous dysplasia, café au lait skin spots, precocious puberty, and overactive endocrinopathies. MAS predisposes to CS in the infantile period that develops from CPAs or nodular adrenal hyperplasia (PBAD, a form of PBMAH) (Kirk et al. 1999; Carney et al. 2011). Clinical manifestations of MAS are highly variable and depend on the distribution of somatic mosaic mutations in the various affected tissues (Carney et al. 2011).

Isolated Micronodular Adrenocortical Disease (iMAD)

Isolated micronodular adrenocortical disease (iMAD) is a rare disorder of the adrenal glands of very early onset that may be caused by mutations in *PDE11A*, *PDE8B*, or germline copy number gain of *PRKACA*. *PRKAR1A* mutations have never been described in iMAD, which is thus differentiated from PPNAD by both its genetics and its lack of pigmentation. On the other hand, iMAD may be associated with a paradoxical rise of glucocorticoid excretion during Liddle's test (1 mg overnight and low- and high-dose dexamethasone suppression tests) as is also observed in patients with PPNAD (Stratakis et al. 1999).

Genetic Counseling of Patients with Disorders of Adrenocortical Function

Genetic testing is a powerful tool in clinical practice for patients and their families. Identification of the underlying genetic etiology will allow estimations of recurrence risk, which will inform family planning decisions, facilitate preimplantation genetic testing, and allow accurate prenatal screening. Additionally, genetic information will allow for the monitoring of disease progression and the introduction of timely treatment regimens to minimize complications and also provides important knowledge of the underlying disease mechanism or mechanisms. One study found that knowledge of carrier status of *SDH* mutations did not deter young couples/patients from having a desire to conceive in the future (Raygada et al. 2014). The complexity of these decisions, with their significant medical and psychosocial implications, is an important aspect of managing patients and their families.

Genetic screening may begin as early as infancy in at-risk individuals, especially with conditions that can manifest with early mortality, such as CNC. Given the complexity of choosing between the multiple candidate genes with overlapping clinical phenotypes, testing genes either singly or in a panel, particularly in patients without known syndromic features, should be considered. Several sequencing technologies exist. The growing availability and use of whole genome sequencing (WGS), whole exome sequencing (WES), whole genome arrays, and multigene panels increase the likelihood of detecting unintentionally or unexpectedly pathogenic mutations or variances of undetermined significance (e.g., detection of *TP53* mutations that predispose to ACC). After identifying a pathogenic mutation, proband's parents, siblings, and offsprings should be tested. If the mutation is transmitted in an autosomal dominant fashion, then each sibling has a 50% risk of having the mutation. In the case of *TP53* and other genes, if neither parent carries the mutation, the risk to siblings is low, but the possibility of germline mosaicism exists.

Early disease screening and intervention in affected or at risk individuals may be associated with better outcomes. A successful patient counseling model would incorporate patient's values and attitudes toward their disease, underscoring the risks and benefits of genetic screening and counseling, psychosocial interventions, and service delivery, see for example in (Raygada et al. 2014). The most important component of the genetic counseling process in patients with adrenocortical disorders is determination and communication of benign and malignant risk. Other aspects of a successful counseling model include a thorough personal medical and family history from at least four generations (with a detailed family pedigree), education regarding the genetics of the condition, and discussions on preventing and screening options that should be carried out by an experienced genetic counselor.

When dealing with a young patient with ACT, genetic counseling regardless of family history should be considered. Many of these conditions (e.g., germline mutations in *ARMC5* in PBMAH) have decreased penetrance, and first-degree relatives that are carriers may not be affected. Moreover, a family history can appear negative due to a limited family structure, incomplete penetrance of the mutation, or presence of *de novo* mutations. Any individual with a positive genetic screen for any of the mutations mentioned herein and without a clear phenotype should be closely monitored by an experienced physician. Further evaluation may be considered based on the type of mutation, disorder, and/or patient's clinical presentation.

Conclusions

Over the past 30 years, the identification of several genetic alterations in the formation of adrenocortical disorders has paved our understanding of adrenocortical development and disease. Causes of CAI are broad and encompass a variety of genetic conditions that present early in infancy. Altered genes in the cAMP, *Wnt*, and other signaling pathways predispose to the development of ACTs of various subtypes. Our knowledge on the diagnosis and management of these conditions is evolving. The use of genetic testing in clinical practice is a powerful tool for patients and their families in the identification of the underlying genetic etiology which will allow estimations of recurrence risk, inform family planning decisions, facilitate preimplantation genetic testing, and allow accurate prenatal screening.

Acknowledgments This work was supported by the intramural program of the *Eunice Kennedy Shriver* National Institute of Child Health and Human Development, National Institutes of Health (NIH), protocol HD008920.

References

Achermann JC, Vilain EJ. In: Pagon RA, Adam MP, Ardinger HH, Wallace SE, Amemiya A, Bean LJH, et al., editors. X-linked adrenal hypoplasia congenita. Seattle: GeneReviews(R); 1993.

Achermann JC, Ito M, Ito M, Hindmarsh PC, Jameson JL. A mutation in the gene encoding steroidogenic factor-1 causes XY sex reversal and adrenal failure in humans. Nat Genet. 1999;22(2):125–6.

Alencar GA, Lerario AM, Nishi MY, Mariani BM, Almeida MQ, Tremblay J, et al. ARMC5 mutations are a frequent cause of primary macronodular adrenal Hyperplasia. J Clin Endocrinol Metab. 2014;99(8):E1501–9.

Almeida MQ, Azevedo MF, Xekouki P, Bimpaki EI, Horvath A, Collins MT, et al. Activation of cyclic AMP signaling leads to different pathway alterations in lesions of the adrenal cortex caused by germline PRKAR1A defects versus those due to somatic GNAS mutations. J Clin Endocrinol Metab. 2012;97(4):E687–93.

Anderson RA, Byrum RS, Coates PM, Sando GN. Mutations at the lysosomal acid cholesteryl ester hydrolase gene locus in Wolman disease. Proc Natl Acad Sci U S A. 1994;91(7):2718–22.

Arboleda VA, Lee H, Parnaik R, Fleming A, Banerjee A, Ferraz-de-Souza B, et al. Mutations in the PCNA-binding domain of CDKN1C cause IMAGe syndrome. Nat Genet. 2012;44(7):788–92.

Arlt W, Biehl M, Taylor AE, Hahner S, Libe R, Hughes BA, et al. Urine steroid metabolomics as a biomarker tool for detecting malignancy in adrenal tumors. J Clin Endocrinol Metab. 2011;96 (12):3775–84.

Assie G, Libe R, Espiard S, Rizk-Rabin M, Guimier A, Luscap W, et al. ARMC5 mutations in macronodular adrenal hyperplasia with Cushing's syndrome. N Engl J Med. 2013;369 (22):2105–14.

Azevedo MF, Faucz FR, Bimpaki E, Horvath A, Levy I, de Alexandre RB, et al. Clinical and molecular genetics of the phosphodiesterases (PDEs). Endocr Rev. 2014;35(2):195–233.

Bachinski LL, Olufemi SE, Zhou X, Wu CC, Yip L, Shete S, et al. Genetic mapping of a third Li-Fraumeni syndrome predisposition locus to human chromosome 1q23. Cancer Res. 2005;65 (2):427–31.

Bertherat J, Groussin L, Sandrini F, Matyakhina L, Bei T, Stergiopoulos S, et al. Molecular and functional analysis of PRKAR1A and its locus (17q22-24) in sporadic adrenocortical tumors: 17q losses, somatic mutations, and protein kinase A expression and activity. Cancer Res. 2003;63(17):5308–19.

Berthon A, Martinez A, Bertherat J, Val P. Wnt/beta-catenin signalling in adrenal physiology and tumour development. Mol Cell Endocrinol. 2012;351(1):87–95.

Beuschlein F, Boulkroun S, Osswald A, Wieland T, Nielsen HN, Lichtenauer UD, et al. Somatic mutations in ATP1A1 and ATP2B3 lead to aldosterone-producing adenomas and secondary hypertension. Nat Genet. 2013;45(4):440–4. 4e1-2.

Beuschlein F, Fassnacht M, Assie G, Calebiro D, Stratakis CA, Osswald A, et al. Constitutive activation of PKA catalytic subunit in adrenal Cushing's syndrome. N Engl J Med. 2014;370 (11):1019–28.

Bezman L, Moser AB, Raymond GV, Rinaldo P, Watkins PA, Smith KD, et al. Adrenoleukodystrophy: incidence, new mutation rate, and results of extended family screening. Ann Neurol. 2001;49(4):512–7.

Bianconi SE1, Conley SK, Keil MF, Sinaii N, Rother KI, Porter FD, Stratakis CA. Adrenal function in Smith-Lemli-Opitz syndrome. Am J Med Genet A. 2011;155A(11):2732–8. doi:10.1002/ajmg.a.34271.

Boikos SA, Xekouki P, Fumagalli E, Faucz FR, Raygada M, Szarek E, et al. Carney triad can be (rarely) associated with germline succinate dehydrogenase defects. Eur J Hum Genet: EJHG. 2016;24(4):569–73.

Boulle N, Baudin E, Gicquel C, Logie A, Bertherat J, Penfornis A, et al. Evaluation of plasma insulin-like growth factor binding protein-2 as a marker for adrenocortical tumors. Eur J Endocrinol. 2001;144(1):29–36.

Bourdeau I, D'Amour P, Hamet P, Boutin JM, Lacroix A. Aberrant membrane hormone receptors in incidentally discovered bilateral macronodular adrenal hyperplasia with subclinical Cushing's syndrome. J Clin Endocrinol Metab. 2001;86(11):5534–40.

Bourdeau I, Antonini SR, Lacroix A, Kirschner LS, Matyakhina L, Lorang D, et al. Gene array analysis of macronodular adrenal hyperplasia confirms clinical heterogeneity and identifies several candidate genes as molecular mediators. Oncogene. 2004;23(8):1575–85.

Brooks BP, Kleta R, Caruso RC, Stuart C, Ludlow J, Stratakis CA. Triple-A syndrome with prominent ophthalmic features and a novel mutation in the AAAS gene: a case report. BMC Ophthalmol. 2004;4:7.

Brooks BP, Kleta R, Stuart C, Tuchman M, Jeong A, Stergiopoulos SG, et al. Genotypic heterogeneity and clinical phenotype in triple A syndrome: a review of the NIH experience 2000–2005. Clin Genet. 2005;68(3):215–21.

Cao Y, He M, Gao Z, Peng Y, Li Y, Li L, et al. Activating hotspot L205R mutation in PRKACA and adrenal Cushing's syndrome. Science. 2014;344(6186):913–7.

Carney JA, Stratakis CA. Familial paraganglioma and gastric stromal sarcoma: a new syndrome distinct from the Carney triad. Am J Med Genet. 2002;108(2):132–9.

Carney JA, Sheps SG, Go VL, Gordon H. The triad of gastric leiomyosarcoma, functioning extra-adrenal paraganglioma and pulmonary chondroma. N Engl J Med. 1977;296(26):1517–8.

Carney JA, Young WF, Stratakis CA. Primary bimorphic adrenocortical disease: cause of hypercortisolism in McCune-Albright syndrome. Am J Surg Pathol. 2011;35(9):1311–26.

Carney JA, Ho J, Kitsuda K, Young Jr WF, Stratakis CA. Massive neonatal adrenal enlargement due to cytomegaly, persistence of the transient cortex, and hyperplasia of the permanent cortex: findings in Cushing syndrome associated with hemihypertrophy. Am J Surg Pathol. 2012;36 (10):1452–63.

Carney JA, Stratakis CA, Young Jr WF. Adrenal cortical adenoma: the fourth component of the Carney triad and an association with subclinical Cushing syndrome. Am J Surg Pathol. 2013;37 (8):1140–9.

Chan LF, Campbell DC, Novoselova TV, Clark AJ, Metherell LA. Whole-exome sequencing in the differential diagnosis of primary adrenal insufficiency in children. Front Endocrinol. 2015;6:113.

Chandrasekharappa SC, Guru SC, Manickam P, Olufemi SE, Collins FS, Emmert-Buck MR, et al. Positional cloning of the gene for multiple endocrine neoplasia-type 1. Science. 1997;276 (5311):404–7.

Chemaitilly W, Goldenberg A, Baujat G, Thibaud E, Cormier-Daire V, Abadie V. Adrenal insufficiency and abnormal genitalia in a 46XX female with Smith-Lemli-Opitz syndrome. Horm Res. 2003;59(5):254–6.

Chen H, Hoffman WH, Kusyk CJ, Tuck-Muller CM, Hoffman MG, Davis LS. De novo dup (5p) in a patient with congenital hypoplasia of the adrenal gland. Am J Med Genet. 1995;55(4):489–93.

Choi M, Scholl UI, Yue P, Bjorklund P, Zhao B, Nelson-Williams C, et al. K+ channel mutations in adrenal aldosterone-producing adenomas and hereditary hypertension. Science. 2011;331 (6018):768–72.

Correa R, Zilbermint M, Berthon A, Espiard S, Batsis M, Papadakis G, et al. The ARMC5 gene shows extensive genetic variance in primary macronodular adrenocortical hyperplasia. Eur J Endocrinol/Eur Fed Endocrine Soc. 2015;173:435.

Couture C, Saveanu A, Barlier A, Carel JC, Fassnacht M, Fluck CE, et al. Phenotypic homogeneity and genotypic variability in a large series of congenital isolated ACTH-deficiency patients with TPIT gene mutations. J Clin Endocrinol Metab. 2012;97(3):E486–95.

Dittmar M, Kahaly GJ. Polyglandular autoimmune syndromes: immunogenetics and long-term follow-up. J Clin Endocrinol Metab. 2003;88(7):2983–92.

Elias LL, Huebner A, Metherell LA, Canas A, Warne GL, Bitti ML, et al. Tall stature in familial glucocorticoid deficiency. Clin Endocrinol. 2000;53(4):423–30.

Else T, Hammer GD. Genetic analysis of adrenal absence: agenesis and aplasia. Trends Endocrinol Metab. 2005;16(10):458–68.

Fassnacht M, Allolio B. Clinical management of adrenocortical carcinoma. Best Pract Res Clin Endocrinol Metab. 2009;23(2):273–89.

Faucz FR, Zilbermint M, Lodish MB, Szarek E, Trivellin G, Sinaii N, et al. Macronodular adrenal hyperplasia due to mutations in an armadillo repeat containing 5 (ARMC5) gene: a clinical and genetic investigation. J Clin Endocrinol Metab. 2014;99(6):E1113–9.

Feigenbaum V, Lombard-Platet G, Guidoux S, Sarde CO, Mandel JL, Aubourg P. Mutational and protein analysis of patients and heterozygous women with X-linked adrenoleukodystrophy. Am J Hum Genet. 1996;58(6):1135–44.

Fernandez-Cuesta L, Oakman C, Falagan-Lotsch P, Smoth KS, Quinaux E, Buyse M, et al. Prognostic and predictive value of TP53 mutations in node-positive breast cancer patients treated with anthracycline- or anthracycline/taxane-based adjuvant therapy: results from the BIG 02-98 phase III trial. Breast Cancer Res: BCR. 2012;14(3):R70.

Ferraz-de-Souza B, Achermann JC. Disorders of adrenal development. Endocr Dev. 2008;13:19–32.

Fienman NL, Yakovac WC. Neurofibromatosis in childhood. J Pediatr. 1970;76(3):339–46.

Forlino A, Vetro A, Garavelli L, Ciccone R, London E, Stratakis CA, Zuffardi O. PRKACB and Carney complex. N Engl J Med. 2014;370(11):1065–7. doi:10.1056/NEJMc1309730. Epub 2014 Feb 26.

Fragoso MC, Domenice S, Latronico AC, Martin RM, Pereira MA, Zerbini MC, et al. Cushing's syndrome secondary to adrenocorticotropin-independent macronodular adrenocortical hyperplasia due to activating mutations of GNAS1 gene. J Clin Endocrinol Metab. 2003;88(5):2147–51.

Francis SH, Blount MA, Corbin JD. Mammalian cyclic nucleotide phosphodiesterases: molecular mechanisms and physiological functions. Physiol Rev. 2011;91(2):651–90.

Fraumeni Jr JF, Miller RW. Adrenocortical neoplasms with hemihypertrophy, brain tumors, and other disorders. J Pediatr. 1967;70(1):129–38.

Gatta-Cherifi B, Chabre O, Murat A, Niccoli P, Cardot-Bauters C, Rohmer V, et al. Adrenal involvement in MEN1. Analysis of 715 cases from the Groupe d'etude des Tumeurs Endocrines database. Eur J Endocrinol. 2012;166(2):269–79.

Gaujoux S, Pinson S, Gimenez-Roqueplo AP, Amar L, Ragazzon B, Launay P, et al. Inactivation of the APC gene is constant in adrenocortical tumors from patients with familial adenomatous polyposis but not frequent in sporadic adrenocortical cancers. Clin Cancer Res: Off J Am Assoc Cancer Res. 2010;16(21):5133–41.

Geller DS, Zhang J, Wisgerhof MV, Shackleton C, Kashgarian M, Lifton RP. A novel form of human mendelian hypertension featuring nonglucocorticoid-remediable aldosteronism. J Clin Endocrinol Metab. 2008;93(8):3117–23.

Giacomazzi J, Selistre SG, Rossi C, Alemar B, Santos-Silva P, Pereira FS, et al. Li-Fraumeni and Li-Fraumeni-like syndrome among children diagnosed with pediatric cancer in Southern Brazil. Cancer. 2013;119(24):4341–9.

Goh G, Scholl UI, Healy JM, Choi M, Prasad ML, Nelson-Williams C, et al. Recurrent activating mutation in PRKACA in cortisol-producing adrenal tumors. Nat Genet. 2014;46(6):613–7.

Goto M, Piper Hanley K, Marcos J, Wood PJ, Wright S, Postle AD, et al. In humans, early cortisol biosynthesis provides a mechanism to safeguard female sexual development. J Clin Invest. 2006;116(4):953–60.

Groussin L, Horvath A, Jullian E, Boikos S, Rene-Corail F, Lefebvre H, et al. A PRKAR1A mutation associated with primary pigmented nodular adrenocortical disease in 12 kindreds. J Clin Endocrinol Metab. 2006;91(5):1943–9.

Haller F, Moskalev EA, Faucz FR, Barthelmess S, Wiemann S, Bieg M, et al. Aberrant DNA hypermethylation of SDHC: a novel mechanism of tumor development in Carney triad. Endocr Relat Cancer. 2014;21(4):567–77.

Hanley NA, Arlt W. The human fetal adrenal cortex and the window of sexual differentiation. Trends Endocrinol Metab. 2006;17(10):391–7.

Hatada I, Nabetani A, Morisaki H, Xin Z, Ohishi S, Tonoki H, et al. New p57KIP2 mutations in Beckwith-Wiedemann syndrome. Hum Genet. 1997;100(5–6):681–3.

Heino M, Scott HS, Chen Q, Peterson P, Maebpaa U, Papasavvas MP, et al. Mutation analyses of North American APS-1 patients. Hum Mutat. 1999;13(1):69–74.

Herrmann LJ, Heinze B, Fassnacht M, Willenberg HS, Quinkler M, Reisch N, et al. TP53 germline mutations in adult patients with adrenocortical carcinoma. J Clin Endocrinol Metab. 2012;97(3): E476–85.

Horvath A, Stratakis CA. Unraveling the molecular basis of micronodular adrenal hyperplasia. Curr Opin Endocrinol Diabetes Obes. 2008;15(3):227–33.

Horvath A, Mericq V, Stratakis CA. Mutation in PDE8B, a cyclic AMP-specific phosphodiesterase in adrenal hyperplasia. N Engl J Med. 2008;358(7):750–2.

Horvath A, Bertherat J, Groussin L, Guillaud-Bataille M, Tsang K, Cazabat L, et al. Mutations and polymorphisms in the gene encoding regulatory subunit type 1-alpha of protein kinase A (PRKAR1A): an update. Hum Mutat. 2010;31(4):369–79.

Hsia YE, Bratu M, Herbordt A. Genetics of the Meckel syndrome (dysencephalia splanchnocystica). Pediatrics. 1971;48(2):237–47.

Hsiao HP, Kirschner LS, Bourdeau I, Keil MF, Boikos SA, Verma S, et al. Clinical and genetic heterogeneity, overlap with other tumor syndromes, and atypical glucocorticoid hormone secretion in adrenocorticotropin-independent macronodular adrenal hyperplasia compared with other adrenocortical tumors. J Clin Endocrinol Metab. 2009;94(8):2930–7.

Husebye ES, Allolio B, Arlt W, Badenhoop K, Bensing S, Betterle C, et al. Consensus statement on the diagnosis, treatment and follow-up of patients with primary adrenal insufficiency. J Intern Med. 2014;275(2):104–15.

Icard P, Goudet P, Charpenay C, Andreassian B, Carnaille B, Chapuis Y, et al. Adrenocortical carcinomas: surgical trends and results of a 253-patient series from the French Association of Endocrine Surgeons study group. World J Surg. 2001;25(7):891–7.

Ikeda M, Hirano M, Shinoda K, Katsumata N, Furutama D, Nakamura K, et al. Triple A syndrome in Japan. Muscle Nerve. 2013;48(3):381–6.

Jackson RS, Creemers JW, Ohagi S, Raffin-Sanson ML, Sanders L, Montague CT, et al. Obesity and impaired prohormone processing associated with mutations in the human prohormone convertase 1 gene. Nat Genet. 1997;16(3):303–6.

James PA, Aftimos S, Hofman P. CHARGE association and secondary hypoadrenalism. Am J Med Genet A. 2003;117A(2):177–80.

Jongmans MC, Admiraal RJ, van der Donk KP, Vissers LE, Baas AF, Kapusta L, et al. CHARGE syndrome: the phenotypic spectrum of mutations in the CHD7 gene. J Med Genet. 2006;43(4):306–14.

Kahaly GJ. Polyglandular autoimmune syndrome type II. Presse Med. 2012;41(12 P 2):e663–70.

Kahana D, Berant M, Wolman M. Primary familial xanthomatosis with adrenal involvement (Wolman's disease). Report of a further case with nervous system involvement and pathogenetic considerations. Pediatrics. 1968;42(1):70–6.

Karpac J, Kern A, Hochgeschwender U. Pro-opiomelanocortin peptides and the adrenal gland. Mol Cell Endocrinol. 2007;265–266:29–33.

Kirk JM, Brain CE, Carson DJ, Hyde JC, Grant DB. Cushing's syndrome caused by nodular adrenal hyperplasia in children with McCune-Albright syndrome. J Pediatr. 1999;134(6):789–92.

Kirschner MA, Powell Jr RD, Lipsett MB. Cushing's syndrome: nodular cortical hyperplasia of adrenal glands with clinical and pathological features suggesting adrenocortical tumor. J Clin Endocrinol Metab. 1964;24:947–55.

Kirschner LS, Carney JA, Pack SD, Taymans SE, Giatzakis C, Cho YS, et al. Mutations of the gene encoding the protein kinase A type I-alpha regulatory subunit in patients with the Carney complex. Nat Genet. 2000;26(1):89–92.

Krude H, Biebermann H, Schnabel D, Tansek MZ, Theunissen P, Mullis PE, et al. Obesity due to proopiomelanocortin deficiency: three new cases and treatment trials with thyroid hormone and ACTH4-10. J Clin Endocrinol Metab. 2003;88(10):4633–40.

Lacroix A. ACTH-independent macronodular adrenal hyperplasia. Best Pract Res Clin Endocrinol Metab. 2009;23(2):245–59.

Lacroix A, Bourdeau I, Lampron A, Mazzuco TL, Tremblay J, Hamet P. Aberrant G-protein coupled receptor expression in relation to adrenocortical overfunction. Clin Endocrinol. 2010;73(1):1–15.

Lafferty AR, Torpy DJ, Stowasser M, Taymans SE, Lin JP, Huggard P, et al. A novel genetic locus for low renin hypertension: familial hyperaldosteronism type II maps to chromosome 7 (7p22). J Med Genet. 2000;37(11):831–5.

Lamolet B, Pulichino AM, Lamonerie T, Gauthier Y, Brue T, Enjalbert A, et al. A pituitary cell-restricted T box factor, Tpit, activates POMC transcription in cooperation with Pitx homeoproteins. Cell. 2001;104(6):849–59.

Lania AG, Mantovani G, Ferrero S, Pellegrini C, Bondioni S, Peverelli E, et al. Proliferation of transformed somatotroph cells related to low or absent expression of protein kinase a regulatory subunit 1A protein. Cancer Res. 2004;64(24):9193–8.

Lefebvre H, Duparc C, Chartrel N, Jegou S, Pellerin A, Laquerriere A, et al. Intraadrenal adrenocorticotropin production in a case of bilateral macronodular adrenal hyperplasia causing Cushing's syndrome. J Clin Endocrinol Metab. 2003;88(7):3035–42.

Lerario AM, Moraitis A, Hammer GD. Genetics and epigenetics of adrenocortical tumors. Mol Cell Endocrinol. 2014;386(1–2):67–84.

Libé R, Horvath A, Vezzosi D, Fratticci A, Coste J, Perlemoine K, Ragazzon B, Guillaud-Bataille M, Groussin L, Clauser E, Raffin-Sanson ML, Siegel J, Moran J, Drori-Herishanu L, Faucz FR, Lodish M, Nesterova M, Bertagna X, Bertherat J, Stratakis CA. Frequent phosphodiesterase 11A gene (PDE11A) defects in patients with Carney complex (CNC) caused by PRKAR1A mutations: PDE11A may contribute to adrenal and testicular tumors in CNC as a modifier of the phenotype. J Clin Endocrinol Metab. 2011;96(1):E208–14. doi:10.1210/jc.2010-1704.

Lifton RP, Dluhy RG, Powers M, Rich GM, Cook S, Ulick S, et al. A chimaeric 11 beta-hydroxylase/aldosterone synthase gene causes glucocorticoid-remediable aldosteronism and human hypertension. Nature. 1992;355(6357):262–5.

Lin L, Gu WX, Ozisik G, To WS, Owen CJ, Jameson JL, et al. Analysis of DAX1 (NR0B1) and steroidogenic factor-1 (NR5A1) in children and adults with primary adrenal failure: ten years' experience. J Clin Endocrinol Metab. 2006;91(8):3048–54.

Lin L, Hindmarsh PC, Metherell LA, Alzyoud M, Al-Ali M, Brain CE, et al. Severe loss-of-function mutations in the adrenocorticotropin receptor (ACTHR, MC2R) can be found in patients diagnosed with salt-losing adrenal hypoplasia. Clin Endocrinol. 2007;66(2):205–10.

Lodish M, Stratakis CA. A genetic and molecular update on adrenocortical causes of Cushing syndrome. Nat Rev Endocrinol. 2016;12(5):255–62.

Louiset E, Duparc C, Young J, Renouf S, Tetsi Nomigni M, Boutelet I, et al. Intraadrenal corticotropin in bilateral macronodular adrenal hyperplasia. N Engl J Med. 2013;369 (22):2115–25.

Mandel H, Shemer R, Borochowitz ZU, Okopnik M, Knopf C, Indelman M, et al. SERKAL syndrome: an autosomal-recessive disorder caused by a loss-of-function mutation in WNT4. Am J Hum Genet. 2008;82(1):39–47.

Matyakhina L, Freedman RJ, Bourdeau I, Wei MH, Stergiopoulos SG, Chidakel A, et al. Hereditary leiomyomatosis associated with bilateral, massive, macronodular adrenocortical disease and atypical cushing syndrome: a clinical and molecular genetic investigation. J Clin Endocrinol Metab. 2005;90(6):3773–9.

McKeever PA, Young ID. Smith-Lemli-Opitz syndrome. II: a disorder of the fetal adrenals? J Med Genet. 1990;27(7):465–6.

Meimaridou E, Hughes CR, Kowalczyk J, Chan LF, Clark AJ, Metherell LA. ACTH resistance: genes and mechanisms. Endocr Dev. 2013;24:57–66.

Melo KF, Martin RM, Costa EM, Carvalho FM, Jorge AA, Arnhold IJ, et al. An unusual phenotype of Frasier syndrome due to IVS9 +4C>T mutation in the WT1 gene: predominantly male ambiguous genitalia and absence of gonadal dysgenesis. J Clin Endocrinol Metab. 2002;87 (6):2500–5.

Menon RK, Ferrau F, Kurzawinski TR, Rumsby G, Freeman A, Amin Z, et al. Adrenal cancer in neurofibromatosis type 1: case report and DNA analysis. Endocrinol Diabetes Metab Case Rep. 2014;2014:140074.

Merke DP, Stratakis CA. The adrenal life cycle: the fetal and adult cortex and the remaining questions. J Pediatr Endocrinol Metab: JPEM. 2006;19(11):1299–302.
Metherell LA, Chapple JP, Cooray S, David A, Becker C, Ruschendorf F, et al. Mutations in MRAP, encoding a new interacting partner of the ACTH receptor, cause familial glucocorticoid deficiency type 2. Nat Genet. 2005;37(2):166–70.
Metherell LA, Chan LF, Clark AJ. The genetics of ACTH resistance syndromes. Best Pract Res Clin Endocrinol Metab. 2006;20(4):547–60.
Muscatelli F, Strom TM, Walker AP, Zanaria E, Recan D, Meindl A, et al. Mutations in the DAX-1 gene give rise to both X-linked adrenal hypoplasia congenita and hypogonadotropic hypogonadism. Nature. 1994;372(6507):672–6.
Nanba K, Omata K, Tomlins SA, Giordano TJ, Hammer GD, Rainey WE, et al. Double adrenocortical adenomas harboring independent KCNJ5 and PRKACA somatic mutations. Eur J Endocrinol. 2016;175(2):K1–6.
Nguyen AD, Conley AJ. Adrenal androgens in humans and nonhuman primates: production, zonation and regulation. Endocr Dev. 2008;13:33–54.
Palmero EI, Achatz MI, Ashton-Prolla P, Olivier M, Hainaut P. Tumor protein 53 mutations and inherited cancer: beyond Li-Fraumeni syndrome. Curr Opin Oncol. 2010;22(1):64–9.
Palsdottir A, Snorradottir AO, Thorsteinsson L. Hereditary cystatin C amyloid angiopathy: genetic, clinical, and pathological aspects. Brain Pathol. 2006;16(1):55–9.
Perry R, Kecha O, Paquette J, Huot C, Van Vliet G, Deal C. Primary adrenal insufficiency in children: twenty years experience at the Sainte-Justine Hospital, Montreal. J Clin Endocrinol Metab. 2005;90(6):3243–50.
Petitjean A, Mathe E, Kato S, Ishioka C, Tavtigian SV, Hainaut P, et al. Impact of mutant p53 functional properties on TP53 mutation patterns and tumor phenotype: lessons from recent developments in the IARC TP53 database. Hum Mutat. 2007;28(6):622–9.
Raygada M, King KS, Adams KT, Stratakis CA, Pacak K. Counseling patients with succinate dehydrogenase subunit defects: genetics, preventive guidelines, and dealing with uncertainty. J Pediatr Endocrinol Metab: JPEM. 2014;27(9–10):837–44.
Reznik Y, Lefebvre H, Rohmer V, Charbonnel B, Tabarin A, Rodien P, et al. Aberrant adrenal sensitivity to multiple ligands in unilateral incidentaloma with subclinical autonomous cortisol hypersecretion: a prospective clinical study. Clin Endocrinol. 2004;61(3):311–9.
Rhayem Y, Perez-Rivas LG, Dietz A, Bathon K, Gebhard C, Riester A, et al. PRKACA somatic mutations are rare findings in aldosterone-producing adenomas. J Clin Endocrinol Metab. 2016;101(8):3010–7.
Ribeiro RC, Sandrini F, Figueiredo B, Zambetti GP, Michalkiewicz E, Lafferty AR, DeLacerda L, Rabin M, Cadwell C, Sampaio G, Cat I, Stratakis CA, Sandrini R. An inherited p53 mutation that contributes in a tissue-specific manner to pediatric adrenal cortical carcinoma. Proc Natl Acad Sci U S A. 2001;98(16):9330–5.
Robinson-White A, Meoli E, Stergiopoulos S, Horvath A, Boikos S, Bossis I, et al. PRKAR1A mutations and protein kinase A interactions with other signaling pathways in the adrenal cortex. J Clin Endocrinol Metab. 2006;91(6):2380–8.
Rump P, Zeegers MP, van Essen AJ. Tumor risk in Beckwith-Wiedemann syndrome: a review and meta-analysis. Am J Med Genet A. 2005;136(1):95–104.
Saeger W, Reinhard K, Reinhard C. Hyperplastic and tumorous lesions of the adrenals in an unselected autopsy series. Endocr Pathol. 1998;9(3):235–9.
Scholl UI, Goh G, Stolting G, de Oliveira RC, Choi M, Overton JD, et al. Somatic and germline CACNA1D calcium channel mutations in aldosterone-producing adenomas and primary aldosteronism. Nat Genet. 2013;45(9):1050–4.
Simonds WF, Varghese S, Marx SJ, Nieman LK. Cushing's syndrome in multiple endocrine neoplasia type 1. Clin Endocrinol. 2012;76(3):379–86.
Sirianni R, Zolea F, Chimento A, Ruggiero C, Cerquetti L, Fallo F, et al. Targeting estrogen receptor-alpha reduces adrenocortical cancer (ACC) cell growth in vitro and in vivo: potential

therapeutic role of selective estrogen receptor modulators (SERMs) for ACC treatment. J Clin Endocrinol Metab. 2012;97(12):E2238–50.
Sorrell AD, Espenschied CR, Culver JO, Weitzel JN. Tumor protein p53 (TP53) testing and Li-Fraumeni syndrome: current status of clinical applications and future directions. Mol Diagn Ther. 2013;17(1):31–47.
Speiser PW, Azziz R, Baskin LS, Ghizzoni L, Hensle TW, Merke DP, et al. Congenital adrenal hyperplasia due to steroid 21-hydroxylase deficiency: an Endocrine Society clinical practice guideline. J Clin Endocrinol Metab. 2010;95(9):4133–60.
Stratakis CA, Boikos SA. Genetics of adrenal tumors associated with Cushing's syndrome: a new classification for bilateral adrenocortical hyperplasias. Nat Clin Pract Endocrinol Metab. 2007;3 (11):748–57.
Stratakis CA, Kirschner LS, Carney JA. Clinical and molecular features of the Carney complex: diagnostic criteria and recommendations for patient evaluation. J Clin Endocrinol Metab. 2001;86(9):4041–6.
Stratakis CA, Sarlis N, Kirschner LS, Carney JA, Doppman JL, Nieman LK, Chrousos GP, Papanicolaou DA. Paradoxical response to dexamethasone in the diagnosis of primary pigmented nodular adrenocortical disease. Ann Intern Med. 1999;131(8):585–91.
Sucheston ME, Cannon MS. Development of zonular patterns in the human adrenal gland. J Morphol. 1968;126(4):477–91.
Suzuki T, Sasano H, Takeyama J, Kaneko C, Freije WA, Carr BR, et al. Developmental changes in steroidogenic enzymes in human postnatal adrenal cortex: immunohistochemical studies. Clin Endocrinol. 2000;53(6):739–47.
Taylor SS, Ilouz R, Zhang P, Kornev AP. Assembly of allosteric macromolecular switches: lessons from PKA. Nat Rev Mol Cell Biol. 2012;13(10):646–58.
Thakker RV, Newey PJ, Walls GV, Bilezikian J, Dralle H, Ebeling PR, et al. Clinical practice guidelines for multiple endocrine neoplasia type 1 (MEN1). J Clin Endocrinol Metab. 2012;97 (9):2990–3011.
Thiel A, Reis AC, Haase M, Goh G, Schott M, Willenberg HS, et al. PRKACA mutations in cortisol-producing adenomas and adrenal hyperplasia: a single-center study of 60 cases. Eur J Endocrinol. 2015;172(6):677–85.
Torpy DJ, Gordon RD, Lin JP, Huggard PR, Taymans SE, Stowasser M, et al. Familial hyperaldosteronism type II: description of a large kindred and exclusion of the aldosterone synthase (CYP11B2) gene. J Clin Endocrinol Metab. 1998;83(9):3214–8.
Tsigos C, Arai K, Hung W, Chrousos GP. Hereditary isolated glucocorticoid deficiency is associated with abnormalities of the adrenocorticotropin receptor gene. J Clin Invest. 1993;92(5):2458–61.
Varley JM, McGown G, Thorncroft M, James LA, Margison GP, Forster G, et al. Are there low-penetrance TP53 Alleles? Evidence from childhood adrenocortical tumors. Am J Hum Genet. 1999;65(4):995–1006.
Vrezas I, Willenberg HS, Bornstein SR. In: De Groot LJ, Beck-Peccoz P, Chrousos G, Dungan K, Grossman A, Hershman JM, et al., editors. Adrenal cortex, development, anatomy, physiology. South Dartmouth: Endotext; 2000.
Weinstein LS, Shenker A, Gejman PV, Merino MJ, Friedman E, Spiegel AM. Activating mutations of the stimulatory G protein in the McCune-Albright syndrome. N Engl J Med. 1991;325 (24):1688–95.
Weksberg R, Shuman C, Beckwith JB. Beckwith-Wiedemann syndrome. Eur J Hum Genet: EJHG. 2010;18(1):8–14.
Williams TA, Monticone S, Schack VR, Stindl J, Burrello J, Buffolo F, et al. Somatic ATP1A1, ATP2B3, and KCNJ5 mutations in aldosterone-producing adenomas. Hypertension. 2014;63 (1):188–95.
Wood MA, Acharya A, Finco I, Swonger JM, Elston MJ, Tallquist MD, et al. Fetal adrenal capsular cells serve as progenitor cells for steroidogenic and stromal adrenocortical cell lineages in M. musculus. Development. 2013;140(22):4522–32.

Zanaria E, Muscatelli F, Bardoni B, Strom TM, Guioli S, Guo W, et al. An unusual member of the nuclear hormone receptor superfamily responsible for X-linked adrenal hypoplasia congenita. Nature. 1994;372(6507):635–41.

Zilbermint M, Xekouki P, Faucz FR, Berthon A, Gkourogianni A, Schernthaner-Reiter MH, Batsis M, Sinaii N, Quezado MM, Merino M, Hodes A, Abraham SB, Libé R, Assié G1, Espiard S, Drougat L, Ragazzon B, Davis A, Gebreab SY, Neff R, Kebebew E, Bertherat J, Lodish MB, Stratakis CA. Primary Aldosteronism and ARMC5 Variants. J Clin Endocrinol Metab. 2015;100 (6):E900–9. doi: 10.1210/jc.2014-4167. Epub 2015 Mar 30.

Targeting of Steroid Hormone Receptor Function in Breast and Prostate Cancer

29

Shilpa Gupta and Douglas Yee

Abstract

Regulation of the normal breast and prostate epithelial cells by steroid hormones has provided important insight into the control of malignant cells derived from these tissues. Over many years, strategies to disrupt ligand levels and block hormone binding to the estrogen receptor and androgen receptor have led to improved outcomes for breast and prostate cancer. Based on our understanding of hormone receptor function, numerous drugs have been approved for risk reduction, adjuvant therapy, and treatment of metastatic disease. In addition, new strategies are moving forward to further target receptor function by disrupting other signaling inputs. This review will address the current therapies and identify strategies for the future.

Keywords

Breast cancer • Prostate cancer • Estrogen receptor • Androgen receptor • Aromatase • Lyase

Contents

S. Gupta • D. Yee (✉)
Division of Hematology, Oncology, and Transplantation, Department of Medicine, Masonic Cancer Center, University of Minnesota, Minneapolis, MN, USA
e-mail: yeexx006@umn.edu

A. Belfiore, D. LeRoith (eds.), *Principles of Endocrinology and Hormone Action*, Endocrinology, https://doi.org/10.1007/978-3-319-44675-2_30

Introduction

Through a series of accumulated genetic aberrations, normal cells gain the "hallmarks of cancer" (Hanahan and Weinberg 2000). These properties, if left unaddressed, can result in the death of the host from metastasis and unregulated growth at local and distant sites. Advances in technology have revealed hundreds of genetic abnormalities associated with these behaviors in cancer. Moreover, careful characterization of cancers has shown substantial heterogeneity in the genetic abnormalities contained within individual tumors and even in tumors obtained from different metastatic sites in the same patient. While treatments based on mutations are currently being developed and tested in clinical trials, the sheer number of genetic abnormalities would seem to make this a daunting approach.

Thus, it is notable that 60 years before the discovery of the structure of DNA was illuminated, an effective therapy for locally advanced breast cancer was described (Beatson 1896). Beatson intuited a connection between ovarian function and breast physiology, and he removed the ovaries of a young woman with inoperable breast cancer. This maneuver proved effective and served as a basis to consider hormonal regulation of cancer. Despite the multiple genetic events leading to the patient's breast cancer, Beatson showed effective therapy did not require any understanding of these genetic events.

In prostate cancer, Charles Huggins provided further insight into the mechanism of cancer cell biology. In a finding parallel to Beatson's, he discovered castration-induced regressions in prostate cancer (Huggins and Hodges 1941a). Testosterone suppression strategies, including surgical or medical castration, have been the standard of care for advanced prostate cancer for over six decades due to this work (Huggins et al. 1941; Huggins and Hodges 1941b). Huggins proposed lowering testosterone by surgical castration or administration of estrogens induces a major regression of prostate cancer (Huggins et al. 1941Huggins and Hodges 1941b). This discovery led to a landmark randomized study organized by the Veterans Administration Cooperative Urologic Research Group (VACURG), which compared the effects of treating prostate cancer patients with the oral estrogen diethylstilbesterol (DES) (1967). This study showed that DES treatment was as effective as surgical castration in treating prostate cancer (1967). With the knowledge that low level of androgens is produced by adrenal glands as well, Huggins and Scott further demonstrated bilateral adrenalectomy was effective in slowing cancer growth in men with prostate cancer who no longer responded to androgen deprivation (Huggins and Scott 1945). In recent years, we have made significant progress developing more specific and novel agents affecting the androgen receptor (AR) and adrenal androgen production and improving outcomes in men with metastatic prostate cancer. Thus, the conceptual idea showing how pathways regulating normal cell growth and function could also function in the biology of the behavior of malignant cells was firmly established.

Subsequent to Beatson's and Huggins' seminal findings, a molecular pathway for their results was discovered. Regulation of end-organ function was elucidated with the demonstration that sex organs (ovaries and testes) produced soluble steroid hormones which were released into the circulation. Interaction with their cognate receptors in target tissues resulted in changes in organ function. These steroid hormone receptors function as ligand-induced transcription factors to regulate expression of the genes responsible for the malignant phenotype including proliferation, survival, and metastasis.

The steroid superfamily has conserved structure. The receptors, including estrogen receptor alpha (ER) and androgen receptor (AR), have common domains. They contain DNA-binding domains and two activation function domains (AF1 and AF2). The AF1 domain contains the hormone-binding pocket. When steroid hormones bind this domain, a conformational change occurs allowing the binding of transcriptional co-activators and in turn initiate gene transcription. In addition to the hormone-dependent activation domain, receptors have a separate activation function (AF2) affecting gene transcription. Once ligand bound, the receptor complex binds palindromic DNA response elements to initiate target gene transcription. Both ER and AR undergo phosphorylation on serine and threonine sites with further affects their transcriptional activity (Becker et al. 2011).

While there are clearly cytoplasmic and membrane functions for the steroid hormone receptors, the clinical advances have exploited the targeting of the nuclear functions of the receptors. Conceptually, the function of ER and AR could be targeted by blocking the production of ligand, interfering with hormone binding, and altering factors affecting the activation function of the receptors. One of the greatest successes of translational research has been the demonstration that all three of these strategies have clinical benefit for the treatment of breast and prostate cancer as shown in Fig. 1. Moreover, these clinical strategies have been effective in cancer risk reduction, adjuvant therapy, and the treatment of advanced disease.

Receptor Antagonists

Breast Cancer

The hormone-binding domain of the steroid hormone receptors provides an attractive target for cancer therapy. Since the specificity of steroid hormone action is dictated by the structure of their cognate ligands, glucocorticoids are poor activators for ER or AR, and then it follows receptor antagonists could also be discovered.

The first of these discoveries was the drug tamoxifen (Jordan 2000). This triphenylethylene compound is not chemically similar to the endogenous steroids, yet tamoxifen binds the hormone-binding domain with high affinity. Originally

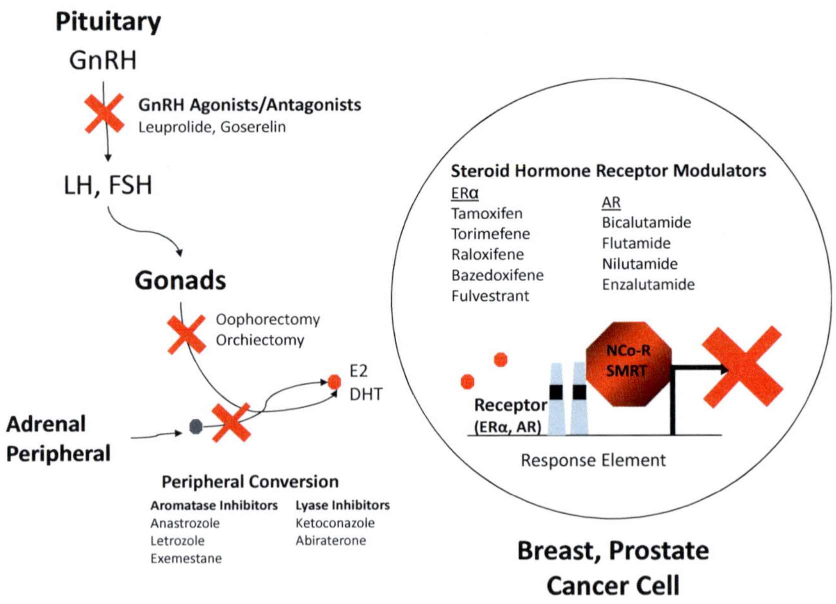

Fig. 1 Inhibition of nuclear steroid hormone receptor function in breast and prostate cancer. The steroid hormone receptors are hormone-dependent nuclear transcription factors. Upon binding of their ligand, they dimerize, enter the nucleus, and bind DNA response elements. To therapeutically inhibit their functions, numerous selective steroid hormone receptor modulators have been developed for breast and prostate cancer therapy. These steroid hormone receptor modulators interfere with the binding of the receptors' cognate ligands (estradiol E2 and dihydrotestosterone DHT) and place the dimerized receptor complex in a transcriptionally inactive form through the binding of nuclear hormone co-repressors (NcoR and SMRT). Receptor hormone function can also be achieved by disrupting the source of hormones. In premenopausal women and men, removal of the gonads via oophorectomy and orchiectomy was the first clinically successful strategies to treat advanced breast and prostate cancer. While these surgical techniques are still frequently used, suppression of pituitary releasing hormones via gonadotropin-releasing hormone (GnRH) agonists/antagonists is also frequently used to suppress sex steroid hormones. In addition, peripheral conversion by aromatase (postmenopausal women) and lyase (men) provides another source of estrogen and androgen. Successful use of all of the inhibitors has led to improvements in breast and prostate cancer outcomes

discovered in an attempt to produce ER antagonists to stimulate ovulation, tamoxifen's intrinsic ability to bind ER was recognized as an effective way to antagonize ER function in breast cancer. While tamoxifen functions as an antagonist in breast cancer, it is a weak estrogen in other organs including the bone and uterus. Thus, the term selective estrogen receptor modulator (SERM) is more appropriate than "antiestrogen."

In breast cancer, the effect of tamoxifen was initially described as an effective inhibitor of an ER-expressing breast cancer cell line (Lippman et al. 1976). Shortly after that description, the clinical utility of tamoxifen was demonstrated in advanced breast cancer (Kiang and Kennedy 1977). This remarkable result was followed by many studies testing the ability of tamoxifen to reduce breast cancer recurrence in the adjuvant setting (Early Breast Cancer Trialists' Collaborative 1998, 2015). These studies are reported in the Oxford overview and show two important findings. First, tamoxifen was effective in reducing breast cancer recurrence at local and distant sites when compared to placebo. Second, the expression of ER predicted benefit of tamoxifen therapy (Davies et al. 2011). While this seems logical, expression of the target was required for drug benefit; this observation sets a basis for the discovery of additional "predictive biomarkers" which can be used to identify the benefit, and lack of benefit, for specific drugs in individual tumors. The success of tamoxifen has led to the development of other SERMs approved for ER targeting including raloxifene, toremifene, bazedoxifene, and fulvestrant. While only toremifene and fulvestrant are used in breast cancer, the related drugs raloxifene and bazedoxifene have found their way into clinical practice for the treatment of osteoporosis and vasomotor symptoms associated with menopause, respectively (Ettinger et al. 1999; Pinkerton et al. 2014).

In many respects, treatment of breast cancer with SERMs has provided an important foundation for the field of "targeted therapies." ER targeting with this class of drugs has provided a conceptual basis for identifying key molecules important in regulating the malignant phenotype and developing mechanism-based drugs to disrupt the function of the target and to use the expression of the target as a way to individualize therapy for patients. In breast cancer, genomic tests to identify patients responsive to ER targeting are increasingly used as decision-making tools for the use of these drugs in women with operable breast cancer (Harris et al. 2016).

Prostate Cancer

Androgen receptor (AR) plays a pivotal role in prostate carcinogenesis and progression to castration-resistant prostate cancer (CRPC) and is a key therapeutic target (Scher and Sawyers 2005). While androgen deprivation therapy (ADT) is effective initially in metastatic hormone-sensitive prostate cancer, the effects are short-lived, and majority of patients progress to CRPC which is inevitably lethal. Adaptive upregulation of AR commonly occurs as prostate cancer transforms from hormone-sensitive to castration-resistant state (Scher and Sawyers 2005). Importantly, prostate cancer cells demonstrate dependence on AR signaling even in castration-resistant stage and the development of novel drugs affecting AR signaling that hinge upon AR being a persistent and critical driver of CRPC growth and progression.

AR is a nuclear transcription factor encoded on the X chromosome at position Xq11-Xq12 (Tan et al. 2015). It contains eight exons and four domains similar to other members of the steroid hormone receptor superfamily: the N-terminal domain (i.e., transcriptional activation domain – AF2), DNA-binding domain, a hinge region, and the ligand-binding domain (LBD; AF-1, C-terminal) (Tan et al. 2015). After androgens bind the AR-AF1 domain, nuclear translocation and dimerization occurs. Once in the nucleus, the dimerized AR binds to androgen response elements

(ARE) to initiate transcription of AR target genes. Subsequently, recruitment of AR co-activators and transcription of AR target genes occur. AR antagonists directly bind to and block the AR LBD and prevent androgens from carrying out their biological activity. AR antagonists can interfere with the required events for activation of AR gene expression by androgens (Koryakina et al. 2014; Tan et al. 2015).

First-generation nonsteroidal AR antagonists such as bicalutamide, flutamide, and nilutamide were developed in the 1970s to avoid the side effects of the steroidal compounds like mifepristone, cyproterone acetate, and spironolactone. Like tamoxifen, the first-generation antiandrogens demonstrate partial agonism of the AR and, thus, may paradoxically elicit an antiandrogen withdrawal prostate-specific antigen (PSA) response in patients upon discontinuation (Kelly et al. 1997). Increased AR levels were implicated in causing resistance to these agents, and AR mutation is one of the mechanisms resulting in conversion of antiandrogens to agonists in prostate cancer cells (Taplin et al. 2003).

The second-generation AR antagonist MDV3100 (enzalutamide) was developed specifically to bind and inhibit AR with no AR agonistic properties (Massard and Fizazi 2011). Enzalutamide inhibits several steps in the AR signaling pathway by competitively inhibiting androgen and AR binding to androgens and inhibiting AR nuclear translocation and interaction with DNA. This makes it a pure AR antagonist. Enzalutamide demonstrated significant preclinical activity in xenograft models, including preclinical models harboring AR amplification (Tran et al. 2009). These findings were confirmed in the phase 1/2 study in patients with metastatic CRPC (Scher et al. 2010). The promising results with enzalutamide from the phase 1/2 study (Scher et al. 2010) led to the landmark phase 3 AFFIRM trial, of men, randomized to receive enzalutamide or placebo, with CRPC following docetaxel chemotherapy, (Scher et al. 2012). Enzalutamide improved overall survival compared to placebo, with a median overall survival of 18.4 months versus 13.6 months, respectively, and was superior in all secondary clinical endpoints, including quality of life (Scher et al. 2012).

The other pivotal study of enzalutamide in metastatic chemotherapy-naive CRPC patients demonstrated a significant 4-month improvement in overall survival compared to placebo in addition to improvement in other clinical outcomes (Beer and Tombal 2014). These results further confirmed metastatic CRPC remains an AR responsive disease. Several next-generation AR antagonists, including ARN-509 and ODM-201, are in late-phase trials in CRPC. AR-509 is another next-generation AR antagonist directly binding to the AR LBD with high affinity inhibiting its nuclear import and transcriptional activity. Data from phase 3 studies in metastatic CRPC is awaited (Clegg et al. 2012; Joseph et al. 2013). ODM-201 is another new-generation full and high-affinity AR antagonist not only inhibiting nuclear translocation of AR but also blocking the activity of the mutant ARs arising in response to antiandrogen therapies including the F876L mutation conferring resistance to enzalutamide and ARN-509 (Moilanen et al. 2015). Primary resistance to enzalutamide was observed in 25% patients in the AFFIRM trial (Scher et al. 2012). Several mechanisms, including AR splice variants, have been implicated in development of enzalutamide resistance (Joseph et al. 2013; Li et al. 2013; Nadiminty et al. 2013). The understanding of mechanisms will further pave the way in development of more effective novel antiandrogens in CRPC.

Ligand Deprivation

Breast Cancer and Aromatase Inhibitors

As noted, Beatson's report of oophorectomy in a premenopausal woman with breast cancer was one of the first systemic treatment strategies. While surgical removal of the ovaries remains an important therapeutic strategy in breast cancer, the development of luteinizing hormone-releasing hormone (LHRH) agonists/antagonists has provided a medical method to suppress ovarian function in premenopausal women (Regan et al. 2016). These drugs can effectively suppress LHRH secretion and substantially lower the circulating estradiol levels.

An important advance in breast cancer was the demonstration postmenopausal women could still produce biologically important levels of estradiol by the aromatization of precursors. The enzymatic pathway catalyzing steroid precursors (androgens) into estradiol can be targeted by inhibitors of aromatase (Santen et al. 2009). Aromatase inhibitors (AIs) result in substantial reductions of estradiol in postmenopausal women, yet they are not potent enough to suppress ovarian-produced estradiol in premenopausal women.

Three separate aromatase inhibitors have been approved: anastrozole, letrozole, and exemestane. In metastatic breast cancer, each drug proved to be effective. Early clinical trials compared the AIs to other second-line therapies for metastatic breast cancer, mostly progestational agents such as megestrol acetate, and were found superior to existing second-line therapies (Gibson et al. 2007). Given the success in this area, the AIs were then tested against tamoxifen as first-line therapy for ER+ metastatic breast cancer. In these trials, there was an advantage to the AIs over tamoxifen when progression-free survival and clinical benefit rate were used as endpoints, but overall survival or objective response differences were not observed in most of the randomized studies. There were some differences in toxicities when tamoxifen was compared to AIs, specifically, and increased arthralgias with AIs, but less vaginal bleeding and thromboembolic disease compared to tamoxifen. AIs became the standard of care in women with ER+ metastatic tumors due to the clinical trials demonstrating efficacy.

Given the clinical activity of AIs in metastatic disease, multiple clinical trials were conducted to evaluate their benefit in the adjuvant therapy of ER+ breast cancer. As 5 years of tamoxifen therapy was the standard of care when these trials began, several different trial designs were created based upon this standard. The first of these trials compared anastrozole versus tamoxifen versus anastrozole plus tamoxifen (ATAC) in operable disease with a duration of therapy of 5 years. This trial showed very early on anastrozole was superior to tamoxifen, while the combination of AI plus tamoxifen was not of benefit (Baum et al. 2002). Additional trials compared switching from tamoxifen to AI after 2–3 years versus AI for 5 years versus starting with an AI and then switching to tamoxifen (Mouridsen et al. 2009; van de Velde et al. 2011). Taken together, these trials suggested AIs were superior to tamoxifen monotherapy when disease-free survival was measured. However, differences in overall survival were not shown. In addition, the trials suggested AIs alone were superior to the switching regimens. Thus, guidelines for treatment of ER+ breast cancer still endorse tamoxifen or AIs (Burstein et al. 2014).

For premenopausal women, the value of ovarian functional suppression (OFS) has recently been shown. A randomized trial comparing OFS in combination with tamoxifen versus exemestane has shown OFS plus exemestane results in reduced recurrences compared to OFS plus tamoxifen (Pagani et al. 2014). These data showing further reduction of ligand levels in premenopausal patients is an aggressive endocrine therapy and superior to OFS plus ER blockade with a SERM.

Risk of recurrence for ER+ disease extends beyond 5 years (Saphner et al. 1996), and this observation led to the idea extending endocrine therapy beyond 5 years would improve outcomes. Since most patients were receiving tamoxifen for a 5-year course of adjuvant therapy, the first studies compared stopping tamoxifen at 5 years or continuing therapy with an AI for an additional 5 years (Goss et al. 2003). This trial, in addition to other studies, has shown extension of endocrine therapy for more than 5 years further reduces the risk of recurrence. Moreover, the extension of tamoxifen therapy for a total of 10 years has shown to be effective at reducing risk when compared to 5 years (Davies et al. 2013). Recently, it has been shown extending ligand deprivation, by aromatase inhibition, for a period of 10 years, is superior to 5 years of therapy in reducing risk of recurrence from breast cancer (Goss et al. 2016).

To date, improved breast cancer outcomes can be achieved by targeting ER. In patients with tumors expressing any level of ER, treatments aimed at receptor targeting by SERMs or ligand deprivation by oophorectomy and AIs are widely used in clinical practice.

Prostate Cancer and Lyase Inhibitors

The 17α-hydroxylase/17,20-lyase (CYP17) is a cytochrome P450 enzyme essential for the biosynthesis of androgens and adrenal hormones and provides the rationale for development of CYP17 inhibitors for treating CRPC (Akhtar et al. 2005). Ketoconazole, an imidazole antifungal agent with CYP17 inhibitory properties, has been used in prostate cancer since the 1980s (De Coster et al. 1987; Witjes et al. 1989). While ketoconazole use achieved PSA response, there was no survival benefit shown in clinical trials (Keizman et al. 2012; Small et al. 2004). Furthermore, ketoconazole use is associated with significant toxicities and poor patient compliance.

Abiraterone acetate was the first-in-class selective and potent CYP17 inhibitor (catalyzes both 17-alpha-hydroxylase and 17,20-lyase reactions) showing promising activity in CRPC in early studies (Attard et al. 2008, 2009; Danila et al. 2010). COU-AA-301 was the landmark randomized controlled phase III trial comparing abiraterone and prednisone versus placebo and prednisone in metastatic CRPC patients who had received prior docetaxel chemotherapy; significant overall survival benefit was seen with abiraterone – 14.8 versus 10.9 months (de Bono et al. 2011). Later, results from the other pivotal trial (COU-AA-301) comparing abiraterone and prednisone to placebo and prednisone in chemotherapy-naive metastatic CRPC patients demonstrated improved overall survival with abiraterone as well (Ryan et al. 2013). The main side effects of abiraterone are excess mineralocorticoid activity, resulting from inhibition of 17-alpha-hydroxylase, which causes a compensatory rise in ACTH. While concomitant use of prednisone is recommended to mitigate these side effects, there is a concern with long-term effects of prednisone use.

Newer CYP17 inhibitors are being developed that are either more selective or with multitarget effects on AR signaling. These include orteronel, galeterone, and seviteronel. Orteronel (TAK-700) is a newer selective inhibitor of CYP17,20-lyase and has a better toxicity profile compared to abiraterone acetate. Orteronel demonstrated promising activity in phase 1/2 studies in CRPC (Agus WMS DB 2011). However, in the phase 3 trial, ELM-PC 4, comparing orteronel and prednisone versus placebo and prednisone in chemotherapy-naive CRPC patients, orteronel improved progression-free survival (PFS) but failed to achieve the primary endpoint of overall survival (Saad et al. 2015). This combination failed to achieve the primary endpoint of overall survival in another phase 3 trial in metastatic CRPC patients who had progressed after docetaxel chemotherapy (Fizazi et al. 2015). Because of these negative findings, further development of orteronel has been terminated in CRPC. However, in hormone-sensitive prostate cancer, an ongoing Southwest Oncology Group study (S1216) is comparing androgen deprivation therapy (ADT) and orteronel at a dose of 300 mg twice daily (without the need for steroids), with ADT and bicalutamide in newly diagnosed metastatic hormone-sensitive prostate cancer and with the primary endpoint of overall survival (NCT01809691).

Galeterone (VN/124-1, TOK-001) is a selective inhibitor of CYP17,20-lyase with multiple targeted effects on AR signaling, including CYP17 inhibition, AR antagonism, and decrease in intratumoral AR level (Vasaitis et al. 2008). Galeterone also behaves as a pure AR antagonist by binding to AR and blocking AR transactivation with a tenfold higher binding affinity for wild-type AR than testosterone (Montgomery et al. 2012). There is preclinical evidence suggesting galeterone is superior to abiraterone (Bruno et al. 2011). Thus, theoretically, galeterone may be able to overcome resistance to abiraterone. Early phase 1/2 studies with galeterone (ARMOR1 and ARMOR2) have shown promising safety and efficacy of galeterone in patients with chemotherapy-naive nonmetastatic or metastatic CRPC. Dose expansion part 2 of ARMOR2 is ongoing with the dose of galeterone at 2,550 mg per day (Montgomery et al. 2016).

Seviteronel (VT-464) is a novel, nonsteroidal, small-molecule CYP17A1 inhibitor with 17,20-lyase selectivity and an AR antagonist effect. In preclinical studies, greater suppression of the AR axis was seen with seviteronel compared to abiraterone likely due to the dual action of seviteronel (Toren et al. 2015). Trials with seviteronel are ongoing in metastatic CRPC patients who have progressed on prior abiraterone, enzalutamide, or both (NCT02130700, NCT02012920).

Mechanisms of Resistance

In breast cancer, several types of resistance to endocrine therapy have been described. In ER+ tumors, patients may never respond to an endocrine agent despite expression of the target. These types of tumors have been called "primary" or "intrinsic" resistance. Molecular profiling is beginning to demonstrate the expression, and mutational patterns of these primary resistant tumors are different from the sensitive tumors (Ellis et al. 2012). Some patients have prolonged benefit (greater than 6 months) to an endocrine agent but then go on to disease progression. These types of tumors have been called "secondary" or "acquired" resistance. It seems very likely the mechanisms of resistance are very different between these two clinical scenarios.

One recently observed mechanism of resistance has been mutation in the target itself. In breast cancer, ER mutations were described many years ago in primary breast cancers (Zhang et al. 1997). With advances in sequencing technology, the ability to detect mutation has improved. It is becoming clearer mutations in ER can be detected especially as seen in patients who have been treated with aromatase inhibitors (Ma et al. 2015). In primary breast cancer, mutation in ER is relatively rare. In several studies following women over time, the appearance of ER mutations occurs after a prolonged clinical course of aromatase inhibitor therapy (Wang et al. 2016). The mutations tend to cluster in the hormone-binding domain resulting in ligand-independent activation of the receptor (Robinson et al. 2013; Toy et al. 2013). Additional genomic abnormalities, such as ER translocation, have been detected in resistant breast cancers. Thus, an important mechanism of resistance is the target gene itself.

In contrast to breast cancer, study of CRPC biology has elucidated several clinically validated mechanisms contributing to transformation of hormone-sensitive prostate cancer to castration-resistant stage. The mechanisms contributing to the development of CRPC include AR amplification and mutation, AR co-activator and co-repressor modifications, aberrant activation (posttranslational modification), altered steroidogenesis, and AR splice variants (Agoulnik and Weigel 2008; Chang et al. 2014; Dehm et al. 2008; Gregory et al. 2001; Hu et al. 2009; Nadiminty et al. 2013; Visakorpi et al. 1995; Wang et al. 2009; Wolf et al. 2008).

Each of these mechanisms ultimately leads to increased AR activation in CRPC and provides the rationale for development of novel treatments targeting the AR signaling pathway. Unfortunately, primary and acquired resistance to AR antagonists and lyase inhibitors is very common in CRPC, and approximately 20–40% patients do not respond to these treatments (de Bono et al. 2011; Scher et al. 2012). Furthermore, patients with metastatic CRPC who initially respond to these agents, eventually, develop resistance. Mechanisms of resistance to these newer drugs are not well understood.

The discovery of alternative mRNA splicing variants of the AR has helped us understand the role of AR signaling in CRPC and an important mechanism of resistance to both enzalutamide and abiraterone (Dehm et al. 2008). Resistance to abiraterone may occur through mechanisms including upregulation of CYP17A1 and/or induction of AR and AR splice variants conferring ligand-independent AR transactivation (Friedlander et al. 2012; Mostaghel et al. 2011). Yamamoto et al. showed AR is key driver of enzalutamide resistance (Yamamoto et al. 2015). Full-length AR and AR variants have been implicated in enzalutamide resistance in CRPC patients (Yamamoto et al. 2015). Among the identified splice variants, variant 7 (AR-V7) has particularly been implicated in drug resistance. Antonarakis et al. showed that AR-V7 expression in patients treated with enzalutamide or abiraterone correlated with poor clinical outcomes compared to those without AR-V7 (Antonarakis et al. 2014). The AR-V7 inhibitor, niclosamide, has been shown to improve enzalutamide sensitivity by inhibiting Stat3 phosphorylation, reducing Stat3 target gene expression, and annulling recruitment of AR to the PSA promoter (Liu et al. 2015).

Autophagy is another mechanism implicated in resistance to enzalutamide (Nguyen et al. 2014). Use of inhibitors of autophagy like metformin combined with enzalutamide may be a potential strategy to overcome resistance to enzalutamide. AR mutation (F876L) has also been shown to drive resistance to AR antagonists, enzalutamide and ARN-509 (Balbas et al. 2013; Korpal et al. 2013). Korpal et al. showed cyclin-dependent kinase (CDK) 4/6 inhibitors effectively antagonized AR (F876L) function (Korpal et al. 2013).

Ongoing efforts to better understand complex molecular and cellular mechanisms of resistance to currently available AR-directed therapies will help us develop novel therapeutic strategies to prevent and overcome drug resistance in CRPC.

New Therapies

While ER activation by ligand results in enhanced transcription of ER-targeted genes, it is also known ER is activated by other cellular signaling pathways. The ability of ER activation by signaling events activating PI3K signaling has been shown (Becker et al. 2011). Strategies to target key signaling molecules have been tested in clinical trials including disruption of the type I insulin-like growth factor receptor, PI3K, Akt, and mTOR. To date, only mTOR targeting has been successful, and the mTORC1 inhibitor everolimus has been shown to be of benefit in combination with AIs (Baselga et al. 2012). The combination of AI plus everolimus improved progression-free survival (PFS) from 10.6 months compared to 4.1 months for AI alone. This result resulted in the approval of this treatment combination in metastatic breast cancer. Combination of everolimus with tamoxifen showed similar benefits for the combination (Bachelot et al. 2012). Studies examining the benefits in the adjuvant therapy of breast cancer are ongoing (NCT01674140).

The use of presurgical treatment (neoadjuvant therapy) of ER-positive breast cancer can also provide insight into the use of targeting this pathway. Pictilisib, a PI3K inhibitor, was studied in a short-term, 2-week window trial with or without anastrozole (Schmid et al. 2016). In this study, the addition of the drug resulted in suppressed proliferation as measured by Ki67 compared to anastrozole alone. Exploratory studies suggested the benefit was primarily in the molecularly defined "luminal B" subgroup. This subgroup tends to be more resistant to endocrine therapy alone, and these data suggest PI3K may specifically benefit a subset of breast cancer patients with primary endocrine resistant tumors. Of course, suppression of Ki67 is only a surrogate marker of clinical benefit (Dowsett et al. 2007), and additional studies will be necessary to determine if inhibition of PI3K signaling will be used in early-stage breast cancer.

One clear effect of estrogen stimulation of ER-positive breast cancer cells is enhanced entry into the cell cycle (Lippman et al. 1977). The mechanisms of estrogen and ER employed to overcome the barriers to active DNA synthesis are complex as many proteins control cell cycle progression. It has long been known cyclins represent barriers to progression from G1-to-S phase which is an important barrier to overcome during proliferation. The cyclins are phosphorylated by cyclin-dependent kinases (CDKs), and one mechanism of estrogen action is to induce CDK4 and CDK6 to phosphorylate cyclin D1 (Hong et al. 1998). Thus, inhibition of the CDKs could enhance the ability of ER targeting to suppress the mitogenic effects of estrogen.

The development of the CDK4/6 inhibitor palbociclib has been tested in combination with AIs and fulvestrant. In both trials, the addition of palbociclib to ER targeting resulted in enhanced benefit (Finn et al. 2015; Turner et al. 2015) and led to the approval of this drug in combination with either ER targeting strategy. Just as everolimus is being tested in earlier-stage disease, palbociclib is being studied in the adjuvant setting (NCT02513394, NCT01864746).

The importance of the everolimus and palbociclib clinical trial results represents a watershed moment in the hormonal targeting of breast cancer. Previous to these findings, the clinical strategies were directed at only improving ER targeting by interfering with its ability to bind estrogens. Using agents that do not affect hormone binding in combination with the traditional agents has identified new pathways to improve clinical outcomes for women with breast cancer.

The Future

It is evident the basic study of steroid hormone receptor function has led to major advances in the treatment of breast and prostate cancer. These original observations, now stretching back over a hundred years, have led to a clearer molecular portrait of the two most common cancers in men and women. Advances in drug therapy have led to the improvement in overall survival for women and men diagnosed with these diseases. Further, the understanding of these pathways has led to several prevention trials using the strategy of targeting ER and AR (Andriole et al. 2010; Fisher et al. 1998; Thompson et al. 2003; Vogel et al. 2006). However, the use of these drug strategies has been limited for several reasons including toxicity and no clear demonstration of improvement in overall survival.

Despite these advances, there are still several important poorly understood areas with a need for better clinical strategies. In breast cancer, it is becoming increasingly clear ER-expressing tumors have a late risk of recurrence. As noted above, the use of endocrine therapy for up to 10 years has been proven to reduce the risk of a breast cancer event compared to 5 years of therapy. While many of the "events" were either ipsilateral or contralateral breast cancer, it is also clear reduction in distant metastasis is seen. For example, in the trial of extended letrozole (MA17R), there were approximately 950 women assigned to either placebo or letrozole for an additional 5 years of therapy (Goss et al. 2016). In that clinical trial, there were 42 women who continued letrozole with distant metastasis compared to 53 women on the placebo arm who developed distant metastasis. Several important lessons can be learned from these results.

First, there is a real, but small, risk of distant recurrence beyond 5 years even when given optimal endocrine therapy for the preceding 5 years. On a biological level, these data highlight the idea ER-expressing tumors can remain dormant for very long periods of time. Moreover, the optimal endocrine therapy does not kill these dormant cells; instead, it appears extended drug therapy works by maintaining tumor dormancy. Currently, we have limited insight into the biology of these dormant cells.

Second, even with extension of endocrine therapy, the majority of these dormant cells are not prevented from recurring. As noted above, only 11 women were spared a distant recurrence by extending their endocrine therapy for out to 10 years. Forty-two women still recurred even though they were receiving extended therapy. These data further support the idea additional mechanisms of resistance must be occurring even when therapy is optimal.

Third, in the MA17R trial, there was toxicity in extending endocrine therapy. In this trial, the women who had extended letrozole therapy had 133 fractures (from 959 treated) compared to 88/954 women who received placebo. Thus, the ability to suppress dormant tumor cells is incomplete, and the strategy is associated with more toxicity.

So how can endocrine therapy be improved? As noted, the ability to target additional pathways inhibiting steroid receptor function has now been shown to be superior to only targeting ER in women with metastatic disease. Similar data are likely to emerge in prostate cancer and AR targeting. It is not clear if these therapies will limit the recurrence of distant metastasis compared to ER-targeted therapies alone, but several clinical trials are underway testing the ability of everolimus or palbociclib to reduce risk of recurrence in the adjuvant setting. Similar data suggesting a role for targeting these signaling pathways has also been recognized.

It is also clear a better understanding of the mechanism of resistance to endocrine therapy is needed. While mutation is the driving factor behind tumor evolution (Shah et al. 2009), it is not clear whether continued mutations occur or if individual clones are selected over the many years of endocrine therapy. Recently, the family of cysteine deaminases has been shown to be a source of mutation in breast cancer (Burns et al. 2013), and ongoing work is underway to determine if activity of the APOBEC3B enzyme contributes to endocrine resistance.

Finally, the complete elimination of dormant tumor cells might be difficult because they are not dividing and therefore are not susceptible to our conventional cytotoxic therapies such as chemotherapy. However, the ability to enhance immune recognition of tumor cells is an active area of clinical research. Certainly, the immune checkpoint inhibitors have been a major advance in some cancers (Harris et al. 2016; Sharma and Allison 2015). The current thinking suggests these tumors have a high mutational load and present neoantigens to the immune center. Once checkpoint inhibition is overcome, then effective cytotoxic immune response will occur. It is also clear mutational load of ER-expressing luminal breast cancers is low compared to other carcinogen-induced cancers (lung, melanoma). Thus, it will be a challenge for us to identify how best to use the immune system to target these indolent tumors. However, it is known ER function drives expression of specific genes, and some of them are expressed as cell surface proteins. It might be possible to develop strategies to use these antigens as "engagers" of the immune system. For example, the monoclonal antibody trastuzumab binds HER2 on breast cancer cells. While there are many functions for trastuzumab, it is becoming increasingly clear trastuzumab could act as an immune engager (Datta et al. 2016).

Beatson's and Huggin's contributions linking steroid hormone activity to cancer pointed the way toward the burgeoning field of "bedside-to-bench-to-bedside" translational research. Clearly, the clinical application of steroid hormone receptor function has improved outcomes for breast and prostate cancer. Certainly, many women and men are alive because of the drugs developed to disrupt steroid hormone receptor function. We need to continue along this pathway to further eliminate mortality from hormone receptor-expressing tumors.

References

Agoulnik IU, Weigel NL. Androgen receptor coactivators and prostate cancer. Adv Exp Med Biol. 2008;617:245–55. doi:10.1007/978-0-387-69080-3_23.

Agus WMS DB SD, Hart L, MacVicar GR, Hamid O, Hainsworth JD, Gross ME, Wang J, de Leon L, MacLean D, Dreicer R. Safety, efficacy, and pharmacodynamics of the investigational agent TAK-700 in metastatic castration-resistant prostate cancer (mCRPC): updated data from a phase I/II study. Safety, efficacy, and pharmacodynamics of the investigational agent TAK-700 in metastatic castration-resistant prostate cancer (mCRPC): updated data from a phase I/II study. 2011.

Akhtar MK, Kelly SL, Kaderbhai MA. Cytochrome b(5) modulation of 17{alpha} hydroxylase and 17–20 lyase (CYP17) activities in steroidogenesis. J Endocrinol. 2005;187:267–74. doi:10.1677/joe.1.06375.

Andriole GL, Bostwick DG, Brawley OW, Gomella LG, Marberger M, Montorsi F, Pettaway CA, Tammela TL, Teloken C, Tindall DJ, Somerville MC, Wilson TH, Fowler IL, Rittmaster RS, Group RS. Effect of dutasteride on the risk of prostate cancer. N Engl J Med. 2010;362:1192–202. doi:10.1056/NEJMoa0908127.

Antonarakis ES, Lu C, Wang H, Luber B, Nakazawa M, Roeser JC, Chen Y, Mohammad TA, Chen Y, Fedor HL, Lotan TL, Zheng Q, De Marzo AM, Isaacs JT, Isaacs WB, Nadal R, Paller CJ, Denmeade SR, Carducci MA, Eisenberger MA, Luo J. AR-V7 and resistance to enzalutamide and abiraterone in prostate cancer. N Engl J Med. 2014;371:1028–38. doi:10.1056/NEJMoa1315815.

Attard G, Reid AH, Yap TA, Raynaud F, Dowsett M, Settatree S, Barrett M, Parker C, Martins V, Folkerd E, Clark J, Cooper CS, Kaye SB, Dearnaley D, Lee G, de Bono JS. Phase I clinical trial of a selective inhibitor of CYP17, abiraterone acetate, confirms that castration-resistant prostate cancer commonly remains hormone driven. J Clin Oncol. 2008;26:4563–71. doi:10.1200/JCO.2007.15.9749.

Attard G, Reid AH, A'Hern R, Parker C, Oommen NB, Folkerd E, Messiou C, Molife LR, Maier G, Thompson E, Olmos D, Sinha R, Lee G, Dowsett M, Kaye SB, Dearnaley D, Kheoh T, Molina A, de Bono JS. Selective inhibition of CYP17 with abiraterone acetate is highly active in the treatment of castration-resistant prostate cancer. J Clin Oncol. 2009;27:3742–8. doi:10.1200/JCO.2008.20.0642.

Bachelot T, Bourgier C, Cropet C, Ray-Coquard I, Ferrero JM, Freyer G, Abadie-Lacourtoisie S, Eymard JC, Debled M, Spaeth D, Legouffe E, Allouache D, El Kouri C, Pujade-Lauraine E. Randomized phase II trial of everolimus in combination with tamoxifen in patients with hormone receptor-positive, human epidermal growth factor receptor 2-negative metastatic breast cancer with prior exposure to aromatase inhibitors: a GINECO study. J Clin Oncol. 2012;30:2718–24. doi:10.1200/JCO.2011.39.0708.

Balbas MD, Evans MJ, Hosfield DJ, Wongvipat J, Arora VK, Watson PA, Chen Y, Greene GL, Shen Y, Sawyers CL. Overcoming mutation-based resistance to antiandrogens with rational drug design. Elife. 2013;2:e00499. doi:10.7554/eLife.00499.

Baselga J, Campone M, Piccart M, Burris 3rd HA, Rugo HS, Sahmoud T, Noguchi S, Gnant M, Pritchard KI, Lebrun F, Beck JT, Ito Y, Yardley D, Deleu I, Perez A, Bachelot T, Vittori L, Xu Z, Mukhopadhyay P, Lebwohl D, Hortobagyi GN. Everolimus in postmenopausal hormone-receptor-positive advanced breast cancer. N Engl J Med. 2012;366:520–9. doi:10.1056/NEJMoa1109653.

Baum M, Budzar AU, Cuzick J, Forbes J, Houghton JH, Klijn JG, Sahmoud T. Anastrozole alone or in combination with tamoxifen versus tamoxifen alone for adjuvant treatment of postmenopausal women with early breast cancer: first results of the ATAC randomised trial. Lancet. 2002;359:2131–9.

Beatson GT. On the treatment of inoperable cases of carcinoma of the mamma. Suggestions for a new method of treatment with illustrative cases. Lancet. 1896;2:104–7.

Becker MA, Ibrahim YH, Cui X, Lee AV, Yee D. The IGF pathway regulates ERalpha through a S6K1-dependent mechanism in breast cancer cells. Mol Endocrinol. 2011;25:516–28. doi:10.1210/me.2010-0373. me.2010-0373 [pii].

Beer TM, Tombal B. Enzalutamide in metastatic prostate cancer before chemotherapy. N Engl J Med. 2014;371:1755–6. doi:10.1056/NEJMc1410239.

Bruno RD, Vasaitis TS, Gediya LK, Purushottamachar P, Godbole AM, Ates-Alagoz Z, Brodie AM, Njar VC. Synthesis and biological evaluations of putative metabolically stable analogs of VN/124-1 (TOK-001): head to head anti-tumor efficacy evaluation of VN/124-1 (TOK-001) and abiraterone in LAPC-4 human prostate cancer xenograft model. Steroids. 2011;76:1268–79. doi:10.1016/j.steroids.2011.06.002.

Burns MB, Lackey L, Carpenter MA, Rathore A, Land AM, Leonard B, Refsland EW, Kotandeniya D, Tretyakova N, Nikas JB, Yee D, Temiz NA, Donohue DE, McDougle RM, Brown WL, Law EK, Harris RS. APOBEC3B is an enzymatic source of mutation in breast cancer. Nature. 2013;494:366–70. doi:10.1038/nature11881.

Burstein HJ, Temin S, Anderson H, Buchholz TA, Davidson NE, Gelmon KE, Giordano SH, Hudis CA, Rowden D, Solky AJ, Stearns V, Winer EP, Griggs JJ. Adjuvant endocrine therapy for women with hormone receptor-positive breast cancer: American society of clinical oncology clinical practice guideline focused update. J Clin Oncol. 2014;32:2255–69. doi:10.1200/JCO.2013.54.2258.

Chang KH, Ercole CE, Sharifi N. Androgen metabolism in prostate cancer: from molecular mechanisms to clinical consequences. Br J Cancer. 2014;111:1249–54. doi:10.1038/bjc.2014.268.

Clegg NJ, Wongvipat J, Joseph JD, Tran C, Ouk S, Dilhas A, Chen Y, Grillot K, Bischoff ED, Cai L, Aparicio A, Dorow S, Arora V, Shao G, Qian J, Zhao H, Yang G, Cao C, Sensintaffar J, Wasielewska T, Herbert MR, Bonnefous C, Darimont B, Scher HI, Smith-Jones P, Klang M, Smith ND, De Stanchina E, Wu N, Ouerfelli O, Rix PJ, Heyman RA, Jung ME, Sawyers CL,

Hager JH. ARN-509: a novel antiandrogen for prostate cancer treatment. Cancer Res. 2012;72:1494–503. doi:10.1158/0008-5472.CAN-11-3948.

Danila DC, Morris MJ, de Bono JS, Ryan CJ, Denmeade SR, Smith MR, Taplin ME, Bubley GJ, Kheoh T, Haqq C, Molina A, Anand A, Koscuiszka M, Larson SM, Schwartz LH, Fleisher M, Scher HI. Phase II multicenter study of abiraterone acetate plus prednisone therapy in patients with docetaxel-treated castration-resistant prostate cancer. J Clin Oncol. 2010;28:1496–501. doi:10.1200/JCO.2009.25.9259.

Datta J, Fracol M, McMillan MT, Berk E, Xu S, Goodman N, Lewis DA, DeMichele A, Czerniecki BJ. Association of depressed anti-HER2 T-helper type 1 response with recurrence in patients with completely treated HER2-positive breast cancer: role for immune monitoring. JAMA Oncol. 2016;2:242–6. doi:10.1001/jamaoncol.2015.5482.

Davies C, Godwin J, Gray R, Clarke M, Cutter D, Darby S, McGale P, Pan HC, Taylor C, Wang YC, Dowsett M, Ingle J, Peto R. Relevance of breast cancer hormone receptors and other factors to the efficacy of adjuvant tamoxifen: patient-level meta-analysis of randomised trials. Lancet. 2011;378:771–84. doi:10.1016/S0140-6736(11)60993-8. doi: S0140-6736(11)60993-8 [pii].

Davies C, Pan H, Godwin J, Gray R, Arriagada R, Raina V, Abraham M, Medeiros Alencar VH, Badran A, Bonfill X, Bradbury J, Clarke M, Collins R, Davis SR, Delmestri A, Forbes JF, Haddad P, Hou MF, Inbar M, Khaled H, Kielanowska J, Kwan WH, Mathew BS, Mittra I, Muller B, Nicolucci A, Peralta O, Pernas F, Petruzelka L, Pienkowski T, Radhika R, Rajan B, Rubach MT, Tort S, Urrutia G, Valentini M, Wang Y, Peto R, Adjuvant Tamoxifen: Longer Against Shorter Collaborative G. Long-term effects of continuing adjuvant tamoxifen to 10 years versus stopping at 5 years after diagnosis of oestrogen receptor-positive breast cancer: ATLAS, a randomised trial. Lancet. 2013;381:805–16. doi:10.1016/S0140-6736(12)61963-1.

de Bono JS, Logothetis CJ, Molina A, Fizazi K, North S, Chu L, Chi KN, Jones RJ, Goodman Jr OB, Saad F, Staffurth JN, Mainwaring P, Harland S, Flaig TW, Hutson TE, Cheng T, Patterson H, Hainsworth JD, Ryan CJ, Sternberg CN, Ellard SL, Flechon A, Saleh M, Scholz M, Efstathiou E, Zivi A, Bianchini D, Loriot Y, Chieffo N, Kheoh T, Haqq CM, Scher HI, Investigators C-A-. Abiraterone and increased survival in metastatic prostate cancer. N Engl J Med. 2011;364:1995–2005. doi:10.1056/NEJMoa1014618.

De Coster R, Mahler C, Denis L, Coene MC, Caers I, Amery W, Haelterman C, Beerens D. Effects of high-dose ketoconazole and dexamethasone on ACTH-stimulated adrenal steroidogenesis in orchiectomized prostatic cancer patients. Acta Endocrinol (Copenh). 1987;115:265–71.

Dehm SM, Schmidt LJ, Heemers HV, Vessella RL, Tindall DJ. Splicing of a novel androgen receptor exon generates a constitutively active androgen receptor that mediates prostate cancer therapy resistance. Cancer Res. 2008;68:5469–77. doi:10.1158/0008-5472.CAN-08-0594.

Dowsett M, Smith IE, Ebbs SR, Dixon JM, Skene A, A'Hern R, Salter J, Detre S, Hills M, Walsh G. Prognostic value of Ki67 expression after short-term presurgical endocrine therapy for primary breast cancer. J Natl Cancer Inst. 2007;99:167–70.

Early Breast Cancer Trialists' Collaborative G. Aromatase inhibitors versus tamoxifen in early breast cancer: patient-level meta-analysis of the randomised trials. Lancet. 2015. doi:10.1016/S0140-6736(15)61074-1.

Early Breast Cancer Trialists' Collaborative Group. Tamoxifen for early breast cancer: an overview of the randomised trials. Lancet. 1998;351:1451–67.

Ellis MJ, Ding L, Shen D, Luo J, Suman VJ, Wallis JW, Van Tine BA, Hoog J, Goiffon RJ, Goldstein TC, Ng S, Lin L, Crowder R, Snider J, Ballman K, Weber J, Chen K, Koboldt DC, Kandoth C, Schierding WS, McMichael JF, Miller CA, Lu C, Harris CC, McLellan MD, Wendl MC, DeSchryver K, Allred DC, Esserman L, Unzeitig G, Margenthaler J, Babiera GV, Marcom PK, Guenther JM, Leitch M, Hunt K, Olson J, Tao Y, Maher CA, Fulton LL, Fulton RS, Harrison M, Oberkfell B, Du F, Demeter R, Vickery TL, Elhammali A, Piwnica-Worms H, McDonald S, Watson M, Dooling DJ, Ota D, Chang LW, Bose R, Ley TJ, Piwnica-Worms D, Stuart JM, Wilson RK, Mardis ER. Whole-genome analysis informs breast cancer response to aromatase inhibition. Nature. 2012;486:353–60. doi:10.1038/nature11143.

Ettinger B, Black DM, Mitlak BH, Knickerbocker RK, Nickelsen T, Genant HK, Christiansen C, Delmas PD, Zanchetta JR, Stakkestad J, Gluer CC, Krueger K, Cohen FJ, Eckert S, Ensrud KE, Avioli LV, Lips P, Cummings SR. Reduction of vertebral fracture risk in postmenopausal women with osteoporosis treated with raloxifene: results from a 3-year randomized clinical trial. Multiple Outcomes of Raloxifene Evaluation (MORE) investigators. JAMA. 1999;282:637–45.

Finn RS, Crown JP, Lang I, Boer K, Bondarenko IM, Kulyk SO, Ettl J, Patel R, Pinter T, Schmidt M, Shparyk Y, Thummala AR, Voytko NL, Fowst C, Huang X, Kim ST, Randolph S, Slamon DJ. The cyclin-dependent kinase 4/6 inhibitor palbociclib in combination with letrozole versus letrozole alone as first-line treatment of oestrogen receptor-positive, HER2-negative, advanced breast cancer (PALOMA-1/TRIO-18): a randomised phase 2 study. Lancet Oncol. 2015;16:25–35. doi:10.1016/S1470-2045(14)71159-3.

Fisher B, Costantino JP, Wickerham DL, Redmond CK, Kavanah M, Cronin WM, Vogel V, Robidoux A, Dimitrov N, Atkins J, Daly M, Wieand S, Tan-Chiu E, Ford L, Wolmark N. Tamoxifen for prevention of breast cancer: report of the National Surgical Adjuvant Breast and Bowel Project P-1 Study. J Natl Cancer Inst. 1998;90:1371–88.

Fizazi K, Jones R, Oudard S, Efstathiou E, Saad F, de Wit R, De Bono J, Cruz FM, Fountzilas G, Ulys A, Carcano F, Agarwal N, Agus D, Bellmunt J, Petrylak DP, Lee SY, Webb IJ, Tejura B, Borgstein N, Dreicer R. Phase III, randomized, double-blind, multicenter trial comparing orteronel (TAK-700) plus prednisone with placebo plus prednisone in patients with metastatic castration-resistant prostate cancer that has progressed during or after docetaxel-based therapy: ELM-PC 5. J Clin Oncol. 2015;33:723–31. doi:10.1200/JCO.2014.56.5119.

Friedlander TW, Roy R, Tomlins SA, Ngo VT, Kobayashi Y, Azameera A, Rubin MA, Pienta KJ, Chinnaiyan A, Ittmann MM, Ryan CJ, Paris PL. Common structural and epigenetic changes in the genome of castration-resistant prostate cancer. Cancer Res. 2012;72:616–25. doi:10.1158/0008-5472.CAN-11-2079.

Gibson LJ, Dawson C, Lawrence DH, Bliss JM. Aromatase inhibitors for treatment of advanced breast cancer in postmenopausal women. Cochrane Database Syst Rev. 2007;CD003370. doi:10.1002/14651858.CD003370.pub2.

Goss PE, Ingle JN, Martino S, Robert NJ, Muss HB, Piccart MJ, Castiglione M, Tu D, Shepherd LE, Pritchard KI, Livingston RB, Davidson NE, Norton L, Perez EA, Abrams JS, Therasse P, Palmer MJ, Pater JL. A randomized trial of letrozole in postmenopausal women after five years of tamoxifen therapy for early-stage breast cancer. N Engl J Med. 2003;349:1793–802.

Goss PE, Ingle JN, Pritchard KI, Robert NJ, Muss H, Gralow J, Gelmon K, Whelan T, Strasser-Weippl K, Rubin S, Sturtz K, Wolff AC, Winer E, Hudis C, Stopeck A, Beck JT, Kaur JS, Whelan K, Tu D, Parulekar WR. Extending aromatase-inhibitor adjuvant therapy to 10 years. N Engl J Med. 2016;375:209–19. doi:10.1056/NEJMoa1604700.

Gregory CW, Johnson Jr RT, Mohler JL, French FS, Wilson EM. Androgen receptor stabilization in recurrent prostate cancer is associated with hypersensitivity to low androgen. Cancer Res. 2001;61:2892–8.

Hanahan D, Weinberg RA. The hallmarks of cancer. Cell. 2000;100:57–70.

Harris LN, Ismaila N, McShane LM, Andre F, Collyar DE, Gonzalez-Angulo AM, Hammond EH, Kuderer NM, Liu MC, Mennel RG, Van Poznak C, Bast RC, Hayes DF. Use of biomarkers to guide decisions on adjuvant systemic therapy for women with early-stage invasive breast cancer: American Society of Clinical Oncology Clinical Practice Guideline. J Clin Oncol. 2016;34:1134–50. doi:10.1200/JCO.2015.65.2289.

Hong J, Shah NN, Thomas TJ, Gallo MA, Yurkow EJ, Thomas T. Differential effects of estradiol and its analogs on cyclin D1 and CDK4 expression in estrogen receptor positive MCF-7 and estrogen receptor-transfected MCF-10AEwt5 cells. Oncol Rep. 1998;5:1025–33.

Hu R, Dunn TA, Wei S, Isharwal S, Veltri RW, Humphreys E, Han M, Partin AW, Vessella RL, Isaacs WB, Bova GS, Luo J. Ligand-independent androgen receptor variants derived from splicing of cryptic exons signify hormone-refractory prostate cancer. Cancer Res. 2009;69:16–22. doi:10.1158/0008-5472.CAN-08-2764.

Huggins C, Hodges CV. Studies on prostatic cancer: effect of castration, of estrogen and of androgen injection on serum phosphtases in metastatic carcinoma of the prostate. Cancer Res. 1941a;1:293–7.

Huggins CB, Hodges C. Studies on prostate cancer: 1. The effects of castration, of estrogen and androgen injection on serum phosphatases in metastatic carcinoma of the prostate. Cancer Res. 1941b;1:203.

Huggins C, Scott WW. Bilateral adrenalectomy in prostatic cancer: clinical features and urinary excretion of 17-ketosteroids and estrogen. Ann Surg. 1945;122:1031–41.

Huggins C, Stevens JR, Hodges CV. The effect of castration on advanced carcinoma of the prostate gland. Arch Surg. 1941;43:209. The effect of castration on advanced carcinoma of the prostate gland. . Arch Surg 1941;43:209.

Jordan VC. Tamoxifen: a personal retrospective. Lancet Oncol. 2000;1:43–9. doi:10.1016/S1470-2045(00)00009-7.

Joseph JD, Lu N, Qian J, Sensintaffar J, Shao G, Brigham D, Moon M, Maneval EC, Chen I, Darimont B, Hager JH. A clinically relevant androgen receptor mutation confers resistance to second-generation antiandrogens enzalutamide and ARN-509. Cancer Discov. 2013;3:1020–9. doi:10.1158/2159-8290.CD-13-0226.

Keizman D, Huang P, Carducci MA, Eisenberger MA. Contemporary experience with ketoconazole in patients with metastatic castration-resistant prostate cancer: clinical factors associated with PSA response and disease progression. Prostate. 2012;72:461–7. doi:10.1002/pros.21447.

Kelly WK, Slovin S, Scher HI. Steroid hormone withdrawal syndromes. Pathophysiology and clinical significance. Urol Clin N Am. 1997;24:421–31.

Kiang DT, Kennedy BJ. Tamoxifen (antiestrogen) therapy in advanced breast cancer. Ann Intern Med. 1977;87:687–90.

Korpal M, Korn JM, Gao X, Rakiec DP, Ruddy DA, Doshi S, Yuan J, Kovats SG, Kim S, Cooke VG, Monahan JE, Stegmeier F, Roberts TM, Sellers WR, Zhou W, Zhu P. An F876L mutation in androgen receptor confers genetic and phenotypic resistance to MDV3100 (enzalutamide). Cancer Discov. 2013;3:1030–43. doi:10.1158/2159-8290.CD-13-0142.

Koryakina Y, Ta HQ, Gioeli D. Androgen receptor phosphorylation: biological context and functional consequences. Endocr Relat Cancer. 2014;21:T131–45. doi:10.1530/ERC-13-0472.

Li Y, Chan SC, Brand LJ, Hwang TH, Silverstein KA, Dehm SM. Androgen receptor splice variants mediate enzalutamide resistance in castration-resistant prostate cancer cell lines. Cancer Res. 2013;73:483–9. doi:10.1158/0008-5472.CAN-12-3630.

Lippman M, Bolan G, Huff K. The effects of estrogens and antiestrogens on hormone-responsive human breast cancer in long-term tissue culture. Cancer Res. 1976;36:4595–601.

Lippman ME, Osborne CK, Knazek R, Young N. In vitro model systems for the study of hormone-dependent human breast cancer. N Engl J Med. 1977;296:154–9.

Liu C, Lou W, Armstrong C, Zhu Y, Evans CP, Gao AC. Niclosamide suppresses cell migration and invasion in enzalutamide resistant prostate cancer cells via Stat3-AR axis inhibition. Prostate. 2015;75:1341–53. doi:10.1002/pros.23015.

Ma CX, Reinert T, Chmielewska I, Ellis MJ. Mechanisms of aromatase inhibitor resistance. Nat Rev Cancer. 2015;15:261–75. doi:10.1038/nrc3920.

Massard C, Fizazi K. Targeting continued androgen receptor signaling in prostate cancer. Clin Cancer Res. 2011;17:3876–83. doi:10.1158/1078-0432.CCR-10-2815.

Moilanen AM, Riikonen R, Oksala R, Ravanti L, Aho E, Wohlfahrt G, Nykanen PS, Tormakangas OP, Palvimo JJ, Kallio PJ. Discovery of ODM-201, a new-generation androgen receptor inhibitor targeting resistance mechanisms to androgen signaling-directed prostate cancer therapies. Sci Rep. 2015;5:12007. doi:10.1038/srep12007.

Montgomery RB EM, Rettig M, Chu F, Pili R, et al. Phase I clinical trial of galeterone (TOK-001), a multifunctional antiandrogen and CYP17 inhibitor in castration resistant prostate cancer (CRPC) (ASCO Meeting Abstr. 2012;30:4665).

Montgomery B, Eisenberger MA, Rettig MB, Chu F, Pili R, Stephenson JJ, Vogelzang NJ, Koletsky AJ, Nordquist LT, Edenfield WJ, Mamlouk K, Ferrante KJ, Taplin ME. Androgen Receptor

Modulation Optimized for Response (ARMOR) phase I and II studies: galeterone for the treatment of castration-resistant prostate cancer. Clin Cancer Res. 2016;22:1356–63. doi:10.1158/1078-0432.CCR-15-1432.

Mostaghel EA, Marck BT, Plymate SR, Vessella RL, Balk S, Matsumoto AM, Nelson PS, Montgomery RB. Resistance to CYP17A1 inhibition with abiraterone in castration-resistant prostate cancer: induction of steroidogenesis and androgen receptor splice variants. Clin Cancer Res. 2011;17:5913–25. doi:10.1158/1078-0432.CCR-11-0728.

Mouridsen H, Giobbie-Hurder A, Goldhirsch A, Thurlimann B, Paridaens R, Smith I, Mauriac L, Forbes JF, Price KN, Regan MM, Gelber RD, Coates AS. Letrozole therapy alone or in sequence with tamoxifen in women with breast cancer. N Engl J Med. 2009;361:766–76.

Nadiminty N, Tummala R, Liu C, Yang J, Lou W, Evans CP, Gao AC. NF-kappaB2/p52 induces resistance to enzalutamide in prostate cancer: role of androgen receptor and its variants. Mol Cancer Ther. 2013;12:1629–37. doi:10.1158/1535-7163.MCT-13-0027.

Nguyen HG, Yang JC, Kung HJ, Shi XB, Tilki D, Lara Jr PN, DeVere White RW, Gao AC, Evans CP. Targeting autophagy overcomes enzalutamide resistance in castration-resistant prostate cancer cells and improves therapeutic response in a xenograft model. Oncogene. 2014;33:4521–30. doi:10.1038/onc.2014.25.

Pagani O, Regan MM, Walley BA, Fleming GF, Colleoni M, Lang I, Gomez HL, Tondini C, Burstein HJ, Perez EA, Ciruelos E, Stearns V, Bonnefoi HR, Martino S, Geyer Jr CE, Pinotti G, Puglisi F, Crivellari D, Ruhstaller T, Winer EP, Rabaglio-Poretti M, Maibach R, Ruepp B, Giobbie-Hurder A, Price KN, Bernhard J, Luo W, Ribi K, Viale G, Coates AS, Gelber RD, Goldhirsch A, Francis PA, the T, Investigators S, the International Breast Cancer Study G. Adjuvant exemestane with ovarian suppression in premenopausal breast cancer. N Engl J Med. 2014;371:107–18. doi:10.1056/NEJMoa1404037.

Pinkerton JV, Harvey JA, Lindsay R, Pan K, Chines AA, Mirkin S, Archer DF, Investigators S. Effects of bazedoxifene/conjugated estrogens on the endometrium and bone: a randomized trial. J Clin Endocrinol Metab. 2014;99:E189–98. doi:10.1210/jc.2013-1707.

Regan MM, Francis PA, Pagani O, Fleming GF, Walley BA, Viale G, Colleoni M, Lang I, Gomez HL, Tondini C, Pinotti G, Price KN, Coates AS, Goldhirsch A, Gelber RD. Absolute benefit of adjuvant endocrine therapies for premenopausal women with hormone receptor-positive, human epidermal growth factor receptor 2-negative early breast cancer: TEXT and SOFT trials. J Clin Oncol. 2016;34:2221–31. doi:10.1200/JCO.2015.64.3171.

Robinson DR, Wu YM, Vats P, Su F, Lonigro RJ, Cao X, Kalyana-Sundaram S, Wang R, Ning Y, Hodges L, Gursky A, Siddiqui J, Tomlins SA, Roychowdhury S, Pienta KJ, Kim SY, Roberts JS, Rae JM, Van Poznak CH, Hayes DF, Chugh R, Kunju LP, Talpaz M, Schott AF, Chinnaiyan AM. Activating ESR1 mutations in hormone-resistant metastatic breast cancer. Nat Genet. 2013;45:1446–51. doi:10.1038/ng.2823.

Ryan CJ, Molina A, Griffin T. Abiraterone in metastatic prostate cancer. N Engl J Med. 2013;368:1458–9. doi:10.1056/NEJMc1301594.

Saad F, Fizazi K, Jinga V, Efstathiou E, Fong PC, Hart LL, Jones R, McDermott R, Wirth M, Suzuki K, MacLean DB, Wang L, Akaza H, Nelson J, Scher HI, Dreicer R, Webb IJ, de Wit R, Investigators E-P. Orteronel plus prednisone in patients with chemotherapy-naive metastatic castration-resistant prostate cancer (ELM-PC 4): a double-blind, multicentre, phase 3, randomised, placebo-controlled trial. Lancet Oncol. 2015;16:338–48. doi:10.1016/S1470-2045(15)70027-6.

Santen RJ, Brodie H, Simpson ER, Siiteri PK, Brodie A. History of aromatase: saga of an important biological mediator and therapeutic target. Endocr Rev. 2009;30:343–75. doi:10.1210/er.2008-0016.

Saphner T, Tormey DC, Gray R. Annual hazard rates of recurrence for breast cancer after primary therapy. J Clin Oncol. 1996;14:2738–46.

Scher HI, Sawyers CL. Biology of progressive, castration-resistant prostate cancer: directed therapies targeting the androgen-receptor signaling axis. J Clin Oncol. 2005;23:8253–61. doi:10.1200/JCO.2005.03.4777.

Scher HI, Beer TM, Higano CS, Anand A, Taplin ME, Efstathiou E, Rathkopf D, Shelkey J, Yu EY, Alumkal J, Hung D, Hirmand M, Seely L, Morris MJ, Danila DC, Humm J, Larson S, Fleisher M, Sawyers CL, Prostate Cancer Foundation/Department of Defense Prostate Cancer Clinical Trials C. Antitumour activity of MDV3100 in castration-resistant prostate cancer: a phase 1–2 study. Lancet. 2010;375:1437–46. doi:10.1016/S0140-6736(10)60172-9.

Scher HI, Fizazi K, Saad F, Taplin ME, Sternberg CN, Miller K, de Wit R, Mulders P, Chi KN, Shore ND, Armstrong AJ, Flaig TW, Flechon A, Mainwaring P, Fleming M, Hainsworth JD, Hirmand M, Selby B, Seely L, de Bono JS, Investigators A. Increased survival with enzalutamide in prostate cancer after chemotherapy. N Engl J Med. 2012;367:1187–97. doi:10.1056/NEJMoa1207506.

Schmid P, Pinder SE, Wheatley D, Macaskill J, Zammit C, Hu J, Price R, Bundred N, Hadad S, Shia A, Sarker SJ, Lim L, Gazinska P, Woodman N, Korbie D, Trau M, Mainwaring P, Gendreau S, Lackner MR, Derynck M, Wilson TR, Butler H, Earl G, Parker P, Purushotham A, Thompson A. Phase II randomized preoperative window-of-opportunity study of the PI3K inhibitor pictilisib plus anastrozole compared with anastrozole alone in patients with estrogen receptor-positive breast cancer. J Clin Oncol. 2016;34:1987–94. doi:10.1200/JCO.2015.63.9179.

Shah SP, Morin RD, Khattra J, Prentice L, Pugh T, Burleigh A, Delaney A, Gelmon K, Guliany R, Senz J, Steidl C, Holt RA, Jones S, Sun M, Leung G, Moore R, Severson T, Taylor GA, Teschendorff AE, Tse K, Turashvili G, Varhol R, Warren RL, Watson P, Zhao Y, Caldas C, Huntsman D, Hirst M, Marra MA, Aparicio S. Mutational evolution in a lobular breast tumour profiled at single nucleotide resolution. Nature. 2009;461:809–13.

Sharma P, Allison JP. The future of immune checkpoint therapy. Science. 2015;348:56–61. doi:10.1126/science.aaa8172.

Small EJ, Halabi S, Dawson NA, Stadler WM, Rini BI, Picus J, Gable P, Torti FM, Kaplan E, Vogelzang NJ. Antiandrogen withdrawal alone or in combination with ketoconazole in androgen-independent prostate cancer patients: a phase III trial (CALGB 9583). J Clin Oncol. 2004;22:1025–33. doi:10.1200/JCO.2004.06.037.

Tan MH, Li J, Xu HE, Melcher K, Yong EL. Androgen receptor: structure, role in prostate cancer and drug discovery. Acta Pharmacol Sin. 2015;36:3–23. doi:10.1038/aps.2014.18.

Taplin ME, Rajeshkumar B, Halabi S, Werner CP, Woda BA, Picus J, Stadler W, Hayes DF, Kantoff PW, Vogelzang NJ, Small EJ, Cancer, Leukemia Group BS. Androgen receptor mutations in androgen-independent prostate cancer: cancer and leukemia group B study 9663. J Clin Oncol. 2003;21:2673–8. doi:10.1200/JCO.2003.11.102.

The Veterans Administration Co-operative Urological Research Group. Treatment and survival of patients with cancer of the prostate. Surg Gynecol Obstet. 1967;124:1011–7.

Thompson IM, Goodman PJ, Tangen CM, Lucia MS, Miller GJ, Ford LG, Lieber MM, Cespedes RD, Atkins JN, Lippman SM, Carlin SM, Ryan A, Szczepanek CM, Crowley JJ, Coltman Jr CA. The influence of finasteride on the development of prostate cancer. N Engl J Med. 2003;349:215–24.

Toren PJ, Kim S, Pham S, Mangalji A, Adomat H, Guns ES, Zoubeidi A, Moore W, Gleave ME. Anticancer activity of a novel selective CYP17A1 inhibitor in preclinical models of castrate-resistant prostate cancer. Mol Cancer Ther. 2015;14:59–69. doi:10.1158/1535-7163. MCT-14-0521.

Toy W, Shen Y, Won H, Green B, Sakr RA, Will M, Li Z, Gala K, Fanning S, King TA, Hudis C, Chen D, Taran T, Hortobagyi G, Greene G, Berger M, Baselga J, Chandarlapaty S. ESR1 ligand-binding domain mutations in hormone-resistant breast cancer. Nat Genet. 2013;45:1439–45. doi:10.1038/ng.2822.

Tran C, Ouk S, Clegg NJ, Chen Y, Watson PA, Arora V, Wongvipat J, Smith-Jones PM, Yoo D, Kwon A, Wasielewska T, Welsbie D, Chen CD, Higano CS, Beer TM, Hung DT, Scher HI, Jung ME, Sawyers CL. Development of a second-generation antiandrogen for treatment of advanced prostate cancer. Science. 2009;324:787–90. doi:10.1126/science.1168175.

Turner NC, Ro J, Andre F, Loi S, Verma S, Iwata H, Harbeck N, Loibl S, Huang Bartlett C, Zhang K, Giorgetti C, Randolph S, Koehler M, Cristofanilli M. Palbociclib in hormone-receptor-positive advanced breast cancer. N Engl J Med. 2015;373:209–19. doi:10.1056/NEJMoa1505270.

van de Velde CJ, Rea D, Seynaeve C, Putter H, Hasenburg A, Vannetzel JM, Paridaens R, Markopoulos C, Hozumi Y, Hille ET, Kieback DG, Asmar L, Smeets J, Nortier JW, Hadji P, Bartlett JM, Jones SE. Adjuvant tamoxifen and exemestane in early breast cancer (TEAM): a randomised phase 3 trial. Lancet. 2011;377:321–31. doi:10.1016/S0140-6736(10)62312-4.

Vasaitis T, Belosay A, Schayowitz A, Khandelwal A, Chopra P, Gediya LK, Guo Z, Fang HB, Njar VC, Brodie AM. Androgen receptor inactivation contributes to antitumor efficacy of 17{alpha}-hydroxylase/17,20-lyase inhibitor 3beta-hydroxy-17-(1H-benzimidazole-1-yl)androsta-5,16-diene in prostate cancer. Mol Cancer Ther. 2008;7:2348–57. doi:10.1158/1535-7163.MCT-08-0230.

Visakorpi T, Hyytinen E, Koivisto P, Tanner M, Keinanen R, Palmberg C, Palotie A, Tammela T, Isola J, Kallioniemi OP. In vivo amplification of the androgen receptor gene and progression of human prostate cancer. Nat Genet. 1995;9:401–6. doi:10.1038/ng0495-401.

Vogel VG, Costantino JP, Wickerham DL, Cronin WM, Cecchini RS, Atkins JN, Bevers TB, Fehrenbacher L, Pajon Jr ER, Wade 3rd JL, Robidoux A, Margolese RG, James J, Lippman SM, Runowicz CD, Ganz PA, Reis SE, McCaskill-Stevens W, Ford LG, Jordan VC, Wolmark N. Effects of tamoxifen vs raloxifene on the risk of developing invasive breast cancer and other disease outcomes: the NSABP Study of Tamoxifen and Raloxifene (STAR) P-2 trial. JAMA. 2006;295:2727–41.

Wang Q, Li W, Zhang Y, Yuan X, Xu K, Yu J, Chen Z, Beroukhim R, Wang H, Lupien M, Wu T, Regan MM, Meyer CA, Carroll JS, Manrai AK, Janne OA, Balk SP, Mehra R, Han B, Chinnaiyan AM, Rubin MA, True L, Fiorentino M, Fiore C, Loda M, Kantoff PW, Liu XS, Brown M. Androgen receptor regulates a distinct transcription program in androgen-independent prostate cancer. Cell. 2009;138:245–56. doi:10.1016/j.cell.2009.04.056.

Wang P, Bahreini A, Gyanchandani R, Lucas PC, Hartmaier RJ, Watters RJ, Jonnalagadda AR, Trejo Bittar HE, Berg A, Hamilton RL, Kurland BF, Weiss KR, Mathew A, Leone JP, Davidson NE, Nikiforova MN, Brufsky AM, Ambros TF, Stern AM, Puhalla SL, Lee AV, Oesterreich S. Sensitive detection of mono- and polyclonal ESR1 mutations in primary tumors, metastatic lesions, and cell-free DNA of breast cancer patients. Clin Cancer Res. 2016;22:1130–7. doi:10.1158/1078-0432.CCR-15-1534.

Witjes FJ, Debruyne FM, Fernandez del Moral P, Geboers AD. Ketoconazole high dose in management of hormonally pretreated patients with progressive metastatic prostate cancer. Dutch South-Eastern Urological Cooperative Group. Urology. 1989;33:411–5.

Wolf IM, Heitzer MD, Grubisha M, DeFranco DB. Coactivators and nuclear receptor trans-activation. J Cell Biochem. 2008;104:1580–6. doi:10.1002/jcb.21755.

Yamamoto Y, Loriot Y, Beraldi E, Zhang F, Wyatt AW, Nakouzi NA, Mo F, Zhou T, Kim Y, Monia BP, MacLeod AR, Fazli L, Wang Y, Collins CC, Zoubeidi A, Gleave M. Generation 2.5 antisense oligonucleotides targeting the androgen receptor and its splice variants suppress enzalutamide-resistant prostate cancer cell growth. Clin Cancer Res. 2015;21:1675–87. doi:10.1158/1078-0432.CCR-14-1108.

Zhang QX, Borg A, Wolf DM, Oesterreich S, Fuqua SA. An estrogen receptor mutant with strong hormone-independent activity from a metastatic breast cancer. Cancer Res. 1997;57:1244–9.

Index

A. Belfiore, D. LeRoith (eds.), *Principles of Endocrinology and Hormone Action*, Endocrinology, https://doi.org/10.1007/978-3-319-44675-2

G

H

Printed by Printforce, the Netherlands